Harley's Pediatric Ophthalmology

Sixth Edition

Harley's Pediatric Ophthalmology

Sixth Edition

Editors

Leonard B. Nelson, MD, MBA

Director, The Wills Eye Strabismus Center
Co-Director, Department of Pediatric Ophthalmology
and Ocular Genetics, Wills Eye Hospital
Associate Professor of Ophthalmology and Pediatrics
Jefferson Medical College
Thomas Jefferson University
Philadelphia, Pennsylvania

Scott E. Olitsky, MD

Professor of Ophthalmology
Children's Mercy Hospitals and Clinics
University of Missouri - Kansas City School of Medicine
Kansas City, Missouri

 Wolters Kluwer | Lippincott Williams & Wilkins
Health

Philadelphia • Baltimore • New York • London
Buenos Aires • Hong Kong • Sydney • Tokyo

Acquisition Editor: *Ryan Shaw*
Product Manager: *Kate Marshall*
Vendor Manager: *Alicia Jackson*
Senior Manufacturing Coordinator: *Beth Welsh*
Marketing Manager: *Alexander Burns*
Designer: *Joan Wendt*
Production Service: *Integra Software Services Pvt. Ltd.*

Library of Congress Cataloging-in-Publication Data
Harley's pediatric ophthalmology. -- Sixth edition / editors, Leonard B. Nelson, Scott E. Olitsky.
    p. ; cm.
  Pediatric ophthalmology
  Preceded by Harley's pediatric ophthalmology / editors, Leonard B. Nelson,
Scott E. Olitsky. 5th ed. c2005.
  Includes bibliographical references and index.
  ISBN 978-1-4511-7283-6
  I. Nelson, Leonard B., editor of compilation. II. Olitsky, Scott E., editor of compilation. III.
Title: Pediatric ophthalmology.
  [DNLM: 1. Eye Diseases. 2. Child. 3. Infant. WW 600]
  RE48.2.C5
  618.92'0977--dc23
                                                                    2013020629

Care has been taken to confirm the accuracy of the information presented and to describe generally accepted practices. However, the authors, editors, and publisher are not responsible for errors or omissions or for any consequences from application of the information in this book and make no warranty, expressed or implied, with respect to the currency, completeness, or accuracy of the contents of the publication. Application of the information in a particular situation remains the professional responsibility of the practitioner.

The authors, editors, and publisher have exerted every effort to ensure that drug selection and dosage set forth in this text are in accordance with current recommendations and practice at the time of publication. However, in view of ongoing research, changes in government regulations, and the constant flow of information relating to drug therapy and drug reactions, the reader is urged to check the package insert for each drug for any change in indications and dosage and for added warnings and precautions. This is particularly important when the recommended agent is a new or infrequently employed drug.

Some drugs and medical devices presented in the publication have Food and Drug Administration (FDA) clearance for limited use in restricted research settings. It is the responsibility of the health-care provider to ascertain the FDA status of each drug or device planned for use in their clinical practice.

To purchase additional copies of this book, call our customer service department at (800) 638-3030 or fax orders to (301) 223-2320. International customers should call (301) 223-2300.

Visit Lippincott Williams & Wilkins on the Internet at LWW.com. Lippincott Williams & Wilkins customer service representatives are available from 8:30 am to 6 pm, EST.

10 9 8 7 6 5 4 3 2 1

*This book is dedicated to our wives, Helene and Andrea,
for their unending understanding patience, support,
and love in pursuit of our academic endeavors.*

*This book is also dedicated to the memory of
Robison D. Harley, MD, who we will forever owe a debt
of profound gratitude for his leadership and mentorship,
and for giving us the opportunity to continue to provide the
pediatric ophthalmology community an outstanding
treatise in the specialty.*

Contributors

Nagham Al-Zubidi, MD
Neuro-Ophthalmology Fellow
Department of Ophthalmology
The Methodist Hospital
Department of Ophthalmology
Well Cornel Medical College
Houston, Texas

J. Bronwyn Bateman
Clinical Professor of Ophthalmology
David Geffen School of Medicine
University of California
Los Angeles, California

William E. Benson, MD
Professor of Ophthalmology
Jefferson Medical College
Thomas Jefferson University
Attending Surgeon
Wills Eye Hospital
Philadelphia, Pennsylvania

Gary C. Brown, MD, MBA
Professor of Ophthalmology
Jefferson Medical College
Thomas Jefferson University
Director of Retina Service
Wills Eye Hospital
*Co-Director of Center for Value-Based
    Medicine*
Adjunct Senior Fellow
Leonard Davis Institute of Health
    Economics
Philadelphia, Pennsylvania

Melissa M. Brown, MD, MN, MBA
Adjunct Professor of Ophthalmology
University of Pennsylvania
*Director of Center for Value-Based
    Medicine*
Adjunct Senior Fellow
Leonard Davis Institute of Health
    Economics
Philadelphia, Pennsylvania

Robert A. Catalano, MD, MBA
Associate Professor of Ophthalmology
Albany Medical College
*Medical Director of Albany Medical
    Center Hospital*
Albany, New York

David K. Coats, MD
*Associate Professor of Ophthalmology and
    Pediatrics*
Baylor College of Medicine
Texas Children's Hospital
Houston, Texas

Forrest J. Ellis, MD
*Assistant Professor of Pediatrics and
    Ophthalmology*
Case Western Reserve University
    School of Medicine
*Co-Director of Pediatric Ophthalmology
    and Strabismus*
Rainbow Babies and Children's Hospital
*Consultant for Ophthalmic Plastic and
    Orbital Surgery*
University Hospitals of Cleveland
    Cleveland, Ohio

Sharon F. Freedman, MD
Professor of Ophthalmology
Professor of Pediatrics
Duke Eye Center
Durham, North Carolina

Nandini G. Gandhi, MD
Assistant Professor of Ophthalmology
University of California
Davis, Sacramento, California

Kammi B. Gunton, MD
Assistant Surgeon of Pediatric Ophthalmology
Wills Eye Hospital
Philadelphia, Pennsylvania

Denise Hug, MD
Assistant Professor of Ophthalmology
University of Missouri
Children's Mercy Hospitals and Clinics
Kansas City, Missouri

Leila M. Khazaeni, MD
Department of Ophthalmology
Loma Linda University Health
Loma Linda, California

Laura Kirkeby, CO
Orthoptist
Scripps Clinic
San Diego, California

Andrew G. Lee, MD
*Professor of Ophthalmology, Neurology,
    and Neurosurgery*
Department of Ophthalmology
Weill Cornell Medical College
Chair
Department of Ophthalmology
The Methodist Hospital
Houston, Texas

Alex V. Levin, MD, MHSc
Pediatric Ophthalmology and Ocular
    Genetics
Wills Eye Institute
Thomas Jefferson University
Philadelphia, Pennsylvania

Timothy P. Lindquist, MD
Department of Ophthalmology
University of Kansas Medicine
Children's Mercy Hospitals and Clinics
Kansas City, Missouri

Grace T. Liu, MD
Pediatric Ophthalmic Consultants
Department of Pediatric Ophthalmology
New York University
New York, New York

David B. Lyon, MD, FACS
Associate Professor
Department of Ophthalmology
Eye Foundation of Kansas City
Vision Research Center, University
    of Missouri-Kansas City School of
    Medicine
Kansas City, Missouri

Leonard B. Nelson, MD
Director
The Wills Eye Strabismus Center
Co-Director
Department of Pediatric
    Ophthalmology and Ocular
    Genetics
Wills Eye Hospital
*Associate Professor of Ophthalmology and
    Pediatrics*
Jefferson Medical College
Thomas Jefferson University
Philadelphia, Pennsylvania

Scott E. Olitsky, MD
Professor of Ophthalmology
Children's Mercy Hospitals and
    Clinics
University of Missouri - Kansas City
    School of Medicine
Kansas City, Missouri

Gregory Ostrow, MD
Director
Pediatric Ophthalmology and Adult
    Strabismus
Scripps Clinic
San Diego, California

Evelyn A. Paysse, MD
Professor of Ophthalmology and
    Pediatrics
Baylor College of Medicine
Physician
Pediatric Ophthalmology
Texas Children's Hospital
Houston, Texas

Christopher J. Rapuano, MD
Professor of Ophthalmology
Jefferson Medical College
Thomas Jefferson University
Director and Attending Surgeon
Cornea Service
Co-Director
Refractive Surgery Department
Wills Eye Institute
Philadelphia, Pennsylvania

Jagadesh C. Reddy, MD
Consultant
Cornea, Anterior and Refractive
    Surgery Services
LV Prasad Eye Institute
Hyderabad, India

Michael X. Repka, MD, MBA
Professor of Ophthalmology and
    Pediatrics
Wilmer Eye Institute
Johns Hopkins University School of
    Medicine
Johns Hopkins Hospital
Baltimore, Maryland

James D. Reynolds, MD
Professor and Chairman of Ophthalmology
University at Buffalo School of Medicine
Department of Ophthalmology
Ross Eye Institute
Buffalo, New York

Donald P. Sauberan, MD
Eye Surgical Associates
Lincoln, Nebraska

Bruce M. Schnall, MD
Associate Surgeon- Pediatric Ophthalmology
Wills Eye Institute
Philadelphia, Pennsylvania

Carol L. Shields, MD
Associate Director
Ocular Oncology Service
Wills Eye Hospital
Professor of Ophthalmology
Jefferson Medical College
Thomas Jefferson University
Consultant
Ocular Oncology
Children's Hospital of Philadelphia
Philadelphia, Pennsylvania

Jerry A. Shields, MD
Director
Ocular Oncology Service
Wills Eye Hospital
Professor of Ophthalmology
Jefferson Medical College
Thomas Jefferson University
Consultant in Ocular Oncology
Children's Hospital of Philadelphia
Philadelphia, Pennsylvania

Arielle Spitze, MD
Department of Ophthalmology
The Methodist Hospital
Houston, Texas

Mitchell B. Strominger, MD
Associate Professor of Ophthalmology
    and Pediatrics
Tufts University School of Medicine
Chief of Pediatric Ophthalmology and
    Ocular Motility Service
Floating Hospital for Children
Boston, Massachusetts

William Tasman, MD
Professor and Chairman of Ophthalmology
Thomas Jefferson Medical College
Ophthalmologist-in-Chief
Wills Eye Hospital
Philadelphia, Pennsylvania

James F. Vander, MD
Clinical Professor of Ophthalmology
Jefferson Medical College
Thomas Jefferson University
Attending Surgeon for Retina Service
Wills Eye Hospital
Philadelphia, Pennsylvania

Rudolph S. Wagner, MD
Clinical Professor of Ophthalmology
University of Medicine and Dentistry
    of New Jersey
Director of Pediatric Ophthalmology
Institute of Ophthalmology and Visual
    Science
University Hospital
Newark, New Jersey

Eric D. Weichel, MD
Director of Vitreoretinal Surgery
Department of Ophthalmology
Walter Reed Army Medical Center
Washington, District of Columbia

Avery H. Weiss, MD
Associate Professor of Ophthalmology
Affiliate Professor of Pediatrics
University of Washington School of
    Medicine
Chief of Division of Ophthalmology
Children's Hospital and Regional
    Medical Center
Seattle, Washington

Sushma Yalamanchili, MD
Department of Ophthalmology
The Methodist Hospital
Houston, Texas

Terri L. Young, MD
Professor of Ophthalmology,
    Pediatrics, and Medicine
Duke Center for Human Genetics
Duke University Medical Center
Durham, North Carolina

Foreword

HARLEY'S *PEDIATRIC OPHTHALMOLOGY* is an essential resource for all pediatric caregivers to provide them with a comprehensive source of information about children's eye problems to enable understanding and excellent clinical care. When first published 38 years ago, it filled a void that was recognized by Dr Harley and Dr Marshall Parks and immediately it became the Bible for their disciples and many trainees who followed these visionary physicians. Writing in the second edition Marshall Parks noted, "Robison Harley has made his mark in medicine through this monumental work, and for this we pediatric ophthalmologists are eternally grateful." Dr Harley recognized the rapid development of new information and procedures in pediatric ophthalmology and encouraged frequent updating of his original classic textbook. He encouraged frequent revisions and would be so delighted with this sixth edition with all its new information and informative illustrations which are so well presented. He recognized the importance of specialization within pediatric ophthalmology and encouraged contributions from many to his book. In the Foreword of the fifth edition, he expressed gratitude "for the expertise of the contributors, the editors, and the publisher for bringing this splendid volume to our profession…"

Dr Robison D. Harley died 6 years ago. When I last visited with him shortly before his passing, we discussed cases and this textbook, the goals for which he was passionate.

Dr Harley was the consummate clinician and teacher. All of us privileged to learn from him and to contribute to this textbook have felt the responsibility to meet his expectations for excellence and his desire to give back in a meaningful way to our colleagues and to our patients.

I was asked recently how I became an ophthalmologist. It is of importance to me to acknowledge that I am indebted completely to Dr Harley for the opportunity and a lifetime of professional and personal fulfillment. I was led by his humanity, love of life, beautiful surgery, humility, tolerance of others less skilled than himself, and constant giving to others. This treasured textbook, *Pediatric Ophthalmology*, has been preserved and rewritten by its very capable and experienced editors Dr Nelson and Dr Olitsky and their carefully selected contributors. Dr Harley gathered and inspired us to fulfill his uncompromising expectations for his *Pediatric Ophthalmology* and we are collectively rewarded by this unique and unrivaled resource to assist all who care for the health of children's eyes.

I am personally very grateful for their work which has made this updated and expanded sixth edition a reality, and which honors Dr Harley and gives back for him a work that I know he would appreciate most in return for his lifetime of mentoring and gifts to each of us.

David S. Walton, MD

Preface

THE SIXTH EDITION of Harley's *Pediatric Ophthalmology* brings a number of changes to the textbook which has served as a benchmark in the subject for more than three decades. Since the publication of the first edition, edited by the late Dr Robison D. Harley in 1975, the field of pediatrics ophthalmology and strabismus has changed markedly. Initially regarded as an unnecessary subspecialty within the field of ophthalmology, pediatric ophthalmology eventually gained acceptance as a fundamental component of the field due to the efforts of early visionaries such as Dr Parks, Dr Costenbader, and Dr Harley. Today, it is regarded as an essential and vital part of both clinical and academic ophthalmology.

The latest edition reflects our desire to create the best educational and teaching treatise in pediatric ophthalmology. With that in mind, the chapters are revised, several previous chapters were eliminated, and all figures are in color. New contributors represent some of the recent leaders in the field and symbolize a "passing of the torch" from one generation of pediatric ophthalmologists to another. Since the first edition, Wills, a rich storehouse of clinical material, has provided a major background for this book. Many of the contributors include a number of outstanding Wills faculty, previous fellows, and residents. In particular, the Pediatric Ophthalmology and Ocular Genetics Department at Wills, which cares for thousands of children each year, provides a rare opportunity for the study of an extremely wide variety of pediatric ocular disorders.

We thank all of our contributing authors for their knowledge and assistance in the preparation of this book. In addition, we are grateful to the publishers at Lippincott Williams & Wilkins who are participating in the fifth decade of a tradition begun by Dr Harley. This textbook, which was one of the first extensive books in pediatric ophthalmology, would not have been possible if it was not for the efforts of Dr Harley, who passed away shortly after the last edition was published. His insight in the ocular problems that occur in children as well as his unique ability to teach those insights to others have benefitted generations of ophthalmologists as well as the patients we treat.

Leonard B. Nelson, MD, MBA
Scott E. Olitsky, MD

Contents

Genetics of Eye Disease

Terri L. Young • *Leila M. Khazaeni* • *J. Bronwyn Bateman*

IN 1903, SUTTON noted parallels between chromosome behavior and Mendel's laws, thus identifying genes with chromosomes and marking the beginning of genetics as a science (1). One hundred years later, the fiftieth anniversary of the publication of the proposed double helical structure of deoxyribonucleic acid (DNA) by Watson and Crick occurred on April 25, 2003 (2). Another monumental undertaking—the Human Genome Project initiative to sequence the entire human genome—was also pronounced as completed in 2003 (www.genome.gov). The Human Genome Project is a joint initiative of the Department of Energy (Washington, DC) and the National Institutes of Health (Bethesda, MD), and was initiated with the major goal of sequencing the DNA that defines the human genome (www.ornl.gov/hgmis/home.shtml). The ultimate goal of the project, the complete sequencing of human DNA, was completed as a first draft both by the government and by the privately funded effort of Celera Genomics (www.celera.com) (now acquired by Quest Diagnostics, Inc., Madison, NJ). The public version of the current sequence is accessible at several web sites including the National Center for Biotechnology Information (http://www.ncbi.nlm.nih.gov) and the genome browser at the University of California at Santa Cruz (http://genome.ucsc.edu). Medicine has benefited immensely from this evolution in scientific discovery. A paradigm shift has occurred in the way diseases are classified, with less emphasis on clinical features as categorical constructs and greater emphasis on gene protein dysfunction due to associated DNA sequence alterations.

Genetics is a universal science that embraces all of biology. Lenz wrote in 1936: "Rules that are obeyed the same way in peas and snapdragons, in flies and butterflies, in mice and rabbits, of course also apply to humans" (3). This has repeatedly played out with the increasing pace of gene discovery in the latter part of the 20th century, and into the 21st century, in large part due to genetic defects found in lower species that were then found to be associatively consistent in humans. Modern genetics has allowed the characterization of mutations that cause congenital human disorders and their comparison to mutations in model organisms. The worm (*Caenorhabditis elegans*), fruit fly (*Drosophila melanogaster*), zebrafish, and mouse all serve the medical community with modules of evolutionary conserved ontogenetic mechanisms that aid in establishing developmental and functional models of human disease (4). With the advent of modern molecular genetics, the medical community has acquired a common language and a new paradigm.

The current statistics of ophthalmic genetic disorders is large and growing. Searching the Online Mendelian Inheritance in Man (OMIM) database (http://www.ncbi.nlm.nih.gov/omim) for the term "eye" yields more than 1,242 entries (5). winter's diagnostic London Dysmorphology Database (LDDB) lists under the general term "eyes, globes" more than 2,900 genetic ophthalmic conditions as part of expanded programmatic database named GENEEYE (6) (www.lmdatabases.com/). This includes many single congenital anomalies both genetic and sporadic, including all the corneal dystrophies, macular dystrophies, the scores of different reo-cone dystrophies. Specific defects found in nearly 192 genes are associated with corneal and retinal dystrophies, eye tumors, retinitis pigmentosa, cataracts, and glaucoma (http://www.sph.uth.tmc.edu/Retnet/disease.htm). Characterization of gene mutations in specific eye diseases aids in the identification of abnormal proteins that cause disease, and expanded definitions of pathologic processes.

Gene mutations have now been identified for several ophthalmic and systemic disorders with significant sight-threatening ophthalmic consequences. Ophthalmologists, and in particular pediatric ophthalmologists, are often on the frontline in assessing patients and families with such disorders. Knowledge of clinical and molecular features of the disease—such as developmental age of onset, heritable probability, DNA testing parameters, and customized treatment options based on molecular insights and strategies—is paramount to customized patient care.

DATABASES FOR CLINICAL USE

Much of the information collected and discussed in this chapter will no doubt be dated even at publication because of the rapid evolution of research discoveries in genetics. For this reason, it is recommended that inquiries regarding specific clinical entities be made consulting online databases that are updated more quickly than any textbook chapter. As mentioned above, the OMIM database is without question the reference of choice of geneticists and genetic counselors for information regarding syndromic and non-syndromic clinical entities for which a genetic basis has been discovered. OMIM's delay of comprehensive coverage of the scientific literature is less than 2 weeks. The LDDB is structured by the symptoms, anatomical sites, or tissues involved. Many genetic and clinical centers also use the Australian Pictures of Standard Syndromes and Undiagnosed Malformation (POSSUM) database at http://www.possum.net.au/, which was launched in March 1987. Similar to LDDB, this program uses a hierarchic trait search list. The syndrome descriptions include the OMIM number, a list of synonyms, pictures of different patients at different ages, clinical and genetic comments, references, and trait lists. The program is continuously updated. The Human Gene Mutation Database (http://www.hgmd.org) at the Institute of Medical Genetics in Cardiff, Wales, curated by Cooper and colleagues since 2000, is at present the most useful general mutation database (7). It covers the scientific literature, references genes (at this writing more than 3,682 genes), and mutations discovered to date of those genes (more than 97,797), with links to approximately 250 open locus-specific databases, such as the retinoblastoma gene *RB1* (http://www.d-lohmann.de/Rb/). The web site of the HUGO (Human Genome Organisation) Mutation Database Initiative (8) at (www.genenames.org) contains a number of links to locus-specific, central, general, national, and ethnic mutation databases. Newer database, such as The 1000 Genomes Project Consortium, is an integrated map of genetic variation from 1,092 individual human genomes from 14 populations, constructed using a combination of low-coverage whole-genome and exome sequencing to provide a validated haplotype map of 38 million single nucleotide polymorphisms, 1.4 million short insertions and deletions, and more than 14,000 larger deletions (www.1000genomes.org/).

BASIC GENETICS CONCEPTS

The eye is affected relatively early in the course of many genetic metabolic diseases; for some disorders, the ocular manifestations are unique and diagnostic. The eye is a complex organ with unique and specialized structures and biochemical functions related to vision. For these reasons, it is particularly vulnerable to genetic mishaps and inborn errors of metabolism.

The hereditary bases of diseases that affect the eye include several broad categories: single-gene mutations consistent with Mendelian inheritance patterns, chromosomal aberrations, cytoplasmic mitochondrial inheritance, and multifactorial inheritance; monogenic disorders can be divided into those that affect only the eye and ocular adnexa, and those that affect other systems in addition to the eye.

The term phenotype is defined as "the entire physical, biochemical, and physiological nature of an individual, as determined by his genetic constitution and the environment in which he develops; or, in a more limited sense, the expression of some particular gene or genes, as classified in some specific way" (9), and usually refers to either a physical feature or features of the individual or the biochemical assay of a gene product. It is a measurable physical or biochemical parameter that is determined by the interaction of the genetic constitution (genotype) with the environment. A wild-type phenotype is considered the normal or standard clinical (physical or biochemical) feature. The genotype may refer to the sum total of an individual's hereditary material (genome) or it may specify a single gene or gene pair.

At the biochemical level, the basic genetic unit for the orchestration of cellular function and transmission of traits from one generation to the next is a macromolecule consisting of DNA; it is self-reproducing and determines the composition of amino acids to form proteins. With rare exceptions, each cell of an organism contains the same DNA as every other cell, and this material encodes the information for the synthesis of proteins that catalyze enzymatic reactions, function as support structures, regulate intra- and intercellular functions, and determine the fate of a cell. The gene is a sequence of DNA that encodes for a single, specific protein or regulates the expression of a gene; just as the DNA is arranged like beads on a necklace, the genes are similarly aligned. The information contained in the DNA is transcribed to ribonucleic acid (RNA), an intermediary template, which is in turn translated to the protein (Fig. 1.1). The four types of RNA that have been identified are messenger RNA (mRNA), transfer RNA (tRNA), ribosomal RNA (rRNA), and heterogeneous RNA (hnRNA). mRNA, which forms the template for protein synthesis in the cytoplasm, is formed in the nucleus of the cell from the DNA; tRNA transfers amino acids from the cytoplasm to the specific positions along the mRNA template. The functions of rRNA and hnRNA are less well understood. rRNA is associated with protein in the ribosomes and carries limited genetic information; hnRNA is an intranuclear RNA that may play a regulatory role. In eukaryotic cells (those with a nucleus and nuclear membrane, including human, plant, and protozoan cells but not bacteria), the DNA segments encoding a protein are interspersed with DNA that does not code for that protein; the coding portions are called exons and the noncoding portions introns. During the processing steps, the introns are removed and the exons are fused to form the mature mRNA, which is translated into the protein.

Both DNA and RNA are arranged in a linear fashion and consist of nucleotides, each of which has a base, pentose

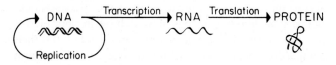

FIGURE 1.1. Relationship between transcription, translation, and replication.

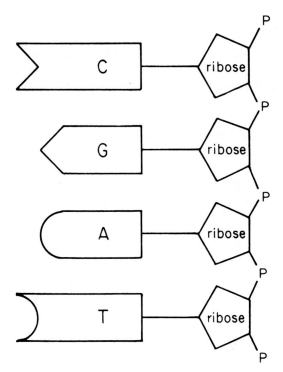

FIGURE 1.2. Nucleic acid structure.

(five-carbon sugar—deoxyribose in the case of DNA and ribose in the case of RNA), and phosphoric acid (Fig. 1.2). The bases are either purines (adenine or guanine) or pyrimidines (cytosine or thymine in DNA, and cytosine or uracil in RNA). The pentose sugar and the phosphoric acid form the macromolecular support. The precise order of the bases within the exons of a gene determines the amino acid sequence of the protein for which it encodes. For each amino acid, a triplet of DNA bases (codon) provides the necessary information for the identification of the amino acid in the protein; many amino acids have several codons that encode for them. For example, the amino acid phenylalanine is encoded by the triplet base sequence uracil–uracil–uracil or uracil–uracil–cytosine.

Genetic disorders may be roughly categorized into those caused by single-gene defects, chromosomal or large DNA abnormalities such as duplications or deletions of large segments, or the effect of more than one gene. For each species, a gene occurs at a particular position (locus) on a specific chromosome. Humans are diploid organisms with two pairs of 22 autosomal chromosomes and two sets of genes—one member of each pair is inherited from each parent. The remaining two chromosomes, X and Y, determine gender. An individual is *homozygous* for a gene pair if the information specified by each member is identical, and *heterozygous* if the two encode for different polypeptides. Alternate forms of a gene are called *alleles*. Some alleles represent common variations not associated with disease (called *polymorphisms*), others represent disease-producing mutations (alterations of the DNA sequence that cause a change in amino acid sequence which alters the actual protein

translated), and others are advantageous to the host under certain conditions. For example, the blood serotypes A, B, and O are common alleles; a normal individual may have AA, AO, BO, AB, or BB blood type. As another example, the genes coding for hemoglobin A (normal), S (sickle), and C are alleles, the hemoglobins S and C being mutations; the end products differ from each other by one amino acid in a chain of 146. Hemoglobin A has the amino acid glutamic acid in the position where valine is found in hemoglobin S and lysine in hemoglobin C. The substitution of glutamic acid alters the function of the protein. Allelism is the source of genetic variation in humans.

Most of the DNA is arranged in discrete chromosomes within the nucleus. A small fraction is within the mitochondria in the cytoplasm of the cell. Different species of animals and plants have different numbers of chromosome pairs; for example, a mouse has 20 pairs and a tomato 12 pairs. As mentioned above, humans have 23 pairs, of which two, X and Y, determine gender. The chromosomes are *homologous*: there are two of each type (autosomes) except the X and Y (sex chromosomes). Each nucleated cell of the organism has the same DNA as every other cell unless a mutation or chromosomal rearrangement occurred after conception.

The chemical bonds of DNA bind each linear strand to the linear strand of the same sequence positioned in the reverse direction. Hydrogen bonding between adenine (A, a purine) from one strand and thymine (T, a pyrimidine) from the other, or guanine (G, a purine) and cytosine (C, a pyrimidine) maintains the alignment of the two strands. The tertiary structure of the double strand is a double helix. Since the pairing of A with T and G with C is essential to the secondary and tertiary structures, the two strands are complementary.

During the process of cell division (*mitosis*), all DNA is duplicated and each daughter cell receives the same information from the parent unless a mutation or chromosomal rearrangement occurs. The process of gamete (spermatozoa or ova) formation (*meiosis*) involves a halving of the number of chromosomes. During meiosis, a single cell forms four gametes, each of which has half the number of chromosomes (haploid). Crossing over (exchange of DNA or *recombination*) occurs during the duplication process between homologous chromosomes (a pair with the same gene loci in the same order), and genetic material is exchanged (Fig. 1.3). This process changes the order of the alleles on a chromosome and increases genetic variability. During fertilization, the two haploid cells (egg and sperm) fuse to form a diploid cell, restoring the normal number of chromosomes.

Single-gene defects may be caused by a point mutation that causes an alteration of an amino acid in the sequence of the protein product or by a deletion or duplication of DNA within the locus of a single gene. Point mutations of functional significance to the organism usually occur in an *exon* or regulatory sequence. Chromosomal abnormalities involve deletions (loss of material) or duplications (extra material) of DNA and can sometimes be identified microscopically.

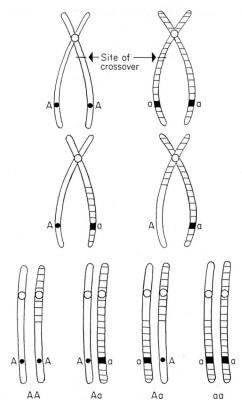

FIGURE 1.3. Crossing over (exchange of genetic material) between homologous chromosomes during meiosis.

Such abnormalities involve a larger segment of DNA or an entire chromosome. *Haploinsufficiency* is a gene-dosage effect that occurs when a diploid requires both functional copies of a gene for a wild-type phenotype. An organism that is heterozygous for a haploinsufficient locus does not have a wild-type phenotype.

Tjio and Levan (10) identified the correct number of human chromosomes as 46; previously the total was thought to be 48. The normal human 22 pairs of autosomal chromosomes and one pair of gender-determining chromosomes (XY for male and XX for female) are divided into seven groups on the basis of length and centromere position. In 1960, the initial Denver classification was developed at a meeting in Colorado and was based on the overall length and centromere position; seven groups, labeled A to G, were created. In 1971, the Paris nomenclature was created, and each chromosome was identified by length, centromere position, and banding. Chromosomes 1, 2, and 3 constituted group A; 4 and 5, group B; 6 to 12 and X, group C; 13 to 15, group D; 16 to 18, group E; 19 and 20, group F; and 21, 22, and Y, group G (Fig. 1.4).

Changes of chromosome structure can involve single chromosomes or an exchange of material between chromosomes. A piece of a chromosome may be lost by deletion or may be duplicated. The former results in *monosomy* for a group of genes and the latter results in *trisomy* for the genes. Chromosome segments can also be *inverted*—flipped 180 degrees from their normal orientation. If no material is gained or lost, the changes may not have a phenotypic effect. There are vast amounts of genetically inert DNA between groups of genes so usually these breaks cause no change in phenotype. Rarely, a gene may be disrupted by the chromosome breakage involved in the inversion. Another intrachromosomal rearrangement is the formation of a *ring*. This usually arises from breakage of the two ends and their subsequent fusion into a ring structure. There may be phenotypic consequences from deletion of chromatin from the two ends, and also from mitotic instability of the rings, resulting in trisomic or monosomic cells.

Translocation involves the exchange of material between chromosomes. Usually, translocations arise as reciprocal exchanges. If no material is lost or gained, the translocation is said to be balanced. Balanced translocations—and inversions for that matter—are occasionally found as variants in

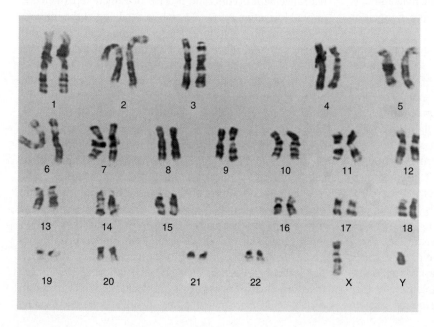

FIGURE 1.4. Karyotype of a normal male, showing banding produced by trypsin treatment of Seabright (11). (Courtesy of Robert S. Sparkes, MD.)

the general population. It is estimated that approximately 0.2% of individuals carry an asymptomatic rearrangement. If one comes to medical attention, it is usually because the unbalanced offspring of an individual with a translocation has congenital anomalies, or the individual has a history of spontaneous abortions.

CYTOGENETIC TESTS

Karyotyping

By synchronizing the reproductive cycle of a group of cells and arresting the progression of the mitotic process, the chromosomes can be visualized microscopically, and specific chromosomal identification can be made on the basis of length and the use of stains such as trypsin-Giemsa (G-banding; Fig. 1.4) (11), quinacrine mustard (Q-banding) (12), "reverse" or R-banding (Giemsa staining following controlled denaturation by heat), silver (staining of nucleolar organizing regions), and C-banding (staining of the condensed chromosome material near the centromere and regions with heterochromatin). All methods identify bands or specific regions and are useful for studying the specific structure of chromosome(s). The number of chromosomes can be counted and the bands of each studied for deletions, duplications, and other rearrangements. This technique is called karyotyping.

Relatively new techniques for arresting the progression of mitosis earlier in the cell cycle have been developed. In late prophase or early metaphase, the chromosomes are longer and less condensed and bands are further subdivided; smaller deletions and/or duplications can be detected. Extended chromosome analysis, termed *high-resolution banding*, is much more time-consuming but is particularly useful if a specific chromosomal abnormality or rearrangement is suspected. As the method is more labor intensive and expensive, one would not order high-resolution banding for a routine sample.

A cytogenetic nomenclature system has been adopted to describe the human chromosomal complement and indicate deviations from normal. An extra chromosome is indicated by a plus (+) and a missing one by a minus (–); thus 47,XX, +21 is a female with trisomy 21 (three copies of chromosome 21). The short arm of a chromosome is called p and the long arm is q. Chromosomal bands are numbered according to landmarks starting from the centromere up the short arm and down the long arm. Chromosomal rearrangements are described by noting the rearrangement and indicating the breakpoint(s). For example, a female with a deletion of the short arm of chromosome 4 with breakpoint at band p15 has the karyotype: 46,XX,del (4)(p15). A ring is indicated as r (e.g., 46,XY,r[13]male with a ring chromosome 13) and translocation as t (e.g., 46,XX,t[3;9][p14; q21] female with a translocation between chromosomes 3 and 9 with breakpoints at band p14 on chromosome 3 and band q21 on chromosome 9). An inversion is indicated as inv (e.g., 46XY,inv[2][p12q12]male with an inversion of chromosome 2 with breakpoints at p12 and q12).

Fluorescent In Situ Hybridization

Recently, DNA probes have become available for all human chromosomes—greatly expanding the field of molecular cytogenetics. If the origin of a duplication or translocation is unknown, the DNA probes can be fluorescently labeled and "painted" onto the metaphase spread or interphase nuclei chromosomal preparation, a technique called fluorescent in situ hybridization (FISH); chromosomal abnormalities can be readily identified under the microscope.

Telomeres, the physical ends of linear eukaryotic chromosomes, are specialized nucleoprotein complexes that have important functions, primarily in the protection, replication, and stabilization of the chromosome ends. In most organisms studied, telomeres contain lengthy stretches of tandemly repeated simple DNA sequences composed of GC-rich strands (called terminal repeats). These terminal repeats are highly conserved; in fact, all vertebrates appear to have the same simple sequence repeat in telomeres: $(TTAGGG)_n$. Often sequences adjacent to the telomeric repeats are highly polymorphic, are rich in DNA repetitive elements (termed subtelomeric repeats), and in some cases, genes have been found in the proterminal regions of chromosomes.

Telomerase is the reverse transcriptase enzyme responsible for the extension of telomeric repeat sequences in most species studied. If telomerase activity is diminished or absent, telomeres will shorten. Shortened telomeres appear to lead to cell senescence (13). Eventually, telomeric sequences can shorten to the point where they are not long enough to support the telomere–protein complex protecting the ends and the chromosomes become unstable. These shortened ends become "sticky" and promote chromosomal rearrangements (14,15). Some rearrangements may contribute to the development of cancers (16,17). Telomere testing has been shown to identify alterations in 7% to 10% of cases with moderate/severe mental retardation and cases of multiple congenital anomalies with mental retardation in the setting of normal karyotype testing (18). The analysis involves the detection of deletions, duplications, or cryptic translocations using subtelomere FISH probes on each chromosome (15).

Comparative Genomic Hybridization

Comparative genomic hybridization (CGH) was developed to screen the entire genome for DNA content differences by comparing a test sample to a control (19,20). Because metaphase chromosomes are used as the substrate for analysis, the detection of unbalanced alterations is limited to the resolution of the metaphase target (at the level of a 450-band karyotype, approximately 5- to 10-Mb change). DNA microarray CGH is a powerful new technology capable of identifying chromosomal imbalance at a high resolution by cohybridizing differentially labeled test and control DNA samples to a microarray chip (21–23). The chip (small metallic platform with applied spots of known large-insert

DNA clones such as bacterial artificial chromosomes) technology offers higher resolution, is faster, and is highly sensitive. Because the DNA clones have a known map location and information, detected alterations are immediately linked to known genetic markers (pieces of DNA with a known chromosomal location and sequence), and the genetic location of a chromosomal abnormality such as a deletion or duplication can be determined by the map distances between known markers or by the length of the clones used.

Whole-Exome and Whole-Genome Sequencing

Newer techniques of producing multiple copies of the coding regions of the genome (exomes), or the entire genome including exons and intronic sequence (whole genome) have revolutionized gene variant detection in disease (www.ambrygen.com/exome-sequencing). There are many factors that make exome sequencing superior to single-gene analysis including the ability to identify mutations in genes that were not tested due to an atypical clinical presentation, or the ability to identify clinical cases where mutations from different genes contribute to the different phenotypes in the same patient. This technology is particularly useful for gene discovery in those conditions in which mapping has been confounded by locus heterogeneity and uncertainty about the boundaries of diagnostic classification. Direct-to-consumer whole exome sequencing services are available to individuals without a physician intermediary through programs such as 23andMe (www.23andme.com/).

SINGLE-GENE MUTATIONS

The substitution, addition, or deletion of one or more of the bases in an exon alters the DNA sequence and results in the formation of a protein with an abnormal amino acid at a specific site or the absence of the protein. Such abnormalities are believed to be common, and each human being is estimated to have three to five such mutations (24). If such a point mutation occurs in a portion of the protein that is not critical to function, the abnormality goes undetected (because it is not evident phenotypically) and does not affect the individual. If the codon error results in an amino acid substitution that changes the formation or function of the protein or truncates the product, the mutation is evidenced by reduced or (rarely) improved function, which would be advantageous to the organism from an evolutionary standpoint.

Autosomal Recessive Inheritance

For some mutations, the loss of a functional protein product from one of the chromosomes is asymptomatic because the gene on the homologous chromosome produces a normal

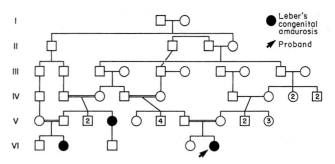

FIGURE 1.5. Pedigree of a family in which Leber congenital amaurosis (LCA) was inherited as an autosomal recessive disorder. Consanguineous matings are indicated by *double lines*.

product. If 50% activity of a protein is sufficient for normal function, the individual with one mutation is called a *carrier*; the signs and symptoms of the disease would be evident only in those who have two abnormal genes. Such a disorder is called *autosomal recessive* and is evident in some (statistically 25%) of the offsprings of two carriers (Fig. 1.5). In general, there is a higher incidence of parental consanguinity associated with rare autosomal recessive disorders. For some diseases, carriers probably have a common ancestor because nearly all affected individuals have the identical mutation; an example of this founder effect is Tay-Sachs disease (OMIM 272800: infantile developmental delay, paralysis, dementia, blindness with lipid-laden ganglion cells leaving a central "cherry-red" spot funduscopically, premature death before the age of 5 years). Mutations of the implicated gene, the enzyme hexosaminidase, occur more commonly in the Ashkenazi Jewish population.

Autosomal Dominant Inheritance

When the protein is structural or the organism requires 100% activity for normal structure or function, phenotypic abnormalities are evident with a mutation of only one of the two homologous chromosomes. Such a disorder is termed *autosomal dominant* because the presence of a mutation on one of the chromosomes results in a phenotypically identifiable disease state. An affected individual with an autosomal dominant trait has a 50% chance of passing the gene to each offspring (Fig. 1.6). Examples of autosomal dominant disorders include Marfan syndrome (OMIM 154700: dislocated lenses, dilated aortic root, increased height, disproportionately long limbs and digits, anterior chest deformity, joint laxity, narrow arched palate, scoliosis due to connective-tissue disorder; caused by mutations of the fibrillin-1 gene); neurofibromatosis type I (OMIM 162200: consistent features of cafe au lait spots, Sakurai-Lisch nodules of the iris, fibromatous skin tumors, occasional hamartomatous tumors found systemically; due to mutations in the neurofibromin gene); and Best disease (OMIM 153700: mutations in the bestrophin gene cause

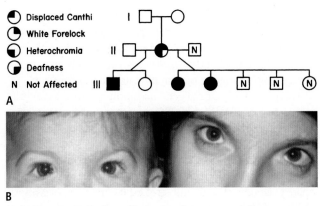

A

B

FIGURE 1.6. A: Pedigree illustrating the autosomal dominant transmission of Waardenburg syndrome. (Adapted from DiGeorge AM, Olmstead RW, Harley RD. Waardenburg's syndrome. A syndrome of heterochromia of the irides, lateral displacement of the medial canthi and lacrimal puncta, congenital deafness, and other characteristic associated defects. *J Pediatr* 1960;57:649–669.) (Figure 1.6 B)

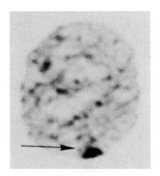

FIGURE 1.7. Barr body (sex chromatin) at the nuclear membrane in a cell from buccal mucosa of a normal female.

juvenile-onset and adult vitelliform macular dystrophy with collections of lipofuscin-like material in the subretinal space creating macular lesions which resemble an egg yolk). Disease-causing genes located on the autosomes occur equally in males and females, regardless of dominant or recessive inheritance.

X-Linked Inheritance

Mutations on the X chromosome are unique, as normal females have a pair, and normal males have only one X chromosome along with an unpaired Y chromosome. X-linked diseases may be recessive or, much less frequently, dominant. Therefore, one abnormal gene for which an individual requires only some of the protein product usually would not cause disease in a female, who is a heterozygote, but would in a male, who is a *hemizygote*. Such disorders are termed X-linked recessive and become clinically evident in the male as he has only one X chromosome copy. Occasionally, a heterozygous female carrier exhibits some manifestations of an X-linked recessive disease. The expression of the single recessive gene on the X chromosome in a female has been explained by the X inactivation theory, or Lyon hypothesis (25). During the second week of embryonic life, one of the two X chromosomes in each cell of the female fetus randomly becomes the "inactive X"; this X chromosome becomes condensed during interphase and appears as a darkly stained mass at the nuclear membrane (Barr body or sex chromatin; Fig. 1.7). Most of the genes on the inactive X are not expressed. Once this differentiation occurs, the same X chromosome continues to be the inactive one in all the linear descendants of that cell. Thus, the female is a mosaic of two cell lines, those in which the genes on the maternally inherited X are active and those in which the paternally inherited X are active. The Lyon hypothesis is invoked to explain the splotchy pigment epithelium and

choroidal pigmentation in the fundus of a female carrier of ocular albinism (OA), or the tapetal reflex in the carrier of X-linked retinitis pigmentosa (ghr.nlm.nih.gov/glossary=xchromsomeinactivation).

The heritable inability to correctly perceive the color green, known as Daltonism (after the English chemist John Dalton, who himself was affected), was the first human trait mapped to the X chromosome (www.colblindor.com/2006/04/09/daltonism). X-linked disorders of the eye for which phenotypic evidence of the carrier state may be present in females include choroideremia (OMIM 303100: degeneration of the choriocapillaris and retina due to mutations in the Rab escort protein-1 gene [*REP1*]); Nance-Horan or cataract-dental syndrome (OMIM 302350: affected males have dense nuclear cataracts and frequent microcornea, and carrier females show posterior Y-sutural cataracts with small corneas and only slightly reduced vision; caused by mutations in the *NHS* gene) (26,27); blue cone monochromatism (OMIM 303700: affected males have poor central vision and color discrimination, infantile nystagmus, and nearly normal retinal appearance due to mutations in the locus control region upstream to the red and green cone pigment gene array) (28); and Lowe syndrome (OMIM 309000: affected males have cataracts, developmental delay, vitamin D–resistant rickets, and aminoaciduria, and carrier females have peripheral cortical lens opacities) (29). A carrier female has a 50% chance of passing a mutant gene on the X chromosome to any offspring; thus, the daughters have that same chance of being carriers and the sons of being affected with the disease (Fig. 1.8). Examples of X-linked recessive disorders include Duchenne muscular dystrophy (OMIM 310200: due to mutations of the dystrophin gene, affected males display progressive proximal muscular dystrophy with characteristic pseudohypertrophy of the calves and severe cardiomyopathy; there is massive elevation of creatine kinase levels in the blood, myopathic changes by electromyography, and myofiber degeneration with fibrosis and fatty infiltration on muscle biopsy); and X-linked juvenile retinoschisis (OMIM 312700: affected males with *RS* gene mutations have intraretinal splitting due to degeneration). If the X-linked gene is dominant, both the heterozygous female and hemizygous male manifest

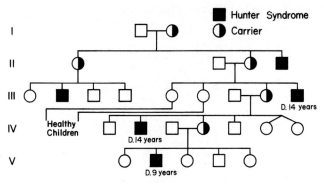

FIGURE 1.8. Pedigree showing X-linked inheritance of Hunter syndrome. Note that affected males are related through their mothers.

the mutant phenotype. It has been observed in the few X-linked dominant traits that a heterozygous female is more likely to have female offspring, and it has been postulated that there is fetal wastage of males. Presumably, the hemizygous state of the mutation may be lethal. Examples of X-linked dominant disorders include familial incontinentia pigmenti type II (OMIM 308300: mutations in the IKK-gamma gene causing skin defects of perinatal inflammatory vesicles, verrucous patches, dermal scarring, and retinal vascular anomalies) and Aicardi syndrome (OMIM 304050: affected females have flexion spasms and lacunar lesions of the choroid and retina).

Mitochondrial Genetics

An additional source of genetic information in the cell lies in the mitochondria (30). Each cell contains hundreds of mitochondria, each of which contains multiple copies of a 16,569-base pair circular, double-stranded DNA molecule. This DNA encodes 13 peptides that are subunits of proteins required for oxidative phosphorylation. In addition, there is a complete set of 22 tRNAs and two rRNAs. These RNAs are involved in translation of mitochondrial-encoded proteins within the mitochondrion. Mitochondria are responsible for the generation of ATP via aerobic metabolism. Most mitochondrial proteins are encoded by nuclear genes; however, some are encoded by mitochondrial genes, and mutations can lead to energy failure. The mitochondrial genome is subject to a number of peculiarities of inheritance including maternal transmission and a phenomenon known as *heteroplasmy*, resulting in distinctive patterns of familial disease. Heteroplasmy determines expression variability of the disease within a family. Different cells in an individual and different individuals in a family contain different proportions of mutant and wild-type mitochondria (31).

Mitochondrial mutation disorders display maternal genetic transmission. There may be the appearance of transmission directly from generation to generation, suggesting dominant inheritance. Both males and females may be affected, but men never transmit the disorder to any of their offspring. Women, on the other hand, pass the trait to all of their children, although expression may be more severe in some than in others. At the time of fertilization, the sperm sheds its tail, including all of its mitochondria. Only the sperm head, containing nuclear DNA, enters the egg. Therefore, all the mitochondria for the next generation are contributed by the egg cell. Hence, mitochondrial genes are exclusively maternally derived, explaining the pattern of maternal transmission.

Major mitochondrial gene mutation syndromes include Kearns-Sayre (OMIM 530000: external ophthalmoplegia, pigmentary retinopathy, heart block, ataxia, increased cerebrospinal fluid protein); myoclonic epilepsy with ragged red fibers or MERRF (OMIM 545000: myoclonic epilepsy, myopathy, dementia); mitochondrial myopathy, encephalopathy, lactic acidosis, and stroke-like episodes or MELAS (OMIM 540000: lactic acidosis, stroke-like episodes, myopathy, seizures, dementia); Leber hereditary optic neuropathy (OMIM 535000: blindness, cardiac conduction defects); and Leigh syndrome (OMIM 256000: movement disorder, respiratory dyskinesia, regression) (32–36).

Penetrance

The clinical features of single-gene mutations vary from one individual to another. *Penetrance* is the percentage of known carriers manifesting the phenotype and reflects our ability to identify an individual with a mutant gene; reduced penetrance means that some individuals with the gene may not exhibit clinical evidence of the disease. Nonpenetrance is defined as the absence of phenotype in a person known to carry a specific mutant gene. Nonpenetrance has been demonstrated to occur with many genetic traits and can be most easily inferred when a grandparent and child have a disorder that does not appear to be expressed in the parent. For example, some individuals without evidence of colobomatous microphthalmia have an affected ancestor and an affected child (Fig. 1.9). The only potential explanation is that the apparently unaffected individual has the mutant gene in his or her genome but that the clinicians cannot find the evidence by ocular examination. If four family members descended from the same affected ancestor had affected progeny but one was free of the disease, the gene would be 75% penetrant.

Expressivity

Expressivity refers to the degree of phenotypic expression of a genetic trait. A disease may exhibit different manifestations among individuals in the same family. Such variable expressivity is common, particularly in autosomal dominant disorders. For example, some individuals with Marfan syndrome (OMIM 154700), an autosomal dominant disease of the connective-tissue gene fibrillin, may be tall and have dislocated lenses; others may be of normal stature and show no evidence of a dislocated lens but have an aneurysm of the ascending aorta.

Autosomal recessive disorders can exhibit variable expressivity, particularly if the mutation occurs at different sites in the protein. For example, there are numerous hemoglobinopathies with distinctive clinical manifestations that are caused by different mutations of the hemoglobin gene.

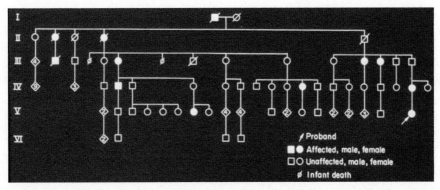

FIGURE 1.9. Multigenerational family with autosomal dominant colobomatous microphthalmia. The proband's (*arrow*) maternal grandfather was examined and showed no evidence of colobomata or microphthalmia. Thus, in this family the gene for colobomatous microphthalmia exhibits reduced penetrance.

Genetic Heterogeneity

Different gene defects, modes of inheritance, and chromosomal abnormalities can produce similar clinical phenotypes, a phenomenon termed *genetic heterogeneity* (ghr.nlm. nih.gov/glossary=geneticheterogeneity). Examples of genetic heterogeneity are common in ophthalmology. Classification of diseases is thus most reliably made on the basis of specific gene mutations or chromosomal aberrations; doing so allows for directed therapies.

Epigenetics

Epigenetics is the study of changes in gene expression or cellular phenotype caused by mechanisms other than changes in the original DNA sequence (www.pbs.org/wgbh/nova/body/epigenetics.html, and learn.genetics.utah.edu/content/epigenetics/). The development and maintenance of an organism is orchestrated by a set of chemical reactions that switch parts of the genome off and on at strategic times and locations. Epigenetics is the study of these reactions and the factors that influence them. In epigenetic modification, a methyl group (–CH3) is added to specific cytosine bases of the DNA. This enzymatic process, called DNA methylation, is known to play a key role in both development and disease. Methylation is a physical modification to the DNA that affects the way the molecule is shaped and, consequently, regulates which genes are transcriptionally active. Another epigenetic modification of DNA is the addition of a hydroxymethyl group (–CH2–OH) to specific cytosine bases of DNA. In eukaryotic cells, genomic DNA is wrapped around histone proteins to form nucleosomes, which together form chromatin fibers that can be further compacted into dense coils. Epigenetic modifications to histone proteins can either inhibit or promote coiling or condensation of the chromatin, leading to chromatin organizational changes, which in turn affects how the associated genes are expressed.

Mucopolysaccharidosis

The autosomal recessive Hurler syndrome or mucopolysaccharidosis type IH (OMIM 607014: corneal clouding, coarse facies, developmental delay, hepatosplenomegaly, and hernia) and X-linked recessive Hunter syndrome or mucopolysaccharidosis type II (OMIM 309900: no corneal clouding, coarse facies, dwarfism, hepatosplenomegaly, and deafness) may be difficult to differentiate clinically on the basis of physical findings in a young boy with no family history. As the inheritance patterns are different, the gene defects are distinctive (http://ghr.nlm.nih.gov/condition/mucopolysaccharidosis-type-i). Conversely, the clinical features of the Hurler and Scheie (OMIM 607016: stiff joints, clouding of the peripheral cornea, and aortic regurgitation) syndromes can be differentiated by the mental retardation and early death that are features of the Hurler syndrome. Life expectancy in the Scheie form is nearly normal and mental retardation is very rare. Originally the two were classified as different diseases. With the identification of the enzymatic defect, it became clear that the disorders were allelic as the same gene is mutated in both, causing a deficiency in the enzyme alpha-l-iduronidase.

Leber Congenital Amaurosis

Leber congenital amaurosis (LCA; OMIM 204000) is a group of autosomal recessive retinal dystrophies. It is the most common genetic cause of congenital retinal disorders in infants and children, and results in significant and often severe vision loss at an early age. Its incidence is 2 to 3 per 100,000 births and it accounts for 10% to 18% of cases of congenital blindness. At least 17 genes contribute to this disorder (37). The observed genetic heterogeneity is the result not only of the number of genes that have been implicated in LCA, but also the consequences of the different mutations in these genes. Mutations in at least two of these genes—*RPE65* and *CRX*—not only cause an LCA clinical presentation, but also lead to other late-onset retinal dystrophies such as retinitis pigmentosa and cone-rod dystrophy (38,39). Gene therapy was used to successfully recover vision in a canine model of LCA (40). The researchers designed an adeno-associated virus vector to use in retinal transgene delivery. This vector was used to carry wild-type canine *RPE65* complementary DNA and was injected into the subretinal space of dog eyes. The LCA dogs showed visual recovery in performing visual function and behavioral tests. Multiple gene therapy trials are in progress to treat humans with the same genetic disease (37).

Albinism

Albinism comprises a group of heterogeneous inherited abnormalities of melanin synthesis characterized by a congenital reduction or absence of melanin pigment associated with specific developmental changes of the visual system (www.albinism.org). Oculocutaneous albinism (OCA) involves two regions of the body: the skin and hair and the optic system, including the eye and optic nerves. Ocular albinism (OA) has similar changes in the visual system by reducing mainly the pigment in the retinal pigment epithelium (RPE) of the eye, usually with no clinical difference in the color of the skin and hair. Ophthalmologic signs, although variable, include nystagmus, hypopigmentation of the uveal tract and RPE, iris transillumination, foveal hypoplasia, and abnormal decussation of the optic nerve fibers at the optic chiasm.

The formation of melanin pigment is a complex event requiring several enzymes and proteins and the pigment-containing subcellular organelle, the melanosome. Melanin pigment is produced in the melanocyte, which is found in the skin, hair follicles, iris, and RPE of the eye. Melanin biosynthesis begins with hydroxylation of the amino acid l-tyrosine to dihydroxylphenylalanine (DOPA) and the oxidation of DOPA to DOPA quinone by the copper-containing enzyme tyrosinase, resulting in either black-brown eumelanin, or in the presence of sulfhydryl compounds, red-yellow pheomelanin. The resulting pigment polymer is deposited on a protein matrix within the melanosome. In the skin and hair follicles, the melanosome is then transferred to keratinocytes via the dendrites of the melanocyte.

At present, four genetic loci responsible for human albinism have been mapped (OCA1: OMIM 203100, OCA2: OMIM 203200, Hermansky-Pudlak syndrome: OMIM 203300, and OA1: OMIM 300500); three of the genes have been isolated and pathologic mutations identified (*OCA1*, *OCA2*, and *OA1*). The classic "tyrosinase-negative" albinism results from tyrosinase gene mutations that inactivate the encoded enzyme and is categorized as OCA1 (41). Mild forms of OCA1, initially described as autosomal recessive OA, result from mutations of the tyrosinase gene that produce an enzyme with residual activity. OCA in which hairbulbs form melanin upon incubation in DOPA or tyrosine (tyrosinase-positive OCA) can be caused by mutations at several loci, including *OCA1*; *OCA2*, which is associated with the human homolog (P) of the mouse p gene—a melanosomal transport protein (42); and the rare Hermansky-Pudlak syndrome (OCA with platelet dysfunction).

Magnetic resonance imaging (MRI) size and configuration comparisons of the optic pathways in normal versus albinism phenotypes revealed significantly smaller optic nerves and tracts, smaller chiasmatic widths, and wider angles between nerves and tracts in the albino group than in the control group (43). The chiasms of the albinos are shaped like an X, whereas the chiasm in the controls was shaped like two back-to-back parentheses, that is, ")(." These differences reflect the atypical crossing of optic fibers. MRI can be an important diagnostic tool in patients with equivocal albinotic presentations.

X-linked OA1 is caused by mutations in the *OA1* gene at chromosome Xp22.3-p22.2, which encodes a membrane glycoprotein localized to melanosomes. Approximately 48% of the reported mutations in the *OA1* gene are intragenic deletions and about 43% are point mutations. Faugere and associates (44) report three *OA1* unrelated families with an initial diagnosis of congenital nystagmus. They identified three novel *OA1* mutations consisting of two intragenic deletions and a point mutation. Direct testing of carrier females is advocated and can be performed by direct sequencing or by scanning methods such as denaturing gradient gel electrophoresis or denaturing high-performance liquid chromatography. The real-time fluorescent PCR gene-dosage assay is an accurate, nonradioactive, and fast method for gene carrier assessment that can be applied to any type of *OA1* gene deletion. A similar two-tiered diagnostic test strategy for mutation screening for *OA1* has been proposed (45).

Examples of Pleiotropic Disorders with Ophthalmic Considerations

A single-gene mutation that is expressed in many different tissues or can affect more than one organ system is termed *pleiotropic*. Waardenburg syndrome (Ptosis-epicanthus syndrome) is an example of a disorder in which the mutation of one gene has multiple organ effects. This dominantly inherited disorder includes displaced canthi, heterochromia of the irides, white forelock, broad nasal root, and deafness (Fig. 1.6); the syndrome is divided into four types (I, II [A, B, and C], III, and IV) with the most severe being associated with upper limb defects (type III; OMIM 148820) and a ganglionic megacolon (Hirschsprung disease) (type IV; OMIM 277580). Dystopia canthorum, the lateral displacement of the inner canthi, distinguishes type I (OMIM 193500) (which shows this clinical phenotype) from type II. Types I and III (OMIM 148820) are caused by mutations in the *PAX3* gene, which was first identified in *Drosophila* (46,47). Mutations in the transcription factor *MITF* have been implicated for Waardenburg syndrome type IIA (OMIM 193510) (48–50); digenic inheritance of type IIA and autosomal recessive OA has been proposed (51). Type IV or Waardenburg-Shah syndrome is a disorder of the embryonic neural crest that combines clinical features of Waardenburg syndrome and Hirschsprung disease with colonic aganglionosis.

Alagille Syndrome

Alagille syndrome (OMIM 118450) is an autosomal dominant disorder characterized by cholestatic liver disease, pulmonic valvular and peripheral arterial stenosis, "butterfly" vertebrae, posterior embryotoxon (anterior displacement of Schwalbe's line) with retinal pigmentary changes in the eye in some individuals, and unusual facies with broad forehead, pointed mandible, and bulbous nose tip (http://digestive.niddk.nih.gov/ddiseases/pubs/alagille/). The syndrome is due to mutations in the Notch signaling *JAG1* gene on chromosome 20p12 (52,53).

Cornelia de Lange Syndrome

Cornelia de Lange syndrome (CDLS; OMIM 122470) is a dominantly inherited multisystem developmental disorder characterized by growth and cognitive retardation, abnormalities of the upper limbs, gastroesophageal dysfunction, hirsutism, cardiac and genitourinary anomalies, and characteristic facial features (54–56) (www.cdlsusa.org/). Ophthalmic features include ptosis, nasolacrimal duct obstruction, arched eyebrows with synophrys, long eyelashes, refractive error, and infrequent glaucoma (57). The prevalence is estimated to be as high as 1 in 10,000. Gene mutations in the *NIPBL* gene on chromosome 5p13.1 have recently been associated with this disorder (58,59). The *fly* homolog of *NIPBL*, Nipped-B, facilitates enhancer-promoter communication and regulates Notch signaling and other developmental pathways in *D. melanogaster* (60).

Marfan Syndrome

Marfan syndrome (OMIM 154700) is an autosomal dominant connective-tissue disorder with an estimated incidence of 1 in 5,000 with approximately 25% being sporadic cases (www.marfan.org/). Three systems are predominantly involved: the skeleton, heart, and eye. Common and major manifestations of the disease include subluxation of the crystalline lens; dilatation of the aortic root and aneurysm of the ascending aorta; and skeletal abnormalities such as pectus excavatum and kyphoscoliosis and an upper segment/lower segment ratio of two standard deviations below the mean for age. Other criteria such as myopia, mitral valve prolapse, arachnodactyly, joint laxity, tall stature, pes planus, pneumothorax, and dural ectasia are also contributory. The diagnostic criteria have been recently revised, requiring involvement of three systems with two major diagnostic manifestations (61). The gene defect has been identified: Fibrillin (*FBN1*) maps to chromosome 15q15–q21.1. It is a large gene of more than 230 kb and highly fragmented with 65 exons. The protein is a 350-kDa glycoprotein and is the principal structural component of connective-tissue microfibrils found ubiquitously in all extracellular matrices. Fibrillin structures serve as scaffolds for the deposition of elastin in elastic tissues (61).

To date, more than 500 mutations have been identified in the *FBN1* gene in Marfan syndrome patients and related diseases (61). Presently, no definite genotype–phenotype correlations have been identified except for neonatal mutations. An association with a subset of mutations in exons 24 to 32 and neonatal MFS appears correlative, thus molecular diagnostic testing can be performed (62). With a few exceptions, almost all mutations found in fibrillinopathies other than classic Marfan syndrome have been unique to one affected individual or family, which has hampered the delineation of potential genotype–phenotype correlations (62).

Comeglio and associates (63) characterized the incidence and class of *FBN1* mutations in the largest series reported to date, a group of 11 consecutive British patients affected predominantly by ectopia lentis (EL). The investigators identified six causative mutations in the fibrillin 1 gene (*FBN1*)—three mutations are novel and one was recurrent in two patients—thus establishing an *FBN1* mutation incidence of 63% (7/11). These results are within the 23% to 86% range of mutation identification rate in Marfan syndrome and related patients in recent investigations. All mutations were within the first 15 exons of the fibrillin gene, while database citations of Marfan mutations are distributed throughout the gene. A different type of *FBN1* mutation presents in this group of patients, with arginine to cysteine substitutions appearing frequently. Patients with predominant EL should be screened for *FBN1* mutations. Echocardiography is recommended initially and at regular intervals throughout the patients' lifetimes, as there is a tendency for late-onset aortic dilatation and/or dissection to develop.

Lens subluxation is the diagnostic ocular abnormality in this disease. It is present in 65% to 70% of patients and varies from a mild superotemporal displacement of the lens seen only in postpupillary dilation to significant subluxation that places the equator of the lens in the pupillary axis. Subluxation of the lens due to stretched or absent zonular fibers is slowly progressive in the first two decades of life. Further displacement at a later age is uncommon. Total dislocation into the vitreous cavity is uncommon and may be complicated by phacolytic uveitis and glaucoma. Anterior displacement of the lens into the anterior chamber or within the pupillary space is rare in Marfan syndrome with EL. Premature cataracts are common, developing 10 to 20 years earlier in patients with Marfan syndrome than in the general population.

MASTER CONTROL GENES

The mature eye is a highly complex organ that develops through a highly organized process during embryogenesis. Alterations in the genetic programming of the eye could lead to outcomes of severe eye disorganization that are apparent at birth or shortly thereafter.

For the past decade, several master-control genes that direct developmental and differential pathways have been identified. *PAX6*, *SOX2*, and *RX* are at the top of the eye developmental hierarchy; mutation or loss of these genes leads mainly to loss of the entire eye. Other genes, such as *FOX*, *PITX*, and *MAF*, are important for the development of particular regions of the eye and are thought to be downstream of the top level of regulation in eye development. These genes are expressed during embryogenesis and initiate a cascade of gene expression responsible for specific cell-lineage commitments. Most genes at the top of the hierarchy of eye development code for transcription factors, although a few code for signaling molecules. The mutant phenotypes that are associated with some of these genes are described below, along with the genetic and molecular interactions that have been inferred between their products.

Paired Box Gene 6

Paired box gene 6 (*PAX6*) is the prototype for an eye master-control gene. It is one of the family of genes that encode transcription factors with a homeodomain and a paired domain. Loss of function leads to the eyeless (ey) phenotype in *Drosophila* and also causes severe ocular defects in many other animals (64). Interestingly, ectopic (at a different location other than normal) expression of *Pax6* in *Drosophila*, mouse, and frog (*Xenopus*) causes the formation of a functional eye. This supports two concepts: (a) homologous genes in different species have the same function—to "switch on" eye development; (b) there is only one way to make the eye, by a cascade of signals initiated by *Pax6* expression (65).

In humans, *PAX6* mutations mainly cause aniridia (OMIM 106210), which is a panocular disorder, and less commonly cause isolated cataracts and macular hypoplasia (failure of retinal foveal development; OMIM 136520), keratitis (OMIM 148190), and Peters' anomaly (central corneal opacity which is frequently associated with adhesion between the cornea and the lens; OMIM 603807) (66). As in the mouse, the homozygous loss (both parental alleles have mutations) of *PAX6* function in humans affecting all expressing tissues is lethal.

Targets of *PAX6* encode other transcription factors or structural proteins of the lens (crystallins) and cornea (keratins 1–12). Many PAX6-regulated transcription factors (such as *SIX3*, *FOXE3*, *MAF*, *MITF*, *PROX1*, *LHX2*, and *PITX3*) are involved in the formation of the cornea and lens; others (such as *PAX2*, *CHX10*, and *EYA1*) are involved in retina and optic nerve development (67).

Only a few transcription factors or signaling molecules (e.g., *BMP4*, *BMP7*, *RX*, and *SHH*) are known to regulate *PAX6*. Among them, *SHH* might be highest in the hierarchy: knockout mice and humans with mutations in *SHH* suffer from holoprosencephaly with ocular manifestations that range from microphthalmia to cyclopia, which indicates a disruption in the earliest event in eye development, separation of the central eye field (68).

Genotype and phenotype information for human *PAX6* mutations is freely available from the *PAX6* mutation database (http://pax6.hgu.mrc.ac.uk).

Sex-Determining Region Y-Related High-Mobility Group Box Gene 2

Sex-determining region Y-related high-mobility group box gene 2 (*SOX2*) is expressed in the developing lens placode, lens pit, optic cup, neural retina, lens, brain, and ear; heterozygous mutations of the gene result in anophthalmia in humans. Interestingly, all of these mutations seem to occur de novo (spontaneously) and are inherited as dominant alleles (69).

Retina and Anterior Neural Fold Homeobox Gene

The retina and anterior neural fold homeobox gene (*RX*) encodes a homeodomain transcription factor and is one of the first retinal patterning genes to be expressed during development (70). Rx-deficient mouse embryos lack eye anlagen (simple preliminary organ structures in the embryo) and do not express *Pax6* in the eye field, which indicates that *Pax6* upregulation in these tissues is dependent on functional *Rx* expression (71). It has recently been shown that the spontaneous mouse mutant *eyeless* (analogous to anophthalmia in humans) is caused by a point mutation in an alternative translation-initiation codon of *Rx* (72).

ISOLATED OCULAR AND PERIOCULAR SYNDROMES

Microphthalmia and Anophthalmia

Microphthalmia (OMIM 309700), a term derived from the Greek *micro* (small) and *ophthalmos* (eye), refers to a congenital malformation in which the volume of the eye is reduced; the spectrum ranges from mild reduction in the anteroposterior axis to histologically documented anophthalmia (OMIM 206900) (www.ncbi.nlm.nih.gov/books/NBK1378/). Nanophthalmia (OMIM 600165 and 605738) is used to describe microphthalmia with normal intraocular structures, and refers to a refractive error of +8.00 D or greater hyperopia. Although microcornea or high hyperopia may be a useful clinical clue, the diagnosis frequently can be made by inspection alone; however, as microcornea can occur in the absence of microphthalmia (73,74) and conversely, microphthalmia in association with a normal-sized cornea (75–77), the clinical diagnosis may be inaccurate (http://eyepathologist.com/disease.asp?IDNUM=308040). As the spectrum of microphthalmia varies from slightly reduced axial length to histologically documented anophthalmia, ultrasonography with precise measurement of the anteroposterior axis is essential for the diagnosis. Since most normal adult eyes range from 21.50 to 27.00 mm, an adult axial length of less than 20 mm should be considered abnormal (78,79). Despite the use of this technologically advanced tool, extreme microphthalmia may be difficult to distinguish from anophthalmia.

Microphthalmia appears to be a relatively common ocular malformation in all races. The high prevalence, which would be unusual for a disorder caused by a single gene, suggests multiple causes. Few studies have documented the prevalence in the general population. In a prospective study of more than 50,000 pregnancies in the United States in the late 1960s, the incidence of anophthalmia or microphthalmia was found to be 0.22 per 1,000 births and that of coloboma to be 0.26 per 1,000 (80). Prevalence among blind adults varies from 0.6% to 1.9% (81,82). In the pediatric age group, it accounts for 3.2% to 11.2% of cases of blindness (82–84). These differences are not readily explainable

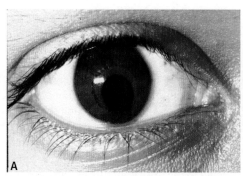
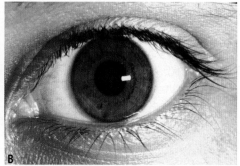

FIGURE 1.10. Right **(A)** and left **(B)** irides of a young man with mental retardation and deletion of the long arm of chromosome 18. Note the asymmetry.

but may reflect the race or population studied; the highest prevalence (11.2%) was found in the 1980 survey on the causes of blindness among Japanese schoolchildren.

Visual impairment in microphthalmia varies from little or no loss to absence of vision, as would be found in cases of anophthalmia. The degree of visual loss best correlates with the associated abnormalities and degree of microphthalmia; cataracts, optic nerve hypoplasia, and/or colobomata of the macula or optic nerve may cause significant visual impairment.

Cases of microphthalmia may be divided into two general forms: colobomatous and noncolobomatous. Although uveal colobomata may occur in the absence of microphthalmia, the two are frequently associated and presumably etiologically related. A coloboma may occur in the iris, choroid, optic nerve, or any combination thereof (Figs. 1.10 and 1.11). The colobomata result from incomplete closure of the fetal fissure, a process normally completed by the 6th week of gestation (85). The embryonic processes that determine the size of the eye are poorly understood. Congenital cystic microphthalmia and anophthalmia are extreme forms of this dysembryogenesis (86,87). As extreme microphthalmia may be difficult to distinguish from anophthalmia, serial sectioning of the orbit may be necessary to differentiate them. The malformation may be unilateral or bilateral, and asymmetry is common.

Microphthalmia, with or without colobomata, may be a manifestation of many different disorders: genetic, environmental, and those of unknown cause. The evaluation of a patient is interdisciplinary. Aside from a complete ocular examination, all patients should have a careful history, including a genetic pedigree and physical examination. In certain cases, family members should also be examined.

Isolated colobomatous microphthalmia (OMIM 300345) may occur as an autosomal dominant disorder with incomplete penetrance; expressivity varies from small colobomata of the eye to microphthalmia and even anophthalmia (Fig. 1.9). Microphthalmia without colobomata also may be inherited as an autosomal dominant disease; more commonly, associated congenital cataracts or other ocular malformations are present (88,89). Microphthalmia with congenital retinal detachment or congenital cataracts may be inherited as an autosomal recessive disorder (90,91).

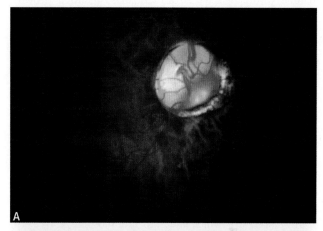
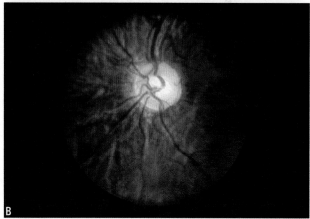

FIGURE 1.11. A: Coloboma of the right optic nerve in an eye with 20/20 vision. **B:** The left eye optic nerve head is normal.

Microphthalmia (Mi) was one of the first mouse mutant genes to be described in which the development of the retina is affected. An interesting allelic series ranging from weak recessive to severe dominant phenotype has been compiled and genetically characterized. The eyes of the mutants develop poorly because of the defects in the RPE. The mutated gene, microphthalmia-associated transcription factor (*Mitf*) is a member of the basic-helix-loop-helix leucine zipper family of transcription factors. Mutations in the human homolog *MITF* (OMIM 156845) cause 20% of cases of Waardenburg syndrome type IIA (OMIM 193510) (92).

Human mutations in *SIX3* lead to holoprosencephaly; in some cases, the phenotype is milder and manifests as microphthalmia and iris coloboma (93). Several reports indicate that *SIX3* might function as a repressor of some developmental processes in the eye (94,95). In the mouse, *Six3* is activated by *Pax6* and *Prox1* (a transcription factor that is important for the differentiation of lens fiber cells and alpha crystalline expression) but is regulated by its own negative feedback loop (96). Transgenic mouse experiments have shown that *Pax6* and *Six3* regulate the transcription of each other (97).

The CHARGE syndrome (OMIM 214800) is characterized by the nonrandom association of colobomatous microphthalmia, heart defects, atresia choanae, retarded growth, genital anomalies, and ear anomalies or deafness; at least two of the features are necessary for the diagnosis (98–104) (www.chargesyndrome.org/). The ocular malformation is a common feature; the cardiac defects described in the syndrome are varied and may be lethal. The phenotypes of the chromosomal trisomy syndromes (13,18), 4p– (Wolf-Hirschhorn; deletion of the short arm of chromosome 4) syndrome, and cat-eye syndrome may be similar to the features of CHARGE association, and chromosomal analysis may be necessary to clarify the diagnosis (see section "Chromosomal Rearrangements").

Two genetic loci have been identified in conjunction with isolated high hyperopia, autosomal dominant nanophthalmos (NNO1; OMIM 600165) on chromosome 11p (105) and NNO2 (OMIM 605738), which maps to chromosome 15q12–15. The phenotype for NNO2, however, is not of isolated, nonsyndromic high hyperopia. Rather it is that of unilateral or bilateral microphthalmos with variable expressivity such as corneal clouding and iridocorneal synechiae resembling Peters' anomaly or no microphthalmia with optic nerve agenesis.

Ocular Adnexa and Eyelid Abnormalities

The development of the eyelids and ocular adnexal structures is closely related to the formation of the eyes themselves. Complete failure of the eyelids to form results in cryptophthalmos (OMIM 123570), a condition in which the skin extends from the forehead to the cheeks uninterrupted, but attached to a usually malformed globe underneath. It may occur in isolation or as part of Fraser syndrome (OMIM 219000), which is autosomal recessive. A review of 27 cases of isolated cryptophthalmos revealed 11 of those to be familial, inherited in a dominant fashion (106). A gene has not yet been identified. Treatment depends upon the functional capability of the underlying globe, and this can be measured using imaging modalities in conjunction with visually evoked response and electroretinogram testing. If visual potential can be demonstrated, surgery may be attempted with the goal of creating a clear visual axis, possibly via a keratoprosthesis, as well as creating functioning lid structures. There is a clinical trial for this and a closely related disorder, Fryns syndrome (clinicaltrials.gov/ct2/show/NCT00032877).

Eyelid formation during development requires the eyelid folds to initially fuse and then to separate into upper and lower lids. The failure of this separation results in ankyloblepharon (OMIM 106250 and 106260), a condition in which the eyelids are completely or partially joined. Filiforme adnatum is a unique condition characterized by multiple strands of tissue connecting the two eyelids.

Structural maldevelopment of the eyelid may result in an eyelid coloboma or a disruption in the margin of the eyelid. Isolated eyelid colobomata range from a near total absence of the lid to the appearance of a small notch in the lateral aspect of the lid. Colobomata of the eyelid may also be part of a syndrome such as Treacher Collins syndrome (OMIM 154500) or Goldenhar syndrome (OMIM 164210) or may occur in association with cleft palate, dermoid, cleft lip, microphthalmia, iris colobomata, brow colobomata, and osseous facial clefts.

Congenital ptosis is due to a deficiency of the striated muscle fibers in the levator muscle. This abnormality may occur in three main forms: simple hereditary ptosis, with external ophthalmoplegia, and in the blepharophimosis syndrome (horizontal narrowing of the palpebral fissure; OMIM 110100). Simple congenital ptosis, unilateral or bilateral, may be inherited in an autosomal dominant fashion with incomplete penetrance (107). A gene for hereditary congenital ptosis type 1 (OMIM 178300) has been mapped to 8q21.12 (108). A case of bilateral isolated ptosis was also reported in a male patient found to have a de novo balanced translocation t(1;8) (p34.3;q21.12). The cytogenetic breakpoints were refined, and the chromosome 8 breakpoint was found to disrupt a gene homologous to the murine *zfh4* gene, which encodes for a transcription factor expressed in muscle and nerve tissue. This suggests the human *ZFH4* may be a candidate gene for congenital bilateral isolated ptosis (109). Analysis of a large white English pedigree revealed an X-linked dominant form of congenital isolated ptosis that mapped to chromosome Xq24–q27.1. This was named hereditary congenital ptosis type 2 (OMIM 300245) (110). Treatment for isolated congenital ptosis is surgical and may be performed on patients at any age; however, if the ptosis is significant, early surgery is necessary to prevent occlusion amblyopia. The choice of surgical procedure is dictated by the degree of ptosis, amount of levator muscle function, and clinical response to 2.5% phenylephrine ophthalmic solution. Patients who have a mild to moderate amount of ptosis which improves within 5 minutes after the administration of 2.5% phenylephrine ophthalmic drops into the upper eyelid fornix may benefit from a Mueller's muscle resection, while those with minimal response may require a levator muscle resection. In the absence or near absence of levator muscle function, a frontalis sling procedure is performed.

The association of blepharophimosis with ptosis and epicanthus inversus (BPES) is usually inherited in an autosomal dominant pattern (111). There are two types of BPES—type I is associated with ovarian failure and type II is not. The gene, *FOXL2*, is a winged helix/forkhead transcription factor and maps to chromosome 3q22–q23 (112–114). *FOXL2* is mutated to produce truncated proteins in type I families and larger proteins in type II. In this disorder, the palpebral fissures are narrowed both horizontally and vertically, and the ptosis is characterized by poor levator muscle function and the absence of a lid crease. Treatment involves correcting the ptosis with a frontalis sling procedure due to the poor levator muscle function. Surgical repair of the epicanthus inversus may also be undertaken in some cases.

Fibrosis of the extraocular muscle syndrome (FEOM) is a congenital disorder of innervation to the extraocular and eyelid muscles, which in turn affects muscular development (115). Affected individuals have a nonprogressive inability to move some or all of the extraocular muscles due to fibrotic and scarred muscles, adhesions between muscles and Tenon's capsule, and adhesions between Tenon's capsule and the globe. The eyes are usually fixed in a downward gaze, and as a result the patient assumes a chin-up head posture. The adhesions may involve the levator muscle, resulting in bilateral ptosis. FEOM1 (OMIM 135700) is caused by a mutation in the *KIF21A* gene (116), typically maps to chromosome 12q12, and shows neuropathologic changes suggesting a primary defect in the development of the superior division of the oculomotor nerve (117,118). FEOM2 (OMIM 602078) is associated with bilateral ptosis, with the eyes fixed in an exotropic position. This autosomal recessive phenotype maps to chromosome 11q13.3–q13.4 and results from mutations of the *ARIX* gene (119). In families with FEOM3 (OMIM 600638), one or more affected individuals do not have the classic findings of the disorder. Their eyes may be not be infraducted or may elevate above midline, or the individual may be unilaterally affected. Ptosis may not be present (120).

Congenital entropion and ectropion refer to a malposition of the eyelid where the eyelashes are rotated towards and away from the globe, respectively. Congenital entropion results from imbalances in preseptal and pretarsal orbicularis. Congenital ectropion may result from inflammatory conditions such as *Chlamydia* infection and may be associated with noninflammatory conditions such as Down syndrome and ichthyosis.

Distichiasis, an anomaly in which two rows (instead of one row) of lashes are present at the lid margin, may be autosomal dominant. During development, eyelashes differentiate in association with the glands of Zeis in the eyelids during the invagination of ectoderm to form pilosebaceous units. Distichiasis results from maldevelopment in which cilia formation occurs in association with Meibomian glands. Treatment is directed toward protecting the corneal epithelium. If the lashes do not touch the epithelium, no treatment is required. Electrolysis, cryotherapy, or a surgical eyelid-splitting procedure to remove the hair follicles may be performed when the lashes contact the corneal epithelial surface.

Conjunctiva

Many genetic disorders manifest themselves in the conjunctiva. Patients with ataxia telangiectasia (OMIM 208900: progressive cerebellar ataxia of childhood, oculomotor apraxia, absent optokinetic nystagmus, oculocutaneous telangiectases, immune defects, and malignancy predisposition) have significant dilatation and tortuosity of the conjunctival vessels. A characteristic oculomotor apraxia, that is, difficulty in the initiation of voluntary eye movements, frequently precedes the development of the telangiectases. The ataxia telangiectasia mutated gene on chromosome 11q23.3 (121) encodes a large protein kinase that regulates the cell cycle (122,123).

Congenital or early adult pterygium of the conjunctiva and cornea (OMIM 178000) is inherited as a dominant trait with 70% penetrance (124,125).

Pingueculae are evident in all forms of Gaucher disease (OMIM 230800, 230900, and 231000), one of the glycogen storage disorders (126).

Cornea
Developmental Corneal Abnormalities

Developmental abnormalities of the cornea include cornea plana, sclerocornea, microcornea, megalocornea, and keratoconus.

Cornea plana (CNA1; OMIM 121400, and CNA2; OMIM 217300) is a condition in which the cornea is flat, with a radius of curvature less than 43 D. A cornea with the same radius of curvature as the adjacent sclera is pathognomonic. This condition results from a failure of formation of the limbus by the second wave of neural crest cells during development. Cornea plana maybe associated with microcornea or sclerocornea, as well as cataracts, anterior or posterior colobomata, and Ehlers-Danlos syndrome. Glaucoma may develop as a result of angle abnormalities (open-angle glaucoma) or due to a morphologically shallow anterior chamber (angle-closure glaucoma). Cornea plana has two subtypes distinguished by their inheritance pattern and severity. CNA1 is autosomal dominant, whereas CNA2 is autosomal recessive and the more severe of the two. Keratocan (*KERA*) mutations are associated with both types, although none were found in the original CNA1 families (127,128). *KERA* codes for a keratin sulfate proteoglycan and is important for the development and maintenance of corneal transparency and structure. *KERA* has restricted expression in early neural crest development and later expression in corneal stromal cells. Treatment includes neutralization of refractive errors and glaucoma management. If central clarity is lost, penetrating keratoplasty may be considered.

Sclerocornea (OMIM 269400) is also characterized by a flat cornea; however, it differs from cornea plana by the partial or complete loss of transparency of the cornea. The limbus may be ill-defined, and scleral, episcleral, and conjunctival vessels extend across the cornea. Half of sclerocornea cases are sporadic, while the other half are either dominant or recessive (129).

Microcornea (OMIM 116150) is a condition in which the cornea is clear and of normal thickness; however, it measures less than 10 mm in diameter (9 mm in a newborn). It is thought to result from either fetal arrest of growth of the cornea or from overgrowth of the anterior tips of the optic cup leaving less space for the cornea to develop. It exists in both autosomal dominant and recessive forms, with the former occurring more commonly. Treatment includes correction of refractive errors and monitoring for the development of glaucoma due to shallow chambers or angle abnormalities.

Megalocornea (OMIM 249300) is a condition in which the corneal diameter is large (13.0 to 16.5 mm), but the cornea is clear and of normal thickness. The enlargement is not a result of congenital glaucoma. This condition represents either a failure of the anterior tips of the optic cup to close, allowing more room for the cornea to grow, or an overgrowth of the cornea in relation to the rest of the eye. It may be associated with a number of ocular abnormalities including miosis, microcoria, goniodysgenesis, cataract, ectopia lentis, central cloudy dystrophy of Francois, and glaucoma. Furthermore, it is associated systemically with disorders of collagen synthesis. It is usually X-linked recessive and located in the Xq21.3–q22 region. There are reports of sporadic, autosomal dominant and recessive cases. A syndromic form of megalocornea, termed megalocornea and mental retardation syndrome (OMIM 249310), was first reported by Neuhauser and associates (130). Children are hypotonic and show mild frontal bossing, antimongoloid slant of the eyes, epicanthal folds, and broad nasal base. Iris hypoplasia may accompany the megalocornea.

Keratoconus (OMIM 148300) can be sporadic or autosomal dominant. The onset is around puberty with a progressive ectatic dystrophy leading to corneal thinning, with induced irregular myopic astigmatism which may be markedly asymmetrical. In advanced cases, anterior corneal scarring is present and hydrops may occur when Descemet's membrane ruptures with subsequent epithelial and stromal edema. Either circumstance may require a corneal graft to attain visual clarity. Keratoconus has been associated with several chromosomal anomalies including trisomy 21, Turner syndrome, ring chromosome 13, and chromosomal 7;11 translocation; connective-tissue disorders such as Ehlers-Danlos, Marfan, and osteogenesis imperfecta syndromes; mitral valve prolapse; Leber congenital amaurosis; and atopy (131,132). Mutations in the *VSX-1* transcription factor gene were identified in 4.7% of patients with isolated keratoconus. This gene also plays a role in posterior polymorphous dystrophy (see below) (133).

Corneal Dystrophies

Hereditary dystrophies affecting all layers of the cornea are numerous; most are rare, and ophthalmologic evaluation is required to distinguish among them. Most of the corneal dystrophies are of Mendelian inheritance with some phenotype diversity and a variable degree of penetrance. The dystrophies involving enzymatic processes tend to be of autosomal recessive inheritance. Corneal clouding may be

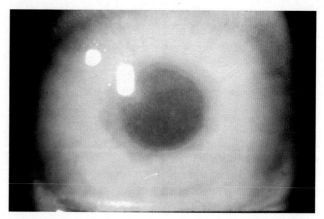

FIGURE 1.12. Opacification of corneal stroma in a 10-year-old patient with Maroteaux-Lamy syndrome (mucopolysaccharidosis VI).

present at birth or is acquired (Fig. 1.12). Presenting signs and symptoms of the corneal dystrophies include cloudiness of the cornea, nystagmus due to poor vision, and photophobia. Corneal transplantation may be performed if vision is seriously reduced.

Meesmann corneal dystrophy (OMIM 122100) has an autosomal dominant inheritance with an onset in early childhood (at approximately 12 months). Formed intraepithelial vesicles and microcysts, which contain periodic acid Schiff-positive "peculiar substances" suggestive of keratin, increase in number throughout life. The symptoms are variable, ranging from asymptomatic to pain and lacrimation associated with corneal erosions. Mutations have been identified in both keratin 12 (OMIM 601687) on chromosome 12q12–q13 and keratin 3 (OMIM 148043) on chromosome 17q12. Both genes, which are expressed in the anterior corneal epithelium, contain a highly conserved helix boundary motif, which plays a role in corneal structural integrity and keratinocyte filament assembly (134).

Defects in the human transforming growth factor β-induced gene (*TGFβI* or *βIGH3*) (135) are associated with multiple "classic" corneal dystrophies: lattice (OMIM 122200), non-classic LCDIIIa, intermediate-type LCDI/LCDIII, and LCD-deep dystrophies; granular (OMIM 121900) and nonclassic granular dystrophies GCDII and GCDIII; Reis-Bucklers (OMIM 608470); Thiel-Behnke dystrophy (OMIM 602082); and Avellino corneal dystrophy. All of the corneal dystrophies show autosomal dominant hereditary transmission with variable penetrance and map to chromosome 5q31 (136–139). *TGFβI* is expressed in keratocytes and encodes for keratoepithelin, a highly conserved 683-amino acid protein. This protein contains an N-terminal secretory signal, four domains of internal homology, and an arginine–glycine–aspartame (RGD) motif at the carboxy terminus, which is found in many extracellular matrix proteins. The RGD motif modulates cell adhesion and acts as a recognition sequence for integrin binding. Gene mutations result in progressive accumulation of keratoepithelin corneal deposits.

Aggregation of abnormal isoforms of keratoepithelin is associated with amyloid or other nonfibrillar deposits depending on the type of mutation (140).

The different subtypes of macular dystrophy, MCDI (OMIM 217800), MCDIa, and MCDII, are genetically and biochemically determined. The dystrophy is inherited in an autosomal recessive fashion, with onset in the first decade of life. Early on, the fine opacities have indistinct edges which start axially in the superficial stroma. The intervening stroma has a ground-glass appearance. Later, the opacities extend peripherally and into the deep stroma. The characteristic accumulation of glycosaminoglycans stains with Alcian blue and colloidal iron. MCDI is characterized by the absence of keratin chain sulfation (KCS) in cornea and cartilage and no appreciable serum KCS. In MCDII, serum and corneal keratin sulfate are detectable. MCD was mapped to chromosome 16q22 and mutations were noted in *CHST6* (OMIM 603797). *CHST6* encodes an enzyme, carbohydrate sulfotransferase, which is expressed in the cornea, spine, and trachea. The gene product initiates sulfation of keratin sulfate in the cornea. Mutations in this gene result in an inactive enzyme with the synthesis and secretion of proteoglycans (corneal structural genes) substituted with polylactosamine instead of keratin sulfate (141–143). Gelatinous drop-like corneal dystrophy (GDLD; OMIM 204870) is an autosomal recessive disorder with clinical onset in the first decade of flat subepithelial nodular deposits similar to early band keratopathy. There is a gradual increase in number and depth of deposits which eventually become raised as yellow-gray gelatinous masses with a mulberry configuration and surrounding dense subepithelial opacities. Recurrent lamellar keratoplasty or penetrating keratoplasty may be required. The gene, *M1S1*, maps to chromosome 1p31 and encodes for a gastrointestinal tumor-associated antigen. The abnormal *M1S1* gene product may affect epithelial cell junctions, resulting in increased cell permeability in GDLD corneas (144,145).

Posterior polymorphous corneal dystrophy (PPCD; OMIM 122000, 120252, and 605020) is an autosomal dominant disorder which shows variable expression and variable age of onset. Although it is usually a disease of adulthood, PPCD can be severe and present at birth. The disorder manifests as variable degrees of vesicular endothelial lesions with or without basement membrane thickening. This may be localized or diffuse, and may be associated with corneal edema. There is an increased risk for glaucoma and keratoconus. The abnormal anterior banded layer of Descemet's membrane is lined posteriorly by an abnormal posterior collagenous layer. PPCD is genetically heterogeneous with mutations identified in the transcription factor *VSX1* (chromosome 20p11.2–20q11.2) and the alpha 2 subunit of type VIII collagen *COL8A2* (chromosome 1p34.3-p32). PPCD is an allelic variant of keratoconus (OMIM 148300) and Fuchs' endothelial dystrophy (FECD; OMIM 136800), as VSX1 appears to play a role in approximately 9% of PPCD cases and 4.5% of keratoconus cases, and *COL8A2* appears

to play a role in approximately 6% of PPCD cases and 3.4% of FECD cases, respectively (133,146).

Congenital hereditary endothelial dystrophy (CHED1; OMIM 121700) is of autosomal dominant inheritance with onset at birth or in the first few months of life up to 8 years of age. CHED2 (OMIM 217700) is of autosomal recessive inheritance with an early onset of signs and symptoms at birth or within the first few weeks of life. The cornea has a ground-glass appearance, and the corneal epithelium may be roughened. There is no guttatae and the corneal sensitivity is normal. The decrease in vision is moderate to severe, and nystagmus is uncommon. The basement membrane is more thickened in CHED2. CHED is genetically heterogeneous, with CHED1 linked to a 2.7-cM locus at chromosome 20p11.2–20q11.2, and CHED2 linked to a chromosome 20p13 locus. No genes have been identified as of yet (147,148).

Anterior Segment Dysgenesis

Malformations of the iris and anterior chamber angle may involve the region responsible for aqueous humor outflow and predispose patients to glaucoma.

As an isolated ocular malformation, aniridia (OMIM 106200) is an autosomal dominant disorder (Fig. 1.3). Visual impairment, which is unrelated to the degree of iris hypoplasia, is caused either by glaucoma or the frequent concomitant malformations of macular or optic nerve hypoplasia. Clinical expressivity can be variable within and among families (149,150). There are multiple reports of aniridia, developmental delays, genitourinary malformations, and Wilms' tumor associated with a deletion of the short arm of chromosome 11 (151–154); one patient had aniridia and Wilms' tumor without a microscopically detectable deletion (155) (see section "Chromosomal Rearrangements"). Autosomal dominant aniridia is due to a mutation in the *PAX6* gene (156,157). Mutations of this gene can cause other disorders, including congenital cataracts, anophthalmia and central nervous system defects (158), Peters' anomaly (159), and keratitis (160).

Axenfeld-Rieger syndrome (OMIM 602482 and 180500) is a spectrum of anterior segment and systemic structural change combinations which may be characterized by a prominent Schwalbe line, iris strands to the cornea, iris hypoplasia, dental abnormalities, characteristic facies, and umbilic defects; it is generally inherited in an autosomal dominant fashion. Associated ocular abnormalities include glaucoma, corectopia, iris pigment epithelial defects, microcornea, corneal opacities, and cataracts (161–166). Uncommonly, chromosomal rearrangements may cause Rieger syndrome, in which case there is usually developmental delay (167–174). Mutations of the eye developmental genes *FOXC1*, a forkhead box transcription factor, and *PITX2*, paired-like class of homeobox transcription factors, cause Axenfeld-Rieger syndrome (175–179). *FoxC1* knockout mice also have anterior segment abnormalities that are similar to those reported in humans. The penetrance of the clinical phenotype varies with the genetic background, which indicates the influence of modulator genes.

In humans, mutations in *PITX3* cause anterior segment mesenchymal dysgenesis (180). In the mouse embryo, *Pitx3* is first expressed in the developing lens, initially in the lens vesicle and later in the anterior epithelium and lens equator. Deletions in the *Pitx3* promoter, which abrogate *Pitx3* expression in the eye, cause the phenotype of the *aphakia* (*ak*) mouse mutant, which lacks lenses and pupils (181).

Peters' anomaly may result from incomplete separation of the cornea and lens during embryogenesis; although evidence supports an autosomal recessive form of inheritance, chromosomal and nongenetic forms may exist (182–185). Mutations in the eye development genes *PAX6*, *PITX2*, *FOXC1*, and *CY1B1* have all been associated with Peters' anomaly (159,178,186,187).

Glaucoma

Glaucoma describes a heterogeneous group of optic neuropathies that lead to optic nerve cell damage, visual field loss, and permanent visual acuity deficits. It is the second most prevalent cause of bilateral blindness in the Western world, and it affects more than 60 million people worldwide. The hereditary forms of glaucoma are genetically heterogeneous. At least eight loci have been linked to glaucoma (GLC1A–F, GLC3A/B), and three genes have been identified to date: *MYOC*, *CYP1B1*, and *OPTN*.

Primary congenital glaucoma (PCG; OMIM 231300) is defined by the onset before 3 years of age. It is often characterized by buphthalmos, or an enlarged eye, as a result of increased intraocular pressure during intrauterine life or infancy when the elasticity of the scleral wall and cornea are greatest. Structurally, these eyes have a normal Schlemm's canal and normal episcleral veins; however, the trabecular meshwork is thought to be abnormal, impeding the drainage of aqueous humor from the anterior chamber. Infants with congenital glaucoma present with the classic triad of epiphora, photophobia, and blepharospasm. On examination, their corneal diameters may be markedly enlarged (greater than 12 mm during the first year of life), and the eye may be buphthalmic. Corneal edema may develop due to increased intraocular pressure, and acute stretching of the cornea may lead to Haab's striae (tears in Descemet's membrane). Inheritance is thought to be recessive with incomplete penetrance, and two loci have been mapped: one to chromosome 2p22-p21 (188,189) and the second to chromosome 1p36.2-p36.1 (190). Mutations of the gene *CYP1B1* (OMIM 601771) on chromosome 2p21 are associated with PCG (191). The gene encodes a 543-amino acid drug-metabolizing enzyme of the cytochrome P_{450} gene superfamily, subfamily I, which is a monooxygenase that is capable of metabolizing various endogenous and exogenous substrates, such as steroids and retinoids. It is expressed in the iris, trabecular meshwork, and ciliary body. Congenital glaucoma has also been reported to occur

in association with deletions of chromosomes 10, 13, and 18; a pericentric inversion of chromosome 11; partial trisomy of chromosomes 3 and 14; and trisomies 13, 18, and 21 (192,193). Treatment is primarily surgical for congenital glaucoma, via a trabeculotomy or goniotomy.

Juvenile-onset open-angle glaucoma (JOAG; OMIM 137750) is defined as glaucoma acquired after birth and thus unaccompanied by buphthalmos. It is dominantly inherited and typically has its onset during the second or third decade of life. There is an association with myopia reported to be as high as 87% (194). Mutations in the myocilin gene (*MYOC*; also known as trabecular meshwork-inducible glucocorticoid response gene; OMIM 601652) are associated with autosomal dominant JOAG (33% of patients) and with primary open-angle glaucoma (POAG; OMIM 137760) (2% to 4% of patients) (195,196). *MYOC* has been mapped to a locus (GLC1A) on chromosome 1q24.3–q25.2. *MYOC* is expressed in almost every ocular tissue, including the optic nerve (197); however, despite considerable effort, the function of MYOC remains obscure.

POAG is a chronic, progressive optic neuropathy characterized by cupping of the optic nerve head and is associated with visual field loss. Intraocular pressure may be elevated. It is insidious in onset and often progresses without symptoms since central visual acuity is relatively unaffected until late in the disease. Inheritance is thought to be multifactorial. In addition to the myocilin gene-associated GLC1A locus on chromosome 1q23–24, POAG has been mapped to several other loci: GLC1B on chromosome 2cen-q13, GLC1C on chromosome 3q21–24, GLC1D on chromosome 8q23, and GLC1F on chromosome 7q35–q36. Recently, mutations in the optineurin gene (*OPTN*), a locus previously designated GLC1E on chromosome 10p14–p15, have been demonstrated in 16.7% of patients with POAG (198). The pathogenic mechanism for glaucoma development due to mutations in *OPTN* is not fully understood—it is speculated that OPTN is operating through an apoptosis (cell death) pathway, playing a neuroprotective role in the eye and optic nerve (198).

Pigment dispersion syndrome (OMIM 600510) is a form of open-angle glaucoma which is characterized by pigment deposition on the corneal endothelium (Krukenberg spindle), trabecular meshwork, and lens periphery. Spoke-like loss of the iris pigment epithelium occurs, resulting in characteristic transillumination defects in the iris midperiphery. This loss of pigment is thought to be due to direct contact between the zonules and iris. Affected individuals are usually myopic men aged 20–50 years. Fluctuations in intraocular pressure are usually wide, and patients are symptomatic with headaches, haloes, intermittent visual blurring, and pain. Medications are often helpful in controlling intraocular pressure; laser iridotomies are often attempted in cases of "reverse pupillary block," and laser trabeculoplasty and filtering surgery are useful in treatment. Inheritance is autosomal dominant (199), and the gene has been mapped to chromosome 7q35–q36 (200).

Lens

Abnormalities of the lens of the eye may be divided into two broad categories: dislocations and opacities. A lens is subluxed if it is not in its proper anatomic location but still retains some zonular attachments to the ciliary body; in a complete dislocation, the lens floats free in the eye. Lens opacities, or cataracts, may occur in different layers of the lens and with varying severity.

The causes of subluxed and dislocated lenses are numerous. Dislocation or subluxation of the lens is a common manifestation of both Marfan syndrome (OMIM 154700) (Fig. 1.13) (201) and homocystinuria (OMIM 236200). Common manifestations in Marfan syndrome include lens subluxation superotemporally, dilatation of the aortic root, aneurysm of the ascending aorta, and skeletal abnormalities such as pectus excavatum, kyphoscoliosis, and an upper segment: lower segment ratio two standard deviations below the mean for age. Pneumothorax, pes planus, dural ectasia, joint laxity, arachnodactyly, and mitral valve prolapse may also occur. The diagnostic criteria require involvement of three systems with at least two major manifestations. As mentioned previously, the basis of Marfan syndrome is a mutation of the fibrillin gene, which maps to chromosome 15q15–q21.1 (202–208).

Homocystinuria is characterized by a deficiency of the enzyme cystathione-β-synthase, resulting in accumulation of homocysteine. Untreated patients present with mental retardation, unusually tall stature, coarse fair hair, cardiac murmurs, and thromboembolic diathesis. These patients have an increased anesthetic risk due to their tendency to develop thrombotic vascular occlusions. Ocular findings include blue irides and progressive myopia, which may be the first sign of lens dislocation. All untreated patients develop inferior or inferonasal dislocation of lenses bilaterally due to deficient zonular fibers. Diagnosis is confirmed by measurement of the serum homocysteine level. Surgery should be avoided if possible, and treatment consists of dietary management

(low methionine and high cysteine) and supplementation of vitamin B6. The gene for cystathione-β-synthase has been mapped to 21q22.3 (209), and it is transmitted in an autosomal recessive fashion.

Ectopia lentis et pupillae (OMIM 225200), an autosomal recessive disorder, is characterized by an eccentric pupil and subluxed lens (usually the lens is dislocated in a direction opposite the pupil) and is slowly progressive (210). Isolated lens subluxation or dislocation is rare, and most reports antedate careful definition of the Marfan syndrome and homocystinuria.

Isolated hereditary cataracts are usually transmitted in an autosomal dominant pattern, although autosomal recessive and X-linked forms have been reported. They may be present at birth or develop over time. Although the severity may vary within a family, the position and patterns are generally consistent. This variability within the same family suggests the importance of additional genes modifying the expression of the primary mutation. Conversely, cataracts with similar or identical clinical presentations can result from mutations in quite different genes. Currently, 27 isolated or primary cataract loci have been identified by linkage analysis or mutational screening, and 13 are associated with specific gene defects. For some α- and β-crystallin mutations, inherited congenital cataracts are associated with microcornea and even microphakia. There are currently no identified developmental lesions causing isolated cataracts. Of those families for whom the mutant gene is known, about half have mutations in crystallins (structural components of the lens nucleus), about one-fourth have mutations in connexins (constituents of gap junctions on which the avascular lens depends for nutrition and intercellular communication), and the remainder are evenly split between aquaporin 0 (an enzyme involved in water-channel activity) and the gene for the beaded filament protein *BFSP2* (structural filament unique to the lens fiber cells that combines with β-crystallin) (158,211–223).

Cataracts are known to occur in association with a large number of metabolic diseases and genetic syndromes. Nance-Horan syndrome (OMIM 302350) is an X-linked recessive congenital cataract-dental disorder associated with microcornea, anteverted and simplex pinnae, brachymetacarpalia, and various dental anomalies; carriers exhibit distinctive sutural opacities (26,27). An isolated X-linked cataract has recently been mapped to chromosome Xp and is possibly allelic with the Nance-Horan syndrome (224).

Galactosemia (OMIM 230400) is an autosomal recessive disorder characterized by the inability to convert galactose to glucose, resulting in the accumulation of galactose and its conversion to galactitol. Classic galactosemia, which is the most common of three forms of the disease, involves a defect in galactose-1-phosphate uridyl transferase (*GALT*) and results in cataract formation during the first few weeks of life in 75% of untreated patients. Two other, less severe forms of the disease involve defects in two other enzymes, galactokinase and UDP-galactose-4-epimerase. Patients

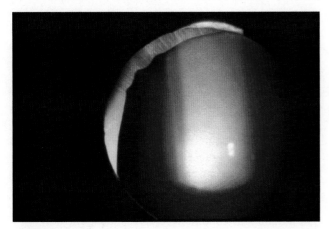

FIGURE 1.13. Superior dislocation of the lens in a young girl with Marfan syndrome.

with classic galactosemia present with malnutrition, hepatomegaly, jaundice, and mental deficiency within the first few weeks of life. The cataract has a very characteristic "oil droplet" appearance on retroillumination due to accumulation of galactose and galactitol within the lens cells causing increased intracellular osmotic pressure and fluid influx into the lens. Diagnosis can be confirmed by testing the urine for reducing substances and demonstrating the presence of the nonglucose reducing substance, galactose. Treatment includes elimination of milk and milk products from the diet. *GALT* has been mapped to chromosome 9p13 (225–227).

Wilson disease, or hepatolenticular degeneration (OMIM 277900), is an autosomal recessive disorder of copper metabolism that results in a characteristic "sunflower cataract" which is not visually significant. This inborn error of metabolism results in excess copper deposition in the liver, kidney, and central nervous system. Systemic features include cirrhosis, renal tubular damage, and a Parkinson-like defect of motor function. Ocular findings include the characteristic sunflower cataract as well as the Kayser-Fleischer ring, a golden brown discoloration around the perilimbal cornea due to copper deposition in Descemet's membrane. The cataract results from the deposition of cuprous oxide in the anterior lens capsule and subcapsular cortex in a stellate pattern resembling the petals of a sunflower. Diagnosis may be confirmed by measuring the serum copper and ceruloplasmin levels, and treatment includes a copper-chelating agent as well as zinc in some cases to preserve hepatic function. Since the cataracts are usually not visually significant, patients may be monitored without the need for surgical intervention. The *WND* gene, in which mutations lead to Wilson disease, has been mapped to chromosome 13q14.3–q21.1 (228) and is a putative copper-transporting P-type ATPase enzyme (229).

Myotonic dystrophy (OMIM 160900) is an autosomal dominant disorder in which patients may develop a characteristic "Christmas tree cataract" due to the deposition of polychromatic iridescent crystals in the lens cortex. Systemic findings usually develop in middle age and include delayed relaxation of contracted muscles, weakness of the facial musculature, frontal balding, and cardiac conduction defects. In addition to the crystalline lens deposits, patients with myotonic dystrophy may develop progressive posterior subcapsular cataract leading to complete cortical opacification. Involvement of the facial muscles and extraocular muscles may lead to ptosis, weakness of eye closure, and ocular motility deficits. Inheritance is autosomal dominant with variable penetrance, and the disease has been mapped to chromosome 19q13.2–q13.3 (230). Boucher and associates (231) identified the gene for myotonic dystrophy type I, called DM locus-associated homeodomain protein.

Vitreous, Retina, and Choroid

Hereditary vitreoretinal and choroidoretinal malformations and degenerations are numerous, and their complete description is beyond the scope of this chapter. Categorization can be difficult, as all three adjacent anatomic regions of the eye (vitreous, retina, and choroid) can be abnormal; classifications are based on clinical features such as funduscopic appearance, color vision tests, electrophysiologic tests, fluorescein angiography, and hereditary patterns. Selected clinical entities will be reviewed in this section.

Color Vision Genetics

Color vision defects are probably the most common abnormality of retinal function and can present at birth or can be acquired. Hereditary congenital color deficiencies are almost always X-linked recessive red–green abnormalities and predominantly affect males. The genes encoding the red and green photopigments are arranged in a head-to-tail tandem array on chromosome Xq28. The normal X-chromosome-linked color vision gene array is composed of a single red pigment gene followed by one or more green pigment genes. The high degree of homology between these genes predisposes them to unequal recombination, leading to gene deletions or the formation of red–green hybrid genes that explain the majority of the common red–green color vision deficiencies. Gene expression studies suggest that only the two most proximal genes of the array are expressed in the retina. The expression of the genes of the array is controlled by a highly conserved sequence of DNA, referred to as the locus control region (LCR), located approximately 3.5 kb upstream of the red pigment gene. Deletion of the LCR was shown to be associated with loss of expression of all the genes of the array, resulting in blue cone monochromacy (BCM; OMIM 303700). The severity of the color vision defect is roughly related to the difference in absorption maxima of the photopigments encoded by the first two genes of the array. The blue pigment gene is located on chromosome 7 (232).

There is wide variation in both normal and defective color vision among humans. The inherited forms of color vision deficiencies are classified into four main categories: (a) the common red–green defects that include the protan type caused by lack of red cones (protanopia) or by replacement of red cones with ones that contain anomalous pigments (protanomaly), and the deutan type caused either by lack of green cones or by replacement of green cones with ones that contain anomalous pigments (deuteranomaly); (b) the blue–yellow or tritan color vision due to nonfunctional blue cones; (c) loss of red and green cone function (BCM); and (d) complete color blindness due to loss of function of all three classes of cone (achromatopsia [ACHM]). The red–green deficiencies, which are inherited as X-chromosome-linked recessive traits, are by far the most common, reaching an incidence of as high as 8% among males of northern European extraction, and approximately 5% among other ethnic groups. The other forms are rare (ghr.nlm.nih.gov/condition=colorvisiondeficiency).

BCM, also known as X-chromosome-linked incomplete achromatopsia, is a rare X-linked ocular disorder, characterized by poor visual acuity, infantile nystagmus (which diminishes with age), and photophobia, together with severely reduced color discrimination capacity. It is sometimes associated with progressive macular atrophy. Deletions encompassing the LCR or point mutations which inactivate both the red and green pigments are responsible for BCM (233,234).

Tritan or blue–yellow color vision deficiency is due to defective blue cones and is characterized by blue–yellow color confusion. It is a rare (less than 1 in 1,000) autosomal dominant trait with severe (tritanopia) and mild (tritanomaly) forms. Mutations in the blue pigment gene on chromosome 7 have been implicated for this disorder (235,236).

ACHM, which is also referred to as total colorblindness or rod monochromacy, is an autosomal recessive congenital and stationary ocular disorder with a prevalence of 1 in 30,000. It is characterized by severe photophobia and nystagmus within the first months of life. Visual acuity is significantly reduced, and there is complete absence of color discrimination. In electroretinogram recordings, rod function is normal, but cone function is absent or strongly reduced. It is due to a genetic dysfunction of all three cone pigment genes. Three genes have been implicated with achromatopsia—two are channel-forming modulatory subunits of the cone photoreceptor cGMP-gated channel *CNGA3* (a subunit) (OMIM 600053) at the ACHM2 (OMIM 216900) locus on chromosome 2q11, and *CGNB3* (p subunit) (OMIM 605080) at the ACHM3 (OMIM 262300) locus on chromosome 8q21. Mutations in the *CGNA3* gene account for 20% to 30% and mutations in the *CNGB3* gene account for 40% to 50% of all achromatopsia patients. Recently, mutations in the cone-specific subunit of the transducin G-protein (*GNAT2*) gene (OMIM 139340) on chromosome 1p13 (ACHM4 locus) were shown to account for approximately 2% of this rare disorder (237–241).

Vitreoretinal Degenerations

Diseases that involve the vitreous and retina predominantly include the X-linked recessive disorder congenital retinoschisis (OMIM 312700). Both the macula and retinal periphery exhibit splitting of the retina, which may be slowly progressive; vision usually is minimally impaired into middle age (242). The gene has been mapped to Xp22.2-p22.1. Familial foveal retinoschisis (OMIM 268080) has been described as an autosomal recessive disorder in one family; macular abnormalities resembled those of congenital retinoschisis (243). A clinical trial is in preparation (www.kellogg.umich.edu).

Familial exudative vitreoretinopathy (FEVR; OMIM 133780 and 305390) is a hereditary ocular disorder characterized by a failure of peripheral retinal vascularization. There is abrupt cessation of growth of peripheral capillaries. This can then lead to compensatory retinal neovascularization, which can secondarily proceed to exudative leakage and bleeding, cicatrization, and tractional retinal detachments. Early diagnosis is essential. FEVR is inherited as an autosomal dominant (244,245) or X-linked recessive condition (246,247). Loci associated with FEVR map to chromosomes 11q13–23, Xp11.4, and 11p13–12. Robitaille and associates (248) confirmed linkage to the chromosome 11q13–23 locus for autosomal dominant FEVR in a large multigenerational family, refined the disease locus, and identified mutations in the frizzled-4 gene (*FZD4*) as causative for this disorder. FZD genes encode Wnt receptors, which are implicated in development and carcinogenesis. Wnts are secreted signaling molecules implicated in various developmental processes, and frizzled proteins are the receptors for these ligands. These processes range from embryonic dorsal-ventral patterning, neural-tube patterning, and limb formation to kidney development. A neovascular inflammatory vitreoretinopathy (OMIM 193235) has been assigned to chromosome 11q13–23 (249) (www.fevr.net/).

The gene (norrin) for Norrie disease (OMIM 310600), an X-linked recessive syndrome of congenital retinal detachment, developmental delay, and hearing loss, has been mapped to the short arm of the X chromosome (250–258) and encodes a nuclear protein (259,260) (www.norriedisease.org/).

Retinal-Choroidal Dystrophies

The term *retinitis pigmentosa* (OMIM 268000) is very general and is applied to conditions in which the retinal deterioration is progressive and characterized by visual field loss, night blindness, and an abnormal or nonrecordable electroretinogram. Ophthalmoscopically, clumping of pigment frequently is present in the retina or adjacent to narrowed retinal vessels giving rise to a "bone-spicule" appearance. The forms of retinitis pigmentosa may be broadly divided into those that affect the cones of the retina initially or predominantly and those that affect the rods initially or predominantly; inheritance may follow autosomal recessive or dominant or X-linked recessive patterns (261). Initial symptoms, progression, and ophthalmoscopic features are not consistent within a given hereditary pattern.

Autosomal dominant retinitis pigmentosa (adRP) may be caused by mutations of the candidate genes for rhodopsin (RP4) (262), peripherin/RDS (RP7) (263), and ROM1 (264); the disease has been linked to loci on chromosomes 7p (RP9) (265), 7q (RP10) (266), 8qll–21 (RP1) (267,268), 17p13.1 (RP13) (269,270), 17p22–24 (271), and 19q13.4 (RP11) (272). Mutations of the peripherin gene can result in a variety of clinical disorders including adRP, retinitis pigmentosa punctata albescens, and macular dystrophy (273–275). Digenic inheritance of a mutation in both peripherin/RDS and *ROM1* has been implicated as another mechanism (276,277).

Autosomal recessive forms of the disease may be caused by mutations of genes encoding for RP4 (278,279), α subunit of rod phosphodiesterase (280), β subunit of rod phosphodiesterase (281,282), and *a* subunit of the cGMP-gated channel CNCG1 (283); additional loci have been mapped to chromosomes 1p13–21 (284), 1q31–q32 (274,285), and 6p (286,287).

At present, there are three X-linked forms of retinitis pigmentosa at chromosomes Xp11 (RP2) (288), Xp21 (RP3) (289,290), and Xp21 (RP6). The gene for RP3 has been identified as having homology with the guanine–nucleotide exchange factor *RCC1* (289,290).

The term *cone-rod degeneration* refers to cases in which central vision is reduced early in the course of the disease; abnormalities in photopic electroretinogram precede alterations in the scotopic response. Mutations of the peripherin/*RDS* gene may cause an autosomal dominant form of the disease (291–293). Genes have been identified on chromosomes 6q16 (294,295), 6q25–q26 (296), 17p (297,298), 17q11 (299), 18q21 (300), 19q13.3–13.4 (301), as well as Xp21.1-p11.3 (302,303) and Xp22.13–11 (304).

Sorsby fundus dystrophy (OMIM 136900) is an autosomal dominant disease with complete penetrance. It is characterized by macular and extramacular chorioretinal neovascularization typically occurring in the fourth and fifth decades of life. Early features consist of small drusenoid lesions (referred to as colloid bodies), pigmentary clumping, and pigment epithelial atrophy, which may extend into the periphery. Visual loss progresses initially peripherally and may deteriorate to hand motion. Color anomalies, night blindness, and diminished electroretinogram responses (rod and cone) are common (305). The disorder is caused by mutations in the tissue inhibitor of metalloproteinases-3 (*TIMP3*) (306). The TIMP3 protein belongs to a family of secreted proteins that play a role in regulating extracellular matrix metabolism. They inhibit matrix metalloproteinases, and thereby determine the extent of matrix degradation during normal tissue remodeling processes.

Dominant Stargardt-like macular dystrophy (OMIM 600110) is an autosomal dominant disorder. Visual loss without apparent fundus lesions is a common first presentation of this disorder, usually in the first or second decade of life. The subtle early changes consist of RPE mottling and slight pallor of the optic nerve. Later, atrophy of the macular RPE occurs, which may or may not be accompanied by yellow flecks. Final visual acuity generally ranges from 20/40 to 20/200, the presence of yellow flecks predicting a more severe visual outcome. The "dark choroid" seen in recessive Stargardt disease is not seen in the dominant form. A photoreceptor-specific gene called *ELOVL4* (elongation factor of very long chain fatty acids) was identified as the responsible gene by Zhang and associates in 2001 (307). It has been hypothesized that the ELOVL4 protein is involved in synthesis of the polyunsaturated fatty acids present in the outer segments, thus playing a critical role in membrane composition and photoreceptor health (308).

Stargardt macular dystrophy (STGD; OMIM 248200) is the most common macular dystrophy with an estimated frequency of 1 in 8,000 to 10,000 in the United States. The age of onset and clinical course are variable. One-third of those affected present symptoms in the first decade of life, and they generally have a more progressive course than those with later onset. Fundus abnormalities include pigmentary changes in the macula, RPE atrophy giving a "bull's eye" appearance, a "beaten bronze" look of the posterior pole, and yellow "fishtail" flecks at the level of the RPE. The latter manifestation is also called fundus flavimaculatus. In a large fraction of STGD patients, a "dark" or "silent" choroid is seen on fluorescein angiography which reflects accumulation of lipofuscin. Electroretinogram findings vary. The causal gene, ATP-binding cassette-transporter *ABCA4* or *ABCR*, was cloned in 1997 and maps to chromosome 1p13–p22. The ABCR protein translocates a precursor of lipofuscin; thus, in a defective state, abnormally high levels of lipofuscin accumulate in the RPE, triggering RPE cell death and causing secondary photoreceptor degeneration (309,310).

Best vitelliform macular dystrophy (OMIM 153700) maps to chromosome 11q13 (311,312), and the gene *VMD2* encodes a protein known as bestrophin, which has been localized to the basolateral plasma membrane of the RPE. Bestrophin is a chloride channel (313,314). The classic clinical presentation is an "egg yolk" appearance of the macula. A diagnostic hallmark is an abnormal electrooculogram with an Arden ratio of less than 1.5, which indicates a lower than normal change in the electric potential derived from the RPE when light is cast on the fundus. Visual symptoms such as blurred vision and metamorphopsia may occur in the first decade, but significant visual decline usually does not happen until the third and fourth decades of life, when subretinal neovascularization and central atrophy may develop.

Gyrate atrophy (OMIM 258870), an autosomal recessive chorioretinal dystrophy associated with hyperornithinemia, is caused by a deficiency of the enzyme ornithine aminotransferase; the gene maps to chromosome 10 (315).

Some retinal dystrophies are relatively stable over time. Congenital stationary night blindness (CSNB; OMIM 310500, 163500, and 300071) is usually divided into complete and incomplete forms; inheritance is autosomal dominant, autosomal recessive, and X-linked recessive. Affected persons have decreased visual acuity and myopia; the defect is related to altered neurotransmission between bipolar cells and photoreceptors (316,317). Autosomal dominant CSNB has been associated with mutations in the rhodopsin (chromosome 3p) (318,319) and p subunit of the rod phosphodiesterase genes (chromosome 3p) (320). The X-linked form has been linked to the Xp11.2-Xp11.23 (321,322); the gene may be allelic with one form of X-linked retinitis pigmentosa (288). A second locus on the X chromosome has been described (323); a third locus near the *RP3* gene region has been reported (324). Aland Island eye disease is a clinical variant of congenital stationary night blindness (325,326). Oguchi disease, a recessively inherited form of stationary night blindness, is caused by defects in the enzyme rhodopsin kinase (327).

Optic Nerve

Congenital Anomalies

Optic nerve hypoplasia (OMIM 165550) is a bilateral or unilateral developmental anomaly characterized by a reduced number of axons in a nerve which otherwise contains the appropriate supportive mesodermal tissue. This abnormality is present at birth and has a clinical spectrum ranging from a subtle segmental reduction in nerve head size to severe, diffuse loss of axons resulting in a small nerve head surrounded by a normal-sized optic canal, the "double-ring sign." Superior segmental optic nerve hypoplasia has been reported in children of insulin-dependent diabetic mothers. Males and females are equally affected, and bilateral disease is more common than unilateral.

Autosomal dominant inheritance of optic nerve hypoplasia has been reported in one family (328). Recently, Azuma and associates (329) reported mutations in the *PAX6* gene of patients with bilateral optic nerve hypoplasia and aplasia. Patients with bilateral, severe optic nerve hypoplasia may present with nonprogressive poor vision and nystagmus. Alternatively, patients with a mild form of optic nerve hypoplasia may be asymptomatic with normal visual acuity, or have only visual field defects in the presence of good visual acuity. Bitemporal visual field defects are commonly found, and these may indicate the presence of midline central nervous system abnormalities. Septooptic dysplasia (OMIM 182230), or De Morsier syndrome, consists of optic nerve hypoplasia and absence of the septum pellucidum or corpus callosum; other associations exist and children with this syndrome are mentally retarded and often have pituitary dysfunction. MRI of the brain is indicated in cases of optic nerve hypoplasia to evaluate associated central nervous system abnormalities.

Optic nerve coloboma (OMIM 120430) is a congenital abnormality resulting from incomplete closure of the embryonic fissure (Fig. 1.11). There is a spectrum of diseases ranging from a small notch inferotemporally to a large excavation of the inferior optic nerve. The superior portion of the nerve is usually unaffected, reflecting the inferotemporal position of the embryonic fissure. Serous detachments of the retina extending to the macula are a common complication. Although most appear to be sporadic, autosomal dominant inheritance has been described in some bilateral cases (330). Azuma reported the association of optic nerve coloboma with a mutation in the *PAX6* gene in a 1-year-old boy with iris anomaly; large coloboma of the optic nerve, retina, and choroid; persistent hyperplastic primary vitreous bilaterally; and growth and mental retardation (329). Mutations in the *PAX2* gene have been reported by several authors in patients with bilateral optic nerve colobomata and renal disease (331–333).

Optic nerve pits are congenital excavations of variable size, shape, depth, and location in the substance of the nerve head. They affect males and females equally and may be bilateral or unilateral, single or multiple. A visual field defect often exists corresponding to the location of the pit. Visual acuity is usually unaffected in the absence of a serous detachment of the retina in the macula, a possible complication which typically occurs in the third or fourth decade of life. Autosomal dominant inheritance has been reported (334).

Hereditary Optic Neuropathies

Dominant optic atrophy (OPA1; OMIM 165500) is a hereditary optic neuropathy with early onset and autosomal dominant inheritance; visual impairment is variable and may be progressive (335,336). Patients typically present with onset of bilateral, although sometimes asymmetric, vision loss in the first decade of life. Progression usually does not occur beyond the second decade of life. A gene was initially localized to chromosome 3q (337) and later identified as *OPA1*, a gene in the optic atrophy-1 candidate region 3q28–3q29; mutations in this gene were identified as the cause of dominant optic atrophy (338,339). A recessive form of optic atrophy also exists, either in isolation or as part of a syndrome. The affected phenotype is more severe than that of dominant optic atrophy.

Wolfram syndrome (OMIM 222300), or DIDMOAD (diabetes insipidus, diabetes mellitus, optic atrophy, and deafness), may present in early childhood or adolescence. Other neurologic abnormalities may also be associated. A gene has been identified, the *WFS1* gene, coding for wolframin on chromosome 4p16.1 (340). This disease maybe sporadic or autosomal recessive in inheritance; a mitochondrial inheritance has also been suggested.

Leber optic atrophy (OMIM 535000) presents as a sudden loss of vision in the second or third decade of life and is characterized by hyperemia of the optic nerve head. The condition predominates in males, most commonly during teenage years or young adulthood. There is no transmission of the disease or the carrier state to the offspring of an affected male; however, female carriers have at least a 50% chance of transmitting the disease to their sons, and most of their daughters are carriers. Some 10% to 20% of female carriers manifest the disease (341). Although nearly all of an individual's DNA is located in the 46 chromosomes in the cell nucleus, a very small amount lies within mitochondria in the cytoplasm and is termed *mtDNA* (see section "Mitochondrial Genetics"). A point mutation of the mtDNA encoding NADH dehydrogenase has been demonstrated in multiple cases of Leber optic atrophy; mutations have been identified as either primary or secondary (342,343). Mutations at codon positions 11778, 14484, or 3460 are considered pathogenic (34,344–350). Secondary mutations, particularly those at 13708 and 15257, appear to contribute to the disease (351–353); these mutations may also occur in the normal population (354–356). An X-linked gene may contribute to the clinical features (357,358). A comprehensive review of optic neuropathies—glaucomatous versus nonglaucomatous, along with current clinical trial information can be found at www.revoptom.com/continuing_education/tabviewtest/lessonid/108438/.

CHROMOSOMAL REARRANGEMENTS

Chromosomal aberrations were first identified in the late 1950s. The bases of Turner syndrome (359), Klinefelter syndrome (360), and Down syndrome (361) were established shortly after Tjio and Levan (10) identified the correct number of human chromosomes. Many other chromosomal diseases have since been delineated. Chromosome studies are now a major diagnostic tool for evaluation of children with congenital malformations, mental retardation, and ambiguous external genitalia. Approximately 1 in every 200 liveborn children and more than half of spontaneously aborted fetuses carry a chromosome abnormality.

Most numerical chromosomal anomalies originate during gametogenesis in a parent (usually the mother) and are due to nondisjunction or anaphase lag. During the first meiotic division, homologous duplicated chromosomes pair and then segregate, migrating to opposite poles independently of their parental origin; 2 cells, each with 23 duplicated chromosomes, are the result. This is followed by a second division of the duplicated chromosomes. Failure of separation of homologous chromosomes may occur in the first division, or failure of chromatid separation of the duplicated chromosomes may occur in the second (Fig. 1.14). In either case, complementary gametes with 24 chromosomes (one present in duplicate) and 22 chromosomes (one missing) result. If the former were fertilized by a normal gamete (23 chromosomes), the zygote would have 47 chromosomes, one being present in triplicate (trisomy); if the latter, the zygote would have 45 chromosomes with one missing (monosomy). The autosomal trisomies compatible with term gestation are those of chromosomes 13, 18, and 21. Full trisomies of other chromosomes are usually lethal in utero and are identified in spontaneous abortions. Autosomal monosomy also is usually lethal, although monosomy 21 has been reported. Mosaicism can occur in such cases.

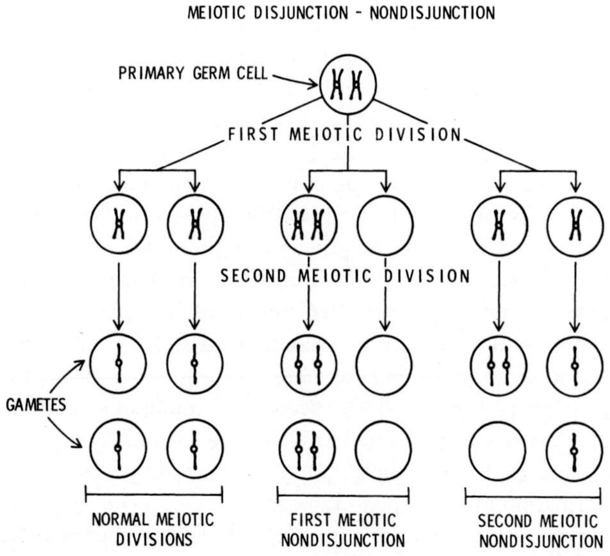

Nondisjunction of sex chromosomes has less severe consequences. Monosomy X is the basis of Turner syndrome, and females with XXX and XXXX have been identified. Males with XXY (Klinefelter syndrome) and XYY are not uncommon and increasing numbers of X and Y to XXXXY or XXYY have been reported.

If nondisjunction occurs after fertilization in an early division of the embryo, mosaicism results. Cell lines with trisomies or monosomies in addition to normal cells may persist in a fetus or an individual. In general, cells with autosomal monosomies are nonviable, but monosomic 9 or X cells may survive. Three cell types—45,X; 46,XX; and 47,XXX—can coexist in females who presumably began life as XX zygotes and developed a single mitotic nondisjunction, producing the X and XXX cells.

The first identified human translocations were centric fusions between two acrocentric chromosomes (centromere near one end of the chromosome), which reduced the chromosome count by 1; the nonessential short arms were lost. Most of the translocations causing Down syndrome and trisomy 13 are due to centric fusions. Reciprocal translocations between biarmed chromosomes alter arm ratios without changing the chromosome number. Carriers of reciprocal translocations are clinically normal and are usually detected because of unbalanced offspring; such carriers may produce a child with multiple anomalies or have a history of spontaneous abortions.

Case reports of familial translocations, deletions, and duplications in which identification of structural abnormalities was possible by use of high-resolution chromosome banding techniques have led to the delineation of many syndromes of partial monosomy or trisomy. Figure 1.15 indicates schematically the chromosome regions involved in some syndromes that have been identified. Many identifiable chromosomal syndromes exhibit ocular manifestations.

Many chromosomal aberrations have ocular involvement, the most common manifestations being hypertelorism, epicanthus, antimongoloid lid slant, ptosis, strabismus, and microphthalmia; however, any and all structures of the eye can be abnormal in a patient with a chromosomal rearrangement. Of the more common manifestations, microphthalmia, a malformation in which the volume of the eye is reduced, is most visually significant; it has been reported to be associated with a variety of chromosomal rearrangements. Usually, an associated coloboma of the uvea (the iris in Fig. 1.10 or the choroid) is evident and is caused by incomplete closure of the fetal fissure; the typical position is inferonasal. Visual impairment may be severe if the eye is significantly decreased in size or completely absent, or if the coloboma involves the macula (the portion of retina responsible for the sharpest

MEIOTIC DISJUNCTION - NONDISJUNCTION

FIGURE 1.14. Diagram of meiosis for one pair of homologous chromosomes. Trisomy and monosomy resulting from nondisjunction in the first and second divisions are shown. (From Nelson WE, Vaughn VC, McKay RJ, eds. *Textbook of pediatrics,* 9th Ed. Philadelphia, PA: WB Saunders, 1969.)

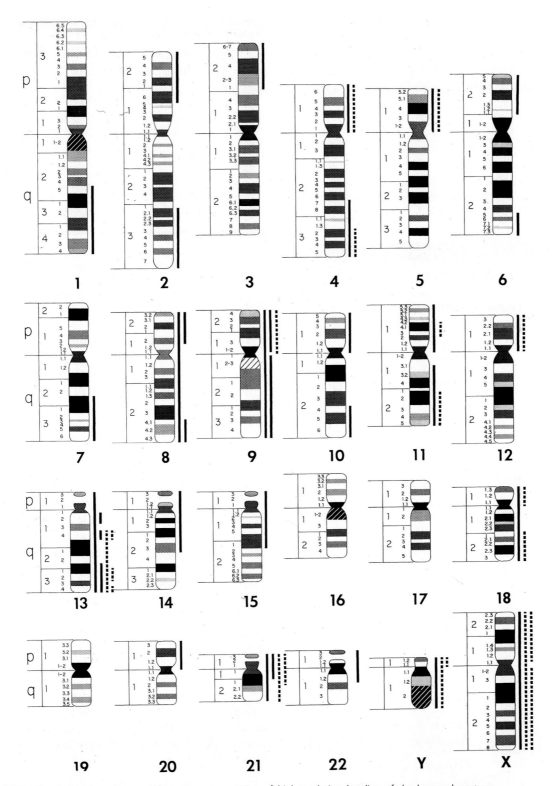

FIGURE 1.15. Chromosomal syndromes. Schematic representation of high-resolution banding of the human karyotype. Subbands are represented by the decimal system recommended by the Paris Conference in 1971. Numbers 1 to 22 represent autosomes, and X and Y sex chromosomes. Letters p and q on the left side of each chromosome row refer to short and long arms, respectively. The variable heterochromatic band q12 of chromosomes 1, 9, 16, and Y is represented with diagonals. To the right of each chromosome, presently known syndromes are represented: trisomic (duplication) syndromes by *solid vertical lines* and deletion (monosomy) syndromes by *dotted lines*. (Adapted from previously unpublished figures, courtesy of Jorge J. Yunis, MD.)

vision) or optic nerve. An isolated iris coloboma does not cause significant visual impairment. Table 1.1 summarizes the chromosomal rearrangements that have been reported in association with colobomatous and noncolobomatous forms of microphthalmia; Table 1.2 describes the associations of cyclopia.

Aneuploidy

Aneuploidy is a state of having a complete diploid set of chromosomes with one or more extra or missing chromosomes. The major chromosomal aneuploidy syndromes compatible with live birth include trisomy 13, 18, and

Table 1.1	
CHROMOSOMAL ABERRATIONS	
Colobomatous Microphthalmia	
Condition	Reference
Triploidy	Cogan (1971) (454) Trisomies
13	Cogan et al. (1964) (455)
18	Mullaney (1973) (456)
Duplications	
4q+	Wilson et al. (1970) (457)
7q+	Vogel et al. (1973) (458)
9p +	Rethore et al. (1970) (459)
9p+q+	Schwanitz et al. (1974) (460)
13q+	Hsu et al. (1973) (461)
22q+	Walknowska et al. (1977) (462)
Deletions	
3q	Alvarado et al. (1987) (463)
4p-	Wilcox et al. (1978) (174)
4r	Carter et al. (1969) (464)
7q–	Taysi et al. (1982) (465)
11q-	Ferry et al. (1981) (466); Bialasiewicz et al. (1987) (467)
13q-	O'Grady et al. (1974) (468)
13r	Saraux et al. (1970) (469)
18q-	Schinzel et al. (1975) (470)
18r	Yanoff et al. (1970) (471)
Microphthalmia duplications	
10q+	Yunis et al. (1976) (472)

Table 1.2	
CHROMOSOMAL REARRANGEMENTS WITH CYCLOPIA AND SYNOPHTHALMIA	
Trisomy 13	Howard (1977) (473)
Trisomy 18	Lang et al. (1976) (474)
18r	Cohen et al. (1972) (475)
18p-	Nitowsky et al. (1966) (476); Faint and Lewis (1964) (477)
3p+	Gimelli et al. (1985) (478)

21 and monosomy X (Turner syndrome), XXY (Klinefelter syndrome), XXX, and XXY. Cat eye syndrome is partial trisomy 22.

Trisomy 13 (Patau Syndrome)

Infants with trisomy 13 (362) usually have normal birth weight and are hypotonic. About half have a cleft lip or palate (Fig. 1.16). Those without clefts have a characteristic face with sloping forehead and bulbous nose (Fig. 1.16B). Perinatal death is common, and survivors are severely retarded; 90% die by 1 year of age.

Anomalies include cardiovascular malformations, polycystic renal cortex, biseptate uterus in females, undescended testes and abnormal insertion of the phallus in males, polydactyly of the hands and feet, hyperconvex nails, capillary cutaneous defects, and cutaneous scalp defects. The central nervous system is markedly affected, degrees of defects ranging from cyclopia (Fig. 1.16C) with absence of rhinencephalon, union of ventricles and thalami, and defects of the corpus callosum, falx cerebri, and commissures to simple arrhinencephaly with absence of olfactory nerves and lobes.

Ocular abnormalities are a cardinal feature of trisomy 13 and include colobomatous microphthalmia, cataracts, corneal opacities, glaucoma, persistent hyperplastic primary vitreous, intraocular cartilage, and retinal dysplasia (Fig. 1.16F,G). Most children with trisomy 13 have 47 chromosomes, but a few have 46 chromosomes with a translocation of two of the D category chromosomes, which usually occurs de novo but rarely is inherited from a carrier parent. Males and females are equally affected.

Trisomy 18 (Edwards Syndrome)

The clinical findings of trisomy 18 are normally related to the presence of an extra chromosome 18 (363). Rarely, an unbalanced translocation involving chromosome 18 may cause the syndrome.

The features that help to differentiate trisomy 18 clinically are microcephaly, characteristic facies (Fig. 1.17), low

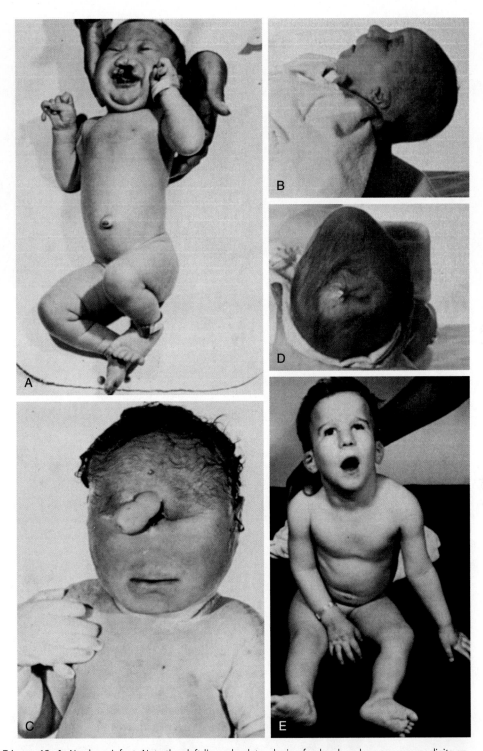

FIGURE 1.16. Trisomy 13. **A:** Newborn infant. Note the cleft lip and palate, sloping forehead, and supernumerary digits on all four extremities. **B:** Characteristic profile in an infant without clefts, showing bulbous nose, sloping forehead, anomalies of the external ear, and micrognathia. **C:** Cyclopia with an extra digit. **D:** Scalp defect. **E:** A 2.5-year-old severely retarded boy with mosaicism for trisomy 13. Characteristic face, with microphthalmia on the left; low-set, abnormal ears; and tapering fingers with hyperconvex fingernails. **F:** Microphthalmic left globe with microcornea. The cataractous lens (L) lies anterior to the detached retina. The persistent hyaloid artery (*arrow*) is surrounded by persistent hyperplastic primary vitreous. **G:** The island of intraocular hyaline cartilage (C) lies in the plane of a uveal coloboma and is surrounded by persistent hyperplastic primary vitreous. Centrally, the embryonal retina shows numerous dysplastic rosettes (**H** and **E:** original magnification × 4). (From Rodrigues MM, Valdes-Dapena M, Kistenmacher M. Ocular pathology in a case of 13 trisomy. *J Pediatr Ophthalmol* 1973;10:54, reproduced with permission from Charles B. Slack, Inc.) **H:** The group D chromosomes, with trisomy 13.

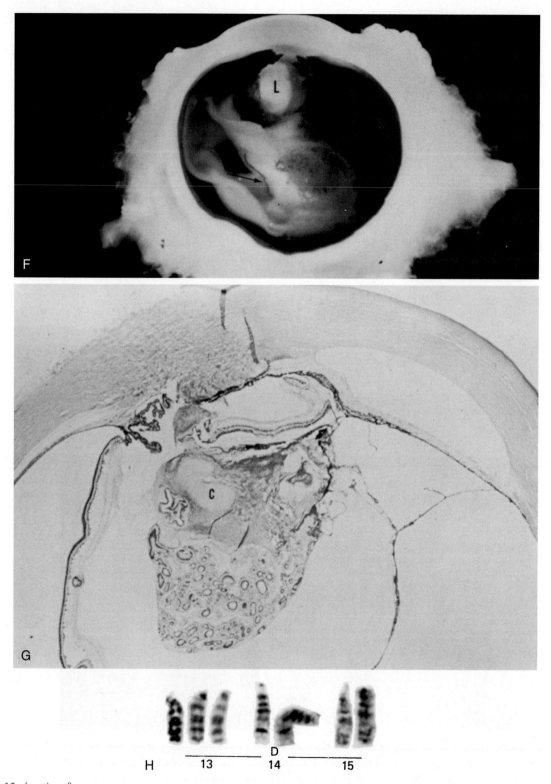

FIGURE 1.16. (*continued*)

birth weight for gestational age, hypertonicity with limbs in flexion, limited hip abduction, apneic spells, and marked failure to thrive. The facial characteristics include a prominent occiput, with narrow bifrontal diameter; receding chin, micrognathia, and high-arched palate; and low-set, large, malformed ears with poor helical development. The hand is usually flexed, with overlapping of the second and fifth fingers and failure of development of interphalangeal creases. Rocker-bottom feet, webbing of toes, and dorsiflexion of a short great toe are common. Arch dermatoglyphic patterns

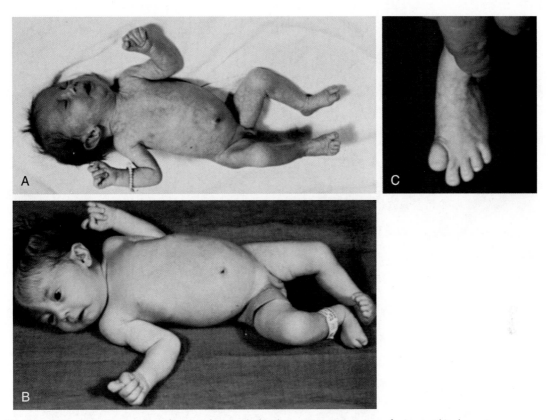

FIGURE 1.17. Trisomy 18. **A, B:** Two newborn female infants with the characteristic appearance of micrognathia, low-set ears, hypoplastic helix, and flexion deformity of the fingers. Note the slightly enlarged clitoris and club feet in **(B)**. **C:** Dorsiflexion of the short great toe. **D:** Retinal pigment epithelium (RPE) displaying marked thickening and hyperpigmentation at the periphery (H and E, original magnification × 256). **E:** Hypopigmentation of the retinal pigmentation (*arrows*) at the posterior pole. **F:** E group chromosomes, with trisomy 18. (**D** and **E** reprinted from Rodrigues MM, Punnett HH, Valdes-Dapena M, et al. Retinal pigment epithelium in a case of trisomy 18. Am J Ophthalmol 1973;76:265–268, with permission from Ophthalmic Publishing Company.)

are seen on most fingertips. These babies have hypoplasia of adipose tissue and poor muscle development.

Renal anomalies and congenital heart disease occur in more than 65% of cases. Pyloric stenosis, eventration of the diaphragm, and Meckel's diverticulum are found in 25% to 50% of cases. The majority (90%) die before 1 year of age.

The most common eye anomalies are orbital and palpebral, including hypertelorism and hypoplastic supraorbital ridges. The less common ocular features of this syndrome include colobomatous microphthalmia, corneal opacities, cataract, microcornea, retinal depigmentation, and congenital glaucoma.

Pathologic studies of the eye in trisomy 18 are limited. In the two cases reported by Ginsberg and coworkers (364), the most significant abnormalities affected the cornea, uveal tract, lens, and retina. Corneal opacities reflected retrograde changes (lamellar disorganization and fibrosis) of stroma. Anomalies of the ciliary process, breaks in the iris sphincter, posterior subcapsular cataract, and muscle abnormalities were described. Rodrigues and colleagues (365) observed abnormalities of the RPE in the patient with trisomy 18 and XY/XXY mosaicism (Fig. 1.17D,E). No abnormalities were

seen in the eyes of one other patient (46,XX/47,XX, + 18) studied by Green (366).

Trisomy 21 (Down Syndrome)

The most common autosomal abnormality in live births is Down syndrome (OMIM 190685), named for Langdon Down, who first described the condition in 1866 (367) (Fig. 1.18). Most children with Down syndrome have 47 chromosomes with an extra chromosome 21 (361); the parents usually have normal chromosomes. Approximately 6% of children with Down syndrome have 46 chromosomes, 1 of which represents the centric fusion of chromosome 21 and a D or G group chromosome. The translocation may have been inherited from a normal parent who has 45 chromosomes (the translocation replacing one 21 and either one D or one G) or may have developed de novo. There is no clinical difference between children with a trisomy and with translocation Down syndrome. The incidence of Down syndrome is 1 in 700 live births and is age dependent. The risk increases with maternal age to 1 in 40 for women over age 44. The risk of having a second child with Down syndrome

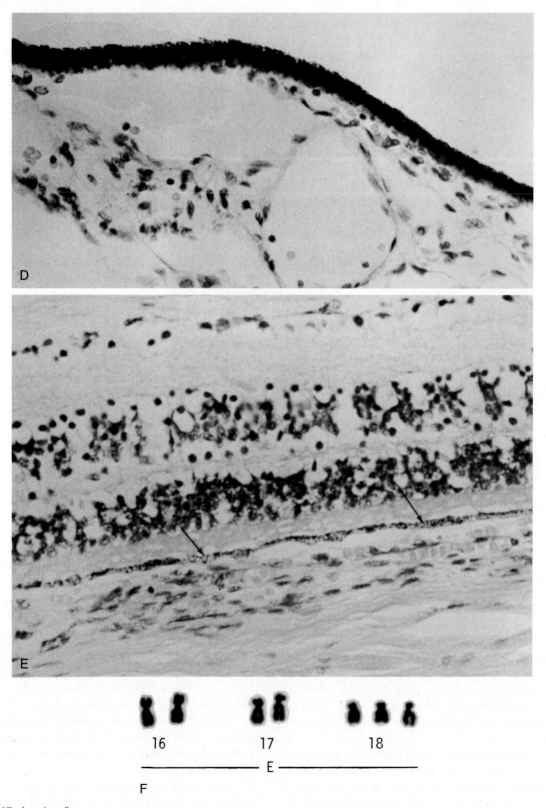

FIGURE 1.17. (continued)

for chromosomally normal parents is 1% to 2%. In the case of a parental translocation, the risk of Down syndrome offspring is 10% to 15% if the mother is the carrier, but only 1% to 2% if the carrier is the father. In the rare case of a 21;21 translocation in a parent, all offsprings have Down syndrome (Fig. 1.19).

Mosaicism for trisomy 21 is not uncommon. The clinical manifestations may vary from a normal phenotype to that

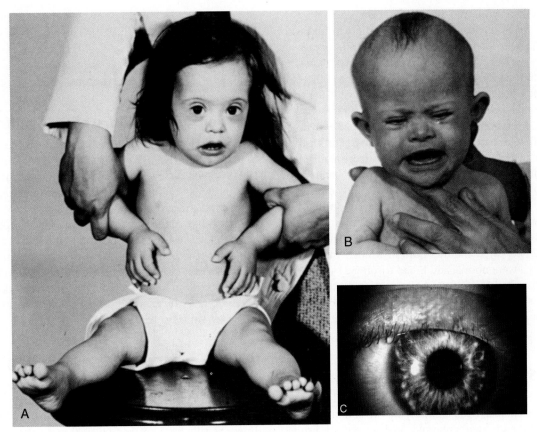

FIGURE 1.18. Down syndrome. **A:** An 11-month-old boy with typical facies, stubby hands, and prominent sandal gap of the feet. **B:** Ectropion of all four eyelids in an infant with Down syndrome. **C:** Iris Brushfield spots in Trisomy 21.

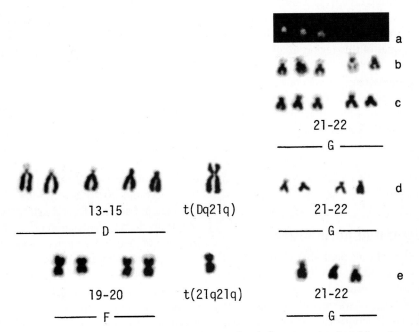

FIGURE 1.19. Chromosomal variations in Down syndrome. Trisomy 21 proved with fluorescent banding (*a*), and trypsin banding *(b)*. Trisomy 21 with karyotyping (c), Centric fusion translocations involving the D and 21 (*d*), and two chromosomes 21 (*e*). In each case the genetic information of chromosome 21 is present in triplicate.

of typical Down syndrome. Physically normal persons with mosaicism are usually detected after the birth of a child with trisomy 21, when chromosomal investigation reveals an abnormal 47,+21 cell line in one parent. The risk of having other children with trisomy 21 may be as high as 50%, but it cannot be calculated with any precision since it depends on knowing the proportion of trisomic cells in the gonad.

Systemic findings of Down syndrome include hypotonia; mental retardation; brachycephaly; large, protruding tongue; small nose with a low, small bridge; small, often poorly defined, ears; short, thick neck; stubby hands with a single palmar crease; clinodactyly of the fifth digit with hypoplasia of the middigital phalanges; short, stubby feet with a wide gap between the first and second toes; and congenital heart disease. Males are usually sterile; females are fertile. Of 21 reported children born to women with Down syndrome, 13 were normal and 8 had trisomy 21 (368).

The characteristic ocular findings are epicanthal folds, mongoloid slant of the eye, hypoplasia of the iris, Brushfield spots, myopia, keratoconus, esotropia, cataracts, and blepharitis. Ectropion of all four eyelids may occur (Fig. 1.18B).

Cat Eye Syndrome

Cat eye syndrome (OMIM 115470), or Schmid-Fraccaro syndrome, is characterized clinically by the combination of coloboma of the iris and/or choroid, anal atresia with fistula, downslanting palpebral fissures, preauricular tags and/or pits, frequent occurrence of heart and renal malformations, and normal or near-normal mental development. A small supernumerary chromosome (smaller than chromosome 21) is present, frequently has two centromeres, is bisatellited, and represents an invdup (22)(q11) (369). The origin of the extra chromosome was identified by DNA probes and is from within the long arm of chromosome 22 (q11 band); there are three or four copies of this region in affected persons (370).

The additional chromosome 22 generally arises de novo from one of the parents. Since cat eye syndrome is a rare chromosome disorder in which transmission is possible through both sexes, chromosome examination should be performed if one of the parents displays characteristic features such as a preauricular pit or downslanting palpebral fissures. Even in nonsymptomatic parents, mosaicism for an extra chromosome is possible.

Cytogenetic Structural Abnormalities

The second group of clinically recognizable chromosomal syndromes have deletions resulting from breaks in a chromosome, usually with loss of a terminal portion. If the deletion occurred de novo in an egg or sperm, only a single child in a family will be affected. Deletions can also be inherited as the unbalanced form of a translocation for which a normal parent has an abnormal but balanced chromosome constitution. Ring chromosomes are formed when the ends of

chromosomes break and fuse to each other, forming a ring. There is a loss of chromatin (DNA) from both ends, and such children may resemble those with simple deletions of the same chromosome. Many partial deletions occur frequently enough to be considered a syndrome.

Deletion 4p– (Wolf-Hirschhorn Syndrome)

The physical findings in partial deletion of the short arm of chromosome 4 (Wolf-Hirschhorn syndrome; OMIM 194190) include severe mental retardation, seizures, prominent glabella, midline scalp defect, preauricular dimple, cleft lip and palate or high-arched palate, deformed nose, hemangiomas of the forehead, internal hydrocephalus, and undescended testes and hypospadias in males (371). Colobomatous microphthalmia is very common, as are ocular hypertelorism, exophthalmos, and strabismus (174). The chromosomal anomaly may be a de novo deletion or may result from an unbalanced segregation in the gamete of a carrier parent (Fig. 1.20).

Deletion 5p– (Cri du Chat Syndrome)

Partial deletion of the short arm of chromosome 5 (Cri du chat syndrome; OMIM 123450) was originally described by Lejeune and colleagues (372). Children with this syndrome usually have low birth weight and a slow growth rate neonatally. They are hypotonic. The infant's cat-like cry that gives the syndrome its name is attributed to an abnormality in laryngeal structure, which is striking in infancy but usually disappears with age. There is severe mental deficiency. Physical findings include microcephaly with a very round face in infancy, micrognathia, low-set ears, and congenital heart disease (Fig. 1.21). Ocular findings are antimongoloid slant, hypertelorism, epicanthal folds, exotropia, myopia, and optic atrophy. Like the syndrome of 4p–, 5p– may represent a new event or be inherited from a carrier parent.

Deletion 11p– (WAGR Syndrome)

WAGR syndrome (OMIM 194072) involves aniridia, mental retardation, and genitourinary anomalies and has been associated with a predisposition to Wilms' tumor. Deletion of the short arm of chromosome 11 involving the llp13 band accounts for this syndrome (151–154) (Fig. 1.22); one patient had aniridia and Wilms' tumor without a microscopically detectable deletion (155). The deletion may occur de novo or as a consequence of meiotic events in a normal carrier parent. Although Wilms' tumor has been the embryonal tumor associated with this triad, benign gonadoblastoma was found in a child with deletion 11p13, aniridia, and mental retardation but who had no evidence of Wilms' tumor on postmortem examination at age of 21 months (154). The gene for catalase is near the aniridia locus in band p13 on the short arm of chromosome 11 (373), and production of this enzyme may be reduced in the presence of some deletions

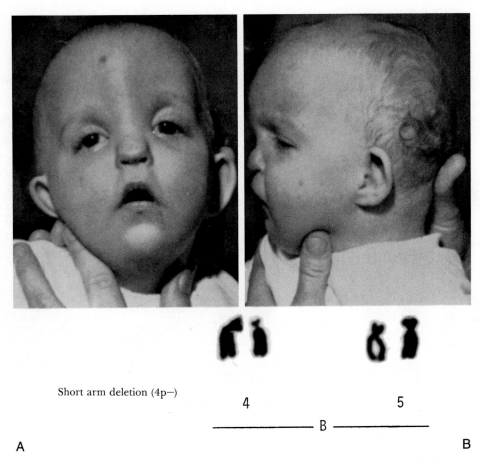

Short arm deletion (4p−)

4   5

——————— B ———————

A   B

FIGURE 1.20. A: A 1-year-old boy with deletion of the short arm of chromosome 4 (4p−). (From Nelson WE, Vaughn VC, McKay RJ, eds. *Textbook of pediatrics*, 9th Ed. Philadelphia, PA: WB Saunders, 1969, with permission.) **B:** Chromosomes of B group with deletion of part of the short arm of 4.

(151). All children with aniridia and this deletion should be followed up carefully by abdominal ultrasonography for the first 4–5 years of life to facilitate early detection of Wilms' tumor.

Deletion 13q–

Partial monosomy for chromosome 13 may be due either to deletion of part of the long arm or to a ring 13. The phenotypes are similar and include microcephaly with trigonocephaly; prominent bridge of the nose; small chin; large, low-set, malformed ears; and facial asymmetry (Fig. 1.23). These children are profoundly retarded. Males have hypospadias and undescended testes. Absent or hypoplastic thumbs are frequent. Ocular findings include hypertelorism, narrow palpebral fissures, epicanthal folds, ptosis, colobomatous microphthalmos, cataract, and retinoblastoma.

In some cases of sporadic retinoblastoma, a deletion of band 13q14 of the long arm of chromosome 13 has been demonstrated; many children with this deletion have dysplastic features and developmental delay. In a few patients, the chromosome deletion was inherited as a consequence of a rearrangement involving chromosome 13 in a parent (374). Most cases arose de novo.

Sporadic retinoblastoma due to deletion of band 13q14 is estimated to account for approximately 2% of all retinoblastomas. The gene for the expression of human esterase D (a ubiquitous enzyme whose biologic function is unknown) is also located at band 13q14. Measurement of esterase D levels is potentially useful for identifying patients with retinoblastoma who have deletions too small to detect cytogenetically.

Deletion 18

Deletions of chromosome 18 may occur in either the short (18p−) or long (18q−) arm, or in both, through ring formation (r18) following fusion of broken chromosome ends with the loss of terminal portions of both arms. Therefore, physical findings of r18 may overlap both the short and long arm deletion syndromes and are not described separately here (Fig. 1.24) (375).

Deletion 18p–

The physical findings associated with the deletion (total or partial) of the short arm of chromosome 18 show a wide range. The mildest expression encompasses microcephaly,

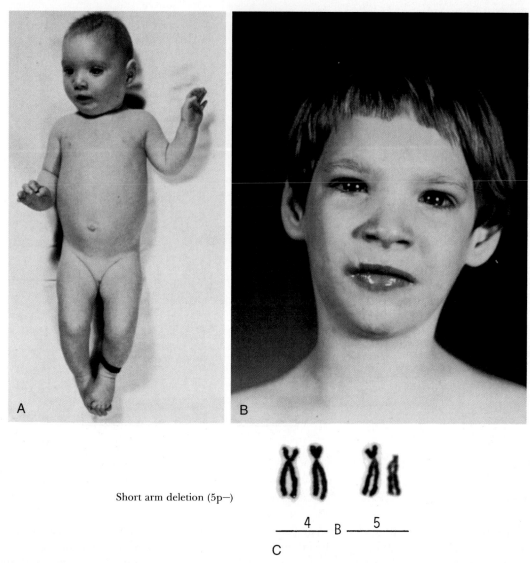

Short arm deletion (5p−)

FIGURE 1.21. Child with deletion of the short arm of chromosome 5 (5p−). **A:** At age 3 months. **B:** At 4 years. She has microcephaly, hypertelorism, epicanthal folds, and severe mental retardation. **C:** Chromosomes of B group with deletion of most of the short arm of 5.

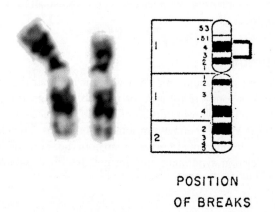

POSITION
OF BREAKS

FIGURE 1.22. Chromosomes 11 in a child with aniridia, hypogonadism, and Wilms' tumor. An interstitial short arm deletion including bands p13-p14 is apparent in the chromosome on the right. The position of breaks giving rise to the deletion is shown schematically. (Courtesy of Laurel Marshall.)

mental retardation, short stature, webbed neck, and immunoglobulin abnormalities (Fig. 1.25) (376).

In its most severe form, the syndrome mimics trisomy 13, with the median facial dysplasia of cebocephaly or cyclopia and incomplete morphogenesis of the brain. Cardiac, renal, and gastrointestinal abnormalities are rarely seen in 18p− syndrome. The eye anomalies of mildly affected children consist of hypertelorism, epicanthal folds, ptosis, and strabismus. Microphthalmia and cyclopia have been reported in the cebocephalic patients.

The only histopathologic study of the eye in an 18p deletion was reported by Yanoff and colleagues (375) in a case of cebocephaly with a ring 18. Bilateral microphthalmia with cyst, intrascleral cartilage, intrachoroidal smooth muscle, and other anomalies were seen. No recognizable components of the optic system could be identified.

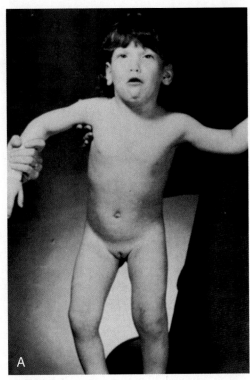

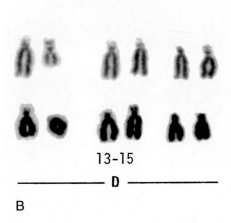

FIGURE 1.23. **A:** A 3-year-old girl with ring chromosome 13, micrognathia, hypertelorism, esotropia, bilateral colobomata of the irides, epicanthal folds, and mongoloid slant of the eyes. (From Kistenmacher ML, Punnett HH. Comparative behavior of ring chromosomes. *Am J Hum Genet* 1970;22:304–318, with permission.) **B:** Chromosomes of the D group, showing long arm deletion (13q–) (*above*) and ring (13r) (*below*).

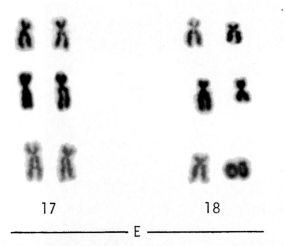

FIGURE 1.24. E group chromosomes 17 and 18, showing normal chromosomes 17 on the left (above, middle, and below). Chromosome 18 on the right with short arm deletion (18p –) (*above*), long arm deletion (18q –) (*middle*), and ring (18r) (*below*).

Deletion 18q–

Partial deletion of the long arm of chromosome 18 (377) produces a syndrome marked by failure of growth and development. The facies is striking: microcephaly, midface hypoplasia, and a carp-like mouth. The ears have a prominent anthelix and/or antitragus. There is a narrow or atretic ear canal and hearing loss.

The fingers taper markedly and have many whorl patterns. Single palmar creases are seen. Toes have abnormal placement, with the third toe placed above the second and fourth. Unusual fat pads occur on the dorsa of the feet. Dimples are prominent on knuckles, knees, elbows, and shoulders (Fig. 1.26). Eye abnormalities include epicanthal folds, slanted palpebral fissures, nystagmus, hypertelorism, microphthalmia, corneal abnormalities, cataracts, and abnormal optic disks. Most cases are sporadic partial deletions of the long arm of chromosome 18, but occasionally a parent carries a balanced translocation.

The ocular features of the trisomy and deletion/duplication syndromes are summarized in Tables 1.3–1.5.

Sex Chromosomes

The syndromes due to aneuploidy of the sex chromosomes were described before the development of modern cytogenetic techniques.

Turner Syndrome

Turner (378) described several patients with infantilism, webbed neck, and cubitus valgus establishing as a clinical syndrome, a previously described endocrine disorder. The absence of sex chromatin (Barr bodies) in most Turner

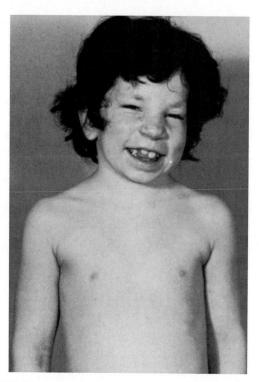

FIGURE 1.25. An 8-year-old girl with deletion of the short arm of chromosome 18, bilateral congenital ptosis, diabetes, and thyroiditis.

syndrome (OMIM 163950) patients was reported independently by three groups in 1954 (379–381). The first published 45,X karyotype (359) was confirmed by many laboratories in the same year. Approximately 80% of girls with Turner syndrome have 44 autosomal chromosomes, a single X, and no sex chromatin. The remaining 20% have other chromosomal variants. The unifying cytogenetic characteristic is the presence of a cell line that does not have two normal X chromosomes. It may lack the second X completely or have an abnormal second X (ring, fragment, deletion). The few patients who have Barr bodies are mosaics (45,X/46,XX) or have a long arm isochromosome—46,X,-i(Xq)—an abnormal chromosome with duplication of one arm forming two arms of equal length.

The typical findings in Turner syndrome, which is now called Noonan syndrome, are sexual infantilism, short stature, webbed neck, broad shield chest with widely spaced nipples, increased carrying angle, small uterus, and multiple pigmented nevi (Fig. 1.27). Recurrent ear infections are common. The ovaries consist of fibrous streaks with few or no follicles, and failure to feminize may be the presenting problem in older girls who have few of the physical stigmata. Coarctation of the aorta is common and may account for some of the early childhood deaths. Autoimmune diseases, particularly Hashimoto thyroiditis and diabetes, have been associated with the syndrome. Turner syndrome in some

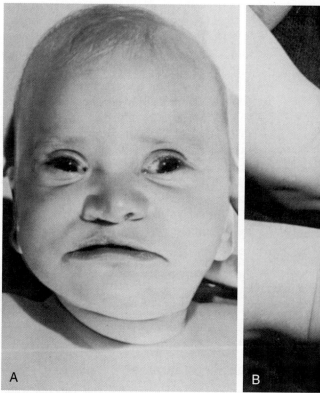
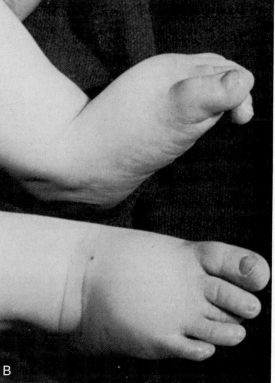

FIGURE 1.26. A: A 10-month-old infant with deletion of the long arm of chromosome 18, cleft lip (repaired) and palate, nystagmus, exotropia, bilateral optic atrophy, and macular anomalies. **B:** Abnormal insertion of the third toe and fat pads on the dorsal aspect of the feet.

Table 1.3

OCULAR MANIFESTATIONS IN TRISOMY SYNDROMES

	Trisomy 13[a]	Trisomy 18[b]	Trisomy 21[c]
Epicanthus	+	+	+
Hypertelorism	+	+	
Hypotelorism			+
Mongoloid lid slant			+
Strabismus	+	+	+
Ptosis		+	
Microphthalmia/ anophthalmia	+	+	
Coloboma	+		
Cataracts			
Juvenile			+
Congenital	+	+	
Corneal opacity	+	+	
Congenital glaucoma	+	+	+
Other			
Brushfield spots			+
Cyclopia	+		
Intraocular cartilage	+		
Absent eyebrows	+		
Congenital retinal detachment	+		

[a]Hoepner and Yanoff (1972) (479); Keith (1966) (480).
[b]Huggert (1966) (481); Rodrigues et al. (1973) (482); Ginsberg et al. (1968) (364).
[c]Ginsberg et al. (1980) (483); Shapiro and France (1985) (484); Caputo et al. (1989) (485).

newborn infants is characterized by lymphedema of the hands and feet, which may persist into adulthood.

Ptosis and strabismus are the most common ocular lesions encountered. Congenital cataracts may occur, as well as those of later onset, particularly in association with diabetes. Refractive errors, corneal scars, blue sclera, and a variety of other anomalies have been reported (382).

The incidence of color blindness in females with 45,X Turner syndrome equals that seen in normal males, since only one X chromosome is present. In informative families, this easily recognized defect may identify the origin of the single X. If the girl with Turner syndrome and her father are discordant (if the child is color blind and the father is normal, or vice versa), the single X must have come from the mother, assuming correct paternity. If both the child and the father are color blind and the mother is normal, the X may be assumed to be from the father.

Ambiguity of the external genitalia is not a feature of Turner syndrome, but it is seen in children with 45,X/46,XY mosaicism in whom the physical findings of Turner syndrome may be combined with varying degrees of masculinization of the genitalia. Some may resemble typical Turner syndrome; others are phenotypic males. Frequently, a unilateral streak gonad is found with a contralateral abdominal testis.

Klinefelter Syndrome

Klinefelter and coworkers (383) described a syndrome of gynecomastia, small testes with hyalinization of seminiferous tubules, absent spermatogenesis but normal Leydig cell complement, and elevated urinary gonadotropins. Patients with this clinical syndrome were shown by Plunkett and Barr (384) to be chromatin positive and by Jacobs and Strong (360) to have 47,XXY chromosome complement. Boys with more severe forms of Klinefelter syndrome (OMIM 278850) may have XXXY sex chromosomes and two Barr bodies, or XXXXY and three Barr bodies. Increasing numbers of X chromosomes cause greater physical and mental impairment. Males with XXXY are mentally retarded and may have radioulnar synostosis, scoliosis, microcephaly, congenital heart disease, and prognathism (Fig. 1.28). The ocular findings include epicanthal folds, hypertelorism, upward slant of the palpebral fissures, strabismus, Brushfield spots, and myopia.

The extra X chromosome may be either maternal or paternal in origin. Mosaicism (46,XY/47,XXY/48,XXXY or 48,XXXY/49,XXXXY) is common and may be explained by two successive nondisjunctions, the initial one in parental gametogenesis and the second in the zygote.

Considerable overlap with Klinefelter syndrome has been seen in boys with 48,XXYY karyotypes. They are unusually tall with eunuchoid proportions and exhibit some degree of mental retardation. Some males have also exhibited the aggressive or bizarre behavior attributed to men with 47,XYY karyotypes. No phenotypic characteristics other than tall stature have been reported with the latter. The physical or behavioral characteristics attributed to XYY males are variable. The first XYY males reported were identified during surveys of persons in British maximum-security hospitals, and their aggressive personalities received considerable publicity. Other XYY males have been identified on the basis of hypogonadism or infertility and are otherwise normal. Structural eye anomalies are not usually seen in the XYY syndrome, although myopia, dislocation of the lens, and bilateral retinal detachments have been reported.

Table 1.4											
CHROMOSOMAL DUPLICATION SYNDROMES											
	4q+	5p+	[c]9p+	[d]10p+	[e]12p+	[f]10q+	[g]11p+	[h]13q+	[i]14q+	[j]18pi[k]	22q	[l]4[b]p+[a]
Epicanthus			+		+							
Blepharophimosis	+		+	+								
Ptosis	+			+							+	
Hypertelorism	+	+		+		+	+				+	
Hypotelorism												
Mongoloid lid slant												
Antimongoloid lid slant							+			+		
Strabismus	+	+		+		+	+			+		
Microphthalmia	+		+	+		+		+	+		+	
Coloboma	+	+		+	+		+	+		+	+	
Cataracts												
Juvenile												
Congenital				+							+	
Corneal opacity								+				
Congenital glaucoma									+			
Brushfield spots				+								

[a]Gustavson et al. (1964) (486).
[b]4q+ : Wilson et al. (1970) (457).
[c]Monteleone et al. (1976) (487).
[d]Rethore et al. (1970) (488).
[e]Yunis et al. (1976) (472).
[f]Rethore et al. (1975) (489).
[g]Orye et al. (1975) (490), Yunis and Sanchez (1974) (491).
[h]Falk et al. (1973) (492).
[i]Hsu et al. (1973) (461).
[j]Raoul et al. (1975) (493).
[k]Supernumery isochromosome 18, Condron et al. (1974) (494).
[l]Cat eye syndrome, Zellweger et al. (1976) (495).

POLYGENIC AND MULTIFACTORIAL INHERITANCE

The concepts of polygenic and multifactorial inheritance provide an explanation for disorders that tend to cluster in families but do not conform to single-gene Mendelian inheritance. The expression of a disease may depend on the presence of a critical number of genes that are inherited independently. Such a disorder would be *polygenic*, and the genetic risk factors would be additive. If environmental factors affect the outcome, the term *multifactorial* is used. The genetic threshold value may differ for the two genders for polygenic and multifactorial disorders. For example, pyloric stenosis occurs more frequently in males than in females, and the risk factors must be greater if a female is to express the anomaly. Therefore, the likelihood of an affected female having affected children is higher than that for an affected male. The gender relationship is reversed for congenitally dislocated hip, which is more common in females. Examples of diseases that cluster in families but are not proven

Table 1.5										
CHROMOSOMAL DELETION SYNDROMES										
	4r[b]	**5p[c]**	**10p[d]**	**11p–[e]**	**11q[f]**	**13q[g]**	**15q–[h]**	**18p–[i]**	**18q–[j]**	**4p–[a]**
Epicanthus	+	+		+	+	+		+	+	
Blepharophimosis										
Ptosis	+				+	+		+		
Hypertelorism	+	+				+		+	+	
Hypotelorism					+					
Mongoloid lid slant					+					
Antimongoloid lid slant									+	
Strabismus	+			+	+				+	
Microphthalmia	+	+				+			+	
Coloboma	+	+	+		+				+	
Cataracts										
Juvenile	+									
Congenital		+		+						
Corneal opacity					+					
Congenital glaucoma		+	+	+						
Aniridia				+						
Retinoblastoma						+				
Ocular albinism									+	

[a]Wolf-Hirschhorn syndrome, Wilcox et al. (1978) (174).
[b]Carter et al. (1969) (464).
[c]Cri du chat syndrome, Breg et al. (1970) (496); Farrell et al. (1988) (497).
[d]Broughton et al. (1981) (498).
[e]Riccardi et al. (1978) (153).
[f]Bateman et al. (1984) (183); Lee and Sciorra (1981) (499).
[g]Allderdice et al. (1969) (500).
[h]Prader-Willi syndrome, Ledbetter et al.(1981, 1982) (501, 502); Hittner et al. (1982) (29); Mattei et al. (1983) (503).
[i]Schinzel et al. (1974) (504).
[j]Schinzel et al. (1975) (470).

to be single-gene defects and are not purely environmental include refractive error, strabismus, diabetes, cleft lip, and spina bifida. We briefly discuss the genetics of myopic refractive error and strabismus below.

Myopia

Myopia is a condition in which the eye is too long for the combined corneal and lens focal lengths, and the plane of sharp focus of the image is therefore in front of the retina. The growth of the eye is controlled by an image-processing feedback mechanism commandeered by the retina. There is no doubt that an environmental component is involved in myopic development, and extended near work appears to be the major risk factor. Inheritance also plays a role, since myopic parents are more likely to have myopic children. Myopia is far more frequent in Asian populations than in the United States or Europe, even if groups are compared that have performed similar amounts of near work.

There are multiple genetic syndromes with systemic findings that have myopia as a consistent clinical feature. For example, Stickler syndrome type I (OMIM 108300) is

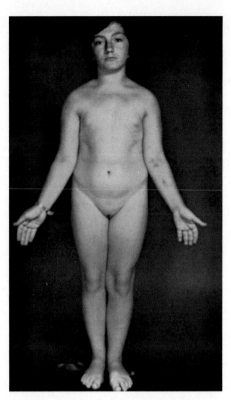

FIGURE 1.27. Turner syndrome in a 15-year-old girl with short stature, cubitus valgus, and a goiter. Her karyotype is 45,X/46,XX. (From Behrman RE, Vaughan VC III, Nelson WE, eds. *Nelson textbook of pediatrics,* 13th Ed. Philadelphia, PA: WB Saunders, 1989, with permission.)

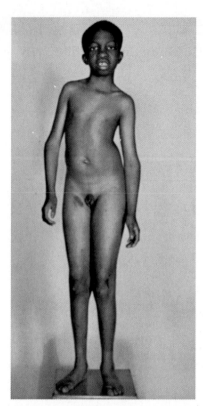

FIGURE 1.28. A 12-year-old boy with 48,XXXY/49,XXXXY mosaicism. He has prognathism, epicanthal folds, scoliosis, hypogonadism, severe mental retardation, clinodactyly, and radioulnar synostosis. (From Behrman RE, Vaughan VC III, Nelson WE, eds. Nelson textbook of pediatrics, 13th Ed. Philadelphia, PA: WB Saunders, 1987.)

an autosomal dominant, type IIa collagen gene mutation, connective-tissue disorder characterized by ocular, orofacial, and skeletal abnormalities. Associated ocular manifestations include high myopia, glaucoma, cataracts, vitreoretinal degeneration, and retinal detachment (385,386). Marfan syndrome (OMIM 154700) is an autosomal dominant, fibrillin-1 gene mutation, connective-tissue disorder with clinical features of myopia, lens dislocation, tall body habitus, and increased aortic wall distensibility (202,387). Knobloch syndrome (OMIM 267750) has an autosomal recessive high myopia presentation with vitreous degeneration and encephalocele, and is due to mutations in the collagen type 18A1 gene on chromosome 21q22.3 (388). Unlike these syndromes, however, the vast majority of individuals with myopia—moderate or severe—have no associated defects.

Determining the role of genetic factors in the development of nonsyndromic myopia has been hampered by the high prevalence, genetic heterogeneity, and clinical spectrum of this condition. The existence of a genetic contribution to any disease is based on evidence of familial aggregation and twin studies (389). In the past, several modes of inheritance for myopia were proposed, with no clear agreement among studies of pedigrees (389–391). Goss and associates (392) reviewed a number of studies, some of which proposed an autosomal dominant mode of inheritance, others autosomal recessive, and still others, an X-linked pattern of inheritance

for myopia. More recently, Naiglin and associates (393) performed segregation analysis on 32 French families with high myopia and determined an autosomal dominant mode of inheritance. The λs for myopia (the increase in risk to siblings of a person with a disease compared to the population prevalence) has been estimated to be approximately 20 for siblings for high myopia, compared to approximately 1.5 for low myopia, suggesting a strong genetic basis for high myopia (394).

Twin studies provide the most compelling evidence that myopia is inherited. Multiple studies note an increased concordance of refractive error and refractive components (axial eye length, corneal curvature, lens power, and anterior chamber depth) in monozygotic twins compared to dizygotic twins (390,395–397). Twin studies estimate a notable heritability value, the proportion of the total phenotypic variance that is attributed to the genome, of between 0.5 and 0.96 (395,396,398).

Many studies report a positive correlation between parental myopia and myopia in their children, indicating a hereditary factor in myopia susceptibility (399–403). Children with a family history of myopia had on average less hyperopia, deeper anterior chambers, and longer vitreous chambers even before becoming myopic. The odds of children with two myopic parents becoming myopic were 6.4

times those of children with one or no myopic parents. The odds of developing myopia for children who had refractions in the lower half of the distribution at 6 to 12 months were 4.3 times those of children who had refractions in the upper half. A pedigree analysis indicated that 63% of individuals at risk for developing juvenile-onset myopia actually became myopic, with an equal number of affected males and females. This implies a strong role for genetics in the initial shape and subsequent growth of the eye in myopia. Assessing the impact of genetic inheritance on myopic development may be confounded by children adopting their parents' behavioral traits, such as higher than average near-work activities (e.g., reading) (404).

In addition to genetics, moderate myopic development can be influenced by environmental factors. This is exemplified by experimental modulation of refractive error in the developing eyes of several mammalian and avian models (405–407), and the development of myopia in young children with media irregularities that prevent a focused retinal image (408–410). Moreover, the prevalence of myopia in some populations appears to have increased dramatically from one generation to the next in increasingly industrialized settings or with increased levels of educational achievement (411–415). The identification of myopia genes may therefore provide insight into genetic–environmental interactions.

The notion that multiple genes may be involved in the pathogenesis of myopia has been supported by the results of recent mapping investigations for high myopia of greater than 6.00 D of spherical refractive error. Three genomic regions on chromosome Xq28 (MYP1 locus; OMIM 310460) (416,417) and autosomal dominant loci on chromosome 18p11.31 (MYP2 locus; OMIM 160700) (418) and chromosome 12q23.1–24 (MYP3 locus; OMIM 603221) (419) have been shown to segregate with myopia in a small number of independent families. The MYP2 locus has been confirmed by two independent laboratories (420,421). Recently, a new locus for autosomal dominant high myopia has been mapped to chromosome 17q21–22 (MYP5; OMIM 608474) (422). A suggestive fourth locus for autosomal dominant high myopia has been reported on chromosome 7q36 (MYP4; OMIM 608367) (423).

An investigation of factors that regulate the rate and duration of eye growth in the mouse has also revealed two loci (Eye1 and Eye2) that may be responsible for genetic factors influencing myopia (424,425). The human homologous regions (*synteny*) are at chromosomes 6p, 16q13.3, and 19q13 for Eye2, and at chromosome 7q for Eye1.

Some forms of severe myopia may be inherited as Mendelian autosomal dominant or recessive traits. However, the majority of myopic individuals have a moderate refractive error that is more likely to be the result of a combination of genetic and environmental influences. Studying the nature of the genes that confer susceptibility for high myopia may provide insights for the development and progression of the common form of myopia, as well as address the interaction of genetic and environmental factors.

Consensus opinion regarding common, juvenile-onset myopia of moderate amounts is that its etiology is influenced by both genetic and environmental factors (403). As a multifactorial, common, complex trait, genes or gene loci for this type of myopia have yet to be identified. Susceptibility loci contributing to common, juvenile-onset myopia may be difficult to map by classic linkage analysis because of the limited power to detect genes of intermediate or small effect using independent pedigrees.

Strabismus

Strabismus (misalignment of the eyes; also referred to as "squint") is one of the most common ocular disorders in humans, affecting 1% to 4% of the population (426). The familial clustering of strabismus has been recognized since antiquity. For example, Hippocrates stated that "children of parents having distorted eyes squint also for the most part" (426). The causes of the common forms of nonsyndromic strabismus, such as concomitant esotropia and exotropia, are likely to be multiple and confounding, and no single malfunction, environmental agent, or gene mutation has been identified (427,428).

Strabismus tends to cluster in families. Population studies support a hereditary component with a sibling prevalence ranging from 11% to 70% (429,430). Francois (431) reported four pedigrees with members affected with esotropic strabismus. He concluded that autosomal dominant inheritance with reduced penetrance accounted for the disease. Dufier and coworkers (432) retrospectively studied the families of 195 persons with isolated esotropia. They found an affected family member of the proband by history or examination in more than 50% and vertical transmission from parents to child in 35%. They performed segregation analysis using a strabismus frequency of 3% in the general population and concluded that an autosomal dominant model with incomplete penetrance was most likely for esotropia and that an autosomal recessive model was most compatible with esotropia with amblyopia.

In a segregation analysis study of 173 pedigrees with infantile nonaccommodative esotropia, Maumenee and colleagues (433) found that the disease best fits a model with either two autosomal dominant genes with incomplete penetrance or multifactorial inheritance. Not included in this analysis are the many genetic conditions that are associated with strabismus via their effect on the development and function of the central nervous system or the anatomy of the eye and orbit.

With respect to overall heritability, the relative risk for first-degree relatives of an affected individual is estimated to be between 3 and 5 (434). Hu (435) found a 9% incidence among first-degree relatives and a 2.2% incidence among second-degree relatives, versus a population incidence of 0.6%. Richter (436) examined and studied the siblings and parents of patients (probands, 697; total, 1,509) and children with strabismus (probands, 136; total, 344) whose condition was ascertained at the time of vaccination. She found that the incidence of strabismus or the various strabismus-associated ocular anomalies among siblings of an affected proband was approximately 20% if both parents were unaffected and 30% to 40% if one or both parents were also affected, versus a population frequency of 4%. Strabismus affects males and females equally.

Studies of families with probands with exotropia are less numerous. Waardenburg (437) reported 18 families who had more than 1 member with exotropia; 13 exhibited vertical transmission from parent to child. He postulated autosomal dominant inheritance with reduced penetrance.

Twin studies further support the concept of a hereditary component predisposing to the development of strabismus (438). Waardenburg (437) combined previous reports of esotropia in twins with his cases and found the concordance rate of strabismus in monozygotic pairs to be approximately 80% (69 sets) and in dizygotic pairs, approximately 12% (101 sets). De Vries and Houtman (439) studied 17 pairs of monozygotic twins in whom 1 of the 2 developed esotropia within the first year of life, and found concordance in 8. Rubin and coworkers (440) questioned 50 ophthalmologists and compiled results on 22 sets of twins, 1 of whom had exotropia, and 122 pairs, and 1 of whom had esotropia; concordance was 77% in monozygotic sets and 50% in dizygotic for exotropia, and 75% in monozygotic and 53% in dizygotic for esotropia, with a heritability of 0.54 for exotropia and 0.47 for esotropia. The authors analyzed esophoria and exophoria separately and found the concordance to be relatively low for both forms of strabismus. Richter (436) also studied strabismus (combining both esotropia and exotropia) in twins and found concordance in 11 or 12 monozygotic pairs and 7 of 27 dizygotic pairs; on the basis of her frequency and twin studies, she concluded that strabismus was multifactorial. If genetic factors alone accounted for strabismus, the concordance of monozygotic twins should be 100%; conversely, if environmental influences alone cause the condition, 4% or less (the prevalence in the general population) of the dizygotic twins of affected persons should be similarly affected.

In 1972, Niederecker and coworkers (441) found that parents of probands with either esotropia or exotropia were less able than controls to maintain ocular alignment (fusional amplitudes). In an assessment of ocular deviation and the relationship of accommodative convergence to accommodation ratio, Mash and coworkers (442) found that certain vergence amplitudes had higher heritability values than others and differed significantly among the strabismus populations.

In a series of large quantitative genetic studies, ocular alignment and other parameters in a group of strabismus patients and their families from Iowa were studied (442,443). The studies assessed the heritability of ocular measurements that might predispose patients to strabismus. They found that ocular alignment (esodeviation or exodeviation) tended to be consistent within a family, with substantial heritability from the female parent at 0.42. Thus, relatives of patients with esodeviations tended also to have esodeviations, and relatives of patients with exodeviations tended to have exodeviations. The mother's ocular alignment correlated best with that of the offspring. These authors calculated the heritability of the relationship of the accommodative convergence to accommodation ratio at 0.38.

A recent study by Parikh and associates (444) identified the linkage of a presumptive strabismus susceptibility locus to chromosome 7p22.1 with a multipoint logarithm of odds score of 4.51 under a model of recessive inheritance in one large family. They also demonstrated the failure to observe significant linkage to chromosome 7p in six other multiplex families, consistent with genetic heterogeneity among families. Their findings suggest that it will be possible to localize and ultimately identify strabismus susceptibility genes by linkage analysis and mutation screening of candidate genes.

In conclusion, isolated strabismus is a common disease in the general population and the causes are poorly understood. Strabismus does not appear to develop as a result of a single-gene mutation; however, all forms cluster in families and there is little evidence to support an environmental cause. Although the evidence is not conclusive, a polygenic and/or multifactorial model is likely with a "threshold" level of many factors such as interpupillary distance, fusional ability, refractive error, and others, with strabismus becoming manifest if the individual has a combination of abnormalities.

GENETIC COUNSELING AND PRENATAL DIAGNOSIS

The recurrence risk for a single-gene disorder depends on whether the mutant gene is located on an autosome or on a sex chromosome, on whether it is manifested in the heterozygous state, and on the penetrance. An individual with a dominantly inherited disease may have a parent with the disorder and a family history of affected individuals in several generations (vertical transmission; Fig. 1.6). An individual with an autosomal dominant disorder mated to a normal partner will pass the gene on to approximately half of his or her offspring, regardless of gender; the other half of the children will receive the normal allele. Thus, the expectation for a child who does not carry the mutation will be 50% for each pregnancy, and the expectation for a child with the abnormal allele will also be 50%, regardless of the outcome of the preceding pregnancies. The likelihood that a child with the abnormal allele will express the disease is a function of its penetrance.

A child with a disorder inherited in a dominant manner may represent a new mutation if the penetrance is high and there is no family history. The recurrence risk for future pregnancies of the mother would be close to zero because most detectable mutations occur in a single gamete. However, a mutation in a tissue sector that includes germ cells could lead to the birth of more than one affected offspring. Documentation of such rare somatic mutations of germ cell lines exists in the case of two achondroplastic children born to normal parents (445). The subsequent birth of an achondroplastic child to one of the affected individuals demonstrated the dominant inheritance of the disorder in this family.

In a mating of two carriers of an autosomal recessive disorder, the probability is equal that each parent will contribute either a normal or an abnormal allele to the zygote for each pregnancy. There are three possible genetic combinations: (a) the homozygous normal child who receives a normal allele from each parent, (b) the heterozygote who receives a normal allele from one parent and the abnormal allele from the other parent, and (c) the affected child who receives an abnormal allele from each parent. The expected ratio is one homozygous clinically normal to two heterozygous clinically normal to one homozygous clinically abnormal (affected) offspring. The probability is 3:1 that the embryo will have received at least one normal allele and be phenotypically normal. Thus, there is a 25% risk of an affected child with each pregnancy.

When the enzyme defect is known and measurable in a recessively inherited metabolic disorder, it is possible to identify which relatives of an affected individual are carriers. The affected individual usually has reduced or absent enzyme activity, whereas the heterozygote has approximately half that of the normal homozygous individual. For example, the clinical manifestations of galactosemia are due to lack of activity of the enzyme galactose-1-phosphate uridyl transferase and accumulation of galactose-1-phosphate. Heterozygotes for galactosemia have approximately half the enzyme activity (as measured in white cells and tissue culture fibroblasts) of individuals with two normal alleles. It is possible to diagnose galactosemia and many other metabolic disorders in utero by measuring the enzyme level in tissue cultures of fetal cells obtained by chorionic villus sampling or by amniocentesis; however, DNA analysis is rapidly supplanting traditional biochemical methods.

In the case of rare recessive disorders, there is an increased incidence of consanguinity between the parents of affected individuals, both parents having received the mutant gene from the same common ancestor (Fig. 1.5). A gene may be relatively rare in one population but common in another. For example, the incidence of OCA in the United States is approximately 1 in 20,000; among the San Blas Indians of Panama, it is 1 in 132. Assuming both diseases are due to a defect in the same gene, the carrier state is more common in the San Blas inhabitants. The genes for Tay-Sachs disease and familial dysautonomia are extremely rare except among Jews who trace their ancestry to Eastern Europe. Cystic fibrosis is almost exclusively a disease of white populations. The high frequency of some recessive genes is attributed to genetic drift within an isolated population, termed the founder effect (as in the San Blas Indians). For other genes, heterozygosity may convey a selective advantage. The increased ability of sickle cell heterozygotes to survive an episode of malaria creates a selective advantage, and the carrier (heterozygous)

state is more frequent in Africa where malaria is more common. It has also been suggested that heterozygosity for Tay-Sachs disease conveys resistance to pulmonary tuberculosis (446).

In the case of an X-linked recessive disorder, the heterozygous female carrier transmits the abnormal allele to half her daughters (who are carriers) and to half her sons, who manifest the disease because they have only one X chromosome (Fig. 1.8). The other 50% of sons and daughters are normal. Affected males transmit their single X chromosome to all their daughters, who are obligate carriers for the X-linked recessive gene and affected for the X-linked dominant gene. Male-to-male transmission of an X-linked gene rarely occurs, since the male transmits his Y chromosome to his son; this phenomenon could occur if a gene were on the X and Y chromosomes. In an X-linked dominant disorder, half the children of an affected female will be affected; usually there is a predominance of females and presumed fetal wastage of males.

In genetic counseling, population genetics is useful for the calculation of a coefficient of inbreeding and a recurrence risk. The coefficient of inbreeding can be calculated for a couple on the basis of their consanguineous relationship. The recurrence risk for a particular disease may be calculated using Bayes' theorem and is based on the ancestral risk and the affected status of the offspring of the individual at risk for being a carrier.

The field of prenatal diagnosis has advanced rapidly in the past decade. The diagnostic use of chorionic villus sampling, amniocentesis, ultrasonography, fetoscopy, and other procedures has dramatically altered the nature of genetic counseling for families with a disease amenable to prenatal detection. Parents now may make a decision whether to continue a pregnancy based on the knowledge of an affected fetus rather than on a statistical risk.

In amniocentesis, amniotic fluid and suspended fetal cells are aspirated transabdominally. Usually, this procedure is performed in the second trimester after the 15th week of gestation. Recently, sophisticated ultrasonography has enabled amniocentesis to be performed as early as 11 to 12 weeks after the last menstrual period.

Chorionic villus sampling involves the removal of cells that are destined to become the placenta from outside the pregnancy sac; these cells are from the fertilized egg from which the embryo develops. The cells are obtained transcervically or transabdominally, using ultrasound monitoring. The procedure is usually performed between the 9th and 12th week after the last menstrual period. The cells can be grown in culture and used for chromosomal analysis and biochemical assay.

The general indications for prenatal diagnostic chorionic villus sampling are (a) an increased risk of having a child with a chromosomal abnormality (i.e., maternal age 35 years or older, previous child with a chromosomal abnormality, or the mother is a known carrier of a chromosomal rearrangement); (b) carrier status in the parents for a diagnosable biochemical disorder; and (c) carrier status of a serious X-linked disorder in the mother. For amniocentesis, the indications are identical. In addition, only amniocentesis is useful for the detection of a neural tube defect such as anencephaly, spina bifida, and encephalocele, and may be indicated if a parent or previous child has been so affected.

Chromosomal abnormalities are detectable by cytogenetic studies. Biochemical disorders are diagnosable in utero if they are expressed in cultured cells or amniotic fluid. Neural-tube defects in the fetus may be detected by elevated alpha-fetoprotein levels in amniotic fluid and altered pseudocholinesterase in the amniotic fluid; pregnancies at high risk are identified by screening of maternal serum. Generally, the neural-tube defect can be characterized by second-trimester ultrasonography. For X-linked diseases, determination of fetal gender is followed by the appropriate diagnostic test. If no test is available, the decision to continue pregnancy may be based solely on the information that a male fetus has a 50% risk of being affected.

Both chorionic villus sampling and amniocentesis have become accepted medical procedures with little risk to the mother or fetus. Ocular trauma to the fetus is an unusual complication. Unilateral hazy cornea with changes suggestive of perforation have been documented and attributed to midtrimester amniocentesis (447–451). This complication should be avoidable by the use of ultrasound-guided procedures.

Prenatal diagnosis is feasible for many diseases with ocular manifestations. Techniques for analysis include ultrasound testing of fetal anatomy and analysis of fetal cells or amniotic fluid. Significant ocular malformations have been diagnosed prenatally by ultrasonography (452,453) as fetal ocular biometry has been established.

REFERENCES

1. Sutton WS. The chromosomes in heredity. *Biol Bull* 1903;4: 231–251.
2. Watson JD, Crick FHC. Molecular structure of nucleic acids: a structure for deoxyribose nucleic acid. *Nature* 1953;171: 737–738.
3. Lenz W. Zukunftsperspektiven in der humangenetik. In: Hammerstein W, Lisch W, eds. *Ophthalmologische genetik.* Stuttgart, Germany: Enke, 1985:384–390.
4. Shin JT, Fishman MC. From zebrafish to human: modular medical models. *Ann Rev Genomics Hum Genet* 2002;3: 311–340.
5. McKusick VA. *Mendelian inheritance in man: a catalog of human genes and genetic disorders*, 11th Ed. Baltimore, MD: Johns Hopkins University Press, 1994.
6. Winter R, Baraister M. *London dysmorphology database,* version 3.0. Oxford: Oxford University Press Electronic Publishing, 2001.
7. Krawczak M, Ball EV, Fenton I, et al. Human gene mutation database—a biomedical information and research resource. *Hum Mutat* 2000;15:45–51.
8. Cotton RGH, McKusick V, Scriver CR. The HUGO mutation database initiative. *Science* 1998;279:10–11.
9. Thompson JS, Thompson MW. *Genetics in medicine,* 3rd Ed. Philadelphia, PA: WB Saunders, 1980:356.
10. Tjio JH, Levan A. The chromosome number of man. *Heredias* 1956;42:1–6.
11. Seabright M. A rapid banding technique for human chromosomes. *Lancet* 1971;2:971–972.
12. Caspersson T, Zech L, Johansson C. Differential binding of alkylating fluorochromes in human chromosomes. *Exp Cell Res* 1970;60:315–319.
13. Prescott JC, Blackburn EH. Telomerase: Dr. Jekyll or Mr. Hyde? *Curr Opin Genet Dev* 1999;9:368–373.
14. Bouffler SD. Involvement of telomeric sequences in chromosomal aberrations. *Mutat Res* 1998;404:199–204.
15. Krejci K, Koch J. An in situ study of variant telomeric repeats in human chromosomes. *Genomics* 1999;58:202–206.
16. Abdulla S. Telomerase as a marker for cancer. *Mol Med Today* 1997;3:187.
17. Albanell J, Lonardo F, Rusch V, et al. High telomerase activity in primary lung cancers: association with increased cell proliferation rates and advanced pathologic stage. *J Natl Cancer Inst* 1997;89:1609–1615.
18. Gendrot C, Ronce N, Raynaud M, et al. X-linked nonspecific mental retardation (MRX16) mapping to distal Xq28: linkage study and neuropsychological data in a large family. *Am J Med Genet* 1999;83:411–418.
19. Lichter P, Joos S, Bentz M, et al. Comparative genomic hybridization: uses and limitations. *Sem Hematol* 2000;37: 348–357.
20. Jeuken JWM, Sprenger SHE, Wesseling P. Comparative genomic hybridization: practical guideline. *Diagn Mol Pathol* 2002;11:193–203.
21. Pinkel D, Segraves R, Sudar D, et al. High resolution analysis of DNA copy number variation using comparative genomic hybridization to microarrays. *Nat Genet* 1998;20: 207–211.
22. Pollack JR, Perou CM, Alizadeh AA, et al. Genome-wide analysis of DNA copy-number changes using cDNA microarrays. *Nat Genet* 1999;23:41–46.
23. Snijders AM, Nowak N, Segraves R, et al. Assembly of microarrays for genome-wide measurement of DNA copy number. *Nat Genet* 2001;29:263–264.
24. Morton NE, Crow JF, Muller HJ. An estimate of the mutational damage in man from data on consanguineous marriages. *Proc Natl Acad Sci USA* 1956;42:855–863.
25. Lyon MF. Gene action in the X-chromosome of the mouse (*Mus musculus* L.). *Naturwissenschaften* 1961;190:372–373.
26. Bixler D, Higgins M, Hartsfield J Jr. The Nance-Horan syndrome: a rare X-linked ocular-dental trait with expression in heterozygous females. *Clin Genet* 1984;26:30–35.
27. Lewis RA, Nussbaum RL, Stambolian D. Mapping X-linked ophthalmic diseases. IV. Provisional assignment of the locus for X-linked congenital cataracts and microcornea (the Nance-Horan syndrome) to Xp22.2–p22.3. *Ophthalmology* 1990;97:110–120.
28. Berson EL, Sandberg MA, Maguire A, et al. Electroretinograms in carriers of blue cone monochromatism. *Am J Ophthalmol* 1986;102:254–261.

29. Hittner HM, Kretzer FL, Antoszyk JH, et al. Variable expressivity of autosomal dominant anterior segment mesenchymal dysgenesis in six generations. *Am J Ophthalmol* 1982;93:57–70.

30. Shoffner JM, Wallace DC. Mitochondrial genetics: principles and practice. *Am J Hum Genet* 1992;51:1179–1186.

31. Wallace DC. Mitochondrial DNA variation in human evolution, degenerative disease, and aging. *Am J Hum Genet* 1995;57:201–223.

32. Bindoff LA, Desnuelle C, Birch-Machin MA, et al. Multiple defects of the mitochondrial respiratory chain in a mitochondrial encephalopathy (MERRF): a clinical, biochemical and molecular study. *J Neurol Sci* 1991;102:17–24.

33. Moraes CT, DiMauro S, Zeviani M, et al. Mitochondrial DNA deletions in progressive external ophthalmoplegia and Kearns-Sayre syndrome. *N Engl J Med* 1989;320:1293–1299.

34. Wallace DC, Singh G, Lott MT, et al. Mitochondrial DNA mutation associated with Leber's hereditary optic neuropathy. *Science* 1988;242:1427–1430.

35. DiMauro S, Moraes CT. Mitochondrial encephalopathies. *Arch Neurol* 1993;50:1197–1208.

36. Shapira AHV, DiMauro S, eds. *Mitochondrial disorders in neurology.* Oxford: Butterworth-Heinemann, 1994.

37. Hufnagel RB, Ahmed ZM, Correa ZM, Sisk RA. Gene therapy for Leber congenital amaurosis: advances and future directions. *Graefes Arch Clin Exp Ophthalmlol* 2012;250:1117–1128.

38. Morimura H, Fishman GA, Grover SA, et al. Mutations in the RPE65 gene in patients with autosomal recessive retinitis pigmentosa or Leber congenital amaurosis. *Proc Natl Acad Sci USA* 1998;95:3088–3093.

39. Sohocki MM, Sullivan LS, Mintz-Hittner HA, et al. A range of clinical phenotypes associated with mutations in CRX, a photoreceptor transcription-factor gene. *Am J Hum Genet* 1998;63:1307–1315.

40. Acland GM, Aguirre GD, Ray J, et al. Gene therapy restores vision in a canine model of childhood blindness. *Nat Genet* 2001;28:92–95.

41. Tomita Y, Takeda A, Okinaga S, et al. Human oculocutaneous albinism caused by a single base insertion in the tyrosinase gene. *Biochem Biophys Res Commun* 1989;164:990–996.

42. Rinchik EM, Bultman SJ, Horsthemke B, et al. A gene for the mouse pink-eyed dilution locus and for human type II oculocutaneous albinism. *Nature* 1993;361:72–76.

43. Schmitz B, Schaefer T, Krick CM, et al. Configuration of the optic chiasm in humans with albinism as revealed by magnetic resonance imaging. *Invest Ophthalmol Vis Sci* 2003;44:16–21.

44. Faugere V, Tuffery-Giraud S, Hamel C, et al. Identification of three novel OA1 gene mutations identified in three families misdiagnosed with congenital nystagmus and carrier status determination by real-time quantitative PCR assay. *BMC Genet* 2003;4:1.

45. Hegde M, Lewis RA, Richards CS. Diagnostic DNA testing for X-linked ocular albinism (OA1) with a hierarchical mutation screening protocol. *Genet Test* 2002;6:7–14.

46. Farrer LA, Arnos K, Asher JH Jr, et al. Locus heterogeneity for Waardenburg syndrome is predictive of clinical subtypes. *Am J Hum Genet* 1994;55:728–733.

47. Zlotogora J. X-linked albinism-deafness syndrome and Waardenburg syndrome type II: a hypothesis. *Am J Med Genet* 1995;59:386–387.

48. Nobukuni Y, Watanabe A, Takeda K, et al. Analysis of loss-of-function mutations of the MITF gene suggests that haploinsufficiency is a cause of Waardenburg syndrome type IIa. *Am J Hum Genet* 1996;59:76–83.

49. Tassabehji M, Newton VE, Liu XZ, et al. The mutational spectrum in Waardenburg syndrome. *Hum Mol Genet* 1995;4:2131–2137.

50. Tassabehji M, Newton VE, Read AP. Waardenburg syndrome type 2 caused by mutations in the human microphthalmia (MITF) gene. *Nat Genet* 1994;8:251–255.

51. Morell R, Spritz RA, Ho L, et al. Apparent digenic inheritance of Waardenburg syndrome type 2 (WS2) and autosomal recessive ocular albinism (AROA). *Hum Mol Genet* 1997;6:659–664.

52. Rand EB, Spinner NB, Piccoli DA, et al. Molecular analysis of 24 Alagille syndrome families identifies a single submicroscopic deletion and further localizes the Alagille region within 20p12. *Am J Hum Genet* 1995;57:1068–1073.

53. Li Y, Bollag G, Clark R, et al. Somatic mutations in the neurofibromatosis 1 gene in human tumors. *Cell* 1992;69:275–281.

54. De Lange C. Sur un type nouveau de degeneration (typus Amsteledamensis). *Arch Med Enfants* 1933;36:713–719.

55. Jackson L, Kline AD, Barr MA, et al. de Lange syndrome: a clinical review of 310 individuals. *Am J Med Genet* 1993;47:940–946.

56. Ireland M, Donnai D, Burn J. Brachmann-de Lange syndrome. Delineation of the clinical phenotype. *Am J Med Genet* 1993;47:959–964.

57. Levin PS, Green WR, Victor DI, et al. Histopathology of the eye in Cockayne's syndrome. *Arch Ophthalmol* 1983;101:1093–1097.

58. Krantz ID, McCallum J, DeScipio C, et al. Cornelia de Lange syndrome is caused by mutations in *NIPLB*, the human homolog of *Drosophila melanogaster Nipped-B. Nat Genet* 2004;36:631–635.

59. Tonkin ET, Wang T-J, Lisgo S, et al. *NIPBL*, encoding a homolog of fungal Scc2-type sister chromatid cohesion proteins and fly Nipped-B, is mutated in Cornelia de Lange syndrome. *Nat Genet* 2004;36:636–641.

60. Rollins RA, Morcillo P, Dorsett D. Nipped-B, a Drosophila homologue of chromosomal adherins, participates in activation by remote enhancers in the *cut* and *Ultrabithorax* genes. *Genetics* 1999;152:577–593.

61. Collod-Beroud G, Boileau C. Marfan syndrome in the third millennium. *Eur J Hum Genet* 2002;10:673–681.

62. Robinson PN, Booms P, Katzke S, et al. Mutations of FBN1 and genotype-phenotype correlations in Marfan syndrome and related fibrillinopathies. *Hum Mutat* 2002;20:153–161.

63. Comeglio P, Evans AL, Brice G, et al. Identification of FBN1 gene mutations in patients with ectopia lentis and marfanoid habitus. *Br J Ophthalmol* 2002;86:1359–1362.

64. Gehrig WJ. The genetic control of eye development and its implications for the evolution of the various eye-types. *Int J Dev Biol* 2002;46:65–73.

65. Halder G, Callaerts P, Gehring WJ. Induction of ectopic eyes by targeted expression of the eyeless gene in Drosophila. *Science* 1995;267:1788–1792.

66. Van Heyningen V, Williamson KA. *PAX6* in sensory development. *Hum Mol Genet* 2002;11:1161–1167.

67. Ashery-Padan R, Gruss P. Pax6 lights up the way for eye development. *Curr Opin Cell Biol* 2001;13:706–714.

68. Chiang C, Litingtung Y, Lee E, et al. Cyclopia and defective axial patterning in mice lacking Sonic hedgehog gene function. *Nature* 1996;383:407–413.

69. Fantes J, Ragge NK, Lynch SA, et al. Mutations in SOX2 cause anophthalmia. *Nat Genet* 2003;33:461–463.

70. Mathers PH, Grinberg A, Mahon KA, et al. The Rx homeobox gene is essential for vertebrate eye development. *Nature* 1997;387:603–607.

71. Zhang L, Mathers PH, Jamrich M. Function of *Rx*, but not *Pax6* is essential for the formation of retinal progenitor cells in mice. *Genesis* 2000;28:135–142.

72. Tucker P, Laemle L, Munson A, et al. The *eyeless* mouse mutation *(ey1)* removes an alternative start codon from the *Rx/Rax* homeobox gene. *Genesis* 2001;31:43–53.

73. Young HB. Microcornea without microphthalmos. Report of a case. *Ann Ophthal* 1904;13:753.

74. Judisch GF, Martin-Casals A, Hanson JW, et al. Oculodentodigital dysplasia. Four new reports and a literature review. *Arch Ophthalmol* 1979;97:878–884.

75. Boynton JR, Purnell EW. Bilateral microphthalmos without microcornea associated with unusual papillomacular retinal folds and high hyperopia. *Am J Ophthalmol* 1975;79:820–826.

76. Spitznas M, Gerke E, Bateman JB. Hereditary posterior microphthalmos with papillomacular fold and high hyperopia. *Arch Ophthalmol* 1983;101:413–417.

77. Uemura Y, Morizane H. The fundus anomalies in high hypermetropic eyes, with particular reference to the interpapillomacular retinal fold. *Rinsho Ganka* 1970;24:15.

78. Francois J, Goes F. Ultrasonographic study of 100 emmetropic eyes. *Ophthalmologica* 1977;175:321–327.

79. O'Malley PF, Allen RA. Peripheral cystoid degeneration of the retina. Incidence and distribution in 1,000 autopsy eyes. *Arch Ophthalmol* 1967;77:769–776.

80. Heinonen OP, Slone D, Shapiro S. *Birth defects and drugs in pregnancy.* Littleton, MA: Publishing Sciences Group, 1977.

81. MacDonald AE. Causes of blindness in Canada: an analysis of 24,605 cases registered with the Canadian National Institute for the Blind. *Can Med Assoc J* 1965;92:264–279.

82. National Society to Prevent Blindness. *Vision problems in the U.S.* (A statistical analysis prepared by the operational research department). New York, NY: National Society to Prevent Blindness, 1980.

83. Fraser GR, Friedman AI. *The causes of blindness in childhood. A study of 776 children with severe visual handicaps.* Baltimore, MD: Johns Hopkins Press, 1967.

84. Fujiki K, Nakajima A, Yasuda N, et al. Genetic analysis of microphthalmos. *Ophthalmic Paediatr Genet* 1992;1:139–149.

85. Mann I. *The development of the human eye.* London: British Medical Association, 1964:277.

86. Pagon RA. Ocular coloboma. *Surv Ophthalmol* 1981;25: 223–236.

87. Bateman JB. Microphthalmos. *Int Ophthalmol Clin* 1984;24: 87–107.

88. Capella JA, Kaufman HE, Lill FJ. Hereditary cataracts and microphthalmia. *Am J Ophthalmol* 1963;56:454–458.

89. Usher CH. A pedigree of microphthalmia with myopia and corectopia. *Br J Ophthalmol* 1921;5:289.

90. Phillips CI, Leighton DA, Forrester RM. Congenital hereditary bilateral non-attachment of retina. A sibship of two. *Acta Ophthalmol (Copenh)* 1973;51:425–433.

91. Temtamy SA, Shalash BA. Genetic heterogeneity of the syndrome: microphthalmia with congenital cataract. *Birth Defects Orig Artic Ser* 1974;10:292–293.

92. Steingrimsson E, Moore KJ, Lamoreux ML, et al. Molecular basis of mouse microphthalmia (mi) mutations helps explain their developmental and phenotypic consequences. *Nat Genet* 1994;8:256–263.

93. Wallis DE, Roessler E, Hehr U, et al. Mutations in the homeodomain of the human *SIX3* gene cause holoprosencephaly. *Nat Genet* 1999;22:196–198.

94. Zhu CC, Dyer MA, Uchikawa M, et al. Six 3–mediated auto repression and eye development requires its interaction with members of the Groucho-related family of co-repressors. *Development* 2002;129:2835–2849.

95. Lengler J, Krausz E, Tomarev S, et al. Antagonistic action of Six3 and Prox1 at the 7-crystalline promoter. *Nucl Acids Res* 2001;29:515–526.

96. Lengler J, Graw J. Regulation of the human SIX3 promoter. *Biochem Biophys Res Commun* 2001;287:372–376.

97. Goudreau G, Petrou P, Reneker LW, et al. Mutually regulated expression of *Pax6* and *Six3* and its implications for the *Pax6* haploinsufficient lens phenotype. *Proc Natl Acad Sci USA* 2002;99:8719–8724.

98. Chemke J, Czernobilsky B, Mundel G, et al. A familial syndrome of central nervous system and ocular malformations. *Clin Genet* 1975;7:1–7.

99. Hall BD. Choanal atresia and associated multiple anomalies. *J Pediatr* 1979;95:395–398.

100. Hittner HM, Hirsch NJ, Kreh GM, et al. Colobomatous microphthalmia, heart disease, hearing loss and mental retardation—a syndrome. *J Pediatr Ophthalmol Strabismus* 1979;16: 122–128.

101. Ho CK, Kaufman RL, Podos SM. Ocular colobomata, cardiac defect, and other anomalies: a study of seven cases including two sibs. *J Med Genet* 1975;12:289–293.

102. Hussels IE. Midface syndrome with iridochoroidal coloboma and deafness in a mother: microphthalmia in her son. *Birth Defects Orig Artic Ser* 1971;8:269.

103. Pagon RA, Graham JM Jr, Zonana J, et al. Coloboma, congenital heart disease, and choanal atresia with multiple anomalies: CHARGE association. *J Pediatr* 1981;99:223–227.

104. Warburg M. Microphthalmos and colobomata among mentally retarded individuals. *Acta Ophthalmol (Copenh)* 1981;59: 665–673.

105. Othman MI, Sullivan SA, Skuta GL, et al. Autosomal dominant nanophthalmos (NNO1) with high hyperopia and angle-closure glaucoma maps to chromosome 11. *Am J Hum Genet* 1998;63:1411–1418.

106. Thomas IT, Frias JL, Felix V, et al. Isolated and syndromic cryptophthalmos. *Am J Med Genet* 1986;25:85–98.

107. Briggs HH. Hereditary congenital ptosis with report of 64 cases conforming to the Mendelian rule of dominance. *Am J Ophthalmol* 1919;2:408–417.

108. Engle EC, Castro AE, Macy ME, et al. Agene for isolated congenital ptosis maps to a 3-cm region within lp32-p34.1. *Am J Hum Genet* 1997;60:1150–1157.

109. McMullan TFW, Crolla JA, Gregory SG, et al. A candidate gene for congenital bilateral isolated ptosis identified by molecular analysis of a de novo balanced translocation. *Hum Genet* 2002;110:244–250.

110. McMullan TFW, Collins AR, Tyers AG, et al. A novel X-linked dominant condition: X-linked congenital isolated ptosis. *Am J Hum Genet* 2000;66:1455–1460.

111. Kohn R, Romano PE. Blepharoptosis, blepharophimosis, epicanthus inversus, and telecanthus—a syndrome with no name. *Am J Ophthalmol* 1971;72:625–632.

112. Amati P, Chomel JC, Nevelon-Chevalier A, et al. A gene for blepharophimosis, ptosis, epicanthus inversus maps to chromosome 3q23. *Hum Genet* 1995;96:213–215.

113. Small KW, Stalvey M, Fisher L, et al. Blepharophimosis syndrome is linked to chromosome 3q. *Hum Mol Genet* 1995;4:443–48.

114. Crisponi L, Deiana M, Loi A, et al. The putative forkhead transcription factor FOXL2 is mutated in blepharophimosis/ ptosis/ epicanthus inversus syndrome. *Nat Genet* 2001;27: 159–166.

115. Engle EC, Goumnerov B, McKeown CA, et al. Oculomotor nerve and muscle abnormalities in congenital fibrosis of the extraocular muscles. *Ann Neurol* 1997;41:314–325.

116. Yamada K, Andrews C, Chan W-M, et al. Heterozygous mutations of the kinesin *KIF21A* in congenital fibrosis of the extraocular muscles type 1 (CFEOM1). *Nat Genet* 2003;35:318–321.

117. Engle EC, Kunkel LM, Specht LA, et al. Mapping a gene for congenital fibrosis of the extraocular muscles to the centromeric region of chromosome 12. *Nat Genet* 1994;7:69–73.

118. Engle EC, Marondel I, Houtman WA, et al. Congenital fibrosis of the extraocular muscles (autosomal dominant congenital external ophthalmoplegia): genetic homogeneity, linkage refinement, and physical mapping on chromosome 12. *Am J Hum Genet* 1995;57:1086–1094.

119. Nakano M, Yamada K, Fain J, et al. Homozygous mutations in *ARIX(PHOX2A)* result in congenital fibrosis of the extraocular muscles type 2. *Nat Genet* 2001;29:315–320.

120. Mackey DA, Chan W-M, Chan C, et al. Congenital fibrosis of the vertically acting extraocular muscles maps to the FEOM3 locus. *Hum Genet* 2002;110:510–512.

121. Gatti RA, Berkel I, Boder E, et al. Localization of an ataxia-telangiectasia gene to chromosome 11q22–23. *Nature* 1988;336: 577–580.

122. Savitsky K, Bar-Shira A, Gilad S, et al. A single ataxia-telangiectasia gene with a product similar to PI-3 kinase. *Science* 1995;268:1749–1753.

123. Savitsky K, Sfez S, Tagle DA, et al. The complete sequence of the coding region of the ATM gene reveals similarity to cell cycle regulators in different species. *Hum Mol Genet* 1995;4:2025–2032.

124. Hecht F, Shoptaugh MG, Winglets of the eye: dominant transmission of early adult pterygium of the conjunctiva. *J Med Genet* 1990;27:392–394.

125. Jacklin HN. Familial predisposition to pterygium formation: report of a family. *Am J Ophthalmol* 1964;57:481–482.

126. Cogan DG, Chu FC, Gittinger J, et al. Fundal abnormalities of Gaucher's disease. *Arch Ophthalmol* 1980;98:2202–2203.

127. Tahvanainen E, Villanueva AS, Forsius H, et al. Dominantly and recessively inherited cornea plana congenital maps to the same small region of chromosome 12. *Genome Res* 1996;6:249–254.

128. Pellegata NS, Dieguez-Lucena JL, Joensuu T, et al. Mutations in *KERA,* encoding keratocan, cause cornea plana. *Nat Genet* 2000;25:91–95.

129. Bloch N. The different types of sclerocornea, their hereditary modes and concomitant congenital malformations. *J Genet Hum* 1965;14:133–172.

130. Neuhauser G, Kaveggia EG, France TD, et al. Syndrome of mental retardation, seizures, hypotonic cerebral palsy and megalocorneae, recessively inherited. *Z Kinderheilk* 1975; 120:1–18.

131. Rabinowitz YS. Keratoconus. *Surv Ophthalmol* 1998;42: 297–319.

132. Edwards M, McGhee CN, Dean S. The genetics of keratoconus. *Clin Exp Ophthalmol* 2001;29:345–351.

133. Heon E, Greenberg A, Kopp KK, et al. VSX1: a gene for posterior polymorphous dystrophy and keratoconus. *Hum Mol Genet* 2002;11:1029–1036.

134. Irvine AD, Corden LD, Swensson O, et al. Mutations in cornea-specific keratin *K3* or *K12* genes cause Meesmann's corneal dystrophy. *Nat Genet* 1997;16:184–187.

135. Munier FL, Korvatska E, Djemai A, et al. Keratoepithelin mutations in four 5831-linked corneal dystrophies. *Nat Genet* 1997;15:247–251.

136. Gregory CY, Evans K, Bhattacharya SS. Genetic refinement of the chromosome 5q lattice dystrophy type 1 locus to within a 2cM interval. *J Med Genet* 1995;32:224–226.

137. Eiberg H, Kjer B, Kjer P, et al. Dominant optic atrophy (OPAL) mapped to chromosome 3q region. *Hum Mol Genet* 1994;3:977–980.

138. Small KW, Mullen L, Barletta J, et al. Mapping of Reis-Bucklers' corneal dystrophy to chromosome 5q. *Am J Ophthalmol* 1996;121:384–390.

139. Stone EM, Mathers WD, Rosenwasser GO, et al. Three autosomal dominant corneal dystrophies map to chromosomes 51. *Nat Genet* 1994;6:47–51.

140. Munier FL, Frueh BE, Othenin-Girard P, et al. pIGH3 mutations in type IIIA and intermediate type I/IIIA of lattice corneal dystrophies are Fas4-specific. *Invest Ophthalmol Vis Sci* 2002;43:949–954.

141. Hassell JR, Newsome DA, Krachmer J, et al. Corneal macular dystrophy: a possible inborn error in corneal proteoglycan maturation. *Fed Proc* 1980;39:2120.

142. Vance JM, Jonasson F, Lennon E, et al. Linkage of a gene for macular corneal dystrophy to chromosome 16. *Am J Hum Genet* 1996;58:757–762.

143. Akama TO, Nishida K, Nakayama J, et al. Macular corneal dystrophy type I and type II are caused by distinct mutations in a new sulphotransferase gene. *Nat Genet* 2000; 25:237–241.

144. Kinoshita S, Nishida K, Dota A, et al. Epithelial barrier function and ultrastructure of gelatinous drop-like corneal dystrophy. *Cornea* 2000;19:551–555.

145. Tasa G, Kals J, Muru K, et al. A novel mutation in the M1S1 gene responsible for gelatinous drop-like corneal dystrophy. *Invest Ophthalmol Vis Sci* 2001;42:2762–2764.

146. Biswas S, Munier FL, Yardley J, et al. Missense mutations in COL8A2, the gene encoding the $\alpha 2$ chain of type VIII collagen, cause two forms of corneal endothelial dystrophy. *Hum Mol Genet* 2001;10:2415–2423.

147. Toma NM, Ebenezer ND, Inglehearn CF, et al. Linkage of congenital hereditary endothelial dystrophy to chromosome 20. *Hum Mol Genet* 1995;4:2395–2398.

148. Hand CK, Harmon DL, Kennedy SM, et al. Localization of the gene for autosomal recessive congenital hereditary endothelial dystrophy (CHED2) to chromosome 20 by homozygosity mapping. *Genomics* 1999;61:1–4.

149. Elsas FJ, Maumenee IH, Kenyon KR, et al. Familial aniridia with preserved ocular function. *Am J Ophthalmol* 1977;83: 718–724.

150. Hittner HM, Riccardi VM, Ferrell RE, et al. Variable expressivity in autosomal dominant aniridia by clinical, electrophysiologic, and angiographic criteria. *Am J Ophthalmol* 1980;89:531–539.

151. Bateman JB, Sparkes MC, Sparkes RS. Aniridia: enzyme studies in an 11p-chromosomal deletion. *Invest Ophthalmol Vis Sci* 1984;25:612–616.

152. Smith ACM, Sujansky E, Riccardi VM. Aniridia, mental retardation and genital abnormality in two patients with 46,XY,11p-. *Birth Defects Orig Artic Ser* 1977;13:257.

153. Riccardi VM, Sujansky E, Smith AC, et al. Chromosomal imbalance in the aniridia-Wilm's; tumor association: 11p interstitial deletion. *Pediatrics* 1978;61:604–610.

154. Warburg M, Mikkelsen M, Anderson SR, et al. Aniridia and interstitial deletion of the short arm of chromosome 11. *Metab Pediatr Ophthalmol* 1980;4:97–102.

155. Riccardi VM, Hittner HM, Strong LC, et al. Wilms tumor with aniridia/iris dysplasia and apparently normal chromosomes. *J Pediatr* 1982;100:574–577.

156. Glaser T, Walton DS, Maas RL. Genomic structure, evolutionary conservation and aniridia mutations in the human *pax6* gene. *Nat Genet* 1992;2:232–239.

157. Jordan T, Hanson I, Zaletayev D, et al. The human *PAX6* gene is mutated in two patients with aniridia. *Nat Genet* 1992;1:328–332.

158. Glaser T, Jepeal L, Edwards JG, et al. *PAX6* gene dosage effect in a family with congenital cataracts, aniridia, anophthalmia and central nervous system defects. *Nat Genet* 1994;7:463–471.

159. Hanson IM, Fletcher JM, Jordan T, et al. Mutations at the *PAX6* locus are found in heterogeneous anterior segment malformations including Peters' anomaly. *Nat Genet* 1994;6:168–173.

160. Mirzayans F, Pearce WG, MacDonald IM, et al. Mutation of the PAX6 gene in patients with autosomal dominant keratitis. *Am J Hum Genet* 1995;57:539–548.

161. Alkemade PPH. *Dysgenesis mesodermalis of the iris and the cornea: a study of Rieger's syndrome and Peters' anomaly.* Assen, The Netherlands: Van Gorcum, 1969.

162. Awan KJ. Peters-Rieger's syndrome. *J Pediatr Ophthalmol* 1977;14:112–116.

163. Crawford RAD. Iris dysgenesis with other anomalies. *Br J Ophthalmol* 1967;51:438–440.

164. Dark AJ, Kirkham TH. Congenital corneal opacities in a patient with Rieger's anomaly and Down's syndrome. *Br J Ophthalmol* 1968;52:631–635.

165. Falls HF. A gene producing various defects of the anterior segment of the eye. *Am J Ophthalmol* 1949;32:41.

166. Henkind P, Sigel IM, Carr RE. Mesodermal dysgenesis of the anterior segment: Rieger's anomaly. *Arch Ophthalmol* 1965;73:810–817.

167. Akazawa K, Yamane S, Shiota H, et al. A case of retinoblastoma associated with Riegers anomaly and 13q deletion. *Jpn J Ophthalmol* 1981;25:321–325.

168. Ferguson JG Jr, Hicks EL. Rieger's anomaly and glaucoma associated with partial trisomy 16q. Case report. *Arch Ophthalmol* 1987;105:323.

169. Heinemann M, Breg R, Cotlier E. Rieger's syndrome with pericentric inversion of chromosome 6. *Br J Ophthalmol* 1979;63:40–44.

170. Herve J, Warnet JF, Jeaneau-Bellego E, et al. Partial monosomy of the short arm of chromosome 10, associated with Riegers syndrome and a Di George type partial immunodeficiency. *Ann Pediatr (Paris)* 1984;31:77–80.

171. Ligutic I, Brecevic L, Petkovic I, et al. Interstitial deletion 4q and Rieger syndrome. *Clin Genet* 1981;20:323–327.

172. Stathacopoulos RA, Bateman JB, Sparkes RS, et al. The Rieger syndrome and a chromosome 13 deletion. *J Pediatr Ophthalmol Strabismus* 1987;24:198–203.

173. Tabbara KF, Khouri FP, der Kaloustian VM. Rieger's syndrome with chromosomal anomaly (report of a case). *Can J Ophthalmol* 1973;8:488–491.

174. Wilcox LM Jr, Bercovitch L, Howard RO. Ophthalmic features of chromosome deletion 4p- (Wolf-Hirschhorn syndrome). *Am J Ophthalmol* 1978;86:834–839.

175. Murray JC, Bennett SR, Kwitek AE, et al. Linkage of Rieger syndrome to the region of the epidermal growth factor gene on chromosome 4. *Nat Genet* 1992;2:46–49.

176. Mears AJ, Mirzayans F, Gould DB, et al. Autosomal dominant iridogoniodysgenesis anomaly maps to 6p25. *Am J Hum Genet* 1996;59:1321–1327.

177. Priston M, Kozlowski K, Gill D, et al. Functional analyses of two newly identified PITX2 mutants reveal a novel molecular mechanism for Axenfeld-Rieger syndrome. *Hum Mol Genet* 2001;10:1631–1638.

178. Nishimura DY, Searby CC, Alward WL, et al. A spectrum of FOXC1 mutations suggests gene dosage as a mechanism for developmental defects of the anterior chamber of the eye. *Am J Hum Genet* 2001;68:364–372.

179. Panicker SG, Sampath S, Mandal AK, et al. Novel mutation in *FOXC1* wing region causing Axenfeld-Rieger anomaly. *Invest Ophthalmol Vis Sci* 2002;43:3613–3616.

180. Semina EV, Ferrell RE, Mintz-Hittner HA, et al. A novel homeobox gene *PITX3* is mutated in families with autosomal-dominant cataracts and ASMD. *Nat Genet* 1998;19:167–170.

181. Semina EV, Murray JC, Reiter R, et al. Deletion in the promoter region and altered expression of Pitx3 homeobox gene in aphakia mice. *Hum Mol Genet* 2000;9:1575–1585.

182. Boel M, Timmermans J, Emmery L, et al. Primary mesodermal dysgenesis of the cornea (Peters' anomaly) in two brothers. *Hum Genet* 1979;51:237–240.

183. Bateman JB, Maumenee IH, Sparkes RS. Peters' anomaly associated with partial deletion of the long arm of chromosome 11. *Am J Ophthalmol* 1984;97:11–15.

184. Kivlin JD, Fineman RM, Crandall AS, et al. Peters' anomaly as a consequence of genetic and nongenetic syndromes. *Arch Ophthalmol* 1986;104:61–64.

185. Mondino BJ, Shahinian L Jr, Johnson BL, et al. Peters' anomaly with the fetal transfusion syndrome. *Am J Ophthalmol* 1976;82:55–58.

186. Doward W, Perveen R, Lloyd IC, et al. A mutation in the REIG1 gene associated with Peters' anomaly. *J Med Genet* 1999;36:152–155.

187. Vincent A, Billingsley G, Priston M, et al. Phenotypic heterogeneity of CYP1B1: mutations in a patient with Peters' anomaly. *J Med Genet* 2001;38:324–326.

188. Plasilova M, Ferakova E, Kadasi L, et al. Linkage of autosomal recessive primary congenital glaucoma to the GLC3A locus in Roms (gypsies) from Slovakia. *Hum Hered* 1998;48:30–33.

189. Sarfarazi M, Akarsu AN, Hossain A, et al. Assignment of a locus (GLC3A) for primary congenital glaucoma (buphthalmos) to 2p21 and evidence for genetic heterogeneity. *Genomics* 1995;30:171–177.

190. Akarsu AN, Turacli ME, Aktan SG, et al. A second locus (GLC3B) for primary congenital glaucoma (buphthalmos) maps to the 1p36 region. *Hum Mol Genet* 1996;5:1199–1203.

191. Stoilov IR, Akarsu AN, Sarfarazi M. Identification of three truncating mutations in cytochrome P_{450}1B1 (CYP1B1) as the principal cause of primary congenital glaucoma (buphthalmos) in families linked to the GLC3A locus on chromosome 2p21. *Hum Mol Genet* 1997;6:641–647.

192. Broughton WL, Rosenbaum KN, Beauchamp GR. Congenital glaucoma and other ocular abnormalities associated with pericentric inversion of chromosome 11. *Arch Ophthalmol* 1983;101:594–597.

193. Chrousos GA, O'Neill JF, Traboulsi EI, et al. Ocular findings in partial trisomy 3q. A case report and review of the literature. *Ophthalmic Paediatr Genet* 1989;9:127–130.

194. Wiggs JL, Del Bono EA Schuman JS, et al. Clinical features of five pedigrees genetically linked to the juvenile glaucoma locus on chromosome 1q21–q31. *Ophthalmology* 1995;102:1782–1789.

195. Stone EM, Fingert JH, Alward WLM, et al. Identification of a gene that causes primary open angle glaucoma. *Science* 1997;275:668–670.

196. Shimizu S, Lichter PR, Johnson AT, et al. Age-dependent prevalence of mutations at the GLC1A locus in primary open-angle glaucoma. *Am J Ophthalmol* 2000;130:165–177.

197. Karali A, Russell P, Stefani FH, et al. Localization of myocilin/ trabecular meshwork—inducible glucocorticoid response protein in the human eye. *Invest Ophthalmol Vis Sci* 2000;41:729–740.

198. Rezaie T, Child A, Hitchings R, et al. Adult-onset primary open-angle glaucoma caused by mutations in optineurin. *Science* 2002;295:1077–1079.

199. Scheie HG, Cameron JD. Pigment dispersion syndrome: a clinical study. *Br J Ophthalmol* 1981;65:264–269.

200. Andersen JS, Pralea AM, DelBono EA, et al. A gene responsible for the pigment dispersion syndrome maps to chromosome 7q35–q36. *Arch Ophthalmol* 1997;115:384–388.

201. Maumenee IH. The eye in the Marfan syndrome. *Trans Am Ophthalmol Soc* 1981;79:684–733.

202. Dietz HC, Cutting GR, Pyeritz RE, et al. Marfan syndrome caused by a recurrent de novo missense mutation in the fibrillin gene. *Nature* 1991;352:337–339.

203. Dietz HC, Pyeritz RE, Hall BD, et al. The Marfan syndrome locus: confirmation of assignment to chromosome 15 and identification of tightly linked markers at 15g15–121.3. *Genomics* 1991;9:355–361.

204. Kainulainen K, Pulkkinen L, Savolainen A, et al. Location on chromosome 15 of the gene defect causing Marfan syndrome. *N Engl J Med* 1990;323:935–939.

205. Lee B, Godfrey M, Vitale E, et al. Linkage of Marfan syndrome and a phenotypically related disorder to two different fibrillin genes. *Nature* 1991;352:330–334.

206. Magenis RF, Maslen KL, Smith L, et al. Localization of the fibrillin (FBN) gene to chromosome 15, band q21.2. *Genomics* 1991;11:346–351.

207. Maslen CL, Corson GM, Maddox BK, et al. Partial sequence of a candidate gene for the Marfan syndrome. *Nature* 1991;352:334–337.

208. Tsipouras P, Del Mastro R, Sarfarazi M, et al. Genetic linkage of the Marfan syndrome, ectopia lentis, and congenital contractural arachnodactyly to the fibrillin genes on chromosomes 15 and 5. *N Engl J Med* 1992;326:905–909.

209. Munke M, Kraus JP, Ohura T, et al. The gene for cystathionine beta-synthase (CBS) maps to the subtelomeric region on human chromosome 21q and to proximal mouse chromosome 17. *Am J Hum Genet* 1988;42:550–559.

210. Diethelm W. Uber ectopia lentis ohne arachnodaktylie und ihre beziehungen zur ectopia lentis et pupillae. *Ophthalmologica* 1947;114:16–32.

211. Brakenhoff RH, Henskens HAM, van Rossum MWPC, et al. Activation of the gamma E-crystallin pseudogene in the human hereditary Coppock-like cataract. *Hum Mol Genet* 1994;3:279–283.

212. Lubsen NH, Renwick JH, Tsui LC, et al. A locus for a human hereditary cataract is closely linked to the gamma-crystallin gene family. *Proc Natl Acad Sci USA* 1987;84:489–492.

213. Rogaev EI, Rogaeva EA, Korovaitseva GI, et al. Linkage of polymorphic congenital cataract to the 7-crystallin gene locus on human chromosome 2q33–35. *Hum Mol Genet* 1996;5:699–703.

214. Kramer P, Yount J, Mitchell T, et al. A second gene for cerulean cataracts maps to the crystallin region on chromosome 22. *Genomics* 1996;38:539–542.

215. Litt M, Carrero-Valenzuela R, LaMorticella DM, et al. Autosomal dominant cerulean cataract is associated with a chain termination mutation in the human 7-crystallin gene CRYBB2. *Hum Mol Genet* 1997;6:665–668.

216. Eiberg H, Lund AM, Warburg M, et al. Assignment of congenital cataract Volkmann type (CCV) to chromosome lp36. *Hum Genet* 1995;96:33–38.

217. Renwick JH, Lawler SD. Probable linkage between a congenital cataract locus and the Duffy blood group locus. *Ann Hum Genet* 1963;27:67–84.

218. Eiberg H, Marner E, Rosenberg T, et al. Maimer's cataract (CAM) assigned to chromosome 16: linkage to haptoglobin. *Clin Genet* 1988;34:272–275.

219. Marner E, Rosenberg T, Eiberg H. Autosomal dominant congenital cataract. Morphology and genetic mapping. *Acta Ophthalmol (Copenh)* 1989;67:151–158.

220. Richards J, Maumenee I, Rowe S, et al. Congenital cataract possibly linked to haptoglobin. *Cytogenet Cell Genet* 1984;37:570.

221. Berry V, Ionides ACW, Moore AT, et al. A locus for autosomal dominant anterior polar cataract on chromosome 17p. *Hum Mol Genet* 1996;5:415–419.

222. Padma T, Ayyagari R, Murty JS, et al. Autosomal dominant zonular cataract with sutural opacities localized to chromosome 17q11–12. *Am J Hum Genet* 1995;57:840–845.

223. Armitage MM, Kivlin JD, Ferrell RE. A progressive cataract gene maps to human chromosome 17q24. *Nat Genet* 1995;9:37–40.

224. Francis PJ, Berry V, Hardcastle AJ, et al. A locus for isolated cataract on human Xp. *J Med Genet* 2002;39:105–109.

225. Shih LY, Rosin I, Suslak L, et al. Localization of the structural gene for galactose-1-phosphate uridyl transferase to band p13 of chromosome 9 by gene dosage studies. (Abstract) *Am J Hum Genet* 1982;34:62A.

226. Shih LY, Suslak L, Rosin I, et al. Gene dosage studies supporting localization of the structural gene for galactose-1-phosphate uridyl transferase (GALT) to band p13 of chromosome 9. *Am J Med Genet* 1984;19:539–543.

227. Kondo I. Nakamura N. Regional mapping of GALT in the short arm of chromosome 9. (Abstract) *Cytogenet Cell Genet* 1984;37:514.

228. Kooy RF, Van der Veen AY, Verlind E, et al. Physical localisation of the chromosomal marker D13S31 places the Wilson

disease locus at the junction of bands q14.3 and q21.1 of chromosome 13. *Hum Genet* 1993;91:504–506.

229. Bull PC, Thomas GR, Rommens JM, et al. The Wilson disease gene is a putative copper transporting P-type ATPase similar to the Menkes gene. *Nat Genet* 1993;5:327–337.

230. Harley HG, Brook JD, Floyd J, et al. Detection of linkage disequilibrium between the myotonic dystrophy locus and a new polymorphic DNA marker. *Am J Hum Genet* 1991;49:68–75.

231. Boucher CA, King SK, Carey N, et al. A novel homeodomain-encoding gene is associated with a large CpG island interrupted by the myotonic dystrophy unstable (CTG)$_n$ repeat. *Hum Mol Genet* 1995;4:1919–1925.

232. Deeb SS, Motulsky AG. Molecular genetics of human color vision. *Behav Genet* 1996;26:195–207.

233. Nathans J, Thomas D, Hogness DS. Molecular genetics of human color vision: the genes encoding blue, green, and red pigments. *Science* 1986;232:193–202.

234. Nathans J, Davenport CM, Maumenee IH, et al. Molecular genetics of human blue cone monochromacy. *Science* 1989;245:831–838.

235. Weitz CJ, Miyake Y, Shinzato K, et al. Human tritanopia associated with two amino acid substitutions in the blue-sensitive opsin. *Am J Hum Genet* 1992;50:498–507.

236. Weitz CJ, Went LN, Nathans J. Human tritanopia associated with a third amino acid substitution in the blue-sensitive visual pigment. *Am J Hum Genet* 1992;51:444–446.

237. Arbour NC, Zlotogora J, Knowlton RG, et al. Homozygosity mapping of achromatopsia to chromosome 2 using DNA pooling. *Hum Mol Genet* 1997;6:689–694.

238. Wissinger B, Jagle H, Kohl S, et al. Human rod monochromacy: linkage analysis and mapping of a cone photoreceptor expressed candidate gene on chromosome 2q11. *Genomics* 1998;51:325–331.

239. Kohl S, Marx T, Giddings I, et al. Total colour blindness is caused by mutations in the gene encoding the a-subunit of the cone photoreceptor cGMP-gated cation channel. *Nat Genet* 1998;19:257–259.

240. Kohl S, Baumann B, Broghammer M, et al. Mutations in the *CNGB3* gene encoding the β-subunit of the cone photoreceptor cGMP-gated channel are responsible for achromatopsia (ACHM3) linked to chromosome 8q21. *Hum Mol Genet* 2000;9:2107–2116.

241. Aligianis IA, Forshew T, Johnson S, et al. Mapping of a novel locus for achromatopsia (ACHM4) to 1p and identification of a germline mutation in the α-subunit of cone transducin (GNAT2). *J Med Genet* 2002;39:656–660.

242. Condon GP, Brownstein S, Wang NS, et al. Congenital hereditary (juvenile X-linked) retinoschisis. Histopathologic and ultrastructural findings in three eyes. *Arch Ophthalmol* 1986;104:576–583.

243. Lewis RA, Lee GB, Martonyi CL, et al. Familial foveal retinoschisis. *Arch Ophthalmol* 1977;95:1190–1196.

244. Criswick VG, Schepens CL. Familial exudative vitreoretinopathy. *Am J Ophthalmol* 1969;68:578–594.

245. Gow J, Oliver GL. Familial exudative vitreoretinopathy: an expanded view. *Arch Ophthalmol* 1971;86:150–155.

246. Clement F, Beckford CA, Corral A, et al. X-linked familial exudative vitreoretinopathy. *Retina* 1995;15:141–145.

247. Fullwood P, Jones J, Bundey S, et al. X-linked exudative vitreoretinopathy: clinical features and genetic linkage analysis. *Br J Ophthalmol* 1993;77:168–170.

248. Robitaille J, MacDonald MEL, Kaykas A, et al. Mutant frizzled-4 disrupts retinal angiogenesis in familial exudative vitreoretinopathy. *Nat Genet* 2002;32:326–330.

249. Stone EM, Kimura AE, Folk JC, et al. Genetic linkage of autosomal dominant neovascular inflammatory vitreoretinopathy to chromosome 11q13. *Hum Mol Genet* 1992;1:685–689.

250. Bleeker-Wagemakers LM, Friedrich U, Gal A, et al. Close linkage between Norrie disease, a cloned DNA sequence from the proximal short arm, and the centromere of the X chromosome. *Hum Genet* 1985;71:211–214.

251. Bleeker-Wagemakers EM, Zweije-Hofman I, Gal A. Norrie disease as part of a complex syndrome explained by a submicroscopic deletion of the X chromosome. *Ophthalmic Paediatr Genet* 1988;9:137–142.

252. Gal A, Stolzenberger C, Wienker T, et al. Norrie's disease: close linkage with genetic markers from the proximal short arm of the X chromosome. *Clin Genet* 1985;27:282–283.

253. Kivlin JD, Sanborn GE, Wright E, et al. Further linkage data on Norrie disease. *Am J Med Genet* 1987;26:733–736.

254. Ngo JT, Spence MA, Cortessis V, et al. Recombinational event between Norrie disease and DXS7 loci. *Clin Genet* 1988;34:43–47.

255. Ngo J, Spence MA, Cortessis V, et al. Duplicate report crossing over in Norrie disease family. *Am J Med Genet* 1989;33:286.

256. Ngo JT, Bateman JB, Cortessis V, et al. Norrie disease: linkage analysis using a 4.2-kb RFLP detected by a human ornithine aminotransferase cDNA probe. *Genomics* 1989;4:539–545.

257. Ngo JT, Bateman JB, Spence MA, et al. Ornithine aminotransferase (OAT): recombination between an X-linked OAT sequence (7.5kb) and the Norrie disease locus. *Genomics* 1990;6:123–128.

258. Sims KB, Ozelius L, Corey T, et al. Norrie disease gene is distinct from the monoamine oxidase genes. *Am J Hum Genet* 1989;45:424–434.

259. Berger W, Meindl A, van de Pol TJ, et al. Isolation of a candidate gene for Norrie disease by positional cloning. *Nat Genet* 1992;1:199–203.

260. Chen ZY, Hendriks RW, Jobling MD, et al. Isolation and characterization of a candidate gene for Norrie disease. *Nat Genet* 1992;1:204–208.

261. Heckenlively JR. The hereditary retinal and choroidal degenerations. In: Rimoin D, Emery A, eds. *Principles and practice of medical genetics*. Edinburgh: Churchill Livingstone, 1983.

262. Kumar-Singh R, Wang H, Humphries P, et al. Autosomal dominant retinitis pigmentosa: no evidence for nonallelic heterogeneity on 3q. *Am J Hum Genet* 1993;52:319–326.

263. Shastry BS. Retinitis pigmentosa and related disorders: phenotypes of rhodopsin and peripherin/RDS mutations. *Am J Med Genet* 1994;52:467–474.

264. Bascom RA, Heckenlively JR, Stone EM, et al. Mutation analyses of the ROM1 gene in retinitis pigmentosa. *Hum Mol Genet* 1995;4:1895–1902.

265. Inglehearn CE, Keen TJ, Al-Maghtheh M, et al. Further refinement of the location for autosomal dominant retinitis pigmentosa on chromosome 7p (RP9). *Am J Hum Genet* 1994;54:675–680.

266. Jordan SA, Farrar GJ, Kenna P, et al. Localization of an autosomal dominant retinitis pigmentosa gene to chromosome 4q. *Nat Genet* 1993;4:54–58.

267. Blanton SH, Heckenlively JR, Conttingham RW, et al. Linkage mapping of autosomal dominant retinitis pigmentosa (RP1)

to the pericentric region of human chromosome 8. *Genomics* 1993;15:376–386.

268. Sadler LA, Gannon AM, Blanton SH, et al. Linkage and physical mapping of the chromosome 8 form of autosomal dominant retinitis pigmentosa (RP1). *Cytogenet Cell Genet* 1993;64:144.

269. Greenberg J, Goliath R, Beighton P, et al. A new locus for autosomal dominant retinitis pigmentosa on chromosome 17p. *Hum Mol Genet* 1995;3:962–965.

270. Kojis TL, Heinzmann C, Flodman P, et al. Map refinement of locus RP13 to human chromosome 17p13.3 in a second family with autosomal dominant retinitis pigmentosa. *Am J Hum Genet* 1996;58:347–355.

271. Bardien S, Ebenezer N, Greenberg J, et al. An eighth locus for autosomal dominant retinitis pigmentosa is linked to chromosome 17q. *Hum Mol Genet* 1995;4:1459–1462.

272. Al-Maghtheh M, Inglehearn CF, Keen J, et al. Identification of a sixth locus for autosomal dominant retinitis pigmentosa on chromosome 19. *Hum Mol Genet* 1994;3:351–354.

273. Kajiwara K, Sandberg MA, Berson EL, et al. A null mutation in the human peripherin/RDS gene in a family with autosomal dominant retinitis punctata albescens. *Nat Genet* 1993;3:208–212.

274. Van Soest S, Vandenborn LI, Gal A, et al. Assignment of a gene for autosomal recessive retinitis pigmentosa (RP12) to chromosome 1q31-q32.1 in an inbred and genetically heterogeneous disease population. *Genomics* 1994;22:499–504.

275. Weleber RG, Carr RE, Murphey WH, et al. Phenotypic variation including retinitis pigmentosa, pattern dystrophy, and fundus flavimaculatus in a single family with a deletion of codon 153 or 154 of the peripherin/RDS gene. *Arch Ophthalmol* 1993;111:1531–1542.

276. Goldberg AFX, Molday RS. Defective subunit assembly underlies a digenic form of retinitis pigmentosa linked to mutations in peripherin/rds and rom-1. *Proc Natl Acad Sci USA* 1996;93:3726–3730.

277. Kajiwara K, Berson EL, Dryja TP. Digenic retinitis pigmentosa due to mutations at the unlinked peripherin/RDS and ROMI loci. *Science* 1994;26:1604–1608.

278. Kumaramanickavel G, Maw M, Denton MJ, et al. Missense rhodopsin mutation in a family with recessive RP. *Nat Genet* 1994;8:10–11.

279. Rosenfeld PJ, Cowley GS, McGee TL, et al. A null mutation I the rhodopsin gene causes rod photoreceptor dysfunction and autosomal recessive retinitis pigmentosa. *Nat Genet* 1992;1:209–213.

280. Huang SH, Pittler SJ, Huang XH, et al. Autosomal recessive retinitis pigmentosa caused by mutations in the alpha subunit of rod cGMP phosphodiesterase. *Nat Genet* 1995;11:468–471.

281. McLaughlin ME, Sandberg MA, Berson EL, et al. Recessive mutations in the gene encoding the beta-subunit of rod phosphodiesterase in patients with retinitis pigmentosa. *Nat Genet* 1994;4:130–134.

282. McLaughlin ME, Ehrhart TL, Berson EL, et al. Mutation spectrum of the gene encoding the beta subunit of rod phosphodiesterase among patients with autosomal recessive retinitis pigmentosa. *Proc Natl Acad Sci USA* 1995;92:3249–3253.

283. Dryja TP, Finn JT, Peng YW, et al. Mutations in the gene encoding the alpha subunit of the rod cGMP-gated channel in autosomal recessive retinitis pigmentosa. *Proc Natl Acad Sci USA* 1995;92:10177–10181.

284. Martinez-Mir A, Bayes M, Vilageliu L, et al. A new locus for autosomal recessive retinitis pigmentosa (RP19) maps to 1p13–1p21. *Genomics* 1997;40:142–146.

285. Leutelt J, Oehlmann R, Younus E, et al. Autosomal recessive retinitis pigmentosa locus maps on chromosome lq in a large consanguineous family from Pakistan. *Clin Genet* 1995;47:122–124.

286. Knowles JA, Shugart Y, Banerjee P, et al. Identification of a locus, distinct from RDS-peripherin, for autosomal recessive retinitis pigmentosa on chromosome 6p. *Hum Mol Genet* 1994;3:1401–1403.

287. Shugart YY, Banerjee P, Knowles JA, et al. Fine genetic mapping of a gene for autosomal recessive retinitis pigmentosa on chromosome 6p21. *Am J Hum Genet* 1995;57:499–502.

288. Thiselton DL, Hampson RM, Nayudu M, et al. Mapping the RP2 locus for X-linked retinitis pigmentosa on proximal Xp: a genetically defined 5-cM critical region and exclusion of candidate genes by physical mapping. *Genome Res* 1996;6:1093–1102.

289. Meindl A, Dry K, Herrmann K, et al. A gene (*RPGR*) with homology to the RCC1 guanine nucleotide exchange factor is mutated in X-linked retinitis pigmentosa (RP3). *Nat Genet* 1996;13:35–42.

290. Roepman R, van Dujnhoven G, Rosenberg T, et al. Positional cloning of the gene for X-linked retinitis pigmentosa 3: homology with the guanine-nucleotide exchange factor RCC1. *Hum Mol Genet* 1996;5:1043–1046.

291. Nakazawa M, Kikawa E, Chida Y, et al. Asn244His mutation of the peripherin/RDS gene causing autosomal dominant cone-rod degeneration. *Hum Mol Genet* 1994;3:1195–1196.

292. Nazawa M, Naoi N, Wada Y, et al. Autosomal dominant cone-rod dystrophy associated with a Val200Glu mutation of the peripherin/RDS gene. *Retina* 1996;16:405–410.

293. Wells J, Wroblewski J, Keen J, et al. Mutations in the human retinal degeneration slow (*RDS*) gene can cause either retinitis pigmentosa or macular dystrophy. *Nat Genet* 1993;3:213–218.

294. Small KW, Weber JL, Roses AD, et al. North Carolina macular dystrophy is assigned to chromosome 6. *Genomics* 1992;13:681–685.

295. Small KW, Weber JL, Roses AD, et al. North Carolina macular dystrophy (MCDR1): a review and refined mapping to 6q14-q16.2. *Ophthalmic Paediatr Genet* 1993;14:143–150.

296. Milosevic J, Kalicamin P. Long arm deletion of chromosome 6 in a mentally retarded boy with multiple physical malformations. *J Ment Def Res* 1975;129:139–144.

297. Balciuniene J, Johansson K, Sandgren O, et al. A gene for autosomal dominant progressive cone dystrophy (CORDS) maps to 17p12–p13. *Genomics* 1995;30:281–286.

298. Kelsell RE, Evans K, Gregory CY, et al. Localisation of a gene for dominant cone-rod dystrophy (CORD6) to chromosome 17p. *Hum Mol Genet* 1997;6:597–600.

299. Kylstra JA, Aylsworth AS. Cone-rod retinal dystrophy in a patient with neurofibromatosis type 1. *Can J Ophthalmol* 1993;28:79–80.

300. Warburg M, Sjo O, Tranebjaerg L, et al. Deletion mapping of a retinal cone-rod dystrophy. Assignment to 18q-211. *Am J Med Genet* 1991;39:288–293.

301. Evans K, Fryer A, Inglehearn C, et al. Genetic linkage of cone-rod retinal dystrophy to chromosome 19q and evidence for segregation distortion. *Nat Genet* 1994;6:210–213.

302. Bartley J, Gies D, Jacobson D. Cone dystrophy (X-linked) (COD1) maps between DXS7 (11.28) and DXS206 (Xj1.1) and is linked to DXS84 (754). *Cytogenet Cell Genet* 1989;51:959.

303. Hong H-K, Ferrell RE, Gorin MB. Clinical diversity and chromosomal localization of X-linked cone dystrophy (COD1). *Am J Hum Genet* 1994;55:1173–1181.

304. McGuire RE, Sullivan LS, Blanton SH, et al. X-linked dominant cone-rod degeneration: linkage mapping of a new locus for retinitis pigmentosa (RP15) to Xp22.13-p22.11. *Am J Hum Genet* 1995;57:87–94.

305. Felbor U, Suvanto EA, Forsius HR, et al. Autosomal recessive Sorsby fundus dystrophy revisited: molecular evidence for dominant inheritance. *Am J Hum Genet* 1997;60:57–62.

306. Weber BH, Vogt G, Pruett RC, Stohr H, Felbor U. Mutations in the tissue inhibitor of metalloproteinases-3 (TIMP3) in patients with Sorsby's fundus dystrophy. *Nat Genet* 1994;8:352–356.

307. Zhang K, Kniazeva M, Han M, et al. A 5-bp deletion in ELOVL4 is associated with two related forms of autosomal dominant macular dystrophy. *Nat Genet* 2001;27:89–93.

308. Stone EM, Nichols BE, Kimura AE, et al. Clinical features of a Stargardt-like dominant progressive macular dystrophy with genetic linkage to chromosome 6q. *Arch Ophthalmol* 1994;112:765–772.

309. Kaplan J, Gerber S, Larget-Piet D, et al. A gene for Stargardt's disease (fundus flavimaculatus) maps to the short arm of chromosome 1. *Nat Genet* 1993;5:308–311.

310. Allikmets R, Singh N, Sun H, et al. A photoreceptor cell-specific ATP-binding transporter gene (ABCR) is mutated in recessive Stargardt macular dystrophy. *Nat Genet* 1997;15: 236–246.

311. Forsman K, Graff C, Nordstrom S, et al. The gene for Best's macular dystrophy is located at 11q13 in a Swedish family. *Clin Genet* 1992;42:156–159.

312. Stone EM, Nichols BE, Streb LM, et al. Genetic linkage of vitelliform macular degeneration (Best's disease) to chromosome 11q13. *Nat Genet* 1992;1:246–250.

313. Petrukhin K, Koisti MJ, Bakall B, et al. Identification of the gene responsible for Best macular dystrophy. *Nat Genet* 1998;19:241–247.

314. Sun H, Tsunenari T, Yau KW, et al. The vitelliform macular dystrophy protein defines a new family of chloride channels. *Proc Natl Acad Sci USA* 2002;99:4008–4013.

315. Barrett DJ, Bateman JB, Sparkes RS, et al. Chromosomal localization of human ornithine aminotransferase gene sequences to l0q26 and Xpll.2. *Invest Ophthalmol* 1987;28:1037–1042.

316. Kato M, Aonuma H, Kawamra H, et al. Possible pathogenesis of congenital stationary night blindness. *Jpn J Ophthalmol* 1987;31:88–101.

317. Rao VR, Cohen GB, Oprain DD. Rhodopsin mutation G90D and a molecular mechanism for congenital night blindness. *Nature* 1994;367:639–642.

318. Dryja TP, McGee TL, Reichel E, et al. A point mutation of the rhodopsin gene in one form of retinitis pigmentosa. *Nature* 1990;343:364–366.

319. Dryja TP, Berson EL, Rao VR, et al. Heterozygous missense mutation in the rhodopsin gene as a cause of congenital stationary night blindness. *Nat Genet* 1993;4:280–283.

320. Gal A, Orth U, Baehr W, et al. Heterozygous missense mutation in the rod cGMP phosphodiesterase beta-subunit gene in autosomal dominant stationary night blindness. *Nat Genet* 1994;7:64–68.

321. Aldred MA, Dry KL, Sharp DM, et al. Linkage analysis in X-linked congenital stationary night blindness. *Genomics* 1992;14:99–104.

322. Bech-Hansen NT, Moore BJ, Pearce WG. Mapping of locus for X-linked congenital stationary night blindness (CSNB1) proximal to DXS7. *Genomics* 1992;12:409–411.

323. Bech-Hansen NT, Pearce WG. Manifestations of X-linked congenital stationary night blindness in three daughters of an affected male: demonstration of homozygosity. *Am J Hum Genet* 1993;52:71–77.

324. Bergen AAB, Brink JB, Riemslag F, et al. Localisation of a novel X-linked congenital stationary night blindness locus: close linkage to the RP3 type retinitis pigmentosa gene region. *Hum Mol Genet* 1995;4:931–935.

325. Glass IA, Good P, Coleman MP, et al. Genetic mapping of a cone and rod dysfunction (AIED) to the proximal short arm of the human X chromosome. *J Med Genet* 1993;30:1044–1050.

326. Schwartz M, Rosenberg T. Aland island eye disease: linkage data. *Genomics* 1991;10:327–332.

327. Yamamoto S, Sippel KC, Berson EL, et al. Defects in the rhodopsin kinase gene in the Oguchi form of stationary night blindness. *Nat Genet* 1997;15:175–178.

328. Hackenbruch Y, Meerhoff E, Besio R, et al. Familial bilateral optic nerve hypoplasia. *Am J Ophthal* 1975;79:314–320.

329. Azuma N, Yamaguchi Y, Handa H, et al. Mutations of the PAX6 gene detected in patients with a variety of optic-nerve malformations. *Am J Hum Genet* 2003;72:1565–1570.

330. Savell J, Cook JR. Optic nerve colobomas of autosomal-dominant heredity. *Arch Ophthalmol* 1976;94:395–400.

331. Schimmenti LA, Pierpont ME, Carpenter BLM, et al. Autosomal dominant optic nerve colobomas, vesicoureteral reflux, and renal anomalies. *Am J Med Genet* 1995;59:204–208.

332. Narahara K, Baker E, Ito S, et al. Localisation of a 10q breakpoint within the PAX2 gene in a patient with a de novo t(10;13) translocation and optic nerve coloboma-renal disease. *J Med Genet* 1997;34:213–216.

333. Amiel J, Audollent S, Joly D, et al. PAX2 mutations in renal-coloboma syndrome: mutational hotspot and germline mosaicism. *Eur J Hum Genet* 2000;8:820–826.

334. Stefko ST, Campochiaro P, Wang P, et al. Dominant inheritance of optic pits. *Am J Ophthalmol* 1997;124:112–113.

335. Kjer P. Infantile optic atrophy with dominant mode of inheritance: a clinical and genetic study of 19 Danish families. *Acta Ophthalmol* 1959;164(Suppl 54):1–147.

336. Brown J Jr, Fingert JH, Taylor CM, et al. Clinical and genetic analysis of a family affected with dominant optic atrophy (OPAl). *Arch Ophthalmol* 1997;115:95–99.

337. Eiberg H, Maoller HU, Berendt II, et al. Assignment of granular corneal dystrophy Groenouw type I (CDGG1) to chromosome 5q. *Eur J Hum Genet* 1994;2:132–138.

338. Alexander C, Votruba M, Pesch UEA, et al. OPA1, encoding a dynamin-related GTPase, is mutated in autosomal dominant optic atrophy linked to chromosome 3q28. *Nat Genet* 2000;26:211–215.

339. Delettre C, Lenaers G, Griffoin J-M, et al. Nuclear gene OPA1, encoding a mitochondrial dynamin-related protein, is mutated in dominant optic atrophy. *Nat Genet* 2000;26:207–210.

340. Hardy C, Khanim F, Torres R, et al. Clinical and molecular genetic analysis of 19 Wolfram syndrome kindreds demonstrating a wide spectrum of mutations in WFS1. *Am J Hum Genet* 1999;65:1279–1290.

341. Rogers JA. Leber's disease. *Aust J Ophthalmol* 1977;5:111–119.

342. Brown MD, Wallace DC. Spectrum of mitochondrial DNA mutations in Lebers hereditary optic neuropathy. *Clin Neurosci* 1994;2:138–145.

343. Howell N. Primary LHON mutations: trying to separate "fruyt" from "chaf." *Clin Neurosci* 1994;2:130–137.

344. Howell N, Bindoff LA, McCullough DA, et al. Leber hereditary optic neuropathy: identification of the same mitochondrial ND1 mutation in six pedigrees. *Am J Hum Genet* 1991;49: 939–950.

345. Huoponen K, Vilkki J, Aula P, et al. A new mtDNA mutation associated with Leber hereditary optic neuroretinopathy. *Am J Hum Genet* 1991;48:1147–1153.

346. Johns DR, Neufeld MJ, Park RD. An ND-6 mitochondrial DNA mutation associated with Leber hereditary optic neuropathy. *Biochem Biophys Res Commun* 1992;187: 1551–1557.

347. Johns DR, Heher KL, Miller NR, et al. Leber's hereditary optic neuropathy: clinical manifestations of the 14484 mutation. *Arch Ophthalmol* 1993;111:495–498.

348. Mackey D, Howell N. A variant of Leber hereditary optic neuropathy characterized by recovery of vision and by an unusual mitochondrial genetic etiology. *Am J Hum Genet* 1992;51:1218–1228.

349. Singh G, Lott MT, Wallace DC. A mitochondrial DNA mutation as a cause of Lebers hereditary optic neuropathy. *N Engl J Med* 1989;320:1300–1305.

350. Vilkki J; Savontaus ML, Kalimo H, et al. Mitochondrial DNA polymorphism in Finnish families with Leber's hereditary optic neuroretinopathy. *Hum Genet* 1989;82:208–212.

351. Brown MD, Voljavec AS, Lott MT, et al. Mitochondrial DNA complex I and III mutations associated with Leper's hereditary optic neuropathy. *Genetics* 1992;130:163–173.

352. Johns DR, Berman J. Alternative, simultaneous complex I mitochondrial DNA mutations in Leber's hereditary optic neuropathy. *Biochem Biophys Res Commun* 1991;174:1324–1330.

353. Johns DR, Smith KH, Savino PJ, et al. Leber's hereditary optic neuropathy: clinical manifestations of the 15257 mutation. *Ophthalmology* 1993;100:981–986.

354. Kellar-Wood H, Robertson N, Govan GG, et al. Leber's hereditary optic neuropathy mitochondrial DNA mutations in multiple sclerosis. *Ann Neurol* 1994;36:109–112.

355. Oostra RJ, Bolhuis PA, Wijburg FA, et al. Leber's hereditary optic neuropathy: correlations between mitochondrial genotype and visual outcome. *J Med Genet* 1994;31:280–286.

356. Oostra RJ, Bolhuis PA, Zorn-Ende G, et al. Leber's hereditary optic neuropathy: no significant evidence for primary or secondary pathogenicity of the 15257 mutation. *Hum Genet* 1994;94:265–270.

357. Chen JD, Cox I, Denton MJ. Preliminary exclusion of an X-linked gene in Leber optic atrophy by linkage analysis. *Hum Genet* 1989;82:203–207.

358. Harding AE, Sweeney MG, Govan GG, et al. Pedigree analysis in Leber hereditary optic neuropathy families with a pathogenic mtDNA mutation. *Am J Hum Genet* 1995;57:77–86.

359. Ford CE, Jones KW, Polani PE, et al. A sex-chromosome anomaly in a case of gonadal dysgenesis (Turner's syndrome). *Lancet* 1959;1:711–713.

360. Jacobs, PA, Strong JA. A case of human intersexuality having a possible XXY sex-determining mechanism. *Nature* 1959;183:302–303.

361. Lejeune J, Gautier M, Turpin R. Human chromosomes in tissue cultures. *C R Hebd Seances Acad Sci* 1959;248:602–603.

362. Patau K, Smith DW, Therman E, et al. Multiple congenital anomaly caused by an extra autosome. *Lancet* 1960;1:790–793.

363. Edwards JH, Harnden DG, Cameron AH, et al. A new trisomic syndrome. *Lancet* 1960;1:787–790.

364. Ginsberg J, Perrin EV, Sueoka WT. Ocular manifestations of trisomy 18. *Am J Ophthalmol* 1968;66:59–67.

365. Rodrigues MM, Punnett HH, Valdes-Dapena M, et al. Retinal pigment epithelium in a case of trisomy 18. *Am J Ophthalmol* 1973;76:265–268.

366. Green WR. Personal communication, 1970.

367. Down JLH. Observations on an ethnic classification of idiots. *Clin Lect Rep Lond Hosp* 1866;3:259–262.

368. Reiss JA, Lovrien EW, Hecht F. A mother with Down's syndrome and her chromosomally normal infant. *Ann Genet* 1971;14:225–227.

369. Schachenmann G, Schmid W, Fraccaro M, et al. Chromosomes in coloboma and anal atresia. *Lancet* 1965;19:290.

370. McDermid HE, Duncan AM, Brasch KR, et al. Characterization of the supernumerary chromosome in cat eye syndrome. *Science* 1986;232:646–648.

371. Wolf U, Reinwein H, Porsch R, et al. Deficiency on the short arms of a chromosome No. 4. *Humangenetik* 1965; 1:397–413.

372. Lejeune J, Lafourcade J, Berger R, et al. 3 cases of partial deletion of the short arm of a 5 chromosome. *C R Hebd Seances Acad Sci* 1963;257:3098–3102.

373. Junien C, Turleau C, de Grouchy J, et al. Regional assignment of catalase (CAT) gene to band 11p13. Association with the aniridia-Wilms' tumor-gonadoblastoma (WAGR) complex. *Ann Genet* 1980;23:165–168.

374. Strong LC, Riccardi VM, Ferrell RE, et al. Familial retinoblastoma and chromosome 13 deletion transmitted via an insertional translocation. *Science* 1981;213:1501–1503.

375. Yanoff M, Rorke LB, Niederer BS. Ocular and cerebral abnormalities in chromosome 18 deletion defect. *Am J Ophthalmol* 1970;70:391–402.

376. Gorlin RJ, Yunis J, Anderson VE. Short arm deletion of chromosome 18 in cebocephaly. *Am J Dis Child* 1968;115: 473–476.

377. De Grouchy J, Royer P, Salmon C, et al. Partial deletion of the long arms of the chromosome 18. *Pathol Biol (Paris)* 1964;12:579–582.

378. Turner HH. A syndrome of infantilism, congenital webbed neck, and cubitus valgus. *Endocrinology* 1938;23:566–574.

379. Decourt L, Sasso WS, Chiorboli E, et al. Genetic sex in Turner's syndrome patients. *Rev Assoc Med Bras* 1954;1:203–206.

380. Polani PE, Hunter WF, Lennox B. Chromosomal sex in Turner's syndrome with coarctation of the aorta. *Lancet* 1954;2: 120–121.

381. Wilkins L, Grumbach MM, van Wyk JJ. Chromosomal sex in ovarian agenesis. *J Clin Endocrinol Metab* 1954;14: 1270–1271.

382. Chrousos GA, Ross JL, Chrousos G, et al. Ocular findings in Turner syndrome. A prospective study. *Ophthalmology* 1984;91:926–928.

383. Klinefelter HF Jr, Reifenstein EC Jr, Albright F. Syndrome characterized by gynecomastia, aspermatogenesis without a-Leydigism, and increased secretion of follicle-stimulating hormone. *J Clin Endocrinol Metab* 1942;2:615–624.

384. Barr ML, Plunkett ER. Testicular dysgenesis affecting the seminiferous tubules principally, with chromatin-positive nuclei. *Lancet* 1956;271:853–856.

385. Knowlton RG, Weaver EJ, Struyk AF, et al. Genetic linkage analysis of hereditary arthro-ophthalmopathy (Stickler syndrome) and the type II procollagen gene. *Am J Hum Genet* 1989;45:681–688.

386. Richards AJ, Yates JRW, Williams R, et al. A family with Stickler syndrome type 2 has a mutation in the COL11A1 gene resulting in the substitution of glycine 97 by valine in alpha-1(XI) collagen. *Hum Mol Genet* 1996;5: 1339–1343.

387. Nijbroek G, Sood S, McIntosh I, et al. Fifteen novel FBN1 mutations causing Marfan syndrome detected by heteroduplex analysis of genomic amplicons. *Am J Hum Genet* 1995;57: 8–21.

388. Sertie AL, Sossi V, Camargo AA, et al. Collagen XVIII, containing an endogenous inhibitor of angiogenesis and tumor growth, plays a critical role in the maintenance of retinal structure and in neural tube closure (Knobloch syndrome). *Hum Mol Genet* 2000;9:2051–2058.

389. Goldschmidt E. On the etiology of myopia: an epidemiological study. *Acta Ophthalmol Suppl* 1968;98:1–172.

390. Teikari JM, O'Donnell J, Kaprio J, et al. Impact of heredity in myopia. *Hum Hered* 1991;41:151–156.

391. Ashton GC. Segregation analysis of ocular refraction and myopia. *Hum Hered* 1985;35:232–239.

392. Goss DA, Hampton MJ, Wickham MG. Selected review on genetic factors in myopia. *J Am Optom Assoc* 1988;59: 875–884.

393. Naiglin L, Clayton J, Gazagne C, et al. Familial high myopia: evidence of an autosomal dominant mode of inheritance and genetic heterogeneity. *Ann Genet* 1999;42:140–146.

394. Guggenheim JA, Kirov G, Hodson SA. The heritability of high myopia: a re-analysis of Goldschmidt's data. *J Med Genet* 2000;27:227–231.

395. Teikari JM, Kaprio J, Koskenvuo M, et al. Heritability of defects of far vision in young adults—a twin study. *Scand J Soc Med* 1992;20:73–78.

396. Sorsby A, Sheriden M, Leary GA. Refraction and its components in twins. Spec Rep Ser Med Res Coun Lond 1962; 303:43, 7s. H.M. Stationery Office (Special Report of the Medical Research Council of London).

397. Lyhne N, Sjolie AK, Kyvik KO, et al. The importance of genes and environment for ocular refraction and its determiners: a population based study among 20–45 year old twins. *Br J Ophthalmol* 2001;85:1470–1476.

398. Hammond CJ, Snieder H, Gilbert CE, et al. Genes and environment in refractive error. The twin eye study. *Invest Ophthalmol Vis Sci* 2001;42:1232–1236.

399. Goss DA, Jackson TW. Clinical findings before the onset of myopia in youth: parental history of myopia. *Optom Vis Sci* 1996;73:279–282.

400. Gwiazda J, Thorn F, Bauer J, et al. Emmetropization and the progression of manifest refraction in children followed from infancy to puberty. *Clin Vis Sci* 1993;8:337–344.

401. Zadnik K, Satariano WA, Mutti DO, et al. The effect of parental history of myopia on children's eye size. *JAMA* 1994;271:1323–1327.

402. Zadnik K. The Glenn A. Fry Award Lecture (1995). Myopia development in childhood. *Optom Vis Sci* 1997;74:603–608.

403. Pacella R, McLellan J, Grice K, et al. Role of genetic factors in the etiology of juvenile-onset myopia based on a longitudinal study of refractive error. *Optom Vis Sci* 1999;76: 381–386.

404. Wallman J: Parental history and myopia: taking the long view. *JAMA* 1994;272:1255–1256.

405. Wallman J, Turkel JI, Trachtman J. Extreme myopia produced by modest change in visual experience. *Science* 1978;201:1249–1251.

406. Weisel TN, Raviola E. Myopia and eye enlargement after neonatal lid fusion in monkeys. *Nature* 1977;266:66–68.

407. Sherman SM, Norton TT, Casagrande VA. Myopia in the lid-sutured tree shrew (Tupaia glis). *Brain Res* 1977;124:154–157.

408. Hoyt CS, Stone RD, Fromer C, et al. Monocular axial myopia associated with neonatal eyelid closure in human infants. *Am J Ophthalmol* 1982;91:197–200.

409. Von Noorden GK, Lewis RA. Ocular axial length in unilateral congenital cataracts and blepharoptosis. *Invest Ophthalmol Vis Sci* 1987;28:750–752.

410. Twomey JM, Gilvarry A, Restori M, et al. Ocular enlargement following infantile corneal opacification. *Eye* 1990;4: 497–503.

411. Lin LLK, Hung PT, Ko LS, et al. Study of myopia among aboriginal school children in Taiwan. *Acta Ophthalmol Suppl* 1988;185:34–36.

412. Zylberman R, Landau D, Berson D. The influence of study habits on myopia in Jewish teenagers. *J Pediatr Ophthalmol Strabismus* 1993;30:319–322.

413. Young FA. Myopia and personality. *Am J Optom Physiol Opt* 1987;64:136–143.

414. Young FA. Reading, measures of intelligence, and refractive errors. *Am J Optom Physiol Opt* 1963;40:257–264.

415. Rosner M, Belkin M. Intelligence, education, and myopia in males. *Arch Ophthalmol* 1987;105:1508–1511.

416. Schwartz M, Haim M, Skarsholm D. X-Linked myopia. Bornholm eye disease. *Clin Genet* 1990;38:281–286.

417. Young TL, Ronan SM, Alvear AB, et al. X-linked high myopia associated with cone dysfunction. *Arch Ophthalmol* 2004;122:897–908.

418. Young TL, Ronan SM, Drahozal LA, et al. Evidence that a locus for familial high myopia maps to chromosome 18p. *Am J Hum Genet* 1998;63:109–119.

419. Young TL, Ronan SM, Alvear A, et al. A second locus for familial high myopia maps to chromosome 12q. *Am J Hum Genet* 1998;63:1419–1424.

420. Lam DSC, Tam POS, Fan, DSP, et al. Familial high myopia linkage to chromosome 18p. *Ophthalmologica* 2003;217:115–118.

421. Heath SC, Robledo R, Beggs W, et al. A novel approach to search for identity by descent in small samples of patients and controls from the same Mendelian breeding unit: a pilot study on myopia. *Hum Hered* 2001;52:183–190.

422. Paluru P, Heon E, Devoto M, et al. A new locus for autosomal dominant high myopia maps to the long arm of chromosome 17. *Invest Ophthalmol Vis Sci* 2003;44:1830–1836.

423. Naiglin L, Gazagne CH, Dallongeville F, et al. A genome wide scan for familial high myopia suggests a novel locus on chromosome 7q36. *J Med Genet* 2002;39:118–124.

424. Zhou G, Williams RW. Mouse models for the analysis of myopia: an analysis of variation in eye size of adult mice. *Optom Vis Sci* 1999;76:408–418.

425. Zhou G, Williams RW. Eye1 and Eye2: gene loci that modulate eye size, lens weight, and retinal area in the mouse. *Invest Ophthalmol Vis Sci* 1999;40:817–825.

426. Von Noorden G. *Binocular vision and ocular motility: theory and management of strabismus*, 5th Ed. St. Louis, MO: Mosby Year Book.

427. Cross HE. The heritability of strabismus. *Am Orthopt J* 1975;25:11–17.

428. Spivey BE. Strabismus: factors in anticipating its occurrence. *Aust J Ophthalmol* 1980;8:5–9.

429. Chimonidou E, Palimeris G, Koliopoulos J, et al. Family distribution of concomitant squint in Greece. *Br J Ophthalmol* 1977;61:27–29.

430. Simpson NE, Alleslev LJ. Association of children's diseases in families from record linkage data. *Can J Genet Cytol* 1972;15:789–800.

431. Francois J. Affections of the ocular muscles. In: Francois J, ed. *Heredity in ophthalmology*. St. Louis: CV Mosby Co, 1961: 239–269.

432. Dufier JL, Briard ML, Bonaiti C, et al. Inheritance in the etiology of convergent squint. *Ophthalmologica* 1979;179:225–234.

433. Maumenee IH, Alston A, Mets MB, et al. Inheritance of congenital esotropia. *Trans Am Ophthalmol Soc* 1986;84:85–93.

434. Podgor MJ, Remaley NA, Chew E. Associations between siblings for esotropia and exotropia. *Arch Ophthalmol* 1996;114: 739–744.

435. Hu DN. Prevalence and mode of inheritance of major genetic eye diseases in China. *J Med Genet* 1987;24:584–588.

436. Richter S. On the heredity of strabismus concomitans. *Humangenetik* 1967;3:235–243.

437. Waardenburg PJ. Squint and heredity. *Doc Ophthalmol Proc Ser* 1954;7:422–494.

438. Reynolds JD, Wackerhagen M. Strabismus in monozygotic and dizygotic twins. *Am Orthopt J* 1986;36:113.

439. De Vries B, Houtman WA. Squint in monozygotic twins. *Doc Ophthalmol* 1979;46:305–308.

440. Rubin W, Helm C, McCormack MK. Ocular motor anomalies in monozygotic and dizygotic twins. In: Reinecke R, ed. *Strabismus: proceedings of the 3rd meeting of the international strabismological association*, Asilomar, CA, 1978. New York, NY: Grune & Stratton, 1978:89.

441. Niederecker O, Mash AJ, Spivey BE. Horizontal fusional amplitudes and versions. Comparison in parents of strabismic and nonstrabismic children. *Arch Ophthalmol* 1972;87:283–285.

442. Mash AJ, Hegmann JP, Spivey BE. Genetic analysis of vergence measures in populations with varying incidences of strabismus. *Am J Ophthalmol* 1975;79.978–984.

443. Mash AJ, Spivey BE. Genetic aspects of strabismus. *Doc Ophthalmol* 1973;34:285–291.

444. Parikh V, Shugart YY, Doheny KF, et al. A strabismus susceptibility locus on chromosome 7p. *Proc Natl Acad Sci USA* 2003;100:12283–12288.

445. Bowen P. Achondroplasia in two sisters with normal parents. *Birth Defects Orig Artic Ser* 1974;10:31–36.

446. Myrianthopoulos NC, Aronson SM. Population dynamics of Tay-Sachs disease. II. What confers the selective advantage upon the Jewish heterozygote? In: *Proceedings of fourth international symposium on sphingolipidoses*. New York, NY: Plenum Press, 1972:561.

447. Cross HE, Maumenee AE. Ocular trauma during amniocentesis. *Arch Ophthalmol* 1973;90:303–304.

448. Broome DL, Wilson MG, Weiss B, et al. Needle puncture of fetus: a complication of second-trimester amniocentesis. *Am J Obstet Gynecol* 1976;126:247–252.

449. Isenberg SJ, Heckenlively JR. Traumatized eye with retinal damage from amniocentesis. *J Pediatr Ophthalmol Strabismus* 1985;22:65–67.

450. Karp LE, Hayden PW. Fetal puncture during midtrimester amniocentesis. *Obstet Gynecol* 1977;49:115–117.

451. Merin S, Beyth Y. Uniocular congenital blindness as a complication of midtrimester amniocentesis. *Am J Ophthalmol* 1980;89:299–301.

452. Elejalde BR, de Elejalde MM, Hamilton PR, et al. Prenatal diagnosis of cyclopia. *Am J Med Genet* 1983;14:15–19.

453. Lev-Gur M, Maklad NF, Patel S. Ultrasonic findings in fetal cyclopia. A case report. *J Reprod Med* 1983;28:554–557.

454. Cogan DG. Congenital anomalies of the retina. *Birth Defects Orig Artic Ser* 1971;7:41–51.

455. Cogan DG, KuwabaraT. Ocular pathology of the 13–15trisomy syndrome. *Arch Ophthalmol* 1964;72:246–253.

456. Mullaney J. Ocular pathology in trisomy 18 (Edwards' syndrome). *Am J Ophthalmol* 1973;76:246–254.

457. Wilson MG, Towner JW, Coffin GS, et al. Inherited pericentric inversion of chromosome no. 4. *Am J Hum Genet* 1970;22:679–690.

458. Vogel W, Siebers JW, Reinwein H. Partial trisomy 7q. *Ann Genet* 1973;16:277–280.

459. Rethore MO, Larget-Piet L, Abonyi D, et al. 4 cases of trisomy for the short arm of chromosome 9. Individualization of a new morbid entity. *Ann Genet* 1970;13:217–232.

460. Schwanitz G, Schamberger U, Rott HD, et al. Partial trisomy 9 in the case of familial translocation 8/9 mat. *Ann Genet* 1974;17:163–166.

461. Hsu LYF, Kim HJ, Sujansky E, et al. Reciprocal translocation versus centric fusion between two no. 13 chromosomes. A case of 46,XX,-13,+t(13;13)(p12;q13) and a case of46,XY,-13, +t(13; 13)(p12;p12). *Cytogenet Cell Genet* 1973;12:235–244.

462. Walknowska J, Peakman D, Weleber RG. Cytogenetic investigation of cat-eye syndrome. *Am J Ophthalmol* 1977;84: 477–486.

463. Alvarado M, Bocian M, Walker AP. Interstitial deletion of the long arm of chromosome 3d: case report, review, and definition of a phenotype. *Am J Med Genet* 1987;27:781–786.

464. Carter R, Baker E, Hayman D. Congenital malformations associated with a ring 4 chromosome. *J Med Genet* 1969;6:224–227.

465. Taysi K, Burde RM, Rohrbaugh JR. Terminal long arm deletion of chromosome 7 and retino-choroidal coloboma. *Ann Genet* 1982;25:159–161.

466. Ferry AP, Marchevsky A, Strauss I. Ocular abnormalities in deletion of the long arm of chromosome 11. *Ann Ophthalmol* 1981;13:1373–1377.

467. Bialasiewicz AA, Mayer UM, Meythaler FH. Ophthalmologic findings in 11 q-deletion syndrome. *Klin Monatsbl Augenheilk* 1987;190:524–526.

468. O'Grady RB, Rothstein TB, Romano PE. D-group deletion syndromes and retinoblastoma. *Am J Ophthalmol* 1974;77:40–45.

469. Saraux H, Rethore MO, Aussannaire M, et al. Ocular abnormalities of phenotype DR (ring D chromosome). *Ann Ocul (Paris)* 1970;203:737–748.

470. Schinzel A, Hayashi K, Schmid W. Structural aberrations of chromosome 18. II. The 18q-syndrome. Report of three cases. *Humangenetik* 1975;26:123–132.

471. Yanoff M, Rorke LB, Niederer BS. Ocular and cerebral abnormalities in chromosome 18 deletion defect. *Am J Ophthalmol* 1970;70:391–402.

472. Yunis E, Silva R, Giraldo A. Trisomy 10p. *Ann Genet* 1976;19:57–60.

473. Howard RO. Chromosomal abnormalities associated with cyclopia and synophthalmia. *Trans Am Ophthalmol Soc* 1977;75:505–538.

474. Lang AF, Schlager FM, Gardner HA. Trisomy 18 and cyclopia. *Teratology* 1976;14:195–203.

475. Cohen MM, Storm DF, Capraro VJ. A ring chromosome (no. 18) in a cyclops. *Clin Genet* 1972;3:249–252.

476. Nitowsky HM, Sindhvananda N, Konigberg UR, et al. Partial 18 monosomy in the cyclops malformation. *Pediatrics* 1966;37:260–269.

477. Faint S, Lewis EJW. Presumptive deletion of the short arm of chromosome 18 in a cyclops. *Hum Chromosome Newsl* 1964;14:5.

478. Gimelli G, Cuoco C, Lituania M, et al. Dup(3) (p2-pter) in two families, including one infant with cyclopia. *Am J Med Genet* 1985;20:341–348.

479. Hoepner J, Yanoff M. Ocular anomalies in trisomy 13–15: an analysis of 13 eyes with two new findings. *Am J Ophthalmol* 1972;74:729–737.

480. Keith CG. The ocular manifestations of trisomy 13–15. *Trans Ophthalmol Soc UK* 1966;86:435–454.

481. Huggert A. The trisomy 18 syndrome. *Acta Ophthalmol (Copenh)* 1966;44:186.

482. Rodrigues MM, Valdes-Dapena M, Kistenmacher M. Ocular pathology in a case of 13 trisomy. *J Pediatr Ophthalmol* 1973;10:54.

483. Ginsberg J, Ballard ET, Buchino JJ, et al. Further observations of ocular pathology in Down's syndrome. *J Pediatr Ophthalmol Strabismus* 1980;17:166–171.

484. Shapiro MB, France TD. The ocular features of Down's syndrome. *Am J Ophthalmol* 1985;99:659–663.

485. Caputo AR, Wagner RS, Reynolds DR, et al. Down syndrome. Clinical review of ocular features. *Clin Pediatr (Phila)* 1989;28:355–358.

486. Gustavson KH, Finley SC, Finley WH, et al. A4–5/21–22 chromosomal translocation associated with multiple congenital anomalies. *Acta Paediatr* 1964;53:172–181.

487. Monteleone P, Monteleone J, Sekhon G, et al. Partial trisomy 5 with a carrier parent t(5p-;9p+). *Clin Genet* 1976;9:437–440.

488. Rethore, MO Larget-Piet, L, Abonyi D, et al. 4 cases of trisomy for the short arm of chromosome 9. Individualization of a new morbid entity. *Ann. Genet* 1970;13:217–232.

489. Rethore MO, Kaplan JC, Junien C, et al. Increase of the LDH-B activity in a boy with 12p trisomy by malsegregation of a maternal translocation t(12;14) (q12;p11). *Ann Genet* 1975;18:81–87.

490. Orye E, Verhaaren H, Samuel K, et al. A46,XX,10q+ chromosome constitution in a girl. Partial long arm duplication or insertional translocation? *Humangenetik* 1975;28:1–8.

491. Yunis JJ, Sanchez O. A new syndrome resulting from partial trisomy for the distal third of the long arm of chromosome 10. *J Pediatr* 1974;84:567–570.

492. Falk RE, Carrel RE, Valente M, et al. Partial trisomy of chromosome 11: a case report. *Am J Ment Defic* 1973;77:383–388.

493. Raoul O, Rethore MO, Dutriliaux B, et al. Partial 14q trisomy. I. Partial 14q trisomy by maternal translocation t(10;14) (p15.2; q22). *Ann Genet* 1975;18:35–39.

494. Condron CJ, Cantwell RJ, Kaufman RL, et al. The supernumerary isochromosome 18 syndrome (+ 18pu). *Birth Defects Orig Artic Ser* 1974;10:36–42.

495. Zellweger H, Ionasescu V, Simpson J, et al. The problem of trisomy 22. A case report and a discussion of the variant forms. *Clin Pediatr (Phila)* 1976;15:601–606.

496. Breg WR, Steele MW, Miller OJ, et al. The cri du chat syndrome in adolescents and adults: clinical finding in 13 older patients with partial deletion of the short arm of chromosome no. 5(5p-). *J Pediatr* 1970;77:782–791.

497. Farrell JW, Morgan KS, Black S. Lensectomy in an infant with cri du chat syndrome and cataracts. *J Pediatr Ophthalmol Strabismus* 1988;25:131–134.

498. Broughton WL, Fine BS, Zimmerman LE. Congenital glaucoma associated with a chromosomal defect. A histologic study. *Arch Ophthalmol* 1981;99:481–486.

499. Lee ML, Sciorra LJ. Partial monosomy of the long arm of chromosome 11 in a severely affected child. *Ann Genet* 1981;24:51–53.

500. Allderdice PW, Davis JG, Miller OJ, et al. The 13q-deletion syndrome. *Am J Hum Genet* 1969;21:499.

501. Ledbetter DH, Riccardi VM, Airhart SD, et al. Deletions of chromosome 15 as a cause of the Prader-Willi syndrome. *N Engl J Med* 1981;304:325–329.

502. Ledbetter DH, Mascarello JT, Riccardi VM, et al. Chromosome 15 abnormalities and the Prader-Willis syndrome: a follow-up of 40 cases. *Am J Hum Genet* 1982;34:278–285.

503. Mattei JF, Mattei MG, Giraud F. Prader-Willi syndrome and chromosome 15. A clinical discussion of 20 cases. *Hum Genet* 1983;64:356–362.

504. Schinzel A, Schmid W, Luscher U, et al. Structural aberrations of chromosome 18. I. The 18p-syndrome. *Arch Genet (Zur)* 1974;47:1–15.

505. DiGeorge AM, Olmstead RW, Harley RD. Waardenburg's syndrome. A syndrome of heterochromia of the irides, lateral displacement of the medial canthi and lacrimal puncta, congenital deafness, and other characteristic associated defects. *J Pediatr* 1960;57:649–669.

506. Nelson WE, Vaughn VC, McKay RJ, eds. *Textbook of pediatrics,* 9th Ed. Philadelphia, PA: WB Saunders, 1969.

507. Kistenmacher ML, Punnett HH. Comparative behavior of ring chromosomes. *Am J Hum Genet* 1970;22:304–318.

508. Behrman RE, Vaughan VC III, Nelson WE, eds. *Nelson textbook of pediatrics,* 13th Ed. Philadelphia, PA: WB Saunders, 1987.

2

Neonatal Ophthalmology: Ocular Development in Childhood

Kammi B. Gunton

THE NEONATAL EYE is one of the most fully developed sensory organs. Despite its similarity to the adult eye, there are tremendous changes that will occur in the refractive correction, axial length, shape of cornea, color of iris, pupillary responses, and retinal and neurologic development during childhood. Understanding this process is vital to the appropriate care of children's eyes. This chapter focuses on the anatomic changes in the eye and orbit during infancy and through adolescence. Intraocularly, the anterior segment, retina, and optic nerve undergo rapid changes within the first year of life to allow the development of clear images on the retina. Neurologic development then allows the subsequent processing of the retinal image. Externally, the bony growth of the orbit and surrounding ocular structures are also influenced by the changes within the eye.

The ophthalmologist caring for the pediatric patient must understand the normal developmental changes so as not to confuse them with pathologic states. In addition, disease states may interfere with normal development. Intervention must occur during critical periods to allow for normal growth of the eye and orbit. Premature infants can exhibit findings normal in the embryonic development consistent with the infant's gestational age and not the chronologic age. This chapter will address the normal changes in the globe, anterior segment, pupil, retina, neurologic development, orbit, and refractive status of the eye from findings in premature infants through to complete maturation of these structures.

GLOBE DIMENSIONS

The weight of the term infant eye varies between 2.3 and 3.4 g (1). The average adult eye weighs 7.5 g. The volume of the infant globe varies between 2.20 and 3.25 cm³. The average axial length of the eye in term infants is between 16.8 and 17.5 mm when measured ultrasonographically (2). The value is slightly less when measurements are obtained through histopathologic studies. Normative data reveal a triphasic pattern of increase in the axial length (2). During the

first year of life, the rate of growth is the greatest. There is on average a 2.5 to 3.8 mm increase in the axial length in the first year of life, making the mean axial length 20.7 mm. The rate of increase then decreases in subsequent years, such that the mean axial length is 21.5 mm in the second year and 21.9 mm in the third year. Thereafter, the rate of growth slows to approximately 0.4 mm/year. The axial length generally reaches adult dimensions by approximately 5 years of age. Between 5 and 15 years of age, there may be small increases in the axial length of usually <1.0 mm without the presence of myopic refractive error. The mean axial length in girls is shorter than boys through adolescence, 23.92 and 24.36 mm, respectively (1).

In pathologic conditions such as congenital glaucoma, cataracts, and retinopathy of prematurity, the axial length measurements vary from these normative values. In a group of 170 children with congenital and infantile cataracts, mean axial length was 17.86 mm between 0 and 3 months of age and 21.96 mm between 30 and 42 months of age (3). The range of axial length in this cohort was 14.22 to 25.98 mm. Another study reported shorter axial lengths in the first year of life for cataractous eyes compared with noncataractous eyes—mean axial lengths of 17.9 and 19.2 mm, respectively (4). The standard deviation in mean axial length in children with cataracts was twice the value in noncataractous eyes. The change in axial length may also vary in children with cataracts. Trivedi reported a 0.19 mm/month change from 6 to 18 months and 0.01 mm/month change from 18 months to 18 years of age (4). In addition, African-American children in the study had statistically significant longer axial lengths than Caucasian children (4). The selection of appropriate intraocular lens correction remains a controversial subject. In children with prematurity, there is greater variability in the axial length compared with age-matched controls (5). Increased axial length in children with retinopathy of prematurity contributed to severe myopia, but changes in refractive parameters in the anterior segment were also significant (5). Finally, measuring axial length changes allows for monitoring of control in congenital glaucoma.

Cornea

The absolute dimensions in the term "newborn eye" are closer to the adult dimensions than nearly any other organ in the body. The cornea undergoes macroscopic and intracellular changes to allow transparency, as well as changes in refractive power postnatally, yet the corneal diameter undergoes only minimal growth. The cornea begins with equal sagittal and transverse diameters. In premature infants, the corneal diameter may be approximated at any gestational age because of its relationship to the child's weight in grams. The corneal diameter in mm equals 0.0014 (weight in grams) plus 6.3 (6). At term, the average corneal diameter horizontally is 9.0 to 10.5 mm, with a mean of 9.8 mm. The vertical diameter may exceed the horizontal with a range of 9.9 to 10.5 mm. In general, a macrocornea is defined as having a horizontal diameter >2 SD from the mean or 11.0 mm in term infants. A microcornea has a diameter < 9.0 mm (Fig. 2.1). This standard range of measurements may help identify children with corneal enlargement secondary to diseases such as infantile glaucoma, once racial variation has been taken into account. The range in corneal diameter was slightly greater in a cohort of African babies, 9.0 to 12.5 mm at 1 week of life, showcasing the importance of evaluating normative data in regard to ethnicity (7).

The growth in corneal diameter is also accompanied by changes in corneal curvature. Since the cornea is instrumental in refraction, the changes in corneal radii of curvature influence the clarity of retinal images. To maintain emmetropia, changes in corneal curvature must be perfectly balanced with changes in the lens and axial length of the eye. The corneal curvature is much steeper in infants than in adults. This observation extends to premature infants as well. In premature infants with a mean gestational age of <32 weeks, the mean keratometry was 63.3 ± 3.3 D in the

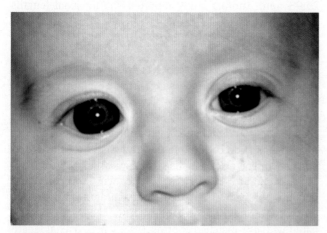

FIGURE 2.1. Megalocornea. The right corneal diameter is 14.0 mm and the left horizontal corneal diameter is 12.0 mm. Each cornea is clear, and there is no evidence of glaucoma. Megalocornea is usually a bilateral condition with corneal horizontal diameter >2 SD from the mean or 11.0 mm in term infants.

horizontal meridian and 57.3 ± 2.6 D in the vertical meridian (8). These values decreased rapidly to 54.0 ± 3.0 D and 50.7 ± 2.4 D, respectively, by 36 weeks of gestational age. The corneal curvature continues to decrease rapidly in the first 2 to 4 weeks of life in term infants and then slows after 8 weeks of life. Keratometry values obtained for term infants range from 48.06 to 47.00 D. In one study of 4,881 children aged 6 to 14, keratometry values in the horizontal median remained stable through childhood, but the vertical meridian power decreased slightly with age (9). Girls had statistically significant greater power in the vertical and horizontal meridian at all ages compared to boys: 44.27 D compared to 43.52 D vertically and 43.17 D compared to 42.49 D horizontally, respectively. Asian children had greater corneal power in the vertical meridian compared to other ethnicities, and white children had greater corneal power in the horizontal meridian. Ethnicity must be taken into account in the interpretation of normative data.

The flattening of the cornea persists into the second and early third decades (10). The average keratometry at age 20 is 42.0 D. The horizontal meridian begins to steepen between the fourth and fifth decades of life and then continues to steepen with age. This results in a gradual change from with-the-rule astigmatism common in youth to against-the-rule astigmatism in 50- to 60-year-old individuals (10). Advances in corneal tomography have lead to greater precision in measuring the cornea in childhood (11).

Histologically, the layers of the cornea develop to attain both the structure and the function needed in mature corneas. The corneal epithelium thickens with successive cellular layers, and there is an increase in cell size within each layer. At 20 weeks' gestational age, the corneal epithelium has only two cellular layers, with the basal cells having a thickness of 20 μm (12). By 6 months of age, the basal cells reach their adult thickness of 18 μm. The desmosomes, which are the intracellular junctions between the corneal epithelial cells, are present in a 20-week gestational-age cornea. They are more abundant in the superficial layer, although thinner and less regularly distributed. Corneal abrasions in the early gestational period would, therefore, be expected to occur more easily. In a study of 1- to 12-week-old children, presenting for well visits, 49% had asymptomatic corneal abrasions (13). Most abrasions in this group resolved within 24 hours. The epithelial basement membrane becomes thicker and more homogenous during the early gestational period. The type IV collagen composition of the infant epithelial basement membrane varies significantly from the adult counterpart (14). The hemidesmosomes anchoring the basal cell layer of the epithelium to the basement membrane increase, and the Bowman's layer becomes compact with more collagen fibrils.

The corneal stroma also becomes thicker during the first several months of life, from 0.229 mm at 20 weeks' gestation to 0.490 mm at 6 months postnatally, at which time the adult thickness has essentially been reached (12). This change in the thickness results from enlargement of the collagen fibrils themselves. Once mature, the collagen fibers no longer thicken during subsequent aging. The average diameter of a collagen fiber is between 250 and 300 Å. Most studies report a slow increase in central corneal thickness until approximately 10 years of age (15,16), although some studies have reported no change (17,18). Some of this discrepancy results from the method of measurement used for central corneal thickness, with specular microscopy yielding lower values than ultrasound pachymetry.

There are small structural changes observed between adolescents' collagen fibers and those from elderly individuals. Adolescent corneal stroma has increased interfibrillary distance compared with samples from elderly individuals. The etiology of the increased cross-sectional area within the corneal collagen fibers has also been investigated. On average, the cross-sectional area increases from approximately 3.04 to 3.46 nm^2 over a 90-year timespan. In contrast, the interfibrillary distance decreases with age. It has been postulated that this change may be due in part to an increase in the nonenzymatic cross-linking between collagen molecules. Biochemical studies have revealed an increase in collagen glycation and its end products within elderly corneal stromal samples resulting in decreased interfibrillary spacing. Counterbalancing the decrease in interfibrillary distance, there is an increased occurrence of water accumulation between collagen fibrils. These "lakes" contribute to light scatter, which may diminish visual clarity with age, and largely account for the overall increased cross-sectional area.

The keratocytes in the corneal stroma decrease in thickness and density during development. One study found a keratocyte density of 6.22×10^4 keratocytes/mm^3 in the first decade of life, decreasing approximately 0.3% per year thereafter (19). This study also found that interindividual keratocyte density was quite variable, while intraindividual density was not. Keratocytes play an important role in corneal stromal wound healing. It has been postulated that the decrease in keratocyte density is due to a combination of environmental and predetermined genetic factors, although the exact mechanism is unknown. The decrease in keratocytes may be partially or completely responsible for the age-related changes within the cornea, including the decrease in central corneal thickness with age, steepening of the cornea with resulting refractive changes through childhood, and increased light scatter noted in the cornea with age. The decline in keratocyte density and the interindividual variability may be of particular importance to refractive procedures where corneal stromal wound healing may affect the outcome of the procedure. An inverse relationship has been noted between the vigor of wound healing with its effect on refractive regression and increasing age.

Like corneal keratocyte density, endothelial cell density also decreases with age. A cornea from a 12-week fetus has an endothelial cell density of 14,000 cells/mm^2 (19). At term, the average endothelial cell density is 6,800 cells/mm^2. This large decline during fetal development may be explained by rapid corneal growth. Yet, the decrease from infancy to

childhood is also rapid, ranging from 1.4% to 4.0%. As mentioned previously, corneal growth has essentially attained adult parameters by 2 years of age. The reason for the further decrease in endothelial cell density is unknown. The annual rate of loss of endothelial cells slows in adulthood to approximately 0.3% per year. This rate of decrease emphasizes the importance of approximate age matching of donor corneas used in corneal transplants in newborns and infants with conditions of visually limiting corneal opacities.

The endothelial cells contribute to the translucent nature of the cornea as well as to the regular spacing of the collagen fibers. The cornea is an intransparent structure in fetuses up to 26 weeks' gestational age (20). The intransparency is mild to moderate, symmetric, and uniform with smooth corneal epithelium. The cornea becomes transparent within 4 to 6 weeks of birth (Fig. 2.2). Most infants >32 weeks' gestational age demonstrate corneal transparency, but any developmental intransparency clears within 1 to 2 days of delivery in term infants.

The etiology for the variability in the structural changes in the cornea has long been sought. Recent studies have identified proteins that may mediate cellular activities in corneal development (21). Tenascin-C (TN-C) mediates several important cellular activities, including cell adhesion, migration, and proliferation and differentiation of stem cells. TN-C is expressed widely in the preterm cornea. TN-C is expressed on both surfaces of Descemet membrane in infant corneas (22). Restriction of expression begins to occur in the neonate, and by adulthood TN-C is expressed only in the limbus. Variants of TN-C caused by alternate splicing of the gene lead to the pleiotropic nature of TN-C. These variants also differ in their expression within the cornea and with age. Rho-mediated signaling in injury can induce expression of TN-C in adult corneas (23). Further studies of proteins that influence growth may lead to development of strategies to effect disease states.

In summary, the corneal diameter increases slightly, especially in the vertical diameter, and the corneal curvature flattens in childhood. Early in the second decade of life,

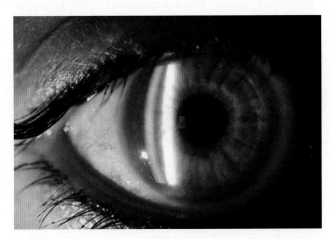

FIGURE 2.2. Slit lamp exam of cornea revealing slight opacity in cornea consistent with very mild congenital hereditary endothelial dystrophy.

the corneal curvature steepens, especially in the horizontal meridian. The corneal layers also mature in the first decade. There is an increase in the size of the epithelial and stromal layers in the early postnatal period, but the endothelial and stromal keratocyte density decreases in the same time period. Nevertheless, there is an increase in the overall corneal thickness.

Corneal thickness influences the measurement of intraocular pressure (24,25). Intraocular pressure measurement may be overestimated as corneal thickness increases. The positive correlation in central corneal thickness and intraocular pressure is generally established in adult populations (26). By extrapolation, thinner corneas in infants <6 months of age would be expected to produce lower intraocular pressures with Goldmann or Schiotz tonometry. Furthermore, the correlation of central corneal thickness and intraocular pressure in children is variable due to variation in central corneal thickness with age and race (18). One study found intraocular pressure varies with age according to the relationship, Ta equals 0.71(age in years) plus 10, until the age of 10 (27). The method of intraocular pressure determination also significantly impacts the value of the intraocular pressure (28). Applanation tonometry underestimates intraocular pressure under general anesthesia and generally underestimates intraocular pressure in childhood according to some studies (27,29). General anesthetics tend to lower intraocular pressure, while infant distress with crying and squeezing of the lids elevates intraocular pressure. Since the Tono-Pen compresses a much smaller corneal area, it is slightly less affected by corneal thickness (30). Some studies have found that intraocular pressure increases 2.1 to 3.5 mmHg with every 100 μm increase in central corneal thickness in children when measured with the Tono-Pen (18,31). These variations in intraocular pressure with corneal characteristics must be incorporated into the management of infantile glaucoma.

Anterior Chamber

The anterior chamber depth is influenced by the growth of the sclera, as well as by factors related to lens movement and thickness. There are many methods to evaluate the anterior chamber including slit-lamp photography, ultrasound biomicroscopy, and anterior segment optical coherence tomography (32). Using some of these methods, estimates of the anterior chamber depth average 2.05 mm with a range of 1.8 to 2.4 mm in depth (33). The depth continues to increase until the end of adolescence, and then it progressively diminishes. In emmetropic patients, the increase in anterior chamber depth appears to stop at an earlier age, compared to patients with myopia (34). This apparent difference is related to the continued changes in the lens and axial length in patients with myopia. The anterior chamber depth appears to vary with ethnicity as well (9). Native American children had the least change in anterior chamber depth from ages 6 to 14 with an average depth of 3.50 mm.

African-American children had the greatest change during this same period, from 3.41 to 3.62 mm. After 12 years of age, the anterior chamber depth appears to be constant regardless of ethnicity.

Care must be taken with the measurement technique as with physiologic accommodation, the anterior chamber depth diminishes approximately 24 μm/D using slit-lamp adapted optical coherence tomography (35). After instillation of mydriatics, the anterior chamber depth may increase (36,37). The difference in the anterior chamber depth between the two eyes does not exceed 0.15 mm in normal individuals (34). The anterior chamber depth is slightly deeper in boys than girls, 3.64 mm compared to 3.56 mm, respectively (9). The volume of the anterior chamber is approximately 64 mm^3 in term infants and 116 mm^3 in adults (34). Adjustments during intraocular surgery in childhood may be necessary based upon these differences in anterior chamber depth.

Iris

The architectural crypts of the iris develop from gestation through the early postnatal period. The primary papillary membrane forms early in gestation and atrophies near term. The color of the iris results from pigmentation of the stromal mesodermal cells and iris blood vessels. At term, the mesodermal stromal cells of the iris continue to develop pigment, which accounts for the darkening of iris color observed in the first few months of life. Researchers have identified many pigment-associated genes that reside on chromosome 15, which contribute to iris color (38). One particular sequence within the regulating element of the HERC2 segment on chromosome 15 accounts for 74% of the variance in human eye color (39). The contour of the iris including Fuchs' crypts, contraction furrows, Wolfflin nodules, and nevi influences the perceived color of the human iris. Separate genes regulate these iris patterns, including SEMA3A and TRAF3IP1, which are also associated with pathways that control neuronal pattern development (40).

Lens

The tunica vasculosa lentis is a plexus of blood vessels that is instrumental in the development and nourishment of the lens in embryonic life. The tunica vasculosa lentis completely regresses after 35 weeks of gestation. Although the exact cellular processes involved in the involution of hyaloid vessels remain unclear, autophagy is thought to play a role (41). The extent of regression can be used to estimate gestation age postnatally as well (42). At 27 to 28 weeks' gestational age, the entire lens surface is covered with vessels. Between 29 and 30 weeks, the central vessels of the tunica begin to atrophy. At 31 to 32 weeks, the central lens is visible, with thinning of the peripheral vessels. Between 33 and 34 weeks of gestation, only thin peripheral vessels remain of the tunica vasculosa lentis.

The crystalline lens is the structure most responsible for adapting to the changing axial length of the eye and its subsequent influence on the refractive needs of the eye. The length of the eye increases rapidly until approximately 3 years of age, followed by slow growth of approximately 1 mm in the next 10 years. The cornea loses approximately 3 to 5 D of power by flattening in the first year of life, leaving the majority of the dioptric change necessary to maintain emmetropia to the lens. A tremendous decrease in dioptric power occurs in the first year of life. The eye's power changes from approximately 90 D at birth to 75 D at 1 year. Despite the axial growth that necessitates this change, the majority of infants maintain emmetropia.

Several authors have attempted to study the structural, molecular, and geometric changes in the lens that allow it to change in power (43–45). New epithelial cells located adjacent to the lens capsule elongate and differentiate into fiber cells throughout life. These cells produce the beta- and gamma-crystallins that make up the body of the lens. These fibers congregate in the nuclear region of the lens with increasing concentration of protein, which increases the refractive index of the lens. Lens growth occurs in two phases. Prenatally, there is a sigmoidal rapid growth rate, which generates approximately 149 mg of the lens tissue (45). This prenatal growth generates the adult nuclear core of the lens (46). Growth continues throughout life, but the growth rate becomes linear after 6 to 9 months of age, approximately 1.38 mg/year (45). There are no gender differences in the rate of growth of the lens, and the lens thickness does not differ between boys and girls regardless of age (9). There is thinning of the lens during the first three years of life due to the equatorial growth of the eye, which essentially stretches the lens (47). Consistent with this change, the anterior and posterior lens radii increase in childhood by 1.0 and 0.2 mm, respectively (44). Equatorial growth would cause passive stretching of the crystalline lens with flattening of the lens surface curvature and reduction of the lens power. Interestingly, the rates of increase of the anterior and posterior lens radii differ. The rate of increase of the anterior lens curvature slows after age 3, whereas the posterior lens curvature rate remains constant throughout childhood. These both contribute to the overall flattening of the lens. At age 6, the lens thickness varies between 3.50 and 3.60 mm depending on ethnicity (9). Hispanic children had the thinnest lenses and African-American children had the greatest thickness. In all ethnicities, the lens decreased in thickness until age 11 to 12 and then began to gradually increase in thickness.

The composition of the lens undergoes molecular changes as well. Fetal lenses have a higher percentage of gamma crystalline protein (21%) compared to adolescents (13%). Gamma crystalline proteins have excellent solubility and stability that prevent the scatter of light (48). The beta and alpha crystalline percentages are similar in childhood. In the elderly on the other hand, the alpha crystalline proportion is greater. The optical density of the lens also increases throughout life, increasing the absorption of light (49). Many proteins play a role in lens formation and in differentiation of lens cells. One of the factors found to influence lens morphology is Epha2. Epha2 is expressed by the epithelial cells of the lens and plays a role in directing lens fibers to the correct location. In the absence of Epha2, fiber cells migrated off the optical axis into new suture lines (50). Further studies will continue to elucidate the proteins involved in lens maturation leading to the possibility of influencing those pathways in the setting of pediatric cataracts.

Sclera

The sclera is predominantly an extracellular collagenous matrix. In adult eyes, the thickness varies from 0.53 ± 0.14 mm at the limbus, 0.39 ± 0.17 mm at the equator, and finally approximately 1.0 mm near the optic nerve (51). The total surface area is 16.3 ± 1.8 cm^2. The collagen in the sclera undergoes developmental changes in the early postnatal period. The sclera is four times as pliable in infants as in adults and has approximately one-half the tensile strength. This pliability explains the buphthalmos seen in infantile glaucoma with elevated intraocular pressure.

The structural changes in the sclera are due to the changing proteoglycan composition of the sclera. There are three major proteoglycans in the sclera: aggrecan, biglycan, and decorin (52). All three are increasingly expressed until the fourth decade. There is an increase in sclera thickness from 0.45 mm in neonates to 1.09 mm in adults. After the fourth decade, decorin and biglycan decrease in expression. Aggrecan has the highest concentration in the posterior sclera and continues to show high expression throughout life. The different expression rates of these proteoglycans may result in the differential growth seen in various portions of the sclera (52). For example, growth of the posterior sclera may result in increases in axial length, which will be discussed in more detail in the refractive section. Certain anatomic relationships confirm the differing growth rates. The posterior portion of the sclera shows greater growth than the equatorial portion in the early postnatal period, resulting in the apparent forward migration of the extraocular muscle insertion sites relative to the equator of the eye (53).

In a primate model, the sclera thinned in older monkeys and became more structurally stiff (54). Collagen fibers with increased stiffness oriented circumferentially around the optic nerve may contribute to the greater sensitivity of nerve fibers to intraocular pressure changes. The sclera also becomes less permeable with age (55). These structural changes arise from changes in the collagen and proteins that compose the sclera. Lumican is a keratin sulfate proteoglycan in the sclera that appears to regulate collagen fiber formation and organization. As the sclera ages, lumican interacts with aggrecan, forming a complex that becomes more abundant with age (56). In addition, glycation end products and advanced lipoxidation end products increase in the sclera with age (57).

PUPIL

Isenberg and associates found that the pupil is proportionally larger in premature infants <26 weeks' gestational age than in adults (58). The size of the pupil is controlled by the actions of the dilator and sphincter muscles of the iris innervated by the sympathetic and parasympathetic nerves, respectively. The larger preterm pupil may be the result of more rapid maturation of the dilator muscle of the iris during gestation. The pupil does not respond to light until approximately 31 weeks' gestational age (59). The presence of the pupillary response may be due to the maturation of the neural pathways at this age, given evidence for retinal photoreceptor function in younger infants (59). It may also be related to the regression of the tunica vasculosa lentis. The level of retinal illuminance, accommodative status of the eye, and sensory and emotional conditions can affect the size of the pupil as well. In addition, the pupil undergoes small, continuous oscillations called hippus which alter the size. Pupillary size decreases linearly with age regardless of gender or iris color (60). Relative atrophy of the dilator muscle compared to the sphincter muscle, iris rigidity, and decreased sympathetic tone relative to parasympathetic tone have also been postulated to cause this decrease.

RETINA

The retina forms from the walls of the optic cup during embryogenesis. The outer layer of the cup forms the retinal pigment epithelium (RPE) and the inner layer differentiates into the neuroretina. Axons of the retinal ganglion cells grow toward the optic stalk becoming the optic nerve. The neural retina is organized into three nuclear layers during development and is composed of seven major cell types: rod and cone photoreceptors, horizontal, bipolar, and amacrine cell interneurons, retinal ganglion cells, and Muller glial cells. These cells arise from common progenitor cells within the inner layer. Four main steps are required for differentiation into one of these cell types. Progenitor cells must expand through cell division, exit the cell cycle, commit to a differentiated cell type, and finally execute the functions of the differentiated cell. The molecular understanding of this process remains largely unknown, but several factors have been identified. Transcription factors of the basic helix-loop-helix (Bhlh) and homeobox families are vital in the differentiation process (61,62). The homeodomain factors regulate specificity into one of the three layers, and the Bhlh factors govern specific cell differentiation within the layer. The first cell type differentiated is the retinal ganglion cell. Growth and differentiation factor 11 (GDF11), a member of the transforming growth factor-β (TGFβ) superfamily, controls the number of each type of retinal cell created. For example, beyond Bhlh factors, expression of Math5 (atonal), shh (sonic hedgehog), and Pax6 in retinal ganglion cells is thought to be vital to their differentiation (63,64). In addition, Iroquois (irx) genes

may be necessary to the function of the shh genes further complicating this delicate cascade (65). GDF11 can downregulate Math5 expression, causing further progenitor cells to form other cell types. For example, Foxn4, Math3, NeuroD expression is involved in the differentiation of horizontal or amacrine cells (66). Amyloid precursor protein is also required for the normal development of the horizontal and amacrine cells (67). Bipolar cells rely on the expression of Chx10 and irx family and Mash1/Math3 (68). Early B-cell factors are also necessary to retinal cell differentiation (69). Several signaling pathways have been identified that are crucial to normal rod and cone development, including fibroblast growth factors (70). The last cell type created, the Muller cells, are governed by repression of Bhlh factors. Pax6 genes are also involved in establishing the nasal–temporal polarity of the retina.

Just as the retinal cells are completing differentiation, the RPE cells are simultaneously finishing development. Ninety-five percent of the RPE is formed at birth, and the remainder is complete by 7 months postnatally (71). RPE genesis begins at the fovea and extends outward. In the central retina, RPE genesis proceeds at a faster rate and for a shorter time than peripheral RPE genesis.

Within the adult fovea, there are no inner retinal layers. This architecture creates a foveal pit with the surrounding retina having the highest concentration of ganglion cells. In addition, there are no rods within 350 μm of the center of the fovea; only cones are found in this area. The neural processing in the fovea allows each cone to communicate through several bipolar cells and at least two ganglion cells. This creates the high visual acuity present in the fovea.

The fovea begins development very early in gestation, and cell division ceases by 14 weeks' gestational age. The foveal pit is appreciable by 32 weeks' gestational age due to the migration of the ganglion cells and subsequently the inner retinal layers. At term, the human fovea is immature, with a single layer of ganglion cells and an inner nuclear layer still present (72). This process of migration is not complete until 11 to 15 months postterm, which may contribute to the relatively low visual acuity of neonates. The foveal cones increase in density by becoming thinner and longer. Rods are pushed peripherally. The cone outer segments develop slowly; this process of cone maturation is not complete until 45 months postterm. The entire process of foveal maturation is not complete until 4 years postnatally. The significant postnatal development of the fovea has implications for the sensitivity in this period to amblyogenic conditions.

In premature infants, the development of the fovea can be monitored and assessed using spectral domain optical coherence tomography (72) (Fig. 2.3). Optical coherence tomography measurements of the foveal region estimate that in children the minimum thickness varies from 140.0 ± 2.3 to 161.1 μm (73,74). Macular measurements are substantially thicker, 326.44 ± 14.17 μm (75). Age and intraocular pressure did not influence macular thickness. The inner fovea was significantly thicker in boys than in girls and in

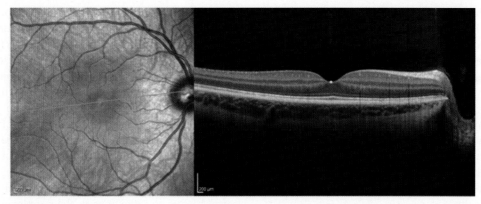

FIGURE 2.3. Optical coherence tomography image through foveal region highlighting foveal depression with lack of nerve fiber layer in fovea.

Caucasians compared to East Asian children. In amblyopic eyes, the central macular thickness may initially be greater, but then decreases by 12 years of age (76).

To evaluate the maturation of the retinal layers, electroretinogram (ERG) analysis in normal individuals at many different ages has been performed (77). ERGs can be performed with corneal, conjunctival, or skin recording electrodes with relatively equal efficacy (78). With skin electrodes though, the ERG responses are much smaller. At term, the full-field cone and rod ERG responses have smaller amplitudes and longer implicit times than adults. The amplitudes and implicit times mature rapidly in the first four months of life. Cone-mediated ERG a-wave and b-wave parameters are more mature than rod-mediated parameters (79). The dark-adapted b-wave amplitude increases with age, and the implicit time decreases. The mixed rod–cone b-wave amplitude reaches one-half maximum value by 1.2 months of age, whereas the rod-mediated responses reach one-half maximum value by 19 months of age. Maximum responses are reached by 37 months and 84 months, respectively (77,80). Oscillatory potentials are unrecordable in the early phase of the b-wave in infants, but they develop faster

than either the a-wave or the b-wave after term. The a-wave correlates with photoreceptor function and the b-wave correlates with second-order neuron maturation in the inner retina. The b-wave is much more pronounced and no a-wave is detectable at 1 month of life. A high-intensity scotopic a-wave is detectable at 3 months. At 6 months, a definitive scotopic a-wave is present. Thus, a ratio of a-wave to b-wave amplitude can be used as an index of the relative maturation of outer and inner retinal elements. The flash intensity required to achieve standard responses normalizes to adult values by 3 years of age (77). By 3 to 5 years of age, the a-wave and b-wave amplitudes and implicit times are comparable to adults (Fig. 2.4).

The reduced sensitivity of the ERG in infancy may be due to rod maturation. Rods are short and immature at birth with reduced outer segment lengths. Although the quality of infant rhodopsin has been shown to be the same as in adults, the net concentration of rhodopsin does increase with age (81). Regeneration of rhodopsin seems to proceed at a similar rate in adults and children; however, responses of temporal and spatial summation differ significantly. These rod-mediated developmental changes are thought to occur

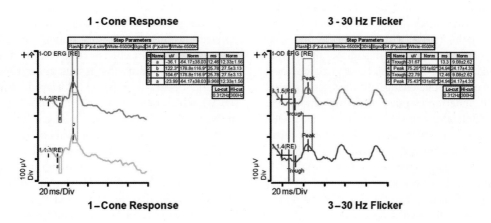

FIGURE 2.4. Electroretinogram showing normal a-wave and b-wave amplitudes in children by 5 years of age.

due to the maturation of processing central to the photo-receptors (82). The elongation of the rod outer segment in infancy is accompanied by an increase in rhodopsin content. At 5 weeks postterm, the rhodopsin content is 50% of the median adult amount (81). The number of rods in an adult retina varies from 78 to 107 million, allowing for a wide range in studies of the total rhodopsin content of an eye (83). In addition, an individual's long-term light exposure history affects rhodopsin content, such that individuals reared in bright habitats have shorter rod outer segments and less rhodopsin than those reared in dark habitats. Therefore, studies of the importance of rhodopsin content are difficult to analyze.

Rods located in different areas of the retina also have different sensitivities during testing. Maturation of the parafoveal rod outer segments (10° eccentric to the fovea) is delayed compared to rod outer segments that are 30° eccentric to the fovea (83,84). Yet, using forced preferential looking techniques and regional ERG to compare parafoveal and peripheral rod responses, Fulton and associates demonstrated concurrent maturation of rod outer segments and rod-mediated visual sensitivity.

In summary, the ERG a-wave and b-wave amplitudes and implicit times mature at different rates. They are sufficiently mature by 3 to 5 years of age to be comparable to adult values. Similarly, oscillatory potential amplitudes are comparable by 2 years of age. This standard of comparison of data can prove useful in the evaluation of retinal disease, often in the absence of visible findings in the retina. In one evaluation of children with nystagmus with no known neurologic disease or visual pathway disease, 56% of children were found to have a sensory deficit, resulting in nystagmus, on ERG testing (85).

The development of the vasculature of the retina will be discussed in the chapter on retinopathy of prematurity.

NEUROLOGIC DEVELOPMENT

The development of the neurologic connections to the eye plays a vital role in visual function. Since the landmark work of Wiesel and Hubel (86,87), there has been an awareness of a critical period of visual development. Disruption of normal visual input during this critical window, whether by ocular media opacities, refractive errors, strabismus, or other visual anomalies, results in decreased visual acuity, or amblyopia. Amblyopia induces anatomic changes in the lateral geniculate nucleus with underrepresentation and atrophy of neurons from the amblyopic eye (88). In the visual cortex, amblyopia causes a decrease in the number of binocularly driven neurons (89) and in the connectivity of the visual pathways (90). The nonamblyopic eye actively inhibits the amblyopic eye even after correction of the process that initiated the amblyopia. Research into the role of dopamine as a mediator in the reversal of amblyopia is ongoing (91). In addition, Otx2 homeoprotein may be the messenger in the visual cortex that signals the extent of sensory stimulus from the eyes in an experience-dependent fashion (92). Amblyopia and its treatment are further covered in other chapters.

Snellen visual acuity is not the only factor reduced by periods of visual deprivation in infancy. Contrast sensitivity, stereopsis, and scotopic and photopic sensitivity are reduced as well (93). These different functions are postulated to have differing critical windows of development (93). The earlier in infancy that visual deprivation occurs, the more profound is the resultant decrease in contrast sensitivity. Stereopsis, which also requires binocular function, has been shown to decrease with early visual deprivation in one eye (93). This may be due to reductions in the population of binocularly driven cortical cells or specific unidentified factors associated with stereopsis. The binocularly driven cortical cells have been shown to become almost exclusively monocular in conditions of monocular visual deprivation (94). In nondeprived monkeys, 81% of cortical neurons are binocularly driven. In contrast, only 25% of cortical neurons were binocularly driven in monocularly visually deprived monkeys. The critical window for this function was also shown to extend to 24 months of age in the monkey model (94). In addition, scotopic sensitivity was reduced in amblyopic monkeys, if visual deprivation occurred from birth to 3 months of age. The critical window for photopic sensitivity is longer, with no reduction detected if visual deprivation occurred after 5 months of age.

Another component of visual function is the interhemisphere integration of visual inputs. One study has shown that this integration occurs in humans after 24 months of age (95). Interhemispheric integration is controlled within the callosal fibers that allow the exchange of information between the left and right hemispheres. This contributes to the "bilateral advantage," which allows increased computing skills when images are presented to both hemifields compared to unilateral hemifield presentation. Another study of infants under 6 months of age reveals some transfer of visual processing of shapes between the hemispheres, but the transfer of learned visual tasks was nonexistent in children under 10 months of age (95,96). The maturation of the visual cortex is controlled by the interplay of molecular components and afferent connections in a precise spatiotemporal sequence (97). In addition, experience-dependent plasticity is incorporated into this model of maturation. With further studies, new insights may be elucidated to help in visual recovery.

Yet another entity that results in decreased visual function and occurs in infancy is delayed visual maturation (DVM), which presents as limited response to visual stimuli in the absence of ocular pathology, cortical pathology, nystagmus, or any other developmental delays. Visual behavior normalizes in these infants by 8 months of age, and when tested in later childhood is within normal ranges (98). Subsequent descriptions of DVM have included children with delays in other developmental milestones. Fielder divided DVM into three subtypes: isolated DVM, DVM associated with neurologic abnormalities, and DVM associated with ocular abnormalities (99). These differing entities have slightly different prognoses. Premature infants <37 weeks of gestation with DVM have a poorer prognosis (100). Cerebral palsy and mental retardation were found much more commonly in preterm infants with DVM than in preterm infants without DVM. Nevertheless, even in this group, 14 of 16 children had normal visual acuity when retested at 3 to 5 years of age, despite their neurologic abnormality (100). The etiology of DVM remains unknown. Studies in monkeys have shown that form vision develops in concert with basic spatial vision. Also, vision that compares local image content matures earlier than visual elements across a larger spatial extent (101). Further understanding of this type of visual processing should help elucidate the abnormalities of DVM.

ORBITAL STRUCTURES

The eyes are a dominant aesthetic feature of the face and are significantly influenced by the dimensions of the structures of the orbit. Several studies using three-dimensional analysis of the orbit have attempted to quantitate the volume and spatial dimensions of the orbit in childhood and adolescence to establish normal parameters (102). In one study, specific landmarks of the orbital region were marked on each subject with a computerized electromagnetic digitizer obtaining the three-dimensional coordinates of these landmarks (103). The exact orbital length and height, intracanthal distance, binocular width from one lateral canthus to the other, and angle of the lid fissure relative to the true horizontal plane were determined. This study revealed that the linear and angular measurements of the orbit continue to change, not only in childhood but also from adolescence to adulthood. Also, a clinically significant difference was found between male and female orbits in all age groups in the linear distances measured (Fig. 2.5). All linear differences were greater in males than in females, except for the height of each orbit. In addition, the age-related differences were more significant in male than in female subjects. For example, the binocular width increased by 4 mm between adolescence and adulthood in males and by only 1.5 mm in females. In male subjects, the greatest change in the dimensions of the orbit took place between adolescence and early adulthood, whereas

females had equally distributed changes from infancy throughout adulthood. Interestingly, the height-to-length ratio of the orbit, which grossly estimates orbital shape, was similar in both males and females despite the linear measurement differences. Farkas and associates revealed that at 1 year of age, the intercanthal width had already reached 84% of its value at 18 years of age (104,105). The intracanthal width increased markedly between 3 and 4 years of age, and reached adult values by 8 years of age in females and 11 years of age in males. The binocular width on the other hand continued to show growth, not reaching full maturation until 13 years of age in females and 15 years of age in males. By 5 years of age, the height and width of the orbit had reached 93% and 88% of their adult values, respectively, leading to the recommendation to delay final corrective craniofacial surgery in this region to 5 years of age in these children (104). With these types of measurements of the orbit, orbital surgeons can more accurately define facial relationships for any age and gender.

In another study, the orbital volume was estimated using magnetic resonance imaging (106). In the first month of life, the orbital volume was found to be 15 cm^3 in males and 13 cm^3 in females. The orbital volume of males was larger than in females at every age measured thereafter as well. The orbital volume grew in a linear pattern in both genders and reached 77% of its adult value by 5 years of age. In patients with craniosynostoses, the restriction on orbital volume loses its major effect within the first few months of life, allowing fronto-orbital advancement surgery to be delayed until the second half of the first year of life to maximize the effect of accelerated orbital growth (106). In addition, understanding normal orbital parameters allows detection of reduced distances in the front ophthalmic length and orbital diameter identifying infants in utero at risk for fetal alcohol syndrome (107).

Understanding these data can also be helpful in planning for enucleation in children. It has long been acknowledged that enucleation during childhood causes retardation of further orbital growth, resulting in facial asymmetry. Fountain and associates found that even if the orbital implant at the time of enucleation was less than 50% of the volume of the globe as an adult, orbital growth was maintained without orbital implant replacement (108). The orbital volume difference between the unaffected orbit and anophthalmic orbit was minimized in patients who used conformers, even without orbital implants (106). Newer studies even question the effect of age at enucleation on volume reduction (109). Reduction of volume is reported as continuous after enucleation, with the mechanism related to volume adaptation more than retardation of growth. In this study, even after the orbit reached adult volumes, enucleation orbital bony volume continued to diminish (109).

In addition to the orbital size and shape, the position of the eyelids relative to the pupil has a large impact on the aesthetics of the eye. The eyelids are fused until the 28th week of gestation. Gentle downward pressure with the fingers on

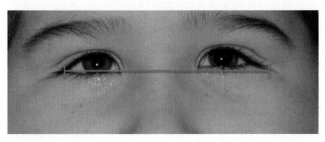

FIGURE 2.5. Binocular width increases in adolescence in males much greater than females.

the lower eyelid accompanied by gentle upward pressure on the upper eyelid will break the epithelial bridge across the lids if examination is required prior to resolution of the fusion. The upper eyelid is in its lowest position relative to the pupil in the first three months of life. Most likely coincident with the development of muscle hyperactivity in the levator or in Muller's muscle, the upper lid achieves its highest position relative to the pupil between 3 and 6 months (110). There is a gradual decrease in the lid position thereafter. In contrast, the distance between the lower eyelid and the center of the pupil linearly increases.

The upper eyelid crease is formed by the superior extension of the levator aponeurosis, which inserts on the pretarsal orbicularis. In non-Asian eyelids, the normal insertion is usually located at the superior margin of the tarsus. In a study of 33 white and African-American children, the normal upper eyelid crease was one-third the distance from the lash line to the lower brow in children 1 year of age (111). The mean distance from the lash line to the lid crease in children less than 4 years of age was 2.6 mm; in children greater than 4 years of age, it was 5.7 mm. In unilateral cases of ptosis with absent eyelid crease, a crease is created to match the contralateral eye; however, in bilateral cases, the above general guidelines may be helpful.

The palpebral fissure width, pretarsal skin height, and crease height vary by gender (112). For example, the adult palpebral fissure length was 23.5 to 29 mm in females and 24.8 and 29.1 mm in males in Caucasian eyes (113). In Asian eyelids, the average palpebral length is 26.8 ± 1.7 mm in females and 27.0 ± 1.8 mm in males horizontally, and 8.0 ± 1.0 mm and 8.2 ± 1.1 mm for males and females vertically, respectively (114). In Asian eyes, the peak level of growth in the vertical dimension of the palpebral fissure height is reached between 10 and 13 years of age. Palpebral fissure length gradually decreased with age (113). In contrast, the distance between the pupil center and the upper eyelid or lower eyelid margin did not change with age. The eyebrow height and eye crease height also remained stable during adulthood. The eyebrow height is greater in females than males at all ages.

Tear production increases with increasing gestational age. The mean total tear production was 7.4 mm by Schirmer testing in preterm infants with a postconceptional age of 32 weeks (115). This study found that total tear production positively correlated with birth weight and postconceptional age in preterm infants. In term infants, the total tear secretion increased at 2 weeks of age to 18.1 mm and by 4 weeks of age to 19.5 mm. Isenberg and associates also studied preterm infants and found a reduction in reflex and basal tearing rates, which gradually increased to reach normal levels at 40 weeks' postconceptional age (116). They found a positive correlation between increasing weight, postconceptional age, and basal tear production. Although the reduction in the aqueous tear component of the preterm infant could put the infant at increased risk of corneal damage from prolonged exposure during exams such as retinopathy of prematurity

screenings, the lipid content of the tear film was found to be much thicker than in adults and presumably protects against tear evaporation (117). The mean tear break-up time in newborns was 32.5 seconds (117). A more stable tear film with prolonged tear break-up time may also explain the prolonged staring of infants. This stable tear film arises from less methylated groups and more saturated carbon groups in the meibum composition than in adults. Infant tears also have increased aldehyde-to-lipid hydroperoxide ratio, leading to a tighter lipid–lipid barrier with reduced evaporation (118). Changes to this composition may lead to pathology in the anterior segment from an altered tear film.

REFRACTIVE ERROR

Refractive errors requiring correction are very common in developing countries. The most common refractive error is myopia. In the Ashton Eye Study group, the incidence of myopia varied by age and ethnicity (119). The incidence of myopia increased from 9.4% in children 6–7 years to 29.4% for children aged 12–13 years. In addition, South Asian children in this population had a higher prevalence of myopia than white European children, 36.8% and 18.6%, respectively (119). The incidence of hyperopia requiring refractive correction is approximately 10% to 15% (120).

In a cross-sectional study of healthy children less than 4 years old, the mean refractive error was +1.4 D with 74% of the children having no significant astigmatism (121). Ninety-five percent of these children had less than 1.50 D of anisometropia, and the same percentage had no greater than +3.25 D of hyperopia (121). In another study in which refractive errors in 514 children were prospectively evaluated, hyperopia was found to decrease with age, as did the high degree of astigmatism found in infants (122). In the majority of children, emmetropia, though, had not been achieved by 4 years of age. Myopia of greater than –0.50 D was found in only 3% of the study population of 514 children. By defining guidelines for normal refractive errors in young children, cross-sectional studies can establish reasonable guidelines for amblyopia screening programs. The American Academy of Pediatric Ophthalmology and Strabismus recommends the following refractive criteria for amblyopia screening: anisometropia > 1.50 D, hyperopia > +3.00 D, myopia > 3.00 D, and astigmatism > 1.50 D or >1.00 D if in an oblique axis (123).

Longitudinal studies of refractive error have supported emmetropization theories. One study of 1,246 children revealed a gradual decrease in refractive error from low hyperopia to emmetropia, resulting from decreased lens power and elongation of the globe as previously discussed in this chapter (43). The evidence for emmetropization lies in the non-Gaussian distribution of refractive errors in the population. Emmetropization appears to have both active and passive components. The increase in axial length, mild reduction in dioptric power of the cornea by lengthening of its radius, reduced power of the lens, and lengthening of the anterior chamber, which further reduces the effective power of the lens, constitute the passive components of emmetropization. The active mechanism of emmetropization hinges on the feedback of image clarity from the retina. The exact mechanism by which this alters growth is yet unknown (124). Many different modulators have been identified. GABA receptor antagonist given intravitreally in chicks prevented myopia development (125). In a Marmoset model, increased levels of all-*trans*-retinoic acid correlated with decreased scleral glycosaminoglycan synthesis (126). This implies that reduced all-trans-retinoic acid may contribute to the active modulation of postnatal eye growth by including changes in scleral extracellular matrix with longer axial length and myopia. In a prospective study of premature and term infants, emmetropization was found to occur by 3 years of age (127).

Animal models of myopia have been used to further evaluate the active feedback mechanism in emmetropization and the causes of ametropia. Several experimental studies have shown that distortion or opacification of visual input during development can result in myopia. Despite the effect of atropine on reducing myopia progression, muscarinic receptors have not been shown to be altered in myopia creating conditions (128). Ocular extensibility in the sclera is increased in myopic eyes with reduced levels of scleral TGFβ (129). Scleral TGFβ causes extracellular matrix remodeling, but scleral stretch is the dominative determinate of increasing the population of contractile cells in the sclera of myopic eyes.

Studies of the characteristics of children with myopia have led to several theories about the mechanical etiology of myopia. Myopia may result when either physical parameters prevent the lens from thinning appropriately or the maximum thinning allowable has occurred but cannot compensate for axial length. In fact, children with myopia in one study were found to have thinner lenses than their hyperopic or emmetropic peers (47). In another proposed passive model, myopia may result from the disassociation of the axial length and biometric lenticular parameter changes. The source of this disassociation may be due to limited equatorial growth compared to axial growth. The discontinuation of equatorial growth could stop the flattening of the lens, decrease the reduction in refractive index, or by some other factor stimulate further axial growth, which ultimately results in myopia.

Myopia is most likely to occur between the ages of 8 and 14 in the United States. Myopic eyes have a prolate shape with greater axial length than equatorial diameter (44). There are two main theories of the etiology of myopia: the genetic predisposition theory and the increased demand of near-work theory. The genetic theory is supported by similar ocular parameters and refractive errors in monozygotic twins (130). There is also an increased prevalence of myopia among children of myopic parents (131). Yet supporting the near-work theory, studies have revealed a greater incidence of myopia in populations with increased near demand and higher education levels (132). Atropine penalization to reduce the near demand has reduced myopia progression prospectively (133). The effect of greater accommodative demand has been simulated by confining animals to small chambers. This resulted in a slight myopia compared to control animals in both monkeys and cats (134). A rabbit model of scleral buckling effects on the eye demonstrated high myopia due to increased axial length in eyes with buckles (135). The axial length in this model increased for 2 weeks postoperatively and then was stabilized. Whether these animal studies are relevant to humans remains to be seen, but there is some evidence supporting the applicability.

Other factors that may be predictive of myopia development include the refractive correction in infancy. Several studies have suggested that cycloplegic refraction in early infancy may be suggestive but not accurately predictive of myopia in later childhood. Myopia in the first year of life correlated with myopia at 3 years of age (136). In early childhood, individuals with emmetropia or low myopia are more susceptible to myopic progression as they do not have a hyperopic buffer (137). Children with greater than +2.50 D of hyperopia at 11 weeks of age were less likely to become myopic at age 7 to 8.

Clearly, an early childhood refractive error is not the only factor predictive of myopia. Myopia is more common in certain ophthalmic disorders known to distort visual input. In one study, greater than 3.00 D of astigmatism was correlated with myopia (138). Even children with 1.00 D of astigmatism become more myopic with age than those children without astigmatism. It is unclear if correction of these astigmatic errors in young children would lessen the overall degree of future myopia. Other factors may play a more important role, given the high percentage (50%) of children less than 3 years old with some astigmatism compared to the lower incidence of myopia in school-age children (138). In addition, the incidence of refractive errors may also be greater in certain medical conditions. In premature infants <36 weeks of gestational age, for example, there is a higher incidence of myopia and astigmatism than in full-term infants (139,140). The etiology of myopia in premature infants is due to steeper corneas, shorter axial lengths, and shallower anterior chamber depths than in full-term infants (141). In addition, children with autism should be screened for significant refractive errors. In a large study, 40% of children with autism had significant ocular pathology, with 29% having significant refractive errors of which the majority were astigmatic (142).

In summary, there are a myriad of changes in ocular features during infancy and early childhood. It appears that these changes are highly orchestrated to result in the appearance of clear retinal images, which are then properly processed to allow vision. Other ocular development proceeds in tandem with the refractive and neurologic changes to result in growth of orbital features, in addition to the intraocular elements. Understanding these normal changes is vital to the care and management of young patients.

REFERENCES

1. Isenberg, SJ. *Physical and refractive characteristics of the eye at birth and during infancy,* 2nd Ed, St. Louis: Mosby, 1994.
2. Gordon RA, Donzis PB. Refractive development of the human eye. *Arch Ophthalmol* 1994;103(6):785–789.
3. Capozzi P, Morini C, Piga S, et al. Corneal curvature and axial length values in children with congenital/infantile cataract in the first 42 months of life. *Invest Ophthalmol Vis Sci* 2008;49(11):4774–4778.
4. Trivedi RH, Wilson ME. Biometry data from Caucasian and African-American cataractous pediatric eyes. *Invest Ophthalmol Vis Sci* 2007;48(10):4671–4678.
5. Chen TC, Tsai TH, Shih YF, et al. Long-term evaluation of refractive status and optical components of eyes in children born prematurely. *Invest Ophthalmol Vis Sci* 2010;51(12):6140–6148.
6. Musarella MA, Morin JD. Anterior segment and intraocular pressure measurements of the unanesthetized premature infant. *Metab Ped Sys Ophthalmol* 1982;8:53–60.
7. Ashaye AO, Olowu JA, Adeoti CO. Corneal diameters in infants born in two hospitals in Ibadan, Nigeria. *East Afr Med J* 2006;83:631–638.
8. Friling R, Weinberger D, Kremer I, et al. Keratometry measurements in preterm and full term newborn infants. *Br J Ophthalmol* 2004;88:8–10.
9. Twelker JD, Mitchell GL, Messer DH, et al. Children's Ocular Components and Age, Gender, and Ethnicity. *Optom Vis Sci* 2009;86:918–935.
10. Hayashi K, Hayahsi H, Hayahsi F. Topographic analysis of the changes in corneal shape during to aging. *Cornea* 1995;14:527–532.
11. Swartz T, Marten L, Wang M. Measuring the cornea: the latest developments in corneal topography. *Curr Opin Ophthalmol* 2007;18:325–333.
12. Lesueur L, Are JL, Mignon-Conte M. et al. Structural and ultrastructural changes in the developmental process of premature infants' and children's corneas. *Cornea* 1994;13:331–338.
13. Shope TR, Reig TS, Kathiria NN. Corneal abrasions in young infants. *Pediatrics* 2010;125:e565–e569.
14. Kabosava A, Azar DT, Bannikov GA, et al. Compositional differences between infant and adult human corneal basement membranes. *Invest Ophthalmol Vis Sci* 2007;48:4989–4999.
15. Muir Kw, Jin J, Freedman SF. Central corneal thickness and its relationship to intraocular pressure in children. *Ophthalmology* 2004;111:2220–2223.
16. Hussein MA, Paysse EA, Bell NP, et al. Corneal thickness in children. *Am J Ophthalmol* 2004;138:744–748.
17. Sauer A, Abry F, Blavin J, et al. Sedated intraocular pressure and corneal thickness in children. *J Fr Ophtalmol* 2011;34:238–242.
18. Heidary F, Gharehaghi R, Wan Hitam WH, et al. G. R. Central corneal thickness and intraocular pressure in Malay children. *PLoS One* 2011;6(10):e25208.
19. Moller-Pedersen, T. A comparative study of human corneal keratocyte and endothelial cell density during aging. *Cornea* 1997;16:333–338.
20. McCormick, AQ. Transient phenomenon of the newborn eye. In: Isenberg SJ, ed., *The eye in infancy,* 2nd Ed. St. Louis: Mosby, 1994;67–72.
21. Maseruka H, Ridgeway A, Tykkim A, et al. Developmental changes in patterns of expression of tenascin-C variants in the human cornea. *Invest Ophthalmol Vis Sci* 2000;41:4101–4107.
22. Kabosova A, Azar DT, Bannikov GA, et al. Compositional differences between infant and adult human corneal basement membranes. *Invest Ophthalmol Vis Sci* 2007;48(11):4989–4999.
23. Chen J, Guerriero E, Sado Y, SundarRaj N. Rho-mediated regulation of TGF-beta1- and FGF-2-induced activation of corneal stromal keratocytes. *Invest Ophthalmol Vis Sci* 2009;50:3662–3670.
24. Gordon MO, Beiser JA, Brandt JD, et al. The ocular hypertension treatment study: baseline factors that predict the onset of primary open-angle glaucoma. *Arch Ophthalmol* 2002;120:714–720.
25. Shih CY, Graff Zivin JS, Trokal LS, Tsai JC. Clinical significance of central corneal thickness in management of glaucoma. *Arch Ophthalmol* 2004;122:1270–1275.
26. Dohadwala AA, Munger R, Damji KF. Positive correlation between Tono-Pen intraocular pressure and central corneal thickness. *Ophthalmology* 1998;105:1849–1854.
27. Eisenberg DL, Sherman BG, McKeown CA, et al. Tonometry in adults and children. A manometric evaluation of pneumatonometry, applanation, and TonoPen in vitro and in vivo. *Ophthalmology* 1998;105:1173–1181.
28. Kim NR, Kim CY, Seong GJ, Lee ES. Comparison of Goldmann applanation tonometer, noncontact tonometer, and TonoPen XL for intraocular pressure measurement in different types of glaucomatous, ocular hypertensive and normal eyes. *Curr Eye Res* 2011;36:395–300.
29. Jaafar MS, Kazi GA. Normal intraocular pressure in children: a comparative study of the Perkins applanation tonometer and the penumatonometer. *J Pediatr Ophthalmol Strabismus* 1993;30:284–287.
30. Sullivan-Mee M, Pham F. Correspondence of Tono-Pen intraocular pressure measurements performed at the central cornea and mid-peripheral cornea. *Optometry* 2004;75:26–32.
31. Yildirim N, Sahin A, Basmak H, Bal C. Effect of central corneal thickness and radius of the corneal curvature on intraocular pressure measured with the Tono-Pen and noncontact tonometer in healthy school children. *J Pediatr Ophthalmol Strabismus* 2007;44:216–222.
32. Mireskandari K, Tehrani NN, Vanderhoven C, et al. Anterior segment imaging in pediatric ophthalmology. *J Cataract Refract Surg* 2011;37:2201–2210.
33. Jeanty P, Dramaix-Wilmet M, Van Gasbeke D, et al. Fetal ocular biometry by ultrasound. *Radiology* 1982;143:513–516.
34. Goes, F. Ocular biometer in childhood. *Bull Soc Belge Ophtalmol* 1982;202:159–193.
35. Yan PS, Lin Ht, Wang QL, Zhang ZP. Anterior segment variation with age and accommodation demonstrated by slit-lamp adapted optical coherence tomography. *Ophthalmology* 2010;117:2301–2307.
36. Tsai IL, Tsai CY, Kuo LL, et al. Transient changes of intraocular pressure and anterior segment configuration after diagnostic mydriasis with 1% tropicamide in children. *Clin Exp Optom* 2011;doi: 10.1111/j.1444-0938.2011.00677.
37. Palamar M, Egrilmez S, Uretmen O, et al. Influences of cyclopentolate hydrochloride on anterior segment parameters with Pentacam in children. *Acta Ophthalmol* 2011;89:e461–e465.
38. Frudakis T, Thomas M, Gaskin Z, et al. Sequences associated with human iris pigmentation. *Genetics* 2003;165:2071–2083.
39. Strum RA, Larsson M. Genetics of human iris colour and pattern. *Pigment Cell Melanoma Res* 2009;22:544–562.

40. Larrson M, Duffy DL, Zhu G, et al. GWAS findings for human iris patterns: associations with variants in genes that influence normal neuronal pattern development. *Am J Hum Genet* 2011;89:334–343.

41. Kim JH, Kim JH, Yu YS, et al. Autophage-induced regression of hyaloid vessels in early ocular development. *Autophagy* 2010;6:922–928.

42. Skapinker R, Rothberg AD. Postnatal regression of the tunica vasculosa lentis. *J Perinatol* 1987;7:279–281.

43. Zadnik K. Myopia development in children. *Optom Vis Sci* 1997;74:603–608.

44. Mutti DO, Sholtz RI, Friedman NE, et al. Peripheral refraction and ocular shape in children. *Invest Ophthalmol Vis Sci* 2000;41:1022–1030.

45. Augusteyn RC. Growth of the human eye lens. *Mol Vis* 2007;23:252–257.

46. Augusteyn RC. On the growth and internal structure of the human lens. *Exp Eye Res* 2010;90:643–654.

47. Zadnik K, Mutti DO, Fusaro RE, et al. Longitudinal evidence of crystalline lens thinning in children. *Invest Ophthalmol Vis Sci* 1998;39:120–133.

48. Zhao H, Brown PH, Magone MT, et al. The molecular refractive function of lens γ-Crystallins. J Mol Biol 2011;411:680–699.

49. Wegener A, Muller-Breitenkamp U, Dragomirescu V, et al. Light scattering in the human lens in childhood and adolescents. Ophthalmic Res 1999;31:104–109.

50. Shi Y, De Maria A, Bennett T, et al. A Role for Epha2 in cell migration and refractive organization of the ocular lens. Invest Ophthalmol Vis Sci 2011;Dec 13 [Epub].

51. Olsen TW, Aaberg SY, Geroski DH, et al. Human sclera: thickness and surface area. Am J Ophthalmol 1998;125:237–241.

52. Rada JA, Achen VR, Penugonda S, et al. Proteoglycan composition in the human sclera during growth and aging. Invest Ophthalmol Vis Sci 2000;41:1639–1648.

53. Swan KC, Wilkins JH. Extraocular muscle surgery in early infancy;anatomical factors. J Pediatr Ophthalmol Strabismus 1984;21:44–49.

54. Girard MJA, Suh JKF, Bottlang M, et al. Scleral biomechanics in the aging monkey eye. Invest Ophthalmol Vis Sci 2009;50:5226–5237.

55. Anderson OA, Jackson TL, Singh JK, et al. Human transscleral albumin permeability and the effect of topographical location and donor age. Invest Ophthalmol Vis Sci 2008;49:4041–4045.

56. Dunlevy JR, Rada AAS. Interaction of lumican with aggrecan in the aging human sclera. Invest Ophthalmol Vis Sci 2009;45:3849–3856.

57. Beattie JR, Pawlak AM, McGarvey JJ, et al. Sclera as a surrogate marker for determining AGE-modification sin Bruch's membrane using a Raman spectroscopy-based index of aging. *Invest Ophthalmol Vis Sci* 2001;52:1493–1598.

58. Isenberg SJ, Dan Y, Jotteran V. The pupils of term and preterm infants. *Am J Ophthalmol* 1989;108:75–79.

59. Robinson J, Fielder AR. Pupillary diameter and reation to light in preterm neonates. *Arch Dis Child* 1990;65:35–38.

60. Winn B, Whitaker D, Elliot DB, et al. Factors affecting light-adapted pupil size in normal human subjects. *Invest Ophthalmol Vis Sci* 1994;35:1132–1137.

61. Marquardt T, Gruss P. Generating neuronal diversity in the retina: one for nearly all. *Trends Neurosci* 2002;25:32–38.

62. Harada T, Harada C, Parada LF. Molecular regulation of visual system development: more than meets the eye. *Genes Dev* 2007;15:367–378.

63. Neumann CJ, Nüsslein-Volhard C. Patterning of the zebrafish retina by a wave of sonic hedgehog activity. *Science* 2000;289:2137–2139.

64. Ferreiro-Galve S, Rodriguez-Moldes I, Candal E. Pax6 expression during retinogenesis in sharks: comparison with markers of cell proliferation and neuronal differentiation. *J Exp Zool B Mol Dev Evol* 2011;Nov 3. [Epub].

65. Choy SW, Cheng CS, Lee ST, et al. A cascade or irx1a and irx2a controls shh expression during retinogenesis. *Dev Dyn* 2010;293:3204–3214.

66. Dyer MA, Livesey FJ, Cepko CL, et al. Prox1 function controls progenitor cell proliferation and horizontal cell genesis in the mammalian retina. *Nat Genet* 2003;34:53–58.

67. Dinet V, An N, Ciccotosto GD, et al. APP involvement in retinogenesis of mice. *Acta Neuropathol.* 2011;121:351–363.

68. Feng L, Xie X, Joshi PS, et al. Requirement for Bhlhb5 in the specification of amacrine and cone bipolar subtypes in mouse retina. *Development* 2006;133:4815–4825.

69. Jin K, Jiag H, Mo Z, et al. Early B-cell factors are required for specifying multiple retinal cell types and subtypes from postmitotic precursors. *J Neurosci* 2010;30:11902–11916.

70. Hochmann S, Kaslin J, Hans S, et al. Fgf signaling is required for photoreceptor maintenance in the adult zebrafish retina. *PLoS One* 2012;7:e30365. Epub 2012 Jan 26.

71. Rapaport DH, Rakic P,Yasamura D, et al. Genesis of the retinal pigment epithelium in the macaque monkey. *J Comp Neurol* 1995;363:359–376.

72. Maldonado RS, O'Connell RV, Sarin N, et al. Dynamics of human foveal development after premature birth. *Ophthalmology* 2011;118:2313–2325.

73. Huynh SC, Wang XY, Rochtchina E, et al. Distribution of macular thickness by optical coherence tomography: findings from a population-based study of 6-year-old children. *Invest Ophthalmol Vis Sci* 2006:47:2351–2357.

74. Zhang Z, He X, Zhu J, et al. Macular measurement using optical coherence tomography in healthy Chinese school age children. *Invest Ophthalmol Vis Sci* 2011;52:6377–6383.

75. Turk A, Ceylan OM, Arici C, et al. Evaluation of the nerve fiber layer and macula in the eyes of healthy children using spectral-domain optical coherence tomography. *Am J Ophthalmol* 2011, Oct 22 [Epub].

76. Huynh SC, Samarawickrama C, Wang XY, et al. Macular and nerve fiber layer thickness in amblyopia: the Sydney Childhood Eye Study. *Ophthalmology* 2009;116:1604–1609.

77. Westall CA, Panton CM, Levin AV. Time courses for maturation of electroretinogram responses from infancy to adulthood. *Doc Ophthalmol* 1999;96:355–379.

78. Pareness-Yossifon R, Mets MB. The electroretinogram in children. *Curr Opin Ophthalmol* 2008;19:398–402.

79. Hansen RM, Fulton AB. Development of the cone ERG in infants. *Invest Ophthalmol Vis Sci* 2005;46:3458–3462.

80. Breton ME, Quinn GE, Schueller AW. Development of electroretinogram and rod phototransduction response in human infants. *Doc Ophthalmol* 1999;96:355–379.

81. Fulton AB, Dodge J, Hansen RM, et al. The rhodopsin content of human eyes. *Invest Ophthalmol Vis Sci* 1999;40:1878–1883.

82. Fulton, AB. The development of scotopic reintal function in human infants. *Doc Ophthalmol* 1988;69:101–109.

83. Hansen RM, Fulton AB. The course of maturation of rod mediated visual thresholds in infants. *Invest Ophthalmol Vis Sci* 1999;40:1883–1885.

84. Hendrickson AE, Ducker D. The development of parafoveal and midperipheral retina. *Behav Brain Res* 1992;19:21–32.

85. Cibis GW, Fitzgerald KM. Electroretinography in congnital idiopathic nystagmus. *Pediatr Neurol* 1993;9:369–371.

86. Wiesel TN, Hubel DH. Comparsion of the effects of unilateral and bilateral eye closure on cortical unit responses in kittens. *J Neurophysiol* 1965;28:1029–1040.

87. Hubel DH, Wiesel TN. The period of susceptibiity to the physiological effects of unilateral eye closure in kittens. *J Physiol* 1970;206:419–436.

88. Wiesel TN, Hubel DH. Effects of visual derivation on morphology and physiology of cells in the cat's lateral geniculate body. *J Neurophysiol* 1963;26:978–993.

89. Wiesel TN, Hubel DH. Single-cell rsponses in striate cortex of kittens deprived of vision in one eye. *J Neurophysiol* 1963;26:1003–1017.

90. Li X, Mullen KT, Thompson B, et al. Effective connectivity anomalies in human amblyopia. *Neuroimage* 2011;54: 505–516.

91. Repka MX, Kraker RT, Beck RW, et al. Pilot study of levodopa dose as treatment for residual amblyopia in children aged 8 years to younger than 18 years. *Arch Ophthalmol* 2010;128:1215–1217.

92. Sugiyama S, Prochiantz A, Hensch TK. From brain formation to plasticity: insights on Otx2 homeoprotein. *Dev Growth Differ* 2009;51:369–377.

93. Crawford MLJ, Harwerth RS. Smith EL, et al. Keeping an eye on the brain: the role of visual experience in monkeys and children. *J Gen Psychol* 1993;120:7–19.

94. Crawford MLJ, von Noorden GK, Meharg LS, et al. Binocular neurons and binocular function in monkeys and children. *Invest Ophthalmol Vis Sci* 1983;24:491–495.

95. Liegeois F, Bentejac L, de Schonen S. When does interhemispheric integration of visual events emerge in infancy? A developmental study on 19- to 28-month-old infants. *Neurophscholgia* 2000;38:1382–1389.

96. Deruelle C, de Schonan S. Hemispheric asymmetries in visual pattern processing in infancy. *Brain Cogn* 1991;16:151–179.

97. Bourne JA. Unraveling the development of the visual cortex: implications for plasticity and repair. *J Anat* 2010;217: 449–468.

98. Cole GF, Hungerford J, Jones RB. Delayed visual maturation. *Arch Dis Child* 1984;59:107–110.

99. Fielder AR, Russell-Eggitt IR, Dodd KL, et al. Delayed visual maturation. *Trans Ophthalmol Soc UK* 1985;104:653–661.

100. Kivlin JD, Bodnar A, Ralston CW, et al. The visually inattentive preterm infant. *J Pediatr Ophthalmol Strabismus* 1990;27: 190–195.

101. El-Shamayleh Y, Movshon JA, Kiorpes L. Development of sensitivity to visual texture modulation in macaque monkeys. *J Vis* 2010;10:11.

102. Saber NR, Phillips J, Looi T, et al. Generatin of normative pediatric skull models for use in cranial vault remodeling procedures. *Childs Nerv Syst* 2011;Nov 17[Epub].

103. Ferrario VF, Sforza C, Colombo A, et al. Morphometry of the orbital region: a soft-tissue study from adolescence to midadulthood. *Plast Reconstru Surg* 2001;108:285–292.

104. Farkas LG, Posnick JC. Growth and development of regional units in the head and face based on anthropometric measurement. *Clef Palate Craniofac J* 1992;29:301–302.

105. Ozturk F, Yavas G, Inan UU. Normal periocular anthropometric measurements in the Turkish population. *Ophthalmic Epidemiol* 2006;13:145–149.

106. Bentley RP, Sgouros S, Natarajan K, et al. Normal changes in orbital volume during childhood. *J Neurosurg* 2002;96: 747–754.

107. Kfir M, Yevtushok L, Onishchenko S, et al. Can prenatal ultrasound detect the effects of inutero alcohol exposure? A pilot study. *Ultrasound in Obstetrics Gynecol* 2009;33:683–689.

108. Fountain TR, Goldberger S, Murphree AL. Orbital development after enucleation in early childhood. *Ophthal Plast Reconstr Surg* 1999;15:32–36.

109. Hintschich C, Zonneveld F, Baldeschi L, et al. Bony orbital development after enucleation in humans. *Br J Ophthalmol* 2001;85:205–208.

110. Paiva RSN, Minare-Filho AM, Cruz AAV. Palpebral fissure changes in early childhood. *J Pediatr Ophthalmol Strabismus* 2002;38:219–223.

111. Zamora RL, Becker WL, Custer PH. Normal eyelid crease position in children. *Ophthal Surg* 1994;25:42–47.

112. Price KM, Gupta PK, Woodward JA, et al. Eyebrow and eyelid dimensions: an anthropometric analysis of African Americans and Caucasians. *Plast Reconstr Surg* 2009;124:615–623.

113. Erbagci I, Erbagci H, Kizilkan N, et al. The effect of age and gender on the anatomic structure of Caucasian healthy eyelids. *Saudi Med J* 2005;26:1535–1538.

114. Park DH, Choi WS, Yoon SH, et al. Anthropometry of Asian eyelids by age. *Plast Reconstr Surg* 2008 121;1405–1413.

115. Toker E, Yenice O, Ogut MS, et al. Tear production during the neonatal period. *Am J Ophthalmol* 2002;133746–749.

116. Isenberg SJ, Apt L, McCarty JA, et al. Development of tearing in preterm and term neonates. *Arch Ophthalmol* 1998;116: 773–776.

117. Isenberg SJ, Del Signore M, Chen A, et al. The lipid layer and stability of the preocular tear film in newborns and infants. *Ophthalmology* 2003;110:1408–1411.

118. Borchman D, Foulks GN, Yappert MC, et al. Changes in human meibum lipid composition with age using nuclear magnetic resonance spectroscopy. *Invest Ophthalmol Vis Sci* 2012;53:475–482.

119. Logan NS, Shah P, Rudnicka AR, et al. Childhood ethnic differences in ametropia and ocular biometry. *Ophthalmic Physiol Opt* 2011;31:550–558.

120. Meyer C, Mueller MF, Duncker GIW, et al. Experimental animal myopia models are applicable to human juvenile onset myopia. *Surv Ophthalmol* 1999;44:S93–S102.

121. Kuo A, Sinatra RB, Donahue SP. Distribution of refractive error in healthy infants. *J AAPOS* 2003;7:174–177.

122. Mayer DL, Hansen RM, Moore BD, et al. Cycloplegic refractions in healthy children aged 1 through 48 months. *Arch Ophthalmol* 2001;119:1625–1628.

123. Donahue SP, Arnold RW, Ruben JB. Preschool vision screening: what should we be detecting and how should we report it? Uniform guidelines for reporting results of preschool vision screening studies. *J AAPOS* 2003;7:314–315.

124. Brown NP, Koretz JF, Bron AJ. The development and maintenance of emmetropia. *Eye* 1999;13:83–92.

125. Chebib M, Hinton T, Schmid KL, et al. Novel, potent, and selective GABAC antagonists inhibit myopia development

and facilitate learning and memory. *J Pharmacol Exp Ther* 2009;328:448–457.

126. Troilo D, Nickla DL, Mertz JR, et al. Change in the synthesis rates of ocular retinoic acid and scleral glycosaminoglycan during experimentally altered eye growth in marmosets. *Invest Ophthalmol Vis Sci* 2006;47:51768–51777.

127. Sharanjeet K, Norlaila MD, Chung KM, et al. Refractive status of children under the age of three years born premature without retinopathy of prematurity. *Clin Ter* 2011;162:517–519.

128. McBrien NA, Jobling AI, Truong HT. Expression of muscarinic receptor subtypes in tree shrew ocular tissues and their regulation during the development of myopia. *Mol Vis* 2009;15:464–475.

129. Jobling AI, Gentle A, Metlapally R, et al. Regulation of scleral cell contraction by transforming growth factor-beta and stress: competing roles in myopic eye growth. *J Biol Chem* 2009;284:2072–2079.

130. Minkovitz JB, Essary LR, Walter RS, et al. Comparative corneal topography and refractive parameters in monozygotic and dizygotic twins. *Invest Ophthalmol Vis Sci* 1993;34:1218.

131. Ip JM, Huynh SC, Robaei D, et al. Ethnic differences in the impact of parental myopia: findings from a population-based study of 12-year-old Australian children. *Invest Ophthalmol Vis Sci* 2007;48:2520–2528.

132. Wallman J. Nature and nuture of myopia. *Nature* 1994;371: 201–202.

133. Chia A, Chua W, Cheung Y, et al. Atropine for the treatment of childhood myopia: safety and efficacy of 0.5%, 0.1% and 0.01% doses (Atropine for the treatment of myopia 2.) *Ophthalmology* 2012;119:347–354.

134. Yinon R, Koslow KC, Goshen S. Eyelid closure effects on the refractive error of the eye in dark and in light reared kittens. The optical effects of eyelid closure on the eyes of kittens reared in light and dark. *Curr Eye Res* 1984;3: 431–439.

135. Choi MY, Yu TS. Effects of scleral buckling on refraction and ocular growth in young rabbits. *Graefes Arch Clin Exp Ophthalmol* 2000;238:774–778.

136. Ehrlich DL, Atkinson J, Braddick O, et al. Reduction of infant myopia: a longitudinal cycloplegic study. *Vision Res* 1995;35:1313–1324.

137. Edwards MJ. Shing FC. Is refraction in early infancy a predictor of myopia at the age of 7 to 8 years? The relationship between cycloplegic refraction at 11 weeks and the manifest refraction at 7 to 8 years in Chinese children. *Optom Vis Sci* 1999;76:272–274.

138. Fulton AB, Hansen RM. Petersen RA. The relation of myopia and astigmatism in developing eyes. *Ophthalmology* 1982;89:298–302.

139. Lavrich JB, Nelson LB, Simon JW, et al. Medium to high grade myopia in infancy and early childhood: frequency, course and association with strabismus and amblyopia. *Binocul Vis Eye Muscle Surg Q* 1993;8:41–44.

140. Davitt BV, Quinn GE, Wallace DK, et al. Astigmatism progression in the early treatment for retinopathy of prematurity study to 6 years of age. *Ophthalmology* 2011;118: 2326–2329.

141. Cook A, White S, Batterbury M, et al. Ocular growth and refractive error development in premature infant without retinopathy of prematurity. *Invest Ophthalmol Vis Sci* 2003;44:953–960.

142. Ikeda J, Davitt BV, Ultmann M, et al. Brief report: incidence of ophthalmologic disorders in children with autism. *J Autism Dev Disord* 2012;Feb 21[Epub].

3

Retinopathy of Prematurity

James D. Reynolds

RETINOPATHY OF PREMATURITY (ROP) is a complex disorder of the developing retinal vasculature in the immature retina of prematurely born infants. A relatively harmless and spontaneously resolving disease in the majority of affected infants, it unfortunately can threaten to cause blindness in a significant minority and even today can still result in blindness despite the best medical care.

ROP was first described in 1942 by Terry. His initial, brief report referred to this new disease as possibly a "fibroblastic overgrowth of the persistent tunica vasculosa lentis" (1). His second report was more extensive and involved several colleagues, one of whom, Messenger, formulated the descriptive term "retrolental fibroplasia" (2). Although not completely endorsed by Terry, the name stuck and the disease was known as retrolental fibroplasia (RLF) for the next 40 years. The second report, containing several pathologic specimens in the cicatricial end stages of the disease with multiple complications, clearly misinterpreted the involved pathophysiology. Terry did not recognize the retina as the source of the problem and still linked it to the rare congenital birth defect of persistence of the hyaloid artery and tunica vasculosa lentis. But he did recognize the salient epidemiology—that "some new factor had arisen" and the condition was occurring much "more frequently in infants born extremely prematurely."

Terry concluded the initial case report with an entreaty to determine the "frequency, cause, and full nature" of the condition to discover "prophylactic treatment and effective therapy." More than half a century of intense clinical and laboratory research efforts have made great strides in developing "effective therapies" for severe stages of ROP, and the understanding of the "nature" of this condition has improved tremendously. But little progress has been made in truly understanding the "cause" of this disease and even less in developing effective "prophylactic treatment." The central mysteries of this disease have not been adequately unraveled to effectively eradicate unfavorable visual outcomes.

Individuals with ROP-induced blindness are far fewer than those afflicted with blindness from macular degeneration or diabetic retinopathy. Nonetheless this is a significant disease to the affected children, their parents, and to society in general. Steinkuller and coworkers (3) analyzed child-

hood blindness in the 10 years preceding their 1999 report. They found the three leading causes of pediatric blindness in the United States were cortical visual impairment, ROP, and optic nerve hypoplasia. Cortical visual impairment results from a variety of brain insults, often in utero, and usually is associated with other global sequelae. Optic nerve hypoplasia is a birth defect in fetal development without a known cause. Neither condition presents an opportunity for treatment. Thus, the leading cause of preventable blindness in children in the United States is ROP. This ongoing problem of ROP-induced infant blindness in the United States is confirmed by the Blind Babies Foundation (4).

Expanding the scope outside the United States finds a worldwide epidemic rivaling the U.S. experience in the 1940s and 1950s. Gilbert and coworkers (5) analyzed ROP throughout the world. They divided the world into three groupings of ROP epidemiology, which correlated highly with national wealth. In high-income countries like the United States, many extremely premature infants are saved, effective ROP treatments are universally applied, and ROP-induced blindness occurs but is limited. In low-income countries like most of those in Africa, extremely premature infants simply do not survive due to a lack of intensive care nursery technology. Hence, ROP blindness does not exist. However, in middle-income countries, such as in Latin America or Asia, intensive care is available, premature infants survive, but adequate means for screening and/or treatment is not available and ROP blindness is epidemic. The World Health Organization (WHO) and various partnering agencies launched the VISION 2020 program, which targeted childhood blindness and confirmed the need for ROP services, especially in middle-income countries (6).

One such middle-income country is Vietnam. A 1-year prospective series at a single maternity hospital in Ho Chi Minh City quantified the assessment of ROP risk (7). This study demonstrated an incidence of any ROP similar to that in the United States. But the incidence of severe ROP was considerably greater, and ROP was present in larger, older babies. Unfortunately, it also demonstrated a high rate of blindness resulting from less-than-ideal management.

In addition to the quantity of the problem, the socioeconomic costs relate to the quality of the problem. Apart from the number of individuals affected, there is a qualitative difference between a lifetime of blindness and end-of-life blindness. Gilbert and Foster refer to this in terms of "blind years" and state that the worldwide number of blind years resulting from childhood blindness is similar to the quantity of blind years resulting from adult cataracts (8).

Another major socioeconomic issue relates to the form of ROP management. Our current understanding of ROP has limited any effective prevention. Treatment regimens have been limited to high technology, high skill, and high-cost interventional therapy. This makes treatment expensive in high-income countries and unaffordable in middle-income countries. This has been changing with the use of intravitreal injections of bevacizumab.

HISTORY

The history of ROP in its early years as a public health epidemic and the scientific investigation involved in the search for answers is fascinating and holds lessons that are still relevant today. This disease seemed to come from nowhere when it burst on the nursery scene in the 1940s. As noted above, it was first described by Terry (1,2). Following this, RLF developed into a full-blown epidemic, blinding 10,000 babies between 1942 and 1954 (9). A frantic search for cause and effect and potential management was initiated. The only sure fact was that RLF occurred with an alarming frequency in premature infants whose lives were being saved for the first time by new approaches to caring for such infants in technologically advanced nurseries. But investigators were beginning to suspect supplemental oxygen administration (10,11).

Jacobson and Feinstein performed a postmortem on the clinical epidemiologic research attempt to solve the RLF puzzle (9). The authors painstakingly described and analyzed a "decade of errors" in this research. Poor methodology, misleading assumptions, reliance on small sample size, empirical methods, investigator bias, lack of controls, and lack of randomization all contributed to dead ends. The story culminates in the success of the multicenter, randomized clinical trial, the National Cooperative Study, in definitively uncovering the correlation between increased exposure to supplemental oxygen and RLF (12,13). These supplementary oxygen revelations resulted in a curtailing of limitless oxygen administration in the nursery. An oxygen policy based on the least amount of inspired oxygen required for survival dramatically lowered the incidence of blind babies. But it did not eliminate them. And unfortunately, it did not minimize mortality and morbidity (14). The oxygen controversy, thought to be put to rest in 1955, still rages today. Silverman states in an editorial that "there has never been a shred of convincing evidence to guide limits for the rational use of supplemental oxygen in the care of extremely premature infants" (15).

In the last half century, in the continuing quest to answer the questions posed by Terry (1), researchers did not always learn from their mistakes. False passages illuminated by poor methodology continued to plague ROP research. Resurrection of perhaps prematurely discarded ideas came into vogue. It required the age of the multicenter randomized trial to arrive in conjunction with basic laboratory investigation to begin to characterize ROP. The rest of this chapter will concentrate on the last 25 years of ROP research, defining what is now known about Terry's "nature, cause, prophylaxis (sic), and therapy."

CLASSIFICATION

An early difficulty in epidemiologic research was the lack of a universal classification of ROP. Investigators were not always speaking the same language, meaning that important elements of the disease could go unrecognized or unappreciated. This serious impediment was removed in 1984 with the publication of the International Classification of Retinopathy of Prematurity (ICROP) (16). This was the key to opening the door to rigorous trials. Its relevance was immediately recognized, and clinicians and researchers alike embraced the classification. Its significance cannot be overstated. Overnight, the epidemiology landscape changed dramatically.

Besides providing this crucial basis for further research, the classification had another, more subtle, much less recognized but still very important benefit. The process of its development and adoption brought many of the central investigators together. It served as a model of cooperation and collaboration and paved the way for the future multicenter trials that would so define this disease. So the classification provided both the scientific foundation and philosophic approach for subsequent investigations.

The core of the classification was defining the stages of the acute disease and presenting a topographic map upon which to locate the disease in the retina. Both have major clinical significance. Staging of ROP relied upon clearly definable and observable structural changes in the retina. The stages proceeded from mildest to most severe disease and were classified as stages 1 through 4. These stages were usually easily recognized by experienced examiners utilizing the indirect ophthalmoscope, which provides the important three-dimensional picture of this disease. The stages of ROP were agreed to be the following:

Stage 1: line of demarcation
Stage 2: ridge of elevated tissue
Stage 3: neovascularization with extraretinal fibrovascular proliferation
Stage 4: retinal detachment
    4a: macula not involved
    4b: macula detached
Stage 5: total retinal detachment

More descriptively, stage 1 is a circumlinear, whitish, thin, flat line distinctly separating normally vascularized retina from as yet unvascularized retina. Stage 2 is present when this circumlinear line becomes thicker and more elevated and forms a true ridge extending out of the plane of the retina. The three-dimensional view of the indirect ophthalmoscope is crucial here. Stage 3 is extraretinal fibrovascular neovascularization. The fibrous component has a very different appearance than the neovascularization in diabetes or sickle cell disease. This neovascularization is more of a continuous sheet of solid pink tissue (Fig. 3.1). Fronds of individual vessels typical of other diseases are not seen in ROP. Stage 4 represents retinal detachment, small or large, shallow or high. The retinal detachment may be exudative, tractional, or both, but is not rhegmatogenous. Stage 5 is an addition to the International Classification used to denote a total retinal detachment, either open funnel or closed (17) (Fig. 3.2).

The topographic map of the retina devised by the International Classification is shown in Figure 3.3. It divides each retina into three zones. The goal of these divisions was to be clinically relevant, yet easily recognized. These zones are defined as follows:

Zone I: a concentric circle, centered on the optic nerve, with a radius of two times the distance from the center of the nerve to the center of the fovea

Zone II: diagrammatically a concentric annular area arising from the outer border of zone I and ending at the ora nasally and just beyond the equator temporally

Zone III: a large temporal crescent arising from the outer border of zone II and terminating at the temporal ora serrata

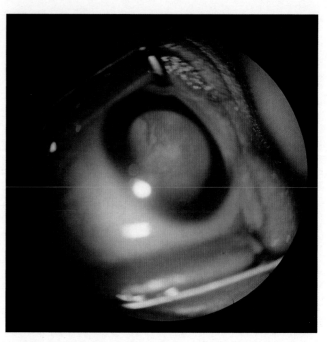

FIGURE 3.2. Stage 5 total retinal detachment with open funnel.

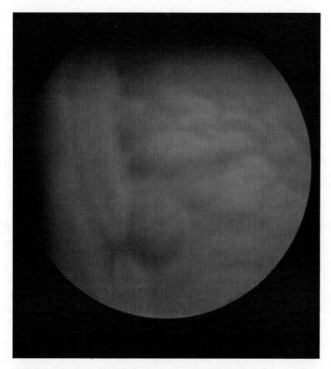

FIGURE 3.1. Typical, moderately severe stage 3 ROP. Note the continuous sheet of extraretinal, fibrovascular tissue. Even in this two-dimensional photo, the elevation is apparent. ROP, retinopathy of prematurity.

There are several very important points to understand about the location classification that have bearing on the way the natural history of this disease plays out on this topography. First, it is an arbitrary classification. The zones were picked to enhance ease of recognition. The optic nerve, macula, and nasal and temporal ora are all distinct and identifiable by indirect ophthalmoscopy. Recognition of the equator, which can be difficult, is irrelevant to the classification. Secondly, the macula is the true anatomic center of the eye, not the optic disc. But vascularization of the retina proceeds centrifugally from the optic disc to the ora. Since the optic disc is in the nasal retina, normal vessel development reaches the nasal ora first, leaving the as yet unvascularized temporal crescent. If observed at just the right moment in time, this temporal crescent can actually extend to well over 300 degrees of the peripheral retina. Thirdly, there is no defined border between zones II and III on the temporal side. Because there is no easily identifiable midperipheral landmark to use as a reference, the temporal location is defined exclusively by the relationship of the normal vessel growth or ROP pathology to the nasal ora. No matter where the real location is temporally, if the vessels have not reached the nasal ora, the location is zone I or II. If the vessels have reached the nasal ora, then the location is defined as zone III. With normal, uninterrupted vascularization, the diagrammatic representation of a concentric zone II reflects reality. But when pathology supervenes, it is possible to have temporal disease in zone II that does not physically move but becomes arbitrarily classified as zone III when nasal vascularization is less impeded by pathology. In other words, nonconcentric ROP can exist in the presence of asymmetric location of disease onset, progression, or involution.

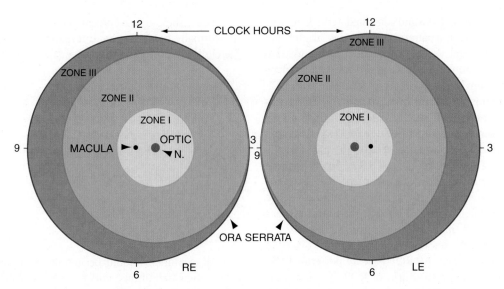

FIGURE 3.3. Schematic representation of the retinas divided into three zones, with the relevant anatomic landmarks. (Reprinted from the Committee for the Classification of Retinopathy of Prematurity: an international classification of retinopathy of prematurity. *Arch Ophthalmol* 1984;102:1130–1134. Copyright American Medical Association, 1984. All rights reserved.)

Although minor, it is a flaw in the classification that the three zones reflect the natural progression of normal vascularization but do not always accurately reflect the true location of temporal disease. A true representation would relate temporal disease to its anatomic proximity to the macula in zone II as it does in zone I. This would realistically predict its ability to impact the macula and central vision. But since temporal disease location is defined by nasal pathophysiology, temporal disease is always, at best, an estimated location. As will be shown in subsequent sections, this has an impact on natural history and screening guidelines. In summary, the location classification is grounded in normal physiology of vascularization, is easily identifiable, and is highly clinically relevant.

By convention, ROP is clinically classified by the highest stage and lowest zone. The retina is imaginarily divided into twelve equal radial segments, commonly referred to as clock hours, and this represents the extent of the disease. Disease can be present for as little as 1 clock hour or as many as 12. But the highest stage and lowest zone of just 1 clock hour determines the disease classification at that time. For example, 1 hour of stage 3, zone I and 11 hours of stage 2, zone II is diagnosed as stage 3, zone I disease.

Finally, the concept of plus disease was introduced (16). Plus disease refers to posterior pole large vessel engorgement and tortuosity. Plus disease occurs in response to a stimulation for increased blood flow. There is usually a neovascular shunt present, which itself has arisen due to ischemia signals within the retina. And plus is more likely to occur when the ROP is more posterior, possibly because the large vessels respond more to an anatomically nearer ischemic microenvironment. Along with flagrant plus disease comes vitreous haze, iris vessel engorgement, and iris resistance to mydriatics. This hemodynamic change is a threshold concept that requires a minimum degree of change before it can be termed plus. Its specific definition is:

Plus disease: posterior venous dilation and arteriolar tortuosity of at least a photographically defined minimum

But the process of developing plus disease is not all-or-none. Posterior pole vessel dilatation and tortuosity can be of gradual onset or to a level not recognized as full plus. Thus, plus disease requires the observer to make a quantifiable judgment of an inherently qualitative clinical sign. This is far different from the other portions of the classification. Stage and location are not a question of degree. Often this judgment is easy with flagrant plus disease being obvious. But borderline plus disease can be difficult. The very word borderline implies the difficulty involved. The minimum level of plus disease required has been traditionally taught to ROP examiners by way of a single standard photograph (16). It has never been put into a prose definition and never been objectively quantified. Various investigators have subdivided pre-plus changes, but they have not been widely accepted (18–20). Additional work has highlighted interobserver disagreement, variability in the nature of dilation versus tortuosity, and the potential of computer-assisted photographic modeling systems (21–24).

Another difficulty in judging plus disease is the impact that the examination has on the clinical picture. Scleral depression can impede blood flow by temporarily raising the intraocular pressure. Reduced blood flow results in reduced dilation. Prolonged examination, perhaps by multiple, sequential observers, can increase blood flow, a kind of rebound effect. Again, a crucial judgment is made more difficult and the observer must be cautious.

The ICROP II described and classified retinal detachments, as well as regression patterns of ROP. Special attention was given to peripheral versus central changes. Regression of acute ROP is synonymous with the onset of cicatricial disease development (17).

The International Classification, parts I and II, was an enormous step forward. It has an ease of use that allows reliable interobserver assignment of disease stage, location, extent, and presence or absence of plus disease. Equally important is its strong clinical relevance. The observer needs only some experience and an awareness of the above caveats.

ICROP was revisited in 2005 (25). This resulted in the addition of "pre-plus" and "AP-ROP." Pre-plus indicates a degree of vascular dilation and/or tortuosity below the minimum needed for plus disease designation. This is an important prognostic sign. AP-ROP is acute posterior ROP, and it describes an aggressive form of ROP that is rapidly progressive and is located in zone I or posterior zone II. It tends to have an earlier onset and can advance to treatable disease surprisingly quickly. This replaces the old term of "rush disease."

Subsequent subsidiary classifications have become clinically universal. These do not alter or depart from the International Classification but have added clinically relevant subclassifications. The Multicenter Trial of Cryotherapy for Retinopathy of Prematurity (CRYO-ROP) developed the concept of assigning clinical significance to a certain level of disease (26). Although arbitrary and developed as a definition to determine study intervention, the concepts proved so clinically useful that they were adopted to define the standard of care. These two ubiquitous definitions are prethreshold ROP and threshold ROP. Prethreshold was defined as a near intervention level of disease severity, and threshold, as the name implies, was a level of disease severity which triggered study intervention. These definitions are:

Prethreshold ROP: any stage ROP in zone I, stage 2 zone II plus, or any stage 3
Threshold ROP: at least 5 contiguous or 8 cumulative clock hours of stage 3 zone I or II with plus

These two concepts are ingrained in clinical parlance, and the terms are always used to mean the exact definitions above. They no longer define the standard of care for disease intervention, but they did so for 15 years.

The Early Treatment of ROP (ET-ROP) trial revisited the concept of threshold ROP and redefined a new treatment standard, replacing threshold (27). Type I ROP became the new intervention point and type 2 ROP designated pre-intervention disease. These are specifically defined as:

Type I ROP: Zone I, any stage ROP, with plus disease,
  Zone I, stage 3 ROP, without plus disease,
  Zone II, stage 2 or 3 ROP, with plus disease.
Type 2 ROP: Zone I, stage 1 or 2 ROP, without plus disease.
  Zone II, stage 3 ROP, without plus disease.

Thus, the current clinical classification system utilizes the formally agreed upon International Classification and the clinically useful modifiers over the years and includes:

Stage
Location
Extent
Pre-plus
Plus disease
AP-ROP
Regression of disease (cicatricial pattern)
Prethreshold ROP
Threshold ROP
Type I ROP
Type II ROP

All examiners should be familiar and facile with these terms, their definitions, and most important, their clinical appearance and relevance.

SCREENING AND EXAMINATION

Screening for ROP is an essential element in the management of ROP. The cardinal rule is that the patient must be examined before the patient can be treated. The cardinal sin is failing to examine the patient within the window of treatment opportunity. Appropriate screening requires not only scientific evidence to outline the screening parameters but also appropriate administrative supervision in applying those screening parameters to each at-risk infant.

An ideal evidence-based screening protocol should detect serious disease in a timely fashion, consistently, reliably, and cost effectively. It should minimize the number of examinations required and maximize the opportunity for intervention. It does not have to account for every conceivable exception. In fact, screening programs by nature must have parameters based in population statistics, not in exceptional circumstance. Risk must be reasonably defined.

Examination of the entire premature infant retina requires a well-dilated pupil and indirect ophthalmoscopy with lid speculum and scleral depression. Minimizing examinations is especially important in premature infants undergoing the stress of pharmacologic pupillary dilation and scleral depression. These tiny infants are especially medically unstable in the early weeks of ROP screening examinations. Reported complications include cardiopulmonary arrest, apnea, bradycardia, tachycardia, alterations in blood pressure, decreased oxygen saturation, inadvertent extubation, gastric reflux, and infection (28–33). In addition, unnecessary examinations add to the expense of care and may inconvenience families and expose infants to infection risk when forced to attend unnecessary outpatient examinations. Thus, ROP screening guidelines should provide for when to appropriately begin examinations, how often to examine, and when to conclude examinations. In addition, the at-risk population needs to be reasonably defined.

Screening guidelines have been developed and updated many times from many sources. These sources include single-center experience, as well as political consensus documents. Utilizing these recommendations, a reasonable conclusion as to the at-risk population would be all premature infants with a birth weight of less than or equal to 1,500 g or with gestational ages of 31 weeks or less. Keep in mind that this represents the at-risk population in high-income countries. The Vietnam series would suggest that larger, older babies are at risk in middle-income countries (7). This is probably due to differences in the standard of care available in the neonatal intensive care nurseries.

The timing of ROP screening no longer needs to rely on single-center data or consensus policy statements.

Reynolds and coworkers utilized the databases from the CRYO-ROP study (34) and the Light Reduction in Retinopathy of Prematurity (LIGHT-ROP) study (35) "to define appropriate ages and retinal ophthalmoscopic signs for the initiation and conclusion of acute-phase ROP screening" (36). The goal was to examine the infant within the window of opportunity for ideal treatment intervention while minimizing exams. An additional goal was to provide for an evolving definition of the ideal point of intervention in the disease spectrum without requiring alteration of the guidelines. Figure 3.3 shows the basic data used by the authors, and Figures 3.4 and 3.5 demonstrate the near identity of CRYO-ROP and LIGHT-ROP despite a decade of separation. This identity of disease

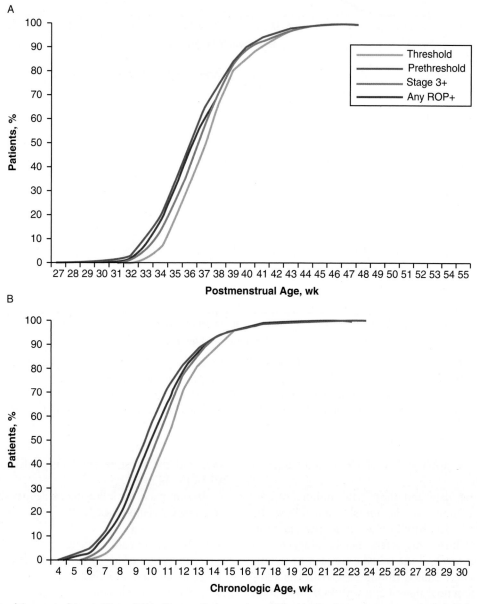

FIGURE 3.4. Timing of the onset of threshold, prethreshold, stage 3 plus, and any ROP with plus disease by postmenstrual age **(A)** and chronologic age **(B)**. ROP, retinopathy of prematurity. (Reprinted from Reynolds JD, Dobson V, Quinn GE, et al. for the CRYO-ROP and LIGHT-ROP Cooperative Groups. Evidence based screening criteria for retinopathy of prematurity. *Arch Ophthalmol* 2002;120:1470–1476. Copyright American Medical Association, 2002. All rights reserved.)

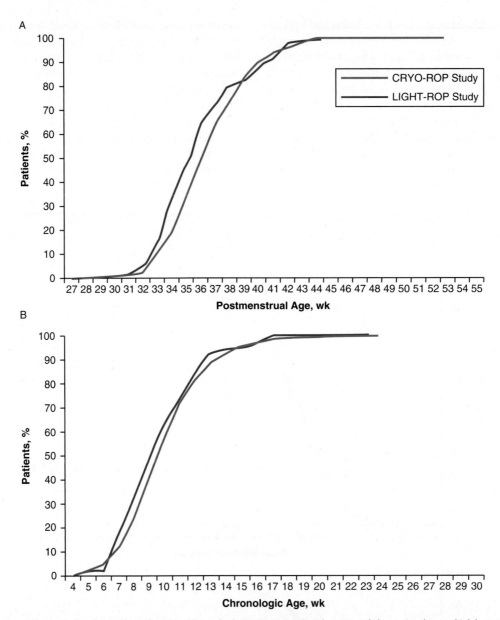

FIGURE 3.5. Timing of the onset of prethreshold ROP for CRYO-ROP and LIGHT-ROP patients less than 31 weeks' gestational age at birth by postmenstrual age **(A)** and chronologic age **(B)**. Note the nearly identical curves. CRYO-ROP, cryotherapy for retinopathy of prematurity; LIGHT-ROP, light reduction in retinopathy of prematurity; ROP, retinopathy of prematurity; (Reprinted from Reynolds JD, Dobson V, Quinn GE, et al. for the CRYO-ROP and LIGHT-ROP Cooperative Groups. Evidence based screening criteria for retinopathy of prematurity. *Arch Ophthalmol* 2002;120:1470–1476. Copyright, American Medical Association, 2002. All rights reserved.)

onset validates the applicability of CRYO-ROP data to today's situation.

Analyzing this data and more, the authors recommended that the timing of the initial exam follow the guidelines in Table 3.1. Based on accurate assessment of gestational age at birth, any infant can be plugged into the table, and the week of the initial exam can be definitively set in advance. Similar timing data, with the addition of prognostic retinal signs along with ROP involution data (37), can be used to determine a safe and appropriate time for the conclusion of screening. This work formed the foundation for the U.S. consensus paper published in

2006 and the most recent U.S. guidelines published in 2013 (38, 39, 40).

In summary, the following guidelines should determine screening for acute-phase ROP:

1. Subjects: premature infants less than or equal to 1,500 g birth weight or less than 31 weeks' gestational age
2. Screening initiation: Table 3.1
3. Screening conclusion
   a. Zone III retinal vascularization attained without previous zone I or II ROP, assuming no examiner error. If there is doubt about the zone or if the

Table 3.1

TIMING OF INITIAL EYE EXAM

Designed to Detect at Least 99% of Serious ROP

Gestational Age at Birth (Weeks)	Age at Initial Examination (Weeks)	
	Postmenstrual	Chronologic
22[a]	31	9
23[a]	31	8
24	31	7
25	31	6
26	31	5
27	31	4
28	32	4
29	33	4
30	34	4
31	35	4
32	36	4

[a]This guideline should be considered tentative rather than evidence based for 22- to 23-week infants owing to the small number of survivors in these gestational age categories.
ROP, retinopathy of prematurity.
Reprinted from Reynolds JD, Dobson V, Quinn GE, et al. for the CRYO-ROP and LIGHT-ROP Cooperative Groups. Evidence based screening criteria for retinopathy of prematurity. *Arch Ophthalmol* 2002;120:1470–1476. Copyright, American Medical Association, 2002. All rights reserved.

postmenstrual age (PMA) is unexpectedly young, confirmatory examinations may be warranted.
  b. Full retinal vascularization
  c. PMA of 45 weeks and no prethreshold ROP or worse present
  d. Definite disease regression signs in compatibly aged infants

In the section on ROP classification, a minor flaw in the system was noted that allowed temporal zone II ROP to be reclassified as zone III ROP without changing its true anatomic location. This is why the above screening conclusion guideline on zone III is qualified by excluding eyes with previous zone II ROP. These latter eyes probably represent most of the uncommon, unfavorable outcomes that occur with zone III ROP. In other words, the poor outcomes that rarely occur in zone III ROP probably had asymmetric temporal vs. nasal disease, and the nasal retina went on to vascularize while the temporal disease progressed without changing its real anatomic location. This is an important caveat for which the examiner must account.

Finally, although the initiation and conclusion of ROP screening exams in an appropriately at-risk population is now known, what about exam frequency and time to treatment? These latter two parameters are still consensus values arising from the conduct of multicenter trials. Exams are thought to be indicated every 2 weeks in infants with retinas showing stage 2 or less disease but should probably be weekly for plus or nearly plus disease, stage 3 disease, zone I disease, rapidly progressive disease, or disease occurring in an atypically young infant. Time from observation of treatable disease to application of treatment should be within 3 days.

This covers the scientific and disease-specific screening guidelines, but what of the administrative component? This is equal in importance. While the goal of evidence-based screening guidelines is to define the 99th percentile parameters, which appropriately exclude consideration of extraordinary events, the goal of the administrative component is the inclusion of 100% of the infants defined as at risk by the 99th percentile parameters. In other words, good science followed by good care. Such inclusive goals do not come easily or casually. All the interested parties must be involved in the attempt to set up a foolproof system of inclusion. Realistically no human activity is foolproof or perfect. But the goals should be set and clearly understood by all. System analysis is the operant process. It does not fall upon any nurse or any physician or any hospital employee to assure success. It is the system that is put in place, conscientiously adhered to by all, modified by the recognition and attempted correction of unforeseen events that will move toward perfection.

The involved parties include neonatologists, primary care pediatricians or family practitioners, nurses, social workers, discharge planners, ophthalmologists, quality assurance officers, clerical workers, and parents. Residents and fellows may also play a role but are appropriately peripheral in responsibility. No single party should accept full responsibility for ensuring inclusion. That is a recipe for disaster without checks and balances. Work as a team, institute the above scientifically based screening protocol, identify responsibilities and responsible parties, monitor progress, utilize system analysis, document the progress, communicate, and finally imbue all concerned with a sense of dedication and determination. The cost of failure is high, in more ways than one (40).

A useful mnemonic summarizes the above:

Delineate responsibility
Develop a process
Discuss frequently with all
Document the entire process
Do it

INCIDENCE

The prevalence of blindness from ROP in the United States appears to be growing despite effective treatments for severe ROP (3,4). The incidence of worldwide ROP blindness is unquestionably on the rise (5). But this could be related to a rise in the number of surviving premature infants and not to a change in the actual incidence or severity of ROP.

Several advances for the care of prematurely born infants have been instituted in neonatal intensive care units in high-income countries. These include surfactant administration, antenatal steroid use, pulse oximetry monitoring, improved nutrition, and others. Have these improvements in systemic care or other, as yet unknown, factors contributed to a change in incidence and severity of ROP as opposed to the prevalence of ROP blindness?

Some studies have suggested at least some type of decrease in ROP. However, these reports have serious flaws. The Vanderbilt experience compared 1995–1996 numbers with the years 1986–1987, when they were part of CRYO-ROP (42). It can be seen that the baseline years of 1986–1987 in Vanderbilt had threshold rates of 19% as compared with overall CRYO-ROP rates of 6%. The 1995–1996 numbers are much closer to both CRYO-ROP and LIGHT-ROP. Although the incidence of threshold ROP went down dramatically in Tennessee, the decrease was from an isolated exorbitant rate to a typical national rate. This study does not prove a decrease in incidence. Rather it proves the aberrations to which single centers with small numbers of babies are prone (43).

A study from an Australian center comparing data between 1988–1991 and 1991–1994 is subject to the same flaws (44). The threshold numbers were 25.0% versus 9.7%, respectively. The first number is extreme, and the second is still higher than the multicenter experience in the United States. This is also probably single-center aberration, but perhaps this is reflective of Australian nursery practices approaching U.S. standards. Conversely, a Danish study found no difference in ROP in high-risk infants (45). Termote and coworkers (46) reported a decrease in ROP in all patients, but an increase in those smaller than 1,000 g at birth.

No independent body of literature has addressed the effects of the previously noted medical advances on ROP incidence except for surfactant use. The prophylactic and therapeutic administration of exogenous surfactant to newborn premature infants has had a dramatic impact on lung disease and survival. Surfactant administration theoretically could increase severe ROP by increasing survival of low-birth-weight infants, decrease ROP by improving the general health of these infants, or impact ROP in other as yet unknown ways. Early studies found conflicting results.

The evidence now seems clear that surfactant administration does not reduce either the incidence or severity of ROP. In a study by Repka and coworkers (47), infants from two CRYO-ROP centers were evaluated in a randomized trial with prospective, serial eye exams. No difference in ROP outcome was noted. With this evidence, the authors postulated that the absolute number of babies with threshold ROP will raise as survival improves and birth-weight-specific incidence of ROP remains the same. Holmes and coworkers (48) also failed to find a statistically significant difference in their randomized trial.

The best way to assess the incidence and severity of ROP over time is to compare multicenter randomized trials. Despite technologic and medical advances in the intervening years, it appears that the rates of ROP are very similar. The CRYO-ROP study enrolled and followed 4,099 patients. Of those, 2,699 (65.8%) developed at least some ROP, 731 (17.8%) developed at least prethreshold ROP, and 245 (6.0%) developed threshold ROP (49). The LIGHT-ROP study enrolled and followed 361 patients. Of those, 251 (69.5%) developed at least some ROP (although only 202 developed the study's minimum definition of at least 3 clock hours of confirmed ROP), 52 (14.5%) developed at least prethreshold ROP, and 18 (4.9%) developed threshold ROP (35). These two studies were conducted in 1986 through 1988 and 1995 through 1997. Table 3.2 shows that even though the enrollment periods were separated by almost a decade, the incidence and severity of ROP is very similar.

What of the more recent Early Treatment for Retinopathy of Prematurity (ET-ROP) randomized trial? Since this was a treatment trial that impacted the incidence of threshold, threshold ROP cannot be used for comparison. But the rate of prethreshold ROP could be used for comparison purposes (27). Utilizing these comparisons, the incidence and severity of ROP were very similar in all three multicenter trials. The one area of sizable difference is in the incidence of zone I disease. ET-ROP had a much higher incidence of zone I disease. While that may represent a true epidemiologic shift, it could also be at least partly explained by the differences in methodology as well as observer bias (50).

It seems safe to conclude that ROP remains a major health issue. The knowledge that ROP rates remain stable despite improvements in neonatal care has a major impact

---

Table 3.2

INCIDENCE AND SEVERITY OF ROP

CRYO-ROP vs. LIGHT-ROP

Patients	4,099	361
Any ROP	2,699 (65.8%)	251 (69.5%)
Prethreshold	731 (17.8%)	52 (14.4%)
Threshold	245 (6.0%)	18 (4.9%)

CRYO-ROP, cryotherapy for retinopathy of prematurity; LIGHT-ROP, light reduction in retinopathy of prematurity; ROP, retinopathy of prematurity.

on the continuing need to be vigilant in screening for this condition. The knowledge that it continues to be a major contributor to childhood blindness despite current interventions is a major reason to continue the unfailing investigation into the basic pathophysiology of ROP and its prevention and treatment.

NATURAL HISTORY AND PROGNOSIS

ROP has traditionally been divided into an acute phase and a cicatricial phase. The acute phase is the period of development and progression of the stages of ROP in ICROP. At some point the disease progression slows and stops, and a transitional period of disease involution or regression occurs. The cicatricial phase begins when the acute phase ends and what could be paraphrased as the regression or scarring phase begins. Most times this scarring phase is clinically insignificant, represented by permanent but minor or subtle changes in the peripheral retina. But occasionally acute fibrovascular severe ROP produces significant scarring and traction, which can ultimately lead to tractional retinal detachment with a fibrous or membranous component. This serious development is usually the definition for which cicatricial disease is reserved. The minor peripheral scarring is appropriately thought of simply as a regression pattern (17).

Attention will be focused on the natural history of acute disease. The empirical knowledge gained from experienced observers added much to the understanding of this disease. But it is the multicenter trials, especially the CRYO-ROP study, on the foundation of ICROP, that have contributed so much epidemiologic science to the understanding.

The primary relevance of the CRYO-ROP study was its proof of the efficacy of cryotherapy in reducing unfavorable anatomic and visual outcomes in severe ROP. But an amazing secondary benefit from this study is the wealth of natural history data and analysis that it produced. It is a testament to the participants in this study that so much has been published on this. The control population and nonrandomized patients have contributed more to the clinical understanding of this disease than the treatment arm (51).

The natural history of a disease is the natural history of a population. It is the defining of the range of potential behaviors. It is governed by the rules of population statistics, i.e., bell curves, standard deviations, etc. As such, it can accurately determine the behavior of the disease in an entire group. But it is difficult to apply such statistics in individuals. Population statistics can predict what an individual's course may be, but the prediction can be right or wrong. Essentially one can predict how likely an individual patient is to behave in a certain pattern. But the exceptional circumstance is by definition not the likely course. Experienced examiners recognize ROP as a disease of individual surprises, and prediction for the individual is imprecise.

For all its twists and turns, ROP is a disease that proceeds acutely in a linear fashion. The ROP screening guidelines are a direct result of this. A major finding of CRYO-ROP was the relation of ROP onset to retinal maturity (49). ROP has always been viewed as resulting from a complex interplay of forces set in motion by exposure of the premature retina to the extrauterine environment. But the length of exposure to this environment, the chronologic age of the infant, is less correlated with ROP onset and progression than the corrected age of the infant, the postgestational age or PMA. The pathophysiologic reasons for this are discussed at length subsequently, but inherent activity in the retina determines the timing of disease expression. Put another way, the youngest infants at birth develop ROP at a later chronologic age, and the infants with the oldest gestational ages at birth develop ROP at an earlier chronologic age. For example, most infants who develop threshold ROP do so between 36 and 38 weeks' postgestational age whether they were born at 25 weeks' gestation and are more than 10 weeks old or they were born at 30 weeks' gestation and are only 6 to 8 weeks old.

We also know many of the prognostic factors in ROP. The specific ROP factors that CRYO-ROP authors considered prognostic were zone, plus disease, stage, circumferential extent of neovascularization, and one not implied above, the rate of progression (49). But these five are not all equal. The presence or absence of plus disease and the presence of zone I disease seem to trump all others (52). The greatest risk of poor outcome was zone I threshold ROP. The unfavorable visual outcome in those patients was close to 90% whether treated or not (53).

The results from the ET-ROP trial essentially confirmed the opinions which arose from CRYO-ROP data analysis (27). Zone I disease and plus disease are the major drivers of unfavorable outcomes. One major difference in the statistics between CRYO-ROP and ET-ROP is appropriately part of the natural history discussion. Zone I disease was found to be much more common in the ET-ROP population and followed a more benign course. The ET-ROP authors appropriately pay special attention to this. They note that it could represent a true change in the natural history of this disease, but more likely it represents observer bias. The heightened knowledge of the importance and relevance of zone I disease to ROP management in general and ET-ROP in particular altered the observational criteria of examiners between CRYO-ROP and ET-ROP. It may represent no more than an excellent example of how even carefully trained and/or instructed study participants can bring their bias to bear.

The natural history of regression or cicatricial disease is less well understood but involves fibrovascular proliferation, contraction, scarring, pigmentary changes, and permanent traction. The CRYO-ROP study again developed a simple but useful way of evaluating cicatricial disease. They used a macular scoring (MS) system, on the premise that the degree of macular damage was the most clinically relevant cicatricial event. They did not classify other changes noted by ICROP II. They classified tractional damage as follows:

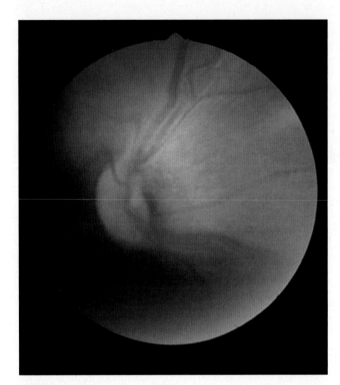

FIGURE 3.6. Macular heterotopia.

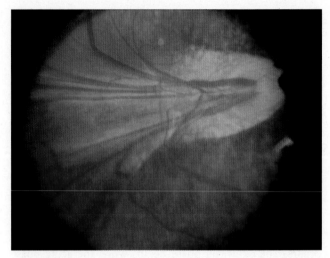

FIGURE 3.7. Macular fold.

MS 0: normal macula
MS 1: macular heterotopia (Fig. 3.6)
MS 2: macular fold (Fig. 3.7)
MS 3: macular retinal detachment

In the presence of normal brain function, a normal macula means normal vision, and a retinal detachment including the macula means very poor vision (54). But macular heterotopia and macular folds yield a surprisingly wide range of visual acuities (55).

RISK FACTORS

Risk factors can be divided into several categories including epidemiologic population, systemic, ambient environment, and retinal signs. The latter are really prognostic natural history signs and were dealt with in the preceding section.

The overwhelming risk factors are birth weight and gestational age at birth. The lower the birth weight and the younger the gestational age, the greater the risk of both mild and severe ROP. In the CRYO-ROP study, for example, the risk of developing prethreshold ROP for the entire population of infants less than 1,251 g was 17.8%. But divided by 250 g increments, the rates were: 1,000 to 1,250 g (equaled 7.3%); 750 to 999 g (equaled 21.4%); and less than 750 g (equaled 39.4%). Gestational age breakdowns were equally impressive. This was true across all subcategories of ROP (49). An additional risk factor in CRYO-ROP was white versus black race (20.5% vs. 13.1% prethreshold).

Over the years many other risk factors have been associated with ROP. McColm and Fleck (56) have reviewed and referenced many of these. Many of those risk factors were reported in single-center studies with small sample sizes and poor controls, utilizing historical and nonrandomized data. Such purported risk factors are not necessarily erroneous but certainly require rigorous confirmation. One of the confounding issues with the epidemiologic investigation of ROP is that it occurs in very sick babies. Their survival may be tenuous, they have multisystem failures, and they are kept alive by vigorous and varied interventions. It is difficult to isolate ROP within this milieu of multiorgan illness and multisystem support. Establishing adequately matched controls is a challenge.

An attempt to assess risk factors with adequately matched controls was reported by Biglan and coworkers (57,58). The group matched an ROP cohort to a no-ROP or minimal-ROP cohort, each with chronic lung disease, an indicator of how sick a baby gets. Although retrospective and from a single center, this attempt at controlling for a baby's acuity of illness level found very few differences between the two groups and hence very few risk factors. The authors suggested many previously reported risk factors were risk factors for severity of general illness level and not ROP. Risk factors that were found were the expected higher levels of inspired oxygen and longer duration of supplemental oxygen. In addition, two other markers of level of illness were also correlated: seizures and intraventricular hemorrhage. A logistic regression analysis by Hammer and coworkers (59) also found the expected oxygen duration risk factor and little else. These two trials, near the end of the single-center era of ROP, approached risk factors in a rigorous epidemiologic fashion and basically confirmed oxygen supplementation as a risk factor, as well as an increased level of general illness. In fact, in a somewhat facetious paraphrase of this reality, Enzenauer (60) noted that ROP correlated with the "smallest and sickest" and speculated that it would also correlate with the weight of the babies' charts.

The ever-present risk factor of oxygen deserves special consideration. All concerned appreciate that oxygen is involved in the pathophysiology of ROP. But how? In what way is it a risk factor? Is timing of administration important? Are fluctuations important? How does the fraction of inspired oxygen (FIO_2), arterial oxygen concentration (PaO_2), transcutaneous monitoring (TcO_2), or oxygen saturation by pulse oximeter relate to retinal tissue oxygen tensions and ROP?

Oxygen was linked to ROP when the work of Patz and the cooperative trial of Kinsey demonstrated that ROP was related to the administration of supplemental oxygen (11,13). This was confirmed repeatedly, but always with duration or with FIO_2, not PaO_2, a supposedly closer approximation to tissue oxygen. Flynn and coworkers (61) finally demonstrated a connection with PaO_2 utilizing TcO_2.

But the debate on the role of oxygen continues. In a dramatic role reversal, the theory that oxygen administration might actually help ROP, at least in its severe acute phase, was resurrected. Interestingly, this concept had been addressed in 1952 as part of the original search for RLF's cause (62). Even more enlightening, the Jacobson and Feinstein review (9) mentioned earlier as addressing the pre-Kinsey study activity ridiculed this concept. But Phelps and Rosenbaum (63) noted a positive effect on serious ROP in animals when the FIO_2 was raised. Gaynon (64) noted similar effects in humans. This led to the Supplemental Therapeutic Oxygen for Prethreshold Retinopathy of Prematurity (STOP-ROP) trial. Unfortunately this study failed to find a definitive therapeutic benefit for oxygen supplementation (64). However, the concept of oxygen manipulation is not dead. Other work has rekindled this idea (66–69).

Another risk factor that fueled a hot debate was ambient light exposure. Discussed as early as 1949 and 1952 (70,71), this debate returned with a vengeance following the 1985 work of Glass and coworkers (72). Supported by some but disputed by others, this question required another multi-center trial to answer (73–75). The LIGHT-ROP study definitively found that ambient light reduction had no impact on ROP (35,76).

Vitamin E supplementation also has been considered and hotly debated, but this is covered in the later section on treatment.

PATHOGENESIS

Recent investigation has shed considerable light on the basic pathogenesis of ROP. Although a cellular understanding of ROP is still lacking, much is known about what is happening at the tissue level. Proper understanding of pathogenesis requires a rudimentary knowledge of normal embryology and physiology of the retina. Not surprisingly, these two paths are deeply intertwined.

Blood supply of the mature retina comes from two distinct sources. The choroidal circulation supplies the outer retina, and the retinal circulation supplies the inner retina.

For example, a central retinal artery occlusion destroys the electroretinogram's b-wave, which arises from the inner retina but leaves the a-wave, generated from the photoreceptors, intact. Embryologically the choroidal circulation is complete prior to 20 weeks' gestational age and therefore prior to survivable premature birth. But the retinal circulation arising from the optic nerve head is just beginning to develop a vascular bed at this time. It is the retinal circulation that is intimately involved with ROP pathogenesis.

By definition, angiogenesis is the formation of endothelial-lined blood vessels. Arteriogenesis is the addition of smooth muscle cells that together with endothelium forms intact arterioles. Vascularization is the new arterialization of a tissue, and vasculogenesis is reserved for the formation of the vascular system, typically embryonic (77). Thus, vasculogenesis of the retinal circulatory system involves the formation of vessels, angiogenesis and arteriogenesis, and the spread of those newly formed vessels throughout the retina, vascularization.

Angiogenesis can occur in different patterns within mammalian systems. In humans, three patterns coexist. The primary pattern in fetal development at least in zone I is via differentiation (78). A primitive mesenchyme spreads over the retina in a centrifugal fashion, originating at the optic nerve. These mesenchymal cells form angioblasts which mature into endothelial cells. These endothelial cells then coalesce into vessels. Periendothelial cells or pericytes add the smooth muscle. This peripherally advancing vascularization requires about 20 weeks of development, reaching the temporal ora at 40 to 42 weeks' gestational age.

The fetal vasculogenesis process is under the control of various factors. The molecule most discussed and widely investigated is vascular endothelial growth factor (VEGF), which is constructed by highly regulated VEGF mRNA (79–82). But this is not the only vasoactive element. VEGF itself comes in several different isoforms (83) and acts in concert with insulin-like growth factor 1 (84–86), basic fibroblast growth factor, and transforming growth factor (77). These various molecules create a complex cocktail of cytokines. Finally, changes in the extracellular matrix are an integral part of regulated cell migration and assembly (87–90). This entire process occurs simultaneously with the development of the structural and functional cells of the retina, some of which undoubtedly interact with the vasculogenesis process, e.g., astrocytes (91–93).

The development of the cellular elements of the retina follows a rigid time schedule in fetal life. It is a system designed to be fully active at or near term gestation. The last trimester is the period in which functional activity of the retina develops. Prior to 32 weeks, the photoreceptors and other cells are minimally electrically active, the retina is thin and immature, retinal metabolic demand is low, and the entire retina's nutrient requirements, both outer and inner, are supplied by the choroid. But on or about 32 weeks, the retinal cells establish connections, begin major metabolic activity, and mature rapidly. The choroid can now only supply the photoreceptors, and the inner retina begins to rely on the developing retinal circulation more and more. This is all evidenced by both anatomic studies and functional electroretinogram and visually evoked response testing (94–98). So anatomic development and a fully functional metabolism are perfectly and rigidly timed to coincide with retinal vasculogenesis.

VEGF production, and that of other regulatory cytokines, are themselves regulated by hyperoxia, normoxia, and hypoxia. The retina is incapable of significant hypoxia prior to the increasing oxygen requirements of very actively metabolizing cells. This connection among vasculogenesis, retinal maturation, and retinal metabolic demand, first hypothesized by Ashton and coworkers (99), interacting with the physiologic perturbations set in motion by premature birth explains the homogeneity of timing of ROP in relation to postgestational age noted in CRYO-ROP (49).

The pathogenesis of ROP begins with premature birth. Exposure to the extrauterine, technologically supportive environment coupled with the inability of the immature lung-oxygen delivery system to adequately supply the needs of the developing retina is the true cause of ROP. The pathogenesis of ROP can be divided into two phases. Phase I is the initial reaction following premature birth and is called the hyperoxia-vasocessation phase. Phase II is the hypoxia-vasoproliferation phase. Phase I is extremely common and ultimately harmless, but phase II can be anatomically and visually threatening. Although these phases are sequential, it is a mistake to think of the pathophysiology as linear. There may be extremely variable retinal oxygenation, especially in the unstable, extremely immature infant. Hyperoxia and hypoxia probably occur in many varied cycles. But for simplicity, they can be considered as single sequential events.

Phase I begins immediately after birth. The in utero retinal microenvironment is habituated to mixed venous blood and its lower PaO_2. At birth, mixed venous blood is transformed into arterial oxygenation levels by the switch from placental oxygenation to lung oxygenation. This alone does not necessarily create an immediate hyperoxic state. The immature lung does not oxygenate efficiently, and the medical response of increasing the FIO_2 and/or utilizing ventilatory support does produce an initial relative hyperoxia. This relative hyperoxia is reinforced by the low metabolism of the retina in very immature infants. This failure to utilize oxygen aids in keeping the initial tissue oxygen tension high.

This relative retinal hyperoxia results in downregulation and diminished production of VEGF. Retinal angiogenesis and retinal vascularization are impaired and vasocessation occurs. Kretzer and Hittner (100) failed to find any evidence of endothelial cell breakdown, which would be present if mature vessels and their endothelial cells were obliterated at the interface. Normal endothelial cell apoptosis would not produce the same degree of very localized endothelial destruction. So vasocessation seems logical and compatible with the evidence.

Phase I then may recede without incident. A more appropriately physiologic state may be achieved, VEGF may be produced in appropriate amounts, normal vasculogenesis is reestablished, and ROP either does not develop or mild ROP regresses and the retina is successfully vascularized. But phase II may supervene.

In phase II, the lungs become damaged and even more unable to oxygenate the blood properly, retinal metabolic demand rises precipitously, and this combination of poor supply and increased demand creates a relative tissue hypoxia. It is easy to understand how this process would be exacerbated in the most ill infants. A return to room air is not the essential element in retinal tissue hypoxia. Weaning high FIO_2 is universal, but only the sickest babies get ROP. A lower FIO_2 may contribute, but it is far too simplistic. VEGF is now upregulated and the vasculogenic system responds. But why doesn't the system respond normally and develop normal vessels? Why does an abnormal fibrovascular component develop? Is it just VEGF gone wild? Or is there an additional cellular component(s)? It is probable that there are other complex factors at work. Oxygen cytotoxicity, either directly or via free radicals, is a possibility, although there is little real evidence beyond speculation for this. It seems likely that increased levels of VEGF act upon somehow abnormal vasoformative elements, either mesenchyme or angioblasts, or perhaps damaged astrocytes or the extracellular matrix contribute. These abnormal elements respond to VEGF by forming abnormal fibrovascular tissue, i.e., neovascularization or stage 3 ROP.

The correlation with ROP onset and gestational age that was discussed in the natural history section has everything to do with the relative retinal hypoxia that can only be produced by poor supply coincident to all the changes wrought by premature birth and exacerbated by the normal increase in retinal metabolic demand, which is rigorously timed by embryologic exigencies. It is not just exposure to a harsh extrauterine environment. It is not just oxygen alternations. It is environment superimposed on the timing of retinal developments.

In summary, the phase I/vasocessation phase is very common in extremely low-birth-weight infants. It can be followed by phase II/revascularization if normal physiology prevails or phase II/vasoproliferation if abnormal physiology triumphs. All of this is mediated by VEGF and other cytokines being down- or upregulated by relative changes in tissue oxygenation levels determined by an interplay of supply and demand on possibly cell-damaged vasoformative elements. If these events are not purely linear but are cycled, as is likely, there is an even greater chance of serious ROP development (101,102).

MANAGEMENT

Management of ROP implies more than just treatment, and indeed there is much more involved with the management of this disease than just treatment intervention. One can divide ROP management into four basic categories: prevention, interdiction, correction, and mitigation.

Prevention involves any means by which ROP may be prevented. Interdiction implies an intervention aimed at halting the progress of ROP. Correction is involved with treatment of cicatricial or end-stage ROP after the acute disease has run its course. And last, mitigation involves appropriate management of all the associated sequelae of ROP, including blindness. Such a broad approach to management will necessarily involve a large variety of professionals, but the ophthalmologist, especially the pediatric ophthalmologist, should be involved in every step—making decisions, aiding and advising decision making, and ensuring proper referrals.

Prevention

The ideal answer to the problem of ROP is complete prevention, and the single best way to achieve that is the prevention of premature birth. The number of premature births is staggering. In 2002 a stable 1.45% of births were very-low-birth-weight infants, i.e., birth weights less than 1,500 g. This means well over 50,000 infants of 1,500 g or less are born annually in the United States (103). All of those survivors are at risk for ROP and require screening. Support of the actions aimed at improving both access to prenatal care and improved obstetric care, via social programs and research, is an appropriate course of action. Reducing ROP in this fashion has the huge advantage of also reducing the other developmental disabilities associated with premature birth. From a public health perspective, this has a large return on investment.

Currently the next best option in preventing ROP is idealized intensive care. As noted previously in this chapter, many of the advances in intensive nursery care have not resulted in diminished ROP. However, as also noted, a rigorous evidence-based approach to infant oxygenation has never been developed. It may be possible, as an outcome of a large, randomized trial, to identify optimal ranges of oxygen saturation that would maximize survival and minimize ROP, cerebral palsy, and developmental disabilities.

Finally, less ideal for the whole patient but still preferable as ROP management is the prevention of ROP itself. This effort has so far been a complete failure. Two major previous attempts at preventing the development of any ROP and/or severe ROP centered on ambient light reduction and pharmacologic vitamin E supplementation. The role of light was discussed in detail in the section "Risk Factors." In short, the LIGHT-ROP cooperative trial found no benefit from ambient light reduction on ROP (35).

Vitamin E supplementation has also had a controversial past. Vitamin E is one of several antioxidant elements involved in normal physiology. One of its purported values is to neutralize free radicals. Acting on the premise that oxygen cytotoxicity, either directly or via free radical production, is an inherent part of the pathogenesis of ROP, vitamin

E supplementation was theorized to be able to prevent or reduce such cytotoxic actions (96). Unfortunately, several randomized clinical trials of pharmacologic doses of vitamin E, as opposed to normal physiologic dose supplements, were contradictory (103–107). Few nurseries have instituted pharmacologic vitamin E protocols (108).

Inositol supplementation in formula may influence ROP. Inositol and phosphoinositides have multiple metabolic actions (109). Hallman and coworkers (110) initially noted a connection between serum inositol concentration and ROP. Detected from a subanalysis of a more global randomized neonatal study, the observation was followed up by subsequent, more focused series (109,111). Again conflicting results were obtained, and no consensus has been reached. A multicenter trial is probably necessary for a definitive answer.

Interdiction

Treatments aimed at interrupting the progression of ROP are currently the mainstay of ROP management and are centered around peripheral retinal ablation with either cryotherapy or laser photocoagulation. The theory behind peripheral retinal ablation is as follows. Applying cryotherapy or laser photocoagulation anterior to the ridge, in nonvascularized ischemic retina, kills the ischemic cells producing the regulatory signals for VEGF production as well as killing the producers of VEGF. This dual effect significantly lowers VEGF (112) and leads to ROP involution rather than progression. Two multicenter randomized clinical trials have fixed the standard of care for this type of intervention. CRYO-ROP was, of course, the landmark study that proved the efficacy of cryotherapy and set the standard for the first widely accepted and instituted interdictory therapy for ROP (26). ET-ROP was a subtle but meaningful refinement of treatment indications for peripheral retinal ablation, although an extra benefit was providing a more recent assessment of overall success rates for this treatment when applied in its now most common method, i.e., laser photocoagulation rather than cryotherapy (27).

The results of CRYO-ROP have been republished so many times in so many venues that repeating them here is redundant. But briefly, cryotherapy applied to the peripheral retina anterior to the fibrovascular ridge of neovascularization when threshold ROP had been reached reduced the unfavorable anatomic outcomes by almost one-half and reduced the unfavorable visual outcomes by almost one-third (113). The difference between anatomic and visual outcomes is notable. This primarily relates to nonocular or subtle ocular differences that can make a significant visual impact (53).

Besides the message of efficacy, there are two important caveats regarding the CRYO-ROP primary results. First, despite application of cryotherapy according to protocol, unfavorable outcomes still occurred in a sizable minority. Second, cryotherapy was proven effective for zone II threshold

ROP, but zone I threshold had a very poor response to protocol treatment, with an unfavorable outcome rate of nearly 90%.

During the decade following the publication of CRYO-ROP results, treatment evolved in two ways. Laser photocoagulation slowly gained widespread predominance over cryotherapy as a retinal ablative technique, and intervention earlier in the course of serious ROP was increasingly utilized, especially for zone I disease. In the first case, laser was simply substituted for cryo as an equivalent or improved way to kill nonvascularized retina (114–119). And in the second case, the shift to earlier treatment occurred because CRYO-ROP protocols did not succeed in zone I disease.

Despite single-center attention to these two evolutions, a multicenter randomized trial was necessary. ET-ROP provided that (27). ET-ROP was successful in its primary goals of refining the level of ROP disease which could benefit significantly from peripheral retinal ablation. Intervention may now be performed on Type I ROP as follows:

Zone I, any stage ROP with plus
Zone I, stage 3 ROP
Zone II, stage 2 or 3 ROP with plus

As noted in the Natural History section, zone I ROP and plus disease are the main signals of poor outcome and were proven to result in better outcomes with early intervention. The extent or clock hours of ROP are irrelevant without plus disease.

But what of the comparison between cryotherapy and laser? Laser is more convenient, more easily applied, especially posteriorly, and better tolerated. But is it more effective? ET-ROP may be able to answer that question indirectly. ET-ROP patients received laser photocoagulation in the overwhelming majority of treated cases. However, the indications for treatment were clearly different. But there was a group of patients in the ET-ROP trial who received laser treatment according to CRYO-ROP guidelines—those with conventionally managed eyes. Comparing only those eyes of ET-ROP with CRYO-ROP can yield valid comparisons, especially since the visual acuity outcomes were tested using similar techniques. CRYO-ROP had an age 9 months unfavorable visual acuity outcome of 35%. ET-ROP had an unfavorable visual acuity outcome rate of 19.6%. The investigators did not address this issue with a separate analysis, the populations were not identical, especially with respect to frequency of zone I disease, and clearly other variables could be contributing. But from this simple comparison of published numbers, it seems that success rates for even conventionally managed ROP improved over 15 years, much as the single-center and anecdotal evidence had been claiming. Whether most of this improvement can be attributed to advantages of laser over cryo is debatable, but it probably is contributory.

While the interdictory treatments of laser and cryotherapy are undoubtedly worthwhile, they do have complications. Minor or transient complications of cryotherapy or laser include lid edema, conjunctival edema and inflammation, retinal or vitreous hemorrhage, diminished peripheral visual fields, and even choroidal or exudative retinal detachments. More serious and vision-threatening complications include cataract, glaucoma, uveitis, anterior segment ischemia, hyphema, macular burn, and occlusion of the central retinal artery (27,53,120–130). Luckily these rates of serious complications are low and do not always produce a loss of vision. However, a reasonable estimate of the visually threatening complication rate from all causes is 2% to 3%.

Another attempt at interdictory therapy was the STOP-ROP trial (65). This trial was based on the theory that increasing the oxygen saturation when serious ROP develops would potentially diminish the relative retinal hypoxia, reduce VEGF levels, and hence prevent progression of serious ROP. Unfortunately, this was not found to be efficacious, although its theoretic potential remains. One indirect message from this study is the difficulty in translating clinical changes in oxygen delivery to the tissue and cellular events of the retina. Relative retinal hypoxia and all that entails undoubtedly is a much more complex series of events to impact than simply monitoring oxygen saturations.

The most recent development is anti-VEGF drug treatment, principally intravitreal bevacizumab. At the time of publication, this form of therapy remains controversial, primarily due to its potential for systemic complications. However, the efficacy of this treatment is established.

As previously noted, there are many angiogenic growth factors. VEGF is one family of such growth factors. VEGF-A appears to be the main culprit in promoting neovascular eye disease, e.g., AMD and diabetes, and there are several isoforms. VEGF-A is a cytokine made up of a dimeric glycoprotein. It achieves isoform status by alternative splicing. These molecules bind to tyrosine kinase and initiate a cascade of signaling events. While VEGF is a necessary physiologic agent, there is no question that it is directly involved in both angiogenesis and vasculogenesis and modulates abnormal neovascularization, all of which are involved in ROP.

There are now four specific molecules that have been clinically proven to have effective anti-VEGF properties: Pegaptanib, an RNA aptamer; Ranibizumab, a partial monoclonal antibody; Bevacizumab, a full monoclonal antibody; and Aflibercept, a recombinant fusion protein and a VEGF (and PGF, placental growth factor) receptor decoy. Pegaptanib was approved for AMD by the FDA in 2004. Bevacizumab obtained FDA approval for cancer treatment in 2004 and widespread off-label use for AMD in 2006. Ranibizumab was approved for AMD in 2005 and aflibercept obtained approval in 2011. Off-label use of intravitreal bevacizumab (IVB) and on-label use of intravitreal ranibizumab (IVR) were demonstrated to be equivalent in nearly all categories in treating AMD in the 2011 CATT Trial (131).

Because of the commonality of VEGF-driven pathophysiology, IVB use in ROP began to be reported in 2007. Since then there have been over a dozen small case series reported, culminating in the BEAT-ROP Trial, a randomized multicenter study published in the NEJM in 2011 (132–137). This study compared outcomes between conventional laser therapy (CLT) and IVB (Table 3.3). The investigators subdivided the severe ROP into Zone I and posterior Zone II. While the results for posterior Zone II were only suggestive of superior efficacy for IVB, the results for Zone I were dramatic. Disease recurrence occurred in 42% of CLT, but only 6% of IVB ($p = 0.0028$). Furthermore, in those patients that had disease recurrence, 18/23 had anatomic abnormalities with CLT as compared to 1/2 with IVB. Clearly IVB has superior efficacy compared to CLT in Zone I disease.

In addition to superior efficacy, IVB is simple to administer and does not require the long sedation or intubation that is necessary for CLT. While IVB is more efficacious for zone I disease and very practical, safety has been a concern. IVB appears to have minimal ocular complications, and none of the published reports show any indication of systemic complications. However, none of the studies were adequately powered to detect small differences in the feared potential complications of negatively impacted organ development, which could produce an increase in the rate of cerebral palsy, paraventricular leukomalacia, bronchopulmonary dysplasia, arteriothrombolic events, etc. Further studies will be needed to answer this most important question. However, the likely dramatic improvement in outcomes for Zone I ROP make a very strong statement for continued use in this very limited subset of treatable ROP that still has a high rate of blindness with CLT.

There are several practical concerns when using IVB. The timing of injections is critical. Injection too early in the disease process can produce a permanently dystrophic retina while injection too late can actually accelerate cicatricial disease. The injection site and technique must be carefully monitored so as to prevent infection and avoid contact with the rounder infant lens. Interestingly, while injection through the ora serrata is optimal, inadvertent penetration through the underdeveloped peripheral retina does not seem to be associated with any untoward effects. These lens and retinal issues have led to some debate regarding the ideal penetration point for the injection. In addition, the drug dosage has not been definitively determined. The most commonly used dose is one half that for the adult disease, namely 0.625 mg. Finally, the patient follow-up is dramatically different. CLT works by eliminating ischemic cell signals to VEGF production and the cells that actually produce VEGF. It does so permanently. Lack of regression is usually from laser skip areas that allow continued production of VEGF. Anti-VEGF drugs work very differently. They bind to and deactivate existing VEGF, but do not eliminate ongoing production. This allows for recurrence of disease, sometimes very late. The BEAT-ROP Study noted recurrences as late as 54 weeks PMA. Such recurrences may require additional treatment, either repeat injection or CLT depending on clinical judgment (138). In a related way, since peripheral retina is not destroyed by IVB and VEGF production is not permanently halted, normal vascularization may resume, decreasing the potential field loss.

There are several major questions that remain as anti-VEGF therapy evolves. What will become the eventual drug of choice? While IVB and IVR are very likely to have equivalent efficacy, perhaps the lower serum concentrations of ranibizumab will prove to be safer systemically, or perhaps intravitreal pegaptanib will be safer due to its limited iso form targeting, i.e., VEGF-A165. Aflibercept is unlikely to be safer since its affinity for VEGF-A molecules is much higher. New drugs are on the horizon whose physiologic action and pharmacokinetics may be superior in efficacy or safety.

In summary, IVB is highly efficacious and practical. It has decidedly superior efficacy for Type I ROP in Zone I. It is likely that all the anti-VEGF agents will have comparable efficacy, but the systemic safety profiles may be very different. Cost is not a scientific question, but is certainly a socioeconomic one.

Given these facts and being cognizant of what can be inferred as well as what is still unknown, IVB seems to be a preferred treatment for Type I, Zone I ROP, AP-ROP, or Zone II ROP with vitreous hemorrhage, media opacity, or insufficient pupillary dilation. To quote the NEJM editorial that accompanied the publication of the BEAT-ROP trial, "Use of [IVB] must include off-label informed consent that is based on a discussion of the known and unknown risks versus the risk of blindness." (139)

Corrective Therapy

Unfortunately, current corrective therapy aimed at correcting visually significant cicatricial disease has been disappointing. The tractional retinal detachments and retinal folds that develop in ROP are difficult surgical problems. This is the most expensive, most heroic, most technically demanding treatment phase of ROP. Yet even hard-won anatomic success yields disappointingly little relevant improvement in vision.

Table 3.3

RESULTS OF THE BEAT-ROP STUDY

Disease Recurrence by Infant

Location	CLT (%)	IVB (%)	P
Zone I	42	6	0.0028
Zone II posterior	12	5	0.2709

Anatomic abnormality (eyes) incidence/recurrence

Zone I	18/23	1/2
Zone II posterior	7/9	2/4

CLT, conventional laser therapy; IVB, intravitreal bevacizumab.

The published results on this phase of therapy in total retinal detachment patients in the CRYO-ROP trial were dismal (140,141). Patients reported by surgeons from single centers often fare better, but the results are still not good (142–145). However, newer, more sophisticated attempts continue to be made and perhaps will slowly improve results. One overriding logic governs almost all of these interventions, i.e., there is no real alternative hope. The key lies in prevention and interdiction, not correction.

Mitigation

This is the final phase of ROP management. It comes into play once the treatment phases for ROP have ended. Mitigation management is aimed at the treatment of all the sequelae that can arise from ROP. Such conditions, escalating in seriousness, include: myopia, anisometropia, amblyopia, strabismus, cataract, glaucoma, phthisis, and blindness. Indirect problems of ophthalmologic concern that result more from intracranial disease than ROP include nystagmus, optic atrophy, and cortical visual impairment. Late-onset rhegmatogenous retinal detachments also occur.

Myopia is by far the most common sequelae of ROP. It correlates highly with increasing severity of ROP. In the CRYO-ROP study, the myopia and high myopia rates were 20% and 5%, respectively, in all ROP eyes less than threshold, and were a dramatic 80% and 54% in stage 3 plus with 9 or more clock hours of disease (146). Early and frequent cycloplegic refractions are essential in this group of patients.

Anisometropia, amblyopia, and strabismus are also common problems. Their incidence also increases with increasing severity of ROP (147–150). Again, early and frequent ophthalmologic exams are critical in detecting these problems. Management may require glasses, amblyopia therapy, possibly superimposed on organic disease, and surgery.

Cataract and glaucoma are thankfully much less common. As noted, each can occur as a complication of ROP treatment but are more common as disease sequelae from severe ROP, usually with visually significant cicatricial disease. Cataracts arise in a wide variety of severely altered ocular physiology states, and ROP cataracts are undoubtedly similar. ROP glaucoma can take various forms (151). Treatment of both of these conditions is complicated by the underlying ROP changes and age of the patient.

Finally, the management of uncorrectable visual impairment and blindness is a necessity. Although at times uncomfortable for the ophthalmologist, it can be of paramount importance to the individual. The role of the ophthalmologist here is often comfort and reassurance coupled with education and advocacy. Proper referral to low-vision specialists, early interventionists, community and government programs, and patient and family support and advocacy groups can make major differences in both the approach to and coping with a blindness disability.

CONCLUSION

It is appropriate to conclude this review of ROP in the same manner as it began. There have been great strides made since Terry's description in 1942 (1). Despite the epidemiologic pitfalls inherent in this disease and in scientific inquiry in general, progress has been dramatic. Basic research offers much promise for the future. But the irrefutable truth is that there are still babies who are blinded by ROP in the United States and throughout the world. There is still much to learn. So this chapter ends with the same plea that Terry made in 1942. Appropriate resources need to be brought to bear to determine the full cause of and discover a prevention for this enigmatic disease.

REFERENCES

1. Terry TL. Extreme prematurity and fibroblastic overgrowth of persistent vascular sheath behind each crystalline lens. I. Preliminary report. *Am J Ophthalmol* 1942;25:203–204.
2. Terry TL. Fibroblastic overgrowth of persistent tunica vasculosa lentis in premature infants. II. Report of cases—clinical aspects. *Arch Ophthalmol* 1943;29:36–53.
3. Steinkuller PG, Du L, Gilbert C, et al. Childhood blindness. *J AAPOS* 1999;3:26–32.
4. Tompkins C. A sudden rise in the prevalence of retinopathy of prematurity blindness? *Pediatrics* 2001;108:526–527.
5. Gilbert C, Rahi J, Eckstein M, et al. Retinopathy of prematurity in middle-income countries. *Lancet* 1997;350:12–14.
6. Pizzarello L, Abiose A, Ffytche T, et al. Vision 2020: the right to sight. A global initiative to eliminate avoidable blindness. *Arch Ophthalmol* 2004;122:615–620.
7. Hong Phan M, Nguyen PN, Reynolds JD. Incidence and severity of retinopathy of prematurity in Vietnam, a developing middle-income country. *J Pediatr Ophthalmol Strabismus* 2003;40: 208–212.
8. Gilbert C, Foster A. Childhood blindness in the context of VISION 2020—the right to sight. *Bull World Health Organ* 2001;79:227–232.
9. Jacobson RM, Feinstein AR. Oxygen as a cause of blindness in premature infants: "Autopsy" of a decade of errors in clinical epidemiological research. *J Clin Epidemiol* 1992;45:1265–1287.
10. Campbell K. Intensive oxygen therapy as a possible cause of retrolental fibroplasia: a clinical approach. *Med J Aust* 1951;2: 48–50.
11. Patz A, Hoeck LE, de la Cruz E. Studies on the effect of high oxygen administration in retrolental fibroplasia. *Am J Ophthalmol* 1952;35:1248–1252.
12. Kinsey VE, Hemphill FM. Etiology of retrolental fibroplasia and preliminary report of the cooperative study of retrolental fibroplasia. *Trans Am Acad Ophthalmol Otolaryngol* 1955; 59:15–24.
13. Kinsey VE. Retrolental fibroplasia: cooperative study of retrolental fibroplasia and the use of oxygen. *AMA Arch Ophthalmol* 1956;56:481–543.

14. Bolton DPG, Cross KW. Further observations on cost of preventing retrolental fibroplasia. *Lancet* 1974;445–448.

15. Silverman WA. A cautionary tale about supplemental oxygen: the albatross of neonatal medicine. *Pediatrics* 2004;113:394–396.

16. Committee for the Classification of Retinopathy of Prematurity. An international classification of retinopathy of prematurity. *Arch Ophthalmol* 1984;102:1130–1134.

17. International Committee for the Classification of the Late Stages of Retinopathy of Prematurity. An international classification of retinopathy of prematurity. II. The classification of retinal detachment. *Arch Ophthalmol* 1987;105:906–912.

18. Wallace DK, Kylstra JA, Chesnutt DA. Prognostic significance of vascular dilation and tortuosity insufficient for plus disease in retinopathy of prematurity. *J AAPOS* 2000;4:224–229.

19. Freedman SF, Kylstra JA, Capowski JJ, et al. Observer sensitivity to retinal vessel diameter and tortuosity in retinopathy of prematurity: a model system. *J Pediatr Ophthalmol Strabismus* 1996;33: 248–254.

20. Saunders RA, Bluestein EC, Sinatra RB, et al. The predictive value of posterior pole vessels in retinopathy of prematurity. *J Pediatr Ophthalmol Strabismus* 1995;32:82–85.

21. Wallace DK, Quinn GE, Freedman SF, et al. Agreement among pediatric ophthalmologists in diagnosing plus and pre-plus disease in retinopathy of prematurity. *J AAPOS* 2008;12:352–356.

22. Yanovitch TL, Freedman SF, Wallace DK. Vascular dilation and tortuosity in plus disease. *Arch Ophthalmol* 2009;127(1): 112–113.

23. Chiang MF, Gelman R, Williams SL, et al. Plus disease in retinopathy of prematurity: development of composite images by quantification of expert opinion. *Invest Ophthalmol Vis Sci* 2008;49:4064–4070.

24. Wallace DK, Zhao Z, Freedman SF. A pilot study using "ROP tool" to quantify plus disease in retinopathy of prematurity. *J AAPOS* 2007;11:381–387.

25. An International Committee for the Classification of Retinopathy of Prematurity. *Arch Ophthalmol.* 2005;123:991–999.

26. Cryotherapy for Retinopathy of Prematurity Cooperative Group. Multicenter trial of cryotherapy for retinopathy of prematurity. Preliminary results. *Arch Ophthalmol* 1988;106: 471–479.

27. Early Treatment for Retinopathy of Prematurity Cooperative Group. Revised indications for the treatment of retinopathy of prematurity. Results of the early treatment for retinopathy of prematurity randomized trial. *Arch Ophthalmol* 2003;121:1684–1696.

28. Young TE. Topical mydriatics: the adverse effects of screening examinations for retinopathy of prematurity. *NeoPreviews* 2003; 4:163–166.

29. Kumar H, Nainiwal S, Singha U, et al. Stress induced by screening for retinopathy of prematurity. *J Pediatr Ophthalmol Strabismus* 2002;36:349–350.

30. Laws DE, Morton C, Weindling M, et al. Systemic effects of screening for retinopathy of prematurity. *Br J Ophthalmol* 1996;80:425–428.

31. Mirmanesh SJ, Abbasi S, Bhutani VK. Alpha-adrenergic bronchoprovocation in neonates with bronchopulmonary dysplasia. *J Pediatr* 1992;121:622–625.

32. Palmer EA. How safe are ocular drugs in pediatrics? *Ophthalmology* 1986;93:1038–1040.

33. Isenberg S, Everett S. Cardiovascular effects of mydriatics in low-birth-weight infants. *J Pediatr* 1984;105:111–112.

34. Cryotherapy for Retinopathy of Prematurity Cooperative Group. Multicenter trial of cryotherapy for retinopathy of prematurity. 3 month outcome. *Arch Ophthalmol* 1990;108: 195–204.

35. Reynolds JD, Hardy RJ, Kennedy KA, et al. for the Light Reduction in Retinopathy of Prematurity (LIGHT-ROP) Cooperative Group. Lack of efficacy of light reduction in preventing retinopathy of prematurity. *N Engl J Med* 1998;338: 1572–1576.

36. Reynolds JD, Dobson V, Quinn GE, et al. for the CRYO-ROP and LIGHT-ROP Cooperative Groups. Evidence-based screening criteria for retinopathy of prematurity. *Arch Ophthalmol* 2002; 120:1470–1476.

37. Repka MX, Palmer EA, Tung B, for the Cryotherapy for Retinopathy of Prematurity Cooperative Group. Involution of retinopathy of prematurity. *Arch Ophthalmol* 2000;118:645–649.

38. Section on Ophthalmology, American Academy of Pediatrics, American Academy of Ophthalmology, and American Association of Pediatric Ophthalmology and Strabismus. Screening examination of premature infants for retinopathy of prematurity. *Pediatrics* 2006;117:572–576.

39. ERRATA. Section on Ophthalmology, American Academy of Pediatrics, American Academy of Ophthalmology, and American Association of Pediatric Ophthalmology and Strabismus. Screening examination of premature infants for retinopathy of prematurity. *Pediatrics* 2006;118:1324.

40. Section on Ophthalmology, American Academy of Pediatrics, American Academy of Ophthalmology, and American Association of Pediatric Ophthalmology and Strabismus. Screening examination of premature infants for retinopathy of prematurity. *Pediatrics* 2013;131:189–195.

41. Reynolds JD. Malpractice and the quality of care in retinopathy of prematurity (An American Ophthalmological Society Thesis). *Trans Am Ophthalmol Soc* 2007;105:461–480.

42. Bullard SR, Donahue SP, Feman SS, et al. The decreasing incidence and severity of retinopathy of prematurity. *J AAPOS* 1999;3:46–52.

43. Reynolds JD, Hardy RJ, Palmer EA. Incidence and severity of retinopathy of prematurity. *J AAPOS* 1999;3:321–322.

44. Kennedy J, Todd DA, Watts J, et al. Retinopathy of prematurity in infants less than 29 weeks' gestation: 3 1/2 years pre- and post-surfactant. *J Pediatr Ophthalmol Strabismus* 1997;34: 289–292.

45. Fledelius HC. Retinopathy of prematurity in a Danish county. Trends over the 12-year period 1982–93. *Acta Ophthalmol Scand* 1996;74:285–287.

46. Termote J, Schalij-Delfos NE, Brouwers HAA, et al. New developments in neonatology: less severe retinopathy of prematurity? *J Pediatr Ophthalmol Strabismus* 2000;37:142–148.

47. Repka MX, Hardy RJ, Phelps DL, et al. Surfactant prophylaxis and retinopathy of prematurity. *Arch Ophthalmol* 1993;111: 618–620.

48. Holmes JM, Cronin CM, Squires P, et al. Randomized clinical trial of surfactant prophylaxis in retinopathy of prematurity. *J Pediatr Ophthalmol Strabismus* 1994;31:189–191.

49. Palmer EA, Flynn JT, Hardy RJ, et al. For the Cryotherapy for Retinopathy of Prematurity Cooperative Group. Incidence and early course of retinopathy of prematurity. *Ophthalmology* 1991;98:1628–1640.

50. Early Treatment of Retinopathy of Prematurity Cooperative Group. The incidence and course of retinopathy of prematurity:

findings from the early treatment for retinopathy of prematurity study. *Pediatrics* 2005;116(1):15–23.

51. Kupfer C, McManus E, Berlage N. *History of the National Eye Institute 1968–2000*. Bethesda, MD: National Eye Institute, 2009.

52. Cryotherapy for Retinopathy of Prematurity Cooperative Group. The natural ocular outcome of premature birth and retinopathy. Status at 1 year. *Arch Ophthalmol* 1994;112:903–912.

53. Cryotherapy for Retinopathy of Prematurity Cooperative Group. Multicenter trial of cryotherapy for retinopathy of prematurity. One year outcome—structure and function. *Arch Ophthalmol* 1990;108:1408–1416.

54. Gilbert WS, Dobson V, Quinn GE, et al. For the Cryotherapy for Retinopathy of Prematurity Cooperative Group. The correlation of visual function with posterior retinal structure in severe retinopathy of prematurity. *Arch Ophthalmol* 1992;110:625–631.

55. Reynolds J, Dobson V, Quinn GE, et al. For the Cryotherapy for Retinopathy of Prematurity Cooperative Group. Prediction of visual function in eyes with mild to moderate posterior pole residua of retinopathy of prematurity. *Arch Ophthalmol* 1993;111:1050–1056.

56. McColm JR, Fleck BW. Retinopathy of prematurity: causation. *Semin Neonatol* 2001;6:453–460.

57. Biglan AW, Brown DR, Reynolds JD, et al. Risk factors associated with retrolental fibroplasia. *Ophthalmology* 1984;91:1504–1511.

58. Brown DR, Milley JR, Ripepi UJ, et al. Retinopathy of prematurity. Risk factors in a five-year cohort of critically ill premature neonates. *Am J Dis Child* 1987;141:154–160.

59. Hammer ME, Mullen PW, Ferguson JG, et al. Logistic analysis of risk factors in acute retinopathy of prematurity. *Am J Ophthalmol* 1986;102:1–6.

60. Enzenauer RW. Retinopathy of prematurity and weight of the baby's chart. *J AAPOS* 2001;5:198.

61. Flynn JT, Bancalari E, Snyder ES, et al. A cohort study of transcutaneous oxygen tension and the incidence and severity of retinopathy of prematurity. *N Engl J Med* 1992;326:1050–1054.

62. Jefferson E. Retrolental fibroplasia. *Arch Dis Child* 1952;27:329–336.

63. Phelps DL, Rosenbaun AL. Effects of variable oxygenation and gradual withdrawal of oxygen during the recovery phase in oxygen induced retinopathy: kitten model. *Pediatr Res* 1987;22:297–301.

64. Gaynon MD. Supplemental oxygen and photopic lighting in the management of retinopathy of prematurity. Presented at: Update on Retinopathy of Prematurity Conference; February 22, 1992; Los Angeles, California.

65. The STOP-ROP Multicenter Study Group. Supplemental therapeutic oxygen for prethreshold retinopathy of prematurity (STOP-ROP), a randomized, controlled trial. I: primary outcomes. *Pediatrics* 2000;105:295–310.

66. Tin W, Milligan DWA, Pennefather P, et al. Pulse oximetry, severe retinopathy, and outcome at one year in babies of less than 28 weeks gestation. *Arch Dis Child Fetal Neonatal Ed* 2001;84:F106–F110.

67. Askie LM, Henderson-Smart DJ, Irwig L, et al. Oxygen-saturation targets and outcomes in extremely preterm infants. *N Engl J Med* 2003;349:959–967.

68. Chow LC, Wright KW, Sola A for the CSMC Oxygen Administration Study Group. Can changes in clinical practice decrease the incidence of severe retinopathy of prematurity in very low birth weight infants? *Pediatrics* 2003;111:339–345.

69. Cole CH, Wright KW, Tarnow-Mordi W, et al. Resolving our uncertainty about oxygen therapy. *Pediatrics* 2003;112:1415–1419.

70. Hepner WR, Krause AC, Davis ME. Retrolental fibroplasia and light. *Pediatrics* 1949;3:824–828.

71. Locke JC, Reese AB. Retrolental fibroplasia. The negative role of light, mydriatics, and the ophthalmoscopic examination in its etiology. *Arch Ophthalmol* 1952;48:44–47.

72. Glass P, Avery GB, Subramanian KNS, et al. Effect of bright light in the hospital nursery on the incidence of retinopathy of prematurity. *N Engl J Med* 1985;313:401–404.

73. Hommura S, Usuki Y, Takei K, et al. Ophthalmic care of very low birthweight infants. Report 4. Clinical studies on the influence of light on the incidence of retinopathy of prematurity. *Nippon Ganka Gakkai Zasshi* 1988;92:456–461.

74. Ackerman B, Sherwonit E, Williams J. Reduced incidental light exposure: effect on the development of retinopathy of prematurity in low birth weight infants. *Pediatrics* 1989;83:958–962.

75. Seiberth V, Linderkamp O, Knorz MC, et al. A controlled clinical trial of light and retinopathy of prematurity. *Am J Ophthalmol* 1994;118:492–495.

76. LIGHT-ROP Cooperative Group. The design of the multicenter study of light reduction in retinopathy of prematurity (LIGHT-ROP). *J Pediatr Ophthalmol Strabismus* 1999;36:257–263.

77. Carmeliet P. Mechanisms of angiogenesis and arteriogenesis. *Nat Med* 2000;6:389–395.

78. Casey R, Li WW. Factors controlling ocular angiogenesis. *Am J Ophthalmol* 1997;124:521–529.

79. Stone J, Itin A, AlonT, et al. Development of retinal vasculature is mediated by hypoxia-induced vascular endothelial growth factor (VEGF) expression by neuroglia. *J Neurosci* 1995;15:4738–4747.

80. Alon A, Hemo I, Itin A, et al. Vascular endothelial growth factor acts as a survival factor for newly formed retinal vessels and has implications for retinopathy of prematurity. *Nat Med* 1995;1:1024–1028.

81. Pierce EA, Foley ED. Smith LEH. Regulation of vascular endothelial growth factor by oxygen in a model of retinopathy of prematurity. *Arch Ophthalmol* 1996;114:1219–1228.

82. Aiello LP. Vascular endothelial growth factor. *Invest Ophthalmol Vis Sci* 1997;38:1647–1652.

83. Robinson CJ, Stringer SE. The splice variants of vascular endothelial growth factor (VEGF) and their receptors. *J Cell Sci* 2001;114:853–865.

84. Hellstrom A, Engstrom E, Hard AL, et al. Postnatal serum insulinlike growth factor I deficiency is associated with retinopathy of prematurity and other complications of premature birth. *Pediatrics* 2003;112:1016–1020.

85. Hellstrom A, Perruzzi C, Ju M, et al. Low IGF-I suppresses VEGF-survival signaling in retinal endothelial cells: direct correlation with clinical retinopathy of prematurity. *Proc Natl Acad Sci USA* 2001;98:5804–5808.

86. Smith LEH, Shen W, Perruzzi C, et al. Regulation of vascular endothelial growth factor-dependent retinal neovascularization by insulin-like growth factor-1 receptor. *Nat Med* 1999;5:1390–1395.

87. McGuire PG, Jones TR, Talarico N, et al. The urokinase/urokinase receptor system in retinal neovascularization: inhibition by A6 suggests a new therapeutic target. *Invest Ophthalmol Vis Sci* 2003;44:2736–2742.

88. Majka S, McGuire PG, Das A. Regulation of matrix metallo-proteinase expression by tumor necrosis factor in a murine model of retinal neovascularization. *Invest Ophthalmol Vis Sci* 2002;43:260–266.

89. Majka S, McGuire PG, Colombo S, et al. The balance between proteinases and inhibitors in a murine model of proliferative retinopathy. *Invest Ophthalmol Vis Sci* 2001;42:210–215.

90. Das A, McLamore A, Song W, et al. Retinal neovascularization is suppressed with a matrix metalloproteinase inhibitor. *Arch Ophthalmol* 1999;117:498–503.

91. Chan-Ling T, Stone J. Degeneration of astrocytes in feline retinopathy of prematurity causes failure of the blood-retinal barrier. *Invest Ophthalmol Vis Sci* 1992;33:2148–2159.

92. Zhang Y, Stone J. Role of astrocytes in the control of developing retinal vessels. *Invest Ophthalmol Vis Sci* 1997;38:1653–1666.

93. Sun Y, Dalal R, Giariano RF. Cellular composition of the ridge in retinopathy of prematurity. *Arch Ophthalmol* 2010;128(5):638–641.

94. Hendrickson AE, Yuodelis C. The morphological development of the human fovea. *Ophthalmology* 1984;91:603–612.

95. Johnson AT, Kretzer FL, Hittner HM, et al. Development of the subretinal space in the preterm human eye: ultrastructural and immunocytochemical studies. *J Comp Neurol* 1985;233:497–505.

96. Taylor MJ, Menzies R, MacMillan LJ, et al. VEPs in normal full-term and premature neonates: longitudinal versus cross-sectional data. *Electroencephalogr Clin Neurophysiol* 1989;68:76–80.

97. Norcia AM, Tyler CW, Piecuch R. Visual acuity development in normal and abnormal preterm human infants. *J Pediatr Ophthalmol Strabismus* 1987;24:70–74.

98. Harding GF, Grose J, Wilton A, et al. The pattern reversal VEP in short-gestation infants. *Electroencephalogr Clin Neurophysiol* 1989;74:76–80.

99. Ashton NA, Ward B, Serpell G. Effect of oxygen on developing retinal vessels with particular reference to the problem of retrolental fibroplasia. *Br J Ophthalmol* 1954;38:397–430.

100. Kretzer FL, Hittner HM. Vitamine E and retrolental fibroplasia: ultrastructural mechanism of clinical efficacy. In: Porter R, Whelan J, eds. *Biology of vitamin E*. London: Pittman Books, 1983:165–185.

101. Penn JS, Henry MM, Wall PT, et al. The range of PaO_2 variation determines the severity of oxygen-induced retinopathy in newborn rats. *Invest Ophthalmol Vis Sci* 1995;36:2063–2070.

102. Penn JS, Tolman BL, Lowery LA. Variable oxygen exposure causes preretinal neovascularization in the newborn rat. *Invest Ophthalmol Vis Sci* 1993;34:576–585.

103. Arias E, MacDorman MF, Strobino DM, et al. Annual summary of vital statistics—2002. *Pediatrics* 2003;112:1215–1230.

104. Hittner HM, Godio LB, Rudolph AJ, et al. Retrolental fibroplasia: efficacy of vitamin E in a double-blind clinical study of preterm infants. *N Engl J Med* 1981;305:1365–1371.

105. Phelps DL, Rosenbaum AL, Isenberg SJ, et al. Tocopherol efficacy and safety for preventing retinopathy of prematurity: a randomized, controlled, double-masked trial. *Pediatrics* 1987;79:489–500.

106. Schaffer DB, Johnson L, Quinn GE, et al. Vitamin E and retinopathy of prematurity. Follow-up at one year. *Ophthalmology* 1985;92:1005–1011.

107. Puklin JE, Simon RM, Ehrenkranz RA. Influence on retrolental fibroplasia of intramuscular vitamin E administration during respiratory distress syndrome. *Ophthalmology* 1982;89:96–103.

108. Fielder AR. Retinopathy of prematurity: aetiology. *Clin Risk* 1997;3:47–51.

109. Carver JC, Stromquist CI, Benford VJ, et al. Postnatal inositol levels in preterm infants. *J Perinatal* 1997;17:389–392.

110. Hallman M, Bry K, Hoppu K, et al. Inositol supplementation in premature infants with respiratory distress syndrome. *N Engl J Med* 1992;326:1233–1239.

111. Friedman CA, McVey J, Borne MJ, et al. Relationship between serum inositol concentration and development of retinopathy of prematurity: a prospective study. *J Pediatr Ophthalmol Strabismus* 2000;37:79–86.

112. Young TL, Anthony DC, Pierce E, et al. Histopathology and vascular endothelial growth factor in untreated and diode laser-treated retinopathy of prematurity. *J AAPOS* 1997;1:105–110.

113. Cryotherapy for Retinopathy of Prematurity Cooperative Group. Multicenter trial of cryotherapy for retinopathy of prematurity. Ophthalmological outcomes at 10 years. *Arch Ophthalmol* 2001;119:1110–1118.

114. Ng EYJ, Connolly BP, McNamara JA, et al. A comparison of laser photocoagulation with cryotherapy for threshold retinopathy of prematurity at 10 years. Part 1. Visual function and structural outcome. *Ophthalmology* 2002;109:928–935.

115. Shalev B, Farr AK, Repka MX. Randomized comparison of diode laser photocoagulation versus cryotherapy for threshold retinopathy of prematurity: seven-year outcome. *Am J Ophthalmol* 2001;132:76–80.

116. Paysse EA, Lindsey JL, Coats DK, et al. Therapeutic outcomes of cryotherapy versus transpupillary diode laser photocoagulation for threshold retinopathy of prematurity. *J AAPOS* 1999;4:234–240.

117. McGregor ML, Wherley AJ, Fellows RR, et al. A comparison of cryotherapy versus diode laser retinopexy in 100 consecutive infants treated for threshold retinopathy of prematurity. *J AAPOS* 1998;2:360–364.

118. White JE, Repka MX. Randomized comparison of diode laser photocoagulation versus cryotherapy for threshold retinopathy of prematurity: 3-year outcome. *J Pediatr Ophthalmol Strabismus* 1997;34:83–87.

119. The Laser ROP Study Group. Laser therapy for retinopathy of prematurity. *Arch Ophthalmol* 1994;112:154–156.

120. Cryotherapy for Retinopathy of Prematurity Cooperative Group. Effect of retinal ablative therapy for threshold retinopathy of prematurity. Results of Goldmann perimetry at the age of 10 years. *Arch Ophthalmol* 2001;119:1120–1125.

121. Fallaha N, Lynn MJ, Aaberg TM, et al. Clinical outcome of confluent laser photoablation for retinopathy of prematurity. *J AAPOS* 2002;6:81–85.

122. Lambert SR, Capone A, Cingle KA, et al. Cataract and phthisis bulbi after laser photoablation for threshold retinopathy of prematurity. *Am J Ophthalmol* 2000;129:585–591.

123. Gold RS. Cataracts associated with treatment for retinopathy of prematurity. *J Pediatr Ophthalmol Strabismus* 1997;34:123–124.

124. Simons BD, Wilson MC, Hertle RW, et al. Bilateral hyphemas and cataracts after diode laser retinal photoablation for retinopathy of prematurity. *J Pediatr Ophthalmol Strabismus* 1998;35:185–187.

125. Noonan CP, Clark DI. Acute serous detachment with argon laser photocoagulation in retinopathy of prematurity. *J AAPOS* 1997;1:183–184.

126. Christiansen SP, Bradford JD. Cataract following diode laser photoablation for retinopathy of prematurity. *Arch Ophthalmol* 1997;115:275–276.

127. Watanabe H, Tsukamoto Y, Saito Y, et al. Massive proliferation of conjunctival tissue after cryotherapy for retinopathy of prematurity. *Arch Ophthalmol* 1997;115:278–279.

128. Saito Y, Hatsukawa Y, Lewis JM, et al. Macular coloboma-like lesions and pigment abnormalities as complications of cryotherapy for retinopathy of prematurity in very low birthweight infants. *Am J Ophthalmol* 1996;122:299–308.

129. Christiansen SP, Bradford JD. Cataract in infants treated with Argon laser photocoagulation for threshold retinopathy of prematurity. *Am J Ophthalmol* 1995;119:175–180.

130. Pogrebniak AE, Bolling JP, Stewart MW. Argon laser-induced cataract in an infant with retinopathy of prematurity. *Am J Ophthalmol* 1994;117:261–262.

131. The CATT Research Group. Ranibizumab and Bevacizumab for Neovascular Age-Related Macular Degeneration. *N Engl J Med* 2011;364(20):1897–1908.

132. Wu WC, Yeh PT, Chen SN, et al. Effects and complications of bevacizumab use in patients with retinopathy of prematurity: a multi-center study in Taiwan. *Ophthalmology* 2011;118:176–183.

133. Nazari H, Modarres M, Parvaresh MM, et al. Intravitreal bevacizumab in combination with laser therapy for the treatment of severe retinopathy of prematurity (ROP) associated with vitreous or retinal hemorrhage. *Graefes Arch Clin Exp Ophthalmol* 2010;248:1713–1718.

134. Lee JY, Chae JB, Yang SJ, et al. Effects of intravitreal bevacizumab and laser in retinopathy of prematurity therapy on the development of peripheral retinal vessels. *Graefes Arch Clin Exp Ophthalmol* 2010;248:1257–1262.

135. Dorta P, Kychenthal A. Treatment of type 1 retinopathy of prematurity with intravitreal bevacizumab (Avastin). *Retina* 2010;30(Suppl):S24–S31.

136. Law JC, Recchia FM, Morrison DG, et al. Intravitreal bevacizumab as adjunctive treatment for retinopathy of prematurity. *J APPOS* 2010:14:6–10.

137. Mintz-Hittner, HA, Kennedy KA, and Chuang AZ for the BEAT-ROP Cooperative Group. Efficacy of intravitreal bevacizumab for stage 3+ retinopathy of prematurity. *N Engl J Med* 2011;364(7):603–615.

138. Hu J, Blair M, Shapiro M, et al. Reactivation of retinopathy of prematurity after bevacizumab injection. *Arch Ophthalmol* Online first: April 9, 2012.

139. Reynolds JD. Bevacizumab for retinopathy of prematurity. *N Engl J Med* 2011;364(7):677–678.

140. Quinn GE, Dobson V, Barr CC, et al. for the Cryotherapy for Retinopathy of Prematurity Cooperative Group. Visual acuity of eyes after vitrectomy for retinopathy of prematurity. Follow-up at 5 1/2 years. *Ophthalmology* 1996;103:595–600.

141. Quinn GE, Dobson V, Barr CC, et al. Visual acuity in infants after vitrectomy for severe retinopathy of prematurity. *Ophthalmology* 1991;98:5–13.

142. Mintz-Hittner HA, O'Malley RE, Kretzer FL. Long-term form identification vision after early, closed lensectomy-vitrectomy for stage 5 retinopathy of prematurity. *Ophthalmology* 1997;104:454–459.

143. Seaber JH, Machemer R, Eliott D, et al. Long-term visual results of children after initially successful vitrectomy for stage V retinopathy of prematurity. *Ophthalmology* 1995;102:199–204.

144. Fuchino Y, Hayashi H, Kono T, et al. Long-term follow-up of visual acuity in eyes with stage 5 retinopathy of prematurity after closed vitrectomy. *Am J Ophthalmol* 1995;120:308–316.

145. Hirose T, Katsumi O, Mehta MC, et al. Vision in stage 5 retinopathy of prematurity after retinal reattachment by open-sky vitrectomy. *Arch Ophthalmol* 1993;111:345–349.

146. Quinn GE, Dobson V, Repka MX, et al. for the Cryotherapy for Retinopathy of Prematurity Cooperative Group. Development of myopia in infants with birth weights less than 1251 grams. *Ophthalmology* 1992;99:329–340.

147. O'Connor AR, Stephenson TJ, Johnson A, et al. Strabismus in children of birth weight less than 1701 g. *Arch Ophthalmol* 2002;120:767–773.

148. Bremer DL, Palmer EA, Fellows RR, et al. For the Cryotherapy for Retinopathy of Prematurity Cooperative Group. Strabismus in premature infants in the first year of life. *Arch Ophthalmol* 1998;116:329–333.

149. Summers G, Phelps DL, Tung B, et al. for the Cryotherapy for Retinopathy of Prematurity Cooperative Group. Ocular cosmesis in retinopathy of prematurity. *Arch Ophthalmol* 1992;110:1092–1097.

150. Reynolds JD. Anisometropic amblyopia in severe posterior retinopathy of prematurity. *Binocul Vis Quarterly* 1990;5:153–158.

151. Reynolds JD, Olitsky SE. Pediatric Glaucoma. In Wright KW, Spiegel PH, eds. Pediatric Ophthalmology and Strabismus Second Ed. New York, NY. Springer-Verlag, 2003:483–498.

4

Pediatric Eye Examination

Gregory Ostrow • *Laura Kirkeby*

INTRODUCTION

The pediatric eye exam is often feared by general ophthalmologists as a difficult, loud, frustrating, and often nonproductive office visit. Unlike adult patients, children often are not able to realize or communicate what is wrong with their eyes. Moreover, they often are not willing participants in the examination and so it requires significant effort to gain all the necessary information. To obtain a good history, we have to ask the right questions to both the parent and child, as well as direct our line of questioning so that the least amount of time is wasted while we have the child's interest. Children must be engaged throughout the visit and the physician must hold their attention and learn how to "play" with them during the exam. Pediatric ophthalmologists are not born with the ability to make an exam fun and interesting for a child. This "art" of medicine requires significant patience, adaptability, and a lot of practice. This chapter will discuss various techniques that can be used to maximize the quality of pediatric eye exams as well as some suggestions to make the exam less tedious and more enjoyable for both the ophthalmologist and the pediatric patient.

Some general considerations to keep in mind throughout the exam:

1. Gather as much information from the chart as possible prior to entering the room. You have limited time when the child is paying attention and every moment counts. If you spend time looking at the chart while you are already in the room you may have lost the chance to complete your exam with the child's cooperation.
2. Even when a child is not cooperative, a considerable portion of the exam can be completed to rule out worrisome pathology.
3. The child is the patient, not the parent. Remember to engage and make eye contact as much as possible with the child. Keeping up to date on current movies or characters or trends that different age children enjoy can allow you to break the ice with some brief conversation prior to the exam. A little small talk and a big smile will go a long way toward a cooperative visit.
4. Begin your examination when you walk into the room and while taking your directed history. Gross abnormalities, torticollis, red eyes, chalazia, strabismus, tearing, or irregular pupils can often be recognized at the onset of the exam while talking to the child and can help you direct your history and exam toward final diagnosis.
5. Speak to children in a language they can understand. Adult words or medical jargon will quickly alienate you from a child (and possibly a parent). Ask the child "Why are you here?" and "Why are we looking at your eyes?" Let children know you will not be doing anything without explaining it to them first. Make them your ally and helper for the exam. Children will respond much better if you ask: "Do you want to play some fun games and shine some cool lights in your eyes?" rather than just examining them without warning. Describe each instrument you use in child-friendly terms: "Can I take a peek at your pretty eyes in my microscope? Do you want to hold on to the handlebars while I look?" helps to make a slit lamp exam less threatening. For the indirect exam, let a child know you are going to put on your funny hat and show some beautiful rainbows. Ask which eye they want you to look at first.
6. Whenever possible, have well-trained staff put your dilating drops in. Try to not be in the room when it occurs. When you return for the dilated exam you can re-earn their trust by letting the child know that you won't be letting anyone else put drops in their eyes today.

HISTORY

For most busy practitioners, a majority of the history is taken by ancillary staff. This can be very helpful for a baseline history but it is usually necessary for the physician to ask further directed questions to aid in diagnosis and treatment. Many practices use intake forms for patients where the parents can fill out some of the history in the waiting room prior to their evaluation. These can be very helpful, but it is imperative that they be pediatric oriented and not a standard adult medical history form that is given to all patients. One recommendation is to have check boxes in the chief complaint section for common pediatric eye complaints and a box for "other" if the patient or parent has something else to add. Some common chief complaints include failed vision screen at school or pediatrician's office, red eyes, itchy eyes, tearing eyes, wandering or lazy eyes, head tilt, shaking or jiggling eyes, bumps on the eyelids, headaches, or trouble with reading. Having one of these complaints checked on an intake sheet can help ancillary staff direct their line of questions and improve workflow significantly. A diagnosis and exam sheet from the referring physician is valuable as well.

The chief complaint should be stated in the child's or parent's own words. This should be elaborated on in the history of present illness. For children with a complaint of tearing, the staff can ask the time of onset, whether it is part-time or full-time tearing, whether the eyes get red, whether there is a green or goopy discharge, or whether it gets worse outdoors or when the child is sick. For strabismus, questions to confirm the time of onset, part-time or full-time symptoms, whether the child closes or covers one eye, whether one eye or both eyes are seen wandering, or whether there is any associated head posturing, are all good questions your staff can ask for you so as not to waste valuable time in the room. If you must take the history yourself, only take what is necessary prior to beginning your exam. You can always ask the parent more questions after you have lost the child's attention.

Past history questions should be directed toward possible contributing factors to the child's diagnosis. This can include prenatal and postnatal history, birth weight, gestational age, history of major trauma, surgery or disease, developmental milestones, and any medical problems. Questions on grade level and school performance are also good questions. These can be included on your intake form along with medications and medication allergies. It is also important to know if the child was prescribed any glasses or patching therapy in the past.

Family history is very important for many pediatric eye diseases. Questions of family history should be directed toward any genetic diseases as well as a family history of pediatric eye diseases like pediatric glaucoma, cataracts, strabismus, or amblyopia (rather than adult onset eye problems like senile cataracts and macular degeneration).

PHYSICAL EXAM

The physical exam begins when you enter the room. Is the child alert? Does he or she hold you or her surroundings in regard? Are there any gross abnormalities to the face or orbit? Is the child adopting any head posturing? Are there any gross ocular alignment abnormalities or ptosis? The information you gain from just looking at the child at the beginning of the exam can help direct the remainder of your examination.

VISUAL ACUITY

Corrected or correctable visual acuity assessment is one of the most important parts of the pediatric eye exam. In a young baby, this may only be measuring visual attention and eye-popping reflex, but as a child matures you can measure vision

in much more detail. Pediatric visual acuity should be measured at the most advanced developmental level for each child. This begins with an eye-popping reflex in very young children, proceeds through fix and follow, Central, Steady and Maintained (CSM), HOTV or pictures, and through to Snellen vision. The ophthalmologist who sees pediatric patients should be adept at measuring visual acuity in children of all ages.

Visual acuity assessment in preverbal children is truly an art but it is an art that can be learned with attention and repetition. There can also be some variability in the measurements of young children based on a child's health and sleep patterns. A baby ready for a nap will be much less visually attentive than a child who is well rested. Pay close attention to how the child views his or her surroundings. Does the child follow faces or bright lights? Is there a good eye-popping reflex (opening his or her eyes widely when the room light is turned off)? Will he or she follow a fixation target with both eyes open? With one eye occluded? These findings can be codified in a young child as either fixes and follows (monocular or binocular) or does not fix and follow. The smallest possible fixation target that a child will regard should be used. Smooth pursuits do not usually develop until 6 to 8 weeks of age and should not be expected prior to that. A child who can fix and follow with one eye occluded can usually have their visual acuity further defined with the CSM measurement.

CSM measurements are a behavioral technique that use central fixation (holding an object of regard aligned with the visual axis), steady fixation (nystagmus or no nystagmus), and maintained fixation (in a strabismic patient this can be measured by a child's ability to hold regard of an object with either eye when both eyes are open). For testing fixation, a distance target is more sensitive than a near target. An eye that will not fixate centrally (eccentric fixation) is assumed to have poor vision, likely worse than 20/200. An eye that is not steady (has nystagmus) usually has reduced vision. Nystagmus can be a good sign in a child where there are concerns of severely decreased vision as an eye with nystagmus is assumed to have at least pattern vision (the ability to see shapes). An eye that will not maintain fixation when the cover is removed is assumed to be amblyopic.

In a non-strabismic patient, the 10 base down prism testing method (or induced tropia test) can be applied to test for asymmetry. This method involves placing a 10 base down prism in front of either eye while the child has both eyes open and is fixating on a target. The prism generally degrades the image slightly and so a child with equal vision would be expected to maintain fixation with the eye that is not covered by the prism. If the child switches fixation with a vertical shift, it is assumed that the eye with prism is stronger (and therefore preferred). In practice, the symmetry of this test is probably more important than whether or not the fixation is shifted. Many children will shift vertically with the prism over either eye, which signifies symmetric vision in the same way as not shifting with both eyes. In a strabismic patient, the inability to hold fixation (not maintained) often signifies amblyopia. Some large-angle infantile esotropic children will fixate with either eye depending on which side of the face the object is held. This phenomenon is called cross fixation and a child who cross fixates presumably has equal vision in each eye.

Many young (and older) children will resist occlusion of a good eye when one eye is amblyopic. Resisting occlusion of an eye should be documented in the chart. Whenever possible, visual acuity should be tested with one eye patched rather than with an occluder. Children will try to peek around an occluder not because they are cheaters but rather they prefer to use their dominant eye. The patch should be well fixed so that the child cannot tilt his or her head to see around it during testing.

Other Testing

In preverbal children, the optokinetic nystagmus (OKN) response can be used to demonstrate visual function. An OKN response can be elicited by rotating a drum with parallel vertical stripes in the child's visual field. The eyes follow the stripes with an involuntary pursuit movement and are brought back to their initial starting point with a saccade. The eyes continue to demonstrate the OKN response while the drum rotates. An OKN response has an estimated visual acuity of counting fingers at 3 to 5 feet. The OKN drum can be very useful when assessing visual function in infants with nystagmus. In children with horizontal nystagmus, the drum must be held so that the lines are horizontal and the drum is rotated vertically in order to elicit vertical eye movements. If a vertical OKN response can be elicited in the presence of horizontal nystagmus, then vision is usually 20/400 or better.

Although quantifying visual function in preverbal children is usually very difficult, there are a few tests that can provide an estimate of their visual acuity in Snellen or logmar equivalents. Preferential looking techniques such as the Teller acuity and Cardiff cards use patterns and pictures to elicit a change in fixation, respectively. The Teller acuity cards are rectangular and have a high contrast pattern stimulus on one side and a plain stimulus on the other side. An examiner presents the card in front of the child without knowing the orientation of the pattern (to prevent bias) and monitors fixation through a small central peephole. If a child looks directly toward the pattern then it is presumed that the child can distinguish that level of spatial frequency. The examiner will then present the next card with gratings that have a higher spatial frequency until the child does not accurately fixate on the pattern. The highest spatial frequency that the child can locate is the grating acuity threshold and can be recorded as a Snellen equivalent. The test may be performed monocularly to detect amblyopia or binocularly to demonstrate the presence of visual ability in infants with neurologic or developmental disorders. Teller acuity cards are known to underestimate strabismic amblyopia.

The functional integrity of the entire visual pathway can be evaluated by measuring the visual evoked potentials

(VEP). VEPs are generated by electroencephalographic activity in the visual cortex in response to a visual stimulus. A normal VEP requires that all components of the visual pathway including the macula, optic nerve, tracts, radiations, and the occipital cortex are functioning properly. The child wears three electrodes, which include an active electrode over the occipital area, a reference electrode on the forehead, and a ground electrode on the earlobe. The stimulus used in VEP testing is usually a pattern checkerboard or diffuse flash. In most cases, pattern-reversal VEP is the preferred stimulus and is elicited by a digital checkerboard with squares that reverse from black to white and back again. Although flash VEP can be less accurate, it can detect visual function in the presence of a media opacity, nystagmus, or when the patient has poor cooperation or is suspected to be malingering. The age-related visual acuity determined by the VEP response is approximately 20/400 in early infancy, which improves to approximately 20/20 by 6 months of age. VEP testing must be performed and analyzed by trained specialists, and uncooperative children may require sedation.

Visual acuity assessment in verbal children, while no less of an art form, is often less difficult for a general ophthalmologist. If a child is able to identify characters but not letters, Lea symbols or Allen cards can be used (Fig. 4.1). Parents can be given these pictures or symbols prior to the exam so that they

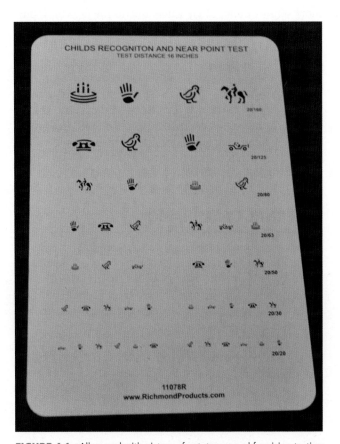

FIGURE 4.1. Allen card with picture of optotypes used for vision testing at near distance.

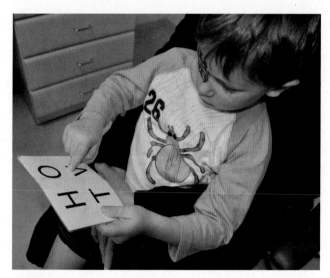

FIGURE 4.2. A child using an HOTV card to match the letters on a screen at distance.

may teach them to the child at home. Many practitioners will use large (20/400) symbols with both eyes open to teach the children what the symbols are and to make the exam more of a game. Both Allen and Lea test only to a 20/30 level, which is adequate for younger children. HOTV is more sensitive than symbols for amblyopia in a preliterate child, and full lines are more sensitive than single letters due to the crowding phenomenon. If a child is shy or does not know the names of the HOTV letters, a card with HOTV in large print can be given to the child, and they can match with their finger what they see on the screen (Fig. 4.2). Parents can be helpful in full line screening as they can point to the letters in order and the child can point to the matching letter on their card in front of them. Tumbling E's are used in a similar fashion to HOTV with a child pointing in the direction of the legs on the E.

When a child is comfortable with his or her letters, vision should be tested with Snellen letters at a distance.

EXTERNAL EXAMINATION

Significant external pathology is often seen in the beginning of the exam when the child is being observed. Significant eyelid pathology, skin tags, growths, chalazia, or dysmorphology can usually be seen with ambient room lighting. In cases where there is some obvious pathology that needs a somewhat enlarged view, a handheld 20D or 28D lens can be used as a magnifier. This is especially helpful when examining the lids or orbits of a young child who may be difficult to examine with a slit lamp.

OCULAR ALIGNMENT AND MOTILITY

A thorough ocular alignment and motility examination is imperative for the pediatric ophthalmic examination. Any

extraocular muscle imbalance in young children can disrupt the binocular visual system and interfere with visual development, which can cause permanent vision loss.

Eye alignment can be tested in a variety of methods ranging from nonspecific screening tests to more extensive tests that can provide angular measurements. The red reflex (Bruckner) test is a widely used screening test that can detect a variety of ocular conditions. The test is performed with a direct ophthalmoscope held approximately one meter from the patient while having them fixate on the light. The examiner can also make sounds or use noise-making toys to acquire the child's attention. The reflection from the retina is observed simultaneously through the ophthalmoscope. The examiner should look for differences in illumination, crescent location, or dark opacities. Conditions such as strabismus, anisometropia, anisocoria, posterior pole anomalies, and media opacities can cause the red reflex to be asymmetric. In patients with strabismus, the red reflex is usually brighter in the deviating eye. The light crescents may be a different size or in opposite locations in patients with anisometropia. Media opacities such as cataracts will block the light from the fundus and present as a darkened or black area. An asymmetric red reflex requires a cycloplegic refraction and fundus exam.

Corneal light reflections can also be used to check ocular alignment. The examiner holds a muscle light while assessing the corneal reflex in each eye, relative to the pupil. Both light reflexes should either be centered in the pupil or at an equal distance from the center of the pupil. Many young children may appear to have a false appearance of an eye turn (pseudostrabismus), due to wide epicanthal skin folds or narrow interpupillary distance but will have central light reflexes with the Hirschberg test (Fig. 4.3). However, if the corneal reflex is asymmetric, then strabismus is suspected. The light reflex of the deviated eye will be perceived more temporally in a patient with esotropia and more nasally in a patient with exotropia. If there is a vertical misalignment, the light reflex will be more inferior in a patient with hypertropia and more superior in a patient with hypotropia. Angle kappa

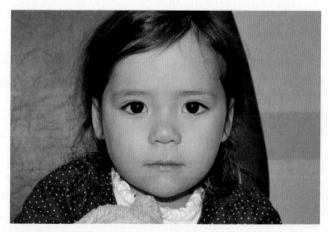

FIGURE 4.3. A child examined for pseudostrabismus showing symmetric corneal light reflexes with the Hirschberg test.

is an exception to this rule and will create an asymmetric reflex that may be present with or without strabismus. Angle kappa occurs if the pupillary axis is not aligned with the visual axis. A light reflex that is displaced nasally represents a positive angle kappa, whereas a light reflex displaced temporally is created by a negative angle kappa. Positive angle kappa is more common than negative angle kappa and can be associated with retinal diseases such as retinopathy of prematurity. Strabismus can be ruled out in patients with angle kappa by performing a cover–uncover test and by demonstrating that they do not have a manifest deviation.

Ocular alignment is more precisely examined by using various cover testing techniques. The cover–uncover test is used to detect a manifest eye misalignment. The test is performed by having the child fixate on a target while the examiner covers one eye with an occluder and observes any movement in the other eye. The occluder is removed and then the cover is placed over the other eye (Fig. 4.4). If either eye has to move to fix on the target when the other eye is covered, then a manifest deviation is present. The eye under the cover may move when the cover is removed if there is a latent deviation that is controlled by binocular fusion. An intermittent strabismus or a large phoria can be detected with the alternate test. The occluder is moved back and forth while alternately occluding either eye. The alternate cover test disrupts fusion and brings out the maximum deviation, which includes both the manifest and latent strabismus.

The size of the eye misalignment can be measured by using a prism with the cover test. The light entering a prism is displaced toward the base of the prism and the image is perceived toward the apex. To measure strabismus, the base of the prism is placed in the direction that the eye moves. For example, if a patient has an esotropia, the eye must move temporally to pick up fixation of the target. Therefore, the base of the prism would be placed temporally and is termed "base-out." The simultaneous prism cover test measures the manifest component of the deviation and is performed by introducing a prism over the deviating eye and an occluder

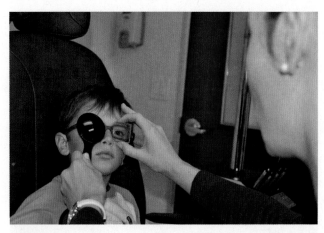

FIGURE 4.5. A base-out prism is placed over the left eye of a child with an esotropia while focusing on a sticker placed on the examiner's nose. The examiner alternates the cover test and increases the prism strength until neutralization is achieved.

over the fixing eye at the same time while the child fixates on a target. The tropia is neutralized when the deviating eye no longer has to move to fixate on the target. The alternate prism cover test is performed by placing a prism over the deviating eye while the patient focuses on a target and the examiner alternates the occluder (Fig. 4.5). As the examiner increases the prism strength, the size of the eye movement needed to regain fixation will decrease. The misalignment is neutralized when there is no shift on alternate cover testing. The alternate prism cover test measurement includes both the manifest and latent components of the eye misalignment. The cover test should be performed at distance and near and if possible in the 9 diagnostic positions of gaze. Strabismus can also be measured by aligning the corneal light reflex of the deviating eye with a prism. This technique is referred to as the Krimsky method and is performed by introducing increasing prism strengths over the deviating eye until the light reflexes are symmetric. This test is very useful in patients who cannot maintain fixation with their deviating eye due to severe vision loss.

Maddox Rods

The double Maddox rods are used to detect torsion from cyclo-vertical deviations. The test is performed by placing two red lenses with linearly grouped cylinders into a trial frame or the phoropter. The cylinders (rods) are vertically aligned at 90 degrees in each frame and the patient fixates on a muscle light or pen light (Fig. 4.6). The high-powered cylinders create a line of light that the patient perceives to be perpendicular to the rods. A cyclo-vertical deviation will cause one or both lines to appear tilted. The patient is asked to rotate the lenses to make the lines parallel. The direction in which the rods are rotated corresponds to the direction of cyclo-rotation of the eye and is measured in degrees. For example, a patient with a superior oblique (SO) weakness

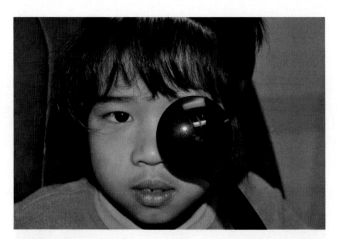

FIGURE 4.4. An occluder is presented in front of the child's eye during a cover–uncover test.

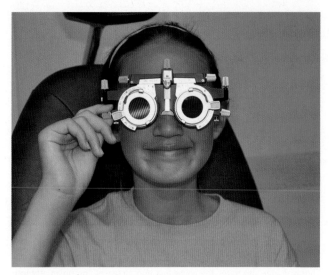

FIGURE 4.6. A child with a superior oblique paresis wearing double Maddox rod lenses in a trial frame to measure the amount of subjective torsion.

will have an eye that is excyclo-rotated due to the decreased ability of the SO to incyclo-rotate the eye. The child will then need to rotate the vertical rods temporally (excyclotorsion) in order to perceive the lines as parallel. If the child is fusing a small intermittent vertical deviation, then a prism can be used to disrupt fusion and vertically displace the two horizontal lines.

Ocular Motility

Extraocular muscle function is tested by having the child fixate on a light or small toy and having the child follow the object into the six cardinal positions (right, right and up, right and down, left, left and up, left and down). All six extraocular muscles can be evaluated for cranial nerve paralysis, muscle restriction, or overaction by moving the eyes into the cardinal positions. This conjugate movement of both eyes together is called a version. If there is a limitation of a muscle on version testing then duction (uniocular) movements should be evaluated. Generally, a paresis of a muscle will improve on duction testing, whereas a restriction will not.

Vergence Movements

Vergence eye movements are disconjugate in direction and are used to maintain or restore binocular fusion. Convergence is when both eyes move inward toward the nose, whereas divergence is when both eyes move temporally. Vertical vergence movements are much smaller but may increase in cases of longstanding vertical deviations, such as superior oblique paresis. Vergence movements are tested binocularly with a prism bar or rotary prism while placing the apex of the prism in the direction that you want the eye to move.

Convergence movements are important for maintaining binocular single vision at near distances, especially while reading. The inability to maintain convergence at near distance is associated with eye strain, diplopia, blurred vision, and headaches. Decreased convergence ability that is associated with the aforementioned symptoms is referred to as convergence insufficiency. Convergence amplitudes are tested by increasing base-out prisms on a horizontal prism bar until the patient can no longer make a convergence movement to maintain fusion (Fig. 4.7). Convergence ability is also tested by examining the near point of convergence (NPC). The NPC is the closest point toward the eye at which a person can maintain binocular single vision. To perform this test, the child focuses on a picture or toy at near distance and the examiner slowly moves the target toward the child's nose (Fig. 4.8). An exotropia will occur when the patient can no longer maintain fusion and is documented as the break point. An NPC distance of less than 10 cm is considered to be within normal limits. Convergence insufficiency can be associated with a moderate to large intermittent exotropia (usually greater than 10 prism diopters). Alternate cover

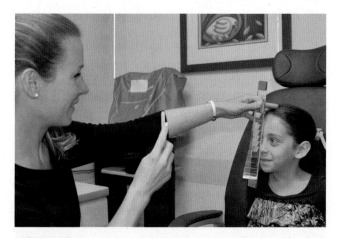

FIGURE 4.7. An examiner testing convergence amplitudes with a horizontal prism bar.

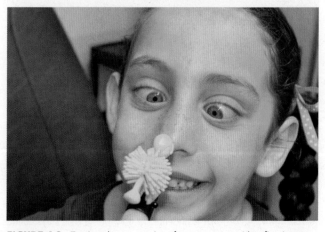

FIGURE 4.8. Testing the near point of convergence with a fixation toy.

needs to be performed at near distance to bring out the maximum deviation. What may initially appear to be a small exophoria can turn out to be a large intermittent exotropia once properly dissociated.

BINOCULAR VISION TESTING

Evaluating the sensory status of children is an essential part of the pediatric eye examination. Testing stereo acuity is an excellent way of screening for various conditions that may interfere with the development of binocular depth perception. Children with strabismus, anisometropia, media opacities, high refractive errors, and other pathologies can have decreased or absent stereo acuity. There are two different types of stereo tests that are commonly used by most ophthalmologists: contour stereopsis tests like the Titmus test and random dot tests like the Randot or Lang tests. The Titmus test consists of slightly disparate images (fly, animals, and circles) that are perceived in depth with polarized glasses. The child is asked to locate the wings on the fly. A child who is able to appreciate depth will attempt to pinch or grasp the wings without touching the page of the book. The child should then be asked to locate the animals or circles that appear to be raised (Fig. 4.9). The Titmus test can measure stereo acuity to a threshold of 40 seconds of arc with the circles. One limitation to the Titmus test is that there are monocular clues that can create a false positive response. Conversely, random dot stereo tests prevent monocular clues by surrounding the images with random dot patterns. The Randot stereo test also uses polarized glasses to enable depth perception. To date, there are three different versions of the Randot test that are commonly used in the ophthalmologist's practice. The standard near test has various geometric shapes, animals, and circles and can test fine stereo acuity up to 20 seconds of arc. The child is asked to name or locate the geometric images or detect which animals and circles are raised. The preschool and distance Randot tests use geometric shapes and can detect up to 40 and 60 seconds of arc, respectively (Fig. 4.10).

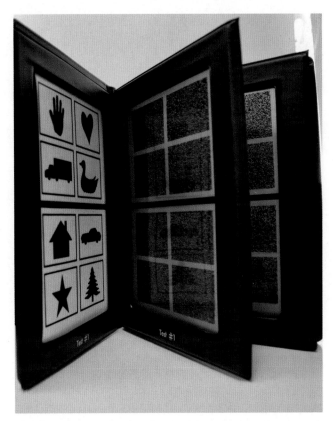

FIGURE 4.10. The preschool Randot test used at near distance with polarized glasses.

The Lang test is also a random dot test that is performed at near distances, but it does not require glasses. There are two versions of the test with 3 or 4 images (Fig. 4.11). This test is very useful in preverbal children or children that refuse to wear the polarized glasses. The child may voluntarily point at the images or glance back and forth between them. Testing fusion with a 20 diopter base-out prism can be used as an alternative method in infants and very young children. The prism is placed over either eye as a child focuses

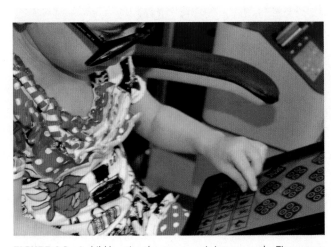

FIGURE 4.9. A child locating the stereoscopic images on the Titmus test.

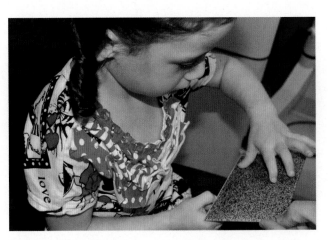

FIGURE 4.11. A child finding a random dot image on the Lang test.

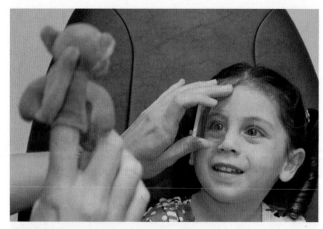

FIGURE 4.12. A child demonstrating fusion and normal binocular vision with the 20 diopter base-out test.

on a target at near. If the child has normal ocular alignment with relatively equal vision, the eyes will make a convergence movement to overcome the base-out prism (Fig. 4.12). Failure to overcome the base-out prism could be indicative of strabismus or amblyopia. Any child with decreased stereo vision needs ocular alignment examination with cover testing, cycloplegic refraction, and a dilated fundus exam.

Further sensory testing to assess fusion and suppression can be performed in children with decreased depth perception. The Worth 4-dot test is commonly used to test for fusion and suppression. A flashlight with 4 circles (2 green, 1 red, 1 white) is viewed with red-green glasses with the right eye looking through a red lens and the left eye looking through a green lens (Fig. 4.13). A child with binocular fusion will see 4 circles at the same time, 2 red and 2 green. If there is suppression, the child will only see the color of the circles that correspond to the dominant eye or may alternate fixation and see the different colors switching. A child who has strabismus and is not suppressing will be diplopic and see 5 circles. Peripheral fusion is assessed when

the flashlight is held near, whereas central fusion is tested when the flashlight is held at distance. A child with mono-fixation syndrome will commonly present with peripheral fusion at near and suppression at distance due to the small area of the suppression scotoma. Another way of testing for a suppression scotoma is by placing a small prism (usually 4 prism diopter base-out) in front of the nondominant eye. Suppression is suspected if the eye does not shift or make a vergence movement.

COLOR VISION TESTING

Color vision testing is important on any male child where there are concerns (either family history or problems with red/green discrimination) of decreased color vision or any patient with suspected loss of color vision. It is not a routine part of every pediatric eye exam. Color vision testing is usually performed with both eyes open. Ishihara pseudo-isochromatic color plates offer an easy to administer, quick screening test that can often be performed by the staff during the workup of the patient. A benefit to the Ishihara plates is that they include tracings that a child who does not know their numbers can follow with his or her finger (Fig. 4.14).

PUPILLARY EXAM

Pupillary size in the pediatric population varies with age. Newborns have very miotic pupils, which gradually enlarge as the child ages and peak at 7 mm average in the early teens before beginning a gradual decline. The pupillary examination on a young baby is often difficult and can be confounded by their accommodative reflex. In older children, the near accommodative response can be controlled by having them fixate on a distant target during the exam. Pupil size should be measured both with the lights on and off. Direct and consensual responses should also be measured. The swinging flashlight test should be performed to check

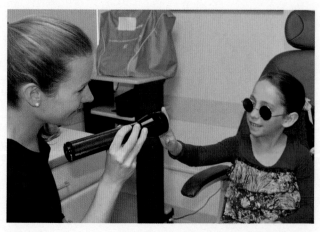

FIGURE 4.13. Testing fusion at near distance with the Worth 4 Dot.

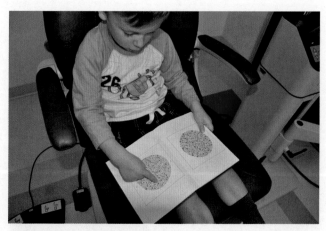

FIGURE 4.14. A boy being tested for color deficiency with the Ishihara pseudo-isochromatic color plates.

for afferent pupillary defects. Care must be taken to ensure the light is pointed at the pupil in cases of strabismus. Children can often have significantly more hippus than adults. Dense amblyopia can cause a small afferent pupillary defect but mild or moderate amblyopia will not. Any pupillary pathology in the setting of presumed amblyopia needs to be further evaluated.

SLIT LAMP EXAMINATION

Slit lamp examination on very young children is often not indicated when an external and anterior segment exam can be performed with either a penlight or an indirect ophthalmoscope using the lens as a magnifier rather than a condensing lens. In cases where anterior segment pathology cannot be adequately evaluated by penlight, a slit lamp exam is indicated. This can often be difficult and frustrating. Babies and infants need to be held in an upright slit lamp often by more than one person, and younger children may be fearful of the instrument. One option, handheld slit lamps, can be used on a supine child; they are portable, and are often less intimidating to a young child. They usually do not offer the quality resolution of an upright slit lamp, so anterior chamber inflammation and subtle corneal changes may be difficult to see.

There are several techniques that can help achieve a good upright slit lamp examination on a child when necessary. For very young children, the parent can hold the child's body at the correct height while an assistant holds the head in the slit lamp. The examiner can then open the child's eyes while viewing through the slit lamp. For older children, positioning is very important. Slit lamp tables and exam chairs generally are not well suited to the pediatric population. Children can be asked to kneel, or move to the edge of the seat with their legs apart so that the chair can be elevated enough for their heads to reach the chin rest (Fig. 4.15). It is beneficial to have them a little higher than is necessary so that they have to lean forward which keeps their heads from drifting back. To lessen the child's fear, the light on the slit lamp should be as dim as possible while still offering a good view. One way to make the slit lamp exam a fun game is have the child "grab the handlebars of the motorcycle" and hold on tightly while the lights are coming. Always look first at what you are most interested in as a slit lamp exam can be cut short quickly by a child's temperament.

TONOMETRY

Tonometry is not part of a routine exam in a child unless there is a concern for increased (or decreased) intraocular pressures. There are several types of tonometers available, each with different strengths and weaknesses. The gold standard of intraocular pressure measurements has long been Goldmann applanation. The main difficulty with Goldmann (or any contact tonometry) is that young children are generally not cooperative, and if it is indicated, exam under anesthesia may be necessary.

The Icare rebound tonometer has shown promise for screening healthy children and has been reported comparable with Goldmann applanation. It is a rebound tonometer that does not require the use of a topical anesthetic drop, is quick, and easy to use (Fig. 4.16). Its drawbacks are that is expensive and still requires some patient cooperation. Similarly the Tonopen is easier to use on a child than Goldmann applanation, but it requires anesthetic and multiple measurements, which can be difficult in a struggling child. We have found that a fixation target or cartoon movie show at the end of the room can often help keep a child's attention long enough to obtain accurate Tonopen readings, although the Tonopen itself is also considered less accurate than the Goldmann. For screening purposes on low-risk older children, pneumotonometry can be performed. Pneumotonometers are easy to use and do not require contact with the cornea; however, they are significantly less accurate and not portable to use on younger children. When accurate intraocular pressure measurements are indicated in an uncooperative child, an exam under anesthesia is indicated.

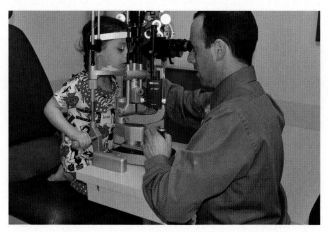

FIGURE 4.15. A young child kneeling for the slit lamp examination.

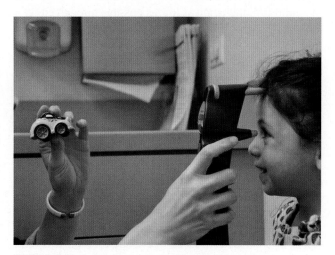

FIGURE 4.16. Icare rebound tonometer.

DILATION

There is a wide variation in dilation practices among pediatric ophthalmologists. Many physicians prefer to have their staff instill the drops in the child so that there is less fear of the doctor for the dilated portion of the exam. For young or premature babies in whom cycloplegia is not necessary, Cyclomydril drops mixed with dilute tropicamide can be used. For any child that needs accurate cycloplegic refraction, cyclopentolate drops should be used, often along with other drops. Cyclopentolate usually achieves full cycloplegia within 30 minutes to 1 hour. For darker irides, many add phenylephrine and or tropicamide drops to improve dilation. Darker irides may require more than one instillation of drops. Some practitioners instill topical anesthetic prior to mydriatics in order to aid penetration and decrease discomfort. For children who do not achieve full cycloplegia from cyclopentolate, atropine drops can be used either in the office, or given to the parent to dilate the patient prior to the exam. For atropine given at home, parents are generally instructed to place one drop, twice a day for 3 days prior to their appointment. Some practitioners prefer mixtures of drops or formulating the drops in a spray bottle so that they can be quickly sprayed into the child's eyes rather than holding them down to instill drops. It is important to remember that unlike adult dilating drops, cyclopentolate can last 24 hours or longer in children and atropine drops can last 1 to 2 weeks.

OPHTHALMOSCOPY

An adequate ophthalmoscopic fundus examination through dilated eyes is an important part of most examinations and can be very difficult for the general ophthalmologist. Slit lamp or direct ophthalmoscope fundus examinations are often impossible in children. Indirect ophthalmoscopy is generally the easiest technique to visualize the fundus in a child. The extent of the examination will vary significantly based on the suspected pathology. Visualization of the posterior pole can be done fairly easily on a cooperative child with the indirect illumination as low as possible through either a 28D or 20D lens. An interesting fixation target can be used to modify the child's gaze in order to visualize any areas of concern. If an adequate fundus examination cannot be performed in the office and posterior pathology is suspected, exam under anesthesia is indicated

REFRACTION

Cycloplegic refraction in a preverbal (and sometimes verbal) child is a mandatory portion of any examination where decreased vision is suspected. It can be a daunting task for non-pediatric ophthalmologists, but with practice and perseverance this "art" can be mastered. Uncorrected refractive errors in children can lead to permanent vision loss, and

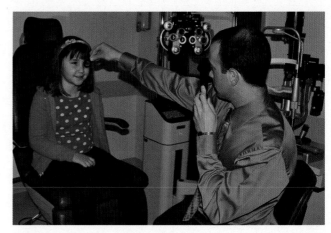

FIGURE 4.17. Retinoscopy with loose lenses.

so it is important to be comfortable and confident in your retinoscopy skills. Expertise with loose lenses and the ability to move fluidly and remain flexible are a must (Fig. 4.17). Remember to keep your working distance stable and engage the child in any way you can. A movie at the end of the room is useful, but the practitioner must remember to stay in line with the pupillary axis in order to get accurate results.

Physicians can use handheld autorefractors to assist with refraction in older children. Many of them have improved accuracy after cycloplegia. If a child can sit upright in an autorefractor, the measurement can be used for more accurate angles of astigmatism than can be measured by handheld lenses. It is important to remember that an autorefractor will frequently over-minus (or under-plus) a child when he or she is not cyclopleged as can manifest refraction.

UNCOOPERATIVE CHILDREN

Some children (usually younger) are uncooperative because they are scared or because they are tired or because they associate doctors' offices with shots or other painful procedures, and no matter how much you smile or laugh or play, they will not warm up to the examiner. In such cases, an adequate examination may still be obtained. If vision can be checked by the CSM method and the pupils can be checked, the patient should then be dilated. After dilation the parent should be enlisted to help in holding the child for the exam. Prior to restraining the child, all necessary instruments should be out on the table including a retinoscope, loose lenses, an indirect ophthalmoscope, and a 20D or 28D lens. One easy technique to perform the examination upright is to have the child sit on a parent's lap facing the physician. The parent's legs should be crossed over the child's legs in order to prevent any kicking injuries. The parent can then hold the child's arms up to secure both the head and the arms at the same time. Assisting staff can then hold the eyes open while the physician performs retinoscopy and fundus exam (Fig. 4.18).

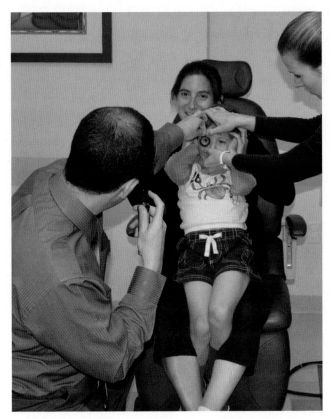

FIGURE 4.18. Retinoscopy on an uncooperative child. The child's legs and arms are restrained by the parent while assisting staff hold the eyes open.

EXAMINATION UNDER ANESTHESIA

Exam under anesthesia is indicated in any child when a necessary part of the exam cannot be performed in the office. Developmentally delayed or combative children that are too strong to be safely held down in the office and require further evaluation should have an exam under anesthesia. This can include tonometry, pachymetry, refraction, gonioscopy, slit lamp, or operating microscope evaluation, and fundus examination (Fig. 4.19). It is important to remember that tonometry should be performed as early as possible during induction as general anesthetics can alter intraocular pressures (Fig. 4.20).

SUMMARY

The pediatric eye examination can be a challenging, time-consuming, and fear-inducing visit for a general ophthalmologist. It requires practice, adaptability, a warm smile, and the ability to engage children and enlist them as allies in the examination. Retinoscopy skills, pediatric vision testing, and motility testing must be practiced regularly to maintain competence. The reward for the general ophthalmologist is the gratification of preventing or treating potentially vision threatening diseases, and offering a child the chance at lifelong excellent vision.

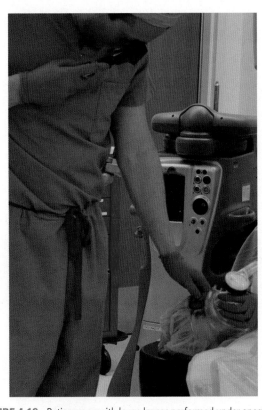

FIGURE 4.19. Retinoscopy with loose lenses performed under anesthesia.

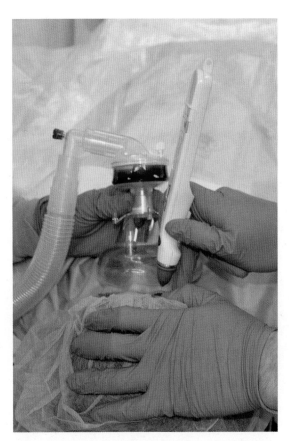

FIGURE 4.20. Measuring intraocular pressure with a tonopen under anesthesia.

REFERENCES

1. American Academy of Ophthalmology. Basic and clinical science course. *Pediatric ophthalmology and strabismus. Section 6.* San Francisco, CA: American Academy of Ophthalmology, 2006.
2. Ansons AM, Davis H. Diagnosis and management of ocular motility disorders, 3rd Ed. Oxford: Blackwell, 2001.
3. Nelson LB, Olitsky S, eds. *Harley's pediatric ophthalmology,* 5th Ed. Philadelphia, PA: Lippincott Williams & Wilkins, 2005.
4. Pratt-Johnson J, Tillson G. *Management of strabismus and amblyopia—a practical guide.* New York: Thieme Medical Publishers, Inc, 1994.
5. von Noorden GK, Campos E. *Binocular vision and ocular motility. Theory and management of strabismus,* 6th Ed. St. Louis, MO: Mosby, 2002.
6. Wright KW, Spiegel PH, eds. *Pediatric ophthalmology and Strabismus,* 2nd Ed. New York: Springer, 2003.

5

Refraction in Infants and Children

Michael X. Repka

THE MANAGEMENT OF refractive error is the most common problem faced by the ophthalmologist examining pediatric patients. Children present with symptoms of blurred vision, inability to read, sitting too close to the television, squinting, or poor performance in school. They may have been referred by a primary care provider or after a failed school screening examination. In addition to subnormal vision, children may complain of ocular fatigue, inability to study, letter reversal while reading and writing, and reading difficulty. Many will have normal eye and ocular motility examinations. For many only reassurance is necessary, while others will have a refractive problem.

DETERMINATION OF VISUAL ACUITY AND REFRACTIVE ERROR

Accurate measurement of refractive error is an essential component of the pediatric eye examination. Refractive error change during childhood mandates frequent rechecks. For instance, an aphakic infant may require monthly examinations, whereas yearly checks are sufficient for most myopic teenagers. Refraction of a child cannot be rushed and should rely on objective techniques rather than on the subjective techniques used in adult practice. The examination is generally carried out with the parents present. It is best for young children to sit on a parent's lap. Older children may prefer to sit alone, as long as a parent or other familiar person is present. The room should not be completely darkened, as this may provoke anxiety (Fig. 5.1).

Visual acuity was considered to be essentially absent at birth, only 6 decades ago (1) Optokinetic nystagmus (OKN) measurements in the late 1950s showed this belief to be erroneous (2). Visual-evoked potential (VEP) acuities have been found to range from 20/200 to 20/100 at birth and to reach 20/20 by 1 year of age. Preferential looking techniques have demonstrated acuities of approximately 1 cycle per degree at birth (20/400), rapidly improving to adult levels of 30 cycles per degree by 30 months (3). Linear letter acuity is normally 20/40 by age 3 and 20/30 by age 4 or 5 years (3). By 7 years of age, most children have achieved 20/20 line acuity.

Acuity in the Preverbal Child

Measurement of visual acuity is normally performed in the course of determining the refractive error. In most children less than 2.5 years of age, preverbal methods must be used (4). Clinical methods for infants involve an estimate of fixation and following behavior (Fig. 5.2). A penlight is never used as a target since it lacks the edge contours necessary for accurate detection. Instead, the test target should incorporate high-contrast edges, e.g., stripes or a checkerboard. Perhaps the best target for an infant is the examiner's face. An infant normally displays a visual preference for the human face. For the child of 6 months and older, an interesting toy should be used. Monocular fixation normally can be demonstrated at term and certainly should be present by the end of the first month of life. Following behavior refers to a qualitative assessment of the competence the infant demonstrates in following a moving target. The smoothness and amplitude of pursuit rapidly improves during the first 6 months of life. Careful observation for the presence of a fine nystagmus should be part of each examination. Some practitioners prefer to describe the quality of the fixation behavior with the terms "central," "steady," and "maintained." Maintained fixation implies that the patient will maintain fixation with the same eye after a blink. No matter how fixation is described, the examiner also assesses the binocular fixation pattern to determine if there is an eye preference. A difference suggests a problem in the less preferred eye. One scheme is listed in Table 5.1, adapted from Zipf (4), in which categories A and B are considered normal, while C and D suggest amblyopia. However, there is considerable overlap between these grades, and the test appears to consistently overdiagnose amblyopia (5,6).

In an attempt to improve upon fixation preference testing with an objective, quantitative method of assessing visual function, techniques utilizing grating targets of varying spatial frequency (stripe width) have evolved. Such methods rely on detection of resolution acuity, a more sophisticated measure of visual performance than mere detection of a target as used for fixation assessment. There are three methods currently used for determining resolution acuity. They rely on preferential looking techniques, eliciting and detecting OKN, or recording a VEP.

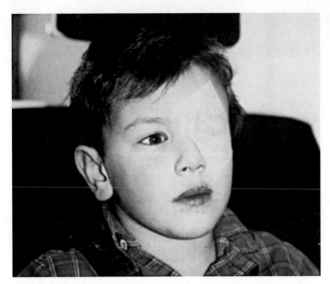

FIGURE 5.1. Examination of the preschooler. The patient is seated comfortably in a partially darkened room. The left eye is occluded with paper tape.

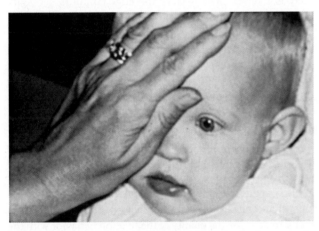

FIGURE 5.2. Fixation preference. The examiner is testing the monocular fixation pattern of an infant by using an attractive toy.

Table 5.1

GRADING SCHEME FOR FIXATION PREFERENCE TESTING[a]

Grade	
A	Spontaneous alternation between the right and left eyes
B (holds well)	Fixation held with non-preferred eye before refixation to preferred eye for:
	≥ 3 s
	during a smooth pursuit
	through a blink
C (holds momentarily)	Fixation held with non-preferred eye for 1–3 s
D (does not hold)	Refixation with preferred eye occurs immediately (<1 s) when the occluder is removed from the preferred eye

[a]12–16 prism diopter placed base-down before one eye to produce a strabismus in the orthotropic patient
Adapted from Zipf RF. Binocular fixation pattern. *Arch Ophthalmol* 1979;94:401–405

The most widely used test is preferential looking. Forced-choice preferential looking (3), operant preferential looking (7), and current variations of the acuity card procedure have been developed to provide a simple, efficient method of assessing visual acuity in infants, young children, and nonverbal patients (Fig. 5.3) (8,9). Each of these methods assumes that the child prefers to look at an area of higher visual interest, the striped grating, rather than a neutral gray field. By determining the smallest width grating on which the patient will fixate, resolution acuity can be determined. Normative data for these tests can be used to translate these spatial resolution values to approximate Snellen acuity (8,10). There are wide ranges in normal, especially among the youngest children.

Preferential looking methods require time and specially trained personnel. These methods are not suitable as screening tools. The acuity card testing required 36 minutes for testing of the monocular and binocular acuity of one patient (9). The acuity card procedure seems most useful for monitoring amblyopia therapy in children with severe unilateral abnormalities (e.g., monocular aphakia).

Visual acuities in infants have also been measured with VEP recordings or eliciting OKN in response to stripes of various widths. These two methods are handicapped by the complicated apparatus necessary for their performance. The OKN method is additionally handicapped by its reliance on a normal ocular motor system for end-point determination. The usefulness of VEP is diminished by its reliance on a dedicated technician. An additional concern with VEP is that acuities determined by it are better than those determined by behavioral methods because VEP bypasses neural processing to determine a response end point. All three resolution methods for assessing visual acuity (forced-choice preferential looking, VEP, and OKN) are further hampered by their overestimation of visual acuity even among normal individuals (10). Unfortunately, this is the exact infant for whom the development of this type of test is most important.

Between 1 and 3 years of age, visual acuity remains difficult to measure. Behavioral techniques are too time consuming to maintain an active toddler's interest, although limited success has been reported with the acuity card procedure (9). Other tests for this age range are reviewed by Simons (11)

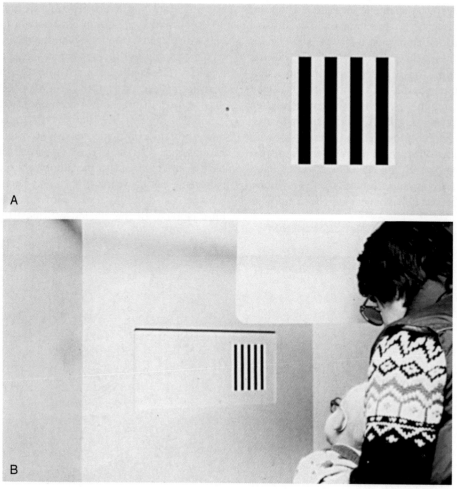

FIGURE 5.3. Teller acuity cards for preferential looking. **A:** Grating card with the largest striped pattern (0.32 cycles/degree) on one side and gray field on the other. **B:** An infant being tested with acuity cards.

and McDonald (12). Most clinicians have found these to be insufficiently reliable, and they continue to rely on assessment of fixation behavior until the child is 3 years old.

Acuity in the Older Child

After the age of 2.5 years, children will increasingly be able to read a chart to determine their visual acuity. These tests measure recognition acuity: the ability to differentiate one stimulus from a group of similar stimuli.

The particular test used, as well as the method of presentation, should be the most complex to which the patient can respond consistently. Comparison of visual acuities from visit to visit must take into account the specific test performed as well as the child's reliability during each examination.

For any test of children's vision, the method of optotype presentation may affect the measured acuity. Give adequate time and remove as much distraction from the exam room as possible. The testing distance should be 3 m rather than 6 m because of better testability. Presentation of a line of characters or surrounded single optotypes (Fig. 5.4) is preferable. These two methods produce similar results (13). Single letter

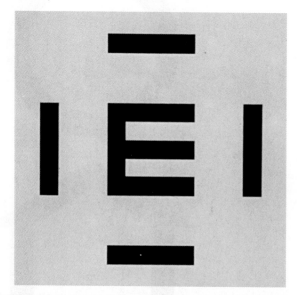

FIGURE 5.4. Letter with "surround" bars. A single letter is used to eliminate recognition confusion from multiple stimuli, while the bars produce the necessary edge interactions to produce good linear acuity. These are positioned one-half symbol width away from the optotype.

presentation eliminates contour interactions around the test optotype, which results in improvement in the measured visual acuity in both normal and amblyopic eyes (11). This effect is clinically termed "the crowding phenomenon." The effect is greater in amblyopic eyes; thus, a patient with amblyopia may not be detected when tested with single optotypes.

The test most commonly used for the youngest children involves picture optotypes (Fig. 5.5A), as they are more easily tested in young children. However, these tests even with surround bars are less sensitive to intereye acuity disparity than letter optotypes, and thus may not detect all cases of decreased vision. Hyvarinen invented a set of symbols (house, square, apple, circle) modeled on the Landolt C (Fig. 5.5B) (14).

Single surrounded HOTV tests are of great utility in the 30 to 54-month age group. The patient matches the letter being displayed to one on a handheld card. Consequently, recognition but not literacy is required for this letter optotype test. The method of presenting the HOTV stimuli has been formalized in a protocol developed for the Amblyopia Treatment Studies (15). An automated version of the Amblyopia Treatment Study HOTV test is being used in many centers to provide consistent visual acuity determinations (Fig. 5.6) (16). The Lea symbols in a chart format have been compared to the automated HOTV test among children 3 to 3.5 years of age (17). Equally high proportions were successfully tested. However, children tested 2.5 lines better with the HOTV test, most likely because the

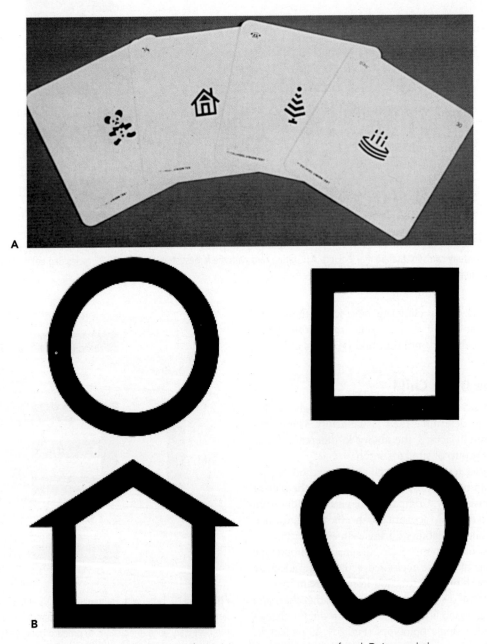

FIGURE 5.5. Picture optotypes. **A:** Traditional Allen pictures. These picture optotypes are not preferred. **B:** Lea symbols.

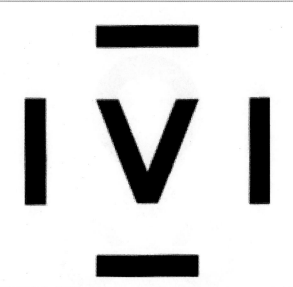

FIGURE 5.6. HOTV optotypes are presented in a single surrounded format in a random sequence on a computer monitor at 3 m. The child should be shown or even can hold a matching card to facilitate the testing. Linear versions of the test are also available.

multiline Lea chart was used. In clinical practice, the Lea symbols have fared much better when tested in a single crowded optotype format (18).

After 4 years of age, the single surrounded HOTV, letters, or tumbling-E test is used (Fig. 5.7). The E test was first devised by Snellen and while widely accepted as a standard, it is not recommended because it tends to be confusing for young children.

The most commonly used letter visual acuity test is one of the modifications of the Snellen chart (Fig. 5.8). The Snellen chart is not ideal as it employs letters of different legibility at the same visual angle and a scale that changes with unequal steps. A better letter test was designed by Sloan consisting of ten letters of approximately equal legibility (Fig. 5.9) (19). These letters have been used in the Early Treatment of Diabetic Retinopathy Study acuity test (20).

A standard optotype test of visual acuity is the Landolt C (Fig. 5.10). The subject identifies the orientation of the opening in the letter. This test, to date has met with limited clinical acceptance and is not useful in young children.

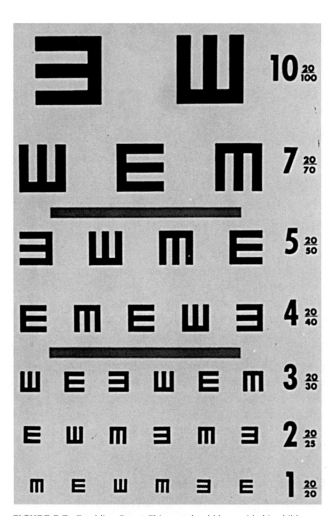

FIGURE 5.7. Tumbling-E test. This test should be avoided in children.

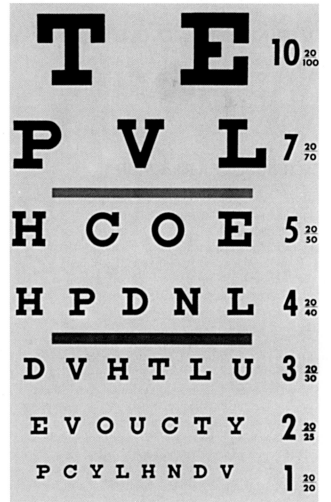

FIGURE 5.8. Snellen chart.

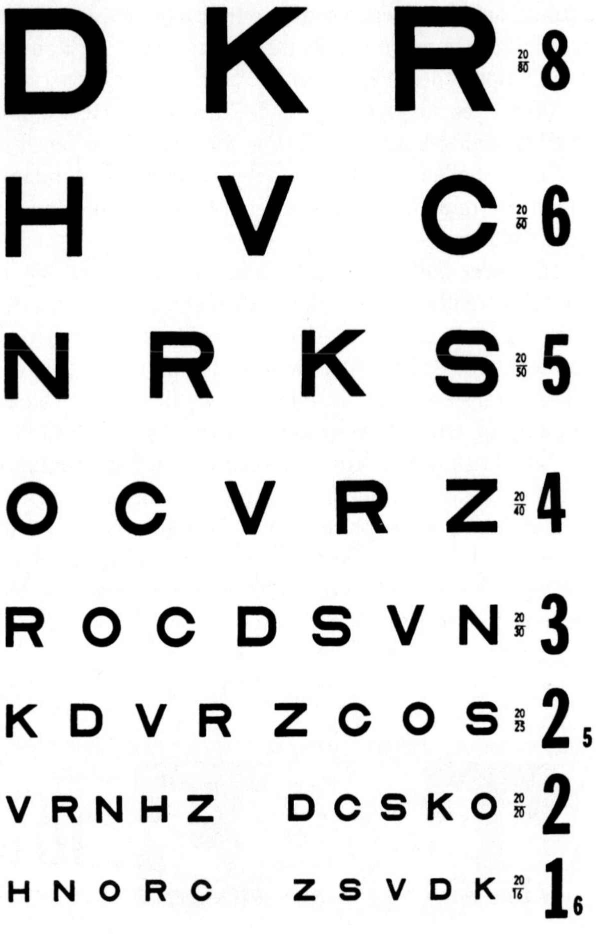

D K R 20/80 8

H V C 20/60 6

N R K S 20/50 5

O C V R Z 20/40 4

R O C D S V N 20/30 3

K D V R Z C O S 20/25 2.5

V R N H Z D C S K O 20/20 2

H N O R C Z S V D K 20/16 1.6

FIGURE 5.9. Sloan letter optotypes.

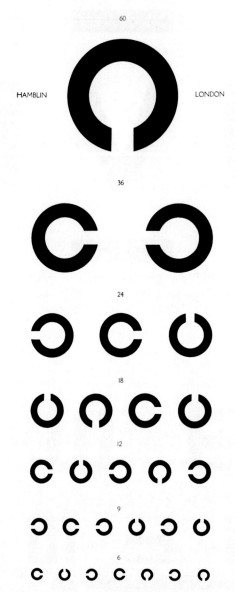

FIGURE 5.10. Landolt C optotype test.

TECHNIQUE OF REFRACTION

Refraction of children is difficult because of their apprehension and brief attention spans. Consequently, the refraction must be both rapid and accurate. Despite the development of objective automatic refracting instruments, objective retinoscopy remains the best method of determining a child's refraction. Retinoscopy is usually performed without sedation or a lid speculum, although conscious sedation or even general anesthesia may be required to perform accurate retinoscopy for some children.

Retinoscopy

The techniques of estimating refractive error taught by Copeland are used infrequently today. Most practitioners prefer neutralization methods using loose lenses in infants and young children, and trial frames or a phoropter in older children and teenagers. Retinoscopy is best performed with cycloplegia. When no cycloplegic agent is used, the retinoscopic refraction is termed "manifest" or dry. For such a refraction to be accurate, the patient's accommodation must be controlled, usually by having them view a distant,

nonaccommodative target such as a target light. Optotypes are unsuitable targets since the accommodative mechanism will respond to retinal blur, constantly adjusting the level of accommodation in an attempt to focus the image.

It is useful to attempt a manifest refraction of school-age children and teenagers before dilation if there is evidence of undiagnosed hypermetropia. If a large hyperopic error is confirmed during the cycloplegic refraction, the examiner will know about how much hyperopic correction the patient will tolerate and prescribe accordingly. This may eliminate the need for the patient to return for a post-cycloplegic manifest refraction.

Cycloplegic Refraction

The cycloplegic refraction is an integral part of the examination of each pediatric patient. In addition to determining refractive error, the instillation of the cycloplegic agent allows a thorough retinal exam. Selection of the cycloplegic agent depends on the age of the patient as well as the pigmentation of the iris. Cycloplegia in children more than 4 months of age is obtained by placing one drop of proparacaine HCl 0.5% in the inferior fornix of each eye, followed by one drop of cyclopentolate 1%. The use of a topical anesthetic before instillation of the cycloplegic drug enhances the cycloplegic effect. This is due to either reduction of reflex tearing and lid squeezing or alteration of the corneal epithelial barrier (21). The refraction is performed 35 to 40 minutes later. For preterm infants, a weaker cycloplegic agent is recommended such as a combination of 0.2% cyclopentolate and 1% phenylephrine. For term to 4-month-old infants, 0.5% cyclopentolate is satisfactory, although phenylephrine is also needed with darker irides. Use of the weaker agents reduces the systemic side effects, especially vomiting. In the case of smaller babies in the neonatal intensive care unit, care should be taken to examine them shortly before a feeding when the stomach is empty.

Many examiners consider atropine the most complete cycloplegic agent for children, especially for those with accommodative forms of esotropia. In a series of 120 patients with accommodative esotropia, Rosenbaum and coworkers found an average of 0.34 diopter more hyperopia with atropine 1% administered over 3 days compared with two drops of 1% cyclopentolate (22). They also noted that the difference between the cyclopentolate and atropine cycloplegic refractions tended to be greater for esotropic patients with hypermetropia greater than 2.00 diopters. Nonetheless, most practitioners continue to reserve atropine for those patients who fail to be adequately cyclopleged, despite two or three doses of cyclopentolate. Because of the potential for under correction with cyclopentolate, any patient who inadequately responds to a hyperopic correction or whose refractive esotropia decompensates should undergo a repeat cycloplegic refraction. It is common to find additional hyperopia at the second refraction.

If the examiner elects to use atropine, care should be taken. Atropine is administered by the parent or guardian usually as 1% ointment or solution twice daily for 3 days before the retinoscopic evaluation. It is important to instruct the parent not to instill the ointment the day of the evaluation, as the ointment vehicle will make retinoscopy nearly impossible. The parents should be instructed to store atropine, especially the solution, well away from children. Each drop of 1% solution contains 0.5 mg of atropine.

Symptoms of atropine toxicity include dryness of the mouth, tachycardia, fever, flushing of the skin, ataxia, disorientation, and even major motor seizures. If the ingestion is recent, milk or water should be administered, and emesis should be induced with syrup of ipecac. Gastric lavage should be performed if the ingestion is recent and emesis cannot be safely induced. Symptoms may persist for hours or even days. If the symptoms or signs are severe (arrhythmia, seizures), they are treated in children with repeated doses of physostigmine 0.25 mg subcutaneously or intramuscularly every 15 minutes. For children under 5 years of age, 0.02 mg/kg physostigmine IV (up to 0.5 mg) every 5 minutes with a maximal dose of 2.0 mg of physostigmine is recommended (23).

Dynamic Retinoscopy

A retinoscopic technique not widely appreciated or used by ophthalmologists is dynamic retinoscopy, which allows a quick assessment of the patient's ability to accommodate without the need for cumbersome laboratory equipment (24). The examiner begins by neutralizing the refractive error while the patient fixates the distant target. The working distance lens is then removed. The patient is asked to look at a near, accommodative target held next to the retinoscope. If the patient is able to accommodate to the near target, the examiner should see the motion of the reflex change to neutralization.

More quantitative techniques are used including automated open-field refractometry, Monocular Estimate Method (MEM), and Nott retinoscopy (25). The accuracy of these techniques to document accommodative lag is reduced.

Patients with high hypermetropia, retinal disease, or amblyopia often have deficient amplitudes of accommodation. When symptomatic accommodative insufficiency is noted, it should be corrected by the prescription of a near correction, which may relieve asthenopia.

Instrument-Based Screening for Refractive Error

Instrument-based screening has been promoted as a means to detect children at risk for amblyopia or having other ocular problems. There are two basic strategies: photoscreening for alignment and significant refractive error, and automated refraction.

Photoscreening, also called photorefraction, describes a screening test designed to detect amblyopiogenic factors, including strabismus, media opacities, and refractive error. These techniques involve simultaneous imaging of the corneal and fundus light reflexes of both eyes.

Two basic methods have been described (26,27). They differ in the relationship of the flash source to the optical axis of the camera. The coaxial method (isotropic) requires three images per patient (26). One is focused at the plane of the pupil, one defocused a fixed number of diopters anteriorly, and one an equal amount posteriorly. Spherical and cylindrical refractive errors can be determined within 0.75 diopter over a range of +4 to −4 diopters. Detection of strabismus is made difficult by the camera defocus necessary to measure the refractive error. This system has been largely supplanted by the off-axis system.

The off-axis system (eccentric photorefraction) provides a clearly focused image of the pupil, fundus red reflex, and corneal light reflex (27). Since the strobe stimulus is linear, each image yields information only along the axis parallel to the flash axis. In the past, two images with the strobe oriented at 90 degrees to each other were necessary. Modifications using two simultaneous flashes have been implemented, thereby requiring a single image (28). The sensitivity of off-axis photorefraction for detection of refractive error is usually greater than 80%, and it is better with cycloplegia and pupillary dilation. This technique can detect hyperopia greater than 1.0 diopter and myopia less than 2.5 diopters. Anisometropia of 1.0 diopter is routinely detected. The actual refractive error, however, can be determined only with cycloplegia because of variable levels of accommodation present during the examination. The corneal light reflex produced by the flash has made it possible to reliably detect strabismic angles as small as 2 degrees. One commercial photorefractor was found to have 91% sensitivity and 74% specificity for abnormal ocular status when tested on a group of patients known to have ocular abnormalities (29).

An important shortcoming remains the absence of demonstrated effectiveness in children under 3 years of age (30). Morgan and Johnson could not test 24% of their patients under 3 years of age (31). Donahue and colleagues did not diagnose strabismus, anisometropia, or astigmatism in children under 2 years of age (31). Further refinement of this method, as well as development of other screening strategies, will ultimately produce an effective screening tool.

Autorefraction instruments utilize optically automated retinoscopy or wavefront technology to evaluate the refractive error of each eye. For screening purposes, these data are analyzed on the basis of preset refractive error criteria to determine whether a child passes or fails a screening. The ability to prescribe from autorefraction in noncyclopleged children younger than 15 years of age has been difficult. This is because of substantial instrument and proximal myopia that is induced by peering into the instrument. Current instruments, which are smaller in size and less threatening, are highly testable and reliable when the testing is performed with cycloplegia. Subjective refractors have largely disappeared from the market. Their utility has been limited by patient cooperation and brief attention spans.

Instrument-based screening is unlikely to replace an exam in the ophthalmologist's office since the standard exam would still be available. Photoscreening and autorefraction have not been shown to be superior or inferior to visual acuity testing using vision charts for children age 4 to 5 years (32). Recent work found fully automated refractometry without cycloplegia to be superior to photoscreening (33).

ANATOMIC COMPONENTS OF REFRACTION

The refractive state of the eye is determined by four variables: corneal curvature, lenticular power, depth of the anterior chamber, and axial length of the globe. Each of these components has been exhaustively studied in an attempt to correlate a particular component to evolution of refractive error. Curtin suggested that axial length is the principal

determinant of refraction (34). During the infantile growth phase of the eye (up to 3 years of age), adjustments of corneal curvature and lens power are capable of producing an emmetropic refraction through a large range of axial lengths. During the juvenile growth period (3 to about 14 years), it appears that corneal curvature and lens power cannot continue compensating for continued axial expansion, resulting in a myopic refractive error.

Each of the components of refraction changes throughout development. Ocular anterior segment growth during infancy is extremely rapid. The newborn cornea of 10 mm attains nearly adult proportions by the end of the second year. At term birth, the mean corneal power is 55.2 diopters, decreasing during the first year of life to 45 diopters (35). The cornea of a premature child is generally steeper than that of a comparable child born at term. The increased corneal power seems to correlate well with the myopic trend observed in premature children (36,37).

The lens, unlike the remainder of the eye, continues to grow throughout life. At birth, a newborn lens is spherical, with a thickness of approximately 4 mm; it doubles in size during the first year of life. Lens power declines from 3 to 14 years of age due to progressive flattening.

The axial length of the eye undergoes two different growth stages, an infantile stage ending at age 3 years and a juvenile stage ending at age 14 years. The average axial length during the infantile stage of growth increases from 18.0 to 22.8 mm (38). During the juvenile growth phase, axial length increases only 1 mm. The eye achieves its full adult size by age 13 years. No spurt of ocular growth has been detected during puberty.

EVOLUTION OF REFRACTIVE ERROR

The natural history of refractive error has been the subject of numerous investigations (34). At birth, the eye is approximately 3 diopters hypermetropic. Cross-sectional studies found that hyperopia increased until 7 years of age, and then declined (39). Other studies have shown a steady decline in hyperopic refraction throughout childhood (35,38,40,41). Among children wearing spectacles, the percentage with correction for hyperopia decreases with age from 66% at 4 to 5 years to 11% at 12 to 17 years (42). The prevalence of myopic correction increases from 30% in the younger group to 87% in the older group. The prevalence of myopia in the general population of the U.S. approaches nearly 27% at 20 years of age.

Emmetropization

Emmetropic refractive error occurs more often than might be expected if refractive error simply followed a normal distribution. This process of emmetropization is a complex interaction of elements that produces near-emmetropia in 97% of the population (+4 to −4 diopters). A wide body of evidence suggests that both hereditary and environmental factors influence each of the components of refraction. Studies of the effect of environment on the refraction of laboratory animals, both primate and nonprimate, have shown that disruption of sensory input can produce an abnormal refractive state, most often myopia (34,43,44). However, hypermetropia can be induced by image defocus in the early postnatal period (45,46). It has been shown that minimal image defocus early in infant nonhuman primate eyes induces a modification in the normal growth pattern of that eye, which would eliminate the induced refractive error (47). Thus, emmetropization in limited instances may be able to compensate for induced refractive error. If this is generalizable to older human children, early correction would not be in the best interest of the child. There is speculation about the theoretical adverse effect of correcting all refractive errors. Such treatment could eliminate the normal emmetropization process. Ingram and coworkers studied fully corrected hypermetropic children with refractive esotropia (48). They found that children treated from 6 months of age had impaired emmetropization.

Etiology of Myopia

Most theories continue to suggest a dominant role for genetic determination of refractive error. This belief is based on twin and genealogic studies reviewed by Curtin (34). No accepted mode of inheritance has been demonstrated. It is not known if each of the refractive components is inherited independently or if the combination of components is the inherited factor.

The role of the environment in producing refractive error has been suggested by the increased frequency of myopia among patients with high intellectual achievement. This finding has been reported multiple times since Cohn's observation in 1907, confirming a strong correlation between myopia and intellectual performance (49). These studies, although suggestive, do not determine if the genetic determination of myopia is expressed because of the superior performance on academic skills (near work theory). It may be that the myopia causes the superior performance, or simply that the two traits are closely linked genetically.

The best conclusion available concerning the etiology of myopia is that the environment alters the penetrance and expressivity of genes, thereby producing the ultimate refractive error.

ACCOMMODATION

Accommodation is the change in dioptric power of the crystalline lens produced by the alteration of its shape in response to ciliary muscle contraction. The neural innervation to the ciliary muscle includes parasympathetic and sympathetic fibers. The parasympathetic fibers stimulate ciliary muscle contraction, while the sympathetic fibers inhibit contraction. A patient typically maintains a "resting" level of accommodation at an intermediate focus, between no accommodation and full accommodation. The position of the resting state varies in response to many factors, including systemic and topical medication use and the amount of near work performed.

The amplitude of accommodation decreases from a high at birth (50). During the second decade of life, the loss of accommodation is very gradual, the patient losing only about 2 diopters. Studies of accommodation in infants, using dynamic accommodation, showed that infants 2 to 10 months of age accommodate in the appropriate direction for changes in target distance, and furthermore accommodate at speeds comparable with those of adults (4.6 diopters/second) (51).

Accommodation is primarily stimulated by retinal image blur. Other factors also play important roles in the control of accommodation, including chromatic aberration, stimulus size, target contrast, and target velocity. Accommodation in normal eyes has the highest gain at the fovea (52). Response amplitude decreases as more eccentric retinal areas are stimulated. This is particularly relevant in the amblyopic eye, in which the amblyopic foveal retinal receptors are less efficient at stimulating accommodation, producing reduced accommodative amplitudes in amblyopic eyes (53). Abnormalities persist in treated amblyopic eyes (54,55). These investigators hypothesized that the unaffected peripheral retina, rather than the amblyopic fovea, was controlling the accommodative response. This resulted in an insufficient response.

Accommodation has also been found to be deficient in children with impaired vision and Down syndrome, as well as in children suffering damage to the ciliary muscle or ciliary ganglion (56,57). Bifocals should be considered for children with these medical conditions.

MANAGEMENT OF REFRACTIVE ERROR

Once the refractive error has been determined with and without cycloplegia, a management decision must be made. Impact-resistant polycarbonate lenses should be prescribed. This material meets most industrial standards and is lightweight. Its drawbacks are that it scratches easily and costs more than other materials.

Glasses are generally worn full-time in school. This facilitates adherence and allows consistency on the part of the patient's teacher. Bifocals are most often prescribed for patients with an esotropia for control of a high accommodative-convergence-to-accommodation ratio and are worn full-time. Bifocals are typically indicated when they provide the patient with the opportunity for fusion; bifocals are not usually employed if they only reduce the strabismic angle to an angle still too large for fusion (greater than 10 prism diopters). It is standard practice to prescribe 30 to 35 mm flat-top-style bifocal lenses, positioned to bisect the pupil. Less commonly, children wear bifocals because of aphakia, premature presbyopia from an ocular injury, or tonic pupil.

Hyperopia is the normal refractive state of the eye in childhood. Hyperopic refractive error may be divided into manifest and latent portions. The latent portion of the hyperopic refractive error is corrected by the patient's tonic accommodation and is not detected during manifest refraction. The latent portion of the hyperopia is uncovered only with a cycloplegic refraction.

Manifest hyperopia is that portion of the hyperopia detected or found in the "dry" or non-cycloplegic portion of the refraction. It may be subdivided into facultative and absolute portions. Facultative hyperopia is the portion that the patient can correct with extreme accommodative effort; such effort often causes asthenopia. Absolute hyperopia represents the portion for which the patient cannot compensate with maximal available accommodative effort, and presents with decreased vision.

Myopia is rare in infants except in those who develop retinopathy of prematurity or who have had severe visual deprivation (36,44). By late adolescence, nearly 27% of the population is myopic. Most have developed simple school-age or physiologic myopia. The only symptom is decreased vision at distance, often asymptomatic. Rarely, protracted squinting may cause asthenopic symptoms that bring the myopic patient to medical attention. Most, however, are detected by routine annual vision tests performed under the school system or by the primary care physician. This type of school-age-onset myopia tends to increase gradually until the child stops growing.

A less common type of myopia presents with poor vision in the first several years of life. This congenital or infantile myopia is generally of large magnitude, 5 diopters and greater, and tends to remain stable throughout life. When this type of myopia is unilateral, it generally leads to amblyopia.

Many therapeutic regimens for relief of myopia have been suggested to prevent or retard the progression of school-age myopia. Since near work has long been considered the etiologic factor in production of myopia, these regimens typically have been aimed at blocking accommodation. These include long-term use of atropine (58–61), the use of bifocals at near ranges, and removing myopic spectacles for near work. Excessive accommodation, according to the nearwork theory of myopia, produces increased refraction power of the anterior segment. This controversial theory remains unproved. A recently completed double-masked randomized clinical trial compared the rate of myopic progression between groups treated with progressive-add bifocals or single-vision lenses (62). These authors evaluated 469 children ages 6 to 11 years. The mean 3-year increases in myopia were –1.28 diopters with the bifocals compared with –1.48 diopters with single-vision myopic spectacles. This difference was statistically significant, but the small magnitude led the authors to conclude that a change in clinical practice to the use of bifocals was not warranted. Pirenzepine, a relatively selective M1 muscarinic antagonist, has been identified and has been found to be safe and effective in slowing myopia progression in a one-year trial (63,64). The magnitude of the effect, however, was modest and additional research is ongoing.

The third type of refractive error is astigmatism, which may be corneal or lenticular. It is important to correct astigmatism to avoid refractive or meridional amblyopia, a form of deprivation amblyopia, especially when the axis is oriented 15 or more degrees away from the vertical or horizontal (65). Although amblyopia usually occurs with large astigmatic errors, errors of 1.5 to 2 diopters may produce a deprivation amblyopia. The full astigmatic correction oriented at the correct axis is prescribed (66). Irregular astigmatism produced by corneal scarring, keratoconus, or other corneal disease is best corrected with a rigid gas-permeable contact lens.

The last major concern in prescribing correction is anisometropia, for which careful attention must be paid to the visual acuity. Anisometropia of 1.0 diopter can produce anisometropic amblyopia in hyperopic patients (67). Myopic patients are more resistant to the development of amblyopia. Any spectacle corrections should take anisometropia into account. If considerable anisometropia is present, the monofixation syndrome may be found. When anisometropia is corrected by spectacles, it is usually well tolerated by children, whereas it would produce symptomatic aniseikonia in adults.

Guidelines

The following guidelines for the correction of refractive error in children should be modified to fit the needs of the individual patient. Usually, such a correction will be worn happily by the child, at least part of the time. However, if glasses are not worn electively by the child, an error has been made somewhere. The error may be in the determination of the refractive state of the eye, but more likely it is an error in judgment regarding the visual demands of the child.

Many children are perfectly content with some distance blur from uncorrected low myopia because so much of interest to them is close. Relatively low myopic correction should be prescribed to be worn for school but may be optional at other times.

The blur from astigmatic errors is present at all distances, unlike the distance blur from uncorrected myopia. Astigmatic errors of more than 2 diopters should be corrected at least part-time to prevent the development of amblyopia. Oblique astigmatic errors of as little as 1 diopter may require correction because of symptoms or the presence of amblyopia. In the presence of hyperopia or myopia of sufficient magnitude to warrant correction, the astigmatism should be fully corrected.

The correction of hyperopic refractive error is dependent on the patient's demonstrated ability to accommodate and the presence of a strabismus. Children have very large amplitudes of accommodation, but they often experience asthenopia from extended periods of accommodation. Thus, it is not surprising that relatively low-power hyperopic corrections are frequently preferred for extended near work, even though sufficient accommodation is present by a near-point method. In the absence of esotropia, the amount of refractive error for which correction of children should be prescribed is uncertain. Some clinicians treat all children over +3.00 diopters with reduced plus lenses, while others individualize based on age, symptoms, and magnitude of the hypermetropic error (65). In addition, in the child without tropia the glasses may be worn part-time. The amount of reduction of plus has not been studied, but ranges in practice from 1 to 2 diopters.

APHAKIA

Contact Lens

The most common method of correcting monocular aphakia in children uses an extended-wear contact lens. A silicon extended-wear lens is often used, which is available in a wide range of powers (up to +320 diopters), base curves (7.3, 7.5, 7.7, 7.9, 8.1, 8.3), and diameter (11.3, 12.5 mm). High plus lenses (more than 20 diopters) are available only in a single 11.3-mm diameter and three base curves: 7.5, 7.7, 7.9. Most aphakic children can be suitably corrected with these lenses (68,69). Rigid gas-permeable lenses are a less costly alternative. Materials that allow extended wear are available, and gas-permeable lenses can be manufactured for especially steep base curves and high powers not available in the silicon extended-wear lenses. An infant contact lens should be adjusted to overcorrect the hypermetropia by approximately 2 diopters. For a toddler, the contact lens correction should be nearly emmetropic for distance or overcorrected by about 1 diopter. This patient should have bifocal spectacles prescribed when near tasks begin. Spectacles will also serve as protection for both eyes.

Epikeratophakia

Epikeratophakia is of historic note as an alternative means of correcting aphakic or other large refractive errors in children (70,71). The correction attained with epikeratophakia in infants has been too variable to be widely used in the management of infantile aphakia. This approach has been abandoned in favor of intraocular lens implantation.

Intraocular Lens

The use of intraocular lens (IOL) implants for aphakia in childhood has become widely accepted for visual rehabilitation in older children and increasingly in infancy (72,73). These lenses are not designed to be interchanged and thus do not keep pace with the myopic shift of the growing eye. In general, a small IOL implant with an optic diameter of 5.0 to 5.5 mm designed for capsular bag fixation is implanted (69,74,75). These lenses have been quite successful in the posttraumatic setting (76). The frequency of visual rehabilitation has been remarkable with the use of implants. The management of the posterior capsule should be planned in advance of the IOL implant surgery, as nearly every capsule opacifies quickly. Primary posterior capsulectomy and anterior vitrectomy is advocated for most children younger than 5 years of age. The lens selected should be implanted with powers predicted to produce hypermetropia. The amount of hypermetropia residual recommended varies widely among experts from 8 diopters in infants, 4 to 5 diopters at age 2 years, and 2 diopters at age 6 years. In the hypermetropic or short eye, the SRK/T, SRKII, or Holladay formulae are preferred (77). The minimum age for implantation in normal children has continued to decline as more experience has been gained and good outcomes have been achieved (73,78,79). Bilateral implantation is routinely considered for children 2 years of age and older, and monocular implants are offered during the first year of life or whenever contact lens use will not be easily achieved. The long-term results of the Infant Aphakia Treatment Study will address the lower age limit for unilateral implantations. The most frequently used implants are acrylic and foldable.

LOW VISION

Uncorrected refractive error is the most common cause of visual impairment in the developed world (80). Children represent a small fraction of patients with low vision (81). The most prevalent causes of visual loss have been congenital cataract, optic atrophy, and albinism. The impact of congenital cataract in the developed world with rubella vaccination is waning, while that of retinopathy of prematurity has become increasingly prevalent.

The physician examining children with impaired vision must perform the routine evaluation, as well as assessments of visual field, ambulatory ability, classroom function, and ability to perform other daily activities. High refractive errors should be corrected at least once. The use of special aids for infants and toddlers is rarely necessary. Early intervention programs for the visually disabled are generally available, and parents should be encouraged to make contact from the time the diagnosis is made. These are generally administered by the local school district. The intention of these programs is to minimize or eliminate any retarding effect on intellectual development that might be caused by subnormal vision.

The print used in books intended for the first three grades is 18-point type (2M), 14 to 16-point type (1.6M) for the fourth grade, and 10 to 12-point type (1M) through high school. Because of a child's high accommodative reserve, the patient with subnormal vision can often gain adequate magnification simply by holding the object close to the eye and accommodating. The use of a hand magnifying lens can help with the occasional need for greater magnification. By having the child bring actual school work to the office or low-vision clinic, an assessment can be made of visual function.

Once approach methods are no longer successful, due to inadequate accommodative capacity, inadequate magnification, need to view distance targets, or the child's self-consciousness, low-vision aids are necessary. These are identical to those available for adults. Spectacles are the first choice for constant use, providing good magnification and ample visual field, but greatly restricting the working distance of the patient. Closed-circuit television (up to 60 X), stand magnifiers, and computer-generated electronic image magnification and/or enhancement are some of the other aids employed. For distant and intermediate-distance tasks, telescopes are necessary. These may be helpful not just for watching sports or catching a bus but for viewing a computer screen or reading music.

The visually impaired child is most often educated within the regular school system, rather than in the residential blind school system. Support for the classroom teacher comes from a specialist in education of the visually impaired, who will provide training and materials for the teacher. The physician should strive to keep the teachers apprised of prognosis, along with important facts about the examination. For example, a patient with a right homonymous hemianopia should be seated on the right side of the classroom so that most of the classroom is within the intact field.

REFERENCES

1. Teller DY, Movshon JA. Visual development. *Vision Res* 1986;26:1483–1506.
2. Gorman JJ, Cogan DG, Gellis SS. An apparatus for grading the visual acuity of infants on the basis of opticokinetic nystagmus. *Pediatrics* 1957;19:1088–1092.
3. Teller DY. The forced-choice preferential looking procedure: a psychophysical technique for use with human infants. *Infant Behav Dev* 1979;2:135–153.
4. Zipf RF. Binocular fixation pattern. *Arch Ophthalmol* 1979;94: 401–405.
5. Atilla H, Oral D, Coskun S, Erkam N. Poor correlation between "fix-follow-maintain" monocular/binocular fixation pattern evaluation and presence of functional amblyopia. *Binoc Vis Strab Quart* 2001;16(2):85–90.
6. Friedman DS, Katz J, Repka MX, et al. Lack of concordance between fixation preference and HOTV optotype visual acuity in preschool children: the Baltimore pediatric eye disease study. *Ophthalmology* 2008;115:1796–1799.
7. Mayer DL, Dobson V. Visual acuity development in infants and young children, as assessed by operant preferential looking. *Vision Res* 1982;22:1141–1151.
8. McDonald MA, Dobson V, Sebris SL, Baitch L, Varner D, Teller DY. The acuity card procedure: a rapid test of infant acuity. *Invest Ophthalmol Vis Sci* 1985;26:1158–1162.
9. Preston KL, McDonald MS, Sebris SL, et al. Validation of the acuity card procedure for assessment of infants with ocular disorders. *Ophthalmology* 1987;94:644–653.
10. McDonald MA, Ankrum C, Preston K, et al. Monocular and binocular acuity estimation in 18- to 36-month-olds: acuity card results. *Am J Physiol Opt* 1986;63:181–186.
11. Simons K. Visual acuity norms in young children. *Surv Ophthalmol* 1983;28(2):84–92.
12. McDonald M. Assessment of visual acuity in toddlers. *Surv Ophthalmol* 1986;31:189–210.
13. Stager DR, Everett ME, Birch EE. Comparison of crowding bar and linear optotype acuity in amblyopia. *Am Orthop J* 1990;40:51–56.
14. Hyvarinen L, Nasanen R, Laurinen P. New visual acuity test for pre-school children. *Acta Ophthalmologica* 1980;58:507–511.
15. Holmes JM, Beck RW, Repka MX, et al. The amblyopia treatment study visual acuity testing protocol. *Arch Ophthalmol* Sept 2001;119(9):1345–1353.
16. Moke PS, Turpin AH, Beck RW, et al. Computerized method of visual acuity testing: adaptation of the amblyopia treatment study visual acuity testing protocol. *Am J Ophthalmol* 2001;132(6):903–909.
17. Vision in Preschoolers (VIP) Study Group. Threshold visual acuity testing of preschool children using the crowded HOTV and Lea symbols acuity tests. *J AAPOS* 2003;7:396–399.
18. Becker R, Hubsch S, Graf, MH, Kaufmann, H. Examination of young children with Lea symbols. *Br J Ophthalmol* 2002;86:513–516.
19. Sloan LL. New test charts for the measurement of visual acuity at far and near distances. *Am J Ophthalmol* 1959;48:807–813.
20. Early Treatment Diabetic Retinopathy Study Research Group. Early treatment diabetic retinopathy study design and baseline patient characteristics. ETDRS report number 7. *Ophthalmology* 1991;98:741–756.
21. Apt L, Henrick A. Pupillary dilatation with single eyedrop mydriatic combinations. *Am J Ophthalmol* 1980;89:553–559.
22. Rosenbaum AL, Bateman JB, Bremer DL, et al. Cycloplegic refraction in esotropic children. *Ophthalmology* 1981;88:1031–1034.
23. Johns Hopkins Hospital, Kristin Arcara K, Tschudy M. *The Harriet Lane handbook*, 19 Ed. St Louis, MO: Mosby, 2012.
24. Guyton DL, O'Connor GM. Dynamic retinoscopy. *Curr Opin Ophthalmol* Feb 1991;2(1):78–80.
25. Correction of Myopia Evaluation Trial 2 Study Group for the Pediatric Eye Disease Investigator Group. Accommodative lag by autorefraction and two dynamic retinoscopy methods. *Optom Vis Sci* 2009;86:233–243.
26. Howland HC, Howland B. Photorefraction: a technique for study of refractive state at a distance. *J Opt Soc Am A Opt Image Sci Vis* 1974;64:240–249.
27. Kaakinen K. A simple method for screening of children with strabismus, anisometropia, or ametropia by simultaneous photography of the corneal and the fundus reflexes. *Acta Ophthalmol* 1979;57:161–171.
28. Kaakinen KA, Kaseua HO, Teir HH. Two-flash photorefraction in screening of amblyogenic refractive errors. *Ophthalmology* 1987;94:1036–1042.
20. Morgan KS, Johnson WD. Clinical evaluation of a commercial photorefractor. *Arch Ophthalmol* 1987;105:1528–1531.
30. US Preventative Services Task Force. Vision Screening for Children 1 to 5 year of age: US preventive services task force recommendation statement. *Pediatrics* 2011;127:340–346.
31. Donahue SP, Johnson TM. Age-based refinement of referral criteria for photoscreening. *Ophthalmology* 2001;108:2309–2314.
32. Schmidt P, Maguire M, Dobson V, et al. Comparison of preschool vision screening tests as administered by licensed eye care professionals in the Vision In Preschoolers Study. *Ophthalmology* Apr 2004;111(4):637–650.

33. Miller J, Dobson V, Harvey, EM, Sherrill, DL,. Comparison of preschool vision screening methods in a population with a high prevalence of astigmatism. *Invest Ophthalmol Vis Sci* 2001;42:917–924.

34. Curtin B. *The myopias: basic science and clinical management.* Philadelphia, PA: Harper and Row, 1985.

35. Grignolo A, Rivara A. Biometry of the eye from the sixth month of pregnancy to the tenth year of life. *Acta Facult Med Brun* 1968;35:251–257.

36. Quinn GE, Dobson V, Repka MX, et al. Development of myopia in infants with birth weights less than 1251g. *Ophthalmology* 1992;99:329–340.

37. Cook A, White S, Batterbury M, et al. Ocular growth and refractive error development in premature infants without retinopathy of prematurity. *Invest Ophthalmol Vis Sci* 2003;44:953–960.

38. Sorsby A, Benjamin B, Sheridan M, et al. Refraction and its components during the growth of the eye from the age of three. *Med Res Counc Annu Rep* 1961;301:1–67.

39. Brown EVL. Net average yearly changes in refraction of atropinized eyes from birth to beyond middle life. *Arch Ophthalmol* 1939;19:719–734.

40. Hirsch MJ. Refraction of children. *Am J Optom Arch Am Acad Optom* 1964;41:395–399.

41. Larsen JS. The sagittal growth of the eye. I. Ultrasonic measurement of the anterior chamber from birth to puberty. *Acta Ophthalmol (Copenh)* 1971;49:239–262.

42. National Center for Health Statistics. Refraction status and motility defects of persons 4–74 years, U. S. 1971–72. In: U.S. Department of Health Education and Welfare, ed. Hyattsville, Maryland, 1978:1–130.

43. Yinon URI. Myopia induction in animals following alteration of the visual input during development: a review. *Curr Eye Res* 1984;3:677–690.

44. Hoyt CS, Stone RD, Fromer C, et al. Monocular axial myopia associated with neonatal eyelid closure in human infants. *Am J Ophthalmol* 1981;91:197–200.

45. Kruther SG, Nathan J, Kiely PM, et al. The effect of defocusing contact lenses on refraction in cynomolgus monkeys. *Clin Vision Sci* 1988;3:221–228.

46. Smith ELI, Hung L, Harwerth RS. Effects of optically induced blur on the refractive status of young monkeys. *Vision Res* 1994;34:290–293.

47. Hung L, Crawford, ML, Smith, EL. Spectacle lenses alter eye growth and the refractive status of young monkeys. *Nat Med* 1995;8:761–765.

48. Ingram R, Arnold, PE, Dally S, Lucas, J. Emmetropization, squint, and reduced visual acuity after treatment. *Br J Ophthalmol* 1991;75:414–416.

49. Rosner M, Belkin M. Intelligence, education, and myopia in males. *Arch Ophthalmol* 1987;105:1508–1511.

50. Duane A. Studies in monocular and binocular accommodation with their clinical applications. *Am J Ophthalmol* 1922;5:865–877.

51. Howland HC, Dobson V, Sayles N. Accommodation in infants measured by photorefraction. *Vision Res* 1987;27:2141–2152.

52. Phillips SR. *Ocular neurological control systems: accommodation in the nearest mons triad.* Berkeley, CA: University of California, 1974.

53. Urist MJ. Primary and secondary deviation in comitant squint. *Am J Ophthalmol* 1959;48:647–656.

54. Abraham SV. Accommodation in the amblyopic eye. *Am J Ophthalmol* Aug 1961;52:197–200.

55. Otto J, Graemiger A. On inexact accommodation of amblyopic eyes with eccentric fixation. *Albrecht Von Graefes Arch Klin Exp Ophthalmol* 1967;173:125–140.

56. Lindstedt E. Failing accommodation in cases of Down's syndrome. A preliminary report. *Ophthalmol Paediatr Genet* 1983;3: 191–192.

57. Lindstedt E. Accommodation in the visually impaired child. In: GC W, ed. *Low vision. Principles and applications.* New York: Springer-Verlag, 1986:424–435.

58. Swann A, Hunter C. A survey of amblyopia treated by atropine occlusion. *Br Orthopt J* 1974;31:65–69.

59. Syniuta L, Isenberg, SJ. Atropine and bifocals can slow the progression of myopia in children. *Binoc Vis Strab Quart* 2001;16:203–208.

60. Chiang M, Kouzis A, Poiter, RW, Repka, MX. Treatment of childhood myopia with atropine eyedrops and bifocal spectacles. *Binoc Vis Strab Quart* 2001;16:209–216.

61. Chia A, Chua W-H, Cheung Y-B, et al. Atropine for the treatment of childhood myopia: safety and efficacy of 0.5%, 0.1%, and 0.01% doses (atropine for the treatment of myopia 2). *Ophthalmology* 2012;119:347–354.

62. Gwiazda J, Hyman L, Hussein M, et al. A randomized clinical trial of progressive addition lens versus single vision lens on the progression of myopia in children. *Invest Ophthalmol Vis Sci* 2003;44:1492–1500.

63. Siatkowski RM, Cotter S, Miller JM, et al. Safety and efficacy of 2% pirenzepine ophthalmic gel in Children With Myopia: a 1-Year, multicenter, double-masked, placebo-controlled parallel study *Arch Ophthalmol* 2004;122:1667–1674.

64. Tan DTH, Lam DS, Chua WH, Shu-Ping DF, Crockett RS, Asian Pirenzepine Study Group. One-year multicenter, double-masked, placebo-controlled, parallel safety and efficacy study of 2% pirenzepine ophthalmic gel in children with myopia. *Ophthalmol* 2005;112(1):84–91.

65. American Academy of Ophthalmology Pediatric Ophthalmology/ Strabismus Panel. *Preferred practice pattern guidelines: pediatric eye evaluations.* San Francisco, CA: American Academy of Ophthalmology, 2012.

66. Guyton DL. Prescribing cylinders: the problem of distortion. *Surv Ophthalmol* 1977;22:177–188.

67. Ingram RM. Refraction as a basis for screening children for squint and amblyopia. *Br J Ophthalmol* 1977;61:8–15.

68. Levin AV, Edmonds SA, Nelson LB, et al. Extended wear contact lenses for the treatment of pediatric aphakia. *Ophthalmology* 1987;94(Suppl):68–69.

69. Infant Aphakia Treatment Study Group. A randomized clinical trial comparing contact lens to intraocular lens correction of monocular aphakia during infancy: grating acuity and adverse events at age 1 year. The Infant Aphakia Treatment Study (IATS) Report 1. *Arch Ophthalmol* 2010;128(7):931–933.

70. Arffa RC, Mavelli TL, Morgan KS. Long-term follow-up of refractive and keratometric results of pediatric epikeratophakia. *Arch Ophthalmol* 1986;104:668–670.

71. Morgan KS, Stephenson GS, McDonald MB, et al. Epikeratophakia in children. *Ophthalmology* 1984;91:780–784.

72. Wilson ME. Intraocular lens implantation: has it become the standard of care for children? *Ophthalmology* 1996;103:1719–1720.

73. Lambert SR, Lynn M, Drews-Botsch C, et al. Intraocular lens implantation during infancy: perceptions of parents and the American Association of Pediatric Ophthalmology and Strabismus members. *J AAPOS* 2003;7:400–405.

74. Brady KM, Atkinson CS, Kiltey L, et al. Cataract surgery and intraocular lens implantation in children. *Am J Ophthalmol* 1995;119:1–9.

75. Crouch ERJ, Pressman SH, Crouch ER. Posterior chamber intraocular lenses: long-term results in pediatric cataract patients. *J Pediatr Ophthalmol Strabismus* 1995;32:210–218.

76. Koenig SB, Ruttum MS, Lewandowski ME, et al. Pseudophakia for traumatic cataracts in children. *Ophthalmology* 1993;100:1218–1224.

77. Nihalani BR, VanderVeen DK. Comparison of intraocular lens power calculation formulae in pediatric eyes. *Ophthalmology* 2010;117(8):1493–1499.

78. Rosenbaum AL, Masket S. Intraocular lens implantation in children. *Am J Ophthalmol* 1995;120:105–107.

79. Repka MX. Monocular infantile cataract: treatment is worth the effort. *Arch Ophthalmol* 2010;129:931–933.

80. Friedman DS, Repka MX, Katz J, et al. Prevalence of decreased visual acuity among preschool-aged children in an American urban population: the Baltimore pediatric eye disease study, methods, and results. *Ophthalmology* 2008;115:1786–1795.

81. Hill AR, Cameron A. Pathology characteristics and optical correction of 900 low vision patients. In: Woo GC, ed. *Low vision. Principles and applications.* New York: Springer-Verlag, 1986:362–385.

6

Amblyopia

Evelyn A. Paysse • *David K. Coats* • *Timothy P. Lindquist*

THE TERM "AMBLYOPIA," derived from Greek, literally means "dullness of vision." Dr. Gunter von Noorden defined amblyopia as a "decrease of visual acuity in one eye when caused by abnormal binocular interaction or occurring in one or both eyes as a result of patterned vision deprivation during immaturity, for which no cause can be detected during the physical examination of the eye(s) and which in appropriate cases is reversible by therapeutic measures" (1).

Ophthalmologic examination of the eye typically reveals no anatomic abnormality. The exact mechanism of vision loss is not known, but it is thought to originate in the visual cortex. Amblyopia results in reduced visual acuity, fusion and stereopsis, and contrast sensitivity.

VISUAL DEVELOPMENT

At birth, the visual system is immature and visual acuity is estimated to be approximately 20/400 (2). Visual acuity improves and stereopsis develops during the first months of life. Myelination of the optic nerves, development of the visual cortex, and growth of the lateral geniculate body occur during the first two years (2). The fovea, the most visually sensitive part of the retina, reaches maturity at approximately 4 years of age. Visual stimuli are critical to the development of normal vision. Development of the visual pathways in the central nervous system requires that the brain receives a similarly clear, focused image from both eyes. Any process that significantly interferes with or inhibits development of the visual pathways in the brain may result in amblyopia.

The period of visual maturation is the critical period during which the visual system is affected by external influences. Most of the maturation of the visual system is thought to occur during the first 3 years of life, although some plasticity remains between 3 and 8 years of age, or even longer to some degree. One author describes three critical periods in the development of visual acuity and amblyopia (3):

- The period of development of visual acuity (from birth to 3 to 5 years of age)
- The period during which deprivation may cause amblyopia (from birth to 7 or 8 years of age)
- The period during which recovery from amblyopia can be achieved (from the time of deprivation to adolescence or possibly young adulthood)

Epidemiologic, Social, and Psychosocial Factors

The prevalence of amblyopia in the United States is estimated between 1% and 3% (4). Using a conservative prevalence estimate of 2%, there are approximately 6 million people with amblyopia living in the United States. Prevalence rates for amblyopia are higher in developing countries. The National Eye Institute has reported that amblyopia is the most common cause of unilateral vision loss in patients under the age of 70 years. Estimates of prevalence, however, are affected by the definition of reduced visual acuity and by the process of early screening and treatment in the population being studied (4,5). Prevalence is not affected by gender. In some series, the left eye was more commonly affected than the right, particularly in cases of anisometropic amblyopia.

The mean age at presentation of amblyopia varies depending on its cause (6). In a series of 961 children with amblyopia, the mean ages at presentation for anisometropic, strabismic, and mixed amblyopia were 5.6, 3.3, and 4.4 years, respectively (6). The upper age limit for the development of amblyopia in children who are exposed to an amblyopia-inducing condition (e.g., traumatic cataract) has been reported to be between 6 to 10 years (7). Individuals with amblyopia are at increased risk for loss of vision and blindness in the nonamblyopic eye (8). In one population-based study of 370 individuals with unilateral amblyopia, the projected lifetime risk of vision loss in the fellow eye was 1.2% (95% CI 1.1 to 1.4) (8). In 16% of patients, vision loss in the nonamblyopic eye was due to orbital or ocular trauma.

Detection and treatment of amblyopia is important for a variety of reasons. Psychosocial effects of amblyopia have been reported by amblyopic children and their parents. Self-image, work, school, and friendships were negatively impacted. Somatization, obsessive-compulsive behavior, interpersonal sensitivity, depression, and anxiety were found to be higher in individuals with amblyopia (9). Vocational opportunities for amblyopic individuals may be limited by requirements for good vision in both eyes.

Amblyopia treatment has been proved to have a positive impact in multiple arenas. Both patching and penalization are well tolerated and well perceived by parents of children undergoing therapy (10). Psychosocial effects are minimized by therapy. Additionally, amblyopia treatment has been shown to be highly cost-effective when evaluating dollars expended to gain a valued commodity (visual acuity) and that impact over the life span of the individual (11).

CLASSIFICATION OF AMBLYOPIA

A distinction must be made between *functional* (potentially reversible) *amblyopia* and *organic* (irreversible) *amblyopia*. Organic amblyopia is a term used to describe visual impairment due to obvious or nonobvious ocular pathology, commonly involving the retina or optic nerve. Examples include optic nerve hypoplasia, optic atrophy, and foveal hypoplasia. Organic amblyopia is not the focus of this chapter. Functional amblyopia occurs in an eye that is anatomically normal. Functional amblyopia can occur concurrently with organic amblyopia and will be discussed later in this chapter.

Amblyopia is most commonly characterized by the clinical associations that initiate the problem. Amblyopia can likewise be classified based upon the causal mechanism. Familiarity with both methods of classification is important for clinicians and can be useful in designing and implementing appropriate treatment strategies.

Clinical Classification
Strabismic Amblyopia
Strabismic amblyopia is one of the most common forms of amblyopia. It results from abnormal binocular interaction that occurs when the visual axes of fellow eyes are misaligned. This abnormal interaction causes the foveae of the two eyes to be presented with different images. Diplopia and visual confusion result. Visual confusion (simultaneous perception of the two different images from the foveae) and diplopia (doubling of perception of the object of regard) stimulate active inhibition of the retinostriate pathways of visual input originating in the fovea and peripheral retina of the deviating eye. The visual cortex then suppresses the image from the deviating eye. Long-term suppression during the sensitive period of visual development results in amblyopia.

Any type of strabismus can be associated with amblyopia. As many as 17% to 40% of children with idiopathic infantile esotropia develop amblyopia. Intermittent exotropia is associated with amblyopia in up to 15% of patients. Paresis and palsy of cranial nerves 3, 4, or 6 may or may not be associated with amblyopia depending upon severity of the defect and the child's ability to maintain fusion by adopting an anomalous head posture.

Strabismus surgery does not treat the associated strabismic amblyopia. Strabismus surgery is usually, though not always, deferred until the amblyopia has been maximally treated, though the success rate of surgery for esotropia is reportedly unaltered by the presence of mild amblyopia (12).

Anisometropic Amblyopia
Anisometropia is the other common cause of amblyopia. Anisometropic amblyopia occurs with hyperopia, myopia, or astigmatism. As a general rule, anisometropic amblyopia occurs more frequently with anisohyperopia (13). This occurs because when viewing binocularly, the fovea of the more ametropic eye in a child with anisohyperopia never receives a clearly focused image than the more hyperopic eye. In mild to moderate anisomyopia, the more myopic eye can be used for near work and the less myopic eye can be used for distance work, providing an important measure of protection against the development of amblyopia. Weakley (13) studied refractive errors likely to produce amblyopia. He noted that as little as one diopter of anisohyperopia and 1.5 diopters of anisoastigmatism were sufficient to produce amblyopia.

Anisometropic amblyopia is typically detected later as the affected child lacks obvious external abnormalities of the eyes (e.g., cataracts, strabismus), and visual function appears normal because the child sees well with the fellow eye.

In a manner thought to be similar to strabismic amblyopia, there is active cortical inhibition of input from the fovea of one eye in a child with anisometropia. This inhibition occurs in order to eliminate sensory misperceptions caused by monocular defocus and aniseikonia.

Visual-Deprivation Amblyopia
Deprivation amblyopia is the least common and most serious form of amblyopia. Visual deprivation is caused by obstruction of the visual axis or severe distortion of the foveal image of one or both eyes. Congenital cataracts, ptosis, congenital corneal opacities, and vitreous hemorrhage can cause deprivation amblyopia. Even transient obstruction of the visual axis, such as that caused by a hyphema or eyelid edema in a very young child can produce visual-deprivation amblyopia. Visual-deprivation amblyopia can be unilateral or bilateral. Sensory strabismus often occurs in children with unilateral vision deprivation. Deprivation amblyopia can result in permanent visual impairment if its cause is not treated urgently in infancy.

Special Forms of Amblyopia
Isoametropic amblyopia is the term used to characterize amblyopia in both eyes due to bilateral uncorrected or improperly corrected high refractive errors. It is most common in children with severe hyperopia, typically greater

than 5 or 6 diopters, but can also occur with high astigmatism and high myopia.

Occlusion amblyopia is an iatrogenic amblyopia caused by obstruction of the visual axis of a sound eye in amblyopia treatment. It is more likely to occur when full-time patching is used. Rapid development of occlusion amblyopia is a sign of continued visual system plasticity and is believed by many ophthalmologists to portend a good visual outcome for both eyes of such patients if detected and corrected promptly.

Idiopathic amblyopia is a diagnosis of exclusion and is typically diagnosed in retrospect when a child with a monocular reduction of visual acuity and no detectable cause responds with improved vision during a trial of treatment for amblyopia. Because of this occasional good visual response, amblyopia treatment is often attempted when visual acuity is reduced in children with no obvious explanation. Presumably, an amblyogenic process was present earlier in the child's life that has since resolved. Detailed history-taking will often identify a history of strabismus or previous occlusion of the visual axis (e.g., prolonged eyelid edema caused by an insect bite or infection of the lids as a young child). Equalization of a previous anisometropic refractive error is another possible explanation cause, although history is unlikely to be helpful in this situation.

Mechanistic Classification

From a mechanistic viewpoint, there are two causes of amblyopia. These include form-vision deprivation and abnormal binocular interaction. Each can occur in isolation or concurrently. Form-vision deprivation refers to amblyopia caused by poor image quality being projected onto the fovea. The visual cortex is thus never allowed to develop the capacity to process a sharply focused image. Form-vision deprivation occurs from conditions that obstruct the visual axis such as cataract, vitreous hemorrhage, corneal opacity, or severe ptosis, but it can also be produced by severe anisometropic hyperopia. For example, a child with an uncorrected refractive error of +10.00 diopters in his right eye and +1.00 diopter in the fellow eye can develop form-vision deprivation in the right eye due to persistent pronounced image blur in the right eye.

Abnormal binocular interaction refers to the condition in which the image projected onto the fovea of each eye is dissimilar enough to preclude fusion, thus prompting suppression and ultimately amblyopia of the suppressed eye. While strabismus may be the most obvious cause of abnormal binocular interaction, unilateral media opacities and severe anisometropia may participate in this mechanism as well. For example, in a child with uncorrected unilateral high myopia, in addition to a blurred image, the size of the image projected onto the fovea of the myopic eye is distinctly different than that projected to the fovea of the contralateral eye, resulting in abnormal binocular interaction in addition to form-vision deprivation.

PATHOPHYSIOLOGY

The mechanism and pathogenesis of amblyopia is an area of vast interest, with hundreds of publications produced on the topic in the last four decades. A common question that remains to be answered fully is the exact location of the disturbance within the visual system that is responsible for ultimately producing amblyopia. Changes have been found in the lateral geniculate nucleus (LGN) and visual cortex. It has been shown that the amblyopic eye functions at its best in mesopic and scotopic conditions and at its worst under photopic conditions. Retinal receptive fields in amblyopic eyes have also been shown to be larger than normal (14). Lastly, contrast-sensitivity function measured at the foveal region in strabismic amblyopes is reduced and similar to contrast-sensitivity function measured from the peripheral retina of a normal eye (15).

While amblyopia is most often detected during visual acuity testing, reduction in visual acuity is not the only visual abnormality that is present in the amblyopic eye. The full range of abnormalities present in the amblyopic eye has probably yet to be identified. Known visual abnormalities include reduced contrast sensitivity, dark adaptation abnormalities, and visual field abnormalities. Even the "sound" eye has been shown to have abnormalities in patients with anisometropic amblyopia. Leguire (16) reported reduced contrast-sensitivity function in both the amblyopic and "sound" eye of amblyopic patients. Kandel (17) reported dark adaptation to be better in the nonamblyopic eye.

Some authors have proposed that most eyes with amblyopia actually have subtle, undiagnosed ocular pathology involving the optic nerves, such as mild optic nerve hypoplasia (18). Certainly, it is true that some children initially diagnosed with amblyopia are later found to have subtle eye pathology when cooperative enough in later life to undergo a more detailed examination. The possibility of occult optic nerve and/or retinal pathology should always be kept in mind during the management of children with amblyopia who are not responding to treatment as anticipated.

Amblyopia is associated with histologic and electrophysiologic abnormalities in the visual cortex. Hubel and Wiesel (19) pioneered methods of studying the effects of changing visual experience in kittens by suturing an eyelid closed. Similar results have been found in a primate model (20). In these and other experiments, amblyopia was produced by suturing the lids closed in one eye and by inducing experimental anisometropia in susceptible animals.

The layers of the LGN corresponding to input from the amblyopic eye have also been shown to be attenuated in monkeys with strabismic, anisometropic, and visual-deprivation amblyopia (Fig. 6.1). Cells from the LGN travel through the parietal or temporal lobes to the visual

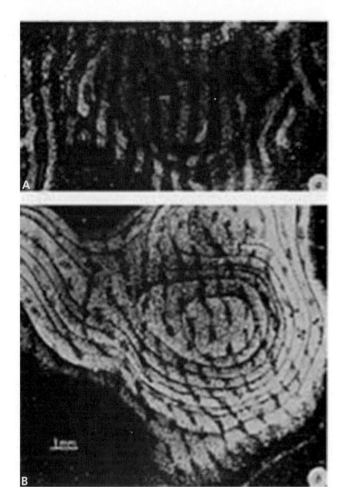

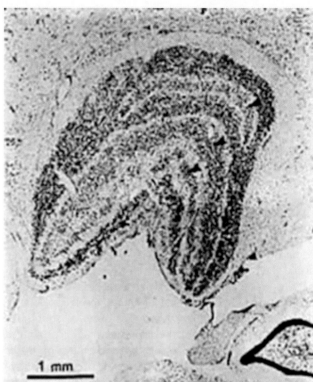

FIGURE 6.2. Coronal section through the right lateral geniculate nucleus of the same monkey. Atrophy in the layers receiving input from the deprived eye is indicated by *arrows* (21). (Reprinted with permission from Amblyopia, in Duane's Ophthalmology.)

FIGURE 6.1. Autoradiographs of monkey visual cortex 2 weeks after injection of a radioactive tracer into the vitreous of one eye. Each figure represents a montage of tangential sections through the cortex. **A:** Normal monkey. The *light stripes*, representing labeled eye columns, are separated by gaps of the same width representing the other eye. **B:** Monocularly deprived monkey, who had the right eye closed at 2 weeks for 18 months. Input from the normal eye is in the form of expanded bands, which in places coalesce, obliterating the narrow gaps that represent the columns connected to the closed eye (21). (Reprinted with permission from Amblyopia, in Duane's Ophthalmology.)

cortex, located in the occipital lobes. Ocular dominance columns representing alternating input from the right and left eyes are present in all portions of the visual cortex that receive binocular input. Notable exceptions are the temporal crescents of retina in each eye and retina corresponding to the position of the optic nerve in the fellow eye, which contribute monocular input. Amblyopia is associated with a decrease in the number of binocularly driven cells in the striate cortex (20,21). In a monkey model with deprivation amblyopia, the ocular dominance columns associated with the amblyopic eye were shown to be markedly attenuated (Fig. 6.2). These cortical changes presumably become irreversible over time. Recently Demer and coworkers (22) demonstrated significant reduction in relative cortical blood flow and glucose metabolism during visual stimulation of the amblyopic eye during a positron emission tomography scan.

VISION SCREENING AND AMBLYOPIA DETECTION

There are both obvious and nonobvious causes of amblyopia from the standpoint of parental perception. Obvious strabismus and dense cataracts are easily detected by parents and pediatricians, resulting in prompt diagnosis and treatment. Less obvious causes of amblyopia, including anisometropia, microstrabismus, posteriorly located cataracts, and vitreous opacities are often associated with later diagnosis and treatment. Amblyopic vision loss associated with these conditions is often not suspected by parents or detected until routine vision screening, which typically occurs when the child is mature enough to undergo formal psychophysical acuity testing (3 to 5 years old).

While it is not the purpose of this chapter to discuss vision screening, a few thoughts on the process of vision screening are in order. While vision screening is recommended for 3- to 5-year-old children, it has been estimated that only 21% of children in the United States actually receive vision screening during this recommended time interval. Snowdon and Smith (23) recently challenged the validity of recommendations on the timing of amblyopia screening, reporting that delay in diagnosis of mild amblyopia (20/40 or better) until age 5 years did not adversely affect the long-term visual outcome.

EXAMINATION OF THE PATIENT WITH AMBLYOPIA

Visual acuity testing protocols used to diagnose amblyopia depend upon the age and cognitive abilities of each individual child. Children under the age of 5 years often fail to achieve better than 20/30 to 20/40 acuity due to inability to concentrate or cooperate for testing with the Snellen visual targets. Amblyopia then should be suspected if the vision in the two eyes is unequal or the visual acuity in both eyes is less than 20/40. While not the only visual abnormality in amblyopia, visual acuity testing is obviously the crux of its diagnosis and the most easily testable aspect of amblyopia. Unfortunately, those children most likely to respond to amblyopia treatment (i.e., younger children) are the most difficult to evaluate.

Assessment of Visual Behavior/Acuity

Assessment of visual behavior is the key critical element in the diagnosis of amblyopia in preverbal children. Assessment of visual behavior begins with evaluation of the child's ability to fixate on and follow an accommodative visual target, such as the examiner's face or a small toy. A child who readily fixates on and follows a toy with one eye but fails to do so with the fellow eye most often has reduced vision in the eye that fails to fixate and/or follow. The examiner must recognize the limited attention span of a young child and assure that failure to fixate and follow the target is not merely due to lack or loss of interest. To guard against this possibility a second or third visually interesting target is often utilized to confirm. Inequality in fixation and following behavior does not necessarily indicate the presence of amblyopia, but may simply indicate the presence of an uncorrected refractive error or other correctable problem.

Fixation Behavior Testing

Fixation behavior testing involves moving a visual target through the child's visual space. Each eye is tested separately by occluding the fellow eye during testing. Occlusion of the fellow eye can be done with an occluder or the examiner's hand and rarely requires use of an eye patch. Accuracy is improved if the test is repeated several times. The eye movements of an infant are expected to be somewhat uncoordinated. The ability to follow past the midline develops at approximately 2 months of age; vertical eye movements typically develop around 3 months.

The Differential Occlusion Objection Test

The differential occlusion objection (DOO) test is a classic visual behavior test for moderate to severe amblyopia. The DOO test involves measuring the child's response to sequential occlusion of the fellow eye. Children with symmetric vision should respond equally to sequential occlusion of the eyes. Children with unequal vision typically become fussy or agitated when the eye with better vision is covered. The test should be repeated several times to improve reliability. A consistently strong preference for one eye, indicated by greater objection to occlusion of that eye, is highly suggestive of amblyopia in the fellow eye.

Fixation Preference Testing

Fixation preference testing is another commonly used procedure to identify amblyopia, especially in children too young to participate in formal psychophysical (quantitative) acuity testing. The test is simple to perform in a patient with strabismus. The examiner simply attempts to demonstrate equal maintenance of fixation with fellow eyes by first occluding one eye and determining if the child can maintain fixation with the currently fixing eye upon removal of the occluder and then repeating the process for the contralateral eye. If the child is able to maintain fixation with either eye upon removal of the occluder, significant amblyopia is probably not present. On the other hand, if the child consistently demonstrates a preference for fixation with one eye when the occluder is removed, amblyopia should be suspected in the nonpreferred eye.

The Vertical Prism Test

The vertical prism test uses a 10- to 14-prism-diopter vertical prism to induce vertical separation of the visual axes to facilitate detection of unequal vision in children with straight eyes (24). The test is performed by first holding the prism base down before the child's right eye, inducing a vertical tropia, shifting the image for the right eye upward, and producing vertical diplopia. The child must then make a decision as to which image he or she is going to fixate. The child with symmetric vision between the two eyes will typically exhibit one of two responses. The majority will show no change in eye position when the prism is sequentially introduced before each eye. Less frequently, a child with symmetric vision will demonstrate an upward movement of the eyes when the prism is placed before either eye as he or she attempts to fixate on the image that has been displaced by the base-down prism. The child with significant amblyopia, on the other hand, will usually have an asymmetric response to sequential placement of the prism before each eye. When the prism is placed before the sound eye, both eyes will move upward as the sound eye attempts to fixate the target that has been displaced upward by the base-down prism. No change in eye position will occur when the prism is placed before the amblyopic eye because the sound eye will continue to maintain fixation on the visual target. The accuracy of the vertical prism test is greatly enhanced by frequent practice and by repeating the test several times during each examination to assure a consistent response.

Visual Acuity Testing

Visual acuity testing should begin as early in life as practical. A child as young as 2 years of age can occasionally participate in psychophysical (quantitative) acuity testing. The examiner should use the most sophisticated psychophysical test possible when assessing a child's vision. Snellen acuity testing is considered optimal, while picture tests, such as Allen figures, are considered the least satisfactory, their use often resulting in overestimation of actual visual acuity. The HOTV, Tumbling E, and Landolt C tests are considered superior to Allen figure testing in this regard. A difference in best-corrected visual acuity difference of two lines between fellow eyes (e.g., 20/20 in the left eye and 20/30 in the right eye) is clinically indicative of amblyopia, though amblyopia may still be present when the acuity difference between fellow eyes is only one line or less. This is an especially important consideration for Allen figure acuity testing. A child with one line difference on Allen figure testing may be found to have several lines of difference with a more sophisticated test. As such, the Allen figure test should always be coupled with a fixation preference test.

Younger children rarely achieve a visual acuity of 20/20 on any test due to limited ability to concentrate. The young child's vision should be considered normal if the visual acuity is equal and in the range of 20/40 to 20/50 or better. Thus, a 3-year-old child who has 20/40 vision in each eye with the Tumbling E test is considered to have normal

vision, but a 3-year-old child with 20/70 vision in each eye, or 20/50 vision in one eye and 20/30 vision in the other eye should undergo further evaluation.

Patients with amblyopia often are noted to have a more severe visual acuity deficit when tested with a full line of optotypes than when tested with isolated optotypes. With full line testing, as acuity limits are approached, figures near the limit of resolution are surrounded by other closely spaced forms, causing contour interaction. This effect, known as the "crowding phenomenon," can be demonstrated in normal eyes as well, but is clinically evident in amblyopic subjects where contour interaction in the fovea extends over increased distances relative to normal subjects. The crowding of visual targets can have a significant impact on visual acuity testing of the amblyopic eye. Ignoring the crowding phenomenon in an amblyopic child by presenting only single optotypes often results in erroneously good acuity scores. Thus, using a row of visual targets provides a more accurate assessment of visual acuity and improved detection of amblyopia.

Spatial summation and lateral inhibition are other features of visual processing that must be considered when testing visual acuity in patients who may have amblyopia. Spatial summation describes the reduction in brightness required for detection of a small spot of light as its area is increased. Lateral inhibition is observed when illumination of the surrounding retina causes an increase in the threshold for detection of a small test light. As with contour interaction, spatial summation and lateral inhibition occur over very short distances in the normal fovea and greater distances in the normal periphery. Lateral inhibition can be demonstrated with a familiar optical illusion called the Hermann grid, which consists of black squares separated by white stripes (Fig. 6.3). The intersections of the stripes appear

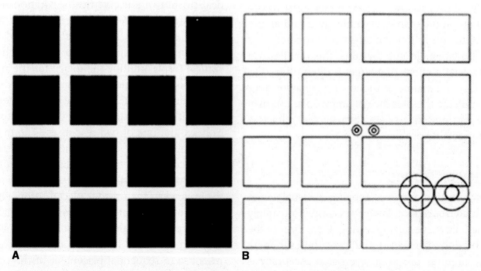

FIGURE 6.3. A: The Hermann grid illusion. **B:** The *unshaded area* of each circle represents the inhibitory zone for the point at the center of the circle. Near fixation the inhibitory zones are small and fit within the boundaries of the white stripes. Points in the intersections and points in the stripes outside the intersections receive the same amount of inhibition. Away from fixation, the larger inhibitory zones extend into the black regions, which do not contribute to lateral inhibition. Points in the intersections receive more inhibition than points outside and therefore appear darker. (Reprinted with permission from Amblyopia, in Duane's Ophthalmology.)

darker than the stripes themselves because the greater area of white surrounding points in the intersections produces greater lateral inhibition. The effect is less near the point of fixation because the smaller foveal zones of inhibition fall entirely within the width of a stripe. Spatial summation and lateral inhibition have both been found to extend over much greater distances than normal in the amblyopic fovea (25).

Testing of isolated letters may have some value in selected situations. Some examiners believe that isolated letter acuity predicts ultimate visual potential after amblyopia therapy. Others have suggested that failure of acuity to improve with conversion to isolated letters is indicative of an organic cause for visual impairment.

VISUAL ACUITY TESTING TIPS

Children have an innate desire to perform well. This drive to do well and please adults stimulates memorization, peeking, and other unwanted behaviors during the vision-testing process. To avoid these potential testing problems, an adhesive patch over the fellow eye is recommended.

The use of a computerized vision-testing device that has the ability to randomly present optotypes is also highly desirable to reduce memorization artifact. Also, it is not uncommon for a child to perform poorly on vision testing of the first eye only to improve with vision testing of the second eye due to a learning-curve effect from practice. If the measured acuity is better in the second eye, the first eye should be retested to guard against this learning-curve artifact.

It is not the purpose of this chapter to review the details of a comprehensive ophthalmologic examination. It is important to note, however, that a comprehensive ophthalmologic examination is required for all children suspected of having amblyopia. Organic causes of vision loss can occasionally be overlooked, especially in active or uncooperative children. Some of the most common causes of undetected organic vision loss include subtle optic nerve hypoplasia (by far the most common), mild optic atrophy, and subtle macular abnormalities. The presence of an afferent pupillary defect, often difficult to identify in the uncooperative child, may be the only clue to the presence of an optic nerve abnormality as the cause of vision loss in the child who is otherwise difficult to evaluate. It is important to consider the possibility of a subtle organic vision abnormality when a child who is compliant with treatment recommendations does not respond as expected to amblyopia therapy.

TREATMENT OF AMBLYOPIA

Management of the patient with amblyopia is less straightforward than the preceding discussions of etiology and detection might imply. The reality is that children are difficult to evaluate, inconsistent in their responses on examination, require continuous reassessment and modification

of assessment techniques, and are often not fully compliant with treatment. The basic treatment recommendations for amblyopia have undergone little change. Occlusion therapy, one of the mainstays of the amblyopia treatment armamentarium, was described as early as 900 AD by Thabit Ibn Qurrah in Mesopotamia. In addition to occlusion therapy, pharmacologic and optical penalization therapies are commonly used treatments for amblyopia. While few effective new treatments have been reported in recent decades, knowledge on timing and treatment strategies utilizing existing treatment methods have significantly expanded.

The literature is replete with recommendations that children be treated as early in life as possible to achieve an optimal outcome. This recommendation has recently been challenged. Several studies have demonstrated less impact of age (up to 6 years) at onset of treatment for strabismic and anisometropic amblyopia of 20/400 or better than previously suspected (26,27). It is important, therefore, for the practicing clinician to remain open-minded about the treatment of amblyopia and be willing to implement new treatment recommendations that are scientifically validated as they become available.

The goal of amblyopia treatment is to maximize the visual acuity for an individual patient. In brief, treatment consists of removing media opacities if present, correcting significant refractive errors with spectacles or contact lenses, encouraging the child to use the amblyopic eye, and monitoring for recurrence . Use of the amblyopic eye is encouraged by using an occluding patch over the sound eye or via penalization using long-acting topical cycloplegic medications or optical blur of the sound eye (28). Some so-called vision therapies, including eye movement exercises, vision training, and methods designed to stimulate or suppress vision using flashing lights or rotating patterns, are not scientifically proven.

While there are a few exceptions, amblyopia treatment measures are usually implemented one at a time. This is done in order to assess each treatment individually. Perhaps an even more important reason to implement only one treatment at a time is to avoid overtaxing the amblyopic child with excessive treatment modalities, which can promote frustration in the child that may lead to more compliance problems.

Optical Correction

The first step in the management of any child with amblyopia involves facilitating projection of a clear image onto the fovea of each eye. Assuring that a clear image is projected onto the fovea requires removal of any significant media opacity (e.g., cataract, corneal opacity) and correction of any significant refractive error with spectacles and/or contact lenses. It has been recently been reported that mild to moderate anisometropic amblyopia can respond completely to refractive correction alone without the need to institute occlusion or penalization therapy (29).

Occlusion Therapy

Occlusion therapy has long been the mainstay of amblyopia treatment. It is preferred by many ophthalmologists because it lacks systemic side effects and is effective and inexpensive. Occlusion therapy involves patching the sound eye to force use of the amblyopic eye. The major disadvantage to occlusion therapy is compliance difficulty. Children can remove the patch to peek, rendering treatment less effective or completely ineffective.

Occlusion therapy recommendations have significantly evolved in the past decade. The schedule of patching varies depending upon the age of the child and the physician's preference. Younger children require less occlusion therapy than older children. In the past, a common treatment recommendation for initial management of amblyopia in the child under 1 year of age was to patch 1 hour per month of life and follow-up initially every 1 to 2 weeks. It has recently been shown, however, that only 2 hours of prescribed patching per day is necessary in most cases of moderate amblyopia in children 3 to 6 years. It is logical to assume that a low-dose patching regimen would be effective in a younger child as well. In older children, past recommendations typically included 6 or more hours of patching per day with initial follow-up at an interval of 1 to 2 weeks per year of life. Follow-up intervals were gradually increased as the child's response to therapy was determined and/or less patching per day was used (30).

A recent series of randomized controlled trials, known collectively as the Amblyopia Treatment Studies, conducted by the Pediatric Eye Disease Investigator Group (PEDIG) have demonstrated that less prescribed occlusion and/or penalization is needed to achieve the same visual improvement in the same amount of time. These studies have changed the way many pediatric ophthalmologists treat amblyopia

Two hours of prescribed daily patching of the sound eye was found to be as effective as 6 hours per day for moderate amblyopia (20/20 to 20/80) and 6 hours of prescribed daily patching of the sound eye was as effective as full-time patching for severe amblyopia (20/100 to 20/ 400) at the 4-month follow-up exam (27). Many have interpreted these results as demonstrating that 2 hours of patching is equal to 6 hours of patching. This, however, may be an erroneous conclusion as the occlusion amount was not monitored. It is however, a "real" life result and what is likely to be achievable.

So the question now arises as to whether 2 hours (or less) of patching per day could be enough for any level of amblyopia. Is there a maximum benefit response of occlusion per day that the visual system can assimilate?

There are several patching alternatives available to facilitate occlusion therapy. Adhesive patches remain the mainstay of treatment. Several commercially available patches have been devised which fully occlude the visual axis and periphery in spectacle-wearing amblyopes and may be preferable, especially in hot, humid climates. In general, devices that clip onto the front of spectacle lenses without fully occluding all sides are not recommended. Such clip-on occluders allow the child to easily peek over or around the glasses and may not be as effective.

An occlusion contact lens is another option in poorly compliant children with amblyopia. This option is usually reserved for noncompliant children with severe amblyopia who have failed all other treatments or children who are aphakic in the amblyopic eye and who have parents who are accustomed to inserting and removing contact lenses. It is imperative that the parents understand the potential complications of contact lenses, which include microbial keratitis, giant papillary conjunctivitis, and corneal scarring. These potential complications along with added cost and parental effort render this option less desirable for most patients and are the major reason why this treatment modality is used sparingly.

Penalization

Penalization is a technique used to temporarily handicap the sound eye, thereby providing a visual advantage to the amblyopic eye. Penalization is blurring of vision in the sound eye through use of medication, spectacle manipulation, or both (28,31).

Pharmacologic penalization is accomplished through the instillation of a cycloplegic ophthalmic drop into the sound eye. Atropine 1% is the most commonly used agent, but homatropine and scopolamine and cyclopentolate are used by some ophthalmologists. All of these topical anticholinergic medications cause temporary pupillary dilation and reduced accommodation, thereby providing the amblyopic eye with a competitive advantage and encouraging its use. Pharmacologic penalization is optimally used in hyperopic eyes, but can be effectively utilized in very low myopia as well. Pharmacologic penalization must be used in conjunction with proper spectacle correction for the amblyopic eye.

Though infrequent, anticholinergic side effects do sometimes occur with use of anticholinergic drops and should be discussed with parents when the drug is prescribed. The most common side effects include flushing of the skin and fever. Irritability, increased aggression, and seizures have rarely been reported.

Atropine penalization may now be gaining increased acceptance and use following the Amblyopia Treatment Study (ATS) that demonstrated that atropine is essentially equally efficacious with regard to effect on visual acuity when compared with occlusion therapy following 6 months of therapy in a group of children with moderate strabismic or anisometropic amblyopia (32). In this large, prospective, masked, multicenter trial, 419 children younger than 7 years with moderate strabismic or anisometropic amblyopia (visual acuity in the range of 20/40 to 20/100) were randomly assigned to receive one drop of 1% atropine sulfate or occlusion for a minimum of 6 hours per day of the sound eye (32). Improvement in visual acuity occurred slightly more rapidly in the occlusion group. After 6 months of treatment, visual acuity in the amblyopic eye improved by three lines or more in similar proportions of both groups (79% of the occlusion group and 74% of the atropine group). Compliance with treatment, however, was better in the atropine group (78% versus 49% completed at least 76% of the prescribed treatment).

Optical penalization involves altering the spectacle or contact lens correction of the sound eye to produce image blur, potentially providing the amblyopic eye a competitive advantage. Optical penalization may be used alone, or more typically, in combination with pharmacologic penalization. The disadvantage to isolated optical penalization is that children can avoid the undesired blur by simply removing or looking over the spectacles. Optical penalization, however, when used in combination with cycloplegic agents, is a powerful adjunct in the management of amblyopia (28).

Care must be taken when reducing the optical correction of the sound eye when used in combination with pharmacologic penalization to assure that penalization amblyopia (similar to occlusion amblyopia) does not occur in the sound eye. Follow-up should occur at frequent-enough intervals to detect and manage penalization amblyopia. Loss of one line of vision in the sound eye was reported in 15% of eyes treated with atropine in the ATS, compared with 7% of eyes randomized to occlusion therapy (32). In both treatment groups, discontinuation of therapy was associated with return of normal vision.

Systemic Treatments

Systemic therapies have been attempted for the treatment of amblyopia with limited success. Levodopa-carbidopa, an agent used to treat Parkinson disease, is one such agent. It works by centrally increasing dopamine availability. Its effect on amblyopia was discovered accidently when some patients with Parkinson's disease and remote amblyopia history reported increased contrast sensitivity and visual acuity after starting levodopa-carbidopa. Levodopa-carbidopa has been found to produce short-term, mild improvement of visual acuity in both the amblyopic and sound eyes of amblyopic patients. The treatment has also been found to be mildly effective in older children with amblyopia who were beyond the standard age range for treatment response (33). The improvement, however, in visual acuity is not always sustained when the drug is discontinued. The addition of occlusion therapy to levodopa-carbidopa therapy has been shown to improve response and maintenance of improvement in visual acuity, although this claim has not been confirmed. Other pharmacologic agents, including citicoline (cytidine-5'-diphosphocholine), are being investigated for the treatment of amblyopia and may prove beneficial in the future (34).

Maintenance Therapy

Once visual acuity has been maximized by treatment, many ophthalmologists recommend maintenance therapy using occlusion therapy several hours per day or periodic penalization for several months to minimize the risk of recurrence (35). A typical protocol is to empirically recommend maintenance occlusion therapy 1 to 2 hours per day or maintenance atropine penalization once every 1 to 2 weeks for a period of 3 to 6 months prior to total cessation of therapy. It has been shown that abruptly discontinuing amblyopia therapy when using more than 2 hours/day occlusion or daily atropine resulted in regression of visual acuity in approximately 40% of patients compared to only 13% of patients using 2 hours/day occlusion or weekend atropine in the sound eye (36).

CESSATION OF THERAPY

Among the most difficult decisions that a physician must make is the decision to discontinue treatment of a chronic condition, especially when response to therapy has not been optimal. This is certainly true for amblyopia. When can the clinician feel both medically and medicolegally comfortable with discontinuing amblyopia therapy? Most of the visual recovery that occurs with amblyopia therapy occurs in the first several months of treatment (32). No validated scientific studies are available to advise clinicians as to when therapy can be safely discontinued. A common practice is to require three consecutive visits, separated by at least 6 to 8 weeks with good treatment compliance and without improvement before considering discontinuation of therapy. Both occlusion and penalization therapies, if applicable, are typically attempted before considering cessation of treatment. Practically speaking, this means that the child who has not equalized vision with treatment will receive 4 to 6 months of therapy with patching or penalization, followed by a similar trial of treatment with the alternate modality before treatment is abandoned. Exceptions to the above practices are not uncommon and depend on a number of factors including compliance, school-related issues, and family stress. A frank discussion with parents prior to discontinuing therapy is recommended, and they should be advised that, although unlikely, continued therapy could result in further improvement. It is essential to have parents participate in the ultimate decision to discontinue therapy when residual amblyopia remains to alleviate current and future guilt parents may feel, believing that they did not do an optimal job in the detection and/or management of their child's amblyopia.

The decision to discontinue treatment of deprivation amblyopia is often the most difficult to make. Such patients are typically patched no more than 6 hours per day because stereopsis has been reported to be better with treatment of 6 hours or less and because it is very difficult to get children with deprivation amblyopia to comply with more extensive patching. Because objective visual acuity cannot be accurately evaluated in preverbal children, amblyopia therapy should be continued until the child is old enough for psychophysical visual acuity testing. Generally a more sophisticated test than picture (Allen) testing is recommended before considering cessation of therapy unless the vision is so poor as to preclude ambulation or other activities of daily living when the sound eye is patched.

PROGNOSIS

The efficacy of the various treatments for amblyopia is difficult to measure and to compare because no standard, accurate, linear test of visual acuity that can be used for children of all ages exists. In addition, many cases are diagnosed and successfully treated before visual acuity can be accurately measured. Treatment that is initiated by the time the child reaches 4 to 5 years of age usually is at least partially successful.

Several factors have been identified that are associated with a high risk of treatment failure, which include poor compliance, age of 6 years or older, astigmatism of at least 1.5 diopters, hypermetropia of more than 3 diopters, and initial acuity of 20/200 or worse (37). ATSs have shown similar VA outcomes in children across the ages of 3 to 6 years (26).

Compliance with the treatment plan, more likely in younger children, is a critical factor in outcome (37,38). Even older children have shown remarkable improvement with amblyopic therapies when they are compliant. In one series of 36 children between the ages of 7 and 10 years who were treated with full-time occlusion (standard occlusion or occlusive contact lens), final best-corrected visual acuity for all patients was between 20/20 and 20/30 (39).

Long-term outcome was studied in a cohort of 94 children who were successfully treated for unilateral amblyopia with occlusion and had 20/20 vision at the end of amblyopia treatment at age 9 years. The patients were examined an average of 6.4 years after cessation of therapy. Deterioration of visual acuity was greater (average deterioration of 1.5 versus 0.6 lines on the Snellen chart) and occurred more often in those with pretreatment visual acuity worse than 20/100 than in those with pretreatment visual acuity between 20/60 and 20/100 (63% versus 42%). Deterioration of visual acuity was related to the type of amblyopia, with deterioration in mixed, strabismic, and anisometropic amblyopia occurring in 79%, 46%, and 36% of patients, respectively. Fifty-four of the patients from this study were reevaluated 21.5 years after cessation of therapy at an average age of 29 years old. Amblyopia had recurred in approximately one-third of the patients.

Amblyopia may have long-term psychosocial consequences. In one survey of 25 patients with a history of amblyopia, approximately 50% responded that amblyopia interfered with their schooling, work, or lifestyle, and approximately 40% responded that it affected their play of sports and/or influenced their job choices (10). In addition, compared to control subjects, patients with amblyopia had a greater degree of somatization, obsessive-compulsive behavior, depression, and anxiety.

SPECIAL ISSUES

Older Children

Recent noncontrolled studies have questioned the belief that treatment of amblyopia beyond the age of 8 or 9 years is of little benefit (39,40). Mintz-Hittner and coworkers (39) reported a dramatic improvement in the Snellen visual acuity in children 7 to 10 years old using full-time occlusion of the sound eye. This study cohort however, may have represented a self-selected group of children who were either likely to respond to therapy or did not perform well on initial visual acuity testing for reasons other than amblyopia. Furthermore, patients who did not comply well with treatment were not included, and there was no control group. Another study demonstrated that approximately 50% of children 7 to 12 years of age would visually improve 2 or more lines of acuity if treated with refractive correction, occlusion 6 hours a day and daily atropine to the sound eye, This same study demonstrated that approximately 50% of previously untreated children 13 to 17 years of age would gain improvement of 2 or more lines of acuity if treated with refractive correction and occlusion of 6 hours a day of the sound eye (29).

Concurrent Ocular Pathology

Amblyopia can coexist with anatomic abnormalities of the retina or optic nerve. Optic nerve hypoplasia, optic atrophy, and retinal colobomata are three examples. Unless it is a clinical certainty that vision loss is irreversible, the clinician should usually assume that there may be a reversible component of amblyopia in eyes with obvious pathology, and a diligent attempt should be made to improve any reversible component of visual impairment.

Children are frequently difficult to examine. It is understandable, therefore, that subtle (and even overt) pathology may be overlooked in the small, uncooperative child. The most commonly overlooked ophthalmologic abnormalities include mild optic nerve hypoplasia, subtle optic atrophy, and subtle foveal hypoplasia. We recommend documenting the level of the child's cooperation during each examination. This alerts the clinician at follow-up visits that the previous examination may have been suboptimal and allows other clinicians to view the clinician's conclusions in the proper perspective. Careful assessment of the pupils for an afferent pupillary defect is recommended at all amblyopia check-ups. When a child fails to respond to amblyopia therapy as expected, the refraction may be incorrect or important pathology may have been overlooked, prompting careful reevaluation.

CONCLUSIONS

In conclusion, amblyopia is a common problem encountered by both pediatric ophthalmologists and practitioners of adult ophthalmology. It is clinically associated with strabismus and anisometropia in the vast majority of cases. Deprivation amblyopia from media opacities is the least common and most severe form of the disease. Amblyopia is a cortical phenomenon with anatomic and functional changes reported in the central nervous system, both in the lateral geniculate body and in the visual cortex. Detection is often difficult, particularly in preverbal and uncooperative children. The psychosocial and socioeconomic benefits of amblyopia treatment are significant. While there is certainly a period of highest response to treatment, the maximum age at which treatment is likely to be ineffective has yet to be determined.

The basic treatment paradigm for amblyopia includes removal of any significant media opacities and correction of any significant refractive errors, followed by treatment designed to encourage utilization of the amblyopic eye.

Long-term follow-up is needed to detect recurrence. Occlusion therapy and atropine penalization are the most common treatments. Optical penalization can be used in selected cases, usually in conjunction with pharmacologic penalization. Systemic treatments have not yet gained widespread acceptance. Maintenance therapy to reduce the risk of recurrence is important, and reducing occlusion to 2 hours/day or atropine penalization to weekend therapy before cessation of treatment will reduce the chance of amblyopia recurrence. When a child fails to respond to therapy, reevaluation for subtle retinal or optic nerve pathology should be performed. Significant and interesting strides have recently been made in the treatment of amblyopia through the Amblyopia Treatment Studies. These studies and hopefully others will eventually lead to improved treatment strategies and overall improved visual outcomes.

REFERENCES

1. vonNoorden GK. Mechanisms of amblyopia. *Adv Ophthalmol* 1977;34:93–115.
2. Boothe RG, Dobson V, Teller DY. Postnatal development of vision in human and nonhuman primates. *Annu Rev Neurosci* 1985;8:495–545.
3. Daw NW. Critical periods and amblyopia. *Arch Ophthalmol* 1998;116:502–505.
4. Thompson JR, Woodruff G, Hiscox FA, et al. The incidence and prevalence of amblyopia detected in childhood. *Public Health* 1991;105:455–462.
5. Eibschitz-Tsimhoni M, Friedman T, Naor J, et al. Early screening for amblyogenic risk factors lowers the prevalence and severity of amblyopia. *J AAPOS* 2000;4:194–199.
6. Woodruff G, Hiscox F, Thompson JR, et al. The presentation of children with amblyopia. *Eye* 1994;8:623–626.
7. Keech RV, Kutschke PJ. Upper age limit for the development of amblyopia. *J Pediatr Ophthalmol Strabismus* 1995;32:89–93.
8. Rahi J, Logan S, Timms C, et al. Risk, causes, and outcomes of visual impairment after loss of vision in the nonamblyopic eye: a population-based study. *Lancet* 2002;360:597–602.
9. Packwood EA, Cruz OA, Rychwalski PJ, et al. The psychosocial effects of amblyopia study. *J AAPOS* 1999;3:15–17.
10. Holmes JM, Beck RW, Kraker RT, et al. Impact of patching and atropine treatment on the child and family in the amblyopia treatment study. *Arch Ophthalmol* 2003;121:1625–1632.
11. Membreno JH, Brown MM, Brown GC, et al. A cost-utility analysis of therapy for amblyopia. *Ophthalmology* 2002;109:2265–2271.
12. Weakley DR Jr, Holland DR. Effect of ongoing treatment of amblyopia on surgical outcome in esotropia. *J Pediatr Ophthalmol Strabismus* 1997;34:275–278.
13. Weakley DR Jr, Birch E. The role of anisometropia in the development of accommodative esotropia. *Trans Am Ophthalmol Soc* 2000;98:71–76.
14. Hommer K, Schubert G. The absolute size of foveal receptive field centers and Panum'sareas. *Albrecht Von Graefe's Arch Ophthalmol* 1963;166:205–210.
15. Thomas J. Normal and amblyopic contrast sensitivity function in central and peripheral retinas. *Invest Ophthalmol Vis Sci* 1978; 17:746–753.
16. Leguire LE, Rogers GL, Bremer DL. Amblyopia: the normal eye is not normal. *J Pediatr Ophthalmol Strabismus* 1990;27:32–38.
17. Kandel GL, Grattan PE, Bedell HE. Are the dominant eyes of amblyopes normal? *Am J Optom Physiol Opt* 1980;57:1–6.
18. Lempert P. The axial length/disc area ratio in anisometropic hyperopic amblyopia: a hypothesis for decreased unilateral vision associated with hyperopic anisometropia. *Ophthalmology* 2004; 111:304–308.
19. Hubel DH, Wiesel TN. Receptive fields and cells in striated cortex of very young, visually inexperienced kittens. *J Neurophysiol* 1963; 26:994–1002.
20. Hubel DH, Wiesel TN, LeVay S. Plasticity of ocular dominance columns in monkey's striate cortex. *Philos Trans R Soc Lond B Biol Sci* 1977;278:377–409.
21. Wiesel TN. Postnatal development of the visual cortex and the influence of environment. *Nature* 1982;299:583.
22. Demer JL, von Noorden GK, Volkow ND, et al. Imaging of cerebral blood flow and metabolism in amblyopia by positron emission tomography. *Am J Ophthalmol* 1988;105:337–347.
23. Snowdon SK, Stewart-Brown SL. Preschool vision screening. *Health Technol Assess* 1997;1:1–83.
24. Wright KW, Walonker F, Edelman P. 10-Diopter fixation test for amblyopia. *Arch Ophthalmol* 1981;99:1242–1246.
25. Lawwill T, Meur G, Howard CW. Lateral inhibition in the central visual field of an amblyopic subject. *Am J Ophthalmol* 1973;76:225–228.
26. Pediatric Eye Disease Investigator Group. A comparison of atropine and patching treatments for moderate amblyopia by patient age, cause of amblyopia, depth of amblyopia, and other factors. *Ophthalmology* 2003;110:1632–1637.
27. Holmes JM, Kraker RT, Beck RW, et al. A randomized trial of prescribed patching regimens for treatment of severe amblyopia in children. *Ophthalmology* 2003;110:2075–2087.
28. France TD, France LW. Optical penalization can improve vision after occlusion treatment. *J AAPOS* 1999;3:341–343.
29. Writing Committee for the Pediatric Eye Disease Investigator Group. Optical treatment of strabismic and combined strabismic-anisometropic amblyopia. *Ophthalmology* 2012;119:150–158.
30. Simon JW, Parks MM, Price EC. Severe visual loss resulting from occlusion therapy for amblyopia. *J Pediatr Ophthalmol Strabismus* 1987;24:244–246.

31. Pediatric Eye Disease Investigator Group. The course of moderate amblyopia treated with atropine in children: experience of the amblyopia treatment study. *Am J Ophthalmol* 2003;136: 630–639.

32. Pediatric Eye Disease Investigator Group. A randomized trial of atropine vs. patching for treatment of moderate amblyopia in children. *Arch Ophthalmol* 2002;120:268–278.

33. Leguire LE, Walson PD, Rogers GL, et al. Levodopa/carbidopa treatment for amblyopia in older children. *J Pediatr Ophthalmol Strabismus* 1995;32:143–151.

34. Campos EC, Schiavi C, Benedetti P, et al. Effect of citicoline on visual acuity in amblyopia: preliminary results. *Graefes Arch Clin Exp Ophthalmol* 1995;233:307–312.

35. Oster JG, Simon JW, Jenkins P. When is it safe to stop patching? *Br J Ophthalmol* 1990;74:709–711.

36. Holmes JM, Beck RW, Kraker RT, et al. Risk of amblyopia recurrence after cessation of treatment. *J AAPOS* Oct 2004;8: 420–428.

37. Lithander J, Sjostrand J. Anisometropic and strabismic amblyopia in the age group 2 years and above: a prospective study of the results of treatment. *Br J Ophthalmol* 1991;75:111–116.

38. Holmes JM, Lazar EL, Melia BM, et al. Effect of age on response to amblyopia treatment in children. *Arch Ophthalmol* Nov 2011;129(11):1451–1457.

39. Mintz-Hittner HA, Fernandez KM. Successful amblyopia therapy initiated after age 7 years: compliance cures. *Arch Ophthalmol* 2000;118:1535–1541.

40. Moseley M, Fielder A. Improvement in amblyopic eye function and contralateral eye disease: evidence of residual plasticity. *Lancet* 2001;357:902–904.

7

Binocular Vision: Adaptations in Strabismus and Monofixation

Bruce M. Schnall

NORMAL BINOCULAR VISION

Single binocular vision is the cortical integration of the similar retinal images produced by each eye into a single unified perception (1). It is important to recognize that binocular vision occurs at a cortical level and any changes or adaptations to binocular vision will occur on a cortical level as well. In children with infantile or congenital strabismus, early surgical alignment of the eyes is needed to either allow the cells for binocular vision to develop in the brain or prevent their loss during the critical period of binocular vision development (2). Cortical changes due to an abnormal visual experience in childhood are not unique to binocular vision. The loss of neurons in the geniculate body due to a unilateral blurred image in childhood is well documented in amblyopia (3).

The first step in understanding binocular vision is to recognize that retinal elements have a visual direction. The visual direction of a retinal element is determined by its relative position to the fovea (4). For example, if the retinal elements inferior to the fovea are stimulated, the visual direction of these retinal elements localize the image to an area in the superior visual field. An object seen by the fovea will localize to an area in space that is straight ahead. If light is shone onto the nasal retina, it will be sensed that this light is in the temporal visual field. An eye with a recent onset sixth nerve palsy will be held in adduction, such that nasal retina lies in the area normally occupied by the fovea. The nasal retina will continue to localize objects to the temporal visual field. In addition, an eye held in adduction is rotated such that the fovea now lies in an area normally occupied by temporal retina. A light shone on this fovea, which is now temporal, will be localized as straight ahead. A representation of the visual direction of retinal elements can be seen when performing visual field testing. Each point of the visual field relates to a specific area in the retina.

Retinal elements of the two eyes that share a common visual direction, or localize to the same area in space are referred to as corresponding retinal points. Similar images falling on corresponding retinal points are localized as coming from the same area in space by both eyes and can be fused and seen as a single image. An image that falls on noncorresponding retinal points are localized to two different areas in space and are seen as double. The horopter is a two-dimensional plane in space of points that fall on corresponding retinal points (Fig. 7.1). Only objects on the horopter will fall on corresponding retinal points. There is a small area in front of and behind the horopter in which the brain can fuse noncorresponding or disparate retinal points. Fusing the images that fall on these noncorresponding or disparate retinal points allows not only single binocular vision but also an individual to order these objects in space, giving rise to stereopsis. This area just in front and behind the horopter is referred to as the Panum's area of single binocular vision (Fig. 7.2). Only within the Panum's area is the retinal disparity small enough to allow the images to be fused into one unified perception. The retinal periphery with its larger receptive fields is able to fuse images with a larger disparity and therefore the Panum's area is larger in the peripheral visual field and smaller centrally. It is only within the limited space of the Panum's area that we can see single. Objects outside of the Panum's area fall on retinal points that are too disparate to be fused and are seen as double.

The horopter and Panum's area are not static but are continually created and recreated with every change in direction of gaze or point of focus. For example, a person looking at a clock on the wall in the distance will create a Panum's area of single binocular vision around the clock. If a person extends their arm and holds their hand out in between themselves and the clock, while focusing on the clock, their hand is seen as double since it lies outside Panum's area. If the focus is shifted to their hand, a Panum's area is created around their hand. The hand will be seen as single and the clock will be seen as double as the clock on the wall now lies outside of the Panum's area of single binocular vision. Normally, the brain intervenes to prevent diplopia that occurs with objects outside of the Panum's area from reaching consciousness. Occasionally, children become aware of this diplopia from objects seen outside Panum's area. This is referred to as physiologic diplopia.

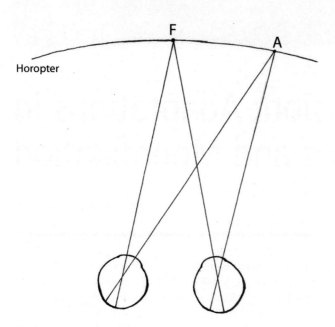

FIGURE 7.1. The horopter. Point F is the fixation point. Point A lies on the horopter and therefore the retinal images will fall on corresponding retinal points.

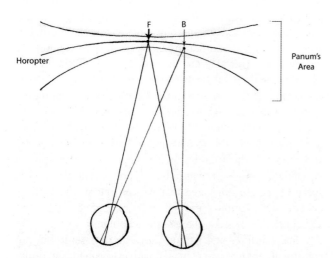

FIGURE 7.2. The Panum's area of single binocular vision is just anterior and posterior to the horopter. Point F is the fixation point. Point B is anterior to the horopter but within the Panum's area. The images of point B will fall on retinal elements that are slightly disparate. Point B would be a single fused image and seen anterior to Point F with stereopsis.

In order to have single binocular vision, the images produced by both eyes must be fused into a single unified perception. This fusion of the images occurs at a cortical level. Fusion has both a sensory and motor component. It is the motor component of fusion that reduces the horizontal, vertical, or torsional disparity of the retinal images making it possible for the images to fuse into a single perception. The motor component of fusion helps maintain ocular alignment and prevent diplopia. A phoria is an example of

motor fusion maintaining ocular alignment. If the amount of the phobia exceeds the abilities of motor fusion, a manifest strabismus or tropia will occur. The eye movements produced by motor fusion to maintain ocular alignment are referred to as vergence movements. It is possible to have fusion with both its sensory and motor components without measurable stereopsis.

Not all individuals will have binocular vision. In order to develop binocular vision, an infant must be capable of seeing with each eye, and the eyes must be aligned, allowing retinal images to project onto corresponding retinal elements during the critical period of binocular vision development (5). This critical period of binocular development is generally accepted to be the first 2 years of life. If binocular vision never develops, this individual will be monocular, viewing with one eye at a time. A monocular patient is incapable of using both eyes simultaneously. It is not possible for a monocular patient to experience diplopia. A monocular patient will not have fusion and therefore will not have the motor component of fusion or vergence movements to help maintain ocular alignment. There are sensory tests that can determine if the patient has monocular or binocular vision (simultaneous perception).

VISUAL SYMPTOMS IN STRABISMUS

A strabismic patient who is monocular is not capable of simultaneous perception and will not experience diplopia. In patients with binocular vision a newly acquired strabismus will produce diplopia. The diplopia results from the simultaneous perception of the images of the object of regard projecting onto noncorresponding retinal points. These noncorresponding retinal points will localize the object to two different areas in space and the object will be seen as doubled. In strabismic eyes two different objects in space that would normally fall on noncorresponding retinal points can fall onto corresponding retinal points. Both of these objects could be localized to the same area in space and would be perceived as two different objects in the same place in space (5). This is referred to as visual confusion. This differs from diplopia, which is one object being seen in two places. When adult patients acquire a new strabismus, they complain of diplopia, an object located in two places at once. They do not complain of seeing one object on top of another, or two objects in one place (visual confusion). Visual confusion is not clinically significant.

Visual confusion does not exist for all portions of the visual field (5). Only similar images projecting on the foveas are perceived simultaneously. From the moment an eye deviates, a macula scotoma exists in one eye. This facultative macula scotoma will occur immediately preventing central confusion. This facultative macula scotoma occurs in all strabismic patients and can be plotted using a binocular perimetric technique (5). The facultative macula scotoma is not an adaptation that slowly develops over time, it occurs immediately in strabismus and is not a suppression scotoma.

CORTICAL ADAPTATIONS IN STRABISMUS

Adaptations can occur to the binocular vision system, which eliminate central and peripheral diplopia in acquired strabismus. These adaptations will only occur only in patients who have preexisting binocular vision. These cortical adaptations that develop gradually over time are suppression and anomalous retinal correspondence (ARC). Suppression and ARC are adaptations that occur in the brain to prevent diplopia from reaching consciousness. Suppression develops to prevent central diplopia. ARC develops to prevent peripheral diplopia. Patients who are monocular are incapable of simultaneous perception (diplopia) and will not develop suppression or ARC. The time needed to develop suppression and ARC is related to the age of the patient. The younger the child, the faster these adaptations will develop.

Suppression is a positive inhibitory reflex (5) that permits the cortex to ignore the images of conscious regard (what is seen centrally in the fixing eye) produced by retinal elements outside the macula in the deviated eye. Unlike the facultative scotoma that occurs in the macula to prevent central confusion, suppression is pathologic and requires time to develop. Suppression only exists when viewing with both eyes. The moment one eye is closed, the suppression scotoma disappears. If either eye can maintain fixation, the suppression scotoma can alternate between eyes, being present in the eye that is nonfixating at that instant. A suppression scotoma will not produce amblyopia because a suppression scotoma involves extramacular retina. It is the facultative macula scotoma that occurs immediately when an eye deviates that causes strabismic amblyopia, not suppression (5).

A suppression scotoma can be measured under binocular conditions with prism or binocular perimetry. In esotropic patients, there is a suppression scotoma nasally of approximately 5 degrees (Fig. 7.3). In exotropia there is a larger hemiretinal scotoma extending to the number of degrees required to include the object of conscious regard (Fig. 7.4). In a strabismic patient with suppression, increasing amounts of prisms can be added until the patient reports diplopia. In an esotropic patient, the amount of prism will generally be smaller than the angle of the esotropia. In an exotropic patient the amount of base-in prism needed to move the image of the object of conscious regard off the suppression scotoma will be slightly greater than the angle of the exotropia. Once the image has been moved off the suppression scotoma, the patient will report diplopia. The patient who reports diplopia once the image of conscious regard has been moved off the suppression scotoma has binocular vision and is capable of having either single binocular vision or diplopia after strabismus surgery. A strabismic patient who does not have diplopia when the strabismus is overcorrected with prism is most likely monocular and not expected to be capable of binocular vision and therefore should not be at risk for diplopia after strabismus surgery.

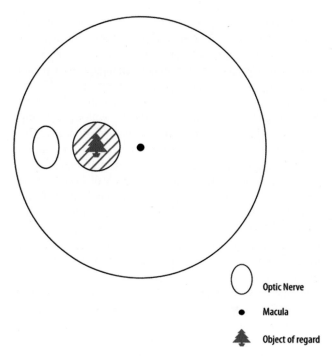

Optic Nerve

Macula

Object of regard

FIGURE 7.3. Suppression scotoma in esotropia.

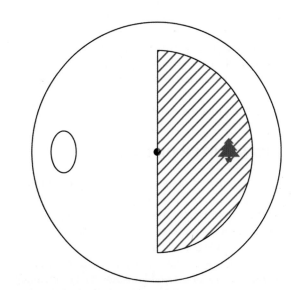

FIGURE 7.4. Suppression scotoma in exotropia.

ARC is a cortical adjustment in a strabismic patient of the normal directional values of the extramacular retinal elements of the nonfixing eye to prevent peripheral diplopia (5). ARC exists only under conditions of binocular viewing. Immediately upon closing the fixing eye the visual direction of the retinal elements of the deviated eye with ARC return to their original directional values.

Suppression and ARC occur at a cortical level and can change rapidly (5). In an A or V pattern strabismus, as the patient changes from down gaze to up gaze, the angle of the horizontal strabismus is continually changing. In a patient with suppression and ARC, each time the angle of the strabismus changes, the suppression scotoma and ARC (visual direction of the extramacular elements) will change. Suppression and ARC are adaptations to prevent diplopia. They do not have an associated motor component. They do not provide vergence amplitudes to help maintain ocular alignment as seen with the motor component of fusion. When the angle of a strabismus changes, a patient with ARC and suppression has a sensory response, rather than a motor response, to prevent diplopia. A new suppression scotoma and ARC pattern will develop to accommodate the new angle of the strabismus. In patients with ARC there is no measurable stereopsis.

Patients with intermittent strabismus may have ARC and a suppression scotoma when the eyes are deviated, but normal retinal correspondence (NRC) when the eyes are straight. A strabismic patient with ARC can convert to NRC if the eyes are aligned within 8 prism diopters or less with glasses, prisms, or strabismus surgery (5). With improved ocular alignment and NRC there can be a return of stereopsis and the motor aspect of fusion, or fusional vergence amplitudes, which can help maintain this improved ocular alignment. The patient who regains NRC can again develop ARC if the angle of the strabismus increases. This can be seen in patients with accommodative esotropia and a history of ARC and suppression. Some patients with accommodative esotropia have stereopsis and NRC when wearing glasses, and ARC and suppression to prevent diplopia when the glasses are removed and they are esotropic.

FIXATION-SWITCH DIPLOPIA

Adults with a history of nonalternating strabismus since childhood will often have a preferred eye with a suppression scotoma in the nonfixing or strabismic eye. These individuals may be capable of suppression and ARC in the nondominant eye only. It is possible that secondary to inadequate refraction, cataract development, or cataract surgery on the nondominate eye, the visual acuity of the nondominate eye becomes superior to the dominant eye. When these individuals view with their nondominant eye, they may incapable of suppression and ARC in the dominant eye and experience diplopia. This diplopia occurs as result of changing fixation from the dominate to nondominate eye, and is referred to as fixation-switch diplopia (6). The angle of the strabismus can be small (under 15 diopters). This diplopia may be present intermittently even if fixation with the nondominant eye is constant.

The treatment for fixation-switch diplopia is to improve the visual acuity in the dominant eye. If the reduced visual acuity is secondary to inadequate refraction, it is best treated by improving the refractive correction in the dominant eye.

Cycloplegic refraction may be needed to determine the best optical correction (6). If the visual acuity is reduced in the dominant eye as a result of cataract, successful cataract surgery and the appropriate optical correction should eliminate the diplopia.

DUALITY OF VISION

An eye has macular and extramacular vision. If a disorder that affects the macula occurs, the high-quality central vision, the ability to read fine print, would be lost in that eye. That eye with macular disease will however retain its peripheral or extramacular vision. There is a macular and an extramacular component to binocular vision. Macular binocular vision is associated with high-grade stereopsis (40 seconds of arc). The foveas must be aligned within two-thirds of a diopter to allow macular binocular vision (7). Macular binocular vision is tenuous and can be lost with a constant strabismus. Once lost, macular binocular vision is rarely regained after the strabismus is corrected. Macular binocular vision is referred to as bifixation, fixating with both eyes at once.

Extramacular binocular vision can exist with deviations up to 8 diopters (8). It is associated with low-grade stereopsis and provides the motor vergence amplitudes that help maintain ocular alignment. Unlike macular binocular vision, extramacular binocular vision is durable. If extramacular binocular vision existed prior to the onset of strabismus, extramacular binocular vision can return with successful treatment of the strabismus even if a constant strabismus has been present for many years. It is possible for an individual to lose their macular binocular vision but retain their extramacular binocular vision. This is common in longstanding acquired strabismus.

MONOFIXATION SYNDROME

The term monofixation was coined by Marshall Parks (8) to describe the syndrome in which extramacular binocular vision exists without macular binocular vision. Preceding Marshall Parks, it was observed that many patients had a small-angle stable strabismus following successful strabismus surgery. These patients had a consistent tropia measuring 8 prism diopters or less and good fusional vergence amplitudes which maintained their ocular alignment. There is a central or macular scotoma in the nonfixing or deviated eye that prevents central diplopia. This small-angle strabismus was referred to as a microtropia or a flick strabismus because of the small flick seen on cover testing as the deviated eye assumed fixation (9). A similar entity was noted in patients without a history of strabismus surgery. These patients either had straight eyes or a microtropia (less than 8 diopters) with a central scotoma in the nonfixing eye with extramacular binocular vision. Marshall Parks united these two entities, one with a history of strabismus and one

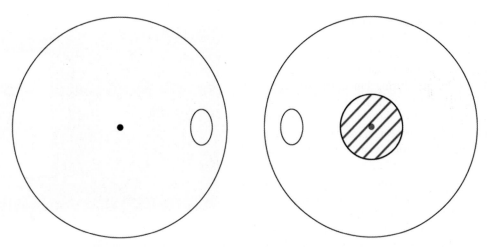

FIGURE 7.5. Monofixation with 8 diopter macular scotoma left eye.

without strabismus into one syndrome, the monofixation syndrome (8). In bifixation, the patient is viewing with the maculas of both eyes. In the monofixation syndrome, there is a scotoma in the macula of one eye and therefore a monofixator is only fixating with one eye (Fig. 7.5).

There are a number of different conditions associated with monofixation, with amblyopia and treated strabismus the being most common. Any condition that is a barrier to macular fusion can cause monofixation. Clear macular images during infancy are required to develop bifixation. Anisometropia of 1.50 diopters spherical equivalent or astigmatism will result in a clear image on one macula and a blurred image on the macula of the other eye (8). This anisometropia may go undetected for the first several year of life, preventing the child from developing bifixation. This anisometropia may also result in amblyopia. Optical correction later in life will aid in the treatment of amblyopia (10), but in all likelihood this child will never develop bifixation. Even with successful treatment of amblyopia, monofixation will remain with rare exceptions. Although a macular scotoma exists in amblyopia under conditions of binocular viewing, spectacle correction without patching will often result in some improvement in the visual acuity in the amblyopic eye (10). All patients with amblyopia will have monofixation. Not all patients with monofixation syndrome will have amblyopia. Parks found that 24% of patients with monofixation syndrome never had amblyopia (11).

Monofixation may be associated with successfully treated infantile and acquired strabismus. Patients with an intermittent strabismus such as intermittent exotropia may fuse and bifixate at near-retaining bifixation. A constant strabismus that prevents bifixation can result in monofixation if the strabismus is not corrected promptly. Monofixation is commonly associated with a strabismus that begins in childhood and has been reported as a result of strabismus acquired as an adult (12). An accommodative esotrope

who is treated shortly after the esotropia began has a greater chance of retaining bifixation than an accommodative esotrope who goes uncorrected for several months. A patient with a constant strabismus that has been present for months or years can develop monofixation if the eyes are aligned within 8 prism diopters with strabismus surgery, lenses, or prisms.

In uncorrected infantile strabismus such as infantile or congenital esotropia, no binocular vision is present. Prior to strabismus surgery these patients are monocular and are not capable of simultaneous perception (diplopia or fusion). Absence of binocular vision in a strabismic patient can be tested for by overcorrecting the angle of the strabismus with prism to determine if the patient is capable of diplopia. A monocular patient would not be diplopic and would not experience any diplopia after strabismus surgery. In congenital or infantile strabismus, aligning the eyes within 8 prism diopters during the critical period would give that child a chance to obtain monofixation. Ing (2) found that children with infantile esotropia have a greater chance of obtaining fusion if the eyes are aligned by 2 years of age and a greater chance of having stereopsis if the eyes are aligned within a year of the onset of the esotropia (13).

Other conditions associated with monofixation include dissociated vertical deviation (DVD) and organic macula lesions. Monofixation can also be idiopathic or not associated with strabismus, anisometropia, amblyopia, or an organic lesion. This has been referred to as primary monofixation. Primary monofixation frequently occurs in a parent, sibling, or child of congenital esotropic patients (14).

Surgery in a child with infantile strabismus at an age young enough to allow development of monofixation gives the child a chance to develop motor vergence amplitudes to help maintain their ocular alignment. A child with infantile strabismus receiving surgery beyond this critical period would be less likely to develop monofixation and its associated vergence amplitudes. Without monofixation and its vergence amplitudes, the chance of an eye becoming strabismic over time is greatly increased (15).

The essential feature of monofixation is a macular scotoma in the nonfixating eye during binocular viewing. A small-angle manifest strabismus (tropia) may be present of 8 prisms diopters or less under conditions of binocular viewing. A latent phoria is often present in excess of the manifest microtropia. A manifest tropia can be tested for with the simultaneous prism cover test and the phoria tested for with the alternate cover test. The simultaneous prism cover test is performed by placing a cover over the fixing eye and a prism over the nonfixing eye simultaneously. The amount of prism resulting in no movement on simultaneous prism cover test is the manifest deviation or tropia. Subsequently, an alternate cover test can be preformed, which will measure the phoria or latent deviation. The vergence amplitudes produced by extramacular binocular vision allows patients with monofixation to have a tropia, which is less than their phoria. These vergence amplitudes are of benefit to the monofixator. They limit the tropia to 8 diopters or less allowing for peripheral NRC, preventing peripheral diplopia. These vergence amplitudes help to maintain a small-angle strabismus, which would not be apparent to others, reducing the risk of developing a significant manifest strabismus (15). Patients with a tropia of greater than 8 diopters may have suppression and ARC, which will prevent diplopia, but no associated motor vergence amplitudes to help maintain their eye alignment. The range of fusional vergence amplitudes for patients with monofixation is similar to that for patients with bifixation (15).

Approximately one third of patients with monofixation will have no strabismus, with no detectable deviation of either eye on cover–uncover test or simultaneous prism cover test (11). In these patients with monofixation without strabismus the image of the object of regard is ignored in one eye as one eye has a macular facultative scotoma. The binocular vision of patients with an organic scotoma from a macular lesion is indistinguishable from the binocular vision of patient with a functional scotoma related to monofixation (11). This macular facultative scotoma is only present when viewing binocularly and can be demonstrated with sensory testing.

SENSORY TESTING

Sensory testing can be used to determine if monofixation or bifixation is present. Most of these tests rely on proving the presence or absence of the macular scotoma that is only present in monofixation when viewing binocularly.

STEREOPSIS

Stereopsis occurs as the slightly disparate images on the retina are cortically fused into a single image. Stereo acuity is a measure of a patient's ability to perceive these slightly

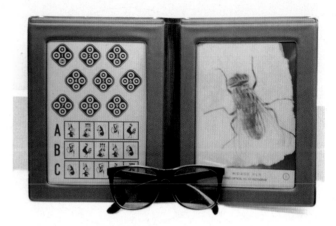

FIGURE 7.6. Titmus Stereo Test.

disparate images. It is measured in seconds of arc. Bifixation allows the patient to perceive very small degrees of retinal image disparity with a stereo acuity of 40 seconds of arc or less. In monofixation the macular scotoma present in one eye limits the stereo acuity to 60 to 3,000 seconds of arc. It is possible in monofixation to have fusion without any measurable stereopsis. Stereo acuity can be measured at near or in the distance. The Titmus Stereo Test (Fig. 7.6) is a widely used simple test to measure stereopsis at near. The patient wears vectographic glasses during testing. Monofixators are usually able to perceive the fly's wings as elevated and may be able to perceive up to 60 seconds of arc. Bifixation is needed to correctly identify which dot is elevated in boxes 8 (50 seconds of arc) and 9 (40 seconds of arc).

WORTH 4-LIGHT TEST

The test target consists of two green lights, one red light, and one white light. The patient wears glasses, which have a red lens in front of one eye and a green lens in front of the other (Fig. 7.7). The eye behind the green lens can see the green light but not the red as the green lens filters out red light (16). The red lens will allow the patient to see the red light but not the two green lights. The white light can be seen by either lens and will appear red when viewed through the red lens and green when viewed through the green lens.

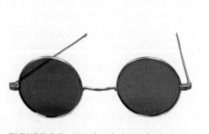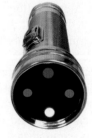

FIGURE 7.7. Worth 4 light with glasses.

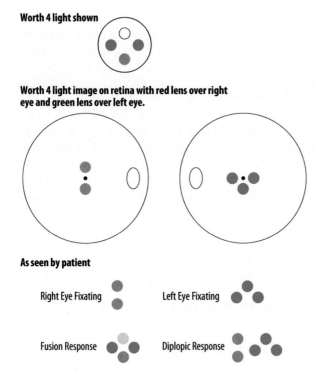

Worth 4 light shown

Worth 4 light image on retina with red lens over right eye and green lens over left eye.

As seen by patient

Right Eye Fixating   Left Eye Fixating

Fusion Response   Diplopic Response

FIGURE 7.8. Possible responses to the Worth 4 light. Note that the images on the retina are inverted from what is projected and what the patient sees.

These lights are on a flashlight, which can be shown to the patient in the distance and at near.

When the Worth 4-light is viewed binocularly in the distance by a patient who has bifixation four lights will be seen. A patient who is diplopic would see five lights in the distance, as the white light would be perceived in two different locations. A patient who is monocular, has strabismus with a suppression scotoma, or has a macular scotoma in one eye related to monofixation, will not see the lights of the Worth 4-light with one eye when viewed in the distance. If the lights are not being seen by the eye behind the green lens, only the l red and white light seen by the eye behind the red lens will be seen. The patient will see two red lights. If the lights are not being seen by the eye behind the red lens, three green lights will be seen (Fig. 7.8).

The key to understanding this test is to recognize that at near the size of the retinal image of these 4 lights is much larger at near than at distance (Fig. 7.9). The Worth 4-light will project an image onto the retina of 1.25 degrees at distance (6 m) and 6 degrees at near (0.33 m). The macular scotoma in monofixation is 3 degrees (11). In monofixation the lights fall within this 3 degree macular scotoma of the nonfixing eye when viewed in the distance and therefore not be seen by the eye with the macular scotoma when viewed binocularly. At near the retinal images are larger projecting an image of approximately 6 degrees, which fall outside of the 3 degree macular scotoma and will be seen by the nonfixing eye in monofixation (Fig. 7.10).

When performing this test if four lights are seen in the distance, the patient is a bifixator and the test does not need to be done at near. If patient sees only two green or three red lights then the test needs to be repeated at near. If the patient does not have a tropia of greater than 8 diopters and sees the four lights only at near, they have monofixation. The ability to see four lights at near but not distance in a patient whose eyes are aligned within 8 diopters is consistent with monofixation. A patient with a manifest strabismus of greater than 8 diopters with suppression and ARC may give a similar response. A monocular patient who never developed binocular vision will continue to see only two or three lights at near.

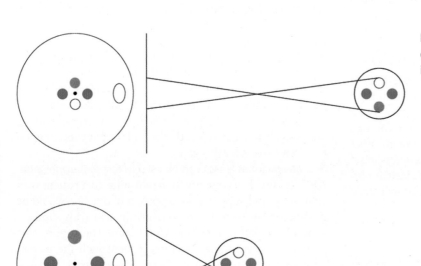

FIGURE 7.9. The Worth 4 lights produce a larger image on the retina when it is brought nearer to the eye as seen in the bottom diagram.

DISTANCE

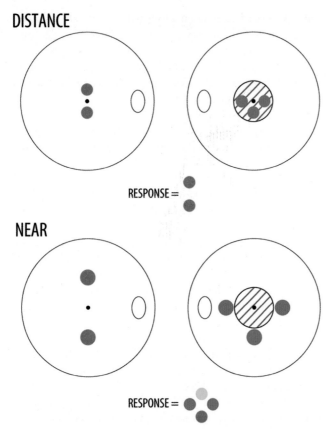

FIGURE 7.10. Monofixation with macular scotoma of the left eye. When viewed in the distance, the green lights fall within the scotoma of the left eye and are not seen. At near the lights project outside the scotoma and 4 lights will be seen.

DISTANCE VECTOGRAPH

The distance vectograph is a quick test to differentiate bifixation from monofixation (11). Letters seen in the distance will create a small image size on the retina and fall within the scotoma in a patient with monofixation. A line of polarized letters is viewed in the distance of 20/40 or 20/50 size print with the appropriate polarized glasses. If using the A-O projection slide, four of the six letters will be polarized. With the appropriate polarized glasses two of the letters are seen through the right lens only, two of the letters are seen through the left lens only, and two of the letters are seen through either lens. A monofixator will only read four of the six letters missing the letters normally seen in the eye with the macular scotoma. A patient with bifixation will see and read all six letters.

4 DIOPTER BASE-OUT TEST

The basis of this test is that the movement of an image 4 diopters within an 8 diopter scotoma is not perceived and would be not cause a compensatory movement by that eye to prevent diplopia. It was initially described by Irvine (17)

as the "image displacement test." It is performed by placing a 4 diopter base-out prism over one eye at a time while the patient is reading letters or viewing an object in the distance. The eye the prism is placed over is viewed carefully for any movement (11). An eye without a macular scotoma will perceive the image being shifted toward the apex of the prism and a movement of that eye inward would be seen. A 4 diopter movement of an image within an eye with an 8 diopter scotoma would not be perceived. Absence of movement of one eye is evidence of a macular scotoma in that eye. The movement of each eye inward with placement of the 4 diopter base-out prim over that eye is consistent with bifixation. Some of the difficulties with this test are that it can be challenging to see a 4 diopter movement of an eye in an uncooperative child. A bifixator may experience diplopia with the 4 diopter prism but not make a convergent movement to eliminate the movement. A movement of an eye may be seen in a patient with monofixation if they switch fixation to the other eye during testing.

BAGOLINI LENSES

Sensory tests that involve viewing through red and green lenses or polarized lenses create an artificial viewing circumstance that may be a hindrance to fusion. The striated lens popularized by Bagolini consists of a clear lens with a faint linear striation that produces a linear streak of light when viewing a bright light. The Bagolini lenses allow the most life-like viewing conditions. In a patient who fuses intermittently the Bagolini striated glasses test is the sensory test most likely to demonstrate fusion. The lenses are placed in a trial frame with the reference line for the right eye at 135 degrees and the left eye at 45 degrees. The patient views a light source through the lenses with the room lights on. A patient with bifixation will see the two sharp perpendicular streaks of light emanating from the light source, one at 135 degrees in the right eye and one at 45 degrees in the left eye, forming an X intersecting at the light. In a patient with bifixation, both of these lines will be fully present passing through the light source without a gap in the line. In monofixation the line seen by the nonfixating eye will have a small gap around the light produced by the 8 diopter macula scotoma (Fig. 7.11). In monofixation this gap or break in the line is small and may be overlooked till the patients attention is drawn to look for this gap.

The Bagolini lenses can be used to test for suppression, NRC, or ARC in a patient with strabismus. In a patient with strabismus and suppression, a portion of one line would be missing or not seen. In an esotropic patient with suppression a large gap in one line would seen. The suppression scotoma is larger in an exotropic patient with the patient observing only a small peripheral streak outside the scotoma or seeing no steak at all. A patient with strabismus and ARC will continue to have the two lines appear to cross in the center. Although one line will have a gap as a result

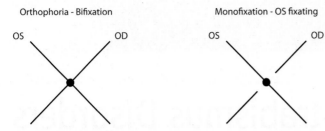

FIGURE 7.11. Streaks of lights seen by a patient when wearing Bagolini lenses. The central dot is the light source. In bifixation, two complete lines will be seen. The scotoma in monofixation will result in gap in the line seen by the eye with the macular scotoma.

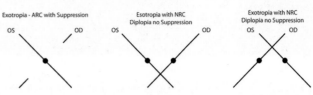

FIGURE 7.12. A strabismic patient will see a gap in one line if a suppression scotoma is present. The lines will appear to cross in the center of the light in strabismus with anomalous retinal correspondence (ARC). In normal retinal correspondence (NRC) with strabismus the lines will cross either below or above the center.

of its suppression scotoma. In a strabismic eye with NRC, these lines will no longer cross in the center (Fig. 7.12). An esotropic patient will experience uncrossed diplopia and see these lines cross below the center. An exotropic patient with NRC will have crossed diplopia and see the lines cross above the center.

REFERENCES

1. Mitchell PR, Parks MM. Sensory tests and treatment of sensorial adaptations. In: Duane TD, Jaeger EJ, eds. *Duane's ophthalmology*, 2011 Ed. Vol. 1, chapter 9. Philadelphia, PA: JB Lippincott Co., 2011:1–16.

2. Ing MR. Early surgical alignment for congenital esotropia. *Trans Am Ophthalmol Soc* 1981;79:625–663.

3. Wiesel T, Hubel D. Single cell response in striate cortex of kittens deprived of vision in one eye. *J Neurophysiol* 1963;26:1003–1017.

4. Burian HM, von Noorden GK. *Binocular vision and ocular motility*. Chapter 2. St Louis, MO: The C.V. Mosby Company, 1974.

5. Parks MM. Binocular vision adaptations in strabismus. In: Duane TD, Jaeger EJ, eds. *Duane's ophthalmology*, 2011 Ed. Vol 1, Chapter 8. Philadelphia, PA: JB Lippincott Co., 2011:1–14.

6. Kushner BJ. Fixation switch diplopia. *Arch Ophthalmol* 1995;113:896–899.

7. Ogle KN. Fixation disparity. *Am Orthoptic J* 1954;4:35–39.

8. Parks MM. Monofixation syndrome. *Trans Am Ophthalmol Soc* 1969;67:609–657.

9. Helveston EM, von Noorden GK. Microtropia. *Arch Ophthalmol* 1967;78:272–281.

10. Cotter SA: Pediatric Eye Disease Investigator Group; Edwards AR, Wallace DK, Beck RW, et al. Treatment of anisometropic amblyopia in children with refractive correction. *Ophthalmology* Jun 2006;113(6):895–903.

11. Parks MM. Monofixation syndrome. In: Duane TD, Jaeger EJ, eds. *Duane's ophthalmology*, 2011 Ed. Vol. 1, Chapter 14. Philadelphia, PA: JB Lippincott Co., 2011:1–12

12. H Eustis HS, Parks MM. Acquired monofixation syndrome. *J Pediatr Ophthalmol Strabismus* 1989;26:169–172.

13. Ing MR, Okino LM. Outcome study of stereopsis in relation to duration of misalignment in congenital esotropia. *J AAPOS* Feb 2002;6(1):3–8.

14. Scott MH, Noble AG Raymond WR 4th, Parks MM. Prevalence of primary monofixation syndrome in parents of children with congenital esotropia. *J Pediatr Ophthalmol Strabismus* 1994;31:298–301.

15. Arthur BW, Smith JT, Scott WE: Long-term stability of alignment in the monofixation syndrome. *J Pediatr Ophthalmol Strabismus* 1989;26:224–231.

16 Rabb EL. Sensory physiology and pathology. In: *Basic and Clinical Science Course, Pediatric Ophthalmology and Strabismus*, 2010–2011 ed. Section 6, chap 4. San Francisco, CA: American Academy of Ophthalmology, 2010:58–63.

17. Irvine SR. Amblyopia ex anopsia: observations on retinal inhibition, scotoma, projections, light difference discrimination and visual acuity. *Trans Am Ophthalmol Soc* 1948;46:527.

8

Strabismus Disorders

Scott E. Olitsky • *Leonard B. Nelson*

STRABISMUS, OR ABNORMAL ocular alignment, is one of the most common eye problems encountered in children. The misalignment may be manifest in any field of gaze, may be constant or intermittent, and may occur at distant or near fixation or both. Strabismus affects between 2% and 5% of the preschool population and is an important cause of visual and psychological disability (1,2). The word "strabismus" derives from the Greek word *strabismos* (meaning a squinting) and probably predates the geographer Strabo, whose "peculiarly horrible and unbecoming squint was famous in Alexandria during the Roman Empire."

Strabismus involves a number of different clinical entities. Knowledge of the terms used to describe a strabismic deviation and the more common patterns of strabismus help to predict the cause of the strabismus and determine proper treatment.

Orthophoria is the condition of exact ocular balance. It implies that the oculomotor apparatus is in perfect equilibrium so that both visual axes always intersect at the object of visual regard.

Heterophoria is a latent tendency for the eyes to deviate. This latent deviation is normally controlled by fusional mechanisms which provide binocular vision or avoid diplopia. The eye deviates only under certain conditions, such as fatigue, illness, stress, or tests that interfere with the maintenance of these normal fusional abilities (such as covering one eye). If the amount of heterophoria is large, it may give rise to bothersome symptoms, such as transient diplopia or asthenopia.

Heterotropia is a misalignment of the eyes that is manifest. The condition may be alternating or unilateral, depending on the vision. In alternating strabismus, either eye may be used for seeing while the fellow eye deviates. Because each eye is used in turn, each develops similar vision. In unilateral strabismus, only one eye is preferred for fixation while the fellow eye deviates consistently. The constantly deviating eye is prone to defective central vision during the visually immature period of life.

A convergent deviation, crossing or turning in of the eyes, is designated by the prefix "eso-" (esotropia, esophoria). Divergent deviation, or turning outward of the eyes, is designated by the prefix "exo-" (exotropia,

exophoria). Vertical deviations are designated by the prefixes "hyper-" and "hypo-" (hypertropia, hypotropia). In cases of unilateral strabismus, the deviating eye is often part of the description of the misalignment (left esotropia). Most vertical deviations are described in terms of the hypertropic eye. An exception to this general rule occurs when the lower, or hypotropic, eye is restricted in its movement. The deviation is then named according to the hypotropic eye.

OCULAR ALIGNMENT IN INFANCY

Ocular deviations during the first months of life do not necessarily indicate an abnormality. Because of oculomotor instability during this time, adequate assessment of alignment usually is not made until the patient is approximately 3 months of age and any angle of strabismus that is present is stable. Infants are often born with their eyes misaligned. During the first month of life, alignment may vary intermittently from esotropia to orthotropia to exotropia. Nixon and coworkers observed 1,219 alert infants in a newborn nursery and found that 40% seemed to have straight eyes, 33% had exotropia, and 3% had esotropia (3). Many had variable alignment and 7% were not sufficiently alert to permit classification. Other large population studies have confirmed that strabismus is common in early infancy (4).

ESODEVIATIONS

Pseudoesotropia

Pseudoesotropia is one of the most common reasons an ophthalmologist is asked to evaluate an infant. This condition is characterized by the false appearance of esotropia when the visual axes are aligned accurately. The appearance may be caused by a flat, broad nasal bridge; prominent epicanthal folds; or a narrow interpupillary distance (Fig. 8.1). The observer sees less sclera nasally than would be expected, which creates the impression that the eye is turned in toward the nose, especially when the child gazes to either side. This might be especially noticeable in

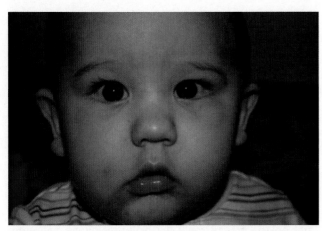

FIGURE 8.1. Pseudoesotropia caused by a wide nasal bridge and epicanthal folds. Note that the light reflex is centered in each pupil. (Reprinted with permission from Olitsky SE, Nelson LB. *Pediatric clinical ophthalmology—A color handbook.* London, UK: Manson Publishing, 2012, ISBN 9781840761511.)

photographs. Pseudoesotropia can be differentiated from a true manifest deviation by use of the corneal light reflex and the cover–uncover test, when possible. Once pseudoesotropia has been confirmed, parents can be reassured that the child will "outgrow" the appearance of esotropia. As the child grows, the bridge of the nose becomes more prominent and displaces the epicanthal folds, so that the sclera medially becomes proportional to the amount visible on the lateral aspect. It should be stressed that it is the appearance of crossing that the child will outgrow. Some parents of children with pseudoesotropia may incorrectly believe that there is an actual esotropia that will resolve on its own. Because true esotropia can develop later in children with pseudoesotropia, parents and pediatricians should be instructed that reassessment is needed if the apparent deviation does not improve.

Congenital Esotropia

Definition

The term congenital esotropia is a confusing one. Few children who are diagnosed with this disorder are actually born with an esotropia. Although parents often give a history of their child's eyes crossing since birth, they rarely remember seeing the deviation in the newborn nursery and will often deny seeing it during the first few weeks of life. Ophthalmologists have also rarely found infants with esodeviations to have been born with the condition. In a prospective study of 3,324 infants, only 3 children developed findings characteristic of congenital esotropia. All of these children were either orthotropic or exotropic at birth (4). Most reports in the literature have therefore considered infants with confirmed onset earlier than 6 months as having the same condition, which some observers have redesignated "infantile" esotropia. The differentiation between these terms may be

important. A child born with a "later onset" infantile esotropia may have a better prognosis for the development of binocular vision than a child with a true "congenital" deviation as he/she would have had an early period of ocular alignment which could provide a stimulus for the early formation of binocular development. The terms congenital and infantile esotropia are used interchangeably by most authors.

Epidemiology

Congenital esotropia is a common form of strabismus. The sex distribution of congenital esotropia is equal. Transmission in many families seems to be as an irregular autosomal dominant trait; however, in others it may be recessive. The reported incidence of affected family members has varied widely (5). It is common to find a history of strabismus in the parents or siblings of affected patients. Reduced binocular function has been reported in parents of patients with congenital esotropia (6). The incidence of congenital esotropia is higher in patients with a history of prematurity, cerebral palsy, hydrocephalus, and other neurologic disorders.

Pathogenesis

Much clinical literature in this century has focused on the implications of two conflicting theories of pathogenesis for congenital esotropia. Worth's "sensory" concept was that congenital esotropia resulted from a deficit in a supposed fusion center in the brain (7). According to his theory, the goal of restoring binocularity was considered hopeless, since there was no way to provide this congenitally absent neural function. Until the 1960s, results of surgical treatment almost universally supported this pessimistic view. Data on these patients were obtained at a time when surgery was rarely performed before 2 years of age.

Chavasse disagreed with Worth's theory. He suggested that normal binocular vision may be achieved through facilitation of conditioned reflexes that depend on early ocular alignment (8). To Chavasse, the primary problem was mechanical. In this view, most children with congenital esotropia were potentially curable if the deviation could be eliminated in infancy. Only theoretical support was available for this "motor" theory until Costenbader, Taylor, Ing and Costenbader, and Parks began to report favorable binocular results in some infants operated on between 6 months and 2 years of age (9–11). These encouraging results became the basis for the theory of early surgery for patients with congenital esotropia.

Even advocates of early surgery have generally found imperfect binocularity in their postoperative patients. Parks defined the monofixation syndrome, in which "peripheral" fusion and vergence amplitudes capable of maintaining alignment within approximately 10 prism diopters (PD) may exist, despite deficient stereopsis and a central suppression scotoma in one eye during binocular viewing (12). Many strabismus surgeons accept this sensory state as the goal of treatment.

Clinical Manifestations

Visual Acuity. The association of amblyopia and congenital esotropia is well known. It is difficult to ascertain the exact incidence, however, especially in preverbal children. The incidence of amblyopia may be as high as 40% to 72%. Many infants spontaneously alternate their fixation and do not develop amblyopia. Others may "cross fixate," using alternate eyes in the opposite fields of gaze, and appear to be protected as well.

Size of Deviation. The characteristic angle of congenital esodeviations is considerably larger than those acquired later in life (Fig. 8.2). Most patients have a deviation in the 40 to 60 PD range (13,14). Measurements tend to be similar at distance and near, although accurate distant fixation is difficult to achieve in the examination of infants. There is little short-term variability in the deviation size; it is generally unaffected by accommodation. Long-term changes may occur: increases seem more frequent than decreases.

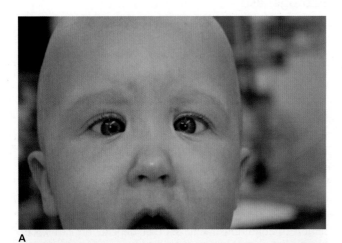

A

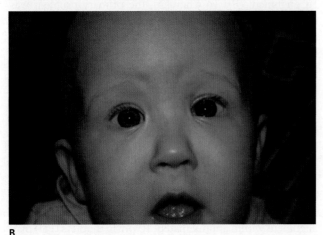

B

FIGURE 8.2. A: Congenital esotropia. **B:** Three days following surgery for congenital esotropia. (Reprinted with permission from Olitsky SE, Nelson LB. *Pediatric clinical ophthalmology—A color handbook.* London, UK: Manson Publishing, 2012, ISBN 9781840761511.)

Refractive Errors. Children with congenital esotropia tend to have cycloplegic refractions similar to those of normal children of the same age. These observations contrast markedly with the characteristic hyperopia associated with accommodative esotropia, especially of the refractive types.

Ocular Rotations. Children with congenital esotropia will often appear to exhibit an apparent abduction deficit. This pseudoparesis is usually secondary to the presence of cross fixation. If the child has equal vision, there is no need to abduct either eye. He/she will use the adducted, or crossed, eye to look to the opposite field of gaze. In this case, he/she will show a bilateral pseudoparesis of abduction. If amblyopia is present, only the better-seeing eye will cross fixate, making the amblyopic eye appear to have an abduction weakness. A true unilateral or bilateral abducens nerve palsy is uncommon in infancy. To differentiate between a true abducens paralysis and a pseudoparalysis, two techniques may be used. The examiner can evaluate ocular rotations by rotating the infant's head, either with the infant sitting upright in a moveable chair or using a doll's head maneuver. Abduction testing can also be examined after covering infant's one eye with a patch for a period of time.

Associated Findings

Dissociated Vertical Deviation. This consists of a slow upward deviation of one or alternate eyes. Occasionally, excyclotorsion can be demonstrated on upward drifting of the eye and incyclotorsion on downward motion. Dissociated vertical deviation (DVD) may be latent, detected only when the involved eye is covered, or manifest, occurring intermittently or constantly (Fig. 8.3). It can be differentiated from a true vertical deviation, because no corresponding hypotropia occurs in the other eye on cover testing. Bielschowsky's phenomenon is another feature of DVD, characterized by downward movement of the occluded eye when filters of increasing density are placed before the fixing eye. The incidence of DVD in patients with congenital esotropia is high, ranging from 46% to 92%, which frequently develops during the second year of life (13,15). DVD appears to be a time-related phenomenon and is not related to successful initial surgery or the development of binocular vision (15,16).

Inferior Oblique Overaction. The incidence of overaction of one or both inferior oblique muscles in patients with congenital esotropia has been reported to be as high as 78%. Studies have shown the onset of inferior oblique overaction (IOOA) to be most frequent during the second and third year of life. There appears to be no correlation between the development of IOOA and age at surgery, time from onset of strabismus to surgery, or decompensation of ocular alignment. The presence of fundus torsion at the time of surgery may help to predict which patients will develop IOOA (17). IOOA and DVD are both conditions that can cause excessive elevation of one or both eyes

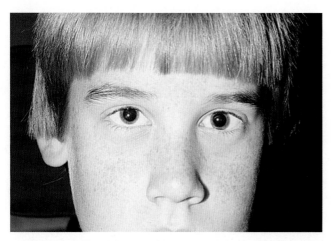 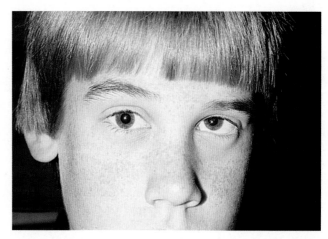

FIGURE 8.3. Bilateral dissociated vertical deviation (DVD). **A**: Right DVD when left eye is fixating. **B**: Left DVD when right eye is fixating. (Reprinted with permission from Tasman W, Jaeger E. *The Wills Eye Hospital atlas of clinical ophthalmology*, 2nd Ed. Philadelphia, PA: Lippincott Williams & Wilkins, 2001.)

in adduction in patients with congenital esotropia. The differentiating features of these two conditions are listed in Table 8.1. IOOA results in elevation of the involved eye as it moves nasally (Fig. 8.4). DVD may also result in

elevation as the eye moves nasally because the nose acts as a cover, dissociating the eyes. However, the vertical misalignment in DVD usually occurs equally in abduction, adduction, and primary position. When the adducting

---

Table 8.1

DISTINGUISHING FEATURES OF DISSOCIATED VERTICAL DEVIATION AND INFERIOR OBLIQUE OVERACTION

Dissociated Vertical Deviation

1. Causes elevation in adduction and abduction

2. Usually comitant, i.e., same in adduction, primary, and abduction

3. Variability of hyperdeviation

4. Usually not associated with a pattern

5. Same amount of hyperdeviation in upgaze and downgaze

6. Hyperdeviation may be associated with torsional movement and abduction

7. No corresponding hypotropia in abducted eye

Inferior Oblique Overaction

1. Causes elevation in adduction, not abduction

2. Incomitant, more in field of action of inferior oblique

3. Not variable

4. Commonly associated with V pattern

5. More hyperdeviation in upgaze than downgaze

6. Hyperdeviation not associated with torsional movement

7. Corresponding hypotropia in abducted eye

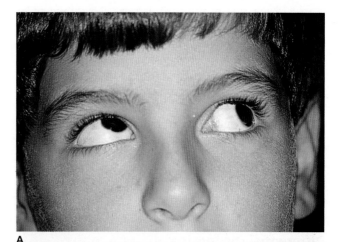

A

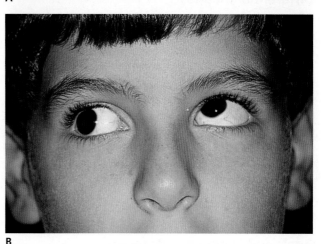

B

FIGURE 8.4. A–B: Overacting inferior oblique muscles. (Reprinted with permission from Tasman W, Jaeger E. *The Wills Eye Hospital atlas of clinical ophthalmology*, 2nd Ed. Philadelphia, PA: Lippincott Williams & Wilkins, 2001.)

eye in IOOA fixates, there is a corresponding hypotropia in the contralateral abducting eye. In DVD, contralateral hypotropia does not occur. IOOA and DVD frequently occur together in these patients. IOOA can be classified as Grades I to IV. Grade I represents 1 mm of higher elevation of the adducting eye in gaze up and to the side. Grade IV indicates 4 mm of higher elevation. These differences in elevation between the two eyes are measured from the 6 o'clock position on each limbus. A measurement of the degree of adduction that is required to elicit the overaction is also helpful when considering treatment. A moderate-size overaction that occurs with limited adduction may be more noticeable than a larger overaction that is seen only in extreme side gaze.

Nystagmus. Rotary nystagmus may occur in children with congenital esotropia and has been reported to be found in 30% of patients with congenital esotropia. In the authors' experience, the incidence of this type of nystagmus is much less.

Latent nystagmus is a predominantly horizontal jerk nystagmus elicited by occluding either eye. The slow phase is toward the side of the occluded eye. Measurement of visual acuity in the uncovered eye while using opaque occlusion of the nonviewing eye produces the maximal nystagmus and the poorest vision. Alternative methods for evaluating visual acuity create a relative binocular state by partially occluding or blurring the image in the non-viewing eye.

Latent nystagmus is more common than rotary nystagmus in congenital esotropia. If a significant latent nystagmus is present, amblyopia treatment using occlusion therapy may be less effective as the nystagmus will decrease the central-vision stimulation. Other forms of amblyopia treatment may be more efficacious if this occurs.

Differential Diagnosis

During the first year of life, a number of conditions can simulate congenital esotropia and cause diagnostic difficulty (Table 8.2). Because the management of these conditions may differ from the treatment of congenital esotropia, their clinical recognition is important. In general, a relatively small-angle deviation should raise doubt in assigning the diagnosis of congenital esotropia. Many of these other disorders can be ruled out following a thorough ophthalmologic evaluation. For this reason, all infants presenting with esotropia require a full evaluation, including a dilated funduscopic examination.

Treatment
Goals and Timing of Treatment

The primary goal of treatment in congenital esotropia is to reduce the deviation at distance and near to orthotropia, or as close to it as possible. Ideally, this results in normal

Table 8.2
DIFFERENTIAL DIAGNOSIS OF CONGENITAL ESOTROPIA
Pseudoesotropia
Duane retraction syndrome
Möbius syndrome
Nystagmus blockage syndrome
Congenital sixth nerve palsy
Early-onset accommodative esotropia
Sensory esotropia
Esotropia in the neurologically impaired

sight in each eye, in straight-looking eyes, and in development of at least a rudimentary form of sensory fusion that will maintain motor alignment. One measurement of long-term success in these patients can be made by the evaluating the number of surgeries required to maintain cosmetically acceptable alignment.

Classically, it has been taught that patients with congenital esotropia never develop bifoveal fixation regardless of their age at surgical alignment. Clinical evidence suggests, however, that alignment within 10 PD of orthotropia before 2 years of age is associated with the attainment of some degree of binocular vision and stereopsis (12,16,18). Conversely, although the chance of developing binocular vision decreases with the patient's age at the time of surgical alignment, even older patients can develop some degree of binocularity later in life once their eyes are aligned.

The most often found sensory result in patients successfully aligned before 2 years of age is the monofixation syndrome, as described by Parks (Table 8.3). The benefit derived from the monofixation syndrome is the development of peripheral normal retinal correspondence and fusional vergence amplitudes which are instrumental in maintaining motor alignment in such patients for the remainder of their lives. Arthur and coworkers showed this to be true (19). In their study, 80 patients who had been treated for congenital esotropia were divided into two groups: those that had obtained monofixation syndrome and those that had not. Over 17.5 years, 74% of patients in the monofixation group had maintained alignment. Over 14 years, only 45% of patients without monofixation had achieved the same outcome. However, the prognosis for long-term alignment is not the same for all patients who achieve the monofixation syndrome. Kushner subdivided these patients into three categories: orthophoria, esotropia up to 8 PD, and exotropia up to 8 PD (20). He found that patients who were orthophoric showed the best long-term stability. Those children with a small-angle esotropia were less stable than those who were orthophoric but more stable than those with a

Table 8.3

CHARACTERISTICS OF THE MONOFIXATION SYNDROME

Manifest horizontal deviation is 8 PD or less

Scotoma under binocular conditions

> Demonstrated by any of several tests: Worth 4 Dot, 4 base-out prism test, Bagolini lenses, binocular perimetry

>> May also be present under monocular conditions, i.e., organic macula lesion

Normal fusional vergences

Stereoacuity is 67–3,000 sec of arc

May also be present as:

> Amblyopia

> Superimposed phoria

> Anisometropia

small-angle exotropia. Because the role of binocular potential at birth could not be eliminated in predicting who would fall into each of these three categories, it is not known if active intervention, that is, further surgery, for small-angle deviations has any role in improving the long-term success rate of maintaining ocular alignment.

Birch et al. demonstrated that surgery prior to 1 year of age increased the level of the binocularity that was obtained (21). In their study, the number of children achieving random dot stereopsis was not significantly different based upon their age at time of surgery. However, there was a statistical significance in the level of stereopsis between groups of these patients. The prevalence of foveal (<60 seconds) or macular stereoacuity (61 to 200 seconds) was 42% in patients who had surgery at 5 to 8 months and 55.6% in patients who had surgery at 9 to 12 months. No patient who underwent surgery at 13 to 24 months achieved this level of binocular vision. The Congenital Esotropia Observational Study (CEOS) showed that patients with a constant and stable esotropia of at least 40 PD and who present between 2 and 4 months of age are unlikely to undergo spontaneous resolution providing another argument for even earlier surgery (22). Other surgeons continue to express concerns over operating at a very early age. These concerns include the documented spontaneous resolution of esotropia in some infants, anesthetic risks, and an unproven influence on long-term horizontal alignment and/or the development of IOOA and DVD.

Parents of children with congenital esotropia often report improvements in their child's fine motor development and visual function after surgery. Rogers and coworkers showed that early alignment is associated with improved fine motor skills and other visually directed tasks (23). The improved appearance of the child can enhance his or her psychological acceptance by the parents. This can be instrumental in the normal development of the parent–child relationship.

Nonsurgical Treatment

Amblyopia. Early and rigorous amblyopia therapy is an important component in the treatment of congenital esotropia. Treatment in older children is more difficult, more time-consuming, and less effective in restoring acuity in the amblyopic eye. Treatment may consist of occlusion or penalization therapy.

Once alternate fixation in the midline can be demonstrated, the child is assumed to have no significant amblyopia. Evaluation for the presence of cross fixation may also be useful in monitoring response to amblyopia treatment. Continued monitoring remains necessary, however. Maintenance treatment may be required for infants who revert to their original fixation preference, and treatment of the previously amblyopic eye may be needed for those who switch fixation preference to the other eye. If treatment has not been successful after several months, reexamination for subtle organic disorders (e.g., optic nerve hypoplasia) is indicated. More often, there has been noncompliance with the recommended therapy. Recurrent and new-onset amblyopia is common in these children during the period of visual immaturity.

Surgery should be performed after amblyopia treatment is completed. Amblyopia management in an infant is easier in the presence of a large esotropia. Judgment concerning fixation preference is difficult in a preverbal child with straight eyes. Amblyopia therapy in children at this young age generally requires only a small amount of time to equalize vision and therefore does not delay surgical correction to a significant degree. Also, parental compliance may be diminished once their child's eyes are straight.

Refractive Errors. Because most children are hyperopic, it may sometimes be difficult to decide which children should be given a trial of antiaccommodative therapy before suggesting surgery. Accommodative esotropia in this age group is uncommon but does occur. The amount of hyperopia relative to the angle of deviation should be considered. Even a moderate level of hyperopia would not be expected to be the cause of a very large esotropia and children with a well-documented history of early crossing may not respond to treatment of even higher levels of hyperopia.

Surgical Treatment

Various surgical techniques have been used for the correction of congenital esotropia. Proponents of two-muscle surgery advocate either symmetric recession of both medial rectus muscles, or monocular medial rectus recession combined with lateral rectus resection, regardless of the size of the preoperative deviation. Both procedures are graded, with more millimeters of surgery performed for larger angles. If a second procedure is required, symmetric resections of both lateral rectus muscles and a recess–resect procedure in the fellow eye are performed.

To increase the success rate in patients with larger deviations, some surgeons operate on three or four horizontal recti muscles at one time. Other surgeons prefer to perform larger bilateral medial rectus recessions instead. These larger recessions provide good results and do not cause a postoperative adduction or convergence deficit (24,25). Two-muscle surgery is a quicker, simpler, and less traumatic procedure. It also leaves the lateral rectus muscle unoperated if further surgeries are required.

Botulinim toxin has been used by some investigators in the treatment of congenital esotropia (26,27). Multiple injections may be necessary and it has not been shown to provide sensory results equal to incisional surgery (28).

Postoperative Management
Over- and Undercorrection

Early successful alignment does not ensure long-term stability. The need for repeating observations throughout the first decade of life cannot be overemphasized.

Reduction of spectacle correction in hypermetropes and overcorrections in myopes has been used to treat small overcorrections. A large overcorrection associated with an adduction weakness in the immediate postoperative period should alert the surgeon to the possibility of a slipped muscle. Exploration of the suspected muscle should be undertaken. Consecutive exotropia > 15 PD approximately 6 weeks after surgery usually requires a secondary procedure.

Undercorrections < 10 PD may respond to correction of hypermetropia > +1.50 D, and a trial of spectacles is indicated. Patients with residual esotropia measuring > 15 PD, unless the deviation is responsive to antiaccommodative therapy, should be evaluated for secondary surgery after 6 weeks' observation.

Accommodative Esotropia Following Congenital Esotropia

Accommodative esotropia may develop in children who were surgically corrected for congenital esotropia. These patients may be prone to the development of an accommodative esotropia secondary to their underlying poor binocular function and may respond to correction of small levels of hyperopia. Consideration for spectacle correction should be given to patients who redevelop esotropia even if the magnitude of their hyperopia is normal.

Dissociated Vertical Deviation

Patients with DVD usually do not complain of diplopia and are often asymptomatic. DVD is less frequently noted in adults with strabismus than in children, suggesting that DVD tends to improve with time. If the disorder is entirely latent, detected by the examiner only on cover testing, surgery is not indicated. If it is intermittent, surgery is dictated by the size and frequency of the deviation as well as the patient's concern regarding its appearance.

Inferior Oblique Muscle Overaction

This rarely, if ever, causes symptoms; it is usually a problem only due to its appearance. Patients usually avoid the extreme lateral gaze necessary to elicit IOOA. Instead, they almost instantaneously turn the face to look laterally, minimizing the cosmetic appearance of IOOA. The indications for surgery for IOOA are different, depending on whether weakening the inferior obliques is the only surgery being contemplated, or whether weakening the inferior obliques in conjunction with horizontal strabismus surgery is being considered. If the inferior obliques alone are weakened, there should be a significant overaction present to justify surgery. When there is an obvious elevation of the adducting eye at about 30 degrees or less of lateral gaze, a reasonable cosmetic defect is present and the option of surgery could be offered. If however, the elevation on adduction is evident only on extreme lateral gaze, this minor cosmetic defect might be best left alone. If horizontal strabismus surgery is performed for congenital esotropia, smaller grades of IOOA may be corrected at the same time.

Surgery for Dissociated Vertical Deviation and Inferior Oblique Muscle Overaction. Three surgical approaches are generally advocated to correct DVD: recession of the superior rectus, recession of the superior rectus combined with a posterior fixation suture, and anterior transposition of the inferior oblique (ATIO).

An overacting inferior oblique muscle may be effectively weakened by recession, disinsertion, myotomy, myectomy, and denervation and extirpation. Inferior oblique recession, as popularized by Parks, is associated with low rates of complications and recurrences (29). The surgeon has the ability to grade the amount of recession according to the extent of overaction.

Scott, using a computer model, described anterior transposition of the inferior oblique muscle (30). Early reports of the procedure showed that it was more effective in treating IOOA, which was noteworthy given the fact that most of these studies utilized anterior transposition for larger degrees of overaction.

One study showed a decreased incidence of DVD development in a group of patients undergoing anterior transposition compared to a group that had undergone standard recession of the inferior oblique. The authors speculated that anterior transposition may decrease the risk for the development of DVD (31). However, the study groups were not comparable and there may have been a degree of bias introduced into the study. ATIO is effective in treating either DVD or IOOA or both when concurrently present (32).

Many surgeons now perform ATIO when either IOOA or DVD occurs alone in patients with a history of congenital esotropia. Many surgeons feel it is the procedure of choice when both motility disorders are present at the same time. It eliminates the need to operate on both the superior rectus and the inferior oblique.

When performing ATIO, placement of the new insertion of the inferior oblique is important. If the new insertion is brought too far anterior or spread too far laterally, the surgeon may induce an anti-elevation syndrome. This syndrome describes the inability to elevate the eye in the abducted position. It is caused by a restriction of the lateral fibers of the inferior oblique muscle when the eye is placed into this position. Because the contralateral adducting eye will demonstrate better elevation in this gaze position, it will appear as if there is an overaction of the inferior oblique muscle. Kushner first described this disorder and demonstrated that the treatment involves correcting the new insertion site so that it is neither too far anterior nor spread too far laterally. Surgery does not need to be directed at the apparent overacting inferior oblique (33).

Amblyopia

Amblyopia occurring postoperatively is common and must always be considered. Fixation preference testing should be performed at each postoperative visit until the visual acuity can be measured. Unfortunately, it is more difficult to recognize a fixation preference, the closer the eyes are to orthotropia. The 10 D fixation test for preverbal children with small angle or no deviation is useful. A 10 D vertical prism is placed in front of one eye to produce a vertical deviation, which facilitates the recognition of a fixation preference (34).

Once recognized, amblyopia should be treated promptly. Some patients may require maintenance therapy until visual maturity is reached, and susceptibility to amblyopia is eliminated as the sensitive period of visual development ends at approximately 9 years of age.

NYSTAGMUS BLOCKAGE SYNDROME

The nystagmus blockage syndrome is characterized by nystagmus that begins in early infancy and is associated with esotropia. The nystagmus is reduced or absent with the fixing eye in adduction. As the fixing eye follows a target moving laterally toward the primary position and then into abduction, the nystagmus increases and the esotropia decreases. A head turn develops in the direction of the uncovered eye when the fellow eye is occluded. This abnormal head posture allows the uncovered eye to persist in an adducted position.

ACCOMMODATIVE ESOTROPIA

Accommodative esotropia is defined as a convergent deviation of the eyes associated with activation of the accommodative reflex. Esotropia that is related to accommodative effort may be divided into three major categories: refractive, nonrefractive, and partial or decompensated.

Refractive Accommodative Esotropia

Refractive accommodative esotropia usually occurs in a child between 2 and 3 years of age with a history of acquired intermittent or constant esotropia. Occasionally, children who are 1 year of age or younger present with all the clinical features of accommodative esotropia (35,36). The refraction of patients with refractive accommodative esotropia averages +4.75 D (37). The angle of esodeviation is the same when measured at distance and near fixation, and is usually moderate in magnitude, ranging between 20 and 40 PD. Amblyopia is common, especially when the esodeviation has become more nearly constant.

Pathogenesis

The mechanism of refractive accommodative esotropia involves three factors: uncorrected hyperopia, accommodative convergence, and insufficient fusional divergence. When an individual exerts a given amount of accommodation, a specific amount of convergence (accommodative convergence) is associated with it. An uncorrected hyperope must exert excessive accommodation to clear a blurred retinal image. This in turn will stimulate excessive convergence. If the amplitude of fusional divergence is sufficient to correct the excess convergence, no esotropia will result. However, if the fusional divergence amplitudes are inadequate or motor fusion is altered by some sensory obstacle, an esotropia will result. Patients with lower levels of hyperopia but with significant anisometropia are also at an increased risk to develop an accommodative esotropia.

Treatment

In refractive accommodative esotropia, the full hyperopic correction, determined by cycloplegic refraction, is initially prescribed (Fig. 8.5). If the child is orthophoric or has a small esophoria while wearing glasses, the child can be followed at regular intervals.

Beginning around age 4 to 5 years, the strength of the hyperopic correction can be reduced gradually to enhance fusional divergence and maximize visual acuity. This can be performed by manifest refraction instead of a cycloplegic refraction. Children with moderate levels of hyperopia may be capable of developing enough fusional divergence to be able to function without their glasses. Children with extreme levels of hyperopia are unlikely to ever "outgrow" their refractive error and will experience asthenopia without their correction. Aggressive reduction of the hyperopic prescription may not be warranted in these children.

It is important to warn parents of children with either refractive or nonrefractive accommodative esotropia that the esodeviation will appear to increase without glasses after the initial correction is worn. Parents frequently state that, before wearing glasses, their child had a small

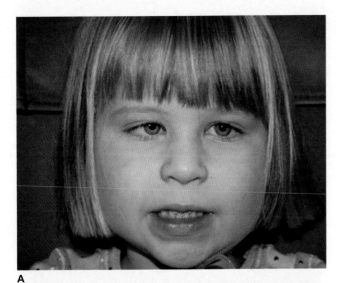

A

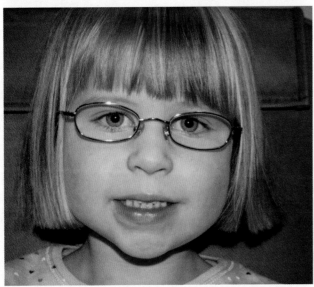

B

FIGURE 8.5. A: Accommodative esotropia. **B:** Glasses eliminate the need to accommodate and therefore the esotropia. (Reprinted with permission from Olitsky SE, Nelson LB. *Pediatric clinical ophthalmology—A color handbook.* London, UK: Manson Publishing, 2012, ISBN 9781840761511.)

esodeviation, whereas after removal of the glasses the esodeviation is now quite large. Parents often blame the increased esodeviation on the glasses and note that their child has become dependent on them. This situation can best be explained on the basis of the child using the appropriate amount of accommodative effort after the glasses have been worn. When the child removes her glasses, she will continue to use an accommodative effort to bring objects into proper focus and increase the esodeviation. The strong desire these children have to wear their new glasses may be secondary to the relief of asthenopia, benefits of single binocular vision, or both. Explaining these phenomena to parents ahead of time is more effective than the same explanation after the fact.

Nonrefractive Accommodative Esotropia

Children with nonrefractive accommodative esotropia usually present between 2 and 3 years of age with an esodeviation that is greater at near than at distance fixation. The refractive error in this condition may be hyperopic or myopic, although the average refraction is +2.25 D.

Pathogenesis

In nonrefractive accommodative esotropia, there is a high accommodative convergence to accommodation (AC:A) ratio: the effort to accommodate elicits an abnormally high accommodative convergence response. There are a number of ways of measuring the AC:A ratio: the heterophoria method, the fixation disparity method, the gradient method, and the clinical evaluation of distance and near deviation. Most clinicians prefer to assess the ratio using the distance–near comparison. This method allows the ratio to be evaluated more easily and quickly, since it employs conventional examination techniques and requires no calculations. The AC:A relationship is derived by simply comparing the distance and near deviation. If the near measurement in an esotropia patient is > 10 D, the AC:A ratio is considered to be abnormally high.

Treatment

The management of nonrefractive accommodative esotropia may involve a variety of modalities. Many pediatric ophthalmologists attempt to correct the esodeviation at near with bifocals, provided that the distance deviation is <10 PD. Initially, a +2.50 executive-type bifocal with the top of the lower segment crossing the lower pupillary border is given. In follow-up, the child should wear the least amount of hyperopic bifocal correction to maintain straight eyes at near fixation.

The use of bifocals in treating the esotropia at near is not without some controversy. Albert and Lederman found no difference in the natural reduction of esotropia in those patients wearing bifocals versus patients who had their bifocal discontinued (38). Only 12% of their group demonstrated bifoveal fixation and none complained of diplopia at near. The reason for the initiation of treatment was the parents' observation of the crossing at near. Because the esotropia at near appeared not to be cosmetically noticeable, the authors questioned the energetic treatment of this disorder. Ludwig, Parks, and coworkers reported on the deterioration rate of patients based on the severity of their distance–near disparity (39). They found that the deterioration rate was proportional to the amount of excess esotropia at near. The authors speculated that these patients continue to experience esotropia at near despite bifocal therapy. Pratt-Johnson and Tillson reviewed the long-term sensory status in 99 patients with excess esotropia at near. Half were treated with bifocals while the others were not. They found no difference in sensory status or deterioration rate between the two groups (40).

Surgery has been found to decrease the AC:A ratio and is usually performed when the esodeviation at near fixation is no longer controlled with bifocals or the distance deviation is higher than an acceptable level. It has also been shown to be an option for the primary treatment of these patients (41). There are two types of surgery that are commonly performed in patients with an excess esotropia at near. O'Hara and Calhoun demonstrated favorable results when operating for the full amount of esotropia at near, even in patients with little or no distance deviation (42). Although many of their patients were orthotropic at distance, there were few overcorrections. However, the concern of producing an exotropia in the distance has lead to the popularization of the posterior fixation, or Faden, suture in the treatment of these patients. Generally, the medial rectus recession is titrated for the distance angle and a posterior fixation suture is performed to decrease convergence at near. Kushner et al. compared these two techniques in a 15-year prospective, randomized study (43). The authors found the use of augmented surgery, taking into account the near deviation, to be more effective than the posterior fixation suture technique. A higher percentage of patients in the augmented surgery group achieved satisfactory alignment and were able to discontinue the use of their bifocal. They also found a trend in this same group toward complete elimination of the glasses.

Partial or Decompensated Accommodative Esotropia

Refractive or nonrefractive accommodative esotropias do not always occur in their "pure" forms. These patients may have a significant reduction in esodeviation when given glasses. However, a residual esodeviation persists in spite of full hyperopic correction, which is the deteriorated or nonaccommodative portion. This condition commonly occurs when there is a delay of months between the onset of accommodative esotropia and antiaccommodative treatment. Sometimes the esotropia may initially be eliminated with glasses but a nonaccommodative portion slowly becomes evident, in spite of the patient's wearing the maximal amount of hyperopic correction consistent with good vision.

The indications for surgery for partial or decompensated accommodative esotropia remain debatable. Some ophthalmologists believe that any esotropia >10 PD warrants surgery to reduce the deviation to <10 PD, in order to enhance the development of the monofixation. These ophthalmologists believe that if the monofixation syndrome develops, the patient will function better because of the advantage of peripheral fusion. Also, the prognosis for the permanency of the surgically created alignment will be enhanced as a result of good motor fusional vergences associated with the monofixation syndrome.

Other ophthalmologists consider that surgery should be performed on the nonaccommodative portion only if it is cosmetically significant as determined by the patient or family, or both. They feel that there is no functional deficit that can be demonstrated consistently in a real-world situation in patients who do not have peripheral fusion, as would be present in the monofixation syndrome.

If surgery is elected, the amount should be determined by the distance deviation with the child's full hyperopic correction. When the near deviation is greater than the distance deviation, it is reasonable to operate for the near deviation. Because of an unacceptable number of undercorrections in some series of patients, other surgical formulas have been advocated. Wright et al. showed that if patients underwent bilateral medial rectus recessions for a target angle halfway between the esotropia that was present at near with glasses and the esotropia that was present at near without glasses, 93% of patients experienced a reduction of their deviation to <10 PD. This was in contrast to a 74% success rate in a group receiving "standard" surgery. Few patients in the augmented study group required a change in their hyperopic prescription following surgery (44). Kushner looked at the effect of surgically overcorrecting patients and then decreasing their hyperopic prescription to maintain alignment (45). He found that this strategy worked for those patients with <2.5 D of hyperopia in their fixating eye. Overcorrections were less likely to be reversible with postoperative reduction in the hyperopic correction in patients with >2.5 D however.

Another method for augmenting surgery is prism adaptation. In prism adaptation, the patient is given press-on base-out prism for any residual esotropia that remains after prescribing the full hyperopic correction. The patient then returns in 2 weeks and if the esotropia has increased, a larger prism is then given. This process continues until the deviation remains stable. The surgeon then operates on the full "prism-adapted" angle. The Prism Adaptation Trial was a multicenter, prospective, and randomized study which looked at this technique (46). Although the study appeared to show an increase in surgical success, patients who were prism adapted may have had better binocular vision potential prior to surgery.

Cyclic (Esotropia) Strabismus

Cyclic strabismus is a relatively rare disorder of ocular motility that is reported to occur in 1 in 3,000 to 5,000 cases of strabismus. A thorough history and repeat examinations are often necessary to elicit the cyclic nature of the deviation. An awareness of the typical characteristics of cyclic strabismus may enable one to make the diagnosis more readily.

Cyclic strabismus is usually an acquired condition with onset at 3 to 4 years of age. Variable presentations with onset at birth and in adult life have been reported. Accidental or surgical trauma has been associated with cyclic strabismus in a few cases.

The type of esodeviation is classically a large-angle esotropia alternating with orthophoria or a small-angle esodeviation on a 48-hour cycle. Variations include vertical deviations, incomitance, and exotropia. Cycles of 1, 3, 4, and 5 days have been reported as well as cycles of 48 hours esotropia and 24 hours orthotropia. The duration of the cycle may be as short as 2 weeks, in which case the diagnosis can be missed, or it may persist for several years before becoming a constant deviation.

Patients with cyclic strabismus often have a family history of strabismus. The fact that most cases occur in the middle preschool may explain the frequency of the mild hyperopic error.

Pathogenesis

Various theories have been proposed to explain cyclic strabismus. It may be the result of an aberration in the biologic clock. One patient with cyclic esotropia underwent a change in the circadian pattern of her esotropia after rapid time travel through six time zones (47). This change would tend to support the biologic clock theory.

Fusion and binocular vision are usually absent or defective on the strabismic day, with marked improvement on the straight day. Diplopia on strabismic days is unusual and has been a prominent symptom only in patients of a relatively older age who are unable to develop suppression.

Treatment

Cyclic esotropia is noted for its unpredictable response to various forms of therapy, with the exception of surgery, which is usually curative. The effectiveness of giving a hyperopic refractive error to reduce the esodeviation is unpredictable. Occlusion therapy has been shown to convert cyclic esotropia into a constant esotropia. Surgical correction of the total esodeviation with either a bilateral medial rectus recession or a monocular medial rectus recession and lateral resection has been the most successful mode of therapy.

Acute Acquired Comitant Esotropia

This condition occurs in older children and adults. It is characterized by the dramatic onset of a relatively large-angle esotropia with diplopia and mild hyperopic refractive error. Although there may be a brief period of intermittency, the esodeviation soon becomes constant.

Pathogenesis

Burian was the first to describe acute acquired comitant esotropia (AACE) in 1945 (48). He divided AACE into two types: Type 1, which becomes apparent immediately after a period of occlusion, and Type 2, which occurs without obvious exogenous cause.

Type 1 occurs after periods of interruption of fusion. It has been reported to follow occlusion therapy for amblyopia in patients in whom no deviation was initially noted. Other cases of Type 1 AACE have occurred after brief occlusion from eyelid swelling, secondary to blunt trauma.

Type 2 has no obvious exogenous cause of precipitating the esotropia.

Treatment

Children and adults who develop an acute esotropia must undergo a careful motility analysis to rule out a paretic deviation, in a search for lateral gaze incomitancy. If the ophthalmic examination is otherwise negative, and a neurologic physical examination is normal, it is still unclear whether further workup, including neuroimaging should be performed. Once an underlying cause has been eliminated and the deviation remains stable, surgery should be considered to restore binocular vision.

EXOTROPIA

Congenital Exotropia

Exotropia occurring under the age of 1 year in an otherwise healthy child is rare (49). Although exotropia before age of 1 year may go through a period of intermittency, many cases progress quickly to a constant alternating exotropia. The angle of deviation is often quite large, averaging 35 PD or greater (Fig. 8.6). Patients with an exotropia of 50 PD or greater often appear to have decreased adduction on side gaze; with gaze right or left, the abducting eye fixates while the opposite eye approaches midline and stops. This is similar to the cross fixation found in congenital esotropes. Occlusion or the doll's head maneuver will demonstrate that good adduction is possible. Amblyopia is not common, as these children typically alternate fixation. The refractive error is similar to that of the general population.

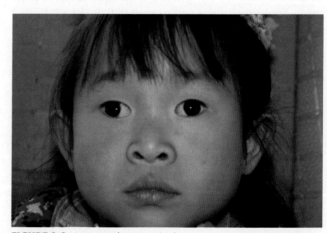

FIGURE 8.6. Large-angle exotropia. (Reprinted with permission from Olitsky SE, Nelson LB. *Pediatric clinical ophthalmology—A color handbook.* London, UK: Manson Publishing, 2012, ISBN 9781840761511.)

Treatment

Patients with congenital constant exotropia are operated early in life in the same manner as those patients with congenital esotropia. Like patients with congenital esotropia, early surgery can lead to gross binocular vision but not bifoveal fixation. In addition, these patients also tend to develop A and V patterns, DVD and IOOA, and should be followed closely for the development of these associated motility disturbances (50).

Intermittent Exotropia

Demographics

Intermittent exotropia is the most common divergent strabismus in childhood (49). The age of onset varies but is often between 6 months and 4 years.

Natural History and Characteristics

The natural history of intermittent exotropia is generally unknown, as most patients inevitably receive therapeutic intervention at some stage of the disease. Although the natural history of this disorder is not well delineated, many pediatric ophthalmologists consider that the frequency or magnitude of the deviation in children with untreated intermittent exotropia is unlikely to improve. An unknown proportion of children with intermittent exotropia decompensate into constant exotropia.

Initially, the deviation is usually intermittent and greater at distance fixation; often, there is no deviation at near fixation in the early stages. Because many non-ophthalmologists examine children only at near, the question of strabismus may be dismissed when a parent first brings this problem to the attention of their pediatrician. Intermittent exotropia may be considered as possibly evolving through following four phases that make useful divisions for discussion and comparison:

Phase I: Exophoria at distance, orthophoria at near.
Phase II: Intermittent exotropia at distance, orthophoria or intermittent exotropia at near.
Phase III: Exotropia at distance, exophoria or intermittent exotropia at near.
Phase IV: Exotropia at distance and near.

In Phase I, in which there is exophoria only at distance, children are asymptomatic and are rarely evaluated by ophthalmologists. In Phase II, an intermittent exotropia is noted by the family when the child views at distance during periods of inattentiveness or fatigue. During this phase, there is no suppression scotoma, so that child may report diplopia or infer it by closing one eye, especially in bright sunlight. When a child in Phase II is examined, the exotropia is easily elicited by the cover test, but the deviating eye returns quickly with a blink or a change of fixation. In Phase III, a suppression scotoma develops to avoid diplopia. Instead of making a correcting fusional convergent movement, the eye remains deviated for longer periods, even through a blink or change in fixation. In Phase IV, the suppression scotoma is firmly set, with constant exotropia at distance and near fixation.

Amblyopia is not common in children with intermittent exotropia. The distribution of refractive errors is similar to that in the general population.

Pathogenesis and Classifications

Exodeviations probably result from a combination of mechanical and innervational factors. Duane proposed a classification system based upon what he believed was an innervational imbalance that upsets the reciprocal relationship between active convergence and divergence mechanisms (51). Based upon this classification system an exodeviation greater at distance than at near fixation is caused by hypertonicity of divergence (divergence excess); a deviation greater at near than at distance is caused by convergence insufficiency and a deviation that is equal at distance and near fixation (basic exotropia) is caused by a divergence excess combined with a convergence insufficiency.

Burian later introduced the term "simulated divergence excess" for those patients with a divergence excess exodeviation where the distance and near deviations become equal after monocular occlusion or when the patient fixates at near through a +3.00 D lens. Kushner introduced the concept of tenacious proximal fusion to describe patients who did not show an increase in their near deviation size through +3.00 D lenses but did do so after a period of occlusion (52).

Intermittent exotropia is commonly a precursor to constant exotropia of both basic and divergence excess types, so it does not seem that entirely different factors are at play among the subtypes of exodeviation. Parks argued that rather than assume that exodeviations which have a distance–near disparity are the result of a faulty divergence or convergence system, these patterns can be explained solely on the basis of the AC:A ratio. A patient with a convergence insufficiency exotropia would then be said to suffer from a low AC:A ratio and a patient with a divergence excess exotropia would have a high AC:A ratio. This may be a compensatory high AC:A ratio which a child develops to maintain fusion at near. This hypothesis would explain why patients with intermittent exotropia tend to have a high AC:A ratio, while patients with a constant exotropia usually have a normal AC:A. With a constant deviation, fusion is lost at distance and near, and there is no longer a reason to maintain a high AC:A ratio. Many clinicians find it difficult to neatly categorize all patients with intermittent exotropia into Duane's system. They find it easier to use the more fluid method of categorization that Parks has devised.

Treatment

Although most pediatric ophthalmologists agree that the treatment for intermittent exotropia is surgical, opinions vary widely regarding the timing of surgical intervention and the preoperative use of nonsurgical methods.

Timing of Surgical Intervention. This is a cause for considerable controversy because of the possible effects on both the immature visual and sensory systems during childhood. The concern is regarding early surgical intervention in a child with intermittent exotropia, in which good preoperative visual acuity and stereopsis could be exchanged for a small-angle esotropia with the threat of amblyopia and decreased stereopsis. However, delaying surgery too long could allow for the development of a suppression scotoma which could increase the risk for a recurrent manifest deviation later in life.

Nonsurgical Management. Nonsurgical treatment of intermittent exotropia includes the use of base-in prisms, overcorrecting minus lenses, occlusion therapy, and orthoptic exercises.

Prisms. The use of prisms in the treatment of exodeviations has been reported primarily in the optometric literature. The success rate of prism therapy varies as reported in these series. Prism therapy consists of two different strategies: "demand-reducing" prisms and full prismatic correction. Demand-reducing prisms correct for a portion of the total deviation and may be useful for presbyopic patients with convergence insufficiency. Full prismatic correction neutralizes the total deviation and is commonly used in children to reestablish "normal" binocular conditions. If possible, the prism power is then gradually reduced as tolerated by the patient. Prism glasses can be very heavy and cause image distortion which makes compliance a problem. In contrast to the support for prisms as an initial treatment in the optometric literature, most ophthalmologists employ the use of prisms in these patients only as a method of postponing surgery until the patient gets older and is at less risk for developing amblyopia in case of a surgical overcorrection.

Overcorrecting Minus Lenses. Overcorrecting with minus lenses to stimulate accommodative convergence has been successfully used by some investigators. Limitations of this therapy include the temporary benefit provided to most patients, possible accommodative asthenopia, and its usefulness only in young patients with a large accommodative amplitude. Patients who do not require optical correction for improvement of their visual acuity may be less compliant with this therapy.

Occlusion Therapy. The objective of occlusion therapy in intermittent exotropia is to eliminate the need for suppression which often occurs in the transition phase between an intermittent deviation and a constant one. There are several small series which evaluate the success rate of occlusion therapy. Most of these studies suffer from a lack of masking and control groups. In addition, most authors limit the use of occlusion to patients with relatively small deviations. Occlusion may have a role in the temporary improvement of fusional control. It does not appear to lead to a long-term benefit. Occlusion therapy may be useful to help postpone surgery in some younger patients until they reach an age when amblyopia following surgery is less likely.

Orthoptics. Although the theoretical basis of using orthoptics to improve fusional convergence amplitudes is appealing, most find the benefits to be limited. Generally, orthoptics consists of diplopia awareness training and improvement in fusional vergence amplitudes. Many patients with intermittent exotropia already experience diplopia as evidenced by their closing of one eye or the fact that the deviation is intermittent. Furthermore, in nearly all patients with intermittent exotropia, the fusional convergence amplitudes are already abnormally large. Many ophthalmologists limit the scope of orthoptic therapy to increasing fusional convergence in patients with convergence insufficiency.

Surgical Management.

Indications for Surgery. When the deviation is intermittent, is eliminated with a blink, and occurs only with fatigue, observation is warranted. In a younger child, if the condition is progressing from Phase II to Phase III, in which the deviation occurs during periods when the child is alert and lasts through a blink or change in fixation, surgery is indicated to try to prevent the development of a suppression scotoma. If the child closes or covers one eye for viewing, the exodeviation is too large for the fusional convergence mechanisms to control. This child has diplopia and compensates by closing or covering one eye. Surgery is indicated in this situation to correct the annoying symptom. In Phase III, with constant exotropia at distant fixation but an exophoria or intermittent exotropia at near, a suppression scotoma is present at distance fixation, because there is no awareness of diplopia or compensation to avoid it. At near, some degree of binocular function can usually be demonstrated with stereoacuity or Worth 4 Dot testing. Surgery should be offered at this stage in order to try and maintain whatever binocular function is present at near, and perhaps regain what has been lost at distance.

In patients older than 10 years of age, symptoms of diplopia and asthenopia and cosmetic concerns are the main indications for surgery, as suppression is unlikely to develop and postponement of surgery will not adversely affect the surgical outcome.

Choice of Surgical Procedure. Some surgeons use the classification system developed by Duane and Burian to decide what type of surgery to perform on patients with intermittent exotropia. They aim to weaken the apparently overacting or strengthen the apparently underacting muscles based upon the distance and near measurements. Therefore, for a basic and "simulated" divergence exotropia, they perform a unilateral recession–resection procedure based upon the assumption that the resultant correction will be the same for both distance and near. A divergence excess deviation is treated with a bilateral lateral rectus recession, and convergence insufficiency is treated with a bilateral medial rectus resection.

In contrast, Parks felt that bilateral lateral rectus recessions and unilateral recess–resect procedures are equivalent in their effect. He felt that a surgeon's confidence in a particular procedure should determine what technique is utilized. Many surgeons prefer doing symmetric surgery and avoiding resections if not necessary.

While bilateral lateral rectus recessions are used by many ophthalmologists in the treatment of intermittent exotropia, unilateral lateral rectus recession has been successfully used for patients with small-to-moderate angles of exotropia. Unilateral surgery has the advantage of requiring less time under anesthesia and limiting the risk of surgery to just one eye.

Goals of Surgery. The surgical success rate in treating intermittent exotropia is difficult to discern from the literature. Reports in the literature are plagued by the variable nature of the disease, a lack of standardized success/failure criteria, and study bias depending on the type of intervention preferred by the authors. It is therefore not surprising that rates of success vary widely in the literature, ranging from 40% to 92%. Most authors define surgical success as a small residual exotropia (<10 PD) or an exophoria/esophoria only.

Surgeons who perform bilateral lateral rectus recessions should anticipate a postoperative esotropia of 10 to 15 PD that may last for the first 10 days to 3 weeks (53). Patients who display this initial overcorrection tend to have the best results once they are fully recovered from surgery although a moderate initial overcorrection does not always predict a good outcome. It may be advisable to warn parents about an initial period where their child's eyes will cross as well as the fact that they may experience diplopia which can be worse than what was present prior to surgery. Patients who undergo unilateral recess–resect procedures do not experience more than a few prism diopters of immediate postoperative overcorrection. Similarly, unilateral lateral rectus recessions show little, if any, initial overcorrection in the immediate postoperative period (54).

The goal for an adult with exotropia should be viewed somewhat differently. In these patients, a persistent consecutive esotropia may cause intractable diplopia. Further surgery may be required to place the patient back into his/her original suppression scotoma. However, a small residual exodeviation will usually provide complete relief of symptoms as well as an improvement in appearance.

CONVERGENCE INSUFFICIENCY

Convergence insufficiency is characterized by an exodeviation that is present only at near or greater than distance fixation. Complaints associated with convergence insufficiency include asthenopia and diplopia during periods of near work. Patients may also complain about blurring of their vision as they attempt to exchange accommodative convergence for fusional convergence and induce an artificial myopia. The symptoms of convergence insufficiency cover a large spectrum, from mild to very severe, and are often extremely annoying in the presence of a small exodeviation at near fixation.

Management

Orthoptic treatment of convergence insufficiency has been successful in improving fusional amplitudes and relieving symptomatology in many cases. The use of base-in prisms may also help alleviate the symptoms of convergence insufficiency.

There is a small, selected group of patients whose symptoms do not respond to orthoptics, prisms, or any other form of medical ophthalmic therapy. These particular patients with intractable and debilitating symptoms may respond to medial rectus resection. An initial overcorrection with diplopia and a need for prismatic treatment may be required for the best long-term result (55). Other authors have had good results using a monocular recess–resect procedure in which the surgery was based upon the near angle and the medial rectus resection was increased with a corresponding decrease in the lateral rectus recession (56).

A and V Patterns

A and V patterns are manifested by a horizontal change of alignment as the eyes move from the primary position to midline upgaze or downgaze. Esotropia with V pattern increases in downgaze and decreases in upgaze. The deviation in V exotropia increases in upgaze and decreases in downgaze. In A esotropia, the deviation increases in upgaze and decreases in downgaze. In A exotropia, the deviation increases in downgaze and decreases in upgaze. Occasionally, a patient may have essentially no deviation or a small one in primary position, although exotropia (X pattern) is present in upgaze and downgaze. Also, exotropia may occur only in upgaze (Y pattern) or in downgaze (λ pattern). The A and V patterns are demonstrated by measuring a deviation in primary position and in approximately 25 degrees of upgaze and downgaze, while the patient fixates on a distant object. An A pattern is said to exist if divergence increases in downgaze by 10 PD or more. A V pattern signifies an increase in divergence of 15 PD or more in upgaze. The smaller amount of change required to make a diagnosis of an A pattern is due to the greater effect of the downgaze deviation on reading and other near tasks. Anomalous head posture is common in patients with A and V patterns. Patients with A esotropia and V exotropia and fusion in downgaze may develop a chin-up position. Conversely, V esotropia and A exotropia may cause chin depression.

Pathogenesis

A number of different theories have been proposed to explain the etiology of A and V patterns. There is no universal agreement of their cause at this time.

One possible cause of A and V patterns is oblique muscle dysfunction. Since the oblique muscles have secondary abducting action, when the superior obliques are overacting, they may cause an A pattern; when the inferior obliques are overacting or the superior obliques are underacting, a V pattern often results. Many patients with oblique dysfunction demonstrate an A or V pattern. However, A and V patterns frequently exist in the absence of demonstrable oblique dysfunction.

Ocular torsion has been proposed as the cause of A and V patterns (57,58). Torsion of the globe results in vertical displacement of the insertions of the horizontal recti and horizontal displacement of the vertical recti. These displacements would then be expected to alter the vectors of the forces exerted on the globe so that the horizontal recti become partial elevators or depressors and the vertical recti become increasing abductors or adductors. This change in force vectors could then produce or enhance an A or V pattern. In the case of excyclotorsion, the superior recti would cause excessive abduction in elevation and the inferior recti would cause adduction in depression, thus producing a V pattern. The cause of the initial torsion that leads to the secondary change in vector forces is unknown. Kushner felt that primary oblique dysfunction was the cause of the ocular torsion, whereas Miller and Guyton felt that a loss of fusion leads to secondary "sensory" torsion of the globe. They observed that patients who were overcorrected following surgery for intermittent exotropia, thereby losing fusion, were more likely to later develop an A or V pattern than those patients who maintained fusion postoperatively.

Treatment

A and V patterns are generally corrected in one of two ways: moving the insertions of the horizontal rectus muscles or weakening or strengthening the oblique muscles.

Vertical transposition of the horizontal rectus muscles is an effective method of treating A and V patterns. Moving or offsetting the horizontal rectus muscle insertion up or down weakens the action of that muscle when the eye is moved in the direction of the offsetting. For example, if the medial rectus muscles are moved up one-half tendon width, their horizontal action further decreases in upgaze. It follows that moving the medial rectus toward the apex of an A and V pattern is appropriate for correcting the incomitant deviation. Conversely, moving the lateral rectus muscle toward the open end of the A or V is also appropriate for correcting the incomitant deviation. This is true regardless of whether recession or resection is performed.

It is generally accepted that offsetting up or down one-half tendon width, irrespective of whether it is performed on the medial rectus or the lateral rectus muscle, or whether it is combined with a recession or resection of that muscle, will correct approximately 15 PD of the A or V pattern when the offsetting is performed on two horizontal rectus muscles. The amount of pattern correction is proportional to the amount of preoperative pattern that was present. Vertical transposition of the horizontal rectus muscles may be performed symmetrically and bilaterally, or may be confined to one eye, with appropriate vertical displacement of the medial and lateral rectus muscles. Surgery on the oblique muscles is another effective method of reducing the vertical incomitancy. Because this procedure has no effect on horizontal alignment in primary or downgaze, a V pattern esotropia with a large deviation in downgaze and underacting superior obliques can also be treated with a bilateral superior oblique tuck as this will increase the abducting force of the superior oblique, and decrease the esotropia, in downgaze. Weakening both overacting superior obliques creates an increase of convergence in downgaze, with little effect in primary position and no effect in upgaze. The effect of a bilateral superior oblique weakening procedure on the downgaze deviation is proportional to the size of the preoperative pattern.

Overacting inferior obliques should not be weakened unless there is some degree of underaction of the superior obliques, and conversely, the superior obliques should not be weakened unless the inferior obliques are underacting. If this advice is ignored, the opposite pattern is likely to develop not too long after surgery, with the unoperated oblique muscles overacting.

If a patient has good binocular function, even if it is intermittent, the superior obliques should be weakened with caution. Typically, this scenario involves a patient with an A pattern intermittent exotropia who demonstrates bifoveal fixation when the deviation is not present. Even with the best surgical technique, weakening of the superior obliques may lead to an asymmetric result with a vertical deviation in primary position occurring postoperatively. This may result in a sustained head tilt to compensate for the vertical tropia. If the superior obliques are to be weakened, a procedure that leaves the tendon available for reoperation may be helpful should an iatrogenic ocular torticollis be produced. Because it may be impossible to reverse a free tenotomy of the superior oblique, some authors have advocated recession of the tendon or placement of an expander between its cut ends. Another option would be to offset the horizontal muscles alone. Although this may not completely correct the pattern, it will diminish it without running the risk of creating torsional diplopia.

CRANIAL NERVE PALSIES

Paralytic strabismus, a motor imbalance caused by paresis or paralysis of an extraocular muscle, is characterized by a deviation that varies according to the direction of gaze and fixation with the involved or uninvolved eye. The diagnosis of paresis of recent onset is suggested by a deviation greatest in the field of action of the paretic muscle, by double vision, and by an increase in the deviation when the patient fixates with the paretic eye. It is important to distinguish paresis or paralysis of one or several extraocular muscles from a comitant form of strabismus, not only because correct identification of the muscle or muscle groups helps the planning of proper therapy, but also because an acquired paresis or paralysis may indicate a systemic or neurologic abnormality.

The treatment of paralytic strabismus, especially in adults with diplopia, can be the most challenging in the field of strabismus. Proper evaluation and treatment strategies are essential in the care of patients with these conditions. It is important that patient and physician alike maintain realistic expectations of the goals in the treatment of these often frustrating disorders.

Third Nerve Palsy

Third nerve palsies in children are frequently congenital. In children with an acquired third nerve palsy, trauma is the most common cause. In contrast, acquired third nerve palsies appear more often in adults.

Congenital

The four extraocular muscles (medial rectus, inferior rectus, superior rectus, and inferior oblique) innervated by the third nerve are affected in various degrees. Typically, the involved eye is hypotropic and exotropic, with varied degrees of limitation of elevation, depression, and adduction (Fig. 8.7). The third nerve also innervates the levator muscle, so that variable degrees of ptosis may also be present. The intraocular musculature is not usually affected in congenital third nerve palsy. However, pupillary constriction may occur on attempted adduction in some cases of aberrant regeneration.

Some patients with congenital third nerve palsy develop binocular vision by maintaining a compensatory head posture. Amblyopia may occur in either eye if the child does not maintain a head posture to compensate for the strabismus.

Congenital third nerve palsies are often benign and isolated. However, because some patients may have other focal neurologic deficits, a consultation with a neurologist may be warranted.

Pathogenesis

There are several possible causes of congenital third nerve palsy. Perinatal trauma to the peripheral oculomotor nerve has been considered the primary mechanism in the development of congenital third nerve palsies. Absence of other brainstem findings in the presence of aberrant regeneration in many patients supports this mechanism. However, other associated neurologic anomalies and brainstem signs sometimes occur in patients with congenital third nerve palsies.

Acquired

Acquired third nerve palsy in children and adults is often an ominous sign. The palsy may be partial or complete, and may involve only the extraocular muscles or both intraocular and extraocular muscles. Aberrant regeneration of the oculomotor nerve is thought to result from extensive and haphazard growth of the regenerated nerve fibers. Signs of aberrant regeneration include those listed in Table 8.4.

Treatment

Initial ophthalmic treatment for patients with acquired third nerve palsy involves relief of diplopia. If there is a complete third nerve palsy, the associated complete ptosis will cover the pupil and prevent diplopia. However, in partial third nerve palsy, the eyelid may not cover the pupillary space, so that diplopia may remain a problem. Occlusion therapy is then the best solution to the diplopia. Surgery to correct an acquired third nerve palsy should be postponed until the deviation is stable.

In congenital third nerve palsy, or an acquired palsy which has not resolved, surgical intervention is indicated in order to allow for the development of binocular vision or to relieve diplopia. If there is significant medial rectus muscle function, the eyes may be aligned in primary position with a lateral rectus muscle recession combined with a medial rectus muscle resection. Ptosis surgery, if necessary, should be performed once the eye alignment is satisfactory. An exception to this rule may occur in a young child where a complete ptosis may produce dense amblyopia. In this case, treatment of the ptosis may need to be performed soon after it occurs. A frontalis suspension procedure is required in patients with poor or absent levator function. Care must be taken not to elevate the eyelid too high as the cornea will be at significant risk for exposure given the inability to elevate the globe. If aberrant regeneration has occurred so that the ptotic eyelid elevates on attempted adduction, it may be possible to operate on the nonparetic eye to force the involved eye into this position and treat the ptosis as well as the strabismus with the same surgery.

In a complete third nerve palsy, the motility of the globe is severely limited, because only the lateral rectus and superior oblique muscles are functional. The eye is fixed in a characteristic down-and-out position. The goal of surgical intervention is to use the two remaining functional muscles in such a way as to achieve a straight-ahead eye with only limited movement of the globe. This goal should be carefully explained to the patient and parents in order to avoid unrealistic postoperative expectations.

In a patient with a complete third nerve palsy, the lateral rectus muscle should be recessed a minimum of 16 mm from its original insertion. It can also be disinserted and attached to the lateral orbital wall (59). Resection of a completely paralyzed medial rectus will add little to the correction of the exotropia. The paralyzed medial rectus will

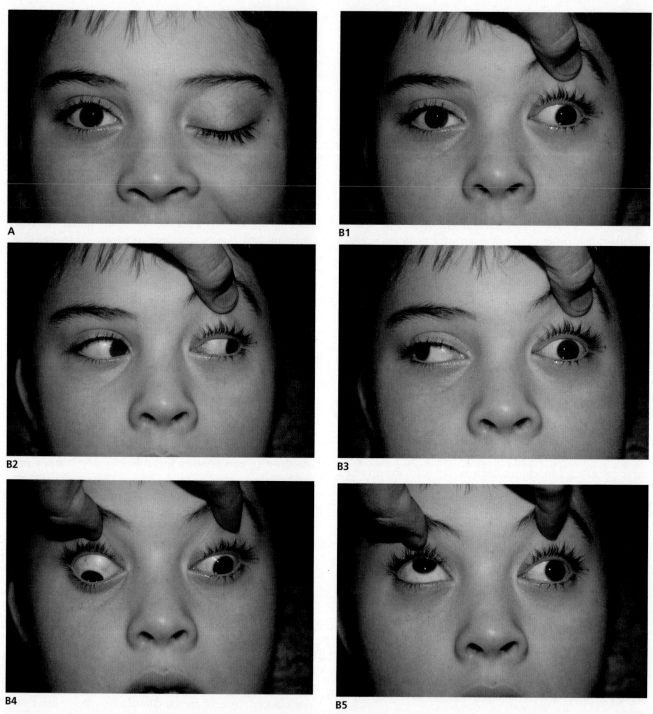

FIGURE 8.7 A: Third cranial nerve palsy with complete ptosis. **B1–B5**: Third nerve palsy demonstrating duction deficits (**B1, B2, B3, B4, B5**). (Reprinted with permission from Olitsky SE, Nelson LB. *Pediatric clinical ophthalmology—A color handbook*. London, UK: Manson Publishing, 2012, ISBN 9781840761511.)

stretch and will not provide any significant tension required to prevent the eye from drifting laterally.

Transposition surgery in the treatment of a third nerve palsy is difficult because the superior and inferior rectus muscles are also paretic. Transposing the superior oblique has been performed with or without fracturing the trochlea.

Limitations of superior oblique transposition include inadequate horizontal alignment, postoperative hyperdeviations, or paradoxical movements. Transposition of the functional lateral rectus can be performed by splitting it in half, bringing it under the vertical rectus muscles, and attaching both halves to the insertion site of the medial rectus (60).

Table 8.4

REGENERATION OF THE THIRD NERVE PALSY

Retraction of the globe on attempted vertical gaze

Adduction of the globe on attempted vertical gaze

Eyelid retraction in downgaze (pseudo-Graefe sign)

Miosis on adduction (pseudo-Argyll Robertson pupil)

Eyelid elevates on adduction

Another surgical option involves fixating the globe to the medial wall of the orbit with a suture or fascia lata (61).

Fourth Nerve Palsy

Fourth nerve palsy is the most common cause of an isolated cyclovertical muscle palsy. Paresis of the fourth nerve can be congenital or acquired. Closed-head trauma is the most common cause of fourth nerve palsy in most cases. A fourth nerve palsy is initially an incomitant hypertropia, greatest in the adducted, depressed position of the involved eye. If the palsy continues, contracture of the ipsilateral inferior oblique occurs and the maximal hyperdeviation is found in the field of action of this muscle. Another sign of contracture of the ipsilateral inferior oblique muscle is overelevation of the adducted palsied eye (Fig. 8.8).

Patients with unilateral fourth nerve palsy often present with torticollis to reduce diplopia. Head tilt to the side of the nonparetic eye is often found in patients with unilateral palsy. Since the superior oblique muscle is a depressor and intortor, its tone is diminished by upgaze and by tilting the head to the shoulder opposite the palsied muscle, patients with unilateral superior oblique palsy can maintain binocular vision. The absence of a head tilt is usually attributed to amblyopia or extremely large amplitude of vertical fusion. Some patients tilt their head to the side of the paretic eye in order to increase the vertical deviation and to make it easier to ignore the second image.

Facial asymmetry has been associated with congenital superior oblique palsy. Typically, this asymmetry is manifested by mid-facial hemihypoplasia on the dependent side, opposite the affected superior oblique. The nose deviates toward the hypoplastic side and the mouth slants so that it approximates a horizontal orientation despite the torticollis. It is thought that the facial asymmetry is secondary to the compensatory head tilt which may lead to secondary gravitational effects, reduced blood flow through a compromised internal carotid artery, or deformational molding of the face and skull during sleep. In muscular torticollis, once facial asymmetry develops, it may persist despite subsequent treatment. To prevent the facial asymmetry from

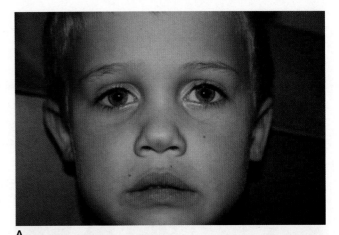

A

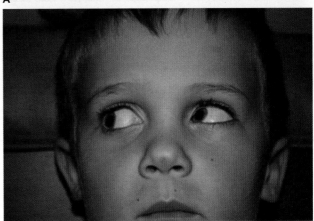

B

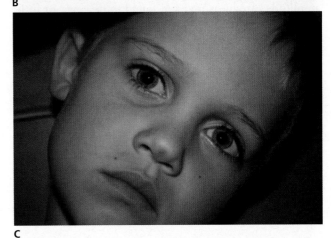

C

FIGURE 8.8 A–C: Left superior oblique palsy. Note the left hypertropia, overaction of the left inferior oblique, and the hypertropia made worse with forced left head tilt. (Reprinted with permission from Olitsky SE, Nelson LB. *Pediatric clinical ophthalmology—A color handbook.* London, UK: Manson Publishing, 2012, ISBN 9781840761511.)

developing, some ophthalmologists recommend early surgery to correct the deviation.

Often an older patient presents with a new onset of diplopia secondary to a fourth nerve palsy. It is important to determine if the palsy has only recently developed

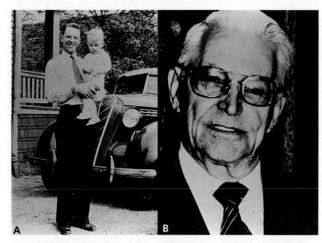

FIGURE 8.9. A: Right head tilt as seen in old photograph of asymptomatic patient. **B**: The same patient who presented with new onset diplopia approximately 40 years later. (Reprinted with permission from Nelson LB, Olitsky SE. *Harley's pediatric ophthalmology*, 5th Ed. Baltimore, MD: Lippincott Williams & Wilkins, 2005:170.)

or if it represents a congenital disorder that has decompensated. A newly acquired fourth nerve palsy may require further evaluation including a detailed neurologic examination and radiographic imaging. Several features may help to determine the acuteness of the deviation. A patient with a congenital superior oblique palsy will often have large vertical fusional amplitudes. If these amplitudes are measured and found to be large, or if the patient experiences only occasional diplopia in the presence of a large vertical deviation, the palsy is most likely long-standing or congenital. Examination of old photographs may show a compensatory head tilt (Fig. 8.9). The presence of facial asymmetry, as described above, would also signify a previous motility disorder. Lastly, patients with congenital superior oblique palsies may not experience subjective torsional diplopia, whereas patients with an acquired palsy generally do complain of tilting of the second image.

In order to evaluate logically any isolated cyclovertical muscle palsy, Parks devised a three-step test which is described below (62).

Step One

Determining whether there is a right hypertropia or left hypertropia in the primary position eliminates four of the eight cyclovertical muscles as possibly palsied. For example, right hypertropia establishes there is possibly.

A. Weak left elevator
1. left superior rectus
2. left inferior oblique

B. Weak right depressor
1. right inferior rectus
2. right superior oblique.

Step Two

Determining whether the vertical deviation increases on right or left gaze eliminates one of the two cyclovertical muscles in each eye. For example,

A. Right hypertropia that increases in left gaze indicates that either
1. the right superior oblique is weak or
2. the left superior rectus is weak.

B. At the end of Step Two, the two possible palsied muscles are always either intortors or extortors.

Step Three

The Bielschowsky head tilt test differentiates which of the two muscles from Step Two is palsied.

The Bielschowsky head tilt test is based on the utricular reflex, which is stimulated by tilting the head. Tilting to the right causes the intortors of the right eye and extortors of the left eye to contract, while the opposite combination contracts on tilting to the left. Of the two extortors and two intortors that are stimulated by head tilting, one muscle in each eye is an elevator and the other a depressor. This balance normally maintains vertical alignment on head tilting. In weakness of a cyclovertical muscle, there is a vertical imbalance with head tilting that is the basis for the Bielschowsky sign, on the third step of the three-step test. If, for example, the right superior oblique is palsied, tilting the head to the right should stimulate the two intortors of the right eye: the superior oblique and superior rectus. Because the superior oblique is palsied, the right superior rectus will be stimulated and increase the right hypertropia.

In addition to the Parks's three-step test, measurement of the deviation in the field of action of the superior oblique (down and in) and inferior oblique (up and in) should be done. This "fourth" step provides information in determining treatment options in patients with superior oblique palsy (see section "Treatment").

In older children and adults who present with hypertropia, the double Maddox rod can be used to detect any torsional component. In children too young for the presence of excyclotropia to be evaluated with the double Maddox rod, indirect ophthalmoscopy and fundus photography are both useful for diagnosing cyclotropia objectively. Anatomically, the fovea is about one-third of a disk diameter below the center of the optic nerve. If the fovea is lower than the expected normal relationship with the optic nerve, excyclotorsion of the retina exists. It should be remembered that the indirect ophthalmoscope inverts and reverses the image of the retina seen by the observer so that the fovea will appear higher than the optic nerve during indirect ophthalmoscopy in the presence of excyclotorsion.

Superior oblique palsy occurs bilaterally in 8% to 29% of cases (Fig. 8.10). In bilateral superior oblique palsy, there is a left hypertropia in right gaze, a right hypertropia in left gaze, a right hypertropia on right head tilt, a left hypertropia

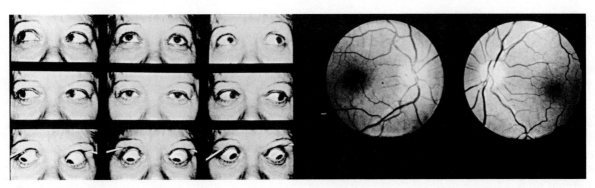

FIGURE 8.10. A: Bilateral fourth nerve palsy. Note the esotropia in downgaze and **(B)** the excyclotorsion of the left eye fundus. (Reprinted with permission from Nelson LB, Olitsky SE. *Harley's pediatric ophthalmology*, 5th Ed. Baltimore, MD: Lippincott Williams & Wilkins, 2005:174.)

on left head tilt, and V-pattern esotropia. The V-pattern eso-tropia is caused by deficient abduction of the palsied superior oblique muscles being offset by the adduction caused by the normally contracting inferior rectus muscles. When the palsies are symmetric, there will be no vertical deviation in primary gaze as the effect of each side will "cancel" the other. However, excyclotorsion will exist and can be measured subjectively or objectively as described previously. If the palsy is asymmetric, the paresis on the lesser affected side may be hidden by the large hypertropia of the more affected eye until after unilateral surgery is performed. The patient will then present postoperatively with a hypertropia of the untreated eye. This phenomenon has been termed a "masked" bilateral superior oblique palsy. Important signs of possible bilaterality include subjective torsion > 10 degrees, bilateral objective fundus torsion, any size reversal of the hypertropia in any gaze position (especially in the field of action of the inferior oblique), or an esodeviation in downgaze.

Treatment

Except for an occasional patient with vertical deviation of 10 PD or less (when prism may be tolerated), most cases of superior oblique palsy require surgery. In general, surgery for superior oblique palsies should be directed to those muscles whose greatest action is in the field when the vertical deviation is the largest.

Patients with congenital palsies will often have a floppy or anomalous superior oblique tendon (63). This can often be suggested with an exaggerated traction test at the time of surgery. If tendon laxity is demonstrated, some surgeons suggest that a superior oblique tuck should be performed. A superior oblique tuck should also be considered when the greatest deviation exists in its field of action. If the deviation is greatest in the field of action of the inferior oblique, this muscle is often weakened. In general, weakening of the inferior oblique or strengthening of the superior oblique will correct up to 15 PD of hypertropia.

For deviations greater than this, surgery on a second muscle is necessary. A simultaneous superior oblique tuck and inferior oblique recession can be performed. Alternatively, either one of these procedures can be combined with a recession of the contralateral inferior rectus or the ipsilateral superior rectus. Care must be taken not to perform too large a recession on the superior rectus if the inferior oblique is also weakened, as a double elevator palsy may result. ATIO has also been used in the treatment of unilateral superior oblique palsy. Because of the risk of primary position hypotropia after this procedure the use of ATIO in the treatment of unilateral superior oblique palsies should generally be reserved for those patients with larger deviations.

Bilateral superior oblique palsies are generally treated by strengthening procedures. If torsional diplopia is the primary problem, a Harada-Ito procedure is indicated. In this procedure, as modified by Fells, the anterior half of the superior oblique tendon is displaced to an anterior and temporal location (64,65). A standard displacement of the tendon is capable of correcting varying degrees of excyclotorsion (66).

Sixth Nerve Palsy

Sixth nerve palsy causes an esotropia in primary position, which increases in the field of action of the paretic lateral rectus muscle. The palsy may be unilateral or bilateral. Continuation of binocular vision is usually possible by maintaining the eyes in the lateral gaze position away from the palsied eye; this results in a compensatory horizontal face turn toward the palsied eye.

Congenital

Congenital sixth nerve palsies are rare. In newborns, a transient lateral rectus paresis may be rarely noted, with resolution by 6 weeks of age (3,4). Most infants with a significant esotropia and reduced lateral gaze are congenital esotropes with a cross-fixation pattern. Others, who have a motility disorder resembling a sixth nerve palsy, may have Duane retraction syndrome or Möbius syndrome.

Acquired

The sixth nerve has a long intracranial course, and there are three anatomic areas where the sixth nerve is most susceptible to injury: as it exits from the pontomedullary junction, where it may be compressed by the anteroinferior cerebellar artery; at its penetration of the dura (Dorello's canal), causing Gradenigo syndrome below the petrous crest; and within the cavernous sinus.

Trauma is probably the most common cause of an acquired sixth nerve palsy in an otherwise healthy child. Nontraumatic acquired sixth nerve palsy is usually a manifestation of a serious intracranial abnormality or increase in intracranial pressure. The diagnosis of a viral sixth nerve palsy is generally made only when other possible causes have been excluded.

Treatment

In a child with an isolated acute sixth nerve palsy without other neurologic signs, including papilledema, headache, or ataxia, further neurologic evaluation, including CT or MRI scanning is usually indicated. If the workup is negative, they should be reexamined at regular intervals and the parents advised to observe for new signs and symptoms.

Management of unilateral sixth nerve palsy should be conservative during the first 6 months after onset. Patients may adopt a compensatory face turn or simply occlude one eye to control the diplopia. Young children who do not develop a compensatory face turn should receive alternate occlusion to prevent the development of amblyopia and suppression. During alternate patching, they should be given full hyperopic correction to prevent accommodative esotropia from developing. In acute sixth nerve palsy, botulinum injection into the ipsilateral medial rectus may permit binocular vision in primary position during recovery. Botulinim injection may also be useful in the treatment of chronic sixth nerve palsies. Although botulinum injection may help eliminate diplopia during the recovery phase of an acute sixth nerve palsy, it has not been shown to prevent the need for future surgery (67). After 6 months of waiting for possible return of sixth nerve function, surgical treatment is appropriate. If the lateral rectus demonstrates some function, a graded medial rectus recession and lateral rectus resection for the appropriate amount of esotropia can be performed. When the lateral rectus has no function, a muscle transfer procedure may be necessary. Three muscle transfer techniques have been popularized. The Hummelsheim procedure consists of transposing the lateral halves of the vertical recti to the lateral rectus. The Jensen procedure involves splitting the vertical and lateral recti, tying the upper half of the lateral rectus to the lateral half of the superior rectus muscles, and doing the same with the inferior rectus. Other surgeons advocate transposing the entire vertical

rectus muscle insertions to the lateral rectus insertion. In addition to the transposition procedure, weakening of the ipsilateral medial rectus is often required to decrease the adduction force. This could lead to anterior segment ischemia, especially in an older patient with poor circulation. Partial tendon transfers (Jensen and Hummelsheim) may decrease this risk. However, anterior segment ischemia has been reported after their use, even in a young child. The use of intraoperative botulinum injection into the medial rectus combined with vertical rectus transposition surgery has been shown to be efficacious and eliminates the need to remove a third rectus muscle. The Hummelsheim procedure can be augmented by resecting the transposed halves of the muscle (68). A non-absorbable suture can also be used in a full or partial transposition to laterally secure the muscles to the sclera near the border of the lateral rectus to augment these procedures as well (69).

Management of bilateral sixth nerve palsy is very similar to that of unilateral sixth nerve palsy. Unfortunately, these patients cannot overcome the diplopia with a compensatory face turn.

STRABISMUS SYNDROMES

Duane Retraction Syndrome

This condition was originally described at the end of the 19th century. In 1905, Duane described 54 cases, summarized all the clinical findings, reviewed previous work, and offered theories on pathogenesis and treatment (70).

Duane retraction syndrome (DRS) more frequently occurs in the left eye than in the right, and in females more than in males. Bilateral involvement is less frequent than unilateral occurrence.

Other ocular or systemic anomalies have been reported in association with DRS. The ocular anomalies include dysplasia of the iris stroma, pupillary anomalies, cataracts, heterochromia, Marcus Gunn jaw winking, coloboma, crocodile tears, and microphthalmos. The systemic anomalies include Goldenhar syndrome, dystrophic defects such as the Klippel-Feil syndrome, cervical spina bifida, cleft palate, facial anomalies, perceptive deafness, malformations of the external ear, and anomalies of the limbs, feet, and hands.

Clinical Manifestations

The most characteristic clinical findings in DRS include an absence of abduction of an eye with slight limitation of adduction, retraction of the globe in attempted adduction, and up- and downshooting, or both in adduction. Huber, with the support of electromyography, provided a useful classification of DRS into three types (71):

Type I: Marked limitation or complete absence of abduction, normal or only slightly restrict adduction, narrowing of the palpebral fissure and retraction of the globe on adduction, and widening of the palpebral fissure on attempted abduction (Fig. 8.11). Electromyography

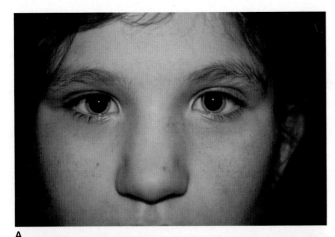

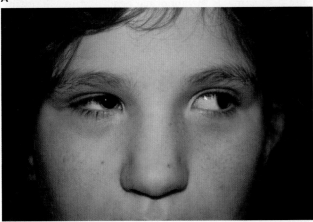

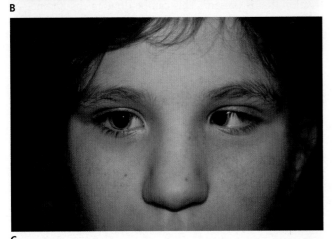

FIGURE 8.11. A–C: Type I Duane retraction syndrome (DRS). Note the limitation of abduction of the right eye with narrowing of the palpebral fissure and retraction of the globe on adduction. (Reprinted with permission from Olitsky SE, Nelson LB. *Pediatric clinical ophthalmology—A color handbook.* London, UK: Manson Publishing, 2012, ISBN 9781840761511.)

shows absence of electrical activity in the lateral rectus muscle on abduction, but paradoxic electrical activity on adduction.

Type II: Limitation or absence of adduction with exotropia of the affected eye, normal or slightly limited abduction, retraction of the globe on attempted adduction (Fig. 8.12). Electromyography reveals electrical activity of the lateral rectus muscle on both abduction and adduction.

Type III: Severe limitation of both abduction and adduction, retraction of the globe, and narrowing of the palpebral fissure on attempted adduction (Fig. 8.13). Electromyography demonstrates electrical activity of both horizontal rectus muscles on both adduction and abduction.

Type I is most common, followed in order of frequency by Types II and III. Most patients with Type I DRS have a small esotropia in the primary position during infancy and childhood, and adopt a compensatory head turn toward the side of the involved eye to maintain normal binocular vision.

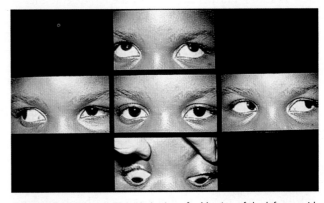

FIGURE 8.12. Type II DRS. Limitation of adduction of the left eye with narrowing of the palpebral fissure and retraction of the globe. Abduction of the left eye is normal. (Reprinted with permission from Tasman W, Jaeger E. *The Wills Eye Hospital atlas of clinical ophthalmology,* 2nd Ed. Philadelphia, PA: Lippincott Williams & Wilkins, 2001.)

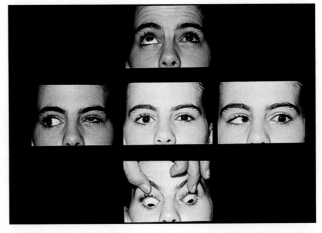

FIGURE 8.13. Type III DRS. Limitation of both abduction and adduction of the left eye. (Reprinted with permission from Tasman W, Jaeger E. *The Wills Eye hospital atlas of clinical ophthalmology,* 2nd Ed. Philadelphia, PA: Lippincott Williams & Wilkins, 2001.)

Pathogenesis

Although DRS has been well described clinically, the etiology remains unclear. Various theories have been formulated on the basis of data collected from surgical, electromyographic, and autopsy studies.

Structural Anomalies

The up- and downshooting that frequently occur in adduction have been blamed on several structural anomalies. Some authors have proposed a "leash" effect to explain these motility patterns. They suggest that during adduction the lateral rectus contracts and may slip vertically over the globe, causing a dynamic up and downshooting of the eye.

An intriguing theory proposed by several investigators to explain the high prevalence of ocular and systemic malformations associated with DRS suggests a common teratogenic stimulus at 8 weeks of gestation may cause these findings. Further support for the teratogenic theory was provided by the fact that a number of patients afflicted with the thalidomide syndrome also had DRS (72).

Innervational Anomalies

In 1957, Breinin, using electromyography, was the first to show paradoxic electric activity of the lateral rectus in a patient with DRS (73). He suggested that the anomalous contraction of the medical and lateral rectus muscles is the cause of retraction in adduction. These findings have been confirmed and expanded on by many other investigators. Abnormal synergistic innervation between the medial rectus and the vertical rectus or oblique muscles has been demonstrated electromyographically, which may explain the up- and downshooting in adduction in DRS.

Treatment

Before surgery is contemplated, coexisting significant refractive errors, anisometropia, and amblyopia must be treated. Indications for surgery for patients with DRS are a significant deviation in primary position, an anomalous head position, a large upshoot or downshoot, or retraction of the globe that is cosmetically intolerable.

In Type I DRS, an esodeviation, usually <30 PD, and a face turn in the direction of the involved eye may develop. In most cases, an ipsilateral medial rectus recession can significantly improve the esodeviation and the face turn. Often the medial rectus of the involved eye is thickened and there is positive forced duction to abduction because of the contracture of the muscle.

Some patients with DRS have markedly reduced adduction saccadic velocities caused by marked lateral rectus cofiring on adduction. There is a risk of severely compromising adduction and causing an exotropia postoperatively after large medial rectus recessions (>6 mm) in such patients. An exotropia that occurs on attempted adduction, caused by cofiring of the lateral rectus, can also be produced in such cases.

Patients with large angles of esotropia in primary position may be especially challenging. Some surgeons utilize muscle transposition procedures for such patients. Transposition of the superior rectus has been shown to be effective and does not produce a postoperative hypertropia (74). Classic teaching has been that resection of the ipsilateral lateral rectus should not be performed, because it will increase retraction of the globe in adduction. However, small resections of the lateral rectus have been safely performed in selected cases where the deviation is large and the globe retraction is minimal (75). Patients who have Type 2 DRS with exotropia in primary position and a face turn away from the involved eye require a recession of the ipsilateral lateral rectus.

The up- or downshooting in DRS can be as cosmetically distracting as the abnormal head posture. Recessing a very stiff, fibrotic lateral rectus may reduce the leash effect if present. However, if there is no deviation in primary position, an ipsilateral medial rectus recession will be necessary to prevent a consecutive esotropia. Splitting of the lateral rectus into a Y configuration or the use of a posterior fixation suture on the lateral rectus has been successful in reducing the leash effect without inducing strabismus in the primary position. Anterior transplantation of the inferior oblique has been successfully used to treat the upshoot.

Patients who suffer from a cosmetically noticeable retraction of the globe in attempted adduction may benefit from recession of both horizontal recti to reduce the co-contraction that is present. This can be done in the absence of a deviation in primary gaze or adjusted to eliminate a deviation if present.

Brown Syndrome

This ocular motility disorder, characterized by an inability to elevate the adducted eye actively or passively, was first described by Brown in 1950 (76). It has since become recognized that there is a variety of causes, that the condition may be congenital or acquired, and that the defect can be permanent, transient, or intermittent.

Clinical Manifestations

Brown syndrome is characterized by a deficiency of elevation in the adducting position (Fig. 8.14). Improved elevation is usually apparent in the midline, with normal or near-normal elevation in abduction. With lateral gaze in the opposite direction, the involved eye may depress in adduction, although no overdepression simulating overaction of the superior oblique muscle occurs on duction testing. Exodeviation (V pattern) often occurs as the eyes are moved upward in the midline. Many patients are orthophoric in the primary position, although with time hypotropia may develop with a compensatory face turn toward the opposite eye. In some cases, there is discomfort on attempted elevation in adduction, the patient may feel or even hear a click under the same

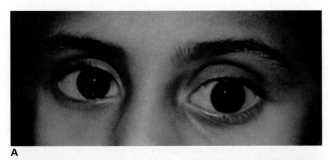

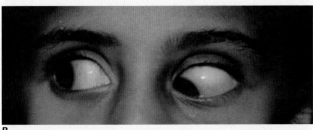

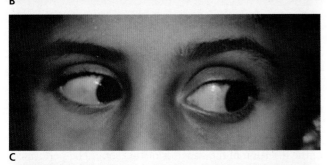

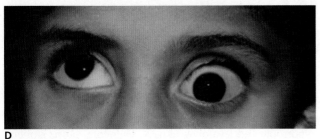

FIGURE 8.14. A–D: Brown syndrome of the left eye.

circumstances, and there may be a palpable mass or tenderness in the trochlear region. A positive forced duction test is the hallmark of Brown syndrome.

Pathogenesis

Brown subsequently redefined the syndrome, recognizing that it is more complex than originally proposed (77). He initially believed that the simulated inferior oblique palsy was due to an innervational disturbance to this muscle, with secondary contracture of the anterior sheath of the superior oblique tendon. Brown attributed the syndrome to congenital shortening of the sheath surrounding the reflected tendon of the superior oblique muscle. However, several investigators were unable to substantiate Brown's theory of a primary congenital anomaly of the

anterior sheath of the superior oblique tendon. Crawford was the first to prove that the cause of the syndrome is a tight superior oblique tendon (78). By cutting the tendon or excising a portion of it, the restricted elevation of the involved eye was cured.

Acquired Brown's syndrome has been attributed to a variety of causes, including superior oblique surgery, scleral buckling bands, trauma, focal metastasis to the superior oblique, and following sinus surgery and inflammation in the trochlear region. An identical motility pattern, as seen in Brown syndrome, can be acquired by patients with juvenile or adult rheumatoid arthritis. It appears that this form of Brown's syndrome represents a stenosing tenosynovitis of the trochlea and shares similar characteristics to inflammatory disorders that affect the tendons of the fingers.

Treatment

If patients with Brown syndrome are orthophoric in primary position and without an anomalous head posture, surgery is not necessary. Such patients may experience diplopia when elevating the involved eye in adduction, but will learn to avoid this position of gaze. However, if the eye is hypotropic in primary position or if a head turn is cosmetically significant, surgery is indicated to attempt to restore binocular function in the primary position.

Tenotomy or tenectomy of the superior oblique will eliminate the restriction to elevation in Brown syndrome. However, these weakening procedures result in superior oblique palsy in some cases. Therefore, some surgeons advocate simultaneous inferior oblique weakening at the time of surgery to reduce the need for later surgery. Others suggest performing a superior oblique recession or inserting a superior oblique expander to provide a graded weakening effect and decrease the risk of iatrogenic superior oblique palsy.

Monocular Elevation Deficiency (Double Elevator Palsy)

Monocular elevation deficiency (MED), previously called double elevator palsy, suggests that both elevator muscles (the superior rectus and inferior oblique muscles) of one eye are weak, with resultant inability or reduced ability to elevate the eye and a hypotropia in the primary position. The term is generally used to describe diminished ocular elevation present in all fields of gaze.

Clinical Manifestations

MED is characterized by reduced elevation in all positions of gaze. When the patient fixates with the nonparetic eye, the paretic eye will become hypotropic and the eyelid may become ptotic. Fixation with the paretic eye will cause a hypertropia of the nonparetic eye (Fig. 8.15). Provided that the elevator muscle is not involved, the ptosis will also disappear. Patients often present with a chin-up position to maintain binocular vision. The Bell's phenomenon is an

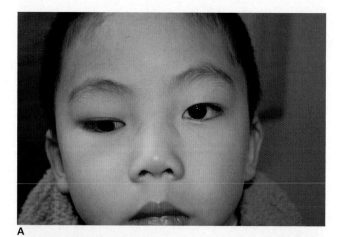

A

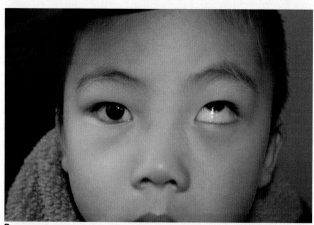

B

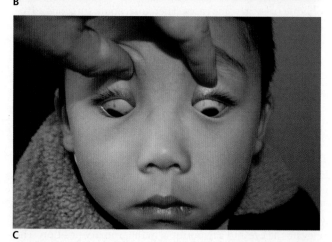

C

FIGURE 8.15. A–C: Double elevator palsy of the right eye. Note the pseudoptosis of the right upper eyelid which disappears when the right eye is fixating. (Reprinted with permission from Olitsky SE, Nelson LB. *Pediatric clinical ophthalmology—A color handbook.* London, UK: Manson Publishing, 2012, ISBN 9781840761511.)

important clinical sign in patients with MED. It will be preserved when the condition is secondary to a supranuclear cause but absent in the presence of a restricted inferior rectus. Rarely, patients with MED have reduced elevation in all positions of gaze but no hypotropia in the primary position.

The absence of elevation in abduction helps differentiate this disorder from Brown syndrome.

Pathogenesis

MED may be due to innervational problems (supranuclear, nuclear, or infranuclear abnormality); mechanical, restrictive conditions in the orbit; or a combination of factors.

Scott and Jackson emphasized the importance of inferior rectus muscle restriction in patients with MED (79). They found 73% of their patients to have restriction of the ipsilateral inferior rectus muscle as determined by the forced duction test. They also noted an accentuated lower eyelid fold associated with inferior rectus restriction. This fold became more prominent with attempted upgaze. They postulated that this eyelid fold was caused by attachments of the capsulopalpebral head of the inferior rectus to the lower eyelid.

Treatment

If a patient with MED is orthophoric in primary position, surgery is not needed. If there is a vertical deviation in primary position, a forced duction test is necessary. In patients with a positive forced duction test, indicating restriction to elevation, an inferior rectus recession is indicated. When the forced duction test is negative, a Knapp procedure (transposing the medial and lateral rectus muscles to the corners of the insertion of the superior rectus) should be performed (80). As much as 35 PD of hypotropia can be corrected with the Knapp procedure. Some patients will require a later recession of the inferior rectus for undercorrections. However, only a modest increase in elevation is usually observed after this procedure.

If a patient has ptosis, the lowered eyelid position may have resulted from the globe's hypotropic position (pseudoptosis), intrinsic levator weakness (true ptosis), or both hypotropic and levator weakness. Therefore, ptosis surgery should be avoided until the hypotropia is corrected. Once the eye alignment is improved, the ptosis can be reevaluated.

Isolated Inferior Oblique Paresis

Isolated paresis of the inferior oblique muscle is a rare entity.

Clinical Manifestations

Patients with an inferior oblique paresis, depending on fixation preference, manifest either a hypotropia of the affected eye or a hypertropia of the unaffected eye. The vertical deviation increases on gaze into the field of action of the involved inferior oblique, but decreases in the opposite gaze. The Bielschowsky head tilt is positive on tilting the head toward the normal side. With time, the superior oblique becomes contracted and shows moderate to marked overaction. Patients characteristically tilt the head toward the side of the paretic eye in an attempt to decrease the vertical deviation and maintain binocular vision.

A forced duction is necessary to differentiate an isolated inferior oblique paresis from Brown syndrome. In inferior oblique paresis, there should not be any substantial restriction to elevation in adduction. Also, with inferior oblique palsy, superior oblique overaction will result in an A pattern. In Brown syndrome, a V pattern will be noted.

Pathogenesis

The cause of isolated inferior oblique palsy is often unknown. In a series of 25 patients with inferior oblique palsy, including 2 with bilateral palsies, no patient had an abnormal neuroimaging study or was found to have myasthenia gravis (81).

Treatment

Tenotomy of the superior oblique can be used to treat inferior oblique paresis but it carries the risk of overcorrection. Contralateral superior rectus recession is another option. When the hyperdeviation is greatest in the field of action of the inferior oblique, recessing the yoke muscle, which is the contralateral superior rectus, makes clinical sense. This procedure works well and decreases the risk for the development of an iatrogenically induced superior oblique palsy.

Möbius Syndrome

Möbius syndrome is a rare congenital disturbance consisting of varying involvement of facial and lateral gaze paresis. In 1888, Möbius first suggested that congenital bilateral abducens–facial paralysis might be an independent pathologic entity, thus gaining eponymic distinction (82).

Clinical Manifestations

Möbius syndrome is characterized by unilateral or bilateral inability to abduct the eyes. Although horizontal movements are usually lacking, vertical movements and convergence are intact. Pupillary constriction, vision, and the retina are generally normal. Congenital esotropia is common in children with Möbius syndrome. The unilateral or bilateral complete or incomplete facial palsy is usually observed during the first few weeks of life because of difficulty with sucking and feeding, and incomplete closure of the eyelids during sleep. These patients typically have masklike faces with an inability to grin and wrinkle the forehead.

Möbius syndrome is frequently associated with paresis of other muscles supplied by the cranial nerves. Often, there is partial atrophy of the tongue with inability to protrude the tongue beyond the lips. Paralysis of the soft palate and muscles of mastication may also occur. Various skeletal and muscle defects are common, including absence or hypoplasia of the pectoral muscles, syndactyly, club feet, and congenital limb amputations.

Pathogenesis

The etiology of Möbius syndrome is presently unknown and is likely multifactorial.

In a small percentage of patients, the condition is predetermined genetically but most cases are sporadic. The occurrence of simultaneous limb malformations have lead some investigators to suggest a disruption of normal morphogenesis during a critical period in the development of the embryonic structures of these regions in patients with Möbius syndrome. This disruption would likely occur at 4 to 7 weeks of gestation.

Vascular interruption is another possible cause of the Möbius syndrome. Possibilities of interruption of blood flow include premature regression of the primitive trigeminal arteries or disruption of flow in the basilar artery or the subclavian artery supply that involves interruption of the embryonic blood supply.

Treatment

Most children with Möbius syndrome who present with early-onset esotropia have a large deviation (Fig. 8.16). Surgery for esotropia is commonly performed in patients of young age, as is advocated for the primary type of congenital esotropia.

Usually the forced duction test and the character of the muscles encountered at surgery in children with Möbius syndrome are abnormal. The forced ductions may be positive to both adduction and abduction, while vertical ductions are typically normal. The horizontal muscles are often thickened, taut, and fibrotic. After surgery for the esotropia, consisting of recession of the taut medial rectus muscles, there is usually little horizontal movement because of the concomitant bilateral gaze palsy.

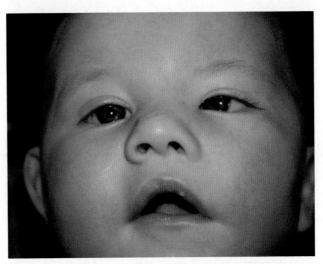

FIGURE 8.16. Möbius syndrome. In the primary position, there is a large-angle esotropia. (Reprinted with permission from Olitsky SE, Nelson LB. *Pediatric clinical ophthalmology—A color handbook*. London, UK: Manson Publishing, 2012, ISBN 9781840761511.)

Congenital Fibrosis of the Extraocular Muscles

Congenital fibrosis of the extraocular muscles (CFEOM) describes a group of disorders that result from the dysfunction of all or part of the muscles innervated by the oculomotor nerve. Patients with CFEOM are typically born with ophthalmoplegia and ptosis (Fig. 8.17). Baumgarten provided the first description of CFEOM in 1840 (83). Brown used the term "generalized fibrosis syndrome" when he described the condition in 1950 (84).

Clinical Manifestations

Three forms of CFEOM have been described. CFEOM 1 is considered the classic form of congenital, restrictive strabismus. The eyes of affected individuals are usually fixed in

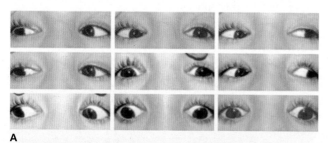

A

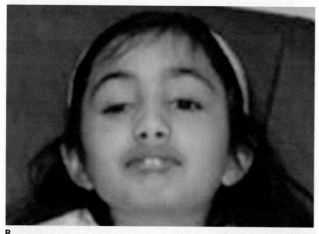

B

FIGURE 8.17. A,B: General fibrosis syndrome. (Reprinted with permission from Cestari DG, Hunter DG. *Learning strabismus surgery: A case-based approach.* Philadelphia, PA: Lippincott Williams & Wilkins, 2012:193–197.)

the infraducted position about 20 to 30degrees below midline. Horizontal movement is absent or severely restricted. Bilateral ptosis is usually present and patients exhibit a marked chin-up head posture. Binocularity is usually absent. Patients with CFEOM 2 demonstrate a nonclassic CFEOM appearance. Like those patients with CFEOM 1, affected individuals present with bilateral ptosis but their eyes are partially or completely fixed in an exotropic position. CFEOM 3 is a clinically heterogenous form of the disease and is usually used to describe individuals who do not meet the criteria for the other two types. Patients with CFEOM have fibrosis of extraocular muscles and Tenon's capsule. Adhesions to the globe and between muscles have been described. Anomalous insertions of the extraocular muscles may also occur.

Pathogenesis

The early reports of affected patients and the use of the term "muscle fibrosis" suggests that these syndromes result from a primary abnormality of muscle. However, evidence suggests that CFEOM results from a primary innervational abnormality with a secondary myopathy (85). The genetic mutations cause abnormal development of the oculomotor nuclei which then lead to the observed changes in the affected extraocular muscles. CFEOM 1 and 3 are inherited in an autosomal dominant fashion and are associated with mutations in the *KIF21A* gene. Mutations in the *PHOX2A* gene have been associated with CFEOM 2 which is inherited in an autosomal recessive fashion.

Treatment

The goal of surgical management in the general fibrosis syndrome is to center the eyes and improve the compensatory head posture. In patients with significant hypotropia, large recession or disinsertion of the inferior rectus muscles is indicated. However, elevation of the hypotropic eye accentuates the ptosis. Bilateral frontalis suspension is required soon after the strabismus surgery. Because these patients often do not have a Bell's phenomenon, corneal drying may occur after ptosis surgery. Therefore, the eyelid should be elevated only to the upper pupillary border. Improvement in the movement of the eyes is not possible.

REFERENCES

1. Olitsky SE, Sudesh S, Graziano A, Hamblen J, Brooks SE, Shaha SH. The negative psychosocial impact of strabismus in adults. *J AAPOS* 1999;3:209–211.
2. Uretmen O, Egrilmez S, Kose S, Pamukcu K, Akkin C, Palamar M. Negative social bias against children with strabismus. *Acta Ophthalmol Scand* 2003;81:138–142.
3. Nixon RB, Helveston EM, Miller K, Archer SM, Ellis FD. Incidence of strabismus in neonates. *Am J Ophthalmol* 1985;100:798–801.
4. Archer SM, Sondhi N, Helveston EM. Strabismus in infancy. *Ophthalmology* 1989;96:133–7.
5. Mohney BG, Erie JC, Hodge DO, Jacobsen SJ. Congenital esotropia in Olmsted County, Minnesota. *Ophthalmology* 1998;105:846–850.
6. Scott MH, Noble AG, Raymond WRT, Parks MM. Prevalence of primary monofixation syndrome in parents of children with congenital esotropia. J Pediatr *Ophthalmol Strabismus* 1994;31:298–301; discussion 302.
7. Worth C. *Squint, its causes and treatment.* London: Bailliere, Tindall, and Cox, 1903.

8. Chavasse FB. *Worth's squint on the binocular reflexes and the treatment of strabismus*, 7th Ed. Philadelphia, PA: P. Blakiston's Son & Co., 1939.

9. Costenbader FD. Infantile esotropia. *Trans Am Ophthalmol Soc* 1961;59:397–429.

10. Taylor DM. How early is early surgery in the management of strabismus? *Arch Ophthalmol* 1963;70:752–756.

11. Ing M, Costenbader FD, Parks MM, Albert DG. Early surgery for congenital esotropia. *Am J Ophthalmol* 1966;61:1419–1427.

12. Parks MM. The monofixation syndrome. *Trans Am Ophthalmol Soc* 1969;67:609–657.

13. Hiles DA, Watson BA, Biglan AW. Characteristics of infantile esotropia following early bimedial rectus recession. *Arch Ophthalmol* 1980;98:697–703.

14. Helveston EM, Ellis FD, Schott J, et al. Surgical treatment of congenital esotropia. *Am J Ophthalmol* 1983;96:218–228.

15. Neely DE, Helveston EM, Thuente DD, Plager DA. Relationship of dissociated vertical deviation and the timing of initial surgery for congenital esotropia. *Ophthalmology* 2001;108:487–490.

16. Vazquez R, Calhoun JH, Harley RD. Development of monofixation syndrome in congenital esotropia. *J Pediatr Ophthalmol Strabismus* 1981;18:42–44.

17. Eustis HS, Nussdorf JD. Inferior oblique overaction in infantile esotropia: fundus extorsion as a predictive sign. *J Pediatr Ophthalmol Strabismus* 1996;33:85–88.

18. Ing MR. Early surgical alignment for congenital esotropia. *Trans Am Ophthalmol Soc* 1981;79:625–663.

19. Arthur BW, Smith JT, Scott WE. Long-term stability of alignment in the monofixation syndrome. *J Pediatr Ophthalmol Strabismus* 1989;26:224–231.

20. Kushner BJ, Fisher M. Is alignment within 8 prism diopters of orthotropia a successful outcome for infantile esotropia surgery? *Arch Ophthalmol* 1996;114:176–180.

21. Birch EE, Stager DR, Everett ME. Random dot stereoacuity following surgical correction of infantile esotropia. *J Pediatr Ophthalmol Strabismus* 1995;32:231–235.

22. Pediatric Eye Disease Investigator G. Spontaneous resolution of early-onset esotropia: experience of the Congenital Esotropia Observational Study. *Am J Ophthalmol* 2002;133:109–118.

23. Rogers GL, Chazan S, Fellows R, Tsou BH. Strabismus surgery and its effect upon infant development in congenital esotropia. *Ophthalmology* 1982;89:479–483.

24. Hess JB, Calhoun JH. A new rationale for the management of large angle esotropia. *J Pediatr Ophthalmol Strabismus* 1979;16:345–348.

25. Weakley DR, Jr, Stager DR, Everett ME. Seven-millimeter bilateral medial rectus recessions in infantile esotropia. *J Pediatr Ophthalmol Strabismus* 1991;28:113–115.

26. Magoon EH. Chemodenervation of strabismic children. A 2- to 5-year follow-up study compared with shorter follow-up. *Ophthalmology* 1989;96:931–934.

27. McNeer KW, Spencer RF, Tucker MG. Observations on bilateral simultaneous botulinum toxin injection in infantile esotropia. *J Pediatr Ophthalmol Strabismus* 1994;31:214–219.

28. Ing MR. Botulinum alignment for congenital esotropia. *Ophthalmology* 1993;100:318–322.

29. Parks MM. The weakening surgical procedures for eliminating overaction of the inferior oblique muscle. *Am J Ophthalmol* 1972;73:107–122.

30. Scott AB. *Planning inferior oblique muscle surgery*. New York: Grune & Stratton, 1978.

31. Mims JL 3rd, Wood RC. Bilateral anterior transposition of the inferior obliques. Arch *Ophthalmol* 1989;107:41–44.

32. Bacal DA, Nelson LB. Anterior transposition of the inferior oblique muscle for both dissociated vertical deviation and/or inferior oblique overaction: results of 94 procedures in 55 patients. *Binocul Vis Eye Muscle Surg* 1992;7:219.

33. Kushner BJ. Restriction of elevation in abduction after inferior oblique anteriorization. *J AAPOS* 1997;1:55–62.

34. Wright KW, Walonker F, Edelman P. 10-Diopter fixation test for amblyopia. *Arch Ophthalmol* 1981;99:1242–1246.

35. Pollard ZF. Accommodative esotropia during the first year of life. Arch *Ophthalmol* 1976;94:1912–1913.

36. Coats DK, Avilla CW, Paysse EA, Sprunger DT, Steinkuller PG, Somaiya M. Early-onset refractive accommodative esotropia. *J AAPOS* 1998;2:275–278.

37. Parks MM. Abnormal accommodative convergence in squint. *AMA Arch Ophthalmol* 1958;59:364–380.

38. Albert DG, Lederman ME. Abnormal distance—near esotropia. Doc *Ophthalmol* 1973;34:27–36.

39. Ludwig IH, Parks MM, Getson PR, Kammerman LA. Rate of deterioration in accommodative esotropia correlated to the AC/A relationship. *J Pediatr Ophthalmol Strabismus* 1988;25:8–12.

40. Pratt-Johnson JA, Tillson G. The management of esotropia with high AC/A ratio (convergence excess). *J Pediatr Ophthalmol Strabismus* 1985;22:238–242.

41. Lueder GT, Norman AA. Strabismus surgery for elimination of bifocals in accommodative esotropia. *Am J Ophthalmol* 2006;142:632–635.

42. O'Hara MA, Calhoun JH. Surgical correction of excess esotropia at near. *J Pediatr Ophthalmol Strabismus* 1990;27:120–123; discussion 4–5.

43. Kushner BJ. Fifteen-year outcome of surgery for the near angle in patients with accommodative esotropia and a high accommodative convergence to accommodation ratio. *Arch Ophthalmol* 2001;119:1150–1153.

44. Wright KW, Bruce-Lyle L. Augmented surgery for esotropia associated with high hypermetropia. *J Pediatr Ophthalmol Strabismus* 1993;30:167–170.

45. Kushner BJ. Partly accommodative esotropia. Should you overcorrect and cut the plus? *Arch Ophthalmol* 1995;113:1530–1534.

46. Efficacy of prism adaptation in the surgical management of acquired esotropia. Prism Adaptation Study Research Group. *Arch Ophthalmol* 1990;108:1248–1256.

47. Metz HS, Bigelow C. Change in the cycle of circadian strabismus. *Am J Ophthalmol* 1995;120:124–125.

48. Burian HM. Motility clinic: sudden onset of comitant convergent strabismus. *Am J Ophthalmol* 1945;28:407.

49. Mohney BG, Huffaker RK. Common forms of childhood exotropia. *Ophthalmology* 2003;110:2093–2096.

50. Hunter DG, Kelly JB, Buffenn AN, Ellis FJ. Long-term outcome of uncomplicated infantile exotropia. *J AAPOS* 2001;5:352–356.

51. Duane A. A new classification of the motor anomalies of the eyes based upon physiological principles, together with their symptoms, diagnosis and treatment. *Ann Ophthalmol Otolaryngol* 1896;5:969–1008.

52. Kushner BJ. Exotropic deviations: a functional classification and approach to treatment. *Am Ortho J* 1988;38:81–93.

53. Raab EL, Parks MM. Recession of the lateral recti. Early and late postoperative alignments. *Arch Ophthalmol* 1969; 82:203–208.

54. Olitsky SE. Early and late postoperative alignment following unilateral lateral rectus recession for intermittent exotropia. *J Pediatr Ophthalmol Strabismus* 1998;35:146–148.

55. Choi DG, Rosenbaum AL. Medial rectus resection(s) with adjustable suture for intermittent exotropia of the convergence insufficiency type. *J AAPOS* 2001;5:13–17.

56. Kraft SP, Levin AV, Enzenauer RW. Unilateral surgery for exotropia with convergence weakness. *J Pediatr Ophthalmol Strabismus* 1995;32:183–187.

57. Kushner BJ. The role of ocular torsion on the etiology of A and V patterns. *J Pediatr Ophthalmol Strabismus* 1985;22:171–179.

58. Miller MM, Guyton DL. Loss of fusion and the development of A or V patterns. *J Pediatr Ophthalmol Strabismus* 1994;31:220–224.

59. Velez FG, Thacker N, Britt MT, Alcorn D, Foster RS, Rosenbaum AL. Rectus muscle orbital wall fixation: a reversible profound weakening procedure. *J AAPOS* 2004;8:473–480.

60. Taylor JN. Surgical management of oculomotor nerve palsy with lateral rectus transplantation to the medial side of globe. *Aust N Z J Ophthalmol* 1989;17:27–31.

61. Sharma P, Gogoi M, Kedar S, Bhola R. Periosteal fixation in third-nerve palsy. *J AAPOS* 2006;10:324–327.

62. Parks MM. Isolated cyclovertical muscle palsy. *AMA Arch Ophthalmol* 1958;60:1027–1035.

63. Plager DA. Tendon laxity in superior oblique palsy. *Ophthalmology* 1992;99:1032–1038.

64. Harada M, Ito, Y. Surgical correction of cyclotropia. *Jpn J Ophthalmol* 1964;8:88–96.

65. Fells P. Management of paralytic strabismus. *Br J Ophthalmol* 1974;58:255–265.

66. Mitchell PR, Parks MM. Surgery of bilateral superior oblique palsy. *Ophthalmology* 1982;89:484–488.

67. Holmes JM, Beck RW, Kip KE, Droste PJ, Leske DA. Botulinum toxin treatment versus conservative management in acute traumatic sixth nerve palsy or paresis. *J AAPOS* 2000;4:145–149.

68. Brooks SE, Olitsky SE, de BRG. Augmented Hummelsheim procedure for paralytic strabismus. *J Pediatr Ophthalmol Strabismus* 2000;37:189–195; quiz 226–227.

69. Foster RS. Vertical muscle transposition augmented with lateral fixation. *J AAPOS* 1997;1:20–30.

70. Duane A. Congenital deficiency of abduction, associated with impairment of adduction, retraction movements, contraction of the palpebral fissure and oblique movements of the eye. *Arch Ophthalmol* 1905;34.

71. Huber A. Electrophysiology of the retraction syndromes. *Br J Ophthalmol* 1974;58:293–300.

72. Maruo T, Kusota N, Arimoto H. Duane's syndrome. *Jpn J Ophthalmol* 1979;23:453.

73. Breinin GM. Electromyography: a tool in ocular and neurologic diagnosis. II. Muscle palsies. *Arch Ophthalmol* 1957;57:165–175.

74. Mehendale RA, Dagi LR, Wu C, Ledoux D, Johnston S, Hunter DG. Superior rectus transposition and medial rectus recession for Duane syndrome and sixth nerve palsy. *Arch Ophthalmol* 2012;130:195–201.

75. Morad Y, Kraft SP, Mims JL 3rd. Unilateral recession and resection in Duane syndrome. *J AAPOS* 2001;5:158–163.

76. Brown HW. *Congenital structural anomalies*. St. Louis, MO: C. V. Mosby Co., 1950.

77. Brown HW. True and simulated superior oblique tendon sheath syndromes. *Aust J Ophthalmol* 1974;2:12–19.

78. Crawford JS. Surgical treatment of true Brown's syndrome. *Am J Ophthalmol* 1976;81:289–295.

79. Scott WE, Jackson OB. Double elevator palsy: the significance of inferior rectus restriction. *Am Orthopt J* 1977;27:5–10.

80. Knapp P. The surgical treatment of double-elevator paralysis. *Trans Am Ophthalmol Soc* 1969;67:304–323.

81. Pollard ZF. Diagnosis and treatment of inferior oblique palsy. *J Pediatr Ophthalmol Strabismus* 1993;30:15–18.

82. PJ M. Uber angeboren doppelseitige abducens-facialis-lahmung. *Munchen Medizinische Wochenschrift* 1888;35:3.

83. Baumgarten M. Erfahrungen uber den strabismus und die Muskeldurchschneidung am Auge in physiologischpathologischer und therapeutischer Beziehung. *Monatsschr Med Augenheilkd Chir* 1840;3(25):474–499.

84. Brown HW. *Congenital structural muscle anomalies*. In: Strabismus Ophthalmic Symposium. St. Louis, MO: C. V. Mosby Co., 1950.

85. Demer JL, Clark RA, Engle EC. Magnetic resonance imaging evidence for widespread orbital dysinnervation in congenital fibrosis of extraocular muscles due to mutations in KIF21A. *Invest Ophthalmol Vis Sci* 2005;46:530–539.

9

Conjunctival Diseases

Rudolph S. Wagner

CONJUNCTIVAL DISEASES

The conjunctiva is a durable mucous membrane composed of bulbar and palpebral components, which provides the primary barrier for protection of the eye. Making a definitive diagnosis for a pediatric patient presenting with signs and symptoms of disease in the conjunctiva can be challenging. This thin membrane is subject to neoplasms, vascular and structural abnormalities, environmental hazards, and is affected in many systemic diseases. Conjunctivitis in the pediatric patient can be mimicked by nasolacrimal duct obstruction and caused by allergies, bacteria, and viruses. Because antimicrobial cultures take time and are not always accurate, the diagnosis and treatment of conjunctivitis are often based on the physician's knowledge regarding the current literature on likely pathogens and clinical experience.

Structure and Function

The conjunctiva originates from the superficial ectoderm of the early embryonic disc, which also gives rise to skin, corneal epithelium, cilia, glands, lacrimal glands, and the nasolacrimal system (1). It is a translucent vascular mucous membrane that is rich in immune components. Being firmly attached to the eyelid along the tarsus (palpebral) starting at the mucocutaneous junction and terminating 1 mm anterior of the corneal limbus (bulbar), the conjunctiva forms a cul-de-sac with its contours, creating the fornices on the superior, inferior, and lateral boundaries. Medially the conjunctiva ends in the caruncle, which contains both skin and conjunctival elements. Tenon's capsule inserts into the bulbar conjunctiva and separates the conjunctiva from underlying tissues. Therefore, the bulbar and forniceal conjunctiva is only loosely attached to the posterior structures, including the levator and rectus muscle fascial tendon sheaths, allowing the motion of tissue upon eye and eyelid movement. The conjunctiva is also attached to the lower eyelid retractor muscles inferiorly and levator aponeurosis and Muller's muscle superiorly. These attachments, in addition to the connections with the canthal ligaments, trochlea, and lacrimal gland, maintain the "suspensory apparatus" (2).

On a cellular level, the conjunctiva is made up of nonkeratinized, stratified columnar epithelium overlying the highly vascular connective tissue, the substantia propria. The columnar cells transition to stratified squamous epithelium continuous with the corneal epithelium (3). Goblet cells populate the conjunctiva in an inferonasal preponderance and are found in greater numbers in children. Limbal stem cells and mucocutaneous junction cells go on to form the bulbar and palpebral epithelial cells. In disease states, the destruction or damage of the limbal stem cells, may allow the conjunctival epithelium to grow onto the cornea creating a pannus.

Mucin, aqueous, and outer lipid layers comprise the tear film. Conjunctival goblet cells produce the mucopolysaccharides that, along with vesicles from the palpebral epithelial cells, form the mucous layer of the tear film (4). The lacrimal and accessory lacrimal gland ducts open to the conjunctival surface and produce the aqueous layer with its multitude of immune factors. The outer lipid layer is produced by the meibomian glands and Zeis' glands. The lipid layer of the tear film is thicker in infants than in adults, with a longer tear breakup time (5). The proportion and interaction of these components create the stability of the tear film.

The conjunctiva protects the eye from pathogens by acting as a physical barrier and contributing immune components into the tear film. The immunologic function occurs in all layers of the conjunctiva: the superficial epithelial goblet cells creating immune protective mucin, the deeper epithelial basal layer infused with Langerhans' cells, and the substantia propria containing mast cells, plasma cells, and neutrophils. The temporal lymphatic vessels transport lymph to the superficial parotid nodes while the nasal vessels drain into the submandibular nodes.

Bulbar innervation is derived from the ophthalmic division of the trigeminal nerve via the long ciliary nerves, branches of the nasociliary nerve. Superior palpebral and forniceal innervation is from the frontal and lacrimal branches of the ophthalmic division of the trigeminal nerve. Inferior palpebral and forniceal innervation is from the lacrimal branch of the ophthalmic division of the trigeminal nerve laterally and from the infraorbital nerve in the maxillary division of the trigeminal nerve.

The bulbar conjunctiva thins with age and loses elasticity as does the subconjunctival connective tissue or Tenon's capsule. The posterior conjunctival arteries are smaller and

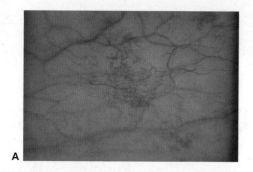

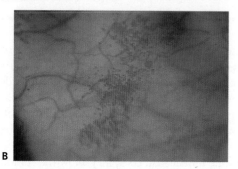

FIGURE 9.1. **(A)** Lissamine green versus rose bengal stain **(B)**.

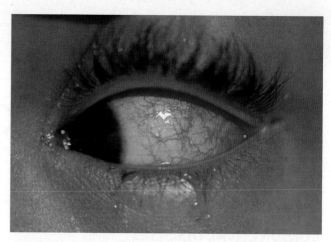

FIGURE 9.2. Actinic episcleritis with conjunctival vascular injection.

less tortuous in childhood. The combination of thinner, straighter blood vessels and a thicker Tenon's capsule create the whiter appearance of young conjunctiva.

Fluorescein is employed routinely to diagnose and differentiate inflammatory states as well as grossly quantitate the tear meniscus and breakup time. Rose bengal stain has been shown to stain damaged cells as well as cells with deficient mucous coating (6). Lissamine green dye stains dead or damaged epithelial cells, producing less stinging sensation than rose bengal (Fig. 9.1).

Pinguecula Pterygium and Actinic Episcleritis

Unlike adults, pinguecula and pterygium are rare in childhood. Children are subject to acute solar ultraviolet (UV) radiation however, which results in basophilic degeneration of the conjunctival substantia propria. Histologically, degeneration of the collagen fibers of the conjunctiva stroma with thinning of the overlying epithelium and occasional calcification occurs. Solar actinic exposure of the thin conjunctiva tissue results in fibroblasts producing more elastin fibers, but they are more twisted than normal, and may lead to the degradation of the collagen fibers. There is a marked decrease in normal elastin fibrils in these tissues (7). Clinically, these appear as a focal area of conjunctival vascular injection with underlying episcleritis (Fig. 9.2). At times, a fleshy elevated central area not contiguous with the limbus appears. Treatment includes lubricating drops and topical steroid.

Invasion of the cornea associated with Bowman's layer destruction by a triangular area of bulbar conjunctiva (pterygium) can disrupt the tear film by creating an area of local drying on the cornea or dellen. Pterygia have increased numbers of mast cells (7). Pseudopterygia, which are usually not firmly adherent to the underlying tissue, can occur following corneal surgery or an inflammatory condition. Removal can be accomplished, as in adults, although recurrence is common.

PIGMENTATION AND PIGMENTED LESIONS

Conjunctival Icterus

Bilirubin has a high affinity for elastin, which is an abundant protein in the conjunctiva as well as the superficial, fibrovascular episclera, but not the sclera proper. An accurate description of the yellow jaundiced appearance of the eyes frequently seen transiently in neonates and chronically in children with hemolytic disorders is conjunctival icterus (8).

Melanocytic Nevi

Nevi are pigmented lesions classified like those of the skin: intraepithelial (junctional), subepithelial, compound (intraepithelial plus subepithelial), blue, and cellular blue (rarely seen in conjunctiva) (9). In adults, most conjunctival nevi are compound or subepithelial. Only in children are the pure intraepithelial (junctional) type observed (10).

Histologically, especially in young individuals, cytologic pleomorphism can be present in conjunctival nevi. A junctional nevus may be indistinguishable from primary acquired melanosis with atypia, a condition of elderly individuals that has a tendency to evolve into melanoma. Large spindle or epithelioid-shaped melanocytes characteristic of Spitz nevi may mimic melanoma (11). Inclusions of conjunctival epithelium in the form of solid islands or cysts are usually observed (12). During puberty, several changes can occur in the conjunctival nevi: the melanocytes may

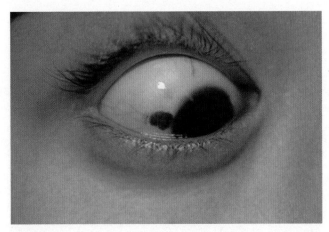

FIGURE 9.3. Nevus with typical inflammatory vascularization of conjunctiva.

proliferate or increase in pigmentation, and the epithelial cells within the inclusions may proliferate and secrete material, causing enlargement of the cysts. As the nevus becomes more prominent, it can cause irritation and inflammation. The inflammatory cell infiltrate can further increase the size, elevation, and vascularity of the nevus (Fig. 9.3). These alterations tend to provoke concern that a malignant melanoma has arisen from the nevus, resulting in excision of a large number of benign conjunctival nevi (9).

Nevus pigmentation is variable, with some devoid of pigment or amelanotic, requiring differentiation from other epithelial lesions. Occasionally, an inflamed nevus may become vascular and be mistaken for an angiomatous tumor (12).

Ocular Melanocytosis

Melanocytosis describes excessive melanotic pigmentation in the absence of a mass causing elevation of the conjunctiva that is typical of a nevus. Melanocytosis can be at the level of the conjunctiva or deeper in the sclera, choroid, or periocular tissues. Heterochromia may be present secondary to diffuse darkly pigmented micropapillae on the iris surface in place of iris crypts.

Epithelial congenital melanocytosis is a stationary lesion present at birth or early childhood. The lesions appear as irregular geographic patches of sclera and episcleral pigmentation that can range from distinct brown to gray in color. It is characterized by melanocytes and excessive melanin mainly in the basal layers of the conjunctival epithelium. It is not a precursor of malignant melanoma (9). Technically, the subepithelial congenital melanocytosis is not a lesion of the conjunctiva, because the abnormal melanocytes are found in the sclera and episclera. The overlying conjunctiva can be moved over the lesion without distorting it (13). There are two forms: (a) "ocular melanocytosis," affecting ocular tissues only, and (b) "oculodermal melanocytosis," or nevus of Ota, associated with ipsilateral melanosis of the lids or periocular facial skin. Most of the cases are unilateral and

ipsilateral iris hyperpigmentation can be observed (14). It is more frequently seen in Asians and African descendants than in Caucasians (15,16) and may also be associated with melanosis of the orbital tissues and the meninges (10). Histologically, nevus of Ota is characterized by a congenital increase in the number, size, and pigmentation of the melanocytes of the uvea associated with increased numbers of pigmented melanocytes in the sclera, episclera, and dermis of the eyelids. Subepithelial congenital melanosis predisposes to the development of malignant melanoma (17,18). Children with oculodermal melanocytosis should be examined periodically because of a risk of pigmentary glaucoma and melanoma (19). Patients with ocular melanosis may also benefit from surveillance of the intraocular pressure (20) (Fig. 9.4). Some children with oculodermal melanocytosis may have pigmented lesions on the tongue and buccal mucosa (13).

Some syndromes and diseases may present with pigmented conjunctival lesions during their course, such as: (a) chronic forms of Gaucher's disease; (b) alkaptonuria, in which the pigmentation can be seen over the horizontal recti insertion; (c) Kartagener's syndrome, with characteristically marked conjunctival melanosis and hypertropia of the plica semilunaris; and (d) Peutz-Jegher's syndrome, in which freckles can be seen over the conjunctiva, lids, and lips (21).

Gaucher's Disease

Gaucher's disease, found most commonly among Ashkenazic Jews, is a hepatorenal syndrome caused by enzyme deficiency of glucocerebrosidase, and is characterized by pinguecula-like lesions, corneal epithelial deposits, vitreous deposits, paramacular ring, white retinal infiltrates, oculomotor apraxia, hepatosplenomegaly, pancytopenia secondary to hypersplenism, bone pain, and accumulation of glucocerebroside. The pinguecula-like lesions can often be differentiated by their tan coloring and histologically contain Gaucher's cells, enlarged lipid-laden macrophages. These lesions usually appear during the teenage years. The gene locus has been found on Chromosome 1.

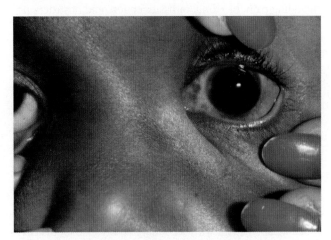

FIGURE 9.4. Ocular melanocytosis; congenital glaucoma.

Alkaptonuria/Ochronosis

Alkaptonuria/ochronosis is a rare disorder of protein metabolism resulting in wasting of homogentisic acid in the urine. An enzyme deficiency of homogentisate-1,2-dioxygenase (ochronosis) results in the accumulation of homogentisic acid. The gene locus has been identified on chromosome 3q21–q23 and is inherited in an autosomal recessive fashion. This leads to pigment deposition in collagenous tissues. The manifestations are pigmented pinguecula, triangular scleral pigmentation near the horizontal rectus muscle insertions, episcleral pigment granules, oil-droplet opacities in the limbal corneal epithelium and Bowman's layer, ochronotic arthropathy, ochronotic calculi in the genitourinary tract, and cardiovascular deposition, including calcification and stenosis in the aortic valve. Treatment is palliative.

Kartagener's Syndrome

Kartagener's syndrome was first described by Siewert in 1904 and later further characterized in the German literature by Kartagener in 1933. It is caused by mutations in the gene encoding the axonemal dynein intermediate chain. It is a rare syndrome associated with *situs inversus* (dextrocardia) and primary ciliary dyskinesia, leading to bronchiectasis and sinusitis. Conjunctival melanosis, hypertrophy of the semilunaris, myopia, and glaucoma have been described.

Peutz-Jegher's Syndrome

Peutz-Jegher's syndrome was initially described by Peutz, a Dutch internist, in 1921, as a familial syndrome. It is caused by mutations in the serine/threonine kinase STK11 gene chromosome locus 19p13.3. Peutz-Jegher's syndrome is characterized by periocular and perioral melanocytic epidermal lesions (freckle-like appearance) in association with gastrointestinal polyps, usually of the small intestine. The macules present mainly on the lips and buccal mucosa but can appear on the palms, soles, and conjunctiva. The hyperpigmented macules precede the onset of gastrointestinal symptoms, including pain, bleeding, intussusception, and obstruction.

TUMORS AND INFILTRATES

Choristomas

Dermoids are the most common choristomas, lesions composed of tissue not normally found in the affected area. These solid, placoid tumors arise from the outer third of the sclera and often contain hair follicles, sebaceous glands, sweat glands, and fat lobules. Commonly occurring at the inferotemporal limbus, they appear as yellowish-white rounded elevations that are sometimes pigmented (Fig. 9.5). Most dermoids do not cause any discomfort but may produce significant astigmatism with secondary amblyopia. Ocular irritation may result from poor lid closure, tear film anomaly, or trauma from the fine hair that may grow from the surface of

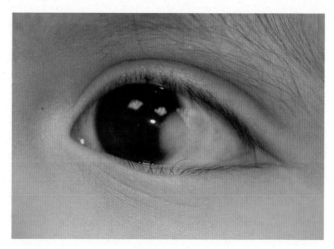

FIGURE 9.5. Limbal epibulbar dermoid choristoma.

these lesions. Dermolipomas are more posterior and are associated with a large amount of fatty tissue. Usually, they arise near the insertion of the lateral rectus and are firmly fixed to the underlying sclera. Rarely, they can form symblepharon-type adhesions, causing restriction of eye movement.

Dermoids and dermolipomas may be present with other systemic malformations, including Goldenhar's syndrome (facio-auricular vertebral syndrome), mandibulofacial dysostosis (Treacher Collins syndrome, Franceschetti's syndrome), and band-like cutaneous nevus and central nervous system dysfunction (Solomon's syndrome, linear sebaceous nevus of Jadassohn). Both tend to grow with the patient and do not usually undergo neoplastic transformation.

Treatment is generally conservative. However, removal is indicated when significant astigmatism, with or without amblyopia, irritation, or cosmetic deformity, occurs. Lamellar excision is usually required because the outer third of the sclera is often involved. When the cornea is more involved, the surgeon should anticipate lamellar or penetrating keratoplasty. Complications of the excision include globe penetration, restriction to motility from scarring or injury of the associated rectus muscle, and increased astigmatism.

Other choristomas include ectopic lacrimal gland, simple and composed choristoma, and osseous choristoma. Ectopic lacrimal gland is the second most common choristoma affecting the epibulbar surface. Osseous choristomas are stationary lesions that resemble conjunctival dermoids; histologically, however, they are composed of mature compact bone surrounded by other choristomatous elements (22,23).

Children with the Organoid Nevus Syndrome present a birth with unilateral or bilateral epibulbar choristomas and raised linear or round lesions on the scalp containing sebaceous skin components (Fig. 9.6). Originally termed "nevus sebaceous of Jadassohn," the skin lesions are now appropriately called organoid nevi because of the breadth of skin abnormalities they include. The most consistent ocular manifestations are epibulbar complex choristomas and posterior scleral cartilaginous choristomas. The epibulbar choristoma

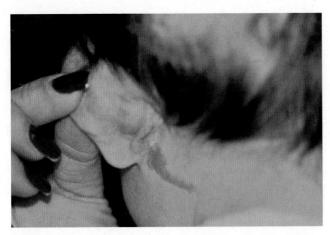

FIGURE 9.6. Posterior scalp and ear of child with organoid nevus syndrome with linear sebaceous nevus.

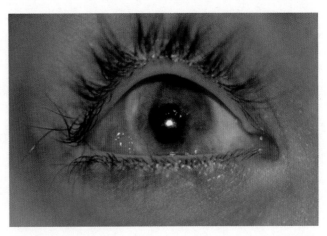

FIGURE 9.8. Progressive infiltration of the cornea by choristoma in organoid nevus syndrome.

is a fleshy pink lesion originating in the bulbar conjunctiva and may contain ectopic lacrimal gland tissue, fat cartilage, bone, nerve, and smooth muscle (Fig. 9.7). The choristoma may grow into the cornea in a progressive pattern after birth, causing partial or complete opacification (Fig. 9.8). These may prove difficult to excise (24).

Hamartomas

Hamartomas are lesions composed of tissue found normally in the affected area. Neurofibromas are solid nodular lesions affecting the bulbar or palpebral conjunctiva. They can be plexiform, solitary, or diffuse type and are almost always associated with neurofibromatosis type 1 or type 2. Type 2B multiple endocrine neoplasia (MEN) is associated with medullary thyroid carcinoma and pheochromocytoma. Ocular abnormalities include mucosal neuroma located on the conjunctiva at the limbus and on the palpebral conjunctiva proximal to the eyelid margin. Prominent medullated corneal nerves occur in 100% of cases. These patients have a marfanoid

habitus including the findings of a high-arched palate, pectus excavatum, bilateral pes cavus, and scoliosis. Neuromas on the eyelids, conjunctiva, nasal and laryngeal mucosa, tongue, and lips are frequent findings. The conjunctival neuromas and neurofibromas appear as yellow-gray sessile or dome-shaped masses located in the stroma. Patients also have prominent, hypertrophied lips leading to a characteristic facial appearance. The male-to-female ratio for MEN is 2:1. The disease may appear in children younger than 10 years. However, all MEN syndromes are rare in children (13).

Fibrous hamartomas are epibulbar lesions that contain abundant mature elastic fibers intermixed with fibrous tissue. They may be seen in patients with Proteus syndrome, a rare syndrome characterized by asymmetrical overgrowth that can affect any structure (bones, skin, viscera) and is generally progressive throughout childhood.

Another hamartomatous lesion that affects the conjunctiva is hemorrhagic lymphangiectasia. These lesions are irregularly dilated lymphatic channels of the bulbar conjunctiva that may sometimes be filled with blood. They may arise as a developmental anomaly or in association with trauma or inflammation (22,23).

Conjunctival Cysts

Conjunctival cysts are stable lesions that can be congenital or acquired. A common cause of acquired conjunctival inclusion cysts is the implantation of conjunctival epithelium islands after surgery or trauma. They may disappear spontaneously, but persistent cases often require surgical excision or diathermy (22).

Pyogenic Granuloma

Pyogenic granuloma is a vasoproliferative inflammatory response composed of granulation tissue. The term "pyogenic granuloma" is a misnomer. The lesion neither causes pus formation nor is a true granuloma. The pathogenesis is

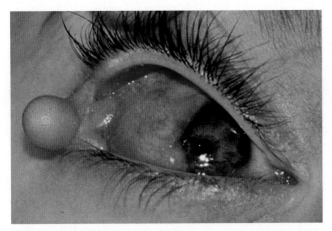

FIGURE 9.7. Epibulbar complex choristoma with skin pedicle containing bone and cartilage in organoid nevus syndrome.

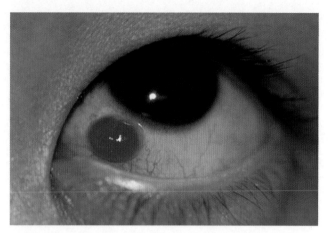

FIGURE 9.9. Post strabismus surgery pyogenic granuloma.

not well understood, but they can develop rapidly and are often associated with previous ocular and adnexal surgery, inflammation, foreign bodies, chemical burns, or phthisis bulbi. Following strabismus surgery these lesions may occur near the sutured margin of the conjunctiva. Spontaneous involution can occur or, if necessary, simple excisional biopsy with cautery of the base can be both diagnostic and curative (22) (Fig. 9.9).

Xeroderma Pigmentosa Syndrome

This disease is a rare autosomal recessive disorder that manifests as an inability to repair deoxyribonucleic acid damage induced by UV radiation. Clinically, this syndrome is characterized by the early development of pigmentary changes, atrophy, keratoses, and skin malignancies (carcinomas, melanomas, sarcomas, angiosarcomas, neuromas), predominantly on light-exposed skin. Some patients may present with recurrent conjunctivitis, dry eyes with areas of pigment deposition and keratin formation, as well as squamous cell carcinomas of the conjunctiva. The syndrome is sometimes associated with slowly progressive neurologic abnormalities that include deafness, ataxia, mental retardation, and cerebellar atrophy. Most patients die of malignancy before age 20 (25). Treatment is avoidance of sunlight and UV exposure by use of sunblock and 100% UV-barrier spectacles with sidearms (23).

Benign Hereditary Epithelial Dyskeratosis

This is a rare disorder that affects primarily members of the Haliwa Indians (Halifax and Washington counties of North Carolina). It is an autosomal dominant disorder with high penetrance characterized by bilateral elevated plaques in the exposed areas of the conjunctiva. Benign hereditary epithelial dyskeratosis has a chronic course of ocular irritation/photophobia and may be associated with dyskeratosis of the oral mucosa. Histologically, the lesions show epithelial acanthosis, parakeratosis, and dyskeratosis, with the stroma

usually containing chronic inflammatory cells. Atypia is absent, and there is no dysplastic potential. Treatment of choice is excision of the lesions, although the recurrence rate is high (22,23).

VASCULAR ABNORMALITIES

Hemangiomas are lesions composed predominantly of blood vessels and may occur as isolated lesions or in association with lid, orbital, or intracranial lesions. Clinically, they appear as red masses on the conjunctival surface and blanch on pressure. Spontaneous hemorrhage is not infrequent and may occur after trivial trauma. Surgical excision is difficult, and recurrences may occur. The surface vasculature in capillary hemangiomas involutes following the application of topical timolol 0.5% in some cases (26).

Lymphangiomas are usually widespread, occasionally affecting an entire hemiface. Clinically, these lesions show clear fluid-filled cystic areas among the blood-filled hemangioma tissue (Fig. 9.10). Surgical excision is difficult due to the diffuse nature of the lesions (13).

Several syndromes can have conjunctival vascular abnormalities among their features. The characteristic feature of Sturge-Weber syndrome is a cutaneous hemangioma, commonly in a trigeminal facial distribution, with the conjunctiva showing only a faint blush on the normal whiteness of the conjunctiva. Klippel-Trenaunay-Weber syndrome, a widespread vascular anomaly causing limb hypertrophy and vascular anomalies of skin, may also have conjunctival angiomas. Conjunctival vascular malformations may be seen associated with racemose angiomatous malformation of the retina in Wyburn-Mason syndrome. Louis-Bar syndrome or ataxia telangiectasia (AT) is an autosomal recessive disorder that presents with a progressive ataxia and degeneration of central nervous system function (choreoathetosis, dysrhythmic speech, aberrant ocular movements and occasional seizures) and presence of extremely tortuous and telangiectatic conjunctival vessels without an associ-

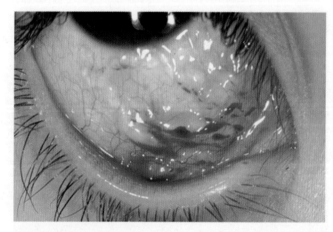

FIGURE 9.10. Lymphangioma with clear fluid-filled cystic areas among the blood-filled hemangioma tissue.

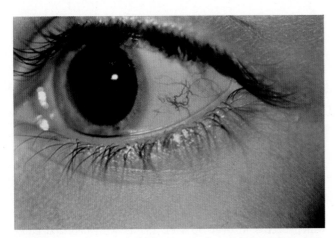

FIGURE 9.11. Tortuous and telangiectatic conjunctival vessels in ataxia telangiectasia (AT).

ated lymphatic component in exposed areas of conjunctiva and skin (Fig. 9.11). In Rendu-Osler-Weber syndrome, conjunctival telangiectases may be seen along with retinal vascular malformation (13).

CONJUNCTIVITIS OF THE NEWBORN

Neonatal conjunctivitis is inflammation of the conjunctiva that affects infants during the first month after birth. It is usually a hyperacute papillary conjunctivitis, because a follicular response is not seen before 6 to 8 weeks of life (27).

The period of time after birth until the onset of the conjunctivitis is variable, but it may be helpful in suggesting the cause by correlating it to the incubation time of the possible etiologic agents.

When the conjunctivitis affects the baby in the first few days after birth, the probable cause is the toxic effect of the prophylactic agent used at birth. It is characterized by mild and transient conjunctival injection and tearing, which usually resolves in 24 to 48 hours. This was more common when silver nitrate was used for prophylaxis.

Conjunctivitis due to *Neisseria gonorrhoeae* typically appears 2 to 5 days after birth. It is still common in developing countries but rare in the most industrialized countries. Clinically, it starts with a serosanguineous discharge that rapidly progresses to a thick purulent discharge associated with markedly edematous eyelids and chemosis. Conjunctival membranes may be seen. This bacteria has the propensity to produce a severe keratitis because of its ability to penetrate intact epithelial cells and replicate rapidly. A delay in diagnosis and treatment may lead to corneal ulceration and perforation.

Historically, the latent period for bacterial conjunctivitis, other than *N. gonorrhoeae* has been 5 to 8 days after birth, but it can occur any time in the immediate postpartum period. Etiologic agents include: *Haemophilus sp.*, *Streptococcus pneumoniae*, *Staphylococcus aureus*, and rarely, *Pseudomonas aeruginosa*. Although rare, this bacteria can rapidly progress from

conjunctivitis to corneal ulceration and perforation. If *Pseudomonas* is not recognized as the etiologic agent, the conjunctival infection may lead to endophthalmitis and possible death.

Chlamydia trachomatis serotype D-K, causing neonatal inclusion conjunctivitis represents the most common isolated pathogen in newborns with conjunctivitis in industrialized countries. The incubation period ranges from 5 to 14 days. Clinically, one sees a mild mucopurulent conjunctivitis associated with moderate lid swelling and mild chemosis typically beginning as unilateral but often becoming bilateral (Fig. 9.12). Although generally considered benign and self-limited with spontaneous resolution in 8 to 12 months, if untreated it may result in the formation of a micropannus and scarring of the tarsal conjunctiva. Systemic spread of this ocular infection can cause disease involving the pharynx, lungs, and/or rectum, which can be fatal. The systemic potential of this disease dictates the need for systemic treatment, generally with a macrolide antibiotic.

Viral neonatal conjunctivitis caused by Herpes simplex virus (HSV) typically occurs within 6 to 14 days afterbirth. Although 80% of the babies affected with HSV have typical herpetic lesions on the skin, eyelids, or mouth, without these lesions the conjunctivitis is indistinguishable from other causes of neonatal conjunctivitis. Signs of corneal involvement include microdendrites or geographical ulcers. Herpetic keratoconjunctivitis is frequently associated with systemic infection, with mortality rates of disseminated disease around 50%.

A less frequent cause of neonatal conjunctivitis is *Candida albicans*. It presents as a pseudomembranous conjunctivitis, with the average time of onset of 5 days after exposure.

Congenital nasolacrimal duct obstruction is also frequently associated with conjunctivitis of the newborn typically caused by *Haemophilus sp.* and *S. pneumoniae*.

Clinically, these differentiation among the various etiologies can be difficult. However, because of the potentially serious complications of an improperly treated conjunctivitis, determination of the causative agent is recommended

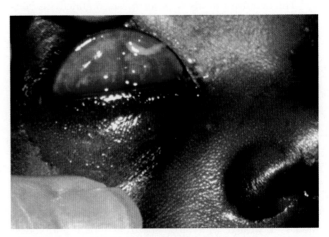

FIGURE 9.12. Neonatal inclusion conjunctivitis caused by *Chlamydia trachomatis* with pseudomembrane formation.

at this age. Conjunctival smears and appropriate cultures should be done in all patients. Scrapings of the conjunctiva should be collected with a spatula and cultures obtained with a calcium-alginate swab, prewetted with sterile liquid culture media. Gram and Giemsa stains should be performed on the conjunctival scraping. Giemsa stain in chemical conjunctivitis shows neutrophils with occasional lymphocytes; in chlamydial infection, neutrophils, lymphocytes, plasma cells, and basophilic intracytoplasmic inclusions in epithelial cells; in viral conjunctivitis, lymphocytes, plasma cells, multinucleated giant cells, and eosinophilic intranuclear inclusions; in fungal infections, neutrophils, and pseudohyphal budding yeast formation; and in bacterial infections, neutrophils, and bacteria. Certain bacteria can be identified on Gram stain. Gram-negative diplococci with polymorphonuclear leucocytes suggest gonococcal infection; Gram-negative coccobacilli correlate with *Haemophilus sp.*; Gram-positive cocci suggest *S. aureus* and *S. pneumoniae.* Recommended medias for culture include: reduced blood agar, thioglycolate, brainheart infusion broth for aerobic bacteria; chocolate agar in CO_2 or Thayer-Martin for *N. gonorrhoeae;* Sabouraud's slant for fungus. McCoy cell culture has been the standard for diagnosing *C. trachomatis* in the past, but this technique is expensive and requires at least 2 to 3 days for results. Polymerase chain reaction (PCR) analysis and direct immunofluorescent monoclonal antibody stain (DFA) have comparable specificity with higher sensitivities and faster results than traditional culture testing. Viral cultures are expensive and take 2 to 4 days to grow. Viral antigens can be detected rapidly, using immunologic tests, such as direct immunofluorescent testing, enzyme-linked immunosorbent assay (ELISA), and immunofiltration method.

Treatment is not required for chemical conjunctivitis caused by prophylactic agents, which typically resolves spontaneously in 24 to 48 hours. According to the World Health Organization (WHO) guidelines, all cases of conjunctivitis in the newborn should be treated for both *N. gonorrhoeae* and *C. trachomatis* because of the possibility of mixed infection.

The treatment of the *N. gonorrhoeae* conjunctivitis consists of intravenous Penicillin G 100,000 units/kg/day for 7 days. *N. gonorrhoeae* resistant to penicillin is found in many urban areas in the United States and worldwide. In this case, the conjunctivitis should be treated with a third-generation cephalosporin. A single intramuscular dose of ceftriaxone 125 mg is highly effective and is the recommended treatment by WHO guidelines (28–30). Intravenous or intramuscular cefotaxime 25 mg/kg every 8 to 12 hours is also effective. In addition to antibiotics, hourly irrigation of the eyes of the infant with gonococcal conjunctivitis with saline is recommended to decrease the intracorneal sequelae. Most ophthalmologists will supplement with topical antibiotic therapy.

Nongonococcal, nonchlamydial bacterial conjunctivitis should be treated with broad-spectrum topical antibiotics. Gram-positive cocci are appropriately treated with tetracycline 1% or erythromycin 0.5% ointment every 4 hours for 7 days. Gram-negative bacilli may be treated with tobramycin 0.3% or ciprofloxacin 0.3% ointment every 4 hours for 7 days (31).

The WHO and American Academy of Pediatrics recommend erythromycin syrup, 50 mg/kg/day orally, in 4 divided doses for 14 days, as treatment for neonatal chlamydial conjunctivitis (32). Although there is no evidence that additional therapy with a topical agent provides further benefit, erythromycin 0.5% ointment 4 times a day is often added. If inclusion conjunctivitis recurs after therapy has been completed, erythromycin treatment should be reinstituted for 2 weeks. Oral erythromycin also treats chlamydial pneumonitis and eradicates nasopharyngeal colonization, which occurs in over 50% of infants with neonatal chlamydial conjunctivitis.

All suspected herpetic simplex infections should be treated with systemic acyclovir or vidarabine to reduce the chance of a systemic infection. An effective acyclovir dose is 30 mg/kg/day, intravenous, divided in 3 doses for 14 days, but higher doses may also be used (45 to 60 mg/kg/day). Infants with HSV keratoconjunctivitis should also receive a topical drug, trifluorothymidine 1% drops or vidarabine 3% ointment for 7 days, or until the cornea has reepithelialized.

Although rare, fungal infection may occur. Treatment should be with natamycin 5% drops or flucytosine 1% drops hourly for 10 to 14 days.

Neonatal conjunctivitis has been a major health problem in many parts of the world for centuries. At the end of the 19th century in Europe, for example, the prevalence of *Ophthalmia neonatorum* among live births in maternity hospitals exceeded 10%, producing corneal damage in 20% and blindness in approximately 3% of affected infants (33). For this reason, ocular prophylaxis is mandatory and widely accepted. Eye prophylaxis involves cleaning the eyes immediately after birth and applying drops or ointment within the first hour of birth. This prophylaxis should be directed primarily against gonococcal ophthalmia because this agent poses the greatest risk of eye injury. The three most frequently applied agents are erythromycin 0.5% ointment, 1% silver nitrate drops, and tetracycline 1% ointment (3). Prophylaxis with erythromycin has resulted in outbreaks of erythromycin-resistant staphylococcal conjunctivitis in neonates (34). Because the most dreaded pathogen of *O. neonatorum* is *N. gonorrhoeae,* the many reports of tetracycline resistance from such countries as the United Kingdom (35), the Netherlands (36), and the United States (37) are alarming. Tetracycline is thus no longer recommended as first-line therapy for gonococcal infections (38). *O. neonatorum* has occurred also after the use of silver nitrate (39,40). Isenberg et al., in 1994, showed that povidone-iodine 2.5% was more effective than silver nitrate or erythromycin against the conjunctival bacteria found in 100 healthy newborns and was less toxic than silver nitrate. It is also active against viruses, at least in vitro, including herpes simplex (41). In another report, Isenberg et al. (42) showed that erythromycin and silver nitrate were not superior to povidone-iodine against any other bacteria encountered in the study. Because of the broad spectrum and exceedingly low cost of povidone-iodine, this agent may become the most widely used for ocular prophylaxis in the future.

ACUTE CONJUNCTIVITIS

Conjunctivitis refers to any inflammatory condition of the conjunctival lining of the eyelids and the exposed surface of the sclera. It is the most common cause of "red or pink eye" and is characterized by cellular infiltration, exudation, and vascular dilation. Chemosis is frequently present. The etiology can usually be determined by a careful history, an ocular examination and knowledge of the most likely pathogens. Cultures or other diagnostic tests are occasionally necessary to establish the diagnosis or to guide therapy.

Five morphologic conjunctival responses can be recognized with slit lamp examination. These are papillary, follicular, membranous/pseudomembranous, cicatrizing, or granulomatous reactions.

Papillae are a nonspecific sign of conjunctival inflammation resulting from edema and polymorphonuclear cell infiltration into the conjunctiva. They are characterized by projections of hypertrophic epithelium that contain a central fibrovascular core whose blood vessels arborize on reaching the surface. True papillae can form only where the conjunctiva is attached to the underlying tissue by anchoring septae, such as over the tarsus or the bulbar limbus. Giant papillae that develop from breakdown of the fine, fibrous strands that make up the anchoring septae are found most commonly in the upper tarsal conjunctiva.

Follicles are discrete round elevations of the conjunctiva produced by a lymphocytic response. The central portion is avascular with blood vessels sweeping up over the convexity from the base. Follicles may be seen in normal conjunctiva, especially temporally in young patients.

Membranes are composed primarily of fibrin that coagulates on the epithelial surface. True membranes are adherent to the underlying epithelium and therefore cause bleeding when debrided. This characteristic differentiates them from nonbleeding pseudomembranes. True membranes represent more intense conjunctival inflammation and may lead to conjunctival scarring.

Cicatricial changes occur only when there is destruction of the stromal tissue. An injury to the conjunctival epithelium does not necessarily lead to scar formation. Cicatrization may cause shortening of the conjunctival fornix and subepithelial fibrosis. Subconjunctival scarring may cause complications, including symblepharon, cicatricial entropion, trichiasis, and in severe cases, obliteration of the conjunctival fornix, keratinization of the epithelium, and fusion of the eyelids (ankyloblepharon).

Granulomas always affect the conjunctival stroma. They may be found in sarcoidosis, related to a retained foreign body or in Parinaud's oculoglandular syndrome.

Papillary Conjunctivitis

Most cases of acute papillary conjunctivitis are bacterial. Recognition of papules at slit lamp examination is often used as the deciding factor for prescribing a topical antibiotic.

N. gonorrhoeae and *Neisseria meningitidis* cause a hyperacute conjunctivitis, with a rapidly progressive course and purulent discharge. This starts usually as a unilateral disease but may rapidly affect the fellow eye. As noted earlier, these aggressive bacteria may also invade intact corneal epithelium and cause corneal ulceration that can lead to corneal perforation in untreated or poorly treated cases. *N. gonorrhoeae* occurs most often in sexually active patients but may be observed occasionally in young children who are the victims of sexual abuse. Rarely, *N. gonorrhoeae* may be transmitted innocently to toddlers who live in close contact with an infected adult (43). It has been suggested that unlike gonococcal infection at other locations, a nonsexual mode of transmission may exist in the eye (44). Although relatively rare, conjunctivitis by *N. meningitidis* has important implications because the conjunctiva is a potential portal of entry leading to meningococcemia and meningitis (45). Diagnosis with Gram stain and culture is mandatory because of the systemic implications. Gram stain will show Gram-negative diplococci. Culture should be done in chocolate agar media with 4% to 8% CO_2 environment. These bacterial infections should be treated with topical and systemic antibiotics. When *N. gonorrhoeae* is isolated, parents of the child with conjunctivitis should be referred for evaluation and treatment. If *N. meningitidis* is identified, close contacts must be treated with a prophylactic oral antibiotic, such as rifampin.

Acute conjunctivitis, the most common ocular infection in childhood, usually affects children younger than 6 years with a peak incidence between 12 and 36 months. Pediatric acute conjunctivitis is diagnosed by clinical signs of purulent ocular discharge, matting of the lids, and/or hyperemia of the bulbar conjunctiva (Fig. 9.13). In children less than 3 years of age, many cases will have hyperemia of the bulbar conjunctiva as the only sign but will grow pathogens. In children under age 2, nasolacrimal duct obstruction can be differentiated from acute conjunctivitis by the absence of hyperemia unless secondarily infected. The etiology of this infection has been documented as bacterial in most (up to 80%) pediatric cases (46,47). Acute conjunctivitis also has a rapid onset, less severe than the *Neisseria sp.* conjunctivitis. Bilateral disease is common with the second eye becoming affected within 1 week after the first symptoms appear. The most common pathogens are *Haemophilus influenza* (non-typeable) *S. pneumoniae, S. aureus,* and anaerobic bacteria (48–50). Non-typeable (non-encapsulated) *S. pneumoniae*

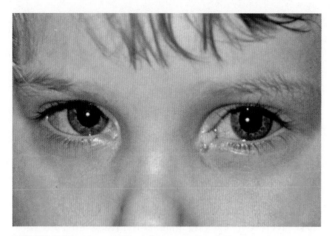

FIGURE 9.13. *Haemophilus influenza* conjunctivitis.

has been implicated in causing outbreaks of conjunctivitis in preschool-aged children and college-aged students (51,52). The same organism causing conjunctivitis in dissimilar age groups substantiates the fact that acute bacterial conjunctivitis occurs in older children and young adults. In the past, such epidemics were usually considered to be caused by adenoviruses. Community-acquired MRSA (methicillin resistant *S. aureus*) has not been implicated as a cause of acute bacterial conjunctivitis in children at this time. Cases of MRSA conjunctivitis in adults are being reported with increasing frequency, so children may be infected (53).

Acute bacterial conjunctivitis is essentially a clinical diagnosis made by observation of signs and symptoms. Most of the cases are self-limited, and symptoms generally subside in about 10 days, even without treatment. However, clinical differentiation between bacterial and other causes of acute conjunctivitis can be difficult (48,54). Laboratory cultures are expensive, time-consuming and should usually be reserved for cases refractory to treatment, severe conjunctivitis, and cases suspected to be caused by *N. gonorrhoeae* and *N. meningitidis*. In a recent prospective observational cohort study at an urban pediatric emergency department, bacterial cultures were isolated from 64.7% of the 368 patients enrolled in the study. *H. influenzae* accounted for 67.6% of positive cultures, *S. pneumoniae* for 19.7%, and *S. aureus* for 8.0% (55). This study investigated how it might be determined when conjunctivitis is not likely to be of bacterial etiology. They found four factors that were likely to be associated with cultures that were negative for bacteria:

- ≥6 years of age
- Presentation in April through November
- Watery or no discharge
- No glued eye in the morning

In this study, 92.2% of patients with all of these factors had cultures that were negative for bacteria and 76.4% of those with 3 factors had negative cultures. These data can help physicians in deciding whether or how to treat a patient in some cases.

Treatment utilizing topical antibiotics with broad-spectrum coverage and low toxicity is recommended. Treatment geared to the most rapid eradication of organisms should be used as first-line treatment, especially considering that bacterial conjunctivitis is usually first encountered by the primary care physician. Newer generation topical fluoroquinolones have been shown to shorten the course of the disease compared to some older antibiotics (56). Short courses of bacteriocidal broad-spectrum antibiotics for bacterial conjunctivitis are unlikely to cause the formation of resistant organisms (57). Moreover, shortening the course of a bacterial conjunctivitis decreases morbidity and allows prompt return to work for the parents and to school or day care provisions for the child. By utilizing an antibiotic expected to work quickly, more worrisome diseases, like herpes, will be unmasked. Systemic antibiotics are rarely used for the treatment of uncomplicated acute conjunctivitis.

In 1982, Bodor (58) brought attention to a clinical syndrome characterized by the combination of conjunctivitis and otitis media: conjunctivitis-otitis media syndrome. This disease usually begins with a low-grade fever and mild respiratory symptoms, including cough and mucopurulent nasal discharge. Simultaneous conjunctival and middle ear exudate cultures have shown concordance (59). *H. influenza* is the most common pathogen, in up to 90% of cases, followed by *S. pneumoniae* (48,58–61). Treatment should first consist of systemic antibiotics, with topical therapy added when the ocular signs and symptoms are extensive (61,62).

Follicular Conjunctivitis

The most common causes of acute follicular conjunctivitis are viral infections. The early phase of chlamydial inclusion conjunctivitis and some topical medications may also present with the same clinical signs.

Adenovirus is by far the most common viral pathogen (48). Adenoviral eye infection can manifest itself in many forms ranging from conjunctivitis that is often self-limiting to keratitis, which can be prolonged. Disease severity similarly can be mild to severely disabling. The usual source of spread is via droplet, person-to-person contact, contaminated ophthalmic instruments, or swimming water. The two most common forms of adenoviral infection are pharyngoconjunctival fever (PCF) and epidemic keratoconjunctivitis (EKC).

EKC is a highly contagious infection that is caused by adenovirus serotypes 8, 11, and 19. Clinical symptoms are typically seen 8 days after contact and include: rapid onset of watery discharge, injection of the conjunctiva, ocular discomfort associated with a foreign body sensation, and mild photophobia. Infection is often bilateral with involvement of the second eye 3 to 7 days after the first. In severe cases, petechial hemorrhages, pseudomembranes, and even true membranes may be present. Associated findings include lid edema and preauricular adenopathy. Conjunctivitis usually resolves in 10 to 14 days, but secondary corneal involvement may last weeks longer. Approximately 1 week after onset, focal epithelial keratitis can coalesce into larger, coarse, epithelial infiltrates with irregular grey-white dots, eventually progressing to the subepithelial layers with increased photophobia and potentially decreased vision. The infiltrates, a delayed hypersensitivity reaction, gradually fade over weeks or months but can persist for years.

PCF is an acute follicular conjunctivitis associated with pharyngitis and fever. It is caused by adenovirus serotypes 3, 4, and 7 and affects children more than adults. Clinical symptoms are similar to those present in EKC. Membrane formation is unusual, and corneal involvement is limited to punctate keratitis. Subepithelial infiltrates are rare (Fig. 9.14).

Treatment for EKC and PCF is palliative and may include compresses, lubrication, topical vasoconstrictors, and cycloplegic drops. Topical steroids are effective in relieving the signs and symptoms of the subepithelial infiltrates; however, the clinical result is probably the same, and weaning may be difficult. Most clinicians limit steroid use to patients who have marked visual changes or in those patients who are unable to perform normal activities. Topical steroids can produce elevation of the intraocular pressure and worsen cases of herpes simplex keratoconjunctivitis.

An antigen-based immunoassay using a direct-sampling microfiltration is available to rapidly confirm the diagnosis of adenoviral conjunctivitis. A Dacron coated sampling tip is dabbed directly on the conjunctiva and provides a positive or negative test result within in 10 minutes (63). The accurate diagnosis of viral conjunctivitis can avoid the prescribing of costly but ineffective topical antibiotics in some cases. Clinical trials for the treatment of adenovirus conjunctivitis with cidofovir are underway (64,65). If effective, this would represent an advance in treating this pathogen, which produces significant ocular morbidity (66).

Many other viruses can cause an acute follicular conjunctivitis and include: HSV, Epstein-Barr virus, *Paramyxoviridae* (measles, mumps, Newcastle disease), *Picornaviridae* (enterovirus, Coxsackie virus), *Orthomyxoviridae* (influenza virus), *Togaviridae* (rubella, arbovirus), and *Poxviridae* (variola, vaccinia).

Acute conjunctivitis caused by HSV is frequently associated with periocular vesicular lesions. Primary HSV infection may include fever, upper respiratory symptoms, and a vesicular stomatitis or dermatitis and may be indistinguishable acute conjunctivitis caused by adenovirus. Within 2 weeks of onset, 50% of patients with primary HSV involving the lid margin will develop corneal epithelial manifestations ranging from fine punctate epithelial staining to dendritic ulcerations. The primary infection typically resolves without scarring. Treatment with vidarabine ointment 5 times a day to the conjunctival sac and eyelids should be used to speed resolution of the infection and prevent spread to the cornea. Neonates who develop primary HSV conjunctivitis should also receive intravenous treatment with vidaribine or acyclovir (67). Recurrent HSV ocular disease usually targets the cornea; however, recurrent conjunctivitis can occur in the absence of corneal disease (Fig. 9.15).

Inclusion conjunctivitis is caused by *C. trachomatis* serotypes D–K. It is a unilateral oculogenital disease that usually affects young, sexually active adults and is rarely transmitted through eye-to-eye contact. Incubation period ranges from 2 to 19 days, but an acute follicular conjunctivitis begins approximately 5 days after exposure. Fully developed follicles do not present until the second or third week of disease and become considerably larger and more opalescent than follicles seen in viral disease. Without treatment, the conjunctivitis can persist for months. Yellowish-white subepithelial infiltrates may be seen in the peripheral cornea. Micropannus may develop at the superior limbus of the cornea, and a superficial punctate epithelial keratitis may be noted. Cultures or direct immunofluorescent antibody (DFA) stains are frequently needed to make a definitive diagnosis, and treatment should consist of systemic antibiotics (doxycycline 100 mg twice a day for 7 to 14 days, or one dose of azithromycin 1,000 mg) (68–70).

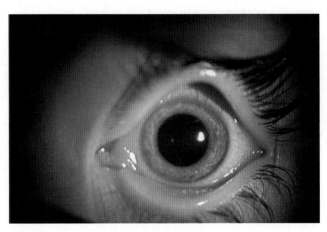

FIGURE 9.14. Pharyngoconjunctival fever (PCF).

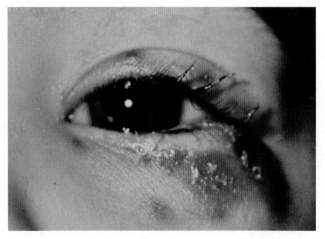

FIGURE 9.15. Herpes simplex virus involving upper and lower eyelid, sparing corneal involvement.

CHRONIC CONJUNCTIVITIS

When the conjunctivitis has an indolent and protracted course, it is classified as chronic disease. Onset is usually insidious and progression may also be slow. Symptoms are variable and include: foreign body sensation, conjunctival injection, minimal discharge, and loss of eyelashes (madarosis).

Blepharitis

The most commonly isolated organism in chronic bacterial conjunctivitis is *S. aureus*. This bacteria causes a blepharoconjunctivitis with loss of eyelashes, trichiasis, and hordeolum. The conjunctival inflammation may be the result of direct infection or release of toxins. The toxins produce the ulcerations surrounding the lash follicles on the eyelid margin and also produce a nonspecific conjunctivitis and superficial punctate keratitis. In severe cases, marginal corneal infiltrates and corneal ulcers may be seen. Symptoms are usually worse in the morning (Fig. 9.16). Treatment includes mechanical cleansing of the eyelids, warm compresses, and topical antibiotics (71).

In some persistent cases, a phlyctenule may develop as an allergic reaction to the endotoxin of *S. aureus*. Typically, a small whitish nodule of degenerated epithelium surrounded by a zone of hyperemia on the bulbar conjunctiva develops. The necrotic epithelial cells and acute inflammatory cells are replaced by lymphocytes and plasma cells (Fig. 9.17). These require topical steroid treatment in addition to treating any concurrent blepharitis or meibomian gland dysfunction (MGD).

Children with chronic blepharitis are prone to develop chalazia, which are lipogranulomas originating from ruptured meibomian glands. These usually erupt through the palpebral conjunctiva. Often the orifices of the meibomian glands are visibly obstructed with white oily plugs. Children with blepharitis and multiple or recurrent chalazia may have MGD or rosacea. Treatment of significant MGD may include dietary supplementation with omega 3 fatty acids (72).

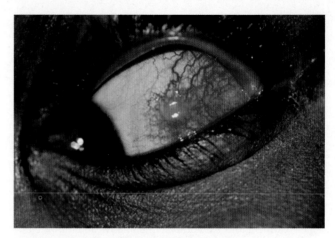

FIGURE 9.17. Phlyctenule on the bulbar conjunctiva.

Other Causes of Chronic Conjunctivitis

Moraxella lacunata causes "external angular conjunctivitis," a chronic follicular conjunctivitis associated with an ulcerative canthal blepharitis (73). Other bacteria that cause chronic conjunctivitis include: *Staphylococcus epidermidis, Proteus sp., Klebsiella pneumoniae, Serratia marcescens,* and *Escherichia coli.*

A chronic unilateral papillary conjunctivitis should arouse the suspicion of a masquerade syndrome caused by an underlying ocular surface malignancy, such as intraepithelial neoplasia, malignant melanoma, or sebaceous cell carcinoma. These conditions fortunately are uncommon in children.

Another important cause of unilateral chronic conjunctivitis is chronic canaliculitis caused by *Actinomyces israelii,* dacryocystitis, or congenital dacryostenosis.

Molluscum contagiosum is a poxvirus that produces a chronic follicular conjunctivitis. Small umbilicated lesions on the eyelids or the periocular skin are the hallmark of this condition. The simple excision of the lesions, including the central plug, will resolve the conjunctivitis (67) (Fig. 9.18).

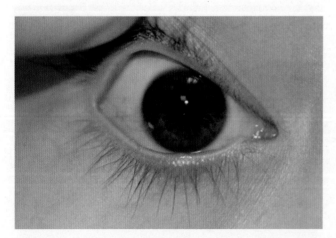

FIGURE 9.16. Marginal corneal infiltrate in child with *Staph* blepharitis and meibomian gland dysfunction (MGD).

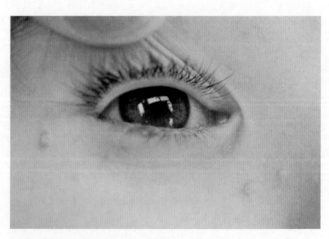

FIGURE 9.18. Chronic conjunctivitis in molluscum contagiosum.

Parinaud oculoglandular syndrome (POS) manifests as a unilateral granulomatous conjunctivitis with preauricular and submandibular adenopathy. Cat-scratch disease, secondary to *Bartonella henselae*, a Gram-negative bacillus, is the most common cause of POS. Treatment is supportive and antibiotics may be effective in severe cases.

Perhaps one of the most concerning chronic infections is trachoma: a bilateral chronic follicular conjunctivitis that is endemic in some developing countries and is the most common cause of preventable blindness. *C. trachomatis* serotypes A–C are transmitted between human beings by intimate social or sexual contact. The incubation period on average is 5 to 10 days. A subsequent self-limited mild mucopurulent conjunctivitis affects the individual and usually heals without any sequelae. Conjunctival scarring and other subsequent complications can result from a chronic, severe conjunctivitis caused by persistent or repeated chlamydial infection. Chronic inflammation is characterized by subepithelial follicles and papillary hypertrophy in the tarsal conjunctiva. Vascular infiltration of the superior portion of the cornea (pannus) is common but rarely progresses to involve the visual axis. These clinical signs of active disease are seen mainly in young children but may also occur in older children and some adults. Conjunctival follicles at the upper limbal margin of the cornea leave characteristic shallow depressions, known as Herbert's pits, after they resolve. Fibrosis and scarring of the upper subtarsal conjunctiva, caused by recurrent infections, is commonly known as Arlt's line. As the scarring progresses, distortion of the lid margin may be seen, causing entropion and trichiasis. Constant trauma to the cornea leads eventually to corneal keratinization, opacification, and blindness. Severe scarring is typically seen in older children, but blindness does not develop until age 40 or 50 (74). Trachoma is, in general, a clinical diagnosis. Laboratory exams, including examination of stained conjunctival scrapings for intracytoplasmic inclusions, tissue culture, immunofluorescence, ELISA, and nucleic-acid-amplification tests, such as PCR, can confirm the diagnosis (75).

Since the 1950s, topical tetracycline has been used widely in trachoma-control programs. The recommended treatment is topical tetracycline, twice a day for 6 weeks. Tetracycline ointment is irritating and difficult to use, particularly in infants, so compliance is poor. Oral antibiotic treatment is more effective than topical treatment because it also eliminates extraocular sites of infection (76). Data from three randomized controlled trials suggest that 1 dose of 20 mg/kg azithromycin (maximum 1 g) is at least as effective in producing resolution of active trachoma as a prolonged course of directly observed topical tetracycline (77–79). Topical 1.5% azithromycin is also effective in treatment (80). The WHO promotes the use of the "SAFE" (Surgery for trichiasis, Antibiotics to reduce the reservoir of infection, Facial cleanliness, and Environmental improvement to reduce transmission of *C. trachomatis)* strategy for trachoma control.

Ocular Allergic Disorders

The most common cause of chronic conjunctivitis is allergy, affecting more than 15% of the world population with a higher prevalence (around 30%) in industrialized countries (81). The eye and the eyelid are common sites of allergic and other hypersensitivity reactions. Patients frequently have a history of atopic diseases, such as eczema, asthma, or rhinitis. Peak age groups are late childhood and young adulthood (82). The ocular allergic response results from the exposure of the conjunctiva to an allergen. Two immune responses may occur. During a type I hypersensitivity ocular reaction (humoral), an environmental allergen binds to the sensitized IgE antibody on the mast cell. The binding of the allergen causes the mast cell (estimated 50 million per eye) to degranulate and release mediators, such as histamine, prostaglandins, and leukotrienes. These mediators, especially histamine, cause itching, vasodilatation, and increased vascular permeability. Type I hypersensitivity ocular reactions include seasonal allergic conjunctivitis and perennial allergic conjunctivitis. In the type IV hypersensitivity reaction (cell-mediated), the delayed allergic reaction is induced by T lymphocytes and macrophages. Contact lens-associated giant papillary conjunctivitis (GPC) is an example of this category, because it involves both types I and IV responses. Atopic keratoconjunctivitis and vernal keratoconjunctivitis are also characterized by both type I and type IV hypersensitivity reactions (83).

Seasonal and perennial allergic conjunctivitis are the most common types of ocular allergy and are typically elicited by airborne allergens, such as pollen, grass, weeds, mold, dust mite, and animal dander (84). Perennial allergic conjunctivitis is distinguished from seasonal allergic conjunctivitis by the presence of symptoms throughout the year and is often considered less severe than the seasonal type. However, almost 80% of the patients with perennial conjunctivitis experience seasonal exacerbations of their symptoms (85,86). Signs and symptoms include bilateral involvement, itching, tearing, mucoid discharge, conjunctival injection, mild eyelid edema, and chemosis. In some cases, a fine conjunctival follicular reaction may also occur. However, corneal involvement is not commonly seen. Treatment should initially be aimed at avoiding or eliminating the causative agent, if possible. Lubricants and cold compress may be helpful in reducing conjunctival irritation in very mild cases but, generally, fail in children. Over-the-counter (OTC) topical antihistamine/vasoconstrictors and nonsteroidal anti-inflammatory agents are generally ineffective for the persistent allergic response. Mast cell stabilizers are also used; however, their treatment lies primarily in the prevention of symptoms by inhibiting the initial release of inflammatory mediators. The delay in their onset limits their effectiveness. Therapy with combination antihistamine/mast cell stabilizer agents, preferably studied in humans, is the most appropriate choice. Human conjunctival mast cells represent a different population of mast cells as compared to lung mast cells and respond to medications differently (87,88). Topical H-1 anatgonists in combination with mast cell inhibitors including alcaftadine, azelastine HCl, bepotastine besilate, epinastine HCl, ketotifen fumerate, and olopatadine HCL 0.1% and 0.2% are available for treatment the signs and symptoms of allergic conjunctivitis. Topical steroids can also be used for the most severe allergies, but their use remains limited and secondary due to their potential adverse effects (81).

Vernal keratoconjunctivitis (VKC) is a vision-threatening, chronic bilateral conjunctival inflammatory disorder that affects mostly young people with a male preponderance. The usual pattern is onset before age 10 and resolves during puberty. Individuals in warm, dry climates tend to be more affected. There is a significant history of other atopic manifestations, such as asthma and eczema (89). Symptoms include pain, itching, conjunctival injection, ptosis, and mucous discharge. Signs of this disease include large (more than 1 mm in diameter), flattened-top papillae on the superior tarsus, gelatinous confluent limbal papillae, conjunctival hyperemia with edema, and Horner-Trantas dots (clumps of eosinophils with dead epithelial cells on the superior limbus) (Figs. 9.19 and 9.20). These changes may lead to superficial corneal neovascularization. In severe cases, corneal ulcers can occur, in addition to epithelial keratitis. The punctate epithelial keratitis may coalesce to an epithelial erosion, leaving Bowman's membrane intact. If treatment is inadequate or no treatment is rendered, a fibrin and mucous plaque is deposited over the defect, delaying the epithelial healing and creating a shield ulcer.

Symptoms can be reduced with conservative measures, such as cold compresses and avoidance or elimination of environmental allergens. Although H1 receptor blockers are used for treatment, topical mast cell stabilizers, like lodoxamide, have been shown to treat VKC more effectively due to its effect on eosinophils (90). Because the complications of VKC can be very serious, topical steroids are almost invariably used at the onset of this disease and then tapered over several weeks while mast cell stabilizers are continued.

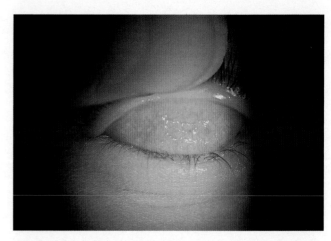

FIGURE 9.20. Palpebral conjunctiva in vernal keratoconjunctivitis.

Atopic keratoconjunctivitis is a bilateral chronic inflammation in individuals, with atopic dermatitis occurring more commonly in men between ages 20 and 50 (83). Up to 40% of the patients with atopic dermatitis have ocular involvement (91,92). The major symptom is itching, and patients often complain of mucous discharge in the morning, blurry vision, photophobia, and pain. At clinical examination, scaling dermatitis of the eyelids, lateral canthal ulceration, madarosis, punctate epithelial keratopathy, papillary reaction, and follicles in the conjunctiva (which are more prominent in the inferior fornix) may be seen. Complications can be severe and include: loss of vision related to the consequences of corneal epithelial defects, keratoconus, cataracts, corneal scarring, and superficial punctate keratitis; lichenified and woody eyelids may lead to cicatricial ectropion and lagophthalmos; and subepithelial fibrosis of the conjunctiva and, rarely, symblepharon (89). The goal in treatment is to prevent visual complications and is similar to vernal conjunctivitis. Topical H1 receptor blockers and mast cell stabilizers are effective. Topical steroids for short periods can help to control symptoms and signs of atopic keratoconjunctivitis. Oral antihistamines and nonsteroidal anti-inflammatory drugs can help to relieve the systemic manifestations. Systemic antihistamines can cause decreased tear production as mucous membrane drying agents and should be used judiciously in all children.

GPC is a noninfectious inflammatory disorder that has been associated with soft contact lens wear, glaucoma filtering blebs, exposed sutures, ocular prosthetics, and extruded scleral buckles (93). GPC may occur with rigid contact lenses but less commonly than with soft (hydrophilic) contact lenses. Symptoms of GPC are low grade at onset. Persistent contact lens wear and/or continued exposure to the inciting material leads to progression of the conjunctivitis with worsening symptoms of itching, blurred vision, mucus production, and lens intolerance. Giant papillae (greater than 0.3 mm) are seen on the superior conjunctival tarsus and, in early cases, are associated with conjunctival injection. The giant papillae appear to manifest increased amounts of

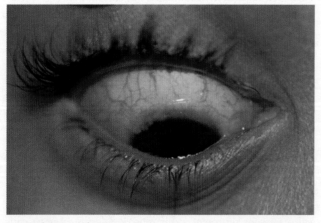

FIGURE 9.19. Vernal keratoconjunctivitis with gelatinous confluent limbal papillae.

mucus-secreting goblet cells with the overlying conjunctiva often thickened and irregular. Corneal involvement in GPC is rare, although pannus formation may occur with persistent soft contact lens wear, despite ocular signs and symptoms. Discontinuation of contact lens or prosthesis use, removal of suture or scleral buckle, helps to reduce, if not eliminate, the clinical manifestations of GPC. However, because many patients do not want to stop wearing contact lenses or prostheses, therapy is directed toward improving lens and prosthesis hygiene by using disposable lenses and finding more compatible lens and prosthesis designs and materials for patients (81). Topical agents, such as histamine antagonists and receptor-blocking agents, have shown limited benefit. Topical steroids help to reduce tarsal hyperemia and inflammation. Mast cell stabilizers have been shown to promote resolution of early GPC when combined with meticulous lens hygiene. Advanced GPC does not respond to mast cell stabilizers, and, in this case, contact lens and prosthesis use should be discontinued for at least several weeks followed by gradual reintroduction of the contact lens with adjuvant mast cell stabilizer treatment (93).

Allergic and Toxic Reactions to Drugs and Other Agents

Allergic reactions to topical ophthalmic medications are not uncommon; however, about 90% of conjunctival drug reactions are toxic (the result of direct chemical irritation) not allergic. In general, allergic reactions are characterized by chronicity (sensitization time is needed for reaction to develop), and a toxic reaction may occur with the first exposure to the agent. Allergies are caused predominantly by active pharmaceutical agents and seldom by preservatives or other additives. Drug-induced ocular allergies are most often the result of type IV hypersensitivity. They result from contact of inciting drugs with the affected tissues. The drug acts as a hapten (incomplete antigen) and becomes immunogenic only after it binds to tissue proteins. The immunologic responses result in conjunctival hyperemia with a papillary reaction and eczema of the skin of the eyelids. Initial sensitization requires at least 5 days and can take months or years of exposure to the hapten. When prior sensitization has occurred, reexposure to the hapten may result in inflammation within 12 to 72 (usually 24 to 48) hours (94).

The earliest sign of allergic and toxic contact reactions is hyperemia; rose bengal dye may reveal punctate staining of the inferonasal bulbar conjunctiva, where topical medications gravitate on their way to the lacrimal outflow system; and eczema of the skin of the eyelids. If the drug is continued, the symptoms and signs worsen. A papillary conjunctivitis with pronounced vasodilation, chemosis, and watery discharge may be seen, although follicles may also be present. In severe cases, keratitis can develop with epithelial defects and, rarely, corneal infiltrates. Corneal involvement is more common in toxic than allergic reactions. Eczema of the skin of the eyelids in the absence of any conjunctival sign indicates that something other than a topical ocular medication is causative, namely, something that has come into contact only with the eyelids (a topical ointment, skin and hair care products, cosmetics, nail polisher, etc.). Misapplication of eye medication should also be considered.

The most common drugs that cause allergy and toxic reactions include atropine, aminoglycoside antibiotics (neomycin in particular), hyoscine (scopolamine), penicillin, apraclonidine, brimonidine, dorzolamide, and older antiviral agents (idoxuridine and, less often, vidarabine) (95). Preservatives and other additives are uncommon causes of allergic contact reactions, except for thimerosal. However, especially with repeated use, preservatives may be quite toxic to the corneal and conjunctival epithelium. Recognition of toxicity is the key to the treatment, which usually involves stopping the causative agent (96).

ERYTHEMA MULTIFORME AND ITS VARIANTS

Erythema multiforme is an acute mucocutaneous hypersensitivity reaction characterized by a symmetrically distributed skin eruption, with or without mucous membrane lesions. It may present within a wide spectrum of severity. The minor form affects primarily the skin and one mucosal surface at most. The major form is known as Stevens-Johnson syndrome. About 20% of cases occur in children and adolescents. It is characterized by involvement of skin and two or more mucosal surfaces with possible internal organ involvement leading to systemic symptoms. There is controversy as to whether toxic epidermal necrolysis is a severe manifestation of erythema multiforme or a distinct entity. The frequent presence of overlapping clinical features in a given patient often makes definitive classification difficult.

Drugs and infections are the most common precipitating factors, but other factors, such as mechanical or physical factors (radiotherapy and sunlight), can also trigger the disease (97). This syndrome presents with a prodrome of fever and influenza-like symptoms, followed by the rapid onset of cutaneous blistering within 1 to 3 weeks after exposure and hours after the reexposure to the inciting agent (98). The initial ocular findings in erythema multiforme is a bilateral nonspecific conjunctivitis with hyperemia and chemosis then progressing to a pseudomembranous conjunctivitis with secondary bacterial conjunctivitis complicating the initial ocular involvement. Anterior uveitis may also occur. The conjunctivitis resolves in 2 to 4 weeks. Pseudomembranous conjunctival erosions may result in scarring and symblepharon formation. These lead to entropion formation, trichiasis, and tear film instability. Persistent corneal defects with scarring and neovascularization can result from the chronic irritation due to eyelid changes. Affected patients can also have severely dry eyes due to cicatrization or stenosis of the lacrimal ducts and destruction of the conjunctival goblet cells responsible for the mucus secretion of the tear film.

Treatment of this ocular disease includes frequent conjunctival irrigation and instillation of prophylactic antibiotic drops and preservative-free artificial tears. Use of topical steroids is controversial because they do not decrease the symblepharon formation and may contribute to secondary infection. Lysis of symblepharon should be performed daily, and a symblepharon ring may also be used. If corneal involvement is severe and there is risk of perforation, a conjunctival flap or penetrating keratoplasty should be performed. Chronic ocular involvement in Stevens-Johnson syndrome is a challenge to most ophthalmologists. Trichiasis and entropion can be corrected surgically with frequent recurrence. Epithelial corneal defects can be treated with a soft contact lens, conjunctival graft, keratoprosthesis, or keratolimbal allograft with limited results. Frequent use of artificial tears, and sometimes tarsorrhaphy, are used to treat keratoconjunctivitis sicca that develops after the acute inflammation (99). The prognosis depends upon the severity of the initial event. Usually, children have the best prognosis (100). Patients should avoid contact with the precipitating agent to decrease the risk of recurrence.

LIGNEOUS CONJUNCTIVITIS

Ligneous conjunctivitis is a rare but devastating form of chronic conjunctivitis characterized by recurrent development of firm fibrin-rich, woody-like pseudomembranous lesions, mainly on the tarsal conjunctiva. It presents in childhood and may affect other mucous membranes of the gastrointestinal, respiratory, and female genital tract. It is more common in women and may be unilateral or bilateral. The initial lesion (raised, friable, and highly vascularized) can be easily removed with forceps. Eventually, this progresses to a white avascular mass that appears above the neovascular membrane. In late stages, this lesion replaces the normal conjunctival mucosa as a thickened, vascularized firm mass with a wood-like consistency. Corneal involvement, occurring in about one third of cases, may lead to blindness as a result of scarring, vascularization, keratomalacia, and corneal perforation. The central features of ligneous conjunctivitis are impaired wound healing, chronic and overwhelming local inflammation, and excessive depositions of fibrin and other plasma proteins, due to an impaired extracellular (plasmin-mediated) fibrinolysis (101).

In predisposed subjects, ligneous conjunctivitis results from an exaggerated inflammatory response to tissue injury and may be triggered by local injuries, local and systemic infections, and surgical procedures to the eyes. The diagnosis is based mainly on the clinical picture. The typical histologic findings are an acellular, eosinophilic, periodic acid-Schiff-positive, hyaline material with areas of granulation tissue, and areas of cellular infiltration (102,103).

Spontaneous resolution of ligneous conjunctivitis has been reported, but these cases are rare (102–104). Local treatment options available for ligneous conjunctivitis are mostly disappointing. Many local drugs have been tried: Topical hyaluronidase (1.5 mg/mL) alone, or in combination with alpha-chymotrypsin (0.2 mg/mL), has been reported to be helpful in some studies but not in others (103,105,106). Limited success was also reported using topical antibiotics, steroids, sodium cromoglycate, and silver nitrate (107).

Some studies have shown that long-term topical treatment with corticosteroids combined with cyclosporine A significantly decreased the frequency and the severity of recurrences after surgical excisions of the pseudomembranes. Systemic side effects of cyclosporine A were not described (108,109). The most promising approach seems to be the initial application of a topical fibrinolytic agent, followed by surgical removal of the pseudomembranes with subsequent intense and long-term topical application of heparin in combination with topical corticosteroids and alpha-chymotrypsin (110). Heparin appears to reduce the otherwise high risk of local recurrence after surgery alone; however, the number of excisions of pseudomembranes and other mechanical manipulations should be kept to a minimum.

SUMMARY

The conjunctiva is a mucous membrane that serves multiple functions for the eye. It provides a smooth surface for appositional motion, immune protection, aids in lubrication, and is resistant to physical trauma. This resilient tissue, more than adequately protects the eye, in a hostile environment.

REFERENCES

1. Torczynski E. Normal development of the eye and the orbit before birth. In: Isenberg SJ, ed. *The eye in infancy.* Chicago: Mosby International, 1988:25–26.
2. Kikkawa DO. Ophthalmic facial anatomy and physiology. In: Kaufman P, Alm A, eds. *Adler's physiology of the eye.* Philadelphia, PA: WB Saunders, 2002:23–25.
3. Lawton A. Structure and function of the eyelids and conjunctiva. In: Kaufman H, Barron B, McDonald M, eds. *The Cornea.* Boston, MA: Butterworth-Heinemann, 1998:51–60.
4. Greiner JV, Kenyon KR, Henriquez AS, et al. Mucus secretory vesicles in conjunctival epithelial cells of wearers of contact lenses. *Arch Ophthalmol* 1980;98(10):1843–1846.
5. Isenberg SJ, Del Signore M, Chen A, et al. The lipid layer and stability of the preocular tear film in newborns and infants. *Ophthalmology* 2003;110(7):1408–1411.
6. Tseng SC, Zhang SH. Interaction between rose bengal and different protein components. *Cornea* 1995;14(4):427–435.
7. Yanoff M, Fine BS. *Ocular pathology,* 5th Ed. Philadelphia, PA: Mosby, 2002:761.
8. Kuiper JJ. Conjunctival icterus. *Ann Intern Med* 2001;134:345–346.

9. Mclean IW. Melanocytic neoplasms of the conjunctiva. In: Krachmer JH, Mannis MJ, Holland EJ, eds. *The Cornea*. St. Louis, MO: Mosby-Year Book, 1997:715–722.

10. Folberg R, Jakobiec FA, Bernardino VB, et al. Benign conjunctival melanocytic lesions: clinicopathologic features. *Ophthalmology* 1989;96(4):436–461.

11. Kantelip B, Boccard R, Nores JM, et al. A case of conjunctival Spitz nevus: review of literature and comparison with cutaneous locations. *Ann Ophthalmol* 1989;21(5):176–179.

12. Jakobiec FA, Folberg R, Iwamoto T. Clinicopathologic characteristics of premalignant and malignant melanocytic lesions of the conjunctiva. *Ophthalmology* 1989;96(2):147–166.

13. Shields JA, Shields CL. *Eyelid, conjunctival, and orbital tumors: an atlas and textbook,* 2nd Ed. Philadelphia, PA: Lippincott Williams & Wilkins, 2008:320,354–358,368.

14. Ticho BH, Tso MO, Kishi S. Diffuse iris nevus in oculodermal melanocytosis: a light and electron microscopic study. *J Pediatr Ophthalmol Strabismus* 1989;26(5):244–250.

15. Gonder JR, Shields JA, Albert DM, et al. Uveal malignant melanoma associated with ocular and oculodermal melanocytosis. *Ophthalmology* 1982;89(8):953–960.

16. Dutton JJ, Anderson RL, Schelper RL, et al. Orbital malignant melanoma and oculodermal melanocytosis: report of two cases and review of the literature. *Ophthalmology* 1984;91(5):497–507.

17. Yamamoto T. Malignant melanoma of the choroid in the nevus of Ota. *Ophthalmologica* 1969;159:1–10.

18. Singh M, Kaur B, Annwar NM. Malignant melanoma of the choroid is a naevus of Ota. *Br J Ophthalmol* 1988;72:131–134.

19. Roldan M, Llanes F, Negrete O, et al. Malignant melanoma of the choroid associated with melanosis oculi in a child. *Am J Ophthalmol* 1987;104(6):662–663.

20. Goncalves V, Sandler T, O'Donnell FE Jr. Open angle glaucoma in melanosis oculi: response to laser trabeculoplasty. *Ann Ophthalmol* 1985;17(1):33–36.

21. Gomi CF, Robbins SL, Heichel CW, et al. Conjunctival diseases. In: Nelson LB, Olitsky SE, eds. *Harley's pediatric oohthalmology*, 5th Ed. Philadelphia, PA: WLippincott Williams & Wilkins, 2005:203–204.

22. Warner M, Jakobiec F. Subepithelial neoplasms of the conjunctiva. In: Krachmer JH, Mannis MJ, Holland EJ, eds. *Cornea-cornea and external disease: clinical diagnosis and management*. St Louis, MO: Mosby, 1997:723–743.

23. Taylor D. Conjunctiva and subconjunctival tissue. In: Taylor D, ed. *Paediatric ophthalmology*. Oxford: Blackwell Science, 1997:237–251.

24. Wagner RS, Facciani JM. Organoid nevus syndrome: manifestations and management. *J Pdiatr Ophthalmol Strabismus* 2003;40:137–141.

25. Kraemer KH, Lee MM, Scotto J. Xeroderma pigmentosum. Cutaneous, ocular, and neurologic abnormalities in 830 published cases. *Arch Dermatol* 1987;123(2):241–250.

26. Ni N, Wagner RS, Langer P, Guo S. New developments in the management of periocular capillary hemangioma in children. *J Pediatr Ophthalmol Strabismus* 2011;48:269–276.

27. Fransen L, Klauss V. Neonatal ophthalmia in the developing world. Epidemiology, etiology, management and control. *Int Ophthalmol* 1988;11(3):189–196.

28. Haase DA, Nash RA, Nsanze H, et al. Single-dose ceftriaxone therapy of gonococcal ophthalmia neonatorum. *SexTransm Dis* 1986;13(1):53–55.

29. Hoosen AA, Kharsany AB, Ison CA. Single low-dose ceftriaxone for the treatment of gonococcal ophthalmia—implications for the national programme for the syndromic management of sexually transmitted diseases. *S Afr Med J* 2002;92(3):238–240.

30. Laga M, Naamara W, Brunham RC, et al. Single-dose therapy of gonococcal ophthalmia neonatorum with ceftriaxone. *N Engl J Med* 1986;315(22):1382–1385.

31. [No authors listed]. Ophthalmia neonatorum. *Afr Health* 1995;17(5):30.

32. AAP, AAOP, Red Book: 2012 Report of the Committee on Infectious Diseases, 29th Ed. Elk Grove Village, IL, 2012.

33. Newel FW. Centenary of Crede' prophylaxis. *Am J Ophthalmol*. 1980;90(6):874–875.

34. Hedberg K, RistinenTL, Soler JT, et al. Outbreak of erythromycin-resistant staphylococcal conjunctivitis in a newborn nursery. *Pediatr Infect Dis J* 1990;9(4):268–273.

35. Ison CA, Terry P, Bendayna K, et al. Tetracycline-resistant gonococci in UK. *Lancet* 1988;1(8586):651–652.

36. van Klingeren B, Dessens-Kroon M, Verheuvel M. Increased tetracycline resistance in gonococci in The Netherlands. *Lancet* 1989;2(8674):1278.

37. Knapp JS, Zenilman JM, Biddle JW, et al. Frequency and distribution in the United States of strains of *Neisseria gonorrhoeae* with plasmid-mediated, high-level resistance to tetracycline. *J Infect Dis* 1987;155(4):819–822.

38. Schwarcz SK, Zenilman JM, Schnell D, et al. National surveillance of antimicrobial resistance in Neisseria gonorrhoeae. The Gonococcal Isolate Surveillance Project. *JAMA* 1990;264(11):1413–1417.

39. Hammerschlag MR, Cummings C, Roblin PM, et al. Efficacy of neonatal ocular prophylaxis for the prevention of chlamydial and gonococcal conjunctivitis. *N Engl J Med* 1989; 320(12): 769–772.

40. Zanoni D, Isenberg SJ, Apt L. A comparison of silver nitrate with erythromycin for prophylaxis against ophthalmia neonatorum. *Clin Pediatr (Phila)* 1992;31(5):295–298.

41. Isenberg SJ, Apt L, Del Signore M, et al. Povidone-iodine for ophthalmia neonatorum prophylaxis. *Am J Ophthalmol* 1994;118(6):701 706.

42. Isenberg SJ, Apt L, Wood M. A controlled trial of povidone-iodine as prophylaxis against ophthalmia neonatorum. *N Engl J Med* 1995;332(9):562–566.

43. Wald ER. Conjunctivitis in infants and children. *Pediatr Infect Dis J* 1997;16[2 Suppl]:S17-S20.

44. Lewis LS, GlauserTA, Joffe MD. Gonococcal conjunctivitis in prepubertal children. *Am J Dis Child* 1990;144(5):546–548.

45. Irani F, Ruddell T. Meningococcal conjunctivitis. *Aust N Z J Ophthalmol* 1997;25(2):167–168.

46. Bodor FF. Diagnosis and management of acute conjunctivitis. *Semin Infect Dis* 1998;9:27–30.

47. Weiss A. Acute conjunctivitis in childhood. *Curr Probl Pediatr* 1994;24(1):4–11.

48. Gigliotti F, Williams WT, Hayden FG, et al. Etiology of acute conjunctivitis in children. *J Pediatr* 1981;98(4):531–536.

49. Brook I. Anaerobic and aerobic bacterial flora of acute conjunctivitis in children. *Arch Ophthalmol* 1980;98(5):833–835.

50. Brook I. Ocular infections due to anaerobic bacteria. *Int Ophthalmol* 2001;24(5):269–277.

51. Martin M, Turco JH, Zegans ME, et al. An outbreak of conjunctivitis due to atypical streptococcus pneumonia. *N Engl J Med* 2003;348:1112–1121.

52. Centers for Disease Control and Prevention. Pneumococcal conjunctivitis at an elementary school—Maine, September 20–December 6, 2002. *MMWR*. 2003;52(4):64–66.

53. Cavuoto K, Zutshi D, Karp CL, et al. Update on bacterial conjunctivitis in South Florida. *Ophthalmology* 2008;115:51–56.

54. Leibowitz HW, Pratt MV, Flagstad IJ, etal. Human conjunctivitis. I. Diagnostic evaluation. *Arch Ophthalmol* 1976;94(10):1747–1749.

55. Meltzer JA, Kunkov S, Crain EF. Identifying children at low risk for bacterial conjunctivitis. *ArchPediatr Adolesc Med* 2010;164(3):263–267.

56. Granet DB, Dorfman M, Stroman D, et al. A multicenter comparison of polymyxin B sulfate/trimethoprim ophthalmic solution and moxifloxacin in speed of clinical efficacy for the treatment of bacterial conjunctivitis. *J Pediatr Ophthalmol Strabismus* 2008;45:340–349.

57. Lichtenstein SJ, DeLeon L, Heller W, et al. Topical ophthalmic moxifloxacin elicits minimal or no selection of fluoroquinolone resistance among bacteria isolated from the skin, nose, and throat. *J Pediatr Ophthalmol Strabismus* 2012;49:88–97.

58. Bodor FF. Conjunctivitis-otitis syndrome. *Pediatrics* 1982;69(6):695–698.

59. Bodor FF, Marchant CD, Shurin PA, et al. Bacterial etiology of conjunctivitis-otitis media syndrome. *Pediatrics* 1985;76(1):26–28.

60. Bodor F. [Purulent conjunctivitis-otitis media syndrome]. *Lijec Vjesn* 1987;109(6):220–223.

61. Bodor FF. Systemic antibiotics for treatment of the conjunctivitis-otitis media syndrome. *Pediatr Infect Dis J* 1989;8(5):287–290.

62. Gigliotti F, Hendley JO, Morgan J, et al. Efficacy of topical antibiotic therapy in acute conjunctivitis in children. *J Pediatr* 1984;104(4):623–626.

63. Sambursky R, Trattler W, Tauber S, et al. Sensitivity and specificity of the adenoplus test for diagnosing adenoviral conjunctivitis. *JAMA Ophthalmol* 2013;131(1):17–22.

64. Hillenkamp J, Reinhard T, Ross RS, et al. The effects of cidofovir 1% with and without cyclosporin 1% as a topical treatment of acute adenoviral keratoconjunctivitis: a controlled clinical pilot study. *Ophthalmology* 2002;109(5):845–850.

65. Hillenkamp J, Reinhard T, Ross RS, et al. Topical treatment of acute adenoviral keratoconjunctivitis with 0.2% cidofovir and 1% cyclosporine: a controlled clinical pilot study. *Arch Ophthalmol* 2001;119(10):1487–1491.

66. Ritterband DC, Friedberg DN. Virus infections of the eye. *Rev Med Virol* 1998;8(4):187–201.

67. Stamler JF. Viral conjunctivitis. In: Krachmer JH, Mannis MJ, Holland EJ, eds. *Cornea—cornea and external disease: clinical diagnosis and management*. St. Louis, MO: Mosby, 1997:773–777.

68. Katusic D, Petricek I, Mandic Z, et al. Azithromycin vs. doxycycline in the treatment of inclusion conjunctivitis. *Am J Ophthalmol* 2003;135(4):447–451.

69. Chandler JW. Chlamydial infections. In: Krachmer JH, Mannis MJ, Holland EJ, eds. *Cornea-cornea and external disease: clinical diagnosis and management*. St. Louis, MO: Mosby, 1997:779–788.

70. Basualdo JA, Huarte L, Bautista E, et al. [Follicular conjunctivitis due to Chlamydia trachomatis]. *Medicina (B Aires)* 2001;61(4):397–400.

71. Soukiasian SH, Baum J. Bacterial conjunctivitis. In: Krachmer JH, Mannis MJ, Holland EJ, eds. *Cornea-cornea and external disease: clinical diagnosis and management*. St. Louis, MO: Mosby, 1997:759–772.

72. Macsai MS. The role of omega-3 dietary supplementation in blepharitis and meibomian gland dysfunction (an AOS thesis). *Trans Am Ophthalmol Soc*. 2008;106:336–356.

73. Taylor D. External eye diseases. In: Taylor D, ed. *Paediatric ophthalmology*. London: Blackwell Science, 1997:185–198.

74. Bowman RJ, Jatta B, Cham B, et al. Natural history of trachomatous scarring in the Gambia: results of a 12-year longitudinal follow-up. *Ophthalmology* 2001;108(12):2219–2224.

75. Mabey DC, Solomon AW, Foster A. Trachoma. *Lancet* 2003;362(9379):223–229.

76. Schachter J, West SK, Mabey D, et al. Azithromycin in control of trachoma. *Lancet* 1999;354(9179):630–635.

77. Bailey RL, Arullendran P, Whittle HC, et al. Randomized controlled trial of single-dose azithromycin in treatment of trachoma. *Lancet* 1993;342(8869):453–456.

78. Dawson CR, Schachter J, Sallam S, et al. A comparison of oral azithromycin with topical oxytetracycline/polymyxin forthe treatment of trachoma in children. *Clin Infect Dis* 1997;24(3):363–368.

79. Tabbara KF, Abu-el-Asrar A, al-Omar O, et al. Single-dose azithromycin in the treatment of trachoma. A randomized, controlled study. *Ophthalmology* 1996;103(5):842–846.

80. Cochereau I, Goldschmidt P, Goepogui A, et al. Efficacy and safety of short duration azithromycin eye drops versus azithromycin single oral dose for the treatment of trachoma in children—a randomised, controlled, double-masked clinical trial. *Br J Ophthalmol* 2007;91(5):667–672.

81. Bielory L, Origlieri , Wagner RS. Allergic and immunologic eye disease. In: Leung DY, Sampson HA, Geha R, et al., eds. *Pediatric allergy: principles and practice 2nd edition*. Edinburgh: Saunders—Elsevier, 2010:600–615.

82. Teoh DL, Reynolds S. Diagnosis and management of pediatric conjunctivitis. *Pediatr Emerg Care* 2003;19(1):48–55.

83. Trocme SD, Sra KK. Spectrum of ocular allergy. *Curr Opin Allergy Clin Immunol* 2002;2(5):423–427.

84. Abelson MB, Schaefer K. Conjunctivitis of allergic origin: immunologic mechanisms and current approaches to therapy. *Surv Ophthalmol* 1993;[38 Suppl]:115–132.

85. Dart JK, Buckley RJ, Monnickendan M, et al. Perennial allergic conjunctivitis: definition, clinical characteristics and prevalence. A comparison with seasonal allergic conjunctivitis. *Trans Ophthalmol Soc U K* 1986;105(Pt 5):513–520.

86. Friedlaender MH. Conjunctivitis of allergic origin: clinical presentation and differential diagnosis. *Surv Ophthalmol* 1993;[38 Suppl]:105–114.

87. Irani AM, Schwartz LB. Mast cell heterogeneity. *Clin Exp Allergy* 1989;19(2):143–155.

88. Irani AM, Butrus SI, Tabbara KF, et al. Human conjunctival mast cells: distribution of MCT and MCTC in vernal conjunctivitis and giant papillary conjunctivitis. *J Allergy Clin Immunol* 1990;86(1):34–40.

89. Barney NP. Vernal and atopic keratoconjunctivitis. In: Krachmer JH, Mannis MJ, Holland EJ, eds. *Cornea-cornea and external disease: clinical diagnosis and management*. St. Louis, MO: Mosby, 1997:811–817.

90. Verin P, Allewaert R, Joyaux JC, et al. Comparison of lodoxamide 0.1% ophthalmic solution and levocabastine 0.05% ophthalmic suspension in vernal keratoconjunctivitis. *Eur J Ophthalmol* 2001;11(2):120–125.

91. Garrity JA, Liesegang TJ. Ocular complications of atopic dermatitis. *Can J Ophthalmol* 1984;19(1):21–24.

92. Rich LF, Hanifin JM. Ocular complications of atopic dermatitis and other eczemas. *Int Ophthalmol Clin* 1985;25(1):61–76.

93. Dunn SP, Heidemann DG. Giant papillary conjunctivitis. In: Krachmer JH, Mannis MJ, Holland EJ, eds. *Cornea-cornea and external disease: clinical diagnosis and management.* St. Louis, MO: Mosby, 1997:819–825.

94. Wilson FI. Toxic and allergic reactions to topical ophthalmic medications. In: Arrffa R, ed. *Grayson's diseases of the cornea.* St. Louis, MO: Mosby, 1997:669–683.

95. Wilson FM II. Allergy to topical medications. *Int Ophthalmol Clin* 2003;43(1):73–81.

96. Chang S. Toxic conjunctivitis. In: Krachmer JH, Mannis MJ, Holland EJ, eds. *Cornea-cornea and external disease: clinical diagnosis and management.* St. Louis, MO: Mosby, 1997:847–856.

97. Pruksachatkunakorn C, Schachner L. Erythema multiforme. In: Farmer E, ed. *Reactive and inflammatory dermatoses.* E-medicine, 2003.

98. Metry DW, Jung P, Levy ML. Use of intravenous immunoglobulin in children with Stevens-Johnson syndrome and toxic epidermal necrolysis: seven cases and review of the literature. *Pediatrics* 2003;112(6 Pt 1):1430–1436.

99. Palmon FE, Webster GF, Holland EJ. Erythema multiforme, Stevens-Johnson syndrome and toxic epidermal necrolysis. In: Krachmer JH, Mannis MJ, Holland EJ, eds. *Cornea-cornea and external disease: clinical diagnosis and management.* St. Louis, MO: Mosby, 1997:835–846.

100. Giannetti A, Malmusi M, Girolomoni G. Vesiculobullous drug eruptions in children. *Clin Dermatol* 1993;11(4):551–555.

101. Schuster V, Seregard S. Ligneous conjunctivitis. *Surv Ophthalmol* 2003;48(4):369–388.

102. Hidayat AA, Riddle PJ. Ligneous conjunctivitis. A clinicopathologic study of 17 cases. *Ophthalmology* 1987;94(8):949–959.

103. Kanai A, Polack FM. Histologic and electron microscope studies of ligneous conjunctivitis. *Am J Ophthalmol* 1971;72(5):909–916.

104. McGrand JC, Rees DM, Harry J. Ligneous conjunctivitis. *Br J Ophthalmol* 1969;53(6):373–381.

105. Francois J, Victoria-Troncoso V. Treatment of ligneous conjunctivitis. *Am J Ophthalmol* 1968;65(5):674–678.

106. Eagle RC Jr, Brooks JS, Katowitz JA, et al. Fibrin as a major constituent of ligneous conjunctivitis. *Am J Ophthalmol* 1986;101(4):493–494.

107. Holland R, Schwartz G. Ligneous conjunctivitis. In: Krachmer JH, Mannis MJ, Holland EJ, eds. *Cornea-cornea and external disease: clinical diagnosis and management.* St. Louis, MO: Mosby, 1997:863–868.

108. Holland EJ, Chan CC, Kuwabara T, et al. Immunohistologic findings and results of treatment with cyclosporine in ligneous conjunctivitis. *Am J Ophthalmol* 1989;107(2):160–166.

109. Rubin BI, Holland EJ, de Smet MD, et al. Response of reactivated ligneous conjunctivitis to topical cyclosporine. *Am J Ophthalmol* 1991;112(1):95–96.

110. De Cock R, Ficker LA, Dart JG, et al. Topical heparin in the treatment of ligneous conjunctivitis. *Ophthalmology* 1995;102(11):1654–1659.

10

Diseases of the Cornea

Jagadesh C. Reddy • *Christopher J. Rapuano*

MANY DISEASES OF the cornea and anterior segment in children do not differ much from diseases in adults, with the exception of congenital and developmental abnormalities. Certain corneal disorders first appear in infancy and childhood, such that careful screening and examination at a young age would have elucidated the nature of disorders recognized later in adulthood.

This chapter delineates the common diseases of the earlier years of life that primarily affect the cornea but may also involve surrounding structures, such as the eyelids, conjunctiva, sclera, anterior chamber, iris, and lens.

EMBRYOLOGY AND DEVELOPMENTAL ABNORMALITIES

The anterior segment of the eye—the cornea, anterior chamber angle, iris, and lens—contains several anatomical and physiologic systems packed into a small space, so that its embryology and malformations are sometimes difficult to understand. The use of multiple names for each malformation further complicates the picture. We can reduce the confusion by reviewing the development of the anterior segment, observing how each abnormality might derive from arrested or aberrant growth, and classifying the abnormalities on a simple anatomical basis.

Congenital anomalies of the anterior segment result from abnormal induction, differentiation, or maturation of the tissues. Abnormalities can be due to inherited genetic defects, new genetic mutations and/or environmental factors. All cells of one individual begin with the same gene pool in their deoxyribonucleic acid (DNA) unless there is a chromosomal abnormality, but each differentiates to manifest a morphology controlled by only a portion of those genes—the genotype. Both internal and environmental influences regulate which genes will express themselves. During differentiation, different tissues are maximally susceptible to injury at different times, so that any agent that interferes during this sensitive period may produce an abnormality. Thus, similar malformations may result from abnormal genes, excessive or inadequate metabolites, viral or other infectious agents, exogenous toxins, hypoxia, or mechanical insults. Similarly, the same agents affecting the developing fetus at different time points produce different abnormalities, depending on which tissues are the most vulnerable at that particular moment. In some instances, such as congenital rubella, we know both the cause of the abnormalities and the approximate time of their development. In most instances, however, these factors are unknown, and we must fall back on more simple anatomical descriptions of the abnormalities, to which we often give eponyms, refining chronology and etiology as more information becomes available.

Developmental Variations in Limbal Anatomy

The limbus is a junctional zone where corneal epithelium and its basement membrane meet stem cells and conjunctival epithelium and its basement membrane. Corneal stroma juxtaposes sclera. Descemet's membrane ends at Schwalbe's ring and the trabecular meshwork. Corneal endothelium becomes continuous with the trabecular endothelium.

These transitional zones form a number of circular structures at the limbus that can be seen on slit-lamp examination (Fig. 10.1), and variations in these structures are common in congenital malformations of the anterior segment (1).

Epithelium

Corneal and conjunctival epithelia are continuous over the limbus. Corneal epithelium, a five- to eight-cell-layered stratified squamous epithelium, attaches to a smooth basement membrane that is supported by the acellular, fibrillar felt-work of Bowman's layer. The conjunctival epithelium, a stratified cuboidal layer that contains goblet cells, lies on an undulating basement membrane, supported by irregular vascular connective tissue. At the limbus, the conjunctival epithelium forms a series of radially arranged extensions into the subepithelial connective tissue, each extension flanked by vascular connective tissue pegs that protrude into the epithelium. Pigmentation of the basal layers makes these epithelial extensions, the limbal palisades of Vogt, visible between the white connective tissue spaces (Figs. 10.1 and 10.2). These limbal palisades have tongue-like epithelial projections into the corneal stroma termed rete ridges. These epithelial rete ridges serve as a repository for corneal epithelial precursor cells.

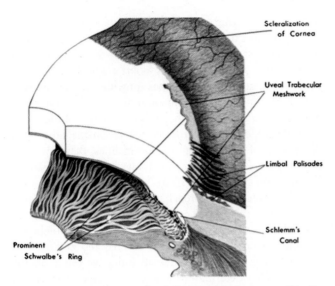

FIGURE 10.1. Developmental variations in limbal anatomy. This diagrammatic representation of limbal structures illustrates the appearance of each structure on the anterior surface and demonstrates its location in cross section.

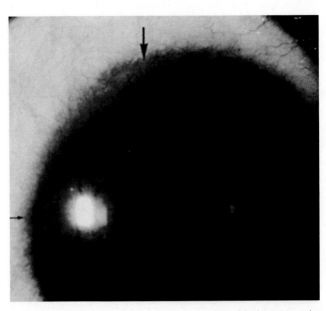

FIGURE 10.3. Scleralization of the cornea. At 12 o'clock position, the sclera and its vessels extend superficially into the cornea, hiding underlying iris and angle details (*area between two large arrows*). Compare the normal extent of sclera over the limbus at 9 o'clock position (*area between two small arrows*).

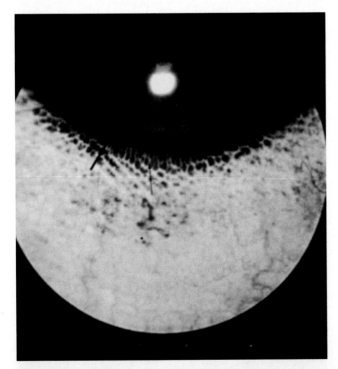

FIGURE 10.2. Limbal palisades of Vogt. This circle of white, fingerlike projections (*small arrow*) that breaks up the limbal pigment ring (*large arrow*) results from subepithelial connective tissue papillae pushing up near the surface, interrupting the pigmentation of the basal conjunctival epithelium.

Corneoscleral Junction

The components of both corneal stroma and sclera are the same: collagen fibrils, proteoglycans (acid mucopolysaccharides), water, and fibrocytes. The tissues appear different because the corneal collagen fibers have a uniform diameter and arrangement, and the proteoglycans are dehydrated,

whereas scleral fibrils vary in size, are randomly oriented, and remain hydrated. At the limbus, the cornea inserts into the sclera as a wedge, like a watch crystal into its casing. Normally, the superficial rim of sclera extends 0.5 mm centrally over the wedge of cornea superiorly and inferiorly as a white, vascularized crescent (Figs. 10.1 and 10.3), so that the vertical corneal diameter is about 1 mm less than the horizontal diameter when measured on the anterior surface. Thus, deeper limbal structures, such as a prominent Schwalbe's ring or uveal trabecular meshwork, are usually visible only medially and laterally. When this scleral tissue extends farther centrally, or when it is present for 360 degrees, the abnormality is called *scleralization* or *scleral overriding*.

Trabecular Meshwork

A thin, translucent, gray band of uveal trabecular meshwork may extend up to and past Schwalbe's line to form a gray arc on the posterior cornea, one sometimes accentuated by a pigmented epithelial ring and a prominent Schwalbe's ring (Figs. 10.4 and 10.5).

Schwalbe's Ring

The corneal endothelium and Descemet's membrane meet the uveal trabecular meshwork at a junction designated as the anterior border ring of Schwalbe, or Schwalbe's line. This ring, part of the uveal meshwork, has a structure similar to a trabeculum, that is, a collagen–proteoglycan core surrounded by thin leaves of the terminal portion of Descemet's membrane and covered on its inner surface by endothelium. With a gonioscope, the clinician sees it as a change from the refractile corneal endothelium to the reticulated translucent trabecular meshwork.

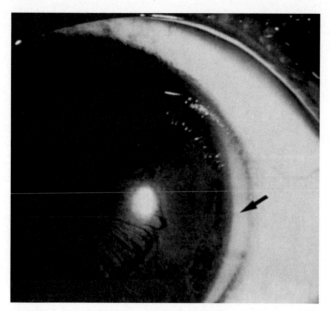

FIGURE 10.4. Prominent uveal trabecular meshwork. The limbus of the eye is demarcated by a pigment ring. Sclera extends up to but not beyond the ring. The light tissue lying central to the pigment ring (*arrow*) is the uveal trabecular meshwork.

Schwalbe's ring may be thickened and positioned centrally, making it visible at the slit lamp as an irregular, refractile, white line lying concentric to the limbus and gonioscopically as a ridge protruding into the anterior chamber. It may be broken or continuous and frequently has pigment spots on its inner surface that represent previous attachment of iris strands. This centrally located prominent Schwalbe's ring is commonly called a *posterior embryotoxon* (Greek, *embryon* ["embryo"] plus *toxon* ["bow"]). It appears in 8% to 15% of normal eyes but is seen this frequently only by those who specifically look for it.

Congenital Anomalies of the Cornea

The clinician confronted with a child who has a developmental anomaly of the ocular anterior segment often has difficulty classifying and naming the disorder. This is an activity of more than academic value, because a precise diagnosis is necessary before the ophthalmologist can predict the natural history of the disorder, look for specific associated ocular or systemic abnormalities, provide genetic counseling, and begin appropriate medical or surgical therapy. It is easiest to describe these abnormalities in terms of their anatomical components. Once clinicians have made a thorough description of the anatomical abnormalities, they can more precisely label the disorder, which may be aided by a simple classification system (Fig. 10.6).

This anatomical approach makes sense embryologically, because it is the neural crest-derived mesenchymal tissue that differentiates into the cornea (except the epithelium), the angle structures, and the iris stroma, and because this mesenchymal tissue may have an inductive effect on the optic cup that determines the size and shape of the pupil and ciliary ring. This approach also makes sense clinically, because many of the abnormalities so easily described in isolation occur in combination with other anomalies. For example, Rieger's anomaly (prominent Schwalbe's ring, iris strands to Schwalbe's ring, and hypoplasia of the anterior iris stroma) is accompanied by megalocornea in about 25% of cases, scleralization of cornea in about 80% of cases, juvenile glaucoma without buphthalmos in about 25% of cases, and one form of Peters' anomaly in occasional cases.

Congenital Corneal Diseases without Corneal Opacification

Abnormalities of Corneal Size and Shape

Megalocornea. The newborn cornea measures approximately 10 mm in horizontal diameter and reaches the average adult measurement of 11.8 mm by age 2. Megalocornea is present if the horizontal diameter of a newborn cornea is 12 mm or more and if an adult cornea is 13 mm or more (Fig. 10.7).

An enlarged cornea occurs in three patterns: (a) megalocornea unassociated with other ocular abnormalities, usually inherited as an autosomal dominant trait; (2,3) (b) X-linked

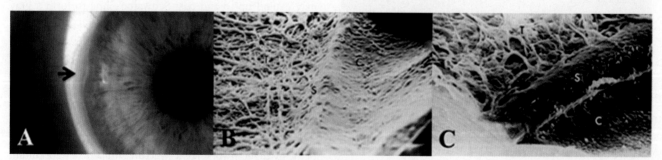

FIGURE 10.5. A: Prominent Schwalbe's ring (posterior embryotoxon). The limbal pigment ring and prominent uveal trabecular meshwork are present. The distinct white ring demarcating the uveal meshwork centrally is the enlarged, displaced Schwalbe's ring (*arrow*), which may be seen in about 10% of normal eyes. **B:** Scanning electron micrograph of normal Schwalbe's ring (*S*), cornea (*C*), and uveal trabecular meshwork (*T*) about at this junction. **C:** Scanning electron micrograph of prominent Schwalbe's ring (posterior embryotoxon). Endothelium covers both cornea (*C*) and elevated Schwalbe's ring (*S*). (Scanning electron micrographs, courtesy of Morton Smith, MD.)

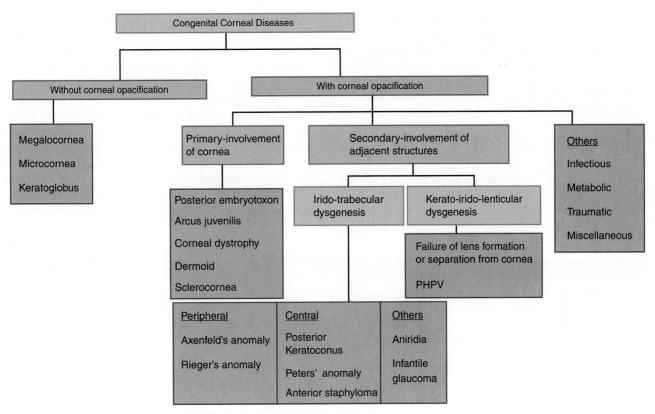

FIGURE 10.6. Flow chart showing clinical classification of congenital corneal diseases.

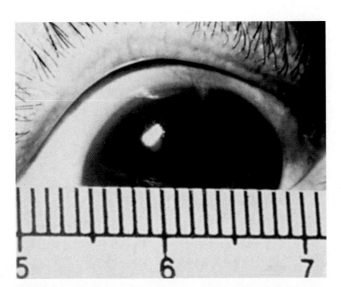

FIGURE 10.7. Anterior megalophthalmos. This cornea measures 15 mm in diameter and has normal thickness and clarity. The disorder is accompanied by transillumination defects in the iris and is associated with lens subluxation and cataract development in the fourth decade.

megalocornea or anterior megalophthalmos, an X-linked recessive trait that consists of megalocornea, iris and angle abnormalities, and lens subluxation with early cataract formation; and (c) buphthalmos in infantile glaucoma (3). In keratoglobus, the protuberant thin cornea appears enlarged clinically but usually has a normal diameter. There seems to be no entity of "megaloglobus" in which the entire globe is congenitally enlarged with a normal intraocular pressure.

Simple Megalocornea. If bilateral clear corneas of normal thickness measure 13 mm or more in diameter without associated ocular abnormalities, the nonprogressive disorder of simple megalocornea exists, and once the diagnosis is clearly made, no other follow-up is necessary (3,4).

X-Linked Megalocornea (Anterior Megalophthalmos). X-linked megalocornea, a recessive disorder, is due to mutation of CHRDL1 gene at locus Xq23. It is the most common type of megalocornea. X-linked megalocornea occurs if the embryonic relationship (bell shaped optic cup) between the diameter of the anterior opening of the cup and the equatorial diameter persists, resulting in an increase in the relative diameter of the anterior segment of the eye compared to the posterior segment (3). It manifests as bilateral, symmetrically enlarged corneas that remain stable throughout life and sometimes contain a stromal mosaic pattern and arcus juvenilis (3,5). The deep anterior chamber occurs because the normal-sized lens, which is too small for the enlarged ciliary ring, subluxates. The iridocorneal angle is open but contains excess mesenchymal tissue, whereas the iris manifests a hypoplastic anterior stroma, transillumination defects, and pigment dispersion. The pupil is occasionally ectopic.

The two associations that threaten vision are the frequently elevated intraocular pressure (often due to pigmentary glaucoma, spherophakia and/or lens subluxation), which requires lifelong annual examinations for early detection, and cataracts, which often appear in the fourth decade and may require the use of vitrectomy-type instruments during extraction, because the lenses are subluxated or dislocated (6,7). Due to enlarged anterior segment, custom-designed intraocular lenses may be required for lens stability and visual rehabilitation (8).

The clinician may have difficulty distinguishing among isolated megalocornea, anterior megalophthalmos, and infantile glaucoma in a young child with an enlarged cornea. Table 10.1 presents the distinctive features of these three disorders.

Keratoglobus. Keratoglobus is a distinct, rare entity that is characterized by generalized thinning and anterior bulging of the cornea. The thinning is greatest in the midperiphery of the cornea (Fig. 10.8A). Keratoglobus may occur as an autosomal recessive disorder that is part of the Ehlers-Danlos syndrome type VIA, in which it is accompanied by hyperextensible joints, blue sclerae, and neurosensory hearing loss. It has also been reported as an acquired condition, associated with various disorders, including vernal keratoconjunctivitis and thyroid ophthalmopathy. In keratoglobus the cornea is one-third normal thickness, usually has a normal diameter, and arcs highly over the iris, creating a very deep anterior chamber. Acute spontaneous breaks in Descemet's membrane

Table 10.1

DIFFERENTIAL DIAGNOSIS OF ENLARGED CORNEA

	Simple Megalocornea	Anterior Megalophthalmos	Primary Infantile Glaucoma with Buphthalmos
Inheritance	Autosomal dominant (?)	X-linked recessive (male preponderance)	Sporadic
Time of appearance	Congenital	Congenital	First year of life
Bilaterality	Bilateral	Bilateral	Unilateral or bilateral
Symmetry	Symmetrical	Symmetrical	Asymmetrical
Natural history	Nonprogressive	Nonprogressive	Progressive
Symptoms	None	None	Photophobia, epiphora
Corneal clarity	Clear	Clear or mosaic dystrophy	Diffuse edema, tears in Descemet's membrane
Intraocular pressure	Normal	Elevated in some adults	Elevated
Corneal diameter	13–18 mm	13–18 mm	13–18 mm
Corneal thickness	Normal	Normal	Thick
Keratometry	Normal	Normal/steep (cornea globosa); ↑ astigmatism (with the rule)	Flat
Gonioscopy	Normal	Excessive mesenchymal tissue	Excessive mesenchymal tissue
Globe diameter (A-scan)	Normal	Normal/increased	Increased and progressive
Anterior chamber depth			
(A-scan)	Presumably normal (3 mm)	Approximately 5 mm	Approximately 4 mm
Vitreous length	Normal	Decreased	Increased
Major ocular complications	None	Lens dislocation, cataract <40 y, secondary glaucoma	Optic disc damage, late corneal edema
Associated systemic disorders	None	Occasionally Marfan's and other skeletal abnormalities	None consistent

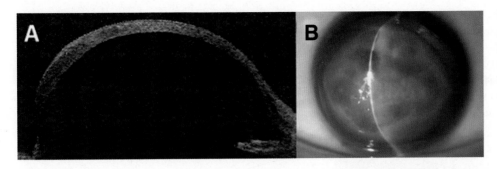

FIGURE 10.8. Keratoglobus **A:** Anterior segment optical coherence tomography showing ectasia of the entire cornea and midperipheral thinning. **B:** Slit-lamp photography demonstrating corneal edema due to corneal hydrops in a patient with keratoglobus.

may produce focal stromal edema (acute hydrops) and heal spontaneously in weeks to months (Fig.10.8B). Minor blunt trauma to the eye or to the head may rupture the thin cornea and sclera, so the ophthalmologist must counsel the parents of these children to provide a safe environment and protective spectacles or eye guards. Amblyopia is often severe because of the high myopia, a problem diminished by carefully fitted spectacles or contact lenses. A scleral lens may be tried if contact lenses are not successful. In patients with severe thinning and anterior bulging of the cornea, surgical treatment may be contemplated. Given the diffuse corneal thinning to the limbus, surgical repair is problematic at best. A large limbus-to-limbus onlay lamellar keratoplasty or epikeratoplasty to both reinforce the corneal integrity and provide a more normal curvature can be performed. A "tuck-in" lamellar keratoplasty (central lamellar keratoplasty with intrastromal tucking of the peripheral flange) is another technique that can be performed in these patients. If the central cornea is scarred, typically from a previous episode of hydrops, a subsequent central visual penetrating keratoplasty can be performed (9–14).

Microcornea. A cornea 7 to 10 mm in diameter occurs in a variety of clinical settings, making classification difficult (Fig. 10.9). Both autosomal dominant and autosomal recessive patterns of inheritance occur, but microcornea may also appear sporadically. Although the exact cause is not known, it is assumed to be due to arrest of the growth of the cornea after differentiation is complete.

Microcornea may be an isolated abnormality in an otherwise normal eye (15,16). It may be associated with nanophthalmos (also called simple microphthalmos), a small, anatomically normal globe; (17–19) or it may be part of microphthalmos (also called complex microphthalmos), a small globe with multiple anomalies (20). A-scan ultrasonography can help distinguish isolated microcornea with normal axial length from microphthalmos with short axial length of the globe (17). All microphthalmic eyes have microcornea but the reverse is not true. Microcornea has syndromic associations with Ehlers-Danlos syndrome (mesodermal), Waardenburg syndrome (craniofacial), Norrie syndrome (neurologic), and Nance-Horan syndrome (osseous).

Management of eyes with microphthalmos varies according to the associated abnormalities. Hyperopia is commonly seen due to the flat cornea (cornea plana) but

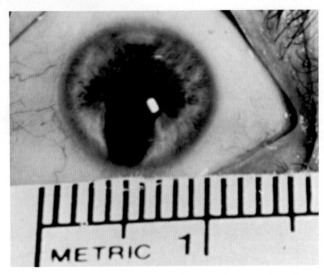

FIGURE 10.9. Microcornea, measuring 9 mm in diameter and accompanied by atypical iris coloboma and congenital cataract. The disorder was inherited as an autosomal dominant trait in this family.

other refractive errors are also seen due to variation in the curvature. Early refraction may help prevent amblyopia. Lifelong examinations will detect intraocular pressure elevation, which occurs more commonly in eyes with microcornea due to associated anomalies of the angle and enlarging lens crowding the small anterior segment. Microcornea is commonly associated with congenital cataracts and is shown to be associated with mutations in various genes. These cataracts should be removed, using special care in eyes manifesting other anomalies (21).

Congenital Corneal Diseases with Corneal Opacification

Anterior Segment Dysgenesis

Abnormal development of the anterior segment structures (cornea, iris, ciliary body and lens) is called anterior segment dysgenesis. It is often difficult to separate abnormalities into individual disease entities. Anterior segment dysgenesis should be considered a heterogeneous clinical spectrum. The terms mesodermal dysgenesis of the iris and stoma (iris and stroma are neuroectoderm elements) and anterior chamber cleavage syndrome (no cleavage plane is formed during the anterior segment development) have been used, but these do not seem to be appropriate in the description of abnormalities that occur during embryogenesis and are of neural crest differentiation (22–25).

Many abnormalities of the cornea, angle, and iris can be classified in an anatomical stepladder fashion, which builds from basic to more complex combinations (26). This approach simplifies our understanding of these anomalies, because the clinician or pathologist needs only to describe the anatomical findings, rather than worry about the proper eponyms or obscure Latin phrases. Unusual anomalies that do not fit into preestablished categories (27) can be inserted into this tabular classification on the basis of their anatomical components. Figure 10.10 represents this classification and includes commonly used eponyms.

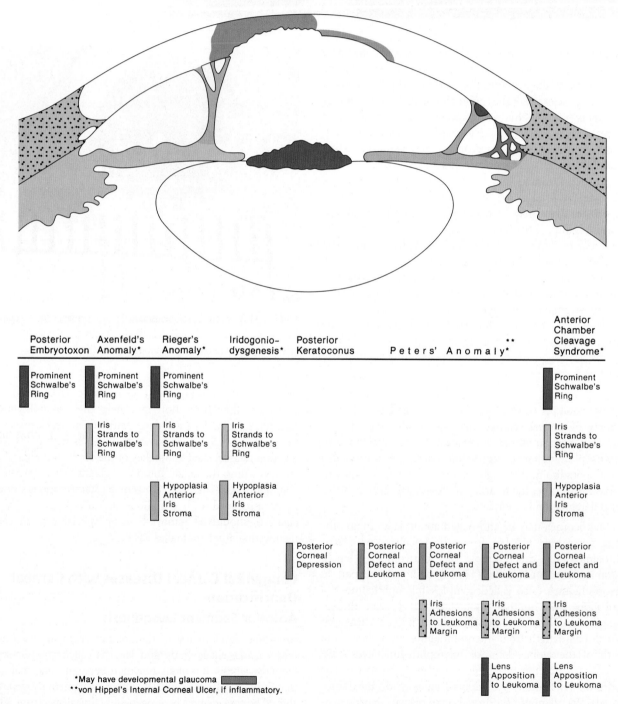

FIGURE 10.10. Composite illustration of the anatomical findings in the anterior chamber cleavage syndrome. The stepladder table demonstrates the spectrum of anatomical combinations and the terms by which they are commonly known. The colored markers in the table indicate the corresponding anatomical component in the illustration. (From Waring GO, Rodrigues M, Laibson PR, et al. Anterior chamber cleavage syndrome: a stepladder classification. *Surv Ophthalmol* 1975;20:5, with permission.)

These malformations conveniently fall into three groups: (a) peripheral (prominent Schwalbe's ring, iris strands to Schwalbe's ring, and hypoplasia of the anterior iris stroma); (b) central (central posterior corneal defect, central iridocorneal adhesions, corneolenticular approximation); and (c) combinations of the peripheral and central components.

Peripheral Anterior Segment Dysgeneses
Prominent Schwalbe's Ring with Attached Iris Strands (Axenfeld's Anomaly)

Iris strands that span the angle to insert on the prominent Schwalbe's ring (Fig. 10.11) display variable morphology: fine threadlike filaments with a terminal knob, broad conical bands, or a confluent, fenestrated, lattice-like membrane. Prominent Schwalbe's ring is usually only partly seen on slit-lamp biomicroscopy but may be seen 360 degrees on gonioscopy. In some cases the pupil is distorted. Axenfeld's syndrome is defined as Axenfeld's anomaly plus glaucoma (26).

Prominent Schwalbe's Ring with Attached Iris Strands and Hypoplastic Anterior Iris Stroma (Rieger's Anomaly)

Eyes with Rieger's anomaly (Figs. 10.12 to 10.17) lack some superficial iris stroma, so that instead of crypts, furrows, and a collarette, the iris manifests a stringy appearance because the delicate radial fibrils of the posterior stroma show through. Abnormally shaped pupils (displaced in the direction of thickened iris band) occur commonly: slit-shaped, pear-shaped, round, ectopic, part of an atypical coloboma, or very large pupils, as in a partial aniridia. In rare cases, the iris atrophy progresses. Contracture of the primordial endothelial layer on the anterior surface of iris leads to these pupillary abnormalities. Rieger's syndrome occurs when systemic anomalies are also present.

Axenfeld's anomaly and syndrome, and Rieger's anomaly and syndrome represent a spectrum of developmental dysgenesis and hence a single diagnostic entity of Axenfeld-Rieger syndrome has been proposed (28,29). Glaucoma is seen in 50% of cases and the onset is delayed compared to infantile glaucoma, and thus lifetime surveillance is required. The pathogenesis of glaucoma is due to improper migration of primordial tissue derived from the neural crest leading to persistence of endothelial layer on the angle and anterior insertion of peripheral iris onto trabecular meshwork leading to impaired aqueous outflow (30). It is inherited as autosomal dominant pattern (70%) with variable expressivity, but sporadic cases are also reported (31). Mutations at locus 4q25 of PITX2 gene and at locus 6p25 of FOXC1 gene are commonly implicated in the pathogenesis of Axenfeld-Rieger syndrome. Corneal endothelium, stroma, iris, ciliary body and sclera express PITX2. Mutations in PITX2 are commonly associated with extraocular systemic abnormalities of Axenfeld-Rieger syndrome. Mutations in FOXC1 are commonly associated with only ocular abnormalities and higher risk for glaucoma (32).

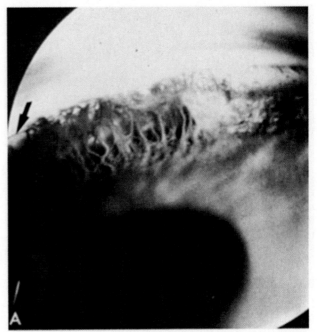

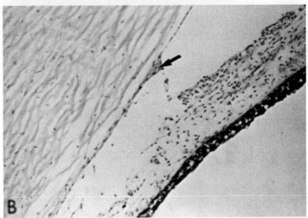

FIGURE 10.11. Axenfeld's anomaly. **A:** Gonioscopic view shows the angle recess filled with dense iris processes (persistent mesenchymal tissue) that extend to a prominent Schwalbe's ring (*arrow*). This configuration may exist alone or as a part of a variety of iridocorneal dysgeneses (Courtesy of Robinson D. Harley, MD). **B:** Histologic section showing the prominent centrally displaced Schwalbe's ring (*arrow*) with iris processes extending to it and across the angle recess (×64). (Courtesy of Merlyn Rodrigues, MD.)

The most common systemic condition associated with Axenfeld-Rieger syndrome is cardiovascular outflow tract abnormalities, but craniofacial and skeletal abnormalities are also seen (33–35).

Iris Strands in Angle and Hypoplasia of Anterior Iris Stroma (Iridogoniodysgenesis)

This abnormality, inherited in an autosomal dominant pattern, resembles Rieger's anomaly without the prominent Schwalbe's ring (36). Affected individuals very commonly have juvenile glaucoma.

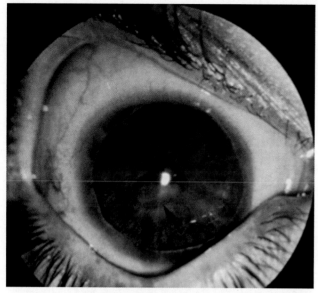

FIGURE 10.12. Rieger's anomaly with central posterior corneal defect. This right eye of a 23-year-old dwarf demonstrates a prominent Schwalbe's ring with the iris process extending to it, an atrophic anterior iris stroma, and a central posterior corneal defect (posterior keratoconus) (*arrow*). Intraocular pressure was normal. The left eye appeared similar.

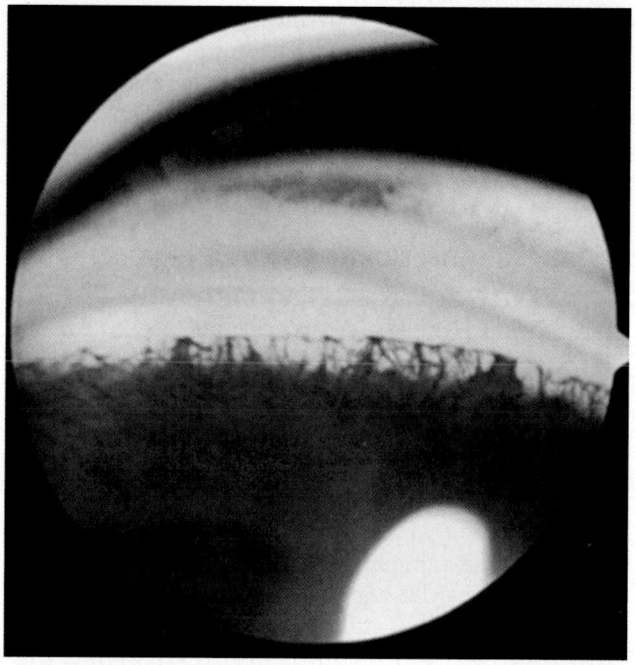

Infantile Glaucoma

If this classification is extended, infantile glaucoma (with or without buphthalmos) can be added, on the basis that it represents a mesenchymal goniodysgenesis. In fact, some authors believe that the megalocornea seen in infantile glaucoma is a result of a primary keratodysgenesis, rather than a result of stretching from increased intraocular pressure (37).

The management of infantile and juvenile glaucoma is discussed in Chapter 12.

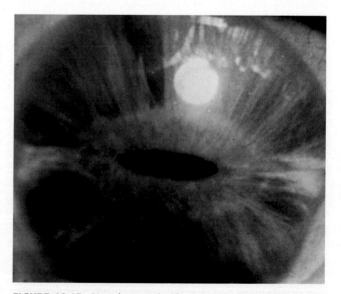

FIGURE 10.14. Angle in Rieger's anomaly. Gonioscopic appearance of eye in Figures 10.12 and 10.13, showing iris processes extending to the prominent Schwalbe's ring.

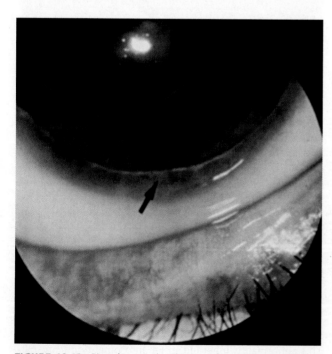

FIGURE 10.13. Rieger's anomaly. Close-up of 6 o'clock limbus of eye in Figure 10.12. Iris processes (*arrow*) extend to the irregular prominent Schwalbe's ring.

FIGURE 10.15. Rieger's anomaly. The right eye shows marked hypoplasia of the anterior iris stroma. The deep stroma is thin and fibrillary, revealing the underlying iris epithelium and pupillary sphincter. The pupil is slit-shaped and central. The prominent Schwalbe's ring is poorly illustrated. (Courtesy of George L. Spaeth, MD.)

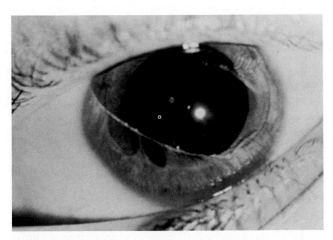

FIGURE 10.16. Rieger's anomaly. This 10-year-old white girl has a centrally displaced prominent Schwalbe's ring with iris processes extending to it from the angle recess and the collarette. Anterior iris stroma is absent at 11 o'clock position. The configuration is accentuated by the dilated pupil. Intraocular pressure was normal. No other ocular anomalies existed. (Courtesy of Harold Koller, MD.)

Central Anterior Segment Dysgenesis: General Features

The basic abnormality in this group is a focal attenuation or absence of the corneal endothelium and Descemet's membrane, usually associated with an overlying corneal opacity. In contrast with the peripheral abnormalities, the central disorders have two separate etiologies, primary dysgenesis and secondary to inflammation, but the clinical and histopathologic distinction between the two is difficult. Presumably, if the cornea is avascular and there are no signs of inflammation, one can assume that the disorder is a primary dysgenesis; however, if the cornea is opaque and vascularized, intrauterine inflammation may have been present. Therefore, these entities are discussed on the basis of their anatomical findings alone, rather than their pathogenesis. Glaucoma is present in about half the cases, usually appearing as a nonbuphthalmic infantile form.

Postnatally, the corneal opacity may clear somewhat, particularly if it is avascular, central, and consists mostly of edema. On the other hand, the opacity may progressively vascularize, particularly if the cornea is ectatic and the anterior segment derangement is severe.

Posterior Corneal Depression (Central Posterior Keratoconus)

This focal, discrete, posterior corneal indentation has a faint overlying stromal haze and is usually central, unilateral, and nonprogressive (Fig. 10.18) (38). In some instances, a ring of pigment clumps surrounds the depression, indicating previous iris contact (39). The anterior corneal curvature is not dramatically irregular, and the disorder is unrelated to the more common form of acquired progressive anterior keratoconus. Visual acuity is only moderately reduced, presumably because of the irregular astigmatism resulting in mild amblyopia. Some authors described a total posterior keratoconus, which may be a variant of the more common progressive

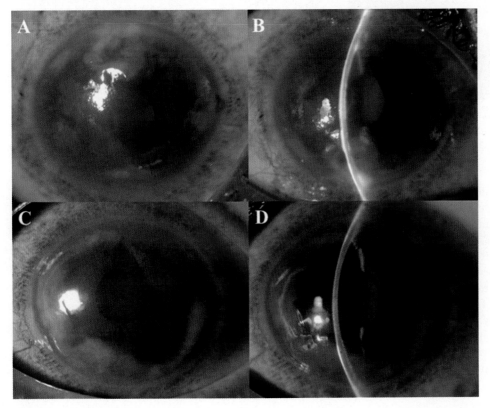

FIGURE 10.17. Rieger's anomaly. **A, B:** The right eye demonstrating a peripheral corneal opacity and edema with iris strands anteriorly with peaking of pupil toward 1 o'clock. **C, D:** The left eye demonstrating peripheral corneal opacity and edema, prominent Schwalbe's ring nasally with iris processes extending to it, atrophic anterior iris stroma (12–3 o'clock) and also inferiorly on gonioscopy. Intraocular pressure was normal.

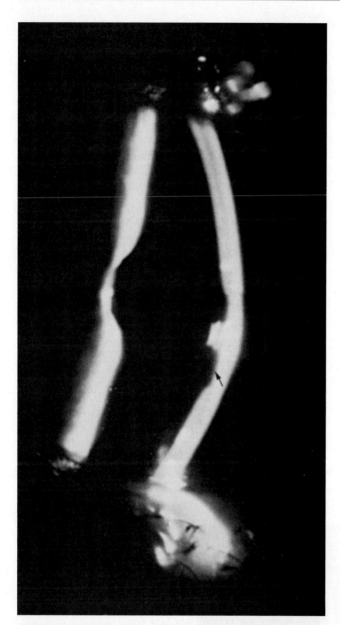

FIGURE 10.18. Posterior keratoconus. Slit-lamp view of the eye in Figure 10.12, showing the depression in the posterior corneal surface (*arrow*). The cornea overlying it is clear, and no iris processes extend to its margin.

degenerative type (40). Histopathologically, abnormalities include an irregularly thickened epithelial basement membrane, focal disruption of Bowman's layer, stromal irregularity, and a multilaminar Descemet's membrane that contains wide-spacing material and focal excrescences (41). Scanning electron microscopy was used to evaluate a cornea with posterior keratoconus, revealing no excrescences of Descemet's membrane or endothelial tags (42). Given these findings, Al-Hazzaa et al. (42) suggest there may be a subset of posterior keratoconus patients who do not fall into the category of anterior segment dysgenesis abnormalities.

The anterior corneal curvature in eyes with posterior keratoconus has generally been described as essentially normal. One problem is that most methods used to evaluate corneal curvature, including the keratometer and keratoscope, do not examine the central few millimeters of cornea well at all. With the advent of computerized corneal topography/tomography, central as well as midperipheral anterior corneal curvature can be effectively analyzed. Computerized corneal videokeratography was performed on an eye with posterior keratoconus, revealing a central steepened "cone" associated with the area of posterior corneal thinning (43).

Posterior Corneal Defect with Overlying Leukoma (Peters' Anomaly)

Peters' anomaly represents a range of features from a simple defect in the posterior cornea producing an overlying opacity to severe ocular and systemic malformations. If the opacity is dense enough, it may obscure the more normal anterior segment anatomy.

Posterior Corneal Defect with Stromal Opacity and Adherent Iris Strands (Peters' Anomaly Type I)

The size and density of the corneal opacity and the depth of the posterior defect can vary widely, from a small, central, focal, ground-glass opacity (Fig. 10.19A); to a dense, round leukoma (Fig. 10.19B); to total corneal vascularization and scarring with an elevated mass (see Fig. 10.21A). The lens is clear and in normal position. The configurations of the iris strands that extend from the collarette to the margin of the posterior defect are as diversified as the opacity and include fine filaments (Fig. 10.19A), broad bands, and fenestrated sheets.

The histopathologic findings are equally varied but usually include thickening or fragmentation of Bowman's layer, disorganization of stromal architecture, central absence of Descemet's membrane and endothelium (both of which are present peripherally), and central iridocorneal adhesions (Figs. 10.20 and 10.21C,D).

Posterior Corneal Defect with Stromal Opacity, Adherent Iris Strands, and Corneolenticular Contact or Cataract (Peters' Anomaly Type II)

In this variant of Peters' anomaly, a variety of lens abnormalities occur (44), including adhesion of lens cortex to the corneal stroma at the site of the posterior defect (Figs. 10.22 and 10.23) (45), approximation to the back of the cornea with an intact lens capsule, displacement into the anterior chamber or into the pupil, or a central cataract with maintenance of a normal position (46). These lens abnormalities occur due to faulty separation of the lens vesicle from the surface ectoderm. It is also associated with other ocular abnormalities such as aniridia, microcornea, microphthalmos (47,48).

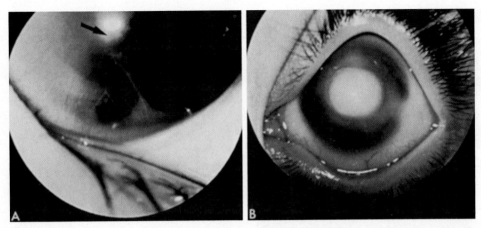

FIGURE 10.19. A: Peters' anomaly. A mild form showing attenuated iris adhesions to the border of a small corneal opacity (*arrow*). This was present bilaterally in this 9-month-old white girl. **B:** Peters' anomaly. This 10-month-old white girl had bilateral congenital central corneal opacities. During penetrating keratoplasty, iris adhesions were found extending from the pupillary margin to the borders of the opacity. An anterior polar cataract was present. (Courtesy of Harold Koller, MD.) The histopathologic findings are equally varied but usually include thickening or fragmentation of Bowman's layer, disorganization of stromal architecture, central absence of Descemet's membrane and endothelium (both of which are present peripherally), and central iridocorneal adhesions (Figs. 10.20 and 10.21C, D).

Peters' anomaly associated with systemic abnormalities such as short stature, developmental delay, and cleft lip/palate is termed as Peters Plus syndrome. Peters' anomaly is usually bilateral. Bilateral Peters' anomaly is associated with more systemic malformations compared to unilateral cases. Peters' anomaly is usually sporadic or autosomal recessive but autosomal dominant patterns have been reported. Peters' anomaly is associated with mutations of homeobox genes PAX6 (locus-11p13), PITX2 (locus-4q25), and FOXC1 (6p25). Peters Plus syndrome is associated with mutation of the gene B3GALTL at locus 13q12.3 (48,49).

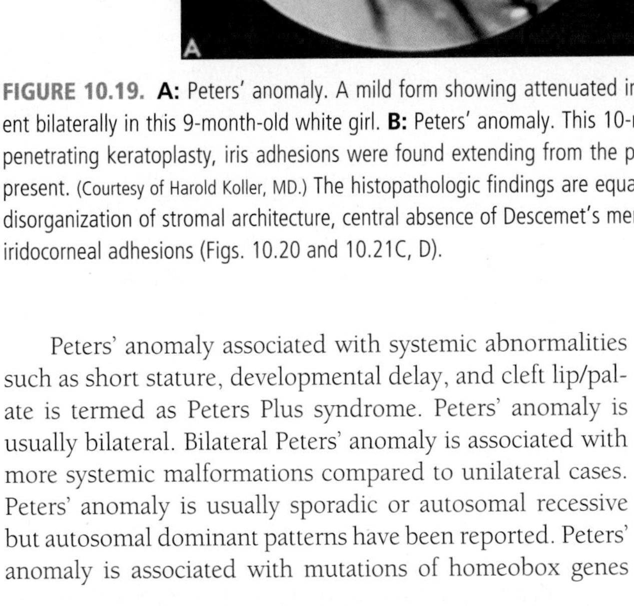

Corneal Staphyloma

In this most severe form of posterior corneal defect, the ectatic, thin, scarred, vascularized cornea is lined by uveal tissue and may protrude between the eyelids (Fig. 10.24) (50). The ectasia may be present at birth but usually becomes worse in the first week of life. Intraocular pressure is usually elevated, and the lens is incorporated into the scarred ectatic cornea. In rare instances, the cornea develops a hypertrophic keloid scar (51).

Pathogenesis of Posterior Corneal Defects

There are four pathogenic theories (44,52,53): (a) intrauterine keratitis, leaving a posterior defect commonly called the *internal corneal ulcer of von Hippel;* (b) incomplete central migration of the neural crest mesenchymal waves that form the corneal endothelium and stroma; (c) improper separation of the lens vesicle from the surface ectoderm, which may produce the central defect by blocking the ingrowth of the neural crest mesenchymal tissue and may result in a persistent keratolenticular adhesion without an intact lens capsule; and (d) secondary anterior displacement of the lens by a vitreoretinal-mass-like persistent hyperplastic primary vitreous or pupillary block from a persistent pupillary membrane. Because none of these four theories adequately explains all the clinical or histopathologic findings, and because there is experimental evidence supporting each one, these congenital anomalies must be regarded as a heterogeneous group with a similar clinical appearance.

FIGURE 10.20. Peters' anomaly. Histologic section demonstrates iris adhesions that extend from the collarette to the margin of a central posterior corneal defect. The overlying cornea is edematous. Descemet's membrane ends abruptly at the margin of the central defect (*arrow*) (×6). (Courtesy of Robert D'Amico, MD.)

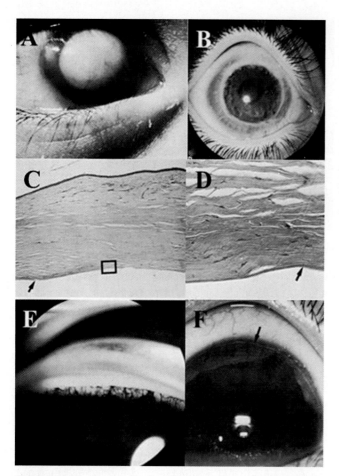

FIGURE 10.21. Anterior chamber cleavage syndrome. **A:** This 7-month-old boy had bilateral megalocornea (13 mm in diameter), **(A–D)** a central posterior corneal defect with corneal leukoma in the right eye (Peters' anomaly), and **(E, F)** Rieger's anomaly of the left eye (Courtesy of Turgut Hamdi, MD). **B:** Keratoplasty for central posterior corneal defect. A penetrating keratoplasty was performed in the right eye at age 22 months, and the graft remained clear for 5 months until graft rejection occurred. No iris processes extended to the corneal leukoma. An anterior polar cataract was discovered postoperatively. **C:** Central posterior corneal defect with scarring. Histopathologically, the corneal button shows superficial fibrovascular invasion and deep stromal edema. In this area, Bowman's layer and Descemet's membrane are absent (*box*). The margin of the button (*left side*) shows more normal cornea with edematous stroma. Descemet's membrane is present in this area (*arrow*) (Periodic acid-Schiff (PAS) ×25). **D:** Central posterior corneal defect. The area in the box shows the transition (*arrow*) from intact Descemet's membrane peripherally to its replacement by fibrous tissue centrally. Only fragments of endothelium were seen (PAS ×250). **E:** Megalocornea and Rieger's anomaly. The left eye of this patient exhibited a 13-mm diameter cornea, a prominent Schwalbe's ring (*arrow*) with iris processes extending to it, and a hypoplastic iris stroma. **F:** Iris processes in Rieger's anomaly. The angle filled with delicate iris processes and mesenchymal tissue extending up to the prominent Schwalbe's ring.

The descriptive anatomical classification is especially helpful in the central–peripheral combinations, because it allows one to see the exact components in each case, instead of resorting to a combination of eponyms.

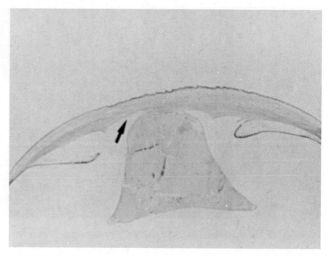

FIGURE 10.22. Congenital lens–corneal adhesion (Peters' anomaly). The eye of this newborn demonstrates irregular and thickened corneal epithelium and stroma, central absence of Bowman's and Descemet's membranes, a central posterior corneal defect (*arrow*) with a lens-corneal adhesion, a conical cataractous lens, and malformation of the anterior chamber angles with adhesion of the iris to the cornea. (PAS ×3) (Courtesy of Charles G. Steinmetz, MD.)

Corneal Keloid

Corneal keloid is a gray-white elevated mass that may present as a localized solitary nodule or diffusely involving the entire cornea (Fig. 10.25). They are congenital or more typically secondary to trauma. Congenital corneal keloids are due to failure of normal differentiation of corneal tissue during embryogenesis. Intrauterine trauma due to amniocentesis may be a cause, but fortunately the incidence of complications due to amniocentesis has decreased due to more advanced ultrasound-guided techniques (54). In posttraumatic cases, a mechanical stimulus triggers a cellular inflammatory response (vasodilation and recruitment of immature fibroblasts). Subsequently, there is regression of blood vessels, myofibroblast proliferation and scar retraction. At times, this response leads to a vigorous fibrocytic response causing formation of an exuberant glistening mass. Diagnosis is confirmed based on histopathologic presence of hyalinized collagen, activated fibroblasts, and myofibroblasts. Congenital keloid may be associated with Lowe syndrome and Rubinstein-Taybi syndrome. Various surgical modalities such as superficial lamellar keratectomy, lamellar keratoplasty or full-thickness keratoplasty have been reported with variable success rates (55–59).

Aniridia

Aniridia is a bilateral congenital disorder associated with panocular abnormalities affecting not only the iris but also the cornea, anterior chamber angle, lens, retina, and optic nerve. It is inherited in an autosomal dominant pattern in most cases, but sporadic and rarely autosomal recessive

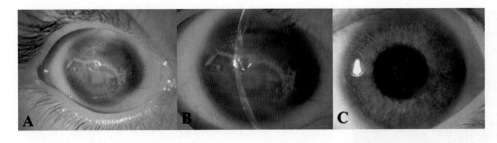

FIGURE 10.23. Peters' anomaly **A, B:** The right eye of this child showing central corneal opacity with relatively clear periphery and iris adhesions to the midperiphery and central cornea. **C:** The left eye of the same patient demonstrating a corneal posterior opacity with an anterior lenticular opacity suggesting a partial dysgenesis.

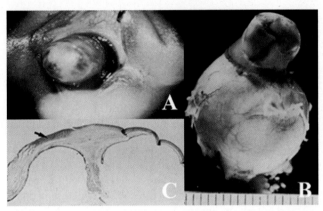

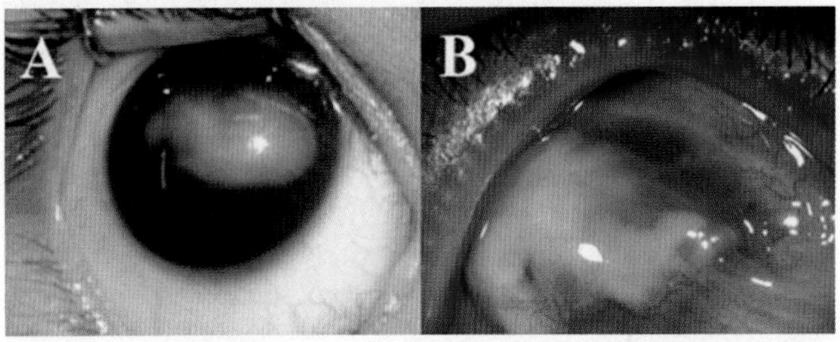

FIGURE 10.25. Congenital corneal keloid. **A:** 3-month-old boy with corneal keloid and normal intraocular structures, **B:** Corneal keloid with vascularization in a child associated with Lowe's syndrome.

FIGURE 10.24. Congenital corneal staphyloma. **A:** This 5-day-old infant was born with a flat opaque right cornea. By age 2 days, the cornea had become blue and ectatic, as shown here. The left eye was normal, except for persistent pupillary membrane (Courtesy of Joseph H. Calhoun, MD). **B:** Gross appearance of the globe. The ectatic area is limited to the cornea (Courtesy of Merlyn Rodrigues, MD). **C:** Histologic section of globe. Areas of the cornea are thin and ectatic. A superficial corneal abscess from exposure is present (*arrow*). Bowman's and Descemet's membranes are absent. A rudimentary lens is adherent to the central posterior cornea, blending with stromal tissue. Uveal tissue is firmly adherent to the posterior cornea, sweeping down along the lens rudiment (Hematoxylin-eosin ×3). (Courtesy of Merlyn Rodrigues, MD.)

inheritance is also seen. Patients with sporadic aniridia are at risk for WAGR syndrome (Wilms tumor, aniridia, genitourinary abnormalities, mental retardation) and should undergo routine surveillance for kidney disorders. Aniridia is due to mutation at locus 11p13 of the paired box gene 6 (PAX6). It is usually associated with keratopathy, cataract, glaucoma, foveal hypoplasia and strabismus. Dental, musculoskeletal and developmental delays are systemic abnormalities frequently associated with aniridia. Keratopathy is thought to be due to an abnormally differentiated epithelium, abnormal cell adhesion, impaired healing response and limbal stem-cell deficiency leading to conjunctivalization of cornea. It begins as vascularized thickening of the cornea at the periphery, which gradually advances centrally. Recurrent corneal erosions lead to subepithelial fibrosis causing corneal opacification. Corneal opacification that occurs due to recurrent erosions is caused by deficiency in matrix metalloproteinase

9 (regulated by PAX6), which is responsible for normal cell remodeling and wound healing. Penetrating keratoplasty for visual rehabilitation is generally unsuccessful because of recurrent surface breakdown. Keratolimbal allograft and Boston keratoprosthesis have proven to be effective for long-term visual rehabilitation (Fig. 10.26) (60–62).

Neonatal Corneal Opacities
Differential Diagnosis

The ophthalmologist often feels stumped when confronted by a child with a neonatal corneal opacity. These feelings provide an apt acronym for the causes of neonatal corneal opacities: STUMPED (Table 10.2) (63).

Sclerocornea (Stumped)

Clinicians often use the term "sclerocornea" as a nonspecific description for any congenitally opaque, vascularized cornea. Too broad a use of the term, however, obscures valuable distinctions. Clinically, sclerocornea denotes a congenital peripheral white vascularized opacity that blends with the sclera, due to anterior displacement of limbal arcades, obliterating the corneoscleral limbus and scleral sulcus.

Previously proposed by Waring and Rodrigues, but recently reclassified by Nischal into three groups (64,65):

1. Isolated sclerocornea (Fig. 10.27A). Patients in this group have no other ocular abnormalities and show either exaggerated scleral extension (scleralization, scleral overriding) or more extensive peripheral corneal opacification and vascularization. It may be associated

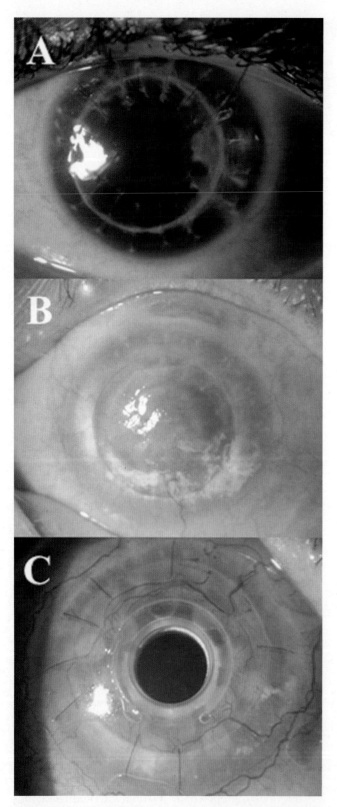

FIGURE 10.26. Aniridia. **A:** Central clear penetrating keratoplasty in a patient with aniridia. **B:** Failed penetrating keratoplasty due to aniridia-induced keratopathy. **C:** Boston keratoprosthesis in a patient with multiple failed grafts. The visual acuity remained 20/400 due to amblyopia and nystagmus.

with cornea plana (<38D) and a slightly shallow anterior chamber, which may be a risk factor for the development of secondary glaucoma (66). It should be differentiated from arcus juvenilis, which is devoid of vessels and has a clear lucid interval between the limbus and the corneal opacification.

2. Complex sclerocornea. It is usually associated with other ocular abnormalities such as microphthalmos, cataract and infantile glaucoma. The central cornea is relatively clear and the corneal thickness is normal or increased (67).

3. Total sclerocornea (Fig. 10.27B). When the cornea is opaque enough to prohibit visualization of the iris and lens, a precise clinical diagnosis is difficult. In some cases, the lens and iris may remain unseparated from the cornea. Limbal anlage that is well defined by the 10th week of gestation distinguishes the cornea and sclera by providing a ring of stability. The absence of this ring leads to corneal curvature similar to that in sclera.

Histopathologically, sclerocornea shows an irregular epithelium with variably thick basement membrane, a fragmented or absent Bowman's layer, and disorganized spindles of vascularized stromal collagenous tissue that contain collagen fibrils. The collagen fibers are of larger diameter in the superficial stroma compared to the deep stroma, similar to the structure of sclera. The random structure of these large fibrils and their attendant blood vessels scatter light and give the cornea its white clinical appearance. Descemet's membrane is abnormal, either being present as a thin irregular layer with collagenous tissue behind it or showing focal dehiscences that may contain fibrous tissue. The endothelium is usually damaged, precluding detailed description (68,69). Syndromic abnormalities inconsistently accompany sclerocornea (70,71).

Tears in Endothelium and Descemet's Membrane (sTumped)

Birth trauma is discussed later in this chapter. Infantile glaucoma is discussed in Chapter 21.

Ulcers (stUmped)

Corneal ulceration in the neonate is extremely rare. It can occur due to a variety of causes including infectious and inflammatory reasons. We have observed one patient with a congenital sensory neuropathy of unknown type who was born with bilateral, shallow, central corneal ulcers. Corneal melting persisted, and in spite of therapy with tarsorrhaphies, soft contact lenses, and keratoplasties, both eyes were finally enucleated.

Viral infections of the cornea are discussed later in this chapter.

Table 10.2

STUMPED: DIFFERENTIAL DIAGNOSIS OF NEONATAL CORNEAL OPACITIES

Diagnosis	Laterality	Opacity	Ocular Pressure	Other Ocular Abnormalities	Natural History	Inheritance
S-Sclerocornea	Unilateral or bilateral	Vascularized, blends with sclera, clearer centrally/total scleralization of the cornea	Normal or elevated	Cornea plana	Nonprogressive	Sporadic
T-Tears in endothelium and Descemet's membrane						
Birth trauma	Unilateral	Diffuse edema	Normal, possibly elevated	Possible hyphema, periorbital ecchymoses	Spontaneous improvement in 1 month	Sporadic
Infantile glaucoma	Bilateral	Diffuse edema	Elevated	Megalocornea, photophobia and tearing, abnormal angle	Progressive unless treated	Autosomal recessive
U-Ulcers						
Herpes simplex keratitis	Unilateral	Diffuse with dendritic or geographical epithelial defect	Normal or elevated	None	Often recurrent	Sporadic
Congenital rubella	Bilateral	Disciform or diffuse edema, no frank ulceration	Normal or elevated	Microphthalmos, cataract, pigment epithelial mottling	Stable, may be clear	Sporadic
Neurotrophic or exposure	Unilateral or bilateral	Central ulcer	Normal	Eyelid anomalies, congenital sensory neuropathy	Progressive unless treated	Sporadic
M-Metabolic (rarely present at birth) (all mucopoly-saccharidoses except II, III; mucolipidosis Type IV)*	Bilateral	Diffuse haze, denser peripherally	Normal	Few	Progressive	Generally autosomal recessive or X-linked recessive
P-Posterior corneal defect (Peters' anomaly)	Unilateral or bilateral	Central, diffuse haze or vascularized leukoma	Normal or elevated	Anterior segment dysgenesis	Stable; sometimes early clearing or vascularization	Sporadic, autosomal recessive
E-Endothelial dystrophy						

(continued)

Table 10.2

(contintued)

Diagnosis	Laterality	Opacity	Ocular Pressure	Other Ocular Abnormalities	Natural History	Inheritance
Congenital hereditary endothelial dystrophy	Bilateral	Diffuse corneal edema, marked corneal thickening	Normal	None	Stable	Autosomal dominant or recessive
Posterior polymorphous corneal dystrophy	Bilateral	Diffuse haze, normal to moderate corneal thickening	Normal or elevated	Occasional peripheral anterior synechiae	Slowly progressive	Autosomal dominant
Congenital stromal corneal dystrophy (more stromal than endothelial)	Bilateral	Flaky, feathery stromal opacities; increased corneal thickness	Normal	None	Stable	Autosomal dominant
D-Dermoid	Unilateral or bilateral	White vascularized mass, hair, lipid arc	Normal	None	Stable	Sporadic

*Mucopolysaccharidosis II (Hunter's syndrome); mucopolysaccharidosis III (Sanfilippo's syndrome).

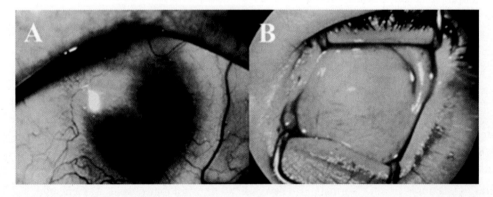

FIGURE 10.27. Sclerocornea. **A:** Scleral tissue extends in a geographical pattern toward the central cornea. Some clear cornea remains centrally. **B:** Total replacement of the cornea by sclera. Penetrating keratoplasty was unsuccessful. The iris and lens were grossly malformed. (Courtesy of Joseph Calhoun, MD.)

Metabolic (stuMped)

Because the fetus has access to maternal enzymes, systemic metabolic disorders, such as the mucopolysaccharidoses, mucolipidosis, and tyrosinosis that later develop corneal opacities, are rarely present at birth. A consistent exception to this is mucolipidosis type IV (ganglioside neuraminidase deficiency). These metabolic disorders are discussed in more detail in Chapter 21.

Posterior Corneal Defect, Peters' Anomaly (stumPed)

These central corneal opacities are discussed earlier in this chapter.

Endothelial Dystrophies (stumpEd)

These dystrophies are discussed later in this chapter.

Dermoid (stumpeD)

A corneal dermoid tumor, classified as a choristoma (Fig. 10.28), is a solid, congenital, rounded mass consisting of keratinized epithelium overlying fibrofatty tissue that contains hair follicles, sebaceous glands, and sweat glands (72,73). Rarely, ectopic lacrimal gland, another choristoma, can appear similar to a dermoid. A dermoid is usually a single unilateral pink-white-gray mass, 1 to 5 mm in diameter, which straddles the limbus inferotemporally. They are usually sporadic but

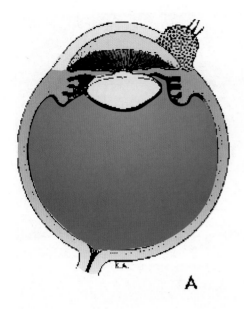

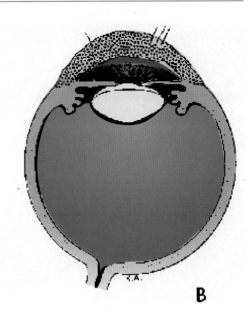

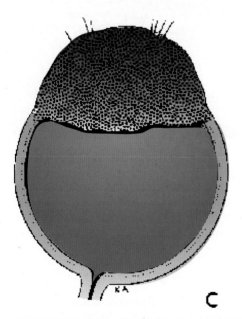

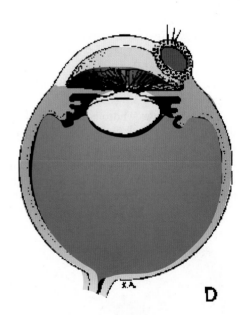

FIGURE 10.28. Corneal dermoids, schematics. **A:** Limbal dermoid tumor. **B:** Dermoid tumor replacing the entire cornea. **C:** Dermoid tumor replacing the entire anterior segment. **D:** Dermoid cyst of cornea (After Ida Mann).

rarely its occurrence in families has been reported. The clinical picture is highly variable, however. The masses may be multiple, bilateral, confined to the cornea alone, minutely small, or large enough to obscure the entire cornea (Fig. 10.29). The dermoid extends into the corneal stroma and sclera but seldom occupies the full thickness and only rarely grows into the angle. Hair is not always present on the surface. Dermoids have been classified into three grades: Grade-1, most frequent type and is small (up to 5 mm) and isolated. Grade-2, is much larger and may cover the entire corneal surface and may extend into deeper layers of the cornea. Grade-3, most severe and rare, it replaces the entire anterior segment (74).

Dermoids may enlarge slowly, especially at puberty or after trauma or irritation. A limbal dermoid may leave visual acuity unaffected, but if it grows over the visual axis or produces significant corneal astigmatism, amblyopia will likely result. Dermoids contain considerable fatty tissue, and a white arcuate haze of lipoid material commonly extends into the corneal stroma in front of the tumor. This lipid may encroach on the visual axis and blur vision.

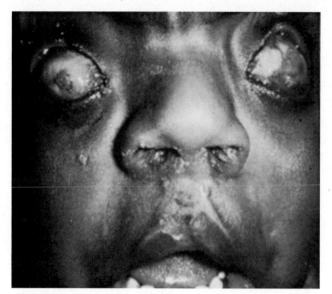

FIGURE 10.29. Bilateral dermoid tumors replacing the entire cornea. This 3-year-old boy was born with masses of vascularized tissue containing surface hair protruding grotesquely between his eyelids. He has had repair of cleft lip and palate. (Courtesy of Robison D. Harley, MD.)

Approximately one-third of patients with limbal dermoids have associated developmental anomalies. Among the most frequent is the constellation of epibulbar dermoids, preauricular appendages, and vertebral anomalies (Goldenhar syndrome [oculoauriculovertebral dysplasia]) (Figs. 10.30 to 10.33) (73,75).

In Goldenhar syndrome the epibulbar dermoid straddles the limbus in the inferotemporal quadrant. It is bilateral in about 25% of cases. A subconjunctival lipodermoid or dermolipoma (lipoma covered by keratinized or nonkeratinized epithelium with hair on the surface) is found in the superotemporal quadrant in about 50% of cases. This

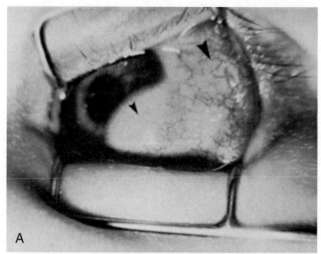

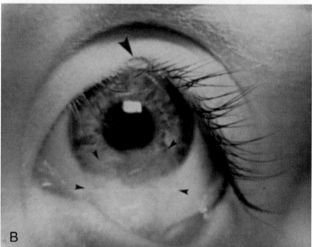

FIGURE 10.31. Goldenhar's (oculoauriculovertebral dysplasia) syndrome. **A:** A lipodermoid of the conjunctiva (*large arrow*) and an epibulbar dermoid of the limbus (*small arrow*) are present concurrently in about half the cases. **B:** A coloboma of the upper eyelid at the junction of the middle and inner thirds is present in about one-fourth of cases (*large arrow*). The limbal dermoid tumor has been excised (*small arrows*). (Courtesy of Jules Baum, MD.)

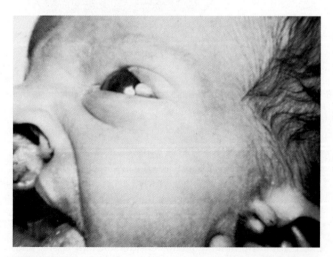

FIGURE 10.30. Goldenhar's (oculoauriculovertebral dysplasia) syndrome. The limbal dermoid and preauricular skin tags are present, in addition to a cleft lip. (Courtesy of Robison D. Harley, MD.)

lipodermoid may blend with the epibulbar dermoid. A coloboma of the upper eyelid is present at the junction of the middle and inner third in about 25% of cases. Other associated ocular anomalies include Duane syndrome, lacrimal duct stenosis, and iris and choroidal colobomas.

Auricular anomalies—usually on the same side as the dermoid—include preauricular appendages, posteriorly placed ears, preauricular sinuses, and stenosis of the external auditory meatus. Vertebral anomalies occur in about two thirds of patients, including fused cervical vertebrae, hemivertebrae, spina bifida, and occipitalization of the atlas. Lumbosacral abnormalities also occur. Facial malformations include micrognathia, macrostomia, dental abnormalities, and facial asymmetry. The diagnosis of Goldenhar syndrome should lead to complete examination for associated

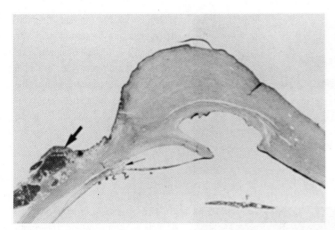

FIGURE 10.32. Corneal dermoid, posterior corneal defect, and Axenfeld's anomaly. In the right eye, cornea is replaced by a mass of vascularized connective tissue. Ectopic lacrimal gland is present at the limbus (*large arrow*). In this area the angle is deep and contains a prominent Schwalbe's ring with iris processes adherent to it (*small arrow*). A central posterior corneal defect is present. On one side, the iris stretches from the angle to the edge of the defect. Descemet's membrane is present in this area. On the opposite side, iris lines the corneal defect and posterior cornea; Descemet's membrane is absent in these areas (Hematoxylin-eosin ×3).

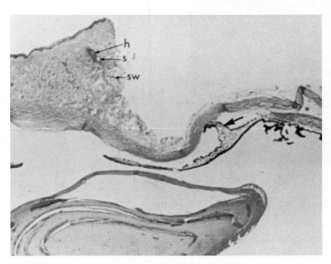

FIGURE 10.33. Corneal dermoid, central posterior corneal defect, and iris-corneal adhesion. The left eye of the patient shown in Figure 10.32. Anterior cornea is replaced by vascularized connective tissue containing hair follicle (*h*), sebaceous gland (*s*), and sweat gland (*sw*). A biopsy has been taken for diagnostic purposes, leaving a defect. Descemet's membrane is present peripherally but absent centrally. An iris adhesion (*arrow*) is present centrally. Angle structures are disorganized (Hematoxylin ×4).

systemic abnormalities, especially cardiovascular, renal, genitourinary, and gastrointestinal defects. Goldenhar syndrome occurs sporadically.

Limbal dermoids should be excised if they produce visual disturbance, are irritated, or are cosmetically embarrassing (see Fig. 10.23). Small asymptomatic tumors may

be observed. Surgical intervention should be tempered by three facts: (a) The attempt to remove all of the dermoid may lead to corneal perforation, (b) the scar remaining after excision is sometimes as unsightly as the original tumor, and (c) astigmatism may not improve significantly postoperatively. Various surgical techniques including lamellar keratectomy with or without amniotic membrane transplantation and lamellar keratoplasty have been performed to remove dermoids and improve the visual and cosmetic outcomes (Figs. 10.34, 10.35, 10.36). Performing a lamellar keratoplasty may help minimize the dangers of ocular perforation and subsequent scar formation. It may be worthwhile to perform gonioscopy on patients before or at the time of surgery to discover possible angle involvement (76–78). A high-frequency ultrasound biomicroscopy (UBM) evaluation can be very helpful in determining the depth and extent of the dermoid preoperatively (79,80). A donor cornea should be available at surgery, in case the anterior chamber is entered. Dermoids rarely recur.

Management of Neonatal Corneal Opacities
Team Approach

The ophthalmologist who takes care of an infant with opaque corneas must decide whether or not keratoplasty is indicated. This complex undertaking is often best managed by subspecialty consultants who form a team to provide optimal management. The team may consist of (a) the coordinating ophthalmologist, who usually practices near the family and is aware of its social and medical circumstances; (b) a social service person, who can look after the details of transportation, economic difficulties, proper delivery of medications at home, and maintenance of appointments; (c) a corneal surgeon, who is experienced in infant keratoplasty and anterior segment reconstruction; (d) a glaucoma consultant, who is experienced in medical and surgical management of infantile and developmental glaucomas; (e) a pediatric ophthalmologist, who is facile in the treatment of amblyopia and strabismus; (f) a contact lens specialist, who has a large inventory of both hard and soft contact lenses, especially those in powers from +20.00 diopters to +30.00 diopters to correct infant aphakia; and (g) motivated parents who understand all of the necessary tasks and are willing and able to perform them before, and for many years after, a corneal transplant in a child. Although the assembly of such an entourage may seem excessive, the complexity and nuances of rehabilitating these eyes over the years of infancy and childhood often require such expertise and dedication.

Preoperative Examination

The preoperative pediatric ophthalmologic examination (81,82) is reviewed briefly here. Thorough history (family and obstetric) from the parents and complete physical examination which play a crucial role in the diagnosis should be completed before ocular examination. Examination under

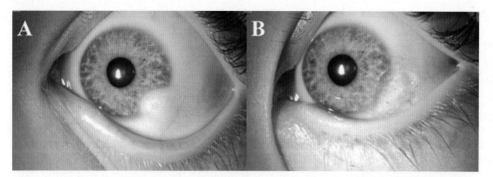

FIGURE 10.34. Corneal dermoid. **A:** Left eye of a 5-year-old child with Goldenhar's (oculoauriculovertebral dysplasia) syndrome with a limbal dermoid (4.8 × 4.5 mm) with visible cilia. **B:** 1 week after superficial keratectomy showing a well-epithelialized wound.

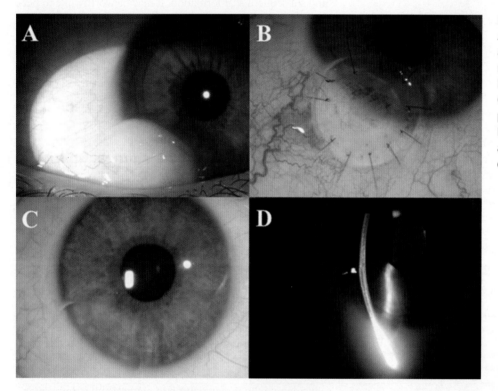

FIGURE 10.35. Corneal dermoid. **A:** Right eye of an 8-year-old child with a limbal dermoid in the inferotemporal quadrant. **B:** 3 weeks after lamellar keratoplasty with intact sutures. **C:** 11 months after lamellar keratoplasty, all sutures have been removed. **D:** Slit-lamp view showing excellent apposition of the graft 11 months postoperatively.

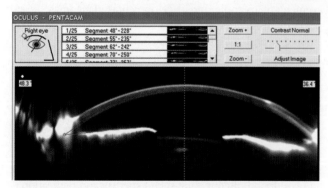

FIGURE 10.36. Scheimpflug photography image of the eye in Figure 10.35 showing the well-apposed lamellar keratoplasty. The interface is at approximately 2/3rd depth and the anterior segment is normal.

anesthesia is often not necessary to evaluate the eyes of infants with corneal opacities, because a hungry child held on the parent's lap and sucking on a bottle will hold still and seldom cry after the instillation of topical anesthetic and the

insertion of an infant eyelid speculum or a Koeppe lens. An examination under anesthesia is typically required as infants get older. Corneal sensation should be checked wherever necessary (herpes simplex keratitis, congenital corneal anesthesia) before inducing the patient. A portable slit lamp provides diagnostic accuracy and the ability to observe structural details, which can be recorded in a color-coded sketch that serves as a basis for planning the surgical approach. A ruler or caliper allows the ophthalmologist to record corneal diameter, to document whether or not the cornea is enlarging as a result of elevated intraocular pressure, and to measure the diameter of the corneal opacity as a basis for selecting the size of the donor button. Measurement of intraocular pressure (IOP) through edematous or scarred corneas in infants is inaccurate with Schiotz and Goldmann applanation tonometers. A handheld applanation tonometer may be used, if the cornea has a regular surface. Most helpful, however, is an electronic Tono-Pen XL (Medtronics, Inc., Minneapolis, MN) or a pneumotonometer (83). If possible the pupil should be dilated and thorough examination of the posterior segment should be done using direct and indirect ophthalmoscopy. High-frequency UBM or handheld anterior segment optical coherence tomography can be extremely helpful in evaluating the anterior segment architecture in the presence of an opacified cornea (69,84,85). A high-resolution B-scan ultrasonogram provides rapid information about the architectural integrity of the vitreous and retina, information in cases with an opaque cornea, small pupil, or cataractous lens. Careful A-scan and B-scan ultrasonographic examination can also help define anterior and posterior segment anatomy.

Indications for Keratoplasty in Infants

A child with dense bilateral corneal opacities should receive a penetrating keratoplasty along with other indicated ocular surgery generally within the first 3 months of life. This surgery, followed by prompt optical correction with contact lenses or spectacles, gives the best chance for prevention of severe amblyopia. For the child with a unilateral neonatal corneal opacity and a contralateral normal eye, the ophthalmologist must weight surgical and social morbidity against the probability of prolonged graft clarity, effective treatment of the amblyopia, and cosmetic improvement. The poor prognosis for prolonged graft clarity also tempers the decision to operate, especially in eyes that are not disfiguring and have only mild corneal opacities. On the other hand, the amblyopia in these eyes, if left untreated, will render them visually useless, so that even if a small percentage retain clear grafts with some improved vision, the effort and risk may be justified, particularly when one considers that trauma may damage the normal eye later in life. For grotesque eyes in which the cornea is ectatic or exhibits a fibrous mass, reconstructive surgery may improve appearance, as well as produce some vision. The team approach and modern microsurgical techniques are improving the prognosis for these grafts—a prognosis that till now has been extremely poor (81,86–96).

Neonatal corneal opacities fall into three groups with different prognosis for successful penetrating keratoplasty: (a) avascular corneas with either diffuse corneal edema or a central corneal opacity and clear periphery, with or without iris adhesions that have about a 50% chance for clarity at 2 years; (b) eyes with dense vascularized corneas, often with keratoiridial and corneolenticular adhesions that have about a 10% chance of success; and (c) eyes with both anterior segment and vitreoretinal disorganization demonstrated by ultrasonography that, in desperation, can be approached with combined keratoplasty, anterior segment reconstruction, open-sky vitrectomy, possible temporary keratoprosthesis, and pars plana vitrectomy and retinal reattachment procedures. These last eyes have an extremely guarded prognosis.

Surgical Techniques and Postoperative Care

High intraocular pressure must generally be controlled surgically. Goniotomy cannot be readily performed in infants with opaque corneas. Trabeculotomy *ab externo* may work, if the surgeon can see the anterior chamber, iris, and lens. Trabeculectomies frequently fail, and cyclocryotherapy is a destructive procedure usually saved until other surgical techniques have failed. An alloplastic tube shunt may be performed prior to the corneal transplant, if there is adequate visualization. An endoscopic cyclophotocoagulation can also be performed before, during or after a corneal transplant. Alternatively, a goniotomy or tube shunt may be performed at the same time or a few weeks after the corneal transplant procedure.

The techniques for neonatal keratoplasty differ little in their broad outline from those used for adults. In general, surgeons search for younger donor tissue for these patients. However, donor tissue less than age 2 years (when combined with 0.5 mm oversized grafts) was associated with abnormally steep corneal transplant curvatures and extremely high postoperative myopia (97). The infant sclera and cornea are much floppier than the adult structures, and therefore a single or double scleral ring, perhaps with an attached blepharostat, secured with 8 to 16 sutures helps prevent collapse of the globe. If multiple anterior segment abnormalities are present, fine intraocular scissors, delicate iris sweeps, and mechanical vitrectomy instruments allow more elegant reconstruction. The surgeon can use viscoelastic agents to dissect iris from cornea, to maintain the anterior chamber, and to prevent rubbing of the donor endothelium on the iris and lens. We prefer interrupted 10-0 nylon sutures with the knots buried in the host, because healing is often irregular in these corneas, requiring early individual suture removal.

Postoperatively, these infants should be examined weekly while sutures are in. The corneas heal rapidly, and sutures often loosen 2 to 6 weeks after surgery. Because these infants cannot communicate any of the symptoms of ocular inflammation, and because most parents are incapable of detecting the minimal red eye or slight graft haze that occurs with loose sutures or immunologic graft rejection, the physician must examine the cornea weekly until all sutures are removed for these phenomena, promptly instituting treatment, if they occur. Social service support is often imperative during these trying times. Examinations under anesthesia are required, if adequate evaluation in the office is not possible. The sutures are removed early compared with adults. In infants, half of the sutures are removed between 4 to 6 weeks and the other half 4 to 6 weeks later, depending on the patient's age.

Management of postoperative elevations of intraocular pressure may require repeated goniotomies, filtering procedures, tube shunts, cyclophotocoagulation and cyclocryotherapies, with the addition of the appropriate doses of topical and oral antiglaucoma medications.

Nonhealing epithelial defects may require lateral tarsorrhaphies, therapeutic soft contact lenses, and vigorous use of artificial teardrops, gels, and ointments.

Prompt contact lens fitting is the cornerstone for prevention of amblyopia. Extended-wear soft contact lenses are most effective, but infants tend to rub them out of their eyes, and an extensive inventory and backup system—including a supply of replacement lenses for parents to keep—will avoid delays in reordering lenses from the manufacturer. This optical correction may also require multiple examinations under anesthesia for refractions, keratometry, and contact lens refitting (98).

Of all the keratoplasties performed in pediatric age group, Peters' anomaly (91,93,96,99) accounts for the most, followed by congenital hereditary endothelial dystrophy (CHED); (90,95) the overall graft survival rate ranges from 47%–80% (86–96) (Table 10.3). The graft survival in patients with Peters' anomaly ranged from 22% to 83% (48,100). This wide range of success is due to the varied spectrum of the disease. Zaidman (101) had a higher success of keratoplasty in Peters' anomaly type 1 compared to studies which have included Peters' anomaly 1 and 2 as a single entity (102,103). In cases of penetrating keratoplasty for CHED, functional success was achieved in 21% to 66% (104,105). The main causes of poor outcome of the grafts in this age group are graft rejection (87–91,93), secondary glaucoma (92,95,96) and infection (94). The advance of surgical techniques for lamellar corneal surgeries have paved the way

Table 10.3

INDICATIONS AND OUTCOMES OF KERATOPLASTY IN CHILDREN

Study	Indication	Grafts (n)	Graft Survival (%)	Follow-up (months)	Complications
Stulting et al. (1984) (86)	Congenital	72	68	12	Unknown
	Nontraumatic	42	74		Sterile ulcer
	Traumatic	38	74		Rejection
Cowden (1990) (87)	Congenital	25	56	1–10 y	Rejection
	Nontraumatic	33	50		Glaucoma
	Traumatic	8	56		Infection
Dana et al. (1995) (88)	Congenital	84	80	12	Rejection
	Nontraumatic	22	76		Glaucoma
	Traumatic	25	84		Infection
Vajpayee et al. (1999) (89)	Congenital	20	80	12	Rejection
	Acquired	20	90		
Aasuri et al. (2000) (90)	Congenital	47	63.8	15	Rejection
	Nontraumatic	85	70.6		Infection
	Traumatic	22	54.5		Glaucoma
Comer et al. (2001) (91)	Congenital	26	61	12	Rejection
					Glaucoma
McClellan et al. (2003) (92)	Congenital	8	71.4	6.6 y	Glaucoma
	Acquired	11	75		
Patel et al. (2005) (93)	Congenital	9	78	12	Rejection
	Nontraumatic	43	85		Primary failure
	Traumatic	6	100		Trauma
Sharma et al. (2007) (94)	Congenital	57	77	24	Infection
	Nontraumatic	87	77		Glaucoma
	Traumatic	24	77		Rejection
Al-Ghamdi et al. (2007) (95)	Congenital	130	47	72 (median)	Glaucoma
	Nontraumatic	18	28	38	Infection
	Traumatic	17	42	14	PED
Huang et al. (2009) (96)	Congenital	64	54	12	Glaucoma
	Nontraumatic	25	53		
	Traumatic	17	48		

for better visual and long-term outcomes in various diseases in adults. Recently, lamellar corneal surgeries have been performed in children with pathologies limited to only anterior or posterior corneal layers. Descemet's stripping endothelial keratoplasty has both intraoperative (closed-globe surgery) and postoperative (less astigmatism, faster visual recovery, no corneal suture related complications) advantages over full thickness penetrating keratoplasty. Busin et al. reported visual acuity of 20/40 or better in 89% of eyes after Descemet's stripping endothelial keratoplasty for CHED (106). Harding et al. reported success with deep anterior lamellar keratoplasty (DALK) in children with pathology limited to the anterior stroma using manual and viscodissection techniques (107). Buzzonetti et al. reported successful DALK assisted by femtosecond laser in children (108). They conclude that DALK is safe and effective and helps in decreasing graft rejection and improving the refractive outcome in eyes with stromal abnormalities.

Traditional corneal transplantation is associated with delayed visual rehabilitation leading to amblyopia, high incidence of allograft rejection, complications (glaucoma and cataract) requiring further surgical intervention thus posing a risk for graft survival. In the recent years, there has been a shift in the trend toward performing a keratoprosthesis as a primary surgical intervention in order to achieve a quiet and comfortable eye with a clear visual axis and stable refraction within days after surgery. The various indications for which keratoprosthesis is performed are Peters' anomaly, multiple failed grafts, congenital glaucoma, spontaneous perforations, limbal stem cell deficiency, and anterior staphyloma. The Boston keratoprosthesis may be appropriate in some pediatric cases to establish a clear optical pathway quickly, and to reduce the potential for reoperation and complications (109–111).

INFECTION

Inflammation and infection of the conjunctiva may extend to the cornea, resulting in a punctate keratitis, corneal ulceration, stromal infiltrate, or combinations of these changes. Once the corneal stroma is affected, a benign conjunctivitis becomes a more serious problem. Corneal infections that occur in the pediatric age group can cause corneal changes ranging from mild punctate keratitis to severe corneal ulceration and permanent opacity. If adequate examination and treatment are performed early in the disease course, corneal involvement may be prevented and subsequent loss of vision may be avoided. If the child is not examined with appropriate thoroughness early in the disease, the diagnosis of infection can be missed or delayed, and serious permanent corneal damage can occur.

It is essential to diagnose a corneal ulcer early and determine its etiology before it spreads and involves the deeper corneal stroma, causing permanent blurred vision from corneal scarring. A thorough history should be obtained

regarding trauma (112–114), contact lens use (114–116), surgical history, use of topical medications, and any systemic illness. Physical examination helps in assessing the nutritional status and any physical abnormalities (117,118).

The ocular examination of an infant or young child is difficult because of the child's pain, fright, and inability to cooperate. Clinical ocular evaluation begins with examining the eyelids for appropriate closure to rule out exposure and lagophthalmos and the blink rate to rule out a neurotrophic cornea. Structural abnormalities of the eyelids or eyelash malposition should be looked for as they may be predisposing factors for infection. When it is necessary to examine such a patient with a slit lamp, sedation or general anesthesia may be needed so that the eye may be adequately seen. A portable or handheld slit lamp may aid in examination but may not provide as accurate details. Heavy sedation or general anesthesia allows for corneal scraping or surface debridement, if necessary. The collected samples are inoculated directly onto culture media including blood agar, chocolate agar, Sabouraud dextrose agar, thioglycollate broth and nonnutrient agar with *E. coli* overlay as needed. Subconjunctival or sub-tenon's injections can be administered when indicated at the conclusion of the examination. This type of examination should be repeated as needed to follow the progress of the disease. If the family socioeconomic situation is not conducive to regular, continuous administration of medication by a parent or guardian, hospitalization may be required.

Application of drops is often difficult for parents, because the child may be struggling and crying, and the drops will be washed out of the lower cul-de-sac with the child's tears. Even if the drops remain in place, they may be diluted with tears. For these reasons, ointments may be preferred in uncooperative infants and children. Once the child is old enough to be annoyed by the blurred vision from ointments, drops should be used instead. Parents must be taught by the ophthalmologist or office staff how to use topical medications properly. Occasionally, we have seen parents who, when asked to demonstrate drug application, place ointment on their fingertip and apply it to the child's closed eyelids. By demonstrating the technique of pulling the lower eyelid down, applying the ointment or drop to the lower cul-de-sac and holding the eye open for several seconds, accurate drug application is achieved. If daily atropine is required in the infant for long-term cycloplegia, digital pressure should be applied over the punctum and canaliculus of the lower eyelid to prevent systemic adsorption and side effects.

An antibiotic should be selected that has the greatest likelihood of controlling the corneal infection as quickly as possible. For that reason, bactericidal rather than bacteriostatic drugs are preferred. Gram-negative organisms, such as *Pseudomonas,* can rapidly destroy corneal stroma and lead to descemetocele formation and corneal perforation within 24 to 48 hours of onset of infection. Another bacterium that may cause severe, rapid corneal melting and perforation is

Neisseria gonorrhoeae (gonococcus). This organism typically causes a hyperacute purulent conjunctivitis. This is a true ocular emergency and must be treated immediately with topical and systemic antibiotics to prevent severe ocular sequelae, such as corneal perforation.

Bacterial Ulceration

Bacteria that cause corneal ulceration in children are similar to those organisms that cause infection in adults (118). The workup and treatment are also similar in children and adults (119). *Staphylococcus aureus* (120,121), Coagulase-negative Staphylococcus (e.g., *Staphylococcus epidermidis*) (112,114,118), *Streptococcus pneumoniae,* and *Pseudomonas* (114,120,122) are the more common bacteria that cause corneal infections in children. *Staphylococcus aureus* is a gram-positive organism that usually causes a punctate keratitis adjacent to the corneal limbus in the lower and upper portions of the cornea (Fig. 10.37). There is almost always concomitant conjunctival inflammation and frequently an associated blepharitis with this corneal infection. The meibomian glands may be infected and serve as a reservoir for continued bacterial release and keratitis. Chronic staphylococcal blepharitis and keratoconjunctivitis in children may be a severe and recurrent problem that requires continued treatment until the source of the infection is eradicated (123,124). In children, the primary treatment is bacitracin or erythromycin ointment or azithromycin gel in conjunction with eyelid hygiene, consisting of warm compresses and eyelid massage. A first-generation cephalosporin agent or a fluoroquinolone in eyedrop form has broad-spectrum effectiveness but is only variably useful against *Streptococcus* and anaerobic species. With more severe staphylococcal infection,

and particularly for recurrent disease that does not respond to this treatment, systemic antibiotics, such as doxycycline, azithromycin or erythromycin, and topical corticosteroids are frequently necessary (125). Doxycycline can cause discoloration of the permanent teeth in children, so they should be avoided until these are developed, usually after age 8 to 12 years. These systemic antibiotics are often started at one half the appropriate dose for the patient's age and weight for several weeks. The dose is then decreased in half and continued for months. Topical application of weak corticosteroids, such as prednisolone 1.8%, loteprednol 0.2% to 0.5%, or fluorometholone 0.1%, is often used in chronic staphylococcal keratitis, because the superficial punctate keratitis, limbal infiltrates, and limbal neovascularization respond well to low doses of topical corticosteroids. Hot compresses for 5 to 10 minutes 1 to 2 times a day also helps decrease eyelid inflammation. In recent years, there has been an increase in methicillin-resistant staphylococcus aureus isolates in pediatric patients with bacterial conjunctivitis, hence there should be a higher suspicion in patients not responding to standard broad-spectrum topical medication (126).

Other bacteria that mainly cause conjunctivitis, but may also cause corneal ulceration, are *Haemophilus influenzae* and *Moraxella* spp. Both are gram-negative organisms, the first a coccobacillus and the second a rod form of bacteria. The incidence of *H. influenzae* ocular infections is lower since the widespread use of vaccination for this bacterium.

Marginal corneal ulcers can be caused by each of these organisms, but *S. aureus* is the most common bacterium causing limbal ulcers. *Moraxella* may produce an angular blepharitis by involving the skin at the lateral canthus, resulting in a serous or mucous discharge accompanied by irritation and pain.

Contact lens use, an important risk factor for bacterial keratitis in adults, is increasingly common in children (116,127). A study highlights the dangers of orthokeratology, the sequential fitting of rigid gas-permeable contact lenses to flatten the cornea to treat myopia, in children. The authors report a series of corneal ulcers in six children, ages 9 to 14, using orthokeratology lenses. Five of the six ulcers were culture-positive for *Pseudomonas aeruginosa,* and all patients suffered a loss of best-corrected visual acuity (127) (Fig. 10.37).

Fungal Keratitis

Fungal keratitis generally occurs in adults but can also occur in children (112,113,118). It is usually associated with trauma from materials, such as wood, vegetables, or plant matter. Fungal infections are also encountered in the compromised host.

Infants rarely develop fungal keratitis, but young children and teenagers may, if they are injured by vegetable material, wood, sticks, dirt, or other outdoor foreign bodies. Additional risk factors include previous systemic illness and prior ocular surgery (113). Fungal keratitis may at first be difficult to distinguish from bacterial keratitis. There is loss

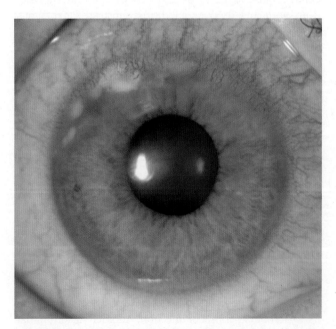

FIGURE 10.37. Peripheral corneal infiltrates from staphylococcal keratitis.

of epithelium and a surface ulcer with white stromal infiltrate. Fungal keratitis is characterized by a slowly advancing stromal ulcer unresponsive to antibiotics. There may be satellite lesions around the edge of the central ulceration or an immune ring around the infected area. Recognition of this depends on a suspicion, based on the history and course of the ulcer, that fungal keratitis may be present.

As in adults, fungal keratitis is often difficult to treat. Pimaricin (5% natamycin) is commercially available and effective against most filamentous fungi (*Fusarium* and *Aspergillus*). Amphotericin 0.15%, voriconazole 1%, and fluconazole 0.3% can be obtained from a compounding pharmacy. Topical voriconazole 1% is being used more and more frequently due to its relatively broad-spectrum antifungal coverage (128). Additionally, a number of oral antifungal agents are used. In general, oral agents should be used with only culture-proved and sensitivity-tested fungal keratitis. Clotrimazole, miconazole, ketoconazole, fluconazole, itraconazole, and voriconazole are oral agents that can be used usually in conjunction with a pediatric infectious disease specialist.

Viral Infections

Corneal infection due to herpes simplex virus (HSV) causes more morbidity and loss of vision than any other corneal infection seen in children. The newborn infant usually has maternal antibodies to HSV for the first 6 months of life, affording temporary protection from infection with this virus. After the maternal antibodies are lost, the infant may acquire HSV infection of the skin or eye, or systemically (see Fig. 10.31). Infection with HSV is probably acquired by close contact (kissing, handling) with someone who has an active lesion either around the lips or fingers (paronychia) or elsewhere on the skin's surface. Inapparent infection with HSV is usually the rule in children. They are exposed to the infection and acquire the disease but do not develop obvious HSV lesions.

Unfortunately, HSV ocular infection is not readily diagnosed early in the disease course. The pediatrician, emergency room physician, or general practitioner usually sees the child first, and treatment is started for what appears to be an obvious red eye on penlight examination. This treatment frequently consists of an antibiotic or antibiotic-steroid combination. Small epithelial corneal or conjunctival dendritic ulcers can be seen only with a slit lamp. If there are dendritic epithelial lesions forming on the cornea or conjunctiva, the use of a topical corticosteroid medication exacerbates the infection and can cause wider spread of viral keratitis in the epithelium and deeper involvement of the corneal stroma, even though the eye appears less inflamed. It is only later that an ophthalmologist is typically consulted.

The ophthalmologist sees an uncooperative infant or child who has been medicated for several days to weeks and has a very uncomfortable eye. Some form of sedation or anesthesia may be necessary to see enough of the cornea to make the proper diagnosis. If the ophthalmologist does not see the child's eye under magnification (with a slit lamp), the diagnosis may be missed. With a history of poor response to previous medication (usually antibiotics or an antibiotic-steroid combination), the index of suspicion for HSV infection should be high. To obtain a satisfactory examination, application of fluorescein or rose bengal dye, examination with a slit lamp or operating microscope (possibly under anesthesia) is generally necessary (Fig. 10.38).

Until several years ago, the choice of an antiviral agent was vidarabine (Vira-A) in ointment form. It was the only available ophthalmic antiviral drug in ointment form in the United States (129), although acyclovir ophthalmic ointment is used overseas (130). Unfortunately, vidarabine ointment is no longer commercially available in the United States. It may be formulated for use by a compounding pharmacy. Trifluorothymidine (e.g., Viroptic) drops, every 2 hours, is an effective antiviral agent against dendritic keratitis in the United States, but it is not overwhelmingly better than vidarabine, and an ointment is preferable in children as a first choice for an antiviral drug. Ganciclovir, a guanosine nucleoside analogue, is a broad-spectrum antiviral agent that inhibits replication of viral DNA and is active against both HSV-1 and -2 (131). Our first choice for infants and children is ganciclovir ophthalmic gel 0.15% (e.g., Zirgan) five times a day for 1 week, then 3 × day for another week. Our second choice is vidarabine ointment 4 to 5 times a day. Our third choice is trifluorothymidine drops 8 to 9 times a day. Topical acyclovir ointment 5 times a day may also be used, if available. In addition to the antiviral drug, a cycloplegic, such as atropine sulfate ½-1% or scopolamine 1/4%, may be used if symptoms such as photophobia or ocular pain are present.

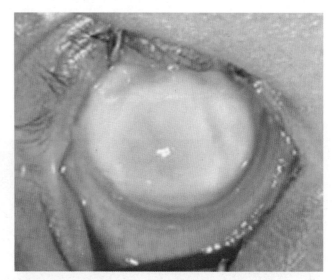

FIGURE 10.38. An 8-month-old child with history of trauma from a wooden stick showing intense collagenolysis and melting due to a severe *Pseudomonas aeruginosa* keratitis.

Primary ocular HSV infection in children is not the most serious form of this disease. Recurrent viral infection is common after the initial bout with ocular herpes simplex virus, and these recurrences are responsible for most of the corneal scarring and visual loss. About 25% of patients with primary ocular herpes develop a recurrent dendritic herpetic infection within 2 years of the initial lesion. Almost 50% of those who have more than one attack of herpetic keratitis have a third or more recurrences within 2 years. Recurrent HSV keratitis may occur after upper respiratory tract infections, fever, minor trauma (e.g., exposure to sunlight at the beach), or other triggering events. Herpetic keratitis in children differs from adults in that they have more simultaneous or sequential bilateral involvement, have robust inflammation in stromal keratitis, and higher number of recurrences (129,130).

When an infant or child who has had HSV keratitis develops any redness or irritation of the previously involved eye, whether or not this is preceded by an initiating event, the parent must suspect recurrent HSV infection and seek ophthalmic care immediately. Reevaluation with careful slit-lamp examination is necessary to determine whether the recurrent red eye is due to conjunctivitis or an actual recurrent dendritic or geographic ulcer of the corneal epithelium, with evidence of active viral replication in the epithelium, or whether this is secondary stromal inflammation or iritis. Parents of children who have HSV infection might benefit from having an antiviral drug available to start using immediately, even before seeing the ophthalmologist, if they note recurrent inflammation. Management of recurrent herpetic dendritic or geographical lesions limited to the epithelium consists of antiviral drugs, such as ganciclovir gel, vidarabine ointment, or trifluorothymidine drops, as for the primary lesion. Toxicity from extended use of topical antiviral drugs is a further problem, so these medications should be tapered and discontinued within 2 to 3 weeks of their initiation.

An oral antiviral drug, such as acyclovir, can be used in infants and children, if they are unable to use topical medication or for preventing recurrent keratitis (132). The dosage (acyclovir syrup-10 mg/kg of body weight, 3 times a day; valacyclovir 500 mg 2 times a day) should be checked with a pediatrician, and kidney disease must be ruled out. Oral antiviral drugs are effective for primary and recurrent dendritic and geographical keratitis. If recurrent infection due to herpes simplex virus is not properly diagnosed, significant corneal scarring, thinning, vascularization, and even perforation can occur. Deeper stromal involvement with corneal vascularization due to disciform keratitis may require use of topical corticosteroids, even though these anti-inflammatory agents are contraindicated in epithelial dendritic herpetic disease (Figs. 10.39 and 10.40).

Ophthalmologists should use the smallest amount of steroid necessary to control the stromal inflammation and should perform frequent examinations. Children should be seen approximately once a week for the first few weeks of this therapy, and the steroid slowly tapered as soon as a response is achieved. Once the steroid dose is down in the once a day range, it should be tapered even more slowly. In conjunction with steroid treatment, either topical or oral antivirals should be used. Prophylactic oral acyclovir is often used in children when treating stromal keratitis with topical steroids in order to prevent recurrent dendritic disease. There have been reports of superinfection with bacteria when steroids and antiviral drugs are used long-term for corneal epithelial infections known to be caused by herpes, emphasizing the need for frequent follow-up visits.

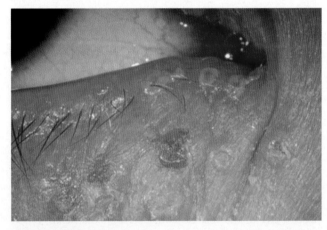

FIGURE 10.39. Primary herpes simplex keratitis involving the skin around the eye in a child.

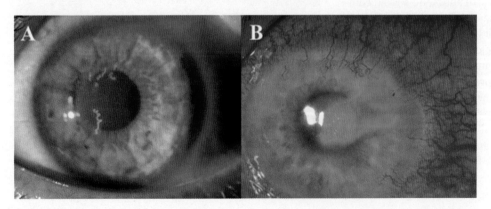

FIGURE 10.40. Herpes simplex epithelial keratitis. **A:** Dendrite. **B:** Geographic ulcer with fluorescein staining.

Oral or intravenous acyclovir is indicated for disseminated neonatal herpes simplex with encephalitis and may be lifesaving in these situations. It can be used in infants and children who are immunocompromised and develop HSV keratitis but should be administered by a pediatrician familiar with its use.

Adenoviral Infections (Epidemic Keratoconjunctivitis)

Childhood adenovirus infections are marked by follicular conjunctivitis with systemic flu-like symptoms and preauricular adenopathy. The adult forms of adenovirus infection are also manifested by marked follicular conjunctivitis, but systemic symptoms are not nearly as common. As in adults, it is extremely contagious, and precautions need to be taken to avoid spreading the infection in the doctor's office and at home and school.

Pseudomembrane formation on the conjunctiva may be seen accompanying adenovirus infection in children. Despite follicular conjunctivitis and pseudomembrane formation, the cornea usually remains clear except for an initial fine, superficial punctate keratitis. Subepithelial changes commonly seen in adults are less often noted in children, which makes the diagnosis more difficult in children (Figs. 10.41 and 10.42).

Numerous adenovirus types, including types 2, 3, 4, 5, 7, 8, 11, and 13, have been isolated in children. The corneal changes seen in adults with adenovirus types 8, 13, and 19 are not usually seen, or are much milder, in infants and children. In one large epidemic of adenovirus type 8, the youngest person involved was 8 years old, and only 3 of 102 persons examined who had the disease were under age 15. In a study of the infantile form of adenovirus type 8, no instance of subepithelial stromal keratitis was noted, although follicular changes and pseudomembranes were prominent in 12 cases (133). If corneal infiltrates do appear

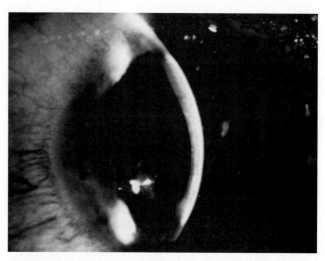

FIGURE 10.42. Slit-lamp view of disciform keratitis in patient.

in children, they are usually transient, leaving no permanent corneal scar. Recently amblyopia and strabismus have been reported in children with unilateral corneal opacity as a consequence of suspected epidemic keratoconjunctivitis (134). In some adults the corneal infiltrates may last for many months or even years, and, rarely, permanent corneal scars remain.

The treatment of adenovirus in children is slightly different from that in adults. Bacterial superinfection of the cornea is very uncommon, and therefore topical therapy with antibiotics is usually unnecessary but there has been an outbreak of bacterial keratitis associated with epidemic keratoconjunctivitis in neonates and children (135). Warm compresses are helpful, if there is much caking or debris from the marked conjunctivitis and clear fluid discharge. Topical corticosteroids, which are often used in severe adenovirus infections in adults, are not indicated in children unless they are very symptomatic from marked follicular conjunctivitis and pseudomembrane formation. In these cases, prednisolone 0.125%, fluorometholone 0.1%, or loteprednol 0.2% to 0.5%, 4 to 5 times a day for a few days and then tapered, may be indicated. The disease in children is self-limited, and no permanent ocular disorder usually results.

Varicella Zoster Keratitis

Chicken pox in children and shingles in adults are caused by the same virus, varicella zoster. This virus is responsible for varicella in children, which is highly contagious, and for herpes zoster (shingles) in adults, which is much less infectious. Shingles in adults is usually a reactivation of latent virus from childhood chicken pox. There are cases of herpes zoster keratoconjunctivitis in children, although this disease is overshadowed by the greater prevalence of chicken pox (varicella) in young people. This disease has been reported more in children after bone marrow transplantation either due to the underlying hematologic

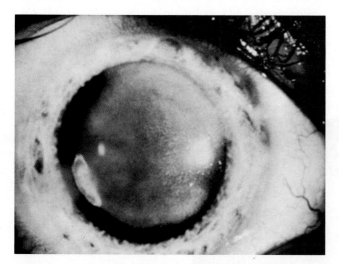

FIGURE 10.41. Disciform keratitis secondary to herpes simplex virus infection and recurrent disease.

malignancy, use of immunosuppressive medications, allogenic transplantation, or radiation in the preparative period (136).

Unilateral clear facial and forehead blisters or similar lesions of the brow may be seen in children without systemic skin involvement. These lesions may be herpes zoster, although they may be a localized varicella infection. When the nasociliary branch of the ophthalmic nerve is involved, there is a greater likelihood that ocular involvement will occur after herpes zoster infection (Hutchinson sign). About half the patients with nasociliary nerve disease develop ocular involvement. With inflammation of the nasociliary branch of this nerve, vesicles may appear on the same side of the nose as the skin vesicles on the brow or forehead.

Various forms of corneal involvement may occur in children with chicken pox. The mildest form is an epithelial keratitis that is self-limited and requires no treatment. The corneal involvement consists of a fine punctate keratitis with some microcystic corneal edema. It is unusual to find more than this. There may be a limbal vesicle with stromal infiltrate and vascularization. This is unusual but has been seen in children. Disciform keratitis or stromal edema may also occur with severe ocular involvement caused by chicken pox. This finding is less common and resembles the disciform keratitis in herpes simplex keratitis. Episcleritis or scleritis may also be seen. There may be phlyctenular limbal and corneal involvement. Varicella zoster infections and ocular sequelae in children are much less common since the widespread use of the chicken pox virus vaccine. However, herpes zoster virus (HZV) sclerokeratitis with anterior uveitis has been reported in a 9-year-old, 3 years after vaccination (137).

Oral acyclovir has been used for herpes zoster infections in adults, 800 mg, 5 times a day for 7 days, if the disease is first detected within 72 hours of disease onset. Valacyclovir 1 gm tid is a prodrug that may have enhanced antiviral action due to better absorption. Famciclovir 500 mg tid is also effective against herpes zoster ophthalmicus in adults.

Oral acyclovir is indicated for children age 2 and older with chicken pox. Intravenous acyclovir is also indicated in the treatment of herpes zoster infections in immunocompromised children and adults. Consultation with a pediatrician or infectious disease specialist may be indicated in these situations. Famciclovir and valacyclovir have not been fully tested in children.

Treatment of herpes zoster keratitis is the same for children and adults. For the milder forms of herpes zoster ocular involvement, such as punctate keratitis, mild stromal edema, and minimal anterior chamber reaction, cycloplegia is all that is necessary. With more severe punctate keratitis, stromal edema, and anterior chamber involvement, the addition of topical corticosteroids is necessary, but this is rare in infants and children. The question of the use of systemic steroids in children who have herpes zoster has not been completely resolved. Because of the concern that the varicella virus may be spread systemically, the use of systemic steroids in children with herpes zoster ocular involvement should be approached with caution; they should be employed only under the joint care of a pediatrician specially trained in infectious diseases and an ophthalmologist. Corticosteroid drops are usually sufficient to quiet the moderate or severe corneal, scleral, and anterior chamber inflammation of herpes zoster and varicella in children. Systemic antiviral drugs are currently used for immunocompromised infants and children with herpes zoster ophthalmicus by pediatric infectious disease specialists.

Other viruses that may cause epithelial keratitis are rubeola, mumps, and molluscum contagiosum. In molluscum contagiosum, the molluscum lesions on the eyelid margins can cause a superficial punctate keratitis but rarely corneal ulcers. Surgical removal is recommended for these eyelid lesions. Epithelial keratitis is the most likely corneal manifestation in mumps, but cases of disciform keratitis have been reported, and local topical steroid therapy is usually all that is required. In most cases there is no residual scarring.

Vaccinia

The increase in terrorism worldwide over the past decade has revived the use of smallpox (vaccinia) vaccine. History of a recent smallpox vaccination or close contact with a recently vaccinated person is usually the way vaccinia blepharitis, conjunctivitis, and keratitis are contracted (Fig. 10.43). Vaccinia may be shed from the vaccination site for approximately 3 weeks. The incubation period from exposure to development of symptoms is 5 to 19 days. It has been estimated

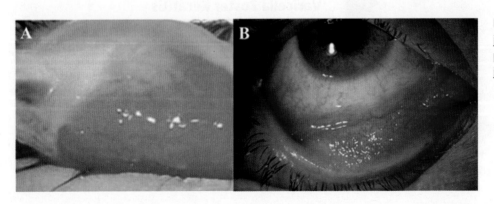

FIGURE 10.43. Epidemic keratoconjunctivitis. **A:** Pseudomembrane being peeled off the superior palpebral conjunctiva. **B:** Follicular conjunctivitis.

that 1 in 40,000 vaccinations leads to ocular vaccinia. It is generally treated similarly to herpes simplex infections with topical ganciclovir ophthalmic gel, trifluorothymidine drops, or vidarabine ointment. Vaccinia immune globulin (available through the Centers for Disease Control [CDC] and Prevention in the United States) may also be used in more severe infections.

Chlamydial Keratitis

Trachoma is endemic in many parts of the world and is the second leading cause of blindness worldwide. In the Far and Middle East there are areas where 90% of the population have trachoma. In endemic areas, it may be possible to control the disease by placing children in an isolated environment (e.g., boarding school), but reinfection is common during visits to the family and local community.

In childhood trachoma, there may be epithelial punctate keratitis in the upper half of the cornea, in addition to superior limbal follicles. With further extension of corneal changes, subepithelial infiltrates at the limbus and pannus may develop as the disease progresses (Fig. 10.44). These limbal inflammatory infiltrates eventually scar and are referred to as Herbert's pits.

Control of this disease is essential, because it is by far the most common worldwide cause of corneal scarring and blindness. Estimates of disease prevalence in child and adult populations are in the range of up to one quarter of a billion people. In a study in Tanzania, children with sustainably clean faces had reduced odds of having severe trachoma. The authors felt that improved face-washing and a reduced fly count on the face plus antibiotic treatment would reduce the risk for blinding trachoma in adulthood (131). In addition to improved hygiene, treatment includes systemic and topical antibiotics (e.g., azithromycin or erythromycin) for several weeks.

Inclusion conjunctivitis (inclusion blennorrhea) of the newborn is seen throughout the United States. The organism responsible is the trachoma-inclusion conjunctivitis (TRIC) agent. This disease should not be confused with gonorrheal ophthalmia, which appears within 2 days of birth. Inclusion conjunctivitis is noted usually between days 4 and 15 after birth. At birth, inclusion conjunctivitis is acquired during passage through the birth canal of infected mothers. Corneal involvement, when keratitis does occur, is limited to the epithelium. There are few, if any, long-lasting corneal changes. The main ocular manifestation of disease is a mucopurulent papillary and follicular conjunctivitis (Fig. 10.45). Treatment for early stages of this disease includes systemic antibiotics (e.g., azithromycin, doxycycline, or erythromycin) for 1 week administered to the patient and parents, and topical antibiotics (e.g., erythromycin, azithromycin) for several weeks. The tetracycline family of medications is contraindicated in children, pregnant women, and nursing mothers. Additional information is covered in Chapter 9.

IMMUNOLOGIC MANIFESTATIONS OF CORNEAL DISEASE

Vernal Keratoconjunctivitis

Vernal keratoconjunctivitis (VKC) is a chronic allergic disease that typically affects younger children and teenagers and exhibits a male preponderance. Although the disease is seen across all continents, its prevalence is higher in the regions with a hot, humid climate or higher load of airborne allergens. Clinically it is characterized by presence of papillary hypertrophy of the palpebral and/or the limbal conjunctiva, bulbar conjunctival pigmentation, limbal thickening, and Horner-Trantas dots. Vernal conjunctivitis, or spring catarrh, is generally more prevalent in the spring but may be symptomatic all year. Although children with vernal conjunctivitis usually have a history of allergy, there is no definite known cause for this disease. The pathogenesis of VKC in the recent years is thought to be due to Th2 driven mechanism which leads to hyperproduction of IgE, and differentiation and activation of mast cells and eosinophils. Common symptoms include itching, tearing, light sensitivity and ropy mucoid discharge (see Figs. 10.46 and 10.47) (139).

VKC can present either as a tarsal form (giant papillary hypertrophy of the upper tarsal conjunctiva), a bulbar form (Trantas dots-aggregates of epithelial cells and eosinophils generally concentrated around the limbus) or mixed form (Fig. 10.48). Complications of VKC can be either disease related (shield ulcer/plaques, corneal scarring, dry eye, limbal stem cell deficiency) or treatment related (steroid-induced cataract and glaucoma) (Fig. 10.49).

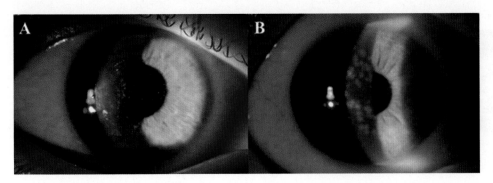

FIGURE 10.44. Epidemic keratoconjunctivitis. **A:** Acute epidemic keratoconjunctivitis showing fine, superficial punctate keratitis and anterior stromal infiltrates. **B:** Subepithelial corneal infiltrates 2 months after resolution of the acute episode.

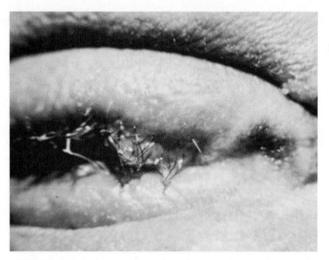

FIGURE 10.45. Vaccinial involvement of the outer canthus with eyelid swelling.

Corneal changes appear as focal (superior) or confluent epithelial punctate keratitis. These confluent microerosions become macroerosions by the mechanical effect of the giant tarsal papillae, subsequently leading to a frank epithelial defect called as shield ulcer. A shield ulcer is a shallow indolent ulcer usually seen on the upper part of the cornea. It is most likely due to abrasion of the corneal surface by the giant papilla on the upper tarsal conjunctiva (mechanical hypothesis) or due to the inflammatory mediators from the eosinophils (toxin hypothesis). Cameron has graded shield ulcers into three grades, grade 1: transparent base, grade 2: translucent base ± opaque white or yellow deposits, grade 3: elevated plaque. Grade 1 shield ulcers usually re-epithelialize with medical therapy (topical steroids, mast cell stabilizers and antibiotics), but grade 2 and 3 shield ulcers require debridement or superficial keratectomy for re-epithelization (140,141).

Treatment for VKC is based on the severity of the disease. Steroids are the first line of treatment to reduce the severity of the acute episode along with a mast cell stabilizer (e.g., cromolyn sodium) or dual-acting (mast cell stabilizer and antihistamine) drugs such as alcaftadine, bepotastine, olopatadine, azelastine, ketotifen or epinastine. The steroids should be tapered rapidly to a maintenance dose to reduce the risk of complications of glaucoma and cataract. If they tolerate the medication satisfactorily, patients may be kept on the mast cell stabilizer for months or years without ocular side effects. Calcineurin inhibitors including cyclosporine and tacrolimus have also been used effectively (139).

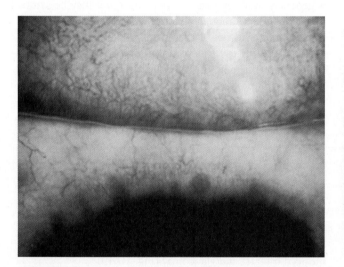

FIGURE 10.46. Superior limbal scarring and Herbert's pits in trachoma.

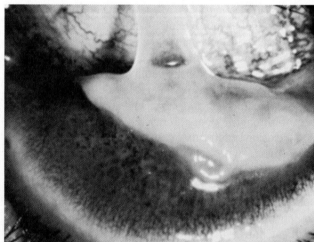

FIGURE 10.47. Purulent conjunctivitis and eyelid erythema in inclusion conjunctivitis.

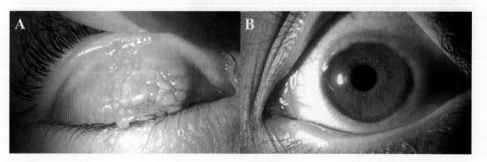

FIGURE 10.48. Vernal keratoconjunctivitis. **A:** Large papillary cobblestone papillae in vernal conjunctivitis involving the upper eyelid. **B:** Limbal form of vernal keratoconjunctivitis with Horner-Trantas dots at the superior limbus.

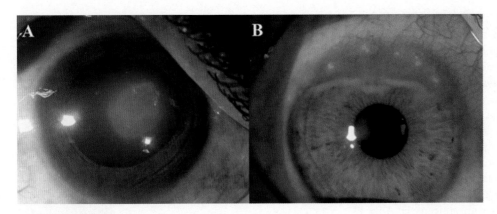

FIGURE 10.49. Vernal keratoconjunctivitis. **A:** Grade-2 shield ulcer in a patient with palpebral form of vernal keratoconjunctivitis. **B:** Superior partial limbal stem cell deficiency in a child with chronic vernal keratoconjunctivitis.

Phlyctenular Keratoconjunctivitis

The phlyctenular changes consist of an elevated, pinkish lymphoid follicle, which invades the cornea at the limbus, leaving a vascularized track behind. Eventually, the phlyctenular appearance is that of a flat or slightly raised gray, vascularized, wedge-shaped area in the cornea with a leash of vessels to the limbus (Fig. 10.50). Occasionally, the corneal involvement is more severe, with catarrhal ulcers and infiltrates, neovascularization, scars, and even perforation (142). Phlyctenular keratoconjunctivitis is not due solely to a hypersensitivity reaction to tuberculin protein but rather the more common underlying mechanism involves type IV Gell and Coombs cell-mediated hypersensitivity to staphylococcal antigens (peptidoglycan and protein A) (143). A small corneal ulcer may occur at the head of the lesion. Phlyctenules may appear around the corneal limbus, but usually only one lesion advances farther into the central cornea. These lesions may cause visual loss when they affect the pupillary area but are usually treated and become quiescent before reaching the pupil.

Staphylococcal infection can also cause phlyctenular conjunctivitis. In these patients, treatment of staphylococcal infection of the eyelid margin, and, particularly, the meibomian gland, quickly quiets the corneal changes, preventing corneal damage. Patients with tuberculosis-associated phlyctenules have more severe lesions and more recurrences (144).

Phlyctenular conjunctivitis may be treated with topical corticosteroids, at first usually prednisolone 1% or loteprednol 0.5% 3 or 4 times a day and then tapering to prednisolone 0.125 %, fluorometholone 0.1%, or loteprednol 0.2% once a day or every other day, over a period of a month or more, once the disease is controlled. The corticosteroids may be discontinued when the eye quiets but may have to be restarted, if there is a flare-up of the phlyctenular conjunctivitis. If staphylococcal infection of the meibomian glands is present, concomitant eyelid hygiene and antibiotic is generally used, either bacitracin or erythromycin ointment or azithromycin gel once or twice a day. The response to steroids is dramatic, and corticosteroids remain the cornerstone of acute ocular treatment for this disease (145). In severe steroid-dependent corneal inflammation, long-term topical cyclosporine 2% therapy is safe and effective in children (146).

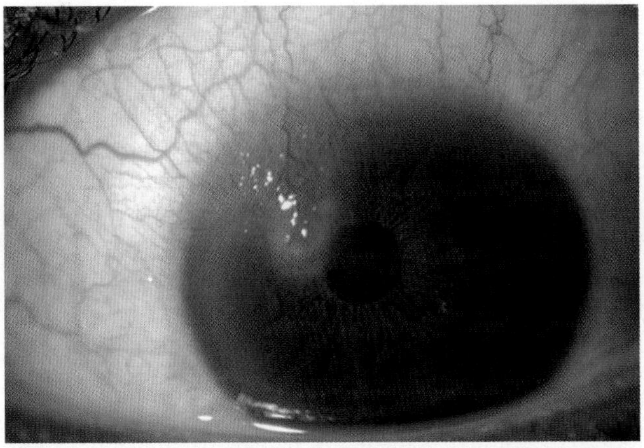

Erythema Multiforme/Stevens-Johnson Syndrome (SJS)/ Toxic Epidermal Necrolysis (TEN)

Erythema multiforme is characterized by skin lesions that are generally palpable "typical targets" or "raised atypical targets," with epidermal detachment for less than 10% of the body's surface area (BSA) and minimal mucous membrane involvement. SJS and TEN are considered to be the same disease entity with different severities. They are characterized by severe mucosal erosions; diffuse, non-palpable, flat atypical targets; and, commonly, a prodrome of fever and flu-like symptoms. The two conditions differ in the extent of epidermal detachment, with SJS limited to less than ~10% of BSA and TEN involving 30%–100% (147,148). There is an overlap in features of the two diseases. The term Stevens-Johnson syndrome will be used here to discuss these entities.

FIGURE 10.50. Phlyctenular keratoconjunctivitis. Raised gray, vascularized, wedge-shaped area in the cornea with a leash of vessels to the limbus.

Stevens-Johnson syndrome (SJS) is an immune-complex–mediated hypersensitivity disorder which typically involves the skin and the mucous membranes. Various etiologic factors have been implicated as causes of SJS. These include infection, vaccination, drugs, systemic diseases, physical agents, and food. Drugs such as antibiotics (sulfonamides, penicillins, cephalosporins), psychoepileptics (carbamazepine, phenytoin, phenobarbital, lamotrigene), nonsteroidal anti-inflammatory drugs (oxicam, ketoprofen, ibuprofen, diclofenac), and antigout (allopurinol, colchicine) medications are the most commonly blamed (149–151). Topical sulfonamides after only a few applications have rarely caused this severe problem. Individuals with antigens HLA-Bw44 and HLA-DQB1*0601 may be more susceptible to developing SJS (152). Clinically vesicular and bullous skin eruptions involving mucous membranes of the mouth and nose, as well as conjunctival eruptions are seen. Mucopurulent and pseudomembranous conjunctivitis may be seen along with ulcerations of the eyelid. There may be corneal involvement secondary to the eyelid reaction. After healing of the eyelid margins, epidermalization occurs on the palpebral surface of the eyelid (Fig. 10.51). With continued irritation from the rough conjunctival surface, the cornea develops superficial punctate keratitis and pannus formation, usually inferiorly or superiorly. In severe cases, cicatrization and symblepharon develop. Epidermalization may involve the corneal epithelium as well as the conjunctival epithelium, so that the end result can be a totally scarred conjunctiva and cornea, with firm adhesion of the eyelid margin to the cornea itself (Fig. 10.52). Corneal transplantation or a keratoprosthesis is the only hope of maintaining vision in some of these patients, but the prognosis is poor. Treatment of the acute disease (2 weeks) is supportive and symptomatic. Systemic and local corticosteroids, and possibly intravenous immunoglobulin offer some hope

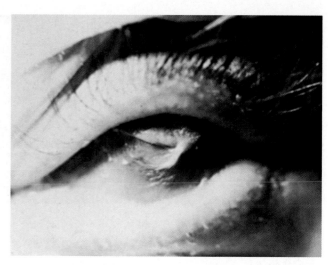

FIGURE 10.52. Eyelid changes in Stevens-Johnson disease with total scarring and symblepharon involving the eyelid and cornea.

of aborting the later, more severe consequences (153). In the acute phase, use of amniotic membrane transplantation has shown to be beneficial (154). When epidermalization occurs, scleral contact lenses or mucous membrane grafting of the eyelids has been shown to be beneficial in reducing the corneal sequelae due to the mechanical friction of the keratinized eyelids (155). Surgical reformation of the inferior cul-de-sac may be necessary when symblepharon develop (156). Amniotic membrane and living related corneal limbal/conjunctival transplantation were successful in only 20% of severe cases of total limbal stem cell deficiency secondary to Stevens-Johnson syndrome (157). Stable ocular surface has been achieved with cultivated oral mucosal epithelial transplantation with ocular surface reconstruction in cases of total limbal stem cell deficiency (158). Boston keratoprosthesis has a reasonable success as a primary or secondary procedure in cases of SJS (159,160).

Graft-Versus-Host Disease (GVHD)

Children who have had bone marrow transplants for aplastic anemia or leukemia may develop graft-versus-host disease and reject their own conjunctiva along with other mucous membranes and their skin. GVHD can be acute or chronic. Chronic graft-versus-host disease (cGVHD) is the most frequent late complication after allogeneic hematopoietic stem cell transplantation (HSCT). It occurs when primarily donor-derived immunocompetent cells are activated by host tissue antigen and initiate consecutive inflammatory processes in numerous target organs. The severity can be graded as follows: limited cGVHD, defined as either or both localized skin involvement and hepatic dysfunction; extensive cGVHD, as generalized, or localized skin involvement or hepatic dysfunction due to cGVHD plus liver histology showing chronic aggressive hepatitis, bridging necrosis or

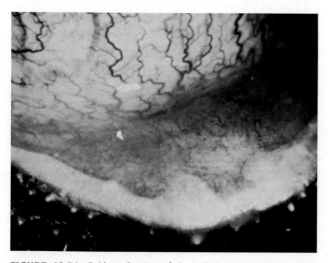

FIGURE 10.51. Epidermalization of the palpebral conjunctiva of the lower eyelid in Stevens-Johnson disease. This is a keratinization of the normal, smooth, glistening palpebral conjunctiva.

cirrhosis, or involvement of the eye or minor salivary glands or oral mucosa, or involvement or any other target organ. Ocular involvement (mostly anterior segment) is seen in 60% to 90% of patients with cGVHD. Ocular features include hyperemia, chemosis, pseudomembranous conjunctivitis, superior limbic keratoconjunctivitis and episcleritis, cicatricial palpebral conjunctival scarring, limbal stem cell deficiency, corneal epithelial sloughing, corneal perforation, lacrimal gland dysfunction ("lacrimal gland stasis"—distended ductules and obliteration of lumina) leading to keratoconjunctivitis sicca and secondary ocular infections. Treatment includes topical steroids and cyclosporine along with systemic management (e.g., steroids, T-cell modulators, rituximab, and photopheresis) (161,162).

Epidermolysis Bullosa

The cornea is involved in the severest form of this disease. There is corneal clouding in the region of Bowman's membrane and epithelium. Bullae similar to those found in the skin result in corneal ulceration, and perforation of the cornea can occur.

CORNEAL DYSTROPHIES AND DEGENERATIONS

Corneal dystrophies are unusual and dramatic when seen against a background of clear corneal tissue. Some degree of corneal opacification or clouding is present in these patients. Dystrophies are bilateral, are hereditary in nature, occur more centrally than peripherally, are nonvascularized, and do not usually manifest inflammatory signs or symptoms. On the other hand, corneal degenerations may be unilateral or bilateral, involve the peripheral as well as the central cornea, and often follow inflammation of the cornea. They are not hereditary and may occur after other ocular or systemic disease.

Over the past several years, many advances have been made in our understanding of the genetics of corneal dystrophies. New classification systems are being developed to incorporate this new information, which will hopefully help in comprehending the pathogenesis of these disorders and in developing new treatment approaches (163).

Corneal dystrophies are not limited to children, and, although they occasionally are noted in early childhood, most are first seen in the adolescent or later years. They become progressively worse during middle adult life. The corneal dystrophies first seen in childhood are emphasized in this section.

Anterior Corneal Dystrophies

The anterior corneal dystrophies include those that involve the epithelium, anterior basement membrane, and Bowman's membrane with *very* superficial stromal changes, but they do not involve primarily the stroma.

Meesmann Corneal Dystrophy (MECD)/ Hereditary Juvenile Epithelial Dystrophy of Meesmann

Meesmann dystrophy is a rare, dominantly inherited epithelial dystrophy seen in early childhood, usually by age 3 or 4 years. It occurs due to mutation in keratin gene K3 (KRT3) at locus 12q13. Symptoms include mild irritation, occasional glare and the visual acuity is not usually seriously affected. The corneal lesions appear as hundreds of tiny cystic changes in the deep epithelium and are noted best during slit-lamp examination by retroillumination. They are concentrated in the interpalpebral zone but can extend to the limbus. Grossly, the cornea may appear slightly hazy, but only on slit-lamp examination is the disease readily evident. On histopathology, the vesicles contain a PAS-positive material known as "peculiar substance", thickened multilaminar basement membrane with projections into the basal epithelium, and the basal epithelium has increased glycogen. Using transmission electron microscopy it has been demonstrated that "peculiar substance" is intracytoplasmic focal collection of fibrogranular material surrounded by tangles of cytoplasmic filaments. The cornea may be slightly thinned and corneal sensation may be reduced. The disease is not progressive; however, if vision is reduced to less than 20/60, epithelial debridement, superficial keratectomy, or excimer laser phototherapeutic keratectomy (PTK) may be performed to replace the abnormal superficial cornea. Unfortunately, when host epithelium grows back, the cystic changes will, eventually, reappear (154) (Fig. 10.53).

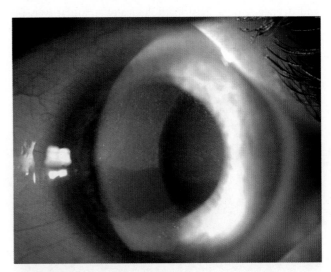

FIGURE 10.53. A patient with Meesmann corneal dystrophy showing recurrence of the dystrophy after epithelial debridement. The central cornea remains relatively clear.

Stocker-Holt Variant of MECD

It is also inherited as dominant pattern and occurs due to a mutation in keratin gene K12 (KRT12) at locus 17q12. Clinically fine, grayish punctate epithelial opacities that may stain with fluorescein and fine linear opacities that may appear in a whorl pattern are seen throughout the cornea. Patients demonstrate more severe signs and symptoms compared with classic Meesmann corneal dystrophy (165).

Corneal Dystrophies of Bowman's Membrane

Corneal epithelial scarring and irregularity accompanied by opacities and scarring in the region of Bowman's membrane, as well as recurrent epithelial erosions, characterize a group of dystrophic corneal changes with various eponyms. In many cases, these corneal changes begin in the first decade of life and are all dominantly inherited. They occur due to a mutation in the gene TGFBI at locus 5q31. Kuchle et al. (166) offered a classification that simplified these dystrophies, based on clinical appearance, as well as light and electron microscopy.

Reis-Bücklers Corneal Dystrophy (RBCD)/ Corneal Dystrophy of Bowman Layer, Type I (CDB I)/Superficial Granular Corneal Dystrophy

Symptoms begin with pain due to recurrent erosions, which resolve with time. Vision is reduced gradually by anterior scarring and surface irregularity (Fig. 10.54). On clinical examination, confluent irregular and coarse geographic-like opacities are seen at the level of Bowman layer and superficial stroma. These may extend to the limbus and deeper stroma. Histopathologically, granular Masson

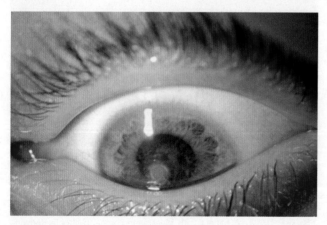

FIGURE 10.54. An 11-year-old child with Reis-Bücklers corneal dystrophy showing central dense scarring as a result of multiple recurrent erosions.

trichrome positive connective tissue layer is seen replacing Bowman layer.

Thiel-Behnke Corneal Dystrophy (TBCD)/ Corneal Dystrophy of Bowman Layer, Type II (CDB2)/Honeycomb-Shaped Corneal Dystrophy

While very similar, recurrent erosions are fewer and visual impairment is delayed compared to RBCD. Initially central subepithelial reticular (honeycomb) opacities are seen which may progress to the periphery and the deeper layers. Irregular epithelial thickening leads to ridges and furrows in the underlying stroma and focal absences of epithelial basement membrane. Histopathologically, saw-toothed fibrocelluler layer (pathognomonic) is seen replacing Bowman layer.

Transmission electron microscopy differentiates these two dystrophies. In CDB-I ultrastructural deposits of rod-like bodies are present, similar to those seen in granular stromal dystrophy. In CDB-II curly fibers (9 to 15nm) are evident, rather than the rod-like granules.

Treatment of RBCD and TBCD has been directed early at correcting the multiple corneal erosions that lead to scarring superficially. As these erosions persist, more scarring occurs, and irregular surface leads to further visual loss. Now, instead of performing a lamellar keratectomy or keratoplasty, or even a penetrating corneal transplantation, excimer laser PTK is used. Eventually, a partial thickness or full-thickness corneal transplant is needed in adulthood, as the opacities slowly progress posteriorly and deeper scars are formed over years of recurrent erosions.

Stromal Corneal Dystrophies

Granular Corneal Dystrophy

Granular dystrophy is inherited as autosomal dominant pattern and mutation is seen in TGFBI gene at locus 5q31. It has two main types:

Granular Corneal Dystrophy, Type 1 (GCD1)

It is usually diagnosed in later childhood but can be seen as early as 2 years of age. The most common presenting features are glare and photophobia. There is relatively good vision in the first few decades of life because the lesions are discrete and sharply outlined, leaving clear cornea around them. With increasing age the opacities progress and the visual acuity decreases (Fig. 10.55). This dystrophy does not usually cause significant epithelial irregularity and does not impair normal corneal sensitivity in the first and second decades of life. It does not lead to corneal vascularization but may be associated with corneal erosions. Histopathologic findings have revealed the presence of Masson-trichrome-stained multiple hyaline, rod-like stromal deposits extending from deep epithelium to Descemet membrane. Excimer

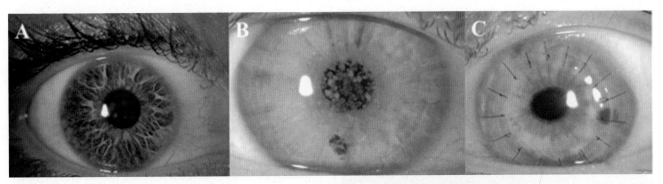

FIGURE 10.55. A: A patient with mild granular dystrophy with centrally located opacities and clear intervening spaces. **B:** A patient with severe granular dystrophy with no clear intervening spaces significantly affecting the visual acuity. **C:** The fellow eye of the same patient after penetrating keratoplasty showing a clear graft.

laser PTK is usually the first line treatment when the superficial opacities become confluent, but that is usually in adulthood. Corneal transplants are rarely performed in children or teenagers with this dystrophy.

Granular Corneal Dystrophy, Type 2 (Granular-Lattice) (GCD2)/Avellino Corneal Dystrophy

It may be diagnosed early (3 years old) in homozygous patients compared with heterozygote patients (8 years old). It has features of both granular and lattice corneal dystrophies. Stellate or snowflake stromal hyaline opacities appear between the anterior and mid stroma. Lattice-like amyloid lines are seen in the deep stromal layers of the cornea. With increasing age, anterior stromal haze develops between the opacities. Visual acuity decreases gradually as the central haze worsens. Opacities stain with either Masson trichrome or Congo red on histopathology.

For superficial granular dystrophy opacities, excimer laser PTK can be performed if there are severe visual symptoms in the teenage years (167,168). Deep anterior lamellar keratoplasty or PK may be performed for deeper lesions. LASIK and LASEK are contraindicated in GCD2 (169).

Classic Lattice Corneal Dystrophy (LCD1)

Lattice dystrophy is also dominant in inheritance and appears at its earliest toward the end of the first decade. The mutation also occurs in the TGFBI gene at locus 5q31. The corneal epithelium is typically spared early on, and therefore vision is good until the third or fourth decade. There is progressive opacification in a linear pattern in the superficial stroma, usually in the central region of the cornea (Fig. 10.42). Corneal sensitivity is decreased when more pathologic changes develop, but this does not occur in adolescence. The lesions appear as irregular, thick, refractile, opacified linear changes that cannot be followed to the limbus and therefore can be differentiated from blood vessels and corneal nerves by careful slit-lamp examination (Fig. 10.56). The stroma around

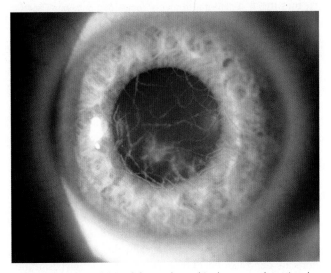

FIGURE 10.56. A child with lattice dystrophic changes and scarring due to recurrent corneal erosions.

these pathologic changes remains clear until later in life, when recurrent erosions and opacifications reduce vision to less than 20/200. Histopathologically, the abnormalities are amyloid material in the stroma distorting the lamellae. The deposits stain positive with Congo red and apple green birefringence is visible with a polarizing filter. In eyes with very superficial opacities, excimer laser PTK may significantly improve vision and recurrent erosion symptoms. A lamellar (DALK) or penetrating corneal transplant is indicated if vision deteriorates and the disease involves most of the corneal stroma. This is rarely necessary in children. Recurrence of lattice dystrophy in grafts is seen about the same time as granular dystrophy and much earlier than macular dystrophy.

Macular Corneal Dystrophy (MCD)

Inherited as an autosomal recessive trait, macular dystrophy is often first noticed early during the first decade and leads to earlier and more corneal opacity than that caused by

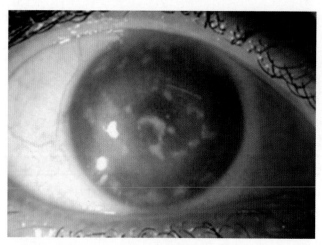

FIGURE 10.57. A patient with macular corneal dystrophy with dispersed opacities and hazy intervening spaces.

granular and lattice dystrophies. The lesions are not as clearly circumscribed as in granular and lattice dystrophies. Mutation of carbohydrate sulfotransferase 6 (CHST6) gene at locus 16q22 leads to deposition of abnormal nonsulfated keratans. In macular dystrophy, the entire cornea appears hazy, with poorly defined margins to the opacities, which blend into more normal-appearing cornea (Fig. 10.57). The lesions vary in size and shape in the stroma. The dense opacities are located anteriorly in the central cornea and posteriorly in the peripheral cornea. Beginning in the second or third decade, the central corneal thickness is typically reduced, often in the range of 400 μm. Histopathologically, the corneal opacifications are deposits of acid mucopolysaccharide (glycosaminoglycan) that stain with colloidal iron and Alcian blue and are seen throughout the stroma, even involving the endothelium. Guttae may be present on Descemet membrane. This dystrophy is much less common in the United States than the dominant corneal dystrophies, lattice and granular.

Patients generally notice decreased vision and may have recurrent erosion symptoms. If the central opacities are very superficial, they may be amenable to treatment with excimer laser PTK. Corneal transplantation is seldom necessary early in life. Recurrent stromal changes similar to those in the original dystrophy often occur after excimer laser PTK and corneal transplantation for the stromal corneal dystrophies,

especially granular and lattice, but less so for macular. Macular dystrophy may rarely be operated on in childhood, and one may expect to eventually see recurrent disease if transplantation is carried out early in life (169,170).

Schnyder Corneal Dystrophy (SCD)

Schnyder corneal dystrophy is an autosomal dominant disorder that may be seen in childhood and, rarely, early in infancy or at birth. It is inherited as autosomal dominant and the mutation is seen in the gene *UBIAD1* (UbiA prenyltransferase domain containing protein 1) at locus 1p36. Intra- and extracellular esterified and unesterified phospholipids and cholesterol are deposited in basal epithelial cells, Bowman layer, and stroma. Special stains such as oil red O or Sudan black are helpful in staining these lipids. The corneal changes are bilateral, although often asymmetrical. Fifty four percent of patients demonstrate corneal crystals (171). Clinically the corneal changes progress with age. In the younger age group only central corneal haze and/or subepithelial crystals are seen. Arcus lipoides develops later and as age advances, midperipheral panstromal haze develops, causing complete corneal opacity (Fig. 10.58). There is slow progression of the dystrophy with no vascularization. Vision remains good throughout early life, despite the crystalline changes in the cornea. There is a disproportionate reduction in photopic vision. Corneal sensitivity decreases with age. Corneal transplantation, when necessary, is usually done at midlife or later because vision is typically satisfactory, despite the opacities in the central cornea. Patients diagnosed with SCD and family members should undergo a lipid workup because it is associated with hyperlipoproteinemia (type IIa, III, or IV).

Congenital Stromal Corneal Dystrophy (CSCD)

It is a rare condition, inherited as autosomal dominant with mutation of the decorin (DCN) gene at locus 12q21.33. Clinically the cornea is thick with diffuse, bilateral clouding, with flake-like whitish stromal opacities seen throughout the stroma. Slowly progressive visual loss is seen. The stromal lamellae are thin and are separated from each other in a regular manner. Amorphous material may be deposited in between the lamellae. In advanced cases PK may be required (172).

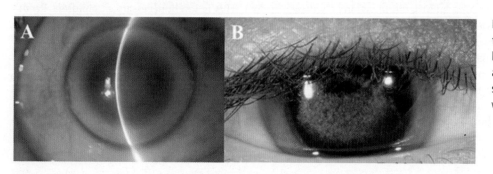

FIGURE 10.58. Schnyder corneal dystrophy. **A:** Slit view showing panstromal haze due to deposition of phospholipids and cholesterol. **B:** Clinical photograph showing subepithelial crystals in a child with Schnyder corneal dystrophy.

Deep Corneal Dystrophies

Dystrophies involving the endothelium are not common in early life. Alterations in Descemet's membrane may be seen at birth, but these are changes from congenital glaucoma or birth injuries, or developmental changes, rather than corneal dystrophies or degenerations.

Congenital Hereditary Endothelial Dystrophy (CHED)

Congenital hereditary endothelial dystrophy is histopathologically characterized by diffuse thickening and lamination of Descemet membrane with few, atrophic endothelial cells. There is deposition of basement membrane-like material on Descemet membrane. Endothelium may be replaced by stratified squamous epithelium. The stroma is grossly thickened with disorganization and disruption of the lamellae.

CHED Type 1

CHED type 1 is autosomally dominantly inherited with the gene unidentified. Patients have decreased vision, photophobia, and tearing that is worse in the morning. It presents at birth or the first few of years of life. Diffuse corneal clouding and thickening is usually seen but in some patients only peau d'orange- like endothelial changes are seen. There may be gradual endothelial decompensation.

CHED Type 2

CHED type 2 is inherited in an autosomal recessive pattern. Mutation is seen at locus 20pl3, sodium borate transporter, member 11 (SLC4A11). It presents at birth with diffuse or ground-glass thickened cornea. Rarely, subepithelial band keratopathy is seen. Patients have more blurring and nystagmus but less photophobia and tearing than seen in CHED type 1.

The corneal appearance of both CHEDs at birth may be mistaken for congenital glaucoma, but the intraocular pressure is normal, and the eye is not enlarged. Full-thickness severe corneal stromal and epithelial edema are present, although the anterior chamber and iris are normal. An interesting finding in this disease is the thickening of collagen fibrils seen histologically. This is not present in any other corneal dystrophy. The endothelium is very attenuated or absent, leading to marked corneal swelling from stromal edema. Corneal sensitivity is normal. Posterior collagenous layer of Descemet membrane contains collagen and laminin on immunohistochemistry. Penetrating corneal transplantation in this disease is successful in 60% to 70% of patients (173). In recent years, DSEK has been performed in CHED patients with good anatomical and functional success (106) (Fig. 10.59).

Posterior Polymorphous Corneal Dystrophy (PPCD)

Posterior polymorphous corneal dystrophy is usually autosomal dominant but may be sporadic.

The mutation occurs on gene PPCD2: collagen type VIII alpha 2 (COL8A2); PPCD3, ZEBl. There may be circular or linear vesicles (railroad tracks) or nodules or blister-like lesions on the posterior surface of the cornea (Fig. 10.60). The changes may be present in the first few years of life and occasionally at birth. There may be peripheral anterior synechiae and iridocorneal adhesions in 25%; glaucoma is found in approximately 15%. Various degrees of corneal abnormality may be present in different members of the same family. The mildest form shows only single or multiple vesicles, sometimes in lines with normal overlying stroma. The severe form shows multiple vesicular changes on the back of the cornea, enough to cause stromal edema and scarring, but seldom requiring corneal transplantation. This disease, unlike endothelial dystrophy and Fuchs dystrophy, is seen in young people, but either is much slower in its progression or does not progress at all. Histopathologically, Descemet membrane is thickened and multilaminated with multilayered endothelial cell with epithelial cell characteristics (microvilli, stain positive for keratin). Very few patients require corneal transplantation. Recently, DESK and Descemet's membrane endothelial keratoplasty have been successfully performed in patients with PPCD (174,175).

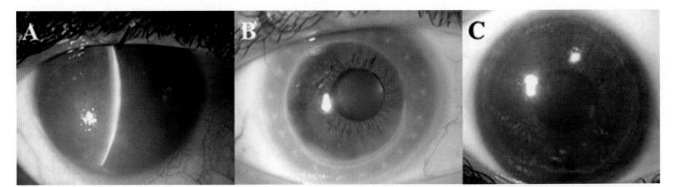

FIGURE 10.59. Congenital hereditary endothelial dystrophy (CHED). **A:** Slit-beam view showing a diffuse hazy and thick cornea in a child. **B:** Clear graft one year after a penetrating keratoplasty for CHED. **C:** Clear cornea 3 months after Descemet's stripping endothelial keratoplasty for CHED.

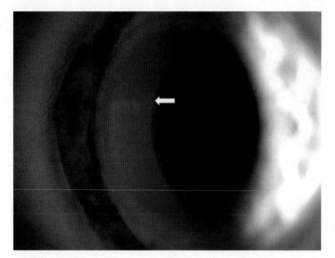

FIGURE 10.60. Slit-beam view showing linear vesicles (railroad tracks) in a patient with posterior polymorphous corneal dystrophy.

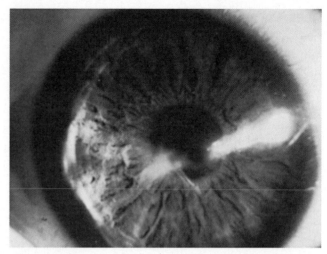

FIGURE 10.61. Keratoconus with abnormal light reflex of the surface of the cornea owing to the central cone.

Corneal Degenerations

Keratoconus

The most common corneal degeneration in early adolescent years is keratoconus, a bilateral, noninflammatory condition that affects both sexes but is slightly more common in women. It often manifests itself at puberty. Keratoconus may be difficult to recognize in the early and middle adolescent years, as it can be very difficult to differentiate from high astigmatism. Progression occurs in the early to late teens and into the 20s and occasionally later. Unilateral keratoconus may also be seen, but bilateral cases are far more frequent. About 10% of patients have other family members with keratoconus. Abnormal computerized corneal topography with inferior steepening has been seen in relatively asymptomatic family members. There is some evidence that keratoconus may develop from long-term contact lens use, but this is controversial. Constant eye rubbing is likely a factor in some patients.

In childhood, the earliest changes are characterized by distorted images at the keratometer or with the Placido disc. With retinoscopy, there is an uneven motion or slit in the reflex that has been described as a scissors motion (Fig. 10.61). One of the earliest ways to diagnose keratoconus is with computerized corneal topography.

With the direct ophthalmoscope, there is a dense, irregular, dark reflex in the center of the reflected red reflex. In the early stages, slit-lamp examination reveals central or paracentral thinning, but this may be hard to detect. There may be fine deep corneal stromal Vogt's striae, and with the slit lamp a Fleischer's iron ring can be found at the upper or lower border of the early cone (Fig. 10.62). Acute hydrops or edema of the cornea following breaks in Descemet's membrane is not usually seen in the first decade but may occur in the middle or late teens (Fig. 10.63). Hydrops is seen only in the more advanced cases of keratoconus and is most common with keratoconus in Down's syndrome. Keratoconus may be

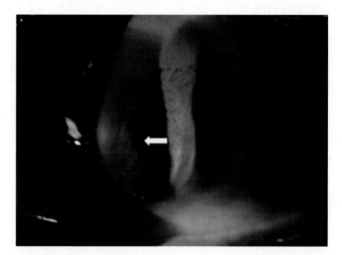

FIGURE 10.62. Slit-beam view of a keratoconus patient with ectasia and Vogt's striae (*arrow*) and a partial superior iron line (Fleischer ring).

seen with other conditions, such as floppy eyelid syndrome, Leber's congenital amaurosis, retinitis pigmentosa, Down's syndrome, and Ehlers-Danlos syndromes. Keratoconus can be associated with atopic disease, and many children with keratoconus have some history of allergy. They often rub their eyes excessively.

Until recently, there has been no successful treatment to prevent progression of keratoconus. A new procedure, corneal collagen crosslinking (CXL) by means of riboflavin (0.1% drops) and ultraviolet-A light (370 nm, irradiance of 3 mW/cm2), has been proposed to strengthen the intrinsic biomechanical properties of corneal collagen and thus improve the biomechanical and biochemical properties. There is growing clinical evidence that CXL halts (at least temporarily) the progression of keratoconus and secondary keratectasia with a small failure rate (3%) and a low complication rate (1%) (176). Although CXL has been shown to be beneficial in adults, there is little to no evidence of its

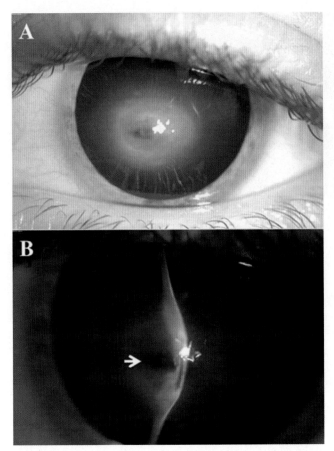

FIGURE 10.63. **A:** Clinical photograph showing a child with corneal edema due to acute hydrops. **B:** Slit-beam view showing fishmouth-shaped break in Descemet's membrane (*arrow*).

outcomes and safety in children. Contact lenses remain the main form of therapy for mild and moderate keratoconus. Corneal transplantation offers the opportunity to restore vision in more severe cases. Corneal transplantation is over 95% successful in appropriate patients but is rarely necessary in childhood. Deep anterior lamellar keratoplasty avoids the problem of endothelial graft rejection and may be successful in many eyes. Intracorneal ring segments may also be of use in some eyes with relatively mild keratoconus (177).

Calcific Corneal Degeneration

Calcific degeneration of the cornea in children is usually secondary to systemic or other corneal diseases. In young children, injuries with alkaline materials, such as cement, lye, lime, and ammonia, are not uncommon, and this severe chemical trauma may quickly lead to secondary calcific changes in the cornea, sometimes within 2 or 3 weeks of the original injury.

Systemic disease associated with hypercalcemia may result in calcium deposits in the cornea. Hyperparathyroidism, vitamin D toxicity, milk-alkali syndrome, renal rickets, and hypophosphatasia, which result in elevations of blood calcium levels, may also induce calcific degeneration in the cornea.

Calcium in the cornea appears either as a paralimbal, slight gray opacification in the region of the basement membrane or Bowman's membrane nasally and temporally, or in a band-shaped distribution across the central cornea. There are small holes in the degenerative area, which are characteristic of calcific degeneration. This corneal degeneration may also result from inflammatory disease of the anterior segment, such as chronic uveitis (as with juvenile rheumatoid arthritis) and trauma.

Debridement with chelating agents, such as ethylenediaminetetraacetic acid (EDTA), enhances removal of the calcium after the overlying epithelium is removed. This is usually better and less expensive than excimer laser PTK for this condition (168).

CORNEAL MANIFESTATIONS OF SYSTEMIC DISEASE

The corneal changes seen in systemic disease of infancy and childhood may or may not affect vision in the young patient. Many of these diseases are rare in children and may have been described in only one or two cases, in either the English or foreign literature. Only the more common systemic conditions seen in infancy and childhood, rather than the adult forms, are discussed in this section.

Diseases of Abnormal Carbohydrate Metabolism

The mucopolysaccharidoses are a group of diseases with definite systemic physical characteristics. They are described in detail in Chapter 21. They are all autosomal recessive, except Hunter's syndrome, which is X-linked recessive.

Hurler's disease, mucopolysaccharidosis (MPS) I-H is important because the disease may be confused with congenital glaucoma and congenital stromal corneal dystrophy, and possibly interstitial keratitis. The cornea is hazy, with a thickened edematous stroma. The disease has many systemic characteristics, and demonstration of mucopolysaccharides in the urine helps in making the diagnosis. The cornea may be clear at first but becomes diffusely clouded in time, without signs of inflammation or vascularization.

In Hunter's disease, MPS II, clouding of the cornea is absent until late in the disease. Pigmentary degeneration of the retina may be responsible for visual loss. Sanfilippo's syndrome, MPS III, does not show corneal changes, whereas Morquio's syndrome, MPS IV, does show corneal clouding.

Scheie's syndrome, MPS I-S, is present in affected children by age 7 or 8. The cornea undergoes progressive clouding and becomes thicker (Fig. 10.64). In Maroteaux-Lamy syndrome, MPS VI, corneal opacities are seen early.

It is evident that with clouded corneas early in life, both urinalysis and testing of the intraocular pressure are essential to rule out a mucopolysaccharidosis or congenital glaucoma

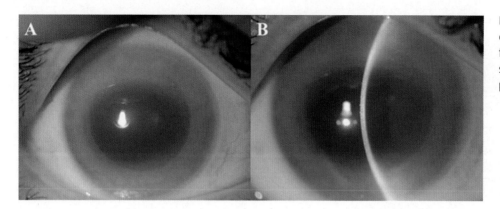

FIGURE 10.64. A: An 11-year-old child with Hurler's disease with a diffusely hazy cornea. **B:** Slit-beam view showing stromal haze more in the periphery than the central cornea.

as soon as the disorder is recognized. While full-thickness corneal transplants have been the main treatment for years, recently good success has been obtained with DALK for MPS I and MPS VI (107).

Diseases of Abnormal Protein Metabolism

Cystinosis is a disease of altered amino acid metabolism, allowing cystine to accumulate in the body. Infantile, adolescent, and adult forms are found. The infantile form (Fanconi's syndrome) is the most severe and is typically fatal early in life without renal transplantation. The adolescent and adult forms are less severe. Growth and development in the infantile form are usually normal until the sixth month of life, when growth fails to continue and muscular weakness develops. Deposits of soluble cystine crystals are found in the conjunctiva, cornea, iris, lens, sclera, and choroid. The cornea is clouded and has very tiny glistening punctate dots, which are the crystals reflecting light from the cornea. They are noted throughout the full thickness of cornea; however, there is a concentration of crystal toward the corneal periphery. The disease is transmitted as an autosomal recessive trait (178). Long-term oral cysteamine can improve renal function but does not seem to improve the corneal opacities. Topical cysteamine has been demonstrated to improve the corneal crystals. Rarely, corneal transplantation may be required to treat severe corneal opacity. Other diseases of the cornea that involve crystals, that is, gout and the dysproteinemias, are not seen in childhood.

Inborn errors of metabolism with corneal changes are rarely seen. In phenylpyruvic oligophrenia, corneal opacities are present, in addition to cataracts. In porphyria, another inborn error of metabolism, the cornea may show ulceration and vascularization as well as keratomalacia. The full-blown picture appears later in life.

Diseases of Abnormal Lipid Metabolism

Corneal changes accompanying abnormal lipid metabolism are not usually seen in infancy and childhood. Arcus juvenilis has previously been described under Embryology and Developmental Abnormalities.

In Fabry's disease, an X-linked, recessively transmitted disorder, abnormal lipid storage, and corneal changes are noted. Fine brown pinpoint opacities may be found in the corneal epithelium. The changes radiate from the inferocentral cornea to the periphery in a fanlike fashion and is termed *cornea verticillata*. The first manifestations of this disease may be the corneal opacities. Although these opacities appear in early childhood and are asymptomatic, they are significant in that systemic changes will later occur and may herald the full-blown disease and early death. There are other ocular signs as well, including focal vascular dilatations of the conjunctival and retinal vessels. Interestingly, the corneal changes are also present in most female carriers of the gene.

Corneal Changes in Avitaminosis

In severe malnutrition, corneal changes from vitamin A deficiency may be seen. Keratomalacia with thickening of the corneal epithelium, epidermalization, and keratinization can occur (Fig. 10.65). In the late stages, Bowman's membrane is replaced by pannus, and the cornea may appear hazy and thickened. Bitot's spot, a foamy surface conjunctival change, nasal or temporal to the limbus, is also seen in vitamin A deficiency .

In riboflavin deficiency, a superficial punctate keratitis may be evident, which causes photophobia. Vascularization of the cornea is seen in the later stages.

Hereditary Benign Intraepithelial Dyskeratosis

Intraepithelial dyskeratosis is a rare disease characterized by plaque-like elevations on the conjunctiva and cornea, as well as on the oral mucous membrane, occurring in the first decade of life. This disease is present only in the descendants of (inbred) triracial group of people of black, white, and American Indian origin, who trace their roots to northeastern North Carolina. The bulbar conjunctiva is involved nasally and temporally, and later corneal changes also occur. There is a dyskeratotic hyperplastic epithelial change on the conjunctiva extending into the cornea, causing blurred vision.

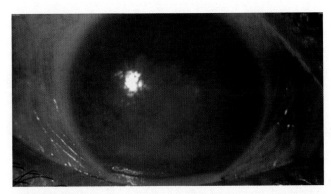

FIGURE 10.65. A patient with xerophthalmia showing conjunctival xerosis and an extremely dry corneal surface.

The thick, opaque, unilateral, and bilateral involvement may cause stromal changes, leading to deep stromal vascularization. Corneal involvement varies and may become apparent in early infancy or even from birth. The plaque-like changes persist throughout life, sometimes worsening and causing severe visual loss (179).

The disease is transmitted as an autosomal dominant trait with a high degree of penetrance. The use of topical corticosteroids is not effective. Except for artificial tears, which may make the patient more comfortable, no topical medication helps. Surgical excision of the corneal lesions later in life, after childhood, usually results in regrowth of similar tissue in the bed of the resection. Surgical excision should be reserved for the most severe cases associated with marked corneal involvement. This is not usually necessary in infancy or childhood (179).

Other hereditary disorders have been associated with hereditary, benign intraepithelial dyskeratosis, including retinitis pigmentosa, Axenfeld's anomaly, and various systemic abnormalities.

Interstitial Keratitis of the Cornea Secondary to Congenital Syphilis

Before the age of penicillin, the most common cause of interstitial keratitis in children was congenital syphilis. The corneal manifestations of this disease acquired in utero occurred in the first decade of life. Corneal changes are uncommon at birth or in early infancy.

Congenital syphilis is first seen in the cornea as a rapid progression of corneal edema diffusely involving the cornea. After this, vascularization of the deep cornea occurs adjacent to Descemet's membrane. The cornea may take on a salmon-pink color because of the marked vascularization, which lasts for several weeks. Later, gradual clearing of these corneal vessels occurs over a period of weeks to many months. These empty deep blood vessels (ghost vessels) remain in the deep cornea. The lines of clearing in the deep cornea are called Fuchs' lines and are characteristic of congenital syphilis.

Treatment in this early stage of corneal involvement consists of topical corticosteroids and systemic therapy for the congenital syphilis. Dilatation of the pupil and antibiotics to prevent secondary infection are also used. During later years, if vision is significantly involved because of the corneal scarring, a corneal transplant may be performed. It is important to examine the lens for opacities and the retina for degenerative changes, which may also cause visual loss.

The ophthalmologist should be aware of the corneal changes in this disease, as well as the Hutchinson's triad (corneal changes, abnormal dentition, and a flat bridge of the nose), all due to congenital syphilis.

Tubercular Interstitial Keratitis

Interstitial keratitis due to tuberculosis was more prevalent in the past when tuberculosis was a common disease. Tuberculosis in children is not rare, although corneal changes from tuberculosis are extremely rare. These corneal changes include nodular corneal lesions with dense residual scarring and opacities, which remain after healing occurs. In children with undiagnosed corneal lesions and midstromal vessels, a tuberculin test and chest x-ray should be obtained if the cause of the corneal disease is unknown. Usually, such corneal disease is due to herpes simplex virus keratitis, rather than tuberculosis.

Viral Interstitial Keratitis

Interstitial keratitis due to herpes simplex virus is much more common than either of the two previously mentioned diseases as described earlier in this chapter. In addition to herpes simplex virus, other viral infections, particularly mumps, measles, and vaccinia, may cause these stromal changes. Herpes zoster and varicella keratitis can also cause interstitial keratitis. Ocular Lyme borreliosis is another infection that can cause interstitial keratitis in children and young adults (180,181).

Wilson's Disease

Wilson's disease (hepatolenticular degeneration) is a disorder of abnormal protein metabolism. There are hepatic and extrapyramidal changes that, if not corrected early in life, lead to permanent brain damage. Decrease in the ceruloplasmin is associated with an increase in the serum copper that is not bound to protein. In addition, there is an increase of copper in the urine as well as copper deposition in various tissues, such as liver and cornea.

The corneal changes are diagnostic of this disease. An orange-brown ring in the periphery of the cornea, called the Kayser-Fleischer ring, is the characteristic feature. The ring is deposited in the deep stroma in and around Descemet's membrane. There is a clear zone separating Descemet's membrane from the limbus. It is essential that all children manifesting undiagnosed progressive mental or hepatic disease be examined with the slit lamp. Gonioscopy may be required to see the earliest changes.

Refsum's Syndrome

Retinitis pigmentosa is part of this autosomal recessive disease along with other findings, such as chronic polyneuritis. The corneal changes may consist of epithelial thickening and degeneration, with pannus formation in the region of Bowman's membrane. Hypertrophy of corneal nerves is present in this disease, but the corneal changes are not the cause of the marked visual loss.

Keratoconjunctivitis Sicca

This is an unusual finding in young children, although dry eyes should not be overlooked in a differential diagnosis of irritative phenomena in older children. Punctate keratitis, and very rarely filamentary keratitis, may be seen in older children with decreased production of tears. In addition, there is an excess of mucus in the precorneal tear film and an increase in viscosity of the tear film itself. Keratoconjunctivitis sicca may be found accompanying Still's disease or rheumatoid arthritis in children and in lupus erythematosus, among other connective tissue diseases (182).

Treatment of keratoconjunctivitis sicca in children is similar to that in adults. The use of artificial tear drops (preferably preservative-free), as frequently as necessary to make the patient comfortable, is recommended. If the patient requires artificial tear drops every 2 hours or more frequently, a solid rod of Lacrisert (Aton Pharma, Lawrenceville, NJ) may be tried. This consists of a hydroxypropyl cellulose small pellet, which is inserted inside the lower eyelid on awakening. The insert gradually melts as the day progresses, reducing the necessity for frequent applications of artificial tears. Because it is sometimes difficult for children to apply artificial tear drops during school hours, the use of the Lacrisert is recommended, at least for a short trial for the unusual child with keratoconjunctivitis sicca. This is also effective in eliminating filamentary keratitis, when this disorder accompanies dry eyes in children. Topical cyclosporine A 0.05% is FDA-approved for the treatment of dry-eye disease, using a twice-a-day regimen. It may be effective in certain children with severe dry eyes.

In more severe keratitis sicca cases, punctal closure is indicated. This can be done on a temporary basis with punctal plugs or permanently with cautery (183). Rarely, a small lateral tarsorrhaphy may be required to decrease ocular surface evaporation.

Congenital Corneal Anesthesia

Congenital corneal anesthesia is a rare clinical entity characterized by punctate keratopathy that can progress to persistent nonhealing epithelial defects and corneal melting in the absence of pain and distress in the child. It leads to abnormal ocular protective mechanisms of the eye. It is associated with decreased basal blink rate, basal tear production, and mucus production. It is usually sporadic but autosomal dominant pattern of inheritance has been reported. It is associated with several neurologic disorders (Mobius syndrome, Riley-Day syndrome), somatic disorders (MURCS-Mullerian duct and renal aplasia, cervical somite dysplasia; Goldenhar syndrome-oculoauriculovertebral dysplasia). Treatment with aggressive lubrication, autologous serum drops, and tarsorrhaphy when indicated are the best options for reducing the risk for corneal damage and visual loss. Recently, custom-designed, fluid-ventilated, rigid gas-permeable scleral lens (e.g., PROSE lens) has been used with good success (184,185). In recalcitrant cases, a conjunctival flap can be performed to stabilize the ocular surface.

CORNEAL INJURIES

Unfortunately, corneal injuries in children may lead to significant or total visual loss as well as psychological problems due to severe corneal scarring and disfigurement (186). An estimated 2.4 million eye injuries occur in the United States each year, with nearly 35% of injuries among persons aged less than 17 years. Incidence of severe visual impairment or blindness caused by ocular trauma in children varies from 2%–14%. As a leading cause of non-congenital unilateral blindness, ocular trauma remains an important cause of ocular morbidity in children. Ocular injuries in adults resulting from accidents may be prevented by the use of safety lenses. In children, these accidents are especially tragic, because they are often preventable by keeping harmful chemicals and sharp-pointed toys and instruments out of reach. Amblyopia is another concern in children under ages 8 to 10 years. This potentially permanent decrease in vision needs to be kept in mind when treating children after trauma.

Corneal lacerations with sharp instruments, such as pencils, darts, and scissors, usually strike the lens also, and the additional problem arises of how to handle the secondary cataract and iris in the corneal wound. The lens material may resorb in children, leaving a thin secondary membrane. If the laceration is paracentral, the visual axis may be clear after injury, allowing a satisfactory image to form on the retina. If the scar is centrally located and the corneal periphery is clear, a rotating autokeratoplasty after the initial trauma may be helpful in rotating the central scar out of the pupillary axis. During initial laceration repair, it is best to attempt removal of anterior synechiae to the back of the cornea. This may best be done by passage of a synechiolysis spatula through a paracentesis to sweep iris or lens remnants from the back of the cornea. It is important to do this to prevent vascularization or retrocorneal membrane formation. Cataract removal at the time of ruptured globe repair is recommended only if the lens capsule is grossly ruptured and lens material is fluffing up into the anterior chamber or out of the wound. Cataract removal at the time of corneal laceration repair is often quite difficult due to poor visualization (Fig. 10.66). Cataract removal at the time of subsequent anterior segment reconstruction or corneal transplantation is generally successful, and an intraocular lens can often be placed. Intraocular lenses for infant traumatic aphakia are controversial. Epikeratophakia for contact-lens–intolerant children with aphakia has been helpful (187), but the commercial manufacturer has stopped making these lenses, and they are rarely used. The various factors associated with decreased final visual acuity after open globe injuries in children include young age at presentation, poor initial visual acuity, presence of a relative afferent pupillary defect, absence of red reflex, cataract, and number of surgeries performed (188).

Ocular burns in children may be due to physical agents (thermal: flames, fireworks, and hot liquids; electrical; microwaved food and drinks), chemical agents (household cleaning agents, industrial chemicals, certain medications, agricultural chemicals), miscellaneous agents—chuna (chewing tobacco, composed of calcium hydroxide) and sodium hydroxide or carbonate (from airbags used in motor vehicles) or biologic agents (millipedes, snake venom, blistering beetles, plant sap from manchineel trees). Chemical injuries may be serious in children, particularly alkali burns of the cornea and sclera. The common household cleaner, ammonia, is exceedingly dangerous and easily accessible to children, because it is usually stored in a cabinet beneath the sink or on a low shelf. Within seconds of splashing ammonia on the eye, the pH in the anterior chamber may climb to 12.0, causing denaturation of stromal protein and inflicting permanent damage to the iris and lens. The iris may balloon forward and touch the back of the cornea. Lens opacities develop rapidly in these accidents, and the healing stage is exceedingly long, frequently years after injury. Calcific degeneration may occur following alkali burns in small children. Alkali burns in children are treated similarly to those in adults, but therapy is often more difficult in children, who

are invariably uncooperative. Examination under anesthesia for removal of toxic chemicals and thorough irrigation of the entire ocular surface may be required to prevent ongoing inflammation and if performed, an amniotic membrane transplantation may be done. Collagenase inhibitors have been used in the past to prevent stromal melting, but the results are equivocal. EDTA is used to remove secondary calcific degeneration. Acids cause corneal burns but are not usually as severe as alkali chemical injuries of the cornea. All chemicals should be kept out of the reach of children, including turpentine, shellac, paints, and other fluids that may be ingested or splashed into the eye (189).

Blast injuries of the cornea, secondary to air guns, such as B-B guns or pellet guns fired at close range, can do great injury to a child's eye. Pellets have considerable range and may cause perforation of the cornea even at 45 m (50 yards). At present, tear gas pen guns are readily available to children and have caused injury to the eyes. Most states have no law prohibiting the sale or use of such guns. Injuries are caused by the blast when the gun is shot within 30 to 60 cm (1 to 2 feet) of the face. The blast comes from the gunpowder used to propel the gas. In addition, the plastic housing may be split, and the plastic itself can also act as a missile at very close range. It is important to recognize that, in addition to corneal lacerations, contusions of the cornea with deep folds in Descemet's membrane and anterior chamber hemorrhage may occur from these injuries (Fig. 10.67). Recession of the angle, macular edema, and retinal hemorrhages have also been found. Airbag-associated ocular injuries (190) and paintball ocular injuries (191) have been reported in children. Injuries to children's eyes are typically handled in the same way as adult ocular injuries. It is important to examine the child's eyes thoroughly. If this is impossible, general anesthesia should be used for careful microscopic examination at the earliest time after injury.

Risk of ocular trauma during birth is due to anatomic abnormalities, extended labor, and the use of obstetric forceps. Compression of the globe between the orbital roof and

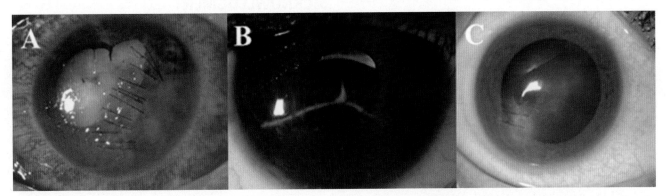

FIGURE 10.66. A: Central repaired corneal laceration with lens opacification and irregular pupil. **B:** Central linear healed laceration in a patient who also had lens aspiration simultaneously for a traumatic cataract. **C:** A peripheral repaired corneal laceration with clear lens and a round pupil.

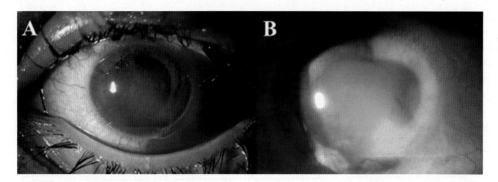

FIGURE 10.67. A: Closed-globe injury in a patient demonstrating corneal edema and hyphema. **B:** Resolving blood staining of the cornea following a total hyphema. Note the clearing peripherally.

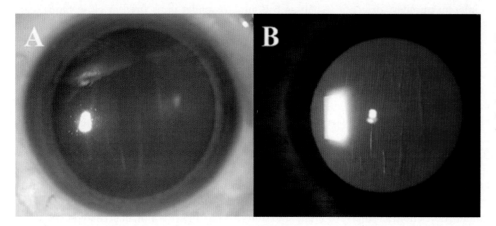

FIGURE 10.68. A: Linear vertical paired ridges of folded Descemet's membrane on the back of the cornea in an adult patient after birth trauma. **B:** The ridges can be better appreciated on retroillumination. The patient developed amblyopia and the vision was 20/400.

the blade of the obstetric forceps results in ocular trauma. Excessive pressure of the blade of the forceps on the cornea results in breaks in Descemet's membrane. These breaks lead to corneal edema at birth, which clears in the first months of life. Unlike congenital glaucoma with diffuse corneal stromal edema, the edema with birth trauma is localized to the area of the break in Descemet's membrane and the intraocular pressure is normal. The breaks in the cornea, which are usually vertical or slightly off the vertical, persist and appear as paired ridges of folded Descemet's membrane attached at both ends to the cornea in later life (Fig. 10.68). Large astigmatic refractive errors may result. These must be recognized and optically treated with spectacles or contact lenses.

Amblyopia from anisometropia or from corneal edema is frequent and must be vigorously treated. Corneal transplantation in infancy and childhood is not usually necessary for this condition. There is generally some visual loss, which is sometimes severe. Corneal edema from endothelial decompensation may occur later in life. Penetrating keratoplasty has been successful in restoring some vision to these eyes. Recently, DSEK has been performed with excellent anatomic and functional outcome (192).

ACKNOWLEDGMENT

Ms. Karen Albert executed the drawings.

REFERENCES

1. Allen L, Burian HM, Braley AE. A new concept of the development of the anterior chamber angle. *Arch Ophthalmol* 1955; 53:783.
2. Topouzis F, Karadimas P, Gatzonis SD, et al. Autosomal-dominant megalocornea associated with ocular hypertension. *J Pediatr Ophthalmol Strabismus* 2000;37:173–175.
3. Meire FM. Megalocornea. Clinical and genetic aspects. *Doc Ophthalmol* 1994;87:1–121.
4. Ho CL, Walton DS. Primary megalocornea: clinical features for differentiation from infantile glaucoma. *J Pediatr Ophthalmol Strabismus* 2004;41:11–17.
5. Meire FM, Delleman JM. Biometry in X-linked megalocornea: pathognomonic findings. *Br J Ophthalmol* 1994;78:781.
6. Turaçli ME, Tekeli O. Anterior megalophthalmos with pigmentary glaucoma. *Graefes Arch Clin Exp Ophthalmol* 2005;243(10): 1066–1068
7. Khan AO, Aldahmesh MA, Alkuraya FS. Congenital megalocornea with zonular weakness and childhood lens-related secondary glaucoma—a distinct phenotype caused by recessive LTBP2 mutations. *Mol Vis* 2011;17:2570–2579
8. Vaz FM, Osher RH. Cataract surgery and anterior megalophthalmos: custom intraocular lens and special considerations. *J Cataract Refract Surg* 2007;33(12):2147–2150.

9. Cameron JA. Keratoglobus. *Cornea* 1993;12:124–130.

10. Judisch GF, Waziri M, Krachmer JH. Ocular Ehlers-Danlos syndrome with normal lysyl hydroxylase activity. *Arch Ophthalmol* 1976;94:1489.

11. McKusick VA. *Mendelian inheritance in man,* 5th Ed. Baltimore, MD: The Johns Hopkins University Press, 1978.

12. Gregoratos ND, Bartsocas CS, Papas K. Blue sclerae with keratoglobus and brittle cornea. *Br J Ophthalmol* 1971;55(6):424–426.

13. Javadi MA, Kanavi MR, Ahmadi M, Yazdani S. Outcomes of epikeratoplasty for advanced keratoglobus. *Cornea* 2007;26(2):154–157.

14. Kaushal S, Jhanji V, Sharma N, Tandon R, Titiyal JS, Vajpayee RB. "Tuck In" lamellar keratoplasty (TILK) for corneal ectasias involving corneal periphery. *Br J Ophthalmol* 2008;92(2):286–290.

15. Batra DV, Paul SD. Microcornea with myopia. *Br J Ophthalmol* 1967;51:57.

16. Tane S, Sakuma Y, Ito S. The studies on the ultrasonic diagnosis in ophthalmology. Report 13. Ultrasonic biometry in microphthalmos and buphthalmos. *Acta Soc Ophthalmol Jpn* 1977;81:1112.

17. Cross HE, Yoder F. Familial nanophthalmos. *Am J Ophthalmol* 1976;81:300.

18. Vignolo EM, Steindl K, Forte R, et al. Autosomal dominant simple microphthalmos. *J Med Genet* 1994;31:721.

19. Reddy MA, Francis PJ, Berry V, et al. A clinical and molecular genetic study of a rare dominantly inherited syndrome (MRCS) comprising of microcornea, rod-cone dystrophy, cataract, and posterior staphyloma. *Br J Ophthalmol* 2003;87:197–202.

20. Elder MJ. Aetiology of severe visual impairment and blindness in microphthalmos. *Br J Ophthalmol* 1994;78:332.

21. Sun W, Xiao X, Li S, Guo X, Zhang Q. Mutational screening of six genes in Chinese patients with congenital cataract and microcornea. *Mol Vis* 2011;17:1508–1513.

22. Sowden JC. Molecular and developmental mechanisms of anterior segment dysgenesis. *Eye (Lond)* 2007;21(10):1310–1318.

23. Reis LM, Semina EV. Genetics of anterior segment dysgenesis disorders. *Curr Opin Ophthalmol* 2011;22(5):314–324.

24. Shigeyasu C, Yamada M, Mizuno Y, Yokoi T, Nishina S, Azuma N. Clinical features of anterior segment dysgenesis associated with congenital corneal opacities. *Cornea* 2012;31(3):293–298.

25. Reese AB, Ellsworth RM. The anterior chamber cleavage syndrome. *Arch Ophthalmol* 1966;75:307.

26. Waring GO, Rodrigues MM, Laibson PR. Anterior chamber cleavage syndrome: a stepladder classification. *Surv Ophthalmol* 1975;20(1):3–27.

27. Jerndal T, Hansson HA, Anders B. *Goniodygenesis.* Copenhagen: Bogtrykkeriet Forum, 1978.

28. Alward WL. Axenfeld-Rieger syndrome in the age of molecular genetics. *Am J Ophthalmol* 2000;130(1):107–115.

29. Shields MB, Buckley E, Klintworth GK, Thresher R. Axenfeld-Rieger syndrome. A spectrum of developmental disorders. *Surv Ophthalmol* 1985;29(6):387–409.

30. Anderson DR. The development of the trabecular meshwork and its abnormality in primary infantile glaucoma. *Trans Am Ophthalmol Soc* 1981;79:458–485.

31. Cunningham ET Jr, Eliott D, Miller NR, Maumenee IH, Green WR. Familial Axenfeld-Rieger anomaly, atrial septal defect, and sensorineural hearing loss: a possible new genetic syndrome. *Arch Ophthalmol* 1998;116(1):78–82.

32. Tümer Z, Bach-Holm D. Axenfeld-Rieger syndrome and spectrum of PITX2 and FOXC1 mutations. *Eur J Hum Genet* 2009;17:1527e39.

33. Tsai JC, Grajewski AL. Cardiac valvular disease and Axenfeld-Rieger syndrome. *Am J Ophthalmol* 1994;118:255e6.

34. Jena AK, Kharbanda OP. Axenfeld-Rieger syndrome: report on dental and craniofacial findings. *J Clin Pediatr Dent* 2005;30:83e8.

35. Chang TC, Summers CG, Schimmenti LA, Grajewski AL. Axenfeld-Rieger syndrome: new perspectives. *Br J Ophthalmol* 2012;96(3):318–322

36. Henkind P, Friedman AH. Iridogoniodysgenesis. *Am J Ophthalmol* 1971;72:949.

37. Barkan O. Pathogenesis of congenital glaucoma. *Am J Ophthalmol* 1955;40:1.

38. Jacobs HB. Posterior conical cornea. *Br J Ophthalmol* 1957;41:31.

39. Donaldson DD. *Atlas of external diseases of the eye,* 1st Ed., Vol I. Congenital anomalies and systemic diseases. St. Louis, MO: Mosby, 1966.

40. Rejdak R, Nowomiejska K, Haszcz D, Jünemann AG. Bilateral circumscribed posterior keratoconus: visualization by ultrasound biomicroscopy and slit-scanning topography analysis. *J Ophthalmol* 2012; Epub 2012 Feb 13.

41. Krachmer JH, Rodrigues MM. Posterior keratoconus. *Arch Ophthalmol* 1978;96:1867.

42. Al-Hazzaa SAF, Specht CS, McLean IW, et al. Posterior keratoconus: case report with scanning electron microscopy. *Cornea* 1995;14:316.

43. Mannis MJ, Lightman J, Plotnik RD. Corneal topography of posterior keratoconus. *Cornea* 1992;11:351.

44. Townsend WM, Font RL, Zimmerman LE. Congenital corneal leukomas. II. Histopathologic findings in 19 eyes with central defect in Descemet's membrane. *Am J Ophthalmol* 1974;77:192.

45. Waring GO, Parks MM. Successful lens removal in congenital corneolenticular adhesion (Peters' anomaly). *Am J Ophthalmol* 1977;83:526.

46. Hamburg A. Incomplete separation of the lens and related malformations. *Am J Ophthalmol* 1967;64:729.

47. Sawada M, Sato M, Hikoya A, et al. A case of aniridia with unilateral Peters anomaly. *J AAPOS* 2011;15(1):104–106.

48. Bhandari R, Ferri S, Whittaker B, Liu M, Lazzaro DR. Peters anomaly: review of the literature. *Cornea* 2011;30(8):939–944.

49. Frydman M, Weinstock AL, Cohen HA, et al. Autosomal recessive Peters anomaly, typical facial appearance, failure to thrive, hydrocephalus, and other anomalies: further delineation of the Krause-Kivlin syndrome. *Am J Med Genet* 1991;40:34–40.

50. Miller MM, Butrus S, Hidayat A, Wei LL, Pontigo M. Corneoscleral transplantation in congenital corneal staphyloma and Peters' anomaly. *Ophthalmic Genet* 2003;24(1):59–63.

51. Eberwein P, Reinhard T, Agostini H, Poloschek CM, Guthoff R, Auw-Haedrich C [Intensive intracorneal keloid formation in a case of Peters plus syndrome and in Peters anomaly with maximum manifestation]. *Ophthalmologe* 2010;107(2):178–181.

52. Townsend WM, Font RL, Zimmerman LE. Congenital corneal leukomas. I. Central defect in Descemet's membrane. *Am J Ophthalmol* 1974;77:80.

53. Waring GO, Laibson PR. Anterior chamber cleavage syndrome: diagnosis and management. *Contact Intraocul Lens Med J* 1979;5:171.

54. Hershey DW. Ocular injury from amniocentesis. *Ophthalmology* 1993;100(11):1601–1602.

55. Weiner MJ, Albert DM. Congenital corneal keloid. *Acta Ophthalmol (Copenh)* 1989;67:188–196.

56. Murray JC. Scars and keloids. *Dermatol Clin* 1993;11:697–708.

57. Mejía LF, Acosta C, Santamaría JP. Clinical, surgical, and histopathologic characteristics of corneal keloid. *Cornea* 2001;20(4):421–424.

58. Rao SK, Fan DS, Pang CP, et al. Bilateral congenital corneal keloids and anterior segment mesenchymal dysgenesis in a case of Rubinsein-Taybi syndrome. *Cornea* 2002;21:126–130.

59. Fukuda K, Chikama T, Takahashi M, Nishida T. Long-term follow-up after lamellar keratoplasty in a patient with bilateral idiopathic corneal keloid. *Cornea* 2011;30(12): 1491–1494.

60. Lee H, Khan R, O'Keefe M. Aniridia: current pathology and management. *Acta Ophthalmol* 2008;86(7):708–715.

61. Holland EJ, Djalilian AR, Schwartz GS. Management of aniridic keratopathy with keratolimbal allograft: a limbal stem cell transplantation technique. *Ophthalmology* 2003;110(1): 125–130.

62. Akpek EK, Harissi-Dagher M, Petrarca R, et al. Outcomes of Boston keratoprosthesis in aniridia: a retrospective multicenter study. *Am J Ophthalmol* 2007;144:227–231.

63. Waring GO,Rodrigues MM: Congenital and neonatal corneal abnormalities. In: Tasman W, Jaeger EA, eds. *Duane's ophthalmology*, CD-ROM. Philadelphia, PA: Lippincott Williams & Wilkins, 2002.

64. Waring GO, Rodrigues MM. Ultrastructure and successful keratoplasty of sclerocornea in Mietens' syndrome. *Am J Ophthalmol* 1980;90:469.

65. Nischal KK. Congenital corneal opacities—a surgical approach to nomenclature and classification. *Eye (Lond)* 2007;21(10): 1326–1337.

66. Waizenegger UR, Kohnen T, Weidle EG, Schutte E. Congenital familial cornea plana with ptosis, peripheral sclerocornea and conjunctival xerosis. *Klin Monatsbl Augenheilkd* 1995;207(2):111–116.

67. Fukuchi T, Ueda J, Hara H, et al. Glaucoma with microcornea; morphometry and differential diagnosis. *Nippon Ganka Gakkai Zasshi* 1998;102(11):746–751.

68. Kanai A, Wood TC, Polack FM, et al. The fine structure of sclerocornea. *Invest Ophthalmol* 1971;10:687.

69. Kim T, Cohen EJ, Schnall BM, Affel EL, Eagle RC Jr. Ultrasound biomicroscopy and histopathology of sclerocornea. *Cornea* 1998;17(4):443–445.

70. Schanzlin DJ, Goldberg DB, Brown SI. Hallermann-Streiff syndrome associated with sclerocornea, aniridia, and a chromosomal abnormality. *Am J Ophthalmol* 1980;90(3):411–415.

71. Harbin RL, Katz JI, Frias JL, Rabinowicz IM, Kaufman HE. Sclerocornea associated with the Smith-Lemli-Opitz syndrome. *Am J Ophthalmol* 1977;84(1):72–73.

72. Dailey EG, Lubowitz RM. Dermoids of the limbus and cornea. *Am J Ophthalmol* 1962;53:661.

73. Shields JA, Laibson PR, Augsburger JJ, et al. Central corneal dermoid: a clinicopathologic correlation and review of the literature. *Can J Ophthalmol* 1986;21:23.

74. Mann I. *Developmental anomalies of the eye*. London: Cambridge University Press, 1957.

75. Mansour AM, Wang F, Henkind P, et al. Ocular findings in the facioauriculovertebral sequence (Goldenhar-Gorlin syndrome). *Am J Ophthalmol* 1985;100:555.

76. Pirouzian A, Holz H, Merrill K, Sudesh R, Karlen K. Surgical management of pediatric limbal dermoids with sutureless amniotic membrane transplantation and augmentation. *J Pediatr Ophthalmol Strabismus* 2012;49(2):114–119

77. Lazzaro DR, Coe R. Repair of limbal dermoid with excision and placement of a circumlimbal pericardial graft. *Eye Contact Lens* 2010;36(4):228–229.

78. Watts P, Michaeli-Cohen A, Abdolell M, Rootman D. Outcome of lamellar keratoplasty for limbal dermoids in children. *J AAPOS* 2002;6(4):209–215.

79. Hoops JP, Ludwig K, Boergen KP, et al. Preoperative evaluation of limbal dermoids using high-resolution biomicroscopy. *Graefes Arch Clin Exp Ophthalmol* 2001;239:459–461.

80. Lanzl IM, Augsburger JJ, Hertle RW, et al. The role of ultrasound biomicroscopy in surgical planning for limbal dermoids. *Cornea* 1998;17:604–606.

81. Waring GO, Laibson PR. Keratoplasty in infants and children. *Trans Am Acad Ophthalmol Otolaryngol* 1977;83:283.

82. Waring GO, Laibson PR. Keratoplasty in young children. In: Kwitko ML, ed. *Surgery of the infant eye*. New York: Appleton-Century-Crofts, 1979:197–215.

83. Uva MG, Reibaldi M, Longo A, et al. Intraocular pressure and central corneal thickness in premature and full-term newborns. *J AAPOS* 2011;15(4):367–369.

84. Nischal KK, Naor J, Jay V, MacKeen LD, Rootman DS. Clinicopathological correlation of congenital corneal opacification using ultrasound biomicroscopy. *Br J Ophthalmol* 2002;86(1):62–69.

85. Gregory-Evans K, Cheong-Leen R, George SM, et al. Non-invasive anterior segment and posterior segment optical coherence tomography and phenotypic characterization of aniridia. *Can J Ophthalmol* 2011;46(4):337–344.

86. Stulting RD, Sumers KD, Cavanagh HD, et al. Penetrating keratoplasty in children. *Ophthalmology* 1984;91:1222–1230.

87. Cowden JW. Penetrating keratoplasty in infants and children. *Ophthalmology* 1990;97(3):324–328; discussion 328–329.

88. Dana MR, Schaumberg DA, Moyes AL, et al. Outcome of penetrating keratoplasty after ocular trauma in children. *Arch Ophthalmol* 1995;113:1503.

89. Vajpayee RB, Ramu M, Panda A, Sharma N, Tabin GC, Anand JR. Oversized grafts in children. *Ophthalmology* 1999;106(4): 829–832

90. Aasuri MK, Garg P, Gokhale N, et al. Penetrating keratoplasty in children. *Cornea* 2000;19:140–144.

91. Comer RM, Daya SM, O'Keefe M. Penetrating keratoplasty in infants. *J AAPOS* 2001;5:285–290.

92. McClellan K, Lai T, Grigg J, et al. Penetrating keratoplasty in children. *Br J Ophthalmol* 2003;87:1212–1214.

93. Patel HY, Ormonde S, Brookes NH, et al. The indications and outcome of pediatric corneal transplantation in New Zealand: 1991–2003. *Br J Ophthalmol* 2005;89:404–408.

94. Sharma N, Prakash G, Titiyal JS, et al: Pediatric keratoplasty in India: indications and outcomes. *Cornea* 2007;26:810.

95. Al-Ghamdi A, Al-Rajhi A, Wagoner MD. Primary pediatric keratoplasty: indications, graft survival, and visual outcome. *J AAPOS* 2007;11(1):41–47.

96. Huang C, O'Hara M, Mannis MJ. Primary pediatric keratoplasty: indications and outcomes. *Cornea* 2009;28(9): 1003–1008.

97. Gloor P, Keech RV, Krachmer JH. Factors associated with high postoperative myopia after penetrating keratoplasties in infants. *Ophthalmology* 1992;99:775.

98. Enoch JM. Fitting parameters which need to be considered when designing soft contact lenses for the neonate. *Contact Intraocul Lens Med J* 1979;5:31.

99. Shi W, Jin H, Li S, Liu M, Xie L. Indications of paediatric keratoplasty in north China. *Clin Experiment Ophthalmol* 2007;35(8):724–727.

100. Rao KV, Fernandes M, Gangopadhyay N, Vemuganti GK, Krishnaiah S, Sangwan VS. Outcome of penetrating keratoplasty for Peters anomaly. *Cornea* 2008;27(7):749–753.

101. Zaidman GW, Flanagan JK, Furey CC. Long-term visual prognosis in children after corneal transplant surgery for Peters anomaly type I. *Am J Ophthalmol* 2007;144(1):104–108.

102. Yang LL, Lambert SR, Lynn MJ, Stulting RD. Long-term results of corneal graft survival in infants and children with Peters anomaly. *Ophthalmology* 1999;106(4):833–848.

103. Dana MR, Schaumberg DA, Moyes AL, Gomes JA. Corneal transplantation in children with Peters anomaly and mesenchymal dysgenesis. Multicenter Pediatric Keratoplasty Study. *Ophthalmology* 1997;104(10):1580–1586.

104. Al-Rajhi AA, Wagoner MD. Penetrating keratoplasty in congenital hereditary endothelial dystrophy. *Ophthalmology* 1997;104(6):956–961.

105. Kirkness CM, McCartney A, Rice NSC, Garner A, Steele AD. Congenital hereditary corneal oedema of Maumenee: its clinical features, management, and pathology. *Br J Ophthalmol* 1987;71(2):130–144.

106. Busin M, Beltz J, Scorcia V. Descemet-stripping automated endothelial keratoplasty for congenital hereditary endothelial dystrophy. *Arch Ophthalmol* 2011;129(9):1140–1146.

107. Harding SA, Nischal KK, Upponi-Patil A, Fowler DJ. Indications and outcomes of deep anterior lamellar keratoplasty in children. *Ophthalmology* 2010;117(11):2191–2195.

108. Buzzonetti L, Petrocelli G, Valente P. Big-bubble deep anterior lamellar keratoplasty assisted by femtosecond laser in children. *Cornea* 2012;31(9):1083–1086.

109. Aquavella JV, Gearinger MD, Akpek EK, McCormick GJ. Pediatric keratoprosthesis. *Ophthalmology* 2007;114(5):989–994.

110. Basu S, Taneja M, Sangwan VS. Boston type 1 keratoprosthesis for severe blinding vernal keratoconjunctivitis and Mooren's ulcer. *Int Ophthalmol* 2011;31(3):219–222.

111. Srinivasan B, Choudhari NS, Neog A, Latka S, Iyer GK. Boston keratoprosthesis and Ahmed glaucoma valve for visual rehabilitation in congenital anterior staphyloma. *Indian J Ophthalmol* 2012;60(3):232–233.

112. Song X, Xu L, Sun S, Zhao J, Xie L. Pediatric microbial keratitis: a tertiary hospital study. *Eur J Ophthalmol* 2011;22(2):136–141.

113. Panda A, Sharma N, Das G, et al. Mycotic keratitis in children: epidemiologic and microbiologic evaluation. *Cornea* 1997;16:295–299.

114. Singh G, Palanisamy M, Madhavan B, et al. Multivariate analysis of childhood microbial keratitis in South India. *Ann Acad Med Singapore* 2006;35(3):185–189.

115. Clinch TE, Palmon FE, Robinson MJ, et al. Microbial keratitis in children. *Am J Ophthalmol* 1994;117:65.

116. Wong VW, Lai TY, Chi SC, Lam DS. Pediatric ocular surface infections: a 5-year review of demographics, clinical features, risk factors, microbiological results, and treatment. *Cornea* 2011;30(9):995–1002.

117. Jhanji V, Naithani P, Lamoureux E, Agarwal T, Sharma N, Vajpayee RB. Immunization and nutritional profile of cases with atraumatic microbial keratitis in preschool age group. *Am J Ophthalmol* 2011;151(6):1035–1040.

118. Kunimoto DY, Sharma S, Reddy MK, et al. Microbial keratitis in children. *Ophthalmology* 1998;105:252–257.

119. Stretton S, Gopinathan U, Willcox MD. Corneal ulceration in pediatric patients: a brief overview of progress in topical treatment. *Paediatr Drugs* 2002;4:95–110.

120. Cruz OA, Sabir SM, Capo H, Alfonso EC. Microbial keratitis in childhood. *Ophthalmology* 1993;100(2):192–196.

121. Ormerod LD, Murphree AL, Gomez DS, Schanzlin DJ, Smith RE. Microbial keratitis in children. *Ophthalmology* 1986;93(4):449–455.

122. Hsiao CH, Yeung L, Ma DH, et al. Pediatric microbial keratitis in Taiwanese children: a review of hospital cases. *Arch Ophthalmol* 2007;125(5):603–609.

123. Hammersmith KM, Cohen EJ, Blake TD, Laibson PR, Rapuano CJ. Blepharokeratoconjunctivitis in children. *Arch Ophthalmol* 2005;123(12):1667–1670.

124. Zaidman GW. The pediatric corneal infiltrate. *Curr Opin Ophthalmol* 2011;22(4):261–266.

125. Meisler DM, Raizman MB, Traboulsi EI. Oral erythromycin treatment for childhood blepharokeratitis. *J AAPOS* 2000;4:379–380.

126. Cavuoto K, Zutshi D, Karp CL, Miller D, Feuer W. Update on bacterial conjunctivitis in South Florida. *Ophthalmology* 2008;115(1):51–56.

127. Young AL, Leung AT, Cheng LL, et al. Orthokeratology lens-related corneal ulcers in children: a case series. *Ophthalmology* 2004;111:590–595.

128. Bunya VY, Hammersmith KM, Rapuano CJ, Ayres BD, Cohen EJ. Topical and oral voriconazole in the treatment of fungal keratitis. *Am J Ophthalmol* 2007;143(1):151–153.

129. Chong EM, Wilhelmus KR, Matoba AY, Jones DB, Coats DK, Paysse EA. Herpes simplex virus keratitis in children. *Am J Ophthalmol* 2004;138(3):474–475.

130. Hsiao CH, Yeung L, Yeh LK, et al. Pediatric herpes simplex virus keratitis. *Cornea* 2009;28(3):249–253.

131. Croxtall JD. Ganciclovir ophthalmic gel 0.15%: in acute herpetic keratitis (dendritic ulcers). *Drugs* 2011;71(5):603–610.

132. Schwartz GS, Holland EJ. Oral acyclovir for the management of herpes simplex virus keratitis in children. *Ophthalmology* 2000;107:278–282.

133. Chiba S, Umetsu M, Yamanaka T, Hori S, Nakao T. An outbreak of epidemic keratoconjunctivitis due to adenovirus type 8 in a babies home. *Tohoku J Exp Med* 1976;119(2):159–163.

134. Gu B, Son J, Kim M. Amblyopia and strabismus by monocular corneal opacity following suspected epidemic keratoconjunctivitis in infancy. *Korean J Ophthalmol* 2011;25(4):257–261.

135. Kim JH, Kim MK, Oh JY, Jang KC, Wee WR, Lee JH. Outbreak of gram-positive bacterial keratitis associated with epidemic keratoconjunctivitis in neonates and infants. *Eye (Lond)* 2009;23(5):1059–1065.

136. Walton RC, Reed KL. Herpes zoster ophthalmicus following bone marrow transplantation in children. *Bone Marrow Transplant* 1999;23(12):1317–1320.

137. Naseri A, Good WV, Cunningham ET Jr. Herpes zoster virus sclerokeratitis and anterior uveitis in a child following varicella vaccination. *Am J Ophthalmol* 2003;135:415–417.

138. West SK, Munoz B, Lynch M, et al. Risk factors for constant, severe trachoma among preschool children in Kongwa, Tanzania. *Am J Epidemiol* 1996;143:73.

139. Bonini S. Coassin M, Aronni S, Lambiase A. Vernal keratoconjunctivitis. *Eye* 2004;18:345–351.

140. Cameron JA. Shield ulcers and plaques of the cornea in vernal keratoconjunctivitis. *Ophthalmology* 1995;102:985–93.

141. Ozbek Z, Burakgazi AZ, Rapuano CJ. Rapid healing of vernal shield ulcer after surgical debridement: A case report. *Cornea* 2006;25(4):472–473.

142. Ostler HB. Corneal perforation in nontuberculous (staphylococcal) phlyctenular keratoconjunctivitis. *Am J Ophthalmol* 1975;79:446–448.

143. Abu el Asrar AM, Geboes K, Maudgal PC, et al. Immunocytological study of phlyctenular eye disease. *Int Ophthalmol* 1987;10:33–39.

144. Rohatgi J, Dhaliwal U. Phlyctenular eye disease: a reappraisal. *Jpn J Ophthalmol* 2000;44:146–150.

145. Mondino BJ, Kowalski RP. Phlyctenulae and catarrhal infiltrates. *Arch Ophthalmol* 1982;100:1968.

146. Doan S, Gabison E, Gatinel D, Duong MH, Abitbol O, Hoang-Xuan T. Topical cyclosporine A in severe steroid-dependent childhood phlyctenular keratoconjunctivitis. *Am J Ophthalmol* 2006;141(1):62–66.

147. Farthing P, Bagan JV, Scully C. Mucosal disease series. Number IV. Erythema multiforme. *Oral Dis* 2005;11:261–267.

148. Auquier-Dunant A, MockenhauptM, Naldi L, Correia O, SchroderW, Roujeau JC. Correlations between clinical patterns and causes of erythema multiforme majus, Stevens-Johnson syndrome, and toxic epidermal necrolysis: results of an international prospective study. *Arch Dermatol* 2002;138:1019–1024.

149. Forman R, Koren G, Shear NH. Erythema multiforme, Stevens-Johnson syndrome and toxic epidermal necrolysis in children: a review of 10 years' experience. *Drug Saf* 2002;25:965–972.

150. Schopf E, Stuhmer A, Rzany B, et al. Toxic epidermal necrolysis and Stevens-Johnson syndrome: an epidemiologic study from West Germany. *Arch Dermatol* 1991;127:839–842.

151. Christou EM, Wargon O. Stevens-Johnson syndrome after varicella vaccination. *Med J Aust* 2012;196(4):240–241.

152. Mondino BJ, Brown SI, Biglan AW, et al. HLA antigens in Stevens-Johnson syndrome with ocular involvement. *ArchOphthalmol* 1982;100:1453–1454.

153. Teo L, Tay YK, Liu TT, Kwok C. Stevens-Johnson syndrome and toxic epidermal necrolysis: efficacy of intravenous immunoglobulin and a review of treatment options. *Singapore Med J* 2009;50(1):29–33.

154. Kobayashi A, Yoshita T, Sugiyama K, et al. Amniotic membrane transplantation in acute phase of toxic epidermal necrolysis with severe corneal involvement. *Ophthalmology* 2006;113(1):126–132.

155. Iyer G, Pillai VS, Srinivasan B, Guruswami S, Padmanabhan P. Mucous membrane grafting for lid margin keratinization in Stevens Johnson Syndrome (SJS): results. *Cornea* 2009;29(2):146–151.

156. Genvert GI, Cohen EJ, Donnenfeld ED, et al. Erythema multiforme following use of topical sulfacetamide. *Am J Ophthalmol* 1985;99:456.

157. Gomes JA, Santos MS, Ventura AS, Donato WB, Cunha MC, Höfling-Lima AL. Amniotic membrane with living related corneal limbal/conjunctival allograft for ocular surface reconstruction in Stevens-Johnson syndrome. *Arch Ophthalmol* 2003;121(10):1369–1374.

158. Satake Y, Higa K, Tsubota K, Shimazaki J. Long-term outcome of cultivated oral mucosal epithelial sheet transplantation in treatment of total limbal stem cell deficiency. *Ophthalmology* 2011;118(8):1524–1530.

159. Sayegh RR, Ang LP, Foster CS, Dohlman CH. The Boston keratoprosthesis in Stevens-Johnson syndrome. *Am J Ophthalmol* 2008;145(3):438–444.

160. Kang JJ, de la Cruz J, Cortina MS. Visual outcomes of Boston Keratoprosthesis implantation as the primary penetrating corneal procedure. *Cornea*; Epub2012 Feb 23.

161. Zecca M, Prete A, Rondelli R, et al. AIEOP-BMT Group. Italian Associationfor Pediatric Hematology and Oncology-Bone Marrow Transplant. Chronic graft-versus-host disease in children: incidence, risk factors, and impact on outcome. *Blood* 2002;100(4):1192–1200.

162. Kim SK. Update on ocular graft versus host disease. *Curr Opin Ophthalmol* 2006;17(4):344–348.

163. Weiss JS, Møller HU, Lisch W, et al. The IC3D classification of the corneal dystrophies. *Cornea* 2008;27(Suppl 2): S1–S83.

164. Fine BS, Yanoff M, Pitts E, et al. Meesmann's epithelial dystrophy of the cornea. *Am J Ophthalmol* 1977;83:633–642.

165. Stocker FW, Holt LB. A rare form of hereditary epithelial dystrophy of the cornea: a genetic, clinical and pathologic study. *Trans Am Ophthalmol Soc* 1954;52:133–144.

166. Kuchle M, Green WR, Volcker HE, et al. Reevaluation of corneal dystrophies of Bowman's layer and the anterior stroma (Reis-Bucklers' and Thiel-Behnke types): a light and electron microscope study of eight corneas and a review of the literature. *Cornea* 1995;14:333–354.

167. Dinh R, Rapuano CJ, Cohen EJ, et al. Recurrence of corneal dystrophy after excimer laser phototherapeutic keratectomy. *Ophthalmology* 1999;106:1490–1497.

168. Rathi VM, Vyas SP, Vaddavalli PK, Sangwan VS, Murthy SI. Phototherapeutic keratectomy in pediatric patients in India. *Cornea* 2010;29(10):1109–1112.

169. Roh MI, Grossniklaus HE, Chung SH, et al. Avellino corneal dystrophy exacerbated after LASIK: scanning electron microscopic findings. *Cornea* 2006;25:306–311.

170. Marcon A, Cohen EJ, Rapuano CJ, et al. Recurrence of corneal stromal dystrophies after penetrating keratoplasty. *Cornea* 2003;22:19–21.

171. Weiss JS. Schnyder corneal dystrophy. *Curr Opin Ophthalmol* 2009;20(4):292–298.

172. Bredrup C, Knappskog PM, Majewski J, et al. Congenital stromal dystrophy of the cornea caused by a mutation in the decorin gene. *Invest Ophthalmol Vis Sci* 2005;46:420–426.

173. Schaumberg DA, Moyes AL, Gomes JA, et al. Corneal transplantation in young children with congenital hereditary endothelial dystrophy. Multicenter Pediatric Keratoplasty Study. *Am J Ophthalmol* 1999;127:373–378.

174. Bromley JG, Randleman JB, Stone D, Stulting RD, Grossniklaus HE. Clinicopathologic findings in iridocorneal endothelial syndrome and posterior polymorphous membranous dystrophy after descemet stripping automated endothelial keratoplasty. *Cornea* 2012; Epub 2012 Feb 13.

175. Studeny P, Jirsova K, Kuchynka P, Liskova P. Descemet membrane endothelial keratoplasty with a stromal rim in the treatment of posterior polymorphous corneal dystrophy. *Indian J Ophthalmol* 2012;60(1):59–60.

176. Wollensak G. Crosslinking treatment of progressive keratoconus: new hope. *Curr Opin Ophthalmol* 2006;17(4):356–360.

177. Khan MI, Muhtaseb M. Intrastromal corneal ring segments for bilateralvkeratoconus in an 11-year-old boy. *J Cataract Refract Surg* 2011;37(1):201–205.

178. Tsilou ET, Rubin BI, Reed GF, et al. Age-related prevalence of anterior segment complications in patients with infantile nephropathic cystinosis. *Cornea* 2002;21:173–176.

179. Reed JW, Cashwell LF, Klintworth GK. Corneal manifestations of hereditary benign intraepithelial dyskeratosis. *Arch Ophthalmol* 1979;97:297.

180. Huppertz HI, Munchmeier D, Lieb W. Ocular manifestations in children and adolescents with Lyme arthritis. *Br J Ophthalmol* 1999;83:1149–1152.

181. Winward KE, Lawton-Smith J, Culbertson WW, et al. Ocular Lyme borreliosis. *Am J Ophthalmol* 1989;108:651.

182. Akinci A, Cakar N, Uncu N, Kara N, Acaroglu G. Keratoconjunctivitis sicca in juvenile rheumatoid arthritis. *Cornea.* 2007;26(8):941–944.

183. Mataftsi A, Subbu RG, Jones S, Nischal KK. The use of punctal plugs in children. *Br J Ophthalmol* 2012;96(1):90–92.

184. Ramaesh K, Stokes J, Henry E, Dutton GN, Dhillon B. Congenital corneal anesthesia. *Surv Ophthalmol* 2007;52(1):50–60.

185. Gungor I, Schor K, Rosenthal P, Jacobs DS. The Boston Scleral Lens in the treatment of pediatric patients. *J AAPOS* 2008;12(3):263–267.

186. Serrano JC, Chalela P, Arias JD. Epidemiology of childhood ocular trauma in a northeastern Colombian region. *Arch Ophthalmol* 2003;121:1439–1445.

187. Morgan KS, McDonald B, Hiles DA, et al. The nationwide study of epikeratophakia for aphakia in children. *Am J Ophthalmol* 1987;103:366.

188. Gupta A, Rahman I, Leatherbarrow B. Open globe injuries in children: factors predictive of a poor final visual acuity. *Eye (Lond)* 2009;23(3):621–625.

189. Ratnapalan S, Das L. Causes of eye burns in children. *Pediatr Emerg Care* 2011;27(2):151–156.

190. Motley WW III, Kaufman AH, West CE. Pediatric airbag-associated ocular trauma and endothelial cell loss. *J AAPOS* 2003;7:380–383.

191. Listman DA. Paintball injuries in children: more than meets the eye. *Pediatrics* 2004;113:e15–e18.

192. Ponchel C, Malecaze F, Arné JL, Fournié P. Descemet stripping automated endothelial keratoplasty in a child with descemet membrane breaks after forceps delivery. *Cornea* 2009;28(3):338–341.

11

Pediatric Cataracts and Lens Anomalies

Denise Hug

ABNORMALITIES OF THE crystalline lens include those that involve opacification, size, shape, location, and development. Cataract (opacification of lens) is a significant cause of preventable visual impairment and blindness in children worldwide. The prevalence of childhood cataracts has been reported between 1.2 and 11 per 10,000 children (1–3). The difference in prevalence can be attributed to the method of data collection and the country in which data are collected. Industrialized nations have a lower prevalence than developing countries. Early detection and prompt treatment remain necessary to avoid permanent vision loss.

ANATOMY AND EMBRYOLOGY

The crystalline lens is a clear, avascular structure suspended behind the iris by the zonules of Zinn. The purpose of the lens is to refract light, accommodate and maintain its own clarity. The lens is comprised of the lens capsule, lens epithelium, cortex, and nucleus.

The lens is derived from surface ectoderm after interacting with the neuroectoderm of the optic vesicle, which occurs at approximately 25 days of gestation. At approximately 27 days of gestation, the surface ectoderm overlying the optic vesicle becomes elongated (columnar) to form the lens plate (also known as the lens placode). By 29 days, the lens pit is formed by indentation of the lens plate. The lens pit continues to invaginate, the stalk of cells connecting the new lens to the surface ectoderm undergoes apoptosis. The resultant structure is a single layer of cuboidal cells encased by a basement membrane, which is referred to as the lens vesicle. This basement membrane is the future lens capsule. The cells in the posterior cellular layer stop dividing, elongate, and lose their organelles. At approximately 40 days, the lumen of the lens vesicle is filled with these primary lens fibers. This structure is now the optically clear embryonic nucleus. The anterior layer of cells remains a monolayer of cuboidal cells referred to as the lens epithelium. The secondary lens fibers originate from the anterior epithelium in the equatorial region. These cells migrate anteriorly and posteriorly beneath the capsule. The fibers meet and interdigitate to form the Y sutures. The anterior suture has the appearance of an upright Y, while the posterior suture

has the appearance of an inverted Y. The secondary lens fibers are formed between 2 and 8 months of gestation and form the fetal nucleus. The adult nucleus and cortex are formed by the continued proliferation of the equatorial lens epithelium.

The lens fibers continue to be added throughout life. At birth, the lens weighs approximately 90 mg and its mass increases by approximately 2 mg per year as new fibers are formed. The average diameter of the lens at birth is 7.0 mm. The most rapid increase in the size of the lens occurs during the first 2 years of life. The average diameter of the lens at age 2 is approximately 9.5 mm (4). Because the diameter of the lens is similar to the adult size early in life and the fact that lens fibers continue to be added throughout life, the density of the lens increases with age. It should also be noted that the lens capsule continues to thicken throughout life.

LENS OPACITIES

The most common lens abnormality in children is opacity (cataract). The visual significance of the cataract depends on several factors including age of onset, location, etiology, and morphology.

Etiology of Childhood Cataracts

The etiology of childhood cataracts is vast (Table 11.1). The historical teaching is that approximately one-third of childhood cataracts are inherited, one-third are associated with other diseases or syndromes, and one-third are idiopathic.

Hereditary Cataract

Hereditary cataracts account for a significant proportion of childhood cataracts. Inheritance patterns that have been reported include autosomal dominant, autosomal recessive, and X-linked recessive. The most common form of inheritance is autosomal dominant. There is often high penetrance with phenotypic variability. These children are usually otherwise normal. Less commonly, autosomal recessive cataracts occur. They are usually bilateral but can also show variability between affected family members.

Table 11.1

POSSIBLE ETIOLOGIES OF CATARACTS IN INFANCY AND CHILDHOOD

I. Intrauterine infection

  A. Viruses

    1. Rubella (61)

    2. Rubeola

    3. Chicken pox/herpes zoster (62)

    4. Poliomyelitis

    5. Herpes simplex (63)

    6. Cytomegalovirus (64)

  B. Protozoa

    1. Toxoplasmosis (64)

II. Prematurity (65)

III. Metabolic disorders

  A. Galactosemia

    1. Galactose-1-phosphate uridyltransferase deficiency (66)

    2. Galactokinase deficiency (67)

  B. Hypoparathyroidism (68)

  C. Pseudohypoparathyroidism

  D. Diabetes mellitus

  E. Refsum's syndrome (69)

  F. Oculocerebrorenal (Lowe's) syndrome (70)

  G. Hypoglycemia (71)

  H. Mannosidosis (72)

  I. Hereditary familial congenital hemorrhagic nephritis (Alport's syndrome) (73)

  J. Wilson's disease

  K. Multiple sulfatase deficiency

  L. Fabry's syndrome

  M. Glucose-6-phosphatase deficiency

IV. Musculoskeletal

  A. Chondrodysplasia punctate (74)

  E. Cerebral giantism (Sotos syndrome) (83)

  F. Batten disease (ceroid lipofuscinosis)

VII. Dermatologic

  A. Cockayne's syndrome (84)

  B. Poikiloderma Atrophicans (Rothmund-Thomson syndrome) (85)

  C. Incontinentia pigmenti (86)

  D. Congenital ichthyosis (87)

  E. Atopic dermatitis (88)

  F. Ectodermal dysplasia (89)

  G. Progeria (90)

VIII. Craniofacial

  A. Hallermann-Streiff syndrome

  B. Rubinstein-Taybi syndrome (91)

  C. Smith-Lemli-Opitz syndrome

  D. Cerebro-oculo-facial-skeletal syndrome (92)

  E. Pierre Robin syndrome

  F. Oxycephaly

  G. Crouzon's syndrome

  H. Apert's syndrome

  I. Congenital cataracts facial dysmorphism neuropathy (93)

  J. Chromosomal disorders

  Trisomy

  21 (Down's syndrome)

  13–15

  18 (Edward's syndrome)

  10q

  20p

  Turner's syndrome

(continued)

Table 11.1

(*contintued*)

B. Myotonic dystrophy (75)	Translocation
C. Albright osteodystrophy	3: 4
	2: 14
D. Potter's syndrome (76)	2 : 16 (94)
	Deletion
	Cri-du-chat syndrome (5p-)
E. Chondrodystrophic myotonia (77)	X. Autoimmune/Inflammatory
F. Smith-Lemli-Opitz syndrome (78)	A. Uveitis
G. Rhizomelic chondrodysplasia punctata	B. Behcet's disease (95)
H. Spondylo-ocular syndrome (79)	XI. Ocular anomalies
	A. Microphthalmia (96)
V. Renal disease	B. Anterior segment dysgenesis
A. Lowe's syndrome	C. Coloboma
B. Alport's syndrome	D. Aniridia
C. Hallermann-Streiff-Francois syndrome (80)	E. Persistent pupillary membrane
	F. Persistent fetal vasculature (97)
VI. Central nervous system	G. Retinitis pigmentosa
A. Marinesco-Sjogren syndrome	XII. Trauma
B. Laurence-Moon-Bardet-Biedl syndrome (81)	A. Laser (98)
C. Sjogren-Larsson syndrome	B. Radiation
D. Peroxisomal disorders	C. Accidental
1. Zellweger's (cerebrohepatorenal) syndrome (82)	D. Lightning (99)

Metabolic Cataract

Errors in metabolism may cause cataracts in neonates, infants and juveniles. Although lens opacities may be permanent, occasionally the early recognition and treatment of underlying disease may reverse the lens damage. It is also critical to recognize and treat the underlying metabolic etiology early for the child's overall health and well-being.

Galactosemia

Galactosemia is an autosomal recessive inherited condition where the child cannot metabolize galactose, a major component of milk. There is a defect in galactokinase, uridine diphosphate galactose-epimerase, or galactose 1-phosphate

uridyltransferase. Because of this defect, galactose is converted to galactitol in the crystalline lens, which makes the lens hyperosmolar, resulting in an influx of water into the lens. The hydration of the lens disrupts the normal packing of the lens fibers, and transparency is lost. The typical lens change described in galactosemia is the "oil droplet," which is not a true cataract but represents refractive change within the lens. The appearance is that of a drop of oil floating in water. If the baby remains untreated, a diffuse white lens will develop. If the baby is diagnosed early, within the first weeks of life, the lens changes are reversible. Unfortunately, this is not always the case, and surgery may be required to treat the cataracts. It is important to note whether the baby has other systemic issues including: vomiting, diarrhea, failure to thrive, and hepatomegaly. If the baby remains untreated, mental retardation and death may occur. Screening for galactosemia is now included in the newborn screening mandatory in many states. Finally, galactosemia is a life long condition, so these children must be followed throughout life for development of cataracts even though they are following dietary restrictions.

Fabry's Disease

Fabry's disease is an uncommon, X-linked recessive metabolic disorder caused by a deficiency of the lysosomal enzyme α-galactosidase A. Abnormal storage of glycosphingolipids causes a chronic progressive painful small-fiber neuropathy, renal dysfunction, heart disease, and stroke. In males, symptoms often start in adolescence with pain in the extremities provoked by exertion or temperature changes. The main life-limiting complications are renal disease and heart disease. Ocular involvement includes the conjunctiva, cornea, lens, and retina. There are two types of lens opacities associated with Fabry's disease. The first is a spoke-like posterior line of spots that radiate and are best seen in retroillumination. The second is an anterior subcapsular, wedge-shaped opacity usually in the inferior lens (5).

Mannosidosis

Mannosidosis is an autosomal recessive disorder resulting from a deficiency in α-mannosidase, which causes defective degradation of lipoproteins. Patients have coarse facies, skeletal abnormalities, deafness, and learning difficulties. Cataracts are common and present early in life. They appear as posterior cortical spokes composed of discrete clear vacuoles (6).

Wilson's Disease

Wilson's disease is an autosomal recessive disorder caused by a deficiency of an ATPase that transports copper into the Golgi apparatus of the hepatocytes. This leads to the toxic accumulation of copper in the hepatocytes and elsewhere. The plasma concentration of non-ceruloplasmin-bound copper is elevated, and copper deposits occur in the liver, brain, and eye. As the lens accumulates copper, a unique sunflower cataract forms, which is a yellowish star like anterior subcapsular discoloration.

Hyperglycemia and Hypoglycemia

Hyperglycemia and hypoglycemia are infrequent causes of cataracts in children. Hypoglycemia in the perinatal period is common in low-birth-weight infants. Lens opacities may result and are often bilateral and lamellar in type. These opacities are often reversible but may progress into total cataracts. Cataracts in diabetic children do occur but often not until the teenage years. They are often diffuse, cortical, or subcapsular in morphology.

Disorders of Cholesterol Synthesis

Because the lens membrane contains the highest cholesterol content of any known membrane, inherited defects in enzymes of cholesterol metabolism are associated with cataracts. Smith-Lemli-Opitz syndrome, mevalonic aciduria, Conradi-Hünermann syndrome, and cerebrotendinous xanthomatosis all have mutations in enzymes of cholesterol metabolism, and cataracts have been reported in all of them. The pathogenesis of the cataracts in this group of disorders remains unknown (7).

Hypocalcemia

Children with hypocalcemia may present with irritability, failure to thrive, and seizures. Cataracts have been reported in children with hypocalcemia and are thought to occur because of altered permeability of the lens capsule. They start as fine white punctuate opacities scattered throughout the lens cortex, which are not visually significant but progression may occur to form lamellar cataracts that become visually significant.

Cataract Associated with Systemic Syndromes

There are many multisystem disorders that have cataracts as part of the syndrome. The incidence of cataracts in this group varies widely. The following text outlines a subset of entities in which cataracts are found in a high percentage of involved patients.

Lowe's Syndrome

Lowe's Syndrome (oculocerebrorenal) is an X-linked recessive condition in which almost 100% of patients have cataracts. Children with Lowe's syndrome have mental retardation, hypotonia, renal aminoaciduria, and typical facies. The lens in Lowe's syndrome is usually a small, flat, disk-like opacified lens. Glaucoma and corneal opacities are common. Of interest, female carriers often have lens opacities that are diffuse punctate opacities or spoke-like opacities in the posterior cortex.

Alport's Syndrome

Alport's syndrome is an X-linked or autosomal recessive disorder consisting of interstitial nephritis, hearing defects, and ocular abnormalities. The lens abnormality is that of anterior lenticonus, which is secondary to an abnormally thin central anterior capsule. Cataract is usually a late finding in anterior lenticonus, but surgery may be required earlier because the thinning of the capsule causes significant aberration of the optics of the natural lens. Rarely, a total cataract may occur if there is spontaneous rupture of the anterior lens capsule.

Chondrodysplasia Punctata

This is a group of disorders, which is broken down into chondrodysplasia punctata and rhizomelic chondrodysplasia punctata. Each of these is then broken down into type one and type two. Chondrodysplasia punctata 1 is X-linked recessive affecting chromosome Xp22.33 and is caused by mutation in the arylsulfatase E gene. These children have short stature, hearing loss, skeletal abnormalities, ichthyosis, and developmental delays. Chondrodysplasia punctata 2 (Conradi's syndrome) is X-linked dominant affecting chromosome Xp11.23 and is caused by defect in cholesterol synthesis. These children have failure to thrive, hearing loss, tracheal stenosis, many skeletal abnormalities, ichthyosis, and mental retardation. The rhizomelic forms are autosomal recessive with defects in the peroxisomal biogenesis pathway. Cataracts are reported in up to 75% of the rhizomelic chondrodysplasia infants, and early death is expected. All of the forms of chondrodysplasia punctata have related cataracts (8).

Myotonic Dystrophy

Myotonic dystrophy is an autosomal dominant muscular dystrophy, which presents with progressive muscle weakness and muscle wasting. Other systemic features include gonadal atrophy, frontal balding, mental deterioration, and cardiac abnormalities. Ocular features include ptosis, progressive external ophthalmoplegia, retinal pigmentary changes, and cataracts. Typical lens changes occur in almost all patients and present as multicolored crystalline iridescent flecks in the cortex and are often referred to as a "Christmas tree" cataract. The lens opacities may also present as small white spherical opacities in the cortex.

Neurofibromatosis Type 2

Neurofibromatosis type 2 is an autosomal dominant trait with high penetrance, which is characterized by vestibular schwannomas and other central nervous system tumors. Cataracts are often present with the most common type being the posterior subcapsular and cortical cataract.

Zellweger Syndrome

Zellweger syndrome is an autosomal recessive disease which consists of abnormal development of the head, face, ears, and feet. These patients also have mental retardation, hypotonia, seizures, and early death. Lamellar cataracts are present in most cases. Other ocular findings include corneal clouding, pigmentary retinopathy, optic atrophy, and glaucoma. Asymptomatic carriers have been found to have curvilinear opacities. This disorder is caused by an error in peroxisome biogenesis involving a defect in the PEX group of genes (9).

Cockayne Syndrome

Cockayne syndrome is an autosomal recessive disorder with a defect of transcription-coupled DNA repair of active genes. The most striking feature of this disorder is premature aging and cachectic dwarfism. Almost all organ systems are affected. There is progressive neurologic deterioration, mental retardation, skeletal abnormalities, skin photosensitivity, and sensorineural hearing loss. Ocular anomalies include cataracts, retinal dystrophy, corneal opacity, decreased lacrimation, optic atrophy (10).

Bloch-Sulzberger Syndrome

Bloch-Sulzberger syndrome (incontinentia pigmenti) is an X-linked dominant disease affecting the skin, bones, teeth, central nervous system, and eyes. The disorder is usually lethal in males. The skin changes go through 4 distinct stages starting with linear bullae and ending in atrophy and scarring. Ocular anomalies are numerous and include cataract, optic atrophy, microphthalmos, retinal changes leading to retinal detachment, and epithelial keratitis. The lens abnormality is reminiscent of that seen with persistent fetal vasculature.

Rothmund-Thomson Syndrome

Rothmund-Thomson syndrome is an autosomal recessive condition consisting of atrophic skin with patches of depigmentation and hyperpigmentation. Patients have telangiectasias, sparse hair, short stature, defective dentition, and hypogonadism. Lamellar cataracts occur in the majority of patients and often have an onset between 3 and 6 years of age.

Hallermann-Streiff Syndrome

Hallermann-Streiff syndrome is an isolated disease, which involves dyscephaly with a beak-shaped nose and micrognathia, short stature, dental abnormalities, respiratory issues, multiple skeletal anomalies, and congenital cataracts. The eyes in Hallermann-Streiff are usually microphthalmic. The lens in Hallermann-Streiff syndrome may be small and has been reported to spontaneously resorb to form a disk-like or membranous type cataract.

Cataract Associated with Chromosomal Anomaly

Cataracts are present in a large number of chromosomal syndromes with the most common being trisomy 21. Cataracts in Down syndrome usually develop later in childhood but they may be present during infancy. Cataracts are also part of the clinical presentation in trisomy 13, trisomy 15, and trisomy 18. Cataracts have also been reported in chromosome deletions with the most common being Turner syndrome (XO) and Cri-du-chat (5p-). Finally, cataracts are part of several translocation defects such as 3:4 translocation, 2:14 translocation, and 2:16 translocation. As genetic mapping continues, the number of known chromosome anomalies associated with cataracts will increase.

Secondary Cataracts

Secondary cataracts can be thought of as lens opacities caused by external forces or secondary to other ocular process.

Maternal Infection

Many intrauterine infections can cause cataracts. The cataracts are usually central and can be bilateral or unilateral. The most common cause of cataract from maternal infection is rubella. Systemic manifestations of congenital rubella infection include cardiac defects, mental retardation, and deafness. The cataract is usually a pearly white nuclear opacity. Sometimes the entire lens is involved and becomes white, the cortex may even liquefy. The lens does contain live virus, and removal is often associated with difficult-to-control postoperative inflammation. Rubella cataracts are still an important cause of cataracts worldwide but are rare in the United States. Cataracts can also occur in toxoplasmosis, varicella, cytomegalovirus, and toxocariasis intrauterine infection.

Drug Toxicity

The lens can be sensitive to both topical and systemic medications. The most common drugs known to cause cataract formation are the corticosteroids. This effect appears to be dose and duration related. The type of cataract is usually posterior subcapsular, but can progress to involve the entire lens.

Iatrogenic Cataracts

Development of cataract related to radiation is seen in children who have had total body radiation in preparation for bone marrow transplant. These cataracts are usually posterior subcapsular and are dose and duration dependent. The incidence of cataract increases with increasing dose of radiation. Cataracts have been reported after laser treatment for threshold of retinopathy of prematurity. Finally, any intraocular surgery increases the risk of cataract formation in children.

Cataract Secondary to Ocular Process

The most common type of secondary cataract related to an intraocular process is uveitis. The uveitis may be anterior, intermediate, or posterior in nature. The cataract may be related to the inflammation or a result of the steroids used to treat the inflammation. Less common associations are with intraocular tumor, intraocular foreign body, or chronic retinal detachment.

Traumatic Cataracts

Traumatic cataracts are a frequent and important cause of cataracts in children. The cataract may be secondary to penetrating, perforating, or blunt trauma. The cataract may form immediately after injury or be delayed in its formation as can be seen in blunt force trauma. Cataracts secondary to trauma may be partial or complete. It is important to be aware that both accidental and inflicted trauma may be the cause. Surgical intervention is only required for visually significant cataracts. The visual prognosis of traumatic cataract is dependent on accompanying ocular injuries.

Cataracts Associated with Ocular Anomalies

Cataracts have been associated with many ocular anomalies including microphthalmia, aniridia, retinitis pigmentosa, and coloboma. The cataract associated with persistent fetal vasculature deserves special mention. This ocular condition is caused by a failure of the primitive hyaloid vascular system to regress and is most commonly unilateral. The ocular abnormalities most commonly consist of a vascularized retrolental plaque in a microphthalmic eye with prominent iris blood vessels, shallow anterior chamber, and elongated ciliary processes. The lens is often clear initially but opacifies with time. The lens may also move forward with time and glaucoma may develop. The retina may be involved in two ways. There may be contraction of the retrolental plaque causing traction on the vitreous base and peripheral retina. If a remnant of the hyaloid vessel is present at the optic nerve, it may become fibrous causing peripapillary retinal folds or detachment. Treatment involves removing the lens and the fibrovascular membrane. It is often difficult to remove the membrane as it is thick and difficult to cut with the vitrector. The hyaloid artery may still have blood in it and may require cauterization at the time of surgery to avoid vitreous hemorrhage. Finally, the peripheral lens material must be removed carefully to avoid damaging the ciliary processes. Visual outcomes may be affected by amblyopia, glaucoma, retinal folds, and retinal detachment.

Cataracts of Unknown Etiology

Many surgeons feel that a majority of nontraumatic unilateral cataracts are idiopathic in nature, but bilateral cataracts may also be idiopathic. A complete ocular history and examination must be performed with detail directed to history and findings consistent with trauma or inflammation. An ocular examination of the parents may reveal visually insignificant cataracts that the parent did not know were present. Further workup may be indicated in some children but should be done with the assistance of a developmental pediatrician or geneticist to focus the testing for improving the likelihood of a positive result (Tables 11.2 and 11.3).

Morphology of Pediatric Cataracts

The morphology of childhood cataracts can be an important tool in determining the age of onset of the cataract, the possible etiology of the cataract, and visual prognosis. The morphology of the cataract is determined by the anatomy of the lens, lens embryology, and the timing and nature of the

Table 11.2

CONGENITAL CATARACTS: DIAGNOSTIC EVALUATION

Condition	Laboratory Test
Galactosemia	Urine reducing substance
	RBC galactokinase activity, RBC galactose-1-phosphate uridyltransferase
Lowe's syndrome	Urine amino acids
Alport's syndrome	Urine microscopy, urine protein
Rubella	Antibody titers
Syphilis	VDRL test
Smith-Lemli-Opitz syndrome	Cholesterol pathway enzymes
Mevalonic aciduria	
Cerebrotendinous xanthomatosis	
Hypoparathyroidism	Serum calcium, phosphorus, alkaline phosphatase
Wilson's disease	Serum ceruloplasmin
Hyperglycemia/hypoglycemia	Blood glucose
Fabry's disease	Urine "Maltese cross" (polarized light)

RBC, red blood cell; VDRL, Venereal Disease Research Laboratories.

insult. Some morphological types have better prognosis, so trying to identify and classify the cataract may be a helpful management tool. The following classification of morphology is broken down into four types mainly based on location of the opacity: total, central, anterior, and posterior.

Cataract Involving the Whole Lens

Total Cataract A total cataract is complete opacification of the whole lens (Fig. 11.1). They can be caused by any number of conditions and is not diagnostic of any one disorder. Many types of cataracts may progress to total

Table 11.3

CONGENITAL CATARACTS: LABORATORY EVALUATION

	Result	Possible Diagnosis
Urine	+ Reducing substance	Galactokinase deficiency
	Aminoaciduria	Lowe's syndrome
	Hematuria, proteinuria	Alport's syndrome
	"Maltese cross" figures	Fabry's disease
Blood	Erythrocyte enzymes	Galactokinase deficiency
	Glucose	Hyperglycemia/hypoglycemia
	TORCH titers, VDRL test	Rubella, toxoplasmosis, CMV, herpes, syphilis
	Calcium, phosphorus	Hypoparathyroidism or pseudohypoparathyroidism

CMV, cytomegalovirus; VDRL, Venereal Disease Research Laboratories.

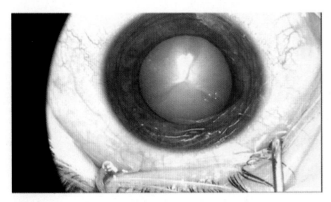

FIGURE 11.1. Total/diffuse cataract.

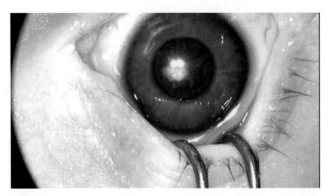

FIGURE 11.2. Fetal nuclear cataract.

cataracts if left untreated. Because no view of structures posterior to the lens is possible, b-scan ultrasonography is recommended to evaluate for retinal detachment, intraocular tumor, or intraocular foreign body. These cataracts require surgical intervention as they are all visually significant.

A special type of total cataract is the Morgagnian cataract. In this cataract the lens fibers liquefy, but the nucleus remains intact. The nucleus will then move within the lens capsule, depending on gravity. These types of cataracts are uncommon in the United States.

Membranous Cataract The membranous cataract is a thin fibrotic lens caused by resorption of the lens material. The anterior and posterior capsules fuse to form a dense white membrane. This type of cataract has been associated with trauma, posterior or anterior capsule defects, congenital rubella, Hallermann-Streiff syndrome, persistent fetal vasculature, Lowe's syndrome, and aniridia (11).

Central Cataracts

Nuclear Cataract These opacities comprise the embryonic and fetal nucleus, between the Y sutures. The fetal nuclear cataract is the most common congenital cataract and presents with a central white opacity approximately 3.5 mm in diameter surrounded by clear cortex. With time, the cortex may become diffusely opacified, or radial opacification (riders) of the cortex may occur. Microphthalmia or microcornea may be present. These cataracts may be unilateral or bilateral. Autosomal dominant inheritance has been reported in the bilateral fetal nuclear form of cataract (11) (Fig. 11.2).

Oil Droplet Cataract This type of cataract is classically seen in galactosemia. It appears as a drop of oil suspended in water. This is caused by the different refractive index within the lens as hydration occurs in response to increased galactitol. If the galactosemia is identified and treated early, resolution of the oil droplet may occur. A similar ophthalmoscopic appearance may also occur in posterior lenticonus but is a result of the thinning of the posterior capsule and the optical distortion of the lens.

Lamellar Cataract The lamellar cataract is an opacification of the lens material between the clear nucleus and cortex. This cataract represents generations of secondary lens fibers that have become opacified in response to an insult when they were metabolically active (11). They can be from an intrauterine event but can be inherited in an autosomal dominant fashion and have been reported in neonatal hypoglycemia. These cataracts are usually bilateral and may be asymmetric. The density of the opacity is quite variable but does tend to progress with time. In general, lamellar cataracts have a better visual prognosis than other morphologic types (11) (Figs. 11.3 and 11.4).

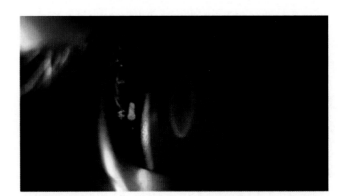

FIGURE 11.3. Lamellar cataract.

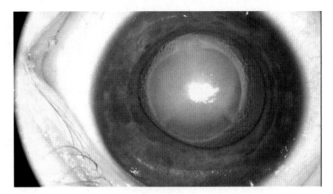

FIGURE 11.4. Dense lamellar cataract.

Central Pulverulent Cataract Central pulverulent cataracts are a unique cataract involving the nucleus of the lens, containing a myriad of tiny dots (pulverized). These cataracts have been historically known as Coppock or Nettleship cataracts but have been renamed. The cataract is usually bilateral, is nonprogressive, and only rarely affects vision. It is most commonly associated with autosomal dominant inheritance and is caused by a mutation in the gamma crystallin. There have been subsequent families that have involvement of the lens cortex. It is important to note that the pulverulent cataract may also occur in transient metabolic changes such as galactosemia, hypoglycemia, and hypocalcemia (11).

"Ant Egg" Cataract An "ant egg" cataract is a rare autosomal dominant lamellar cataract composed of dense pearl-like structures confined to the perinuclear and fetal nucleus. Analysis has shown that these structures are composed mainly of calcium and phosphorus. These calcified white dots may escape during lens aspiration and may be seen in the anterior chamber of the aphakic eye (12).

Sutural Cataract Sutural cataracts are opacities involving the Y sutures of the lens. They may be unilateral or bilateral, are often stationary and are usually not visually significant. Inheritance may be X-linked recessive or autosomal dominant. They have been found in female carriers of Nance-Horan syndrome. An atypical sutural cataract has been described in Fabry disease. It has spoke-like, feathery white lines radiating from the posterior pole along the posterior capsule.

Cortical Cataract Cortical cataracts are unusual in children. The nucleus is not involved and the opacity is limited to the cortex. Autosomal dominant inheritance has been described (11).

Cerulean Cataract Cerulean cataracts are bilateral, small, blue-white opacities found in the peripheral cortex of the lens. Patients are usually asymptomatic. These cataracts are usually inherited in autosomal dominant fashion. Cerulean cataracts that are elongated or club-shaped and concentrated in a ring around the equator of the lens are referred to as coronary cataracts (11).

Anterior Cataracts

Anterior Polar Cataract Anterior polar cataracts present as a small white dot on the central anterior lens capsule (Fig. 11.5). They are thought to arise from abnormal separation of the lens vesicle during embryonic lens development. These cataracts are often bilateral, hereditary, and visually insignificant. Rarely, an adjacent subcapsular/cortical cataract may form and progress to visual significance. Anterior polar cataracts may be associated with significant

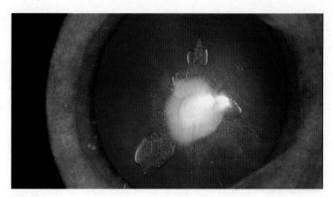

FIGURE 11.5. Anterior polar cataract with duplication.

astigmatism, which causes loss of vision from resultant amblyopia. Anterior pyramidal cataracts are a more severe form of anterior polar cataracts. They are similar to anterior polar cataracts but are shaped like a pyramid on the anterior lens capsule. They tend to be larger and more visually significant. They are usually bilateral, symmetrical, and inherited in an autosomal dominant fashion. If surgery is required for visual rehabilitation, the fibrous tissue is difficult to remove with a vitreous cutter.

Anterior Subcapsular Cataract Anterior subcapsular cataract in childhood is usually associated with acquired disease such as trauma, uveitis, irradiation, Alport syndrome, or atopic skin disease. The opacities vary between very subtle to dense (12).

Posterior Cataracts

Mittendorf's Dot Mittendorf's dot is the remnant of the anterior end of the hyaloid artery. It appears as a small axial or nasally paraxial white dot at the posterior apex of the lens (12). It is visually insignificant. Occasionally, it may be associated with a persistent hyaloid artery. Rarely, it has been associated with posterior lenticonus (11).

Posterior Lenticonus Posterior lenticonus is a thinning of the posterior capsule that results in the adjacent lens material bulging posteriorly. The distorted posterior lens cortex may then opacify (Fig. 11.6) Rarely, the posterior capsule may rupture causing a total white cataract. Prior to cataract formation, vision may be significantly affected because the posterior capsule defect tends to cause a large amount of astigmatism, which may be irregular in nature. Most cases are unilateral and thought to be sporadic. Autosomal dominant inherited bilateral form does occur. X-linked and autosomal recessive inheritance also exists. Posterior lenticonus has been associated with microcornea, hyperglycinuria, and Duane syndrome (11).

Posterior Subcapsular Cataracts Posterior subcapsular cataracts often have a frosted glass appearance, which occurs

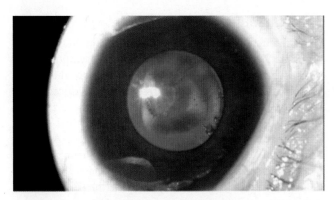

FIGURE 11.6. Posterior lenticonus with opacity.

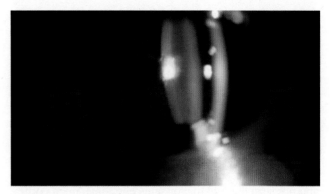

FIGURE 11.8. Posterior polar cataract.

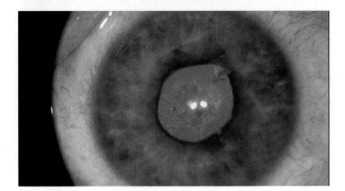

FIGURE 11.7. Posterior subcapsular cataract.

immediately anterior to the posterior capsule (Fig. 11.7). The remainder of the lens is clear. There is usually no associated weakness or defect in the adjacent capsule. Posterior subcapsular cataracts may be idiopathic, related to inflammatory conditions, secondary to steroid use, secondary to trauma, associated with Down syndrome, associated with neurofibromatosis type 2, or may occur after radiation. Because of their location near the nodal point of the eye, posterior subcapsular cataracts are often visually significant. Even a small opacity located in the visual axis can have a profound effect on vision.

Posterior Polar Cataracts Posterior polar cataracts are usually a small, dense, white, central opacity of the posterior lens (Fig. 11.8). These opacities are often associated with posterior capsule weakness. The weakened posterior capsule may spontaneously rupture. Because of their posterior location, a small opacity can result in a significant reduction in vision. The cataract may be unilateral or bilateral and the size and density is variable. They may be familial or sporadic with the familial form usually being bilateral and inherited in an autosomal dominant fashion. If surgery is required for visual rehabilitation, special attention must be paid to the fragility of the posterior capsule.

Genetics of Childhood Cataracts

Hereditary cataracts are most frequently inherited as autosomal dominant traits but may also be inherited in

an autosomal recessive or X-linked fashion. It is interesting to note that phenotypically identical cataracts can result from mutations at different genetic loci and may have different inheritance patterns. The opposite is also true. There can be significant phenotypic variability in families with a known genetic defect. This suggests that additional genes or environmental factors might modify the expression of the primary mutation. There are at least 39 genetic loci to which primary or isolated cataracts have been mapped (13). Twenty-six of the 39 mapped loci for isolated congenital or infantile cataracts have been associated with mutations in specific genes. In the families with at known mutant gene, approximately half have mutations in the crystallins, approximately a quarter have mutations in connexins, with the remainder divided among the genes for heat shock transcription factor-4, aquaporin-0, and beaded filament structural protein-2 (13, 14). When looking at childhood cataracts in a broader form, the genetic mutations multiply. There have been mutations reported in transcription factors (FOXE3, Maf, and PITX 3), enzymes (mainly sugar pathway), axon guidance molecules (ephrins), and proteins. The proteins can be broken down into the crystallins, gap junction proteins (connexins), and membrane proteins (aquaporins). As our understanding of the genetics of childhood cataracts continues to improve, our knowledge of the etiology and pathophysiology should expand.

Evaluation

The evaluation of a child with cataracts should begin with a thorough history. Onset of the cataract is important to ultimate visual prognosis. Care should be taken to ask about possible family history, general development, overall health, and a complete review of systems. This information will help guide whether further workup is necessary. Next, a general assessment should occur. Does the child have any subtle dysmorphy? Is the developmental behavior appropriate? Does growth appear to be normal? Then a complete ophthalmic examination is performed. It is extremely important to determine vision and to determine what impact the lens opacity may have on normal visual development. Evaluation of the red reflex in both the undilated and dilated states may provide valuable information about the obstruction of the visual axis. The retinoscopy reflex is also quite valuable when trying to evaluate the functional impact of the cataract. Pupil examination is important because it may be a clue of associated pathology. Assessment of ocular alignment should be performed. If the child presents with a unilateral cataract and strabismus, this is often a sign of decreased vision and may be a clue to the time of onset. Manifest or latent nystagmus should be noted if present. Examination of all structures of the anterior segment looking for signs of trauma, microcornea, iris abnormalities, and signs of glaucoma should be performed. Unilateral cataracts may be from trauma or associated with other ocular anomalies, so it is important to try to establish one of these etiologies because of the possible impact on visual prognosis. The lens should be examined in detail looking at laterality and morphology. Most unilateral cataracts do not require further systemic workup. Bilateral cataracts are usually idiopathic, hereditary, or secondary to systemic disease. The association with systemic disease is the concern in bilateral cataracts and the morphology may be important in guiding whether further workup is needed. For example, if a baby has bilateral anterior polar cataract, no further workup is necessary. A baby with bilateral, total cataract may warrant further systemic evaluation. A thorough retinal and optic nerve examination should occur, as this may play a role in determining etiology and will have an impact on visual prognosis. If the fundus is not visible, b-scan utrasonography should be performed to evaluate for retinal detachment, intraocular tumor, and persistent hyaloid stalk. Axial length measurement might be helpful in determining whether microphthalmia is present. If systemic evaluation is necessary, it should be performed in a focused manner with a pediatrician or geneticist.

MANAGEMENT

Nonsurgical Management

Not all cataracts need surgical intervention, but they do need to be monitored, especially if the child is in the amblyogenic age group. Nearly all cataracts have an impact on vision at some point whether it is secondary to progression, from refractive error or from amblyopia.

Glasses should be prescribed for any significant refractive error. Amblyopia is a common cause of decreased vision in the childhood cataract population even when the cataract is small. Patching or penalization therapy should be performed to manage this issue. If a small, central opacity is present, pupillary dilation may be performed. Ideally, phenylephrine 2.5% is used 2 to 3 times daily. If adequate dilation is not achieved, a weak cycloplegic agent, such as mydriacyl, may be used. Age of the child, character of the cataract and presence of amblyopia will determine how closely to follow the child.

Surgical Management

Determining visual significance in older children is straightforward. Snellen visual acuity and visual symptoms will direct whether surgery is necessary. It is more difficult in preverbal children. If a child presents with reduced visual behavior, strabismus, or nystagmus and the size, density and morphology fit the clinical picture, then surgical removal of the cataract should be performed. Assessing visual significance in babies is the most difficult scenario. Most clinicians feel that if the cataract is greater than 3 mm, dense, central, and posteriorly located, then it is visually significant.

Once the cataract is determined to be visually significant, prompt surgical intervention is planned. The surgical procedure in children has been refined over the past three decades. Unlike in adults, surgery is usually performed under general anesthesia in an operating room.

Wound Construction

The placement of the wound is the first consideration. Most pediatric ophthalmic surgeons place the wound at the temporal or superior position. If a clear corneal incision is to be used then the either position is fine. If a sclera tunnel is to be used, then the superior position is preferred. The superior placement of the wound gives the added advantage of protection of the wound by the eyelid, brow, and Bell's phenomenon. At times, the location of the wound is directed by unusual facial anatomy or previous or future intraocular surgery. Next is the type of wound used. Both corneal and scleral incisions are used widely in the pediatric population. Advantages to the corneal incision are: avoidance of conjunctival peritomy, ease of intraoperative maneuvering, and reduced potential for bleeding. Disadvantages of the corneal incision are increased risk of endophthalmitis (15,16), higher rate of endothelial cell loss (17), delayed healing compared to the vascular sclera tunnel, and limited wound size. The scleral tunnel has the advantage of minimizing corneal scarring, improved wound security, increased wound size if needed, and wound stability. Two main disadvantages of the scleral wound are the disruption of the conjunctiva, which may impact future surgery and the need for suture.

Anterior Capsule Management

Management of the anterior capsule is one of the key steps to successful cataract surgery in children. The anterior capsulotomy must be done in a fashion that does not compromise the remaining structure or stability of the capsule. The anterior capsule in children makes this act uniquely difficult because of its reduced thickness, exceptional elasticity, and higher tensile strength. Most pediatric cataract surgeons perform either a continuous curvilinear capsulorrhexis (CCC) or vitrectorrhexis. The CCC is favored in children over 2 years of age and the vitrectorrhexis is favored in children younger than 2 years of age (18). To perform a CCC in children, a high-viscosity cohesive viscoelastic agent is recommended. These agents help maintain anterior chamber depth, flatten the anterior capsule, and provide some counter to the positive vitreous pressure seen in young children. The flap is regrasped multiple times to help control the tearing edge and the force is directed to the center of the pupil. The vitrectorrhexis is preferred in infants and young children by some surgeons because of the difficulty performing a CCC as well as the fact that the pupil may be quite small. Wilson reported that the manual CCC produces the best and most stable edge but that the vitrectorrhexis produces a quite acceptable anterior capsule opening (19). The size of the capsulotomy is mainly dependent on the use of an intraocular lens (IOL). If an IOL is to be placed, the anterior capsule opening should be slightly smaller than the size of the optic. If no IOL is to be used, a larger opening should be used to try to minimize secondary membrane formation. No matter the technique, care must be taken in managing the anterior capsule as it is recognized that its shape, size, and edge integrity are important in the long-term success, especially in IOL placement.

Lens Material Removal

The lens material in children is very different from adults. The lens is often quite soft and can be aspirated easily. Therefore, phacoemulsification is not routinely used in pediatric cataract surgery. The technique of aspiration is variable. A vitrectomy handpiece, irrigation/aspiration handpiece, or phacoemulsification handpiece may be used. Most surgeons prefer the vitrectomy handpiece because of its versatility. These systems can be effectively used as single-port systems or bimanual systems. The 20-gauge vitrectomy system was the standard for many years, but smaller gauge systems have been shown to be safe and effective (20). Meticulous, thorough removal of all of the lens material possible is very important to prevent future complications such as visual axis opacification and IOL decentration.

Posterior Capsule Management

Perhaps one of the most difficult and controversial questions related to pediatric cataract surgery involves the appropriate time to perform a posterior capsulotomy. There are benefits to leaving the capsule intact: maintains physiologic barrier, prevents vitreous from entering the anterior chamber, and helps preserve anatomic relationships. Unfortunately, the posterior capsule has an unacceptably high tendency to opacify, with up to 100% posterior capsule opacification (PCO) rates reported (21). Because of the tendency of the posterior capsule to opacify, it is usually recommended to perform a primary posterior capsulotomy during the amblyogenic years or when it is known that YAG laser cannot be performed. Other conditions where primary posterior capsulotomy may be required include posterior capsule tear and posterior capsule plaque. There are several techniques that may be used to make an acceptable posterior capsule opening. The manual

posterior continuous curvilinear capsulorrhexis has been well described (22). This procedure is difficult in the very young but results in a smooth, round edge of the capsule. When using this technique, an anterior vitrectomy must also be performed in young children. If the anterior vitreous face remains intact, secondary opacification often occurs. The posterior capsule opening may also be performed using the vitrector. This may be done by either the anterior, limbal approach or by the pars plana approach. Each technique has its pros and cons. In a randomized, controlled, double-masked clinical trial, Ahmadieh et al. found no statistically significant difference in outcome between the two approaches (23). Therefore, the technique used should be based on the surgeon's skill and experience. It is also important to note that with either method, adequate removal of anterior vitreous must be achieved to help prevent secondary opacification of the visual axis. The size of the posterior capsulotomy also depends on the placement of an IOL. If an IOL is placed, the opening should be slightly smaller than the optic. If no IOL is placed, a larger opening is recommended.

Wound Closure

If a scleral tunnel incision is used, suturing is necessary. A clear cornea incision may not require suturing, but it is important to realize that these incisions do not always self-seal as would be expected in an adult. Basti et al. found self-sealing wounds failed to remain secure in children less than 11 years old, especially in children who had anterior vitrectomy at the time of their cataract extraction (24). Additional reasons to suture the surgical incision in children include increased elasticity of the sclera, higher doses of steroid use, difficulties in examining young children postoperatively, vitrectomy that may further reduce scleral rigidity, and the potential for ocular trauma in the postoperative period. Many types of suture have been used in the past. Bar-Sela et al. reported decreased complications including corneal vascularization, endophthalmitis, and early astigmatism in Vicryl compared to Mersilene suture (25). 10-0 Vicryl (polyglactic acid) suture does not have to be removed, has an in vivo half-life tensile strength of 2 weeks (26) and resorbs between 60 and 90 days. Because of these attributes, many pediatric cataract surgeons prefer 10-0 Vicryl suture for wound closure.

Primary Intraocular Lens Implantation

Placing primary intraocular lenses in children has become widely accepted. There are many issues related to primary IOL implantation including anatomic placement, type of material used, optic edge design, and power of the IOL. These issues are all critically important as children will have these IOLs in their eye for decades of life and often these children are in their visual developmental age.

Placement of the IOL into the capsular bag is the preferred anatomic position. This is the most anatomically accurate placement available. It decreases the potential of the IOL to contact vascularized tissue as well as improves long-term centration of the IOL. If it is not possible to place the IOL in the capsular bag, some lens designs do allow placement within the ciliary sulcus. When no capsular support is available, other methods for IOL placement may be possible but should be approached cautiously (27).

When IOLs were first used in children, polymethylmethacrylate (PMMA) was the only material used. With the development of small incision foldable lenses and the demonstration that other materials are well tolerated in the eye (28), more choices are now available. The most common IOLs, other than PMMA, used include hydrophobic acrylic, hydrophilic acrylic, and silicone lenses. Wilson and Trivedi (29) surveyed pediatric ophthalmologists and found that most surgeons prefer the hydrophobic acrylic lenses for implantation into children. There are many reasons for this. PMMA lenses are rigid; therefore, a larger incision is needed. Since children with cataracts are at higher risk for retinal issues, silicone lenses may be a concern if future retinal surgery may be required. Hydrophilic acrylic lenses have been shown to have lens epithelial cell ongrowth and more issues with optic calcification (28).

Since posterior capsule opacification is a significant problem in pediatric pseudophakia, the design of the IOL is also important. There are some differences in the types of material used but for prevention of PCO, the edge design seems to be the most important factor (28). The square posterior optic edge is the preferred design.

The most difficult issue with placement of primary intraocular lenses is power determination. Multiple issues arise, including the ability to measure corneal curvature and axial length accurately, IOL formulas used, and target refraction. If possible, keratometry and axial length measurements should be performed in the office. In infants and young children, this is not possible and is performed in the operating room while the child is under general anesthesia. An automated keratometer is very useful in this situation. Contact or immersion A-scan ultrasound may be performed in the operating room. Care must be taken to not indent the cornea and to remain on the visual axis for an accurate axial length measurement. There are two basic types of IOL power calculation formulas used in adults. The empiric formulas were the first ones used and are linear formulas. These formulas work well for eyes with normal anatomy and average axial lengths. In eyes that are either short or long, or have abnormal anterior segment anatomy, the accuracy of the formula decreases. The newer theoretic formulas were developed to help take these issues into account. The problem occurs in that these are adult formulas being applied to the pediatric population and larger errors occur compared to the adult population. Andreo et al. (30) compared the actual initial postoperative pseudophakic refraction to the predicted refraction of 4 different formulas including both empiric and theoretic ones. He found no statistical difference in the accuracy between the formulas with the average difference being between 1.2 and 1.4 diopters. No formula

has been proven to be more accurate for all children, so the choice of the formula to be used becomes dependent on the surgeon's experience. In terms of determining optimal target refraction, there is no agreement. It is much easier in older children as a majority of their eye growth has occurred, although Wilson et al. (31) have shown that a significant amount of growth may occur in the second decade of life. Most surgeons target emmetropia or attempt to match the refraction of the other eye in older children. In children that are in the amblyogenic period, the question is even more complicated. Some surgeons feel that the target refraction should be emmetropia in order to try to maximize visual rehabilitation. Other surgeons believe the best target refraction should match the normal eye if unilateral cataract is present. Still others suggest that the target refraction should be hyperopic in an attempt to avoid myopia in adulthood. The amount of recommended hyperopia is dependent on age and the surgeon.

Complications
Intraoperative Complications

Many intraoperative complications may be avoided by meticulous formation of the entrance wound. The wound should not be too small as a very tight fit of the handpiece through the wound may cause corneal opacification. In the eye of infants and small children, reduced sclera rigidity and positive vitreous pressure can make the maintenance of the anterior chamber difficult. If the wound is too large, fluid escapes the eye and can lead to collapse of the anterior chamber. In turn, this can cause prolapse of the iris from the wound and iris damage. If the posterior capsule is open, vitreous may also come forward. The use of smaller wounds and tunnel configurations can also be helpful in avoiding prolapse of intraocular tissue. Direct damage to the iris may occur if the iris is engaged in the vitrector port in cutting mode. One of the most frustrating issues is poor pupillary dilation, especially in infants or trauma. Many infants with congenital cataracts have underdeveloped iris dilator muscles with other iris abnormalities, so even after aggressive pharmacologic dilation, the pupil remains small. In these cases, iris hooks, sphincterotomies, pupilloplasty, or sector iridectomy may be helpful. Any time an injury to the iris occurs, hyphema or vitreous hemorrhage may occur. It is best to respect the iris, but at times it is necessary to enlarge the pupil to aide in intraoperative and postoperative visualization. Radial tears in the anterior capsule may occur and should be managed by stopping, inflating the anterior chamber and redirecting by pulling to the center of the pupil. If unable to redirect, stop before the tear get to equator and convert to vitrectorrhexis. Posterior capsule tears may occur at any time during removal of lens material. The vitrectomy handpiece may be used to round out the tear. Viscoelastic may be used to try to keep the vitreous posterior and the remaining lens material may be removed. Care must be taken not to engage vitreous in irrigation/aspiration mode. Any vitreous that has prolapsed forward must be meticulously removed. Complications relating to IOL use mainly involve malpositioning. Care must be taken to watch the trailing haptic and make sure it is placed within the capsular bag. If one haptic is in the bag and one is in the ciliary sulcus, the chance of future iris capture is higher. Because the posterior capsule is sometimes open in pediatric cataract surgery, inadvertent placement of the IOL into the vitreous may occur. The most common intraoperative and postoperative complications are listed in Table 11.4.

Postoperative Complications

Postoperative complications may be divided into early onset and late onset complications. The most common postoperative complications are listed in Table 11.4 but several should be mentioned.

Early Onset Postoperative Complications

Postoperative inflammation in children after cataract surgery is significantly greater than that seen in adults and may be severe. Steps taken during surgery to help minimize postoperative inflammation include avoiding iris manipulation, meticulous removal of lens material and placement of the IOL in the capsular bag. Aggressive topical steroids are often still required and occasionally systemic steroids may be necessary. Endophthalmitis is potentially the most serious complication as it can result in permanent significant loss of vision or loss of the eye. The incidence of endophthalmitis after intraocular surgery in the pediatric population is approximately 0.71% (32) with most of the cases being diagnosed between 48 and 96 hours after surgery. Gram positive organisms in the *Staphylococcus* and *Streptococcus* family are the most common etiologic agents. Wheeler et al. (32) reported concurrent risk factors including nasolacrimal duct obstruction and upper respiratory infection in 47% of pediatric postoperative endophthalmitis. Preventive measures should include minimizing these risks. Some surgeons use topical antibiotics for 24 to 72 hours before surgery but it is unclear whether this decreases the rate of endophthalmitis. Trinavarat et al. (33) did show a reduction of postoperative endophthalmitis from 0.199% to 0.097% in adults after instilling 5% povidone-iodine solution onto the ocular surface immediately prior to surgery. Finally, the wound should be secure to try to prevent endophthalmitis.

Late Onset Postoperative Complications

The most common postoperative complication in pediatric cataract surgery is obstruction of the visual axis, which may occur secondary to posterior capsule opacification (PCO), secondary membrane formation, or proliferation of lens material. Fastidious removal of the cortex at the time of surgery will help avoid proliferation of lens material postoperatively. Posterior capsule opacification is a significant problem in pediatric cataract surgery as it occurs in nearly 100%

Table 11.4

COMPLICATIONS OF CATARACT SURGERY

Intraoperative

Pupil miosis

Hyphema

Iris damage

Retinal hemorrhage

Vitreous hemorrhage

Retinal detachment

Corneal edema/opacification

Vitreous prolapse

Postoperative (IOL)

Posterior capsule opacification

Secondary membrane

Lens reproliferation

Glaucoma

Inflammation

Cystoid macular edema

Pupillary abnormalities

Retained cortical material

Vitreous to wound

Wound leak

Endophthalmitis

Iris to wound

Corneal edema

IOL decentration

Refractive surprises

Wound-induced astigmatism

Iris synechiae

Iris color change/heterochromia

Hemorrhagic retinopathy

of children over time (34). Nd:YAG laser is often the preferred method of treating PCO in older children. At times, the opacified capsule is too dense and thick for the laser to cut and a surgical posterior capsulotomy and anterior vitrectomy may be required. Posterior capsule opacification is amblyogenic so primary posterior capsulotomy should be considered in children during their visual developmental years. Secondary membrane occurs when a previously open space is closed. Ways to try to avoid secondary membrane formation include making the anterior and posterior capsulotomy adequate size, complete removal of lens material, performing anterior vitrectomy, controlling postoperative inflammation, and maintaining adequate pupil size.

Postoperative glaucoma remains a challenging issue. The mechanism of this type of glaucoma remains unclear. The reported incidence of aphakic/pseudophakic glaucoma is variable and has been reported to range between 3% and 41% (35,36). Microcornea, young age at the time of surgery, poor pupil dilation, and congenital rubella syndrome have been reported as risk factors for developing postoperative glaucoma (37). The risk of developing glaucoma after pediatric cataract surgery is lifelong.

Cataract surgery is a known risk factor for the development of retinal detachment. The incidence of retinal detachment after cataract surgery in the pediatric population is approximately 1% (38). This may in fact may be an underestimation of the true incidence, as retinal detachment has been reported to occur decades after pediatric cataract surgery (39).

Late onset postoperative complications related to IOLs are largely due to malposition. Decentration in the horizontal and vertical plane may occur. If significant reduction in vision or symptoms related to aberration occur, repositioning or explantation may be required. Decentration of the IOL in the anterior/posterior plane is more complicated. If the IOL dislocates posteriorly, removal is required to avoid retinal damage. Anterior dislocation often results in pupil capture. Pupil capture should be surgically treated if reduced vision or glaucoma results. Placing the IOL within the capsular bag minimizes IOL malposition.

Optical Correction/Prognosis

The function of the natural crystalline lens is to bend light to allow the optical image to be focus on the retina. When the natural lens is removed, the power of the natural lens must be replaced to allow for visual rehabilitation. This is particularly difficult in children because they continue to grow, which causes continual changes in the optics of the eye and the fact that children have intact accommodation. There are three methods to address replacement of the natural lens power: spectacles, contact lenses, and IOLs.

Spectacles

Aphakic spectacles are the least invasive method for correcting the resultant refractive error after cataract surgery. They can be used for visual rehabilitation in bilateral as well as unilateral aphakia. In addition to being safe, another advantage is that the power of the lens is easily changed to allow for the variation in refraction that occurs as the child grows. Lens thickness, weight and optical distortions are disadvantages of aphakic spectacles. Bifocals are recommended for older children. In infants and young children, the power of the lens should be selected to allow clear focus of near objects. Most of the infant's world is quite close to them, but they will not be able to use a bifocal add. As the child becomes ambulatory, the child may be moved to a bifocal, or a reduction in the amount of overcorrection should occur.

Contact Lenses

Contact lenses can be used for visual rehabilitation in both bilateral and unilateral aphakia. Advantages of contact lenses include improved optics and the ability to change the power and fit of the lens as the child grows. Disadvantages include cost and corneal complications including infections and ulcers. Contact lenses can be a source of frustration for the parents who have to be able to put them in and take them out. The lenses also have a tendency to be lost as they are relatively thick and the child may be able to rub them out. Because of these issues, back-up spectacles are often recommended. Fitting an aphakic contact lens is a challenge in any age group. Infants pose a special problem because the eyes are small and the power required in the lens is high. In this group, silicone lenses are often used because of their availability and relatively high oxygen permeability. The power of the lens should be over plussed to allow focusing of near objects. As the child grows, bifocal spectacles may be worn over the contact lens. As the child continues to mature and is out of the amblyogenic age, additional contact lens options become available including toric contact lenses, bifocal contact lenses and possibly monovision.

IOLs

Intraocular lens placement is an attractive option for replacing the natural power of the lens. The glasses that may be required over the IOL are much less cumbersome. The difficulties involved with contact lenses are avoided. But, IOLs are not a perfect solution because of the issue of eye growth. Some practitioners may leave infants and young children aphakic and choose to place a secondary IOL at a later date in an effort to avoid this issue. Most pediatric ophthalmologists are comfortable placing intraocular lenses in slightly older children. IOL placement in infants and very young children is more controversial. Some ophthalmologists feel that IOLs should be placed in this group of children because they predict that visual acuity will be improved because of the better optics of an IOL compared to aphakic glasses and contact lenses. The opposing group responds that this has not been proven to be true and is concerned about the significantly higher complication rate in this age group when an IOL is placed. A recent study verified that the complication rate in this age group is significantly higher in the IOL group as compared to the contact lens group (40). The most common intraoperative complication was iris prolapse/damage. The most common postoperative complication was obstruction of the visual axis with the reoperation rate of 70% in the IOL group and 2% in the contact lens group for this complication (40). Early visual acuity data show no statistically different outcome between the two groups when looking at the median visual acuity (0.80 log MAR in contact lens group and 0.97 log Mar in IOL group) (41). Seventy-seven percent of the IOL group had visual acuity of 1.05 log Mar (approximately 20/200) or better compared to 86% of the contact lens group (41). There does not seem to be a clear advantage to either group in terms of postoperative visual acuity. Long-term data are needed to help clarify the issue.

Prognosis

Visual outcome in children who develop cataracts that require surgery after the amblyogenic age generally do very well. In younger children, timely surgery is only the first step in a long process to obtain excellent visual outcomes. Early surgery, early optical correction, and aggressive amblyopia therapy are all required to maximize vision but good outcome is certainly achievable.

DISLOCATED LENSES IN CHILDREN

When the crystalline lens is not located in its normal anatomic position, it is referred to as being dislocated, subluxated, luxated, or ectopic. A luxated lens is completely detached from the ciliary body. A subluxated or ectopic lens is still partially attached to the ciliary body. Children with dislocated lenses usually present with the complaint of blurred vision. As the zonules weaken, the lens curvature increases causing a myopic shift. If the zonules weaken in a segmental fashion, irregular myopic astigmatism occurs. When the lens sublaxation is great enough, the pupil may be bisected, which increases the amount of aberration caused by the lens. Rarely, if the lens completely dislocates into the anterior chamber, the child may present with acute glaucoma.

Etiology

The etiology of dislocated lenses may be broken down into three categories: those associated with ocular anomalies, those associated with system conditions, and trauma (Table 11.5).

Etiology Associated with Ocular Anomalies

All of the ocular anomalies associated with lens dislocation have abnormalities with either the anterior chamber angle or the iris.

Aniridia is a panocular, bilateral disorder caused by a haploinsufficiency of PAX6 gene (42). The iris is always hypoplastic, but the extent of involvement is variable. Foveal hypoplasia, optic nerve hypoplasia, cataracts, and glaucoma are common in aniridia. Zonular weakness and dehiscence leads to lens subluxation.

Table 11.5	
SUBLUXED LENSES: ASSOCIATED CONDITIONS	
Systemic Condition	**Ocular Condition**
Marfan syndrome	Ectopia lentis et pupillae
Metabolic disorders	Aniridia
Homocystinuria	Iris coloboma
Sulfite oxidase deficiency	Glaucoma (congenital)
Hyperlysinemia	**Other**
Weill-Marchesani syndrome	Trauma
Ehlers-Danlos syndrome	Hereditary ectopialentis

Coloboma is a defect in the closure of the embryonic fissure and may involve the iris, fundus, and optic nerve. Depending on the extent of involvement, the zonules adjacent to the iris coloboma may be affected. Flattening of the lens in this area occurs, and if the area involved is large enough, dislocation superotemporally may occur. This is a developmental disorder and the lens subluxation is not progressive.

Ectopia lentis et papillae is an uncommon autosomal recessive condition where there is bilateral displacement of the pupil, usually temporally, with lens dislocation in the opposite direction. The patients may also have microspherophakia, peripheral iris transilluminating defects, miosis, and poor response to mydriatics (43). Significant axial myopia, retinal detachment, increased corneal diameters, and cataract has also been reported in these patients (44).

Rarely, infantile glaucoma can cause lens subluxation. If buphthalmos occurs and there is expansion of the ciliary body ring, stretching of the zonules will occur and the lens may subsequently dislocate.

Etiology Associated with Systemic Conditions

Marfan syndrome is a multisystem disorder mainly affecting the cardiovascular, musculoskeletal, and ocular systems. It is inherited in an autosomal dominant fashion and has been mapped to chromosome 15q21.1 (45). Mutation in the fibrillin 1 gene is responsible for the clinical picture seen in Marfan syndrome. The typical cardiovascular abnormalities include dilation of the aortic root, aortic regurgitation, mitral valve prolapse, and aortic aneurysm. Associated musculoskeletal abnormalities include but are not limited to tall stature, arachnodactyly, and chest wall deformities (45). The most common ocular finding is dislocated lenses, which is seen in approximately 60% of patients (46) (Fig. 11.9). The zonular fibers are fewer in number, stretched, thin, and irregular in diameter (47). Other associated ocular findings include increased axial length, myopia, corneal flattening, iris hypoplasia, retinal detachment, cataract, and glaucoma (45).

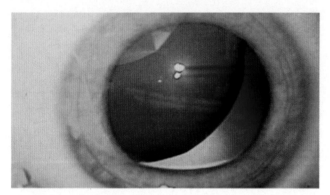

FIGURE 11.9. Subluxed lens in Marfan's patient.

Metabolic disorders may also be associated with lens dislocation. The most common of these is homocystinuria which is a rare autosomal recessive condition caused by a disorder in the methionine catabolism. A mutation in the cystathionine beta-synthase gene is present resulting in a deficiency of the enzyme. Because of the deficiency of this enzyme, the degradation of methionine is interrupted and an intermediate compound, homocysteine, accumulates. The child may be normal early in life or show signs of developmental delay or failure to thrive, making delayed diagnosis common (48). Patients with homocystinuria are often tall with fair hair and blue irides. The musculoskeletal abnormalities include kyphoscoliosis, chest wall abnormalities, arachnodactyly, decreased joint mobility, and osteoporosis. Significant neurologic abnormalities commonly occur including mental retardation, seizures, psychiatric disorders, and cerebrovascular accident. Thromboembolic disease may affect any vessel and may complicate anesthesia. The most common ocular finding is dislocated lenses and in the untreated homocystinuric population may be as high as 90% (49). The lens dislocation is a progressive phenomenon because the zonules tend to break with time. If zonule breakage is complete, the lens may dislocate into the anterior chamber, which may then cause acute glaucoma. The zonular abnormalities may also cause poor accommodation. Myopia is often associated and retinal detachment may occur. Early diagnosis and treatment significantly improves outcome. Approximately 40% to 50% of individuals respond to high doses of pyridoxine (vitamin B6). Dietary restriction of methionine and supplementation of cysteine to help control plasma homocystine helps prevent lens dislocation and mental retardation (50).

Sulfite oxidase is the terminal enzyme in the oxidative degradation pathway of sulfur-containing amino acids. Sulfite oxidase deficiency is a very rare disorder resulting in increased sulfite as it is not converted to sulfate. The location of the defect has been mapped to chromosome 12q13.2 (51). Of interest, this is a more complicated biochemical issue than originally thought. Many patients who were originally diagnosed with sulfite oxidase deficiency actually have been shown to have a deficiency in molybdenum cofactor, which is necessary for the normal function of the

sulfite oxidase. Errors in synthesis of this cofactor have been mapped to chromosomes 14q24, 6p21.3, and 5q11 (52). The clinical presentation for both is similar. The infant has ectopic lenses as well as seizure disorder and severe neurodevelopmental delay. Affected children often die during early childhood (53).

Weill-Marchesani and Ehlers-Danlos syndromes are connective tissue disorders in which lens dislocation occurs. Weill-Marchesani syndrome is actually composed of two phenotypically similar syndromes (WMS1 and WMS2). WMS1 is inherited in an autosomal recessive fashion and the mutation is on chromosome 19p13.2. The defect is in a disintegrin-like and metalloproteinase with thrombospondin type 1 motif (ADAMTS10) (54). WMS2 is inherited in an autosomal dominant fashion and the mutation in the fibrillin 1 gene mapped to chromosome 15q21.1 (55). Phenotypically, these children are of short stature, have brachydactyly, joint stiffness, and lens abnormalities. The most common lens abnormalities are lens dislocation and microspherophakia, which occurs in 64% to 94% of patients, depending on type (54,55). The lens may dislocate into the anterior chamber and a secondary glaucoma may occur. Myopia and cataract may also be present.

Ehlers-Danlos syndrome is a complex group of genetically heterogeneous connective tissue disorders. The essential defect is a deficiency of fibrillar collagen. Ehlers-Danlos syndrome is classified into 6 clinical forms, but skin hyperelasticity, fragility of skin and blood vessels, delayed wound healing, and joint hypermobility are present in most of the forms. Lens dislocation occurs mainly in Ehlers-Danlos syndrome type 1.

Other Causes of Dislocated Lenses

There are two forms of familial ectopia lentis. The most common form is the autosomal dominant inheritance, which has been shown to be a defect in the fibrillin 1 gene found on chromosome 15q21.1 (56). Even though the involved chromosome anomaly is the same as that seen in Marfan syndrome, the lens subluxation occurs in isolation. The dislocation is bilateral and usually upward (57). The autosomal recessive form is secondary to a mutation in the ADAMTSL4 gene on chromosome 1q21 (58). The lens subluxation is not well described but is bilateral (59).

Trauma may also cause lens dislocation. The force involved is usually great. Both penetrating and blunt trauma may cause the dislocation. In penetrating trauma, the lens is often completely lost. The blunt trauma is often secondary to a direct hit to the eye by a high energy projectile. The dislocation is often accompanied by other ocular injury such as hyphema, iris sphincter tears, anterior chamber angle recession, vitreous hemorrhage, and choroidal rupture.

Management of Dislocated Lenses

The management of dislocated lenses involves maximizing vision, avoiding/treating amblyopia, and managing secondary complications. Initially, glasses should be tried. The success of glasses depends mostly on the amount of dislocation present. If the dislocation is small and symmetric, glasses should provide satisfactory results. If the dislocation is asymmetric, contact lenses may be a better choice to minimize the effects of aniseikonia. When larger dislocations are present and the edge of the lens is adjacent to the center of the pupil but the visual axis is still phakic, it is difficult to adequately optically correct for acceptable vision (60). In the larger dislocations where the visual axis is mainly aphakic, glasses or contact lenses for the aphakic portion can give adequate results.

Anteriorly luxated lenses often require surgical removal because of the risk of secondary glaucoma. Posteriorly luxated lenses are better tolerated and may be monitored. If signs of glaucoma, uveitis, or retinal changes occur, the posteriorly dislocated lenses should be surgically removed. Partially dislocated lenses should be surgically removed if adequate visual rehabilitation is not possible with glasses or contact lenses. Subluxated lenses may be removed by either the anterior limbal approach or the posterior pars plana approach. Either approach is effective and the selection of the technique depends on the surgeon's comfort with the technique. Postoperative visual rehabilitation is managed using glasses or contact lenses. Use of intraocular lens implants remains controversial in these cases because of the lack of capsule support. Sutured IOLs, iris claw IOLs, and anterior chamber IOLs have all been used with variable results.

REFERENCES

1. Prakalapakorn SG, Rasmussen SA, Lambert SR, Honein MA. Assessment of risk factors for infantile cataracts using a case-control study: national birth defects prevention study, 2000–2004. *Ophthalmology* 2010;117:1500–1505.
2. Bhatt TR, Dott M, Yoon PW, et al. Descriptive epidemiology of infantile cataracts in metropolitan Atlanta, Ga, 1968–1998. *Arch Pediatr Adolesc Med* 2003;157:341–347.
3. Foster A, Gilbert C. Epidemiology of childhood blindness. *Eye* 1992;6:173–176.
4. Bluestein EC, Wilson ME, Wang XH, et al. Dimensions of the pediatric crystalline lens: implications for intraocular lenses in children. *J Pediatr Ophthalmol Strabismus* 1996;33:18–20.
5. Sher NA, Letson RD, Desnick RJ. The ocular manifestations in Fabry's disease. *Arch Ophthalmol* 1979;97:671–676.
6. Murphree AL, Beaudet AL, Palmer EA, et al. Cataract in mannosidosis. *Birth Defects Orig Artic Ser* 1976;12:319–25.
7. Cenedella RJ. Cholesterol and cataracts. *Surv Ophthalmol* 1996;40:320–327.
8. OMIM chondrodysplasia punctate.
9. OMIM zellweger.
10. OMIM #216400 Cockayne Syndrome.
11. Luis A, Taylor D, Russell-Eggitt I, et al. The morphology and natural history of childhood cataracts. *Surv Ophthalmol* 2003;48:125–144.
12. Hansen L, Wenliang Y, Eiberg H, et al. The congenital "ant egg" cataract phenotype is caused by missense mutation in connexin 46. *Mol Vis* 2006;12:1033–1039.
13. Hejtmancik JF. Congenital cataracts and their molecular genetics. *Semin Cell Dev Biol* 2008;19:134–149.
14. Huang B, He W. Molecular characteristics of inherited congenital cataracts. *Eur J Med Genet* 2010;53:247–257.
15. Cooper BA, Holekamp NM, Bohigian G, Thompson PA. Case-control study of endophthalmitis after cataract surgery comparing sclera tunnel and clear corneal wounds. *Am J Ophthalmol* 2003;136:300–305.
16. Nagaki Y, Hayasaka S, Kadoi C, et al. Bacterial endophthalmitis after small incision cataract surgery. Effect of incision placement and intraocular lens type. *J Cataract Refract Surg* 2003;29:20–26.
17. Beltrame G, Salvetat ML, Driussi G, Chizzolini M. Effect of incision size and site on corneal endothelial changes in cataract surgery. *J Cataract Refract Surg* 2002;28:118–125.

18. Bartholomew LR, Wilson ME, Trivedi RH. Pediatric anterior capsulotomy preferences of cataract surgeons worldwide: comparison of 1993, 2001 and 2003 surveys. *J Cataract Refract Surg* 2007;33:893–900.
19. Wilson ME. Anterior lens capsule management in pediatric cataract surgery. *Trans Am Ophthalmol Soc* 2004;102:391–422.
20. Chee KYH, Lam GC. Management of congenital cataract in children younger than 1 year using a 25-gauge vitrectomy system. *J Cataract Refract Surg.* 2009;35:720–724.
21. Vasavada AR, Praveen MR, Tassignon MJ, et al. Posterior capsule management in congenital cataract surgery. *J Cataract Refract Surg* 2011;37:173–193.
22. Gimbel HV. Posterior continuous curvilinear capsulorrhexis and optic capture of the intraocular lens to prevent secondary opacification in pediatric cataract surgery. *J Cataract Refract Surg* 1997;23:652–656.
23. Ahmadieh H, Javadi MA, Ahmady, M, et al. Primary capsulectomy, anterior vitrectomy, lensectomy, and posterior chamber lens implantation in children: limbal versus pars plana. *J Cataract Refract Surg* 1999;25:768–775.
24. Basti S, Krishnamachary M, Gupta S. Results of sutureless wound construction in children undergoing cataract extraction. *J Pediatr Ophthalmol Strabismus* 1996;33:52–54.
25. Bar-Sela SM, Spierer O, Spierer A. Suture-related complications after congenital cataract surgery: Vicryl versus Mersilene sutures. *J Cataract Refract Surg* 2007;33:301–304.
26. Bourne RB, Bitar H, Andreae PR, et al. In-vivo comparison of four absorbable sutures: Vicryl, Dexon Plus, Maxon and PDS. *Can J Surg* 1988;31:43–45.
27. Hug D. Intraocular lens use in challenging pediatric cases. *Curr Opin Ophthalmol* 2010;21:345–349.
28. Werner L. Biocompatibility of intraocular lens materials. *Curr Opin Ophthalmol* 2008;19:41–49.
29. Wilson ME, Trivedi RH. Choice of intraocular lens for pediatric cataract surgery: survey of AAPOS members. *J Cataract Refract Surg* 2007;33:1666–1668.
30. Andreo LK, Wilson ME, Saunders RA. Predictive value of regression and theoretical IOL formulas pediatric intraocular lens implantation. *J Pediatr Ophthalmol Strabismus* 1997;34:240–243.
31. Wilson ME, Trivedi RH, Burger BM. Eye growth in the second decade of life: implications for the implantation of a multifocal intraocular lens. *Trans Am Ophthalmol Soc* 2009;107:120–124.

32. Wheeler DT, Stager DR, Weakley DR Jr. Endophthalmitis following pediatric intraocular surgery for congenital cataracts and congenital glaucoma. *J Pediatr Ophthalmol Strabismus* 1992;29:139–141.

33. Trinavarat A, Atchaneeyasakul LO, Nopmaneejumruslers C, Inson K. Reduction of endophthalmitis rate after cataract surgery with preoperative 5% povidone-iodine. *Dermatology* 2006;212(suppl 1):35–40.

34. Plager DA, Lipsky SN, Snyder SK, et al. Capsular management and refractive error in pediatric intraocular lenses. *Ophthalmology* 1997;104:600–607.

35. Magnusson G, Abrahamsson M, Sjostrand J. Glaucoma following congenital cataract surgery: an 18-year longitudinal follow up. *Acta Ophthalmol Scand* 2000;78:65–70.

36. Rabiah PK. Frequency and predictors of glaucoma after pediatric cataract surgery. *Am J Ophthalmol* 2004;137:30–37.

37. Mills MD, Robb RM. Glaucoma following childhood cataract surgery. *J Pediatr Ophthalmol Strabismus* 1994;31:355–360.

38. Keech RV, Tongue AC, Scott WE. Complications after surgery for congenital and infantile cataracts. *Am J Ophthalmol* 1989;108:136–141.

39. Algvere PV, Jahnberg P, Textorius O. The Swedish Retinal Detachment Register. I. A database for epidemiological and clinical studies. *Graefes Arch Clin Exp Ophthalmol* 1999;237:137–144.

40. Plager DA, Lynn MJ, Buckley EG, et al. Complications, adverse events, and additional intraocular surgery 1 year after cataract surgery in the infant aphakia treatment study. *Ophthalmology* 2011;118:2330–2334.

41. The Infant Aphakia Treatment Study Group. A randomized clinical trial comparing contact lens with intraocular lens correction of monocular aphakia during infancy: grating acuity and adverse events at age 1 year. *Arch Ophthalmol* 2010;128:810–818.

42. Muto R, Yamomori S, Ohashi H, et al. Prediction by FISH analysis of the occurrence of Wilms tumor in aniridia patients. *Am J Med Genet* 2002;108:285–289.

43. Luebbers JA, Goldberg MF, Herbst R, et al. Iris transillumination and variable expression in ectopialentis et papillae. *Am J Ophthalmol* 1977;83:647–656.

44. Goldberg MF. Clinical manifestations of ectopialentiset papillae in 16 patients. *Ophthalmology* 1988;95:1080–1087.

45. OMIM #154700 Marfan Syndrome.

46. Maumenee IH. The eye in Marfan syndrome. *Trans Am Ophthalmol Soc* 1981;79:684–733.

47. Ashworth JL, Kielty CM, McLeod D. Fibrillin and the eye. *Br J Ophthalmol* 2000;84:1312–1317.

48. Cruysberg JR, Boers GH, Trijbels JM, et al. Delay in diagnosis of homocystinuria: retrospective study of consecutive patients. *BMJ* 1996;313:1037–1040.

49. Cross HE, Jensen AD. Ocular manifestations in the Marfan syndrome and homocystinuria. *Am J Ophthalmol* 1973;75:405–420.

50. Yap S, Rushe H, Howard PM, et al. The intellectual abilities of early treated individuals with pyridoxine-nonresponsive homocystinuria due to cystathionine beta-synthase deficiency. *J Inherit Metab Dis* 2001;24:436–447.

51. OMIM #606887 Sulfite Oxidase.

52. OMIM #252150 Molybdenum Cofactor Deficiency.

53. Edwards MC, Johnson JL, Marriage B, et al. Isolated sulfite oxidase deficiency: review of two cases in one family. *Ophthalmology* 1999;106:1957–1961.

54. OMIM #277600 Weill-Marchesani Syndrome 1.

55. OMIM #608328 Weill-Marchesani Syndrome 2.

56. OMIM #129600 Ectopia Lentis, Isolated, Autosomal Dominant.

57. Casper DS, Simon JW, Nelson LB, et al. Familial simple ectopia lentis: a case study. *J Pediatr Ophthalmol Strabismus* 1985;22:227–230.

58. OMIM #225100 Ectopia Lentis, Isolated, Autosomal Recessive.

59. Greene VB, Stoetzel C, Pelletier V, et al. Confirmation of ADAMTSL4 mutations for autosomal recessive isolated bilateral ectopialentis. *Ophthalmic Genet* 2010;31:47–51.

60. Romano PE, Kerr NC, Hope GM. Bilateral ametropic functional amblyopia in genetic ectopialentis: its relation to the amount of subluxation, an indicator for early surgical management. *Binocul Vis Strabismus* 2002;17:235–241.

61. Zimmerman LE. Histopathologic basis for ocular manifestations of congenital rubella syndrome. *Am J Ophthalmol* 1968;65:837–862.

62. Cotlier E. Congenital varicella cataract. *Am J Ophthalmol* 1978;86:627–629

63. Nahmias AJ, Visintine AM, Caldwell DR. Eye infections with herpes simplex viruses in neonates. *Surv Ophthalmol* 1976;21:100.

64. Stago S, Reynolds DW, Amos CS. Auditory and visual defects resulting from symptomatic and subclinical congenital cytomegaloviral and toxoplasma infections. *Pediatrics* 1977;59:669.

65. Liebman SD. Postnatal development of lamellar cataracts in premature infants. *Arch Ophthalmol* 1955;54:257.

66. Cordes FC. Galactosemia cataract: a review. *Am J Ophthalmol* 1960;50:1151

67. Stambolian D. Galactose and cataract. *Surv Ophthalmol* 1988;32:333.

68. Gass JDI. The syndrome of keratoconjunctivitis, superficial moniliasis, idiopathic hypoparathyroidism and Addison's disease. *Am J Ophthalmol* 1962;54:660.

69. Toussaint D, Davis P. An ocular pathologic study of Refsum's syndrome. *Am J Ophthalmol* 1971;72:342.

70. Wilson WA, Richards W, Donnell GN. Oculo-cerebral-renal syndrome of Lowe. *Arch Ophthalmol* 1963;70:5.

71. Merin S, Crawford JS. Hypoglycemia and infantile cataracts. *Arch Ophthalmol* 1971;86:495.

72. Letson RD, Desnick RJ. Punctate lenticular opacities in type II mannosidosis. *Am J Ophthalmol* 1978;85:218–224.

73. Nielson CE. Lenticonus anterior and Alport's syndrome. *Acta Ophthalmol* 1978;56:518.

74. Levine RE, Snyder AA, Surgarman GI. Ocular involvement in chondrodysplasia punctata. *Am J Ophthalmol* 1974;77:851–858.

75. Simon KA. Diabetes and lens changes in myotonic dystrophy. *Arch Ophthalmol* 1962;67:312.

76. Brownstein S, KirkhamTH, Kalousek DK. Bilateral renal agenesis with multiple congenital ocular anomalies. *Am J Ophthalmol* 1976;82:770.

77. Keating PD, Hepler RS. Blepharophimosis and acquired somato-facial dysmorphism associated with congenital cataracts. *Arch Ophthalmol* 1969;82:1.

78. Cotlier E, Rice P. Cataracts in the Smith-Lemli-Opitz syndrome. *Am J Ophthalmol* 1971;72:955–959.

79. Rudolph G, Kalpadakis P, Bettecken T, et al. Spondylo-ocular syndrome: a new entity with crystalline lens malformation, cataract, retinal detachment, osteoporosis, and platyspondyly. *Am J Ophthalmol* 2003;135:681–687.

80. Soriano JM, Funk J. Bilateral spontaneous reabsorption of a rubella cataract: a case of Hallerman-Streiff syndrome. *Win Mbl Augenheilkd* 1991;199:195–198.

81. Green JS, Parfrey PS, Harnett JD, et al. The cardinal manifestations of Bardet-Biedl syndrome, a form of Laurence-Moon-Biedl syndrome. *N Engl J Med* 1989;321:1002–1009.

82. Moser HW. Peroxisomal diseases. *Adv Pediatr* 1989;36:1.

83. Yeh H, Price RL, Lonsdale D. Cerebral gigantism (Sotos syndrome) and cataracts. *J Pediatr Ophthalmol Strabismus* 1978;15:231.

84. Ferreira RC, Roeder ER, Bateman JB. Cataract in early onset and classic Cockayne syndrome. *Ophthalmic Genet* 1997;18:193–197.

85. Wahl JW, Ellis PP. Rothmund-Thomson syndrome. *Am J Ophthalmol* 1965;60:722–726.

86. Scott JG, Friedmann AI, Chitters M. Ocular changes in the Bloch-Sulzberger syndrome (incontinentia pigmenti). *Br J Ophthalmol* 1955;30:276–292.

87. Jay B, Black RK, Wells RS. Ocular manifestations in ichthyosis. *Br J Ophthalmol* 1968;52:217–226.

88. Bair B, Dodd J, Heidelberg K, Krach K. Cataracts in atopic dermatitis: a case presentation and review of literature. *Arch Dermatol* 2011;147:585–588.

89. Marshall D. Ectodermal dysplasia. *Am J Ophthalmol* 1958;45:143–156.

90. Megarbane A, Loiselet J. Clinical manifestation of a severe neonatal progeroid syndrome. *Clin Genet* 1997;51:200–204.

91. Roy FH, Summitt RL, Hiatt RL. Ocular manifestations of the Rubinstein-Taybi syndrome. *Arch Ophthalmol* 1968;79:272.

92. Insler MS. Cerebro-oculo-facio-skeletal syndrome. *Ann Ophthalmol* 1987;19:54–55.

93. Tournev I, Kalaydjieva L, Youl B, et al. Congenital cataracts facial dysmorphism neuropathy syndrome: a novel complex genetic disease in Balkan Gypsies: clinical and electrophysiological observations. *Ann Neurol* 1999;45:742–750.

94. Yokoyama Y, Uchida M, Matsumoto S, et al. Autosomal dominant congenital cataract and microphthalmia associated with a familial t(2;16) translocation. *Hum Genet* 1992;90:177–178.

95. Tugal-Tutkun I, Urgancioglu M. Childhood-onset uveitis in Behcet disease: a descriptive study of 36 cases. *Am J Ophthalmol* 2003; 136:1114–1119.

96. Zeiter HJ. Congenital microphthalmos. *Am J Ophthalmol* 1963;55:910.

97. Reese AB. Persistent hyperplastic primary vitreous. *Am J Ophthalmol* 1955;40:317.

98. Christiansen SP, Bradford JD. Cataract in infants treated with argon laser photocoagulation for threshold retinopathy of prematurity. *Am J Ophthalmol* 1995;119:175–180.

99. Dinakaran S, Desai SP, Elsom DM. Ophthalmic manifestations of lightning strikes. *Surv Ophthalmol* 2002;47:292.

Glaucoma in Infants and Children

Nandini G. Gandhi • *Sharon F. Freedman*

THE CHILDHOOD GLAUCOMAS constitute a rare, heterogeneous, and vision-threatening group of disorders. Pediatricians and eye care providers are often the first health care professionals to encounter children with glaucoma. Familiarity with the clinical features of this disease, and with the children most at risk for developing glaucoma, may increase correct diagnosis and timely treatment for affected children. In adults, glaucoma is often occult; however, in children, strong suggestive signs of glaucoma are present more often. While there is considerable common ground, children with glaucoma often require examination techniques and treatment strategies, which differ markedly from those most appropriate for their adult counterparts. Genetic, pharmacologic, and technologic advances in the diagnosis and treatment of glaucoma raise the hope that this disease will one day (some day) no longer cause visual impairment in either adults or children.

Many classification systems have been proposed for the childhood glaucomas, and most subdivide them into those of primary and secondary origin (1). Hence, a primary glaucoma is one caused by an intrinsic disease of the aqueous outflow mechanism and is often of genetic origin, whereas a secondary glaucoma is one caused by another ocular disease, injury, drug, or systemic disease (Table 12.1). Both primary and secondary pediatric glaucomas may be associated with significant systemic conditions. It is therefore important for the ophthalmologist to accurately interpret eye signs as clues for the diagnosis and classification of both the glaucoma and associated systemic disease (2). Continued elucidation of the genetic underpinnings of many childhood glaucomas may someday facilitate a classification relying more on underlying genetic abnormalities rather than phenotypically driven diagnostic labels.

SIGNS AND SYMPTOMS OF GLAUCOMA IN CHILDREN

The signs and symptoms of glaucoma vary greatly among children, according to the age of the child and the suddenness and severity of the intraocular pressure (IOP) elevation. During the first year of life, glaucoma is commonly suspected because of signs and symptoms related to secondary corneal changes. Older children are seen more often with loss of vision from chronic glaucoma or with symptoms of pain and vomiting related to acute glaucoma. Elevation of IOP is required to confirm the diagnosis of childhood glaucoma, although its presence (past or present) may be strongly suspected on the basis of classic symptoms and other signs of the disease (see below). While somewhat lower in young infants than in school age children and adults, the range of normal IOP in childhood approximates the normal adult range; rarely are normal measurements above 22 mmHg or below 10 mmHg. Accurate IOP measurements are essential not only to the diagnosis but also to the management of children with glaucoma (see later under Examination).

Infants and young children with glaucoma usually present for ophthalmologic evaluation because the pediatrician or parents have noted something unusual about the appearance of the child's eyes or behavior. Corneal opacification and/or enlargement (a response to elevated IOP) are the signs most commonly heralding glaucoma in the infant; both may progress over the first 2 years of life if IOP remains elevated (Figs. 12.1 and 12.2). At other times, the child's glaucoma may manifest itself as one or more of the "classic triad" of findings: epiphora, photophobia, and blepharospasm (Fig. 12.3) (3). Photophobia and epiphora result from corneal edema (often with associated breaks in Descemet membrane called Haab Striae). The baby may be noted to withdraw from light or to bury his head against his parent or bedding to prevent exposure to light; eye rubbing may also be noted. Even indoors, the infant may show an apparent reluctance to face upward, and may mistakenly be considered shy (Fig. 12.4).

These corneal signs and symptoms of glaucoma in early life may be of sudden onset, with dramatic opacification of the cornea and onset of photophobia occurring over a few hours. Such an acute onset of signs is probably related to initial or additional breaks in Descemet membrane (Figs. 12.5 and 12.6). The occurrence of breaks appears to be confined to the first 2 years of life, when rapid expansion of the cornea may occur secondary to glaucoma. Breaks are permanent and remain as important evidence of early glaucoma; although some are subtle, at other times significant associated corneal scarring may result (Fig. 12.7). The defects appear as wavy parallel lines on

Table 12.1

PRIMARY AND SECONDARY CHILDHOOD GLAUCOMAS

I. Primary glaucomas

A. Primary congenital open-angle glaucoma

1. Newborn congenital glaucoma (iridotrabeculo dysgenesis)

2. Infantile glaucoma (trabeculo dysgenesis)

3. Late recognized

B. Autosomal dominant juvenile (open-angle) glaucoma

C. Primary angle-closure glaucoma

D. Associated with ocular abnormalities

1. Iridodysgenesis

   a. Aniridia

   b. Congenital iris ectropion syndrome

   c. Iridotrabecular dysgenesis (iris hypoplasia)

2. Corneodysgenesis (or iridocorneal dysgenesis)

   a. Axenfeld-Rieger anomaly

   b. Peters anomaly/syndrome

   c. Congenital microcornea with myopia

   d. Sclerocornea

   e. Congenital hereditary endothelial dystrophy

   f. Posterior polymorphous dystrophy

   g. Anterior corneal staphyloma

   h. Iridocorneal endothelial syndrome

3. Other

   a. Idiopathic or familial elevated episcleral venous pressure

E. Associated with systemic abnormalities

1. Chromosomal abnormalities:

   a. Trisomy 13 (Patau syndrome)

   b. Trisomy 18 (Edward syndrome)

   c. Trisomy 21 (Down syndrome)

   d. Turner syndrome (XO)

2. Connective tissue abnormalities:

   a. Stickler syndrome

   b. Marfan syndrome

3. Metabolic disorders:

   a. Hepatocerebrorenal syndrome

   b. Oculocerebrorenal (Lowe) syndrome

   c. Mucopolysaccharidosis

4. Phacomatoses:

   a. Sturge-Weber syndrome

   b. Neurofibromatosis Type 1 (NF-1)

   c. Nevus of Ota (congenital ocular melanosis)

   d. von-Hippel-Lindau syndrome

5. Other:

   a. Rieger syndrome (Axenfeld-Rieger syndrome)

   b. SHORT syndrome

   c. Rubinstein-Taybi syndrome

   d. Infantile glaucoma with mental retardation and paralysis

   e. Oculodentodigital dysplasia

   f. Open-angle glaucoma associated with microcornea and absence of frontal sinuses

   g. Caudal regression syndrome

   h. Cutis marmorata telangiectasia congenita

   i. Warburg syndrome

   j. Kniest syndrome (skeletal dysplasia)

   k. Michel syndrome

   l. Nonprogressive hemiatrophy

   m. PHACE syndrome

   n. Soto syndrome

   o. Linear scleroderma

   p. GAPO syndrome

   q. Roberts pseudothalidomide syndrome

   r. Wolf-Hirschhorn (4p-) syndrome

   s. Rainbow syndrome

   t. Nail-patella syndrome

   u. Proteus syndrome

   v. Fetal hydantoin syndrome

   w. Cranio-cerebello-cardiac (3C) syndrome

   x. Brachmann-deLange syndrome

   y. Hallerman–Streiff syndrome

(continued)

Table 12.1

(continued)

II. Secondary glaucomas

A. Traumatic glaucoma

1. Acute glaucoma

   a. Angle concussion

   b. Hyphema

   c. Ghost cell glaucoma

2. Late-onset glaucoma with angle recession

3. Arteriovenous fistula

B. Secondary to intraocular neoplasm

1. Retinoblastoma

2. Juvenile xanthogranuloma

3. Leukemia

4. Melanoma

5. Melanocytoma

6. Iris rhabdomyosarcoma

7. Aggressive nevi of the iris

C. Secondary to uveitis

1. Open-angle glaucoma

2. Angle-blockage glaucoma

   a. Synechial angle closure

   b. Iris bombe with pupillary block

   c. Trabecular endothelialization

D. Lens-induced glaucoma

1. Subluxation-dislocation and pupillary block

   a. Marfan syndrome

   b. Homocystinuria

   c. Weill-Marchesani

2. Spherophakia and pupillary block

3. Phacolytic glaucoma

E. Following surgery for congenital cataract (Aphakic)

1. Lens tissue trabecular obstruction

2. Pupillary block

3. Chronic open-angle glaucoma associated with angle abnormalities

F. Steroid-induced glaucoma

G. Secondary to rubeosis

1. Retinoblastoma

2. Coats disease

3. Medulloepithelioma

4. Familial exudative vitreoretinopathy

5. Chronic retinal detachment

H. Secondary angle-closure glaucoma

1. Retinopathy of prematurity

2. Microphthalmos

3. Nanophthalmos

4. Retinoblastoma

5. Persistent hyperplastic primary vitreous

6. Congenital pupillary iris-lens membrane

7. Topiramate use

8. Ciliary body cysts

I. Malignant glaucoma (aqueous misdirection)

J. Glaucoma associated with increased venous pressure

1. Cavernous or dural-venous fistula

2. Orbital disease

K. Secondary to maternal rubella

L. Secondary to intraocular infection

1. Acute recurrent toxoplasmosis

2. Acute herpetic iritis

3. Endogenous endopthalmitis

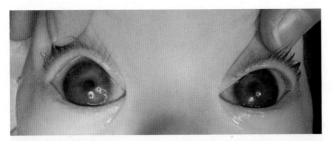

FIGURE 12.1. Corneal enlargement bilaterally, with corneal haze. This infant was 11 months old and had persistent severe corneal enlargement (corneal diameters 14.5 mm both eyes), and corneal edema and opacity with multiple Haab Striae in both eyes. Intraocular pressures were 40 mmHg under anesthesia, on topical medical therapy. Glaucoma was diagnosed at 2 months of age but inadequately treated.

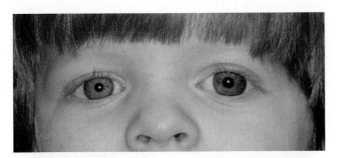

FIGURE 12.2. Corneal enlargement of the left eye that developed slowly over a period of 1 year. Primary infantile glaucoma responded well to angle surgery and medical therapy, and vision improved with glasses for unilateral myopia and patching.

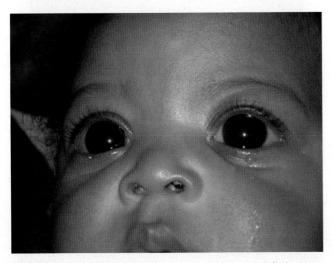

FIGURE 12.3. Tearing of both the eyes caused by uncontrolled primary infantile glaucoma. Note the increased corneal diameter and corneal haze of both eyes.

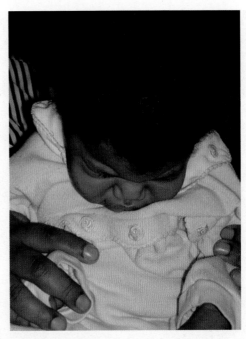

FIGURE 12.4. Hiding of the face caused by photophobia secondary to congenital glaucoma.

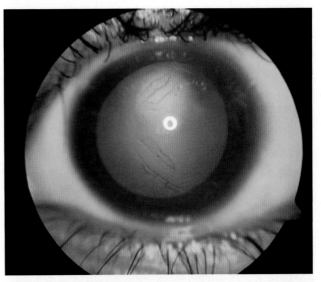

FIGURE 12.5. Haab Striae are seen in retroillumination in the left eye of a teenage girl with advanced primary congenital glaucoma. These marks persist despite her controlled intraocular pressure and resolution of associated corneal edema.

the inner side of the cornea and are usually curvilinear and horizontal. They represent the separated edges of Descemet membrane. Breaks with more vertical orientation may be seen secondary to the acute bending of the cornea rarely occurring with delivery using forceps (Fig. 12.8) (4).

If glaucoma in infancy and early childhood is not treated, progressive enlargement of the cornea may occur throughout the first 2 years of life. The corneal diameter may in extreme cases enlarge to 17 to 18 mm; in these cases, concordant enlargement of the ciliary ring often results in iridodenesis and lens subluxation (Fig. 12.9). Stretched, buphthalmic eyes are easily traumatized, even to the point of rupture.

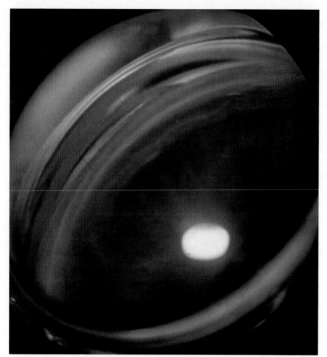

FIGURE 12.6. Haab Striae seen through a Koeppe lens in a child with congenital glaucoma. Note the curvilinear shape to the break.

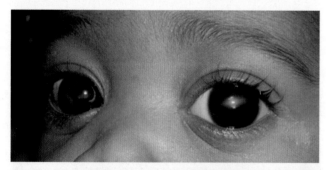

FIGURE 12.7. Corneal scarring in a striking pattern, correlating with the presence of Haab Striae. The associated corneal edema has cleared, and the pressure is normalized after goniotomy surgery, but the visually significant corneal opacities remain in both eyes.

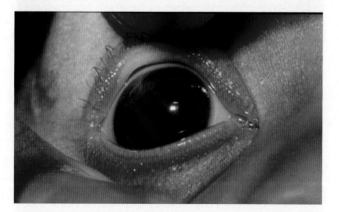

FIGURE 12.8. Forceps injury to the right cornea at birth resulted in two parallel linear breaks in Descemet membrane running in an oblique direction across the visual axis; this eye showed high astigmatism and best corrected vision of 20/80, despite aggressive patching.

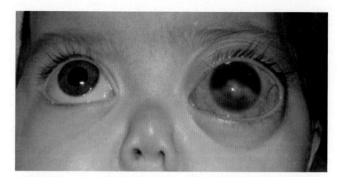

FIGURE 12.9. Hugely enlarged, buphthalmic left eye, in a 6 month old infant with Pierre Robin syndrome and uncontrolled, congenital glaucoma in that eye. Corneal scarring has resulted from exposure, corneal diameter is 17 mm on the left, and spontaneous posterior lens dislocation has occurred. The eye is blind.

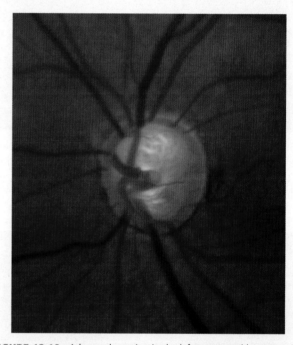

FIGURE 12.10. Advanced cupping in the left eye caused by congenital glaucoma in a 4-year-old girl; vision is preserved at 20/25.

Additional nonspecific signs of glaucoma in early life include the presence of a deep anterior chamber and optic nerve cupping. The extent of optic nerve cupping does not always correlate closely with the anterior segment signs of glaucoma. In the absence of optic atrophy, the optic cup may decrease greatly in size with IOP reduction, and will enlarge again if control of IOP is lost. By contrast, the optic atrophy that may result from chronic or severe IOP elevation is irreversible (Fig. 12.10).

In older children, the anterior segment signs of glaucoma play a less important role in the recognition of this disorder. Of greater importance is the evaluation of the eyes because of decreased vision (usually from induced myopia) or circumstances in which secondary glaucoma might be suspected, such as chronic iridocyclitis, blunt trauma to the anterior segment, neoplasm, or as a consequence of surgery. The presence or absence of optic nerve head cupping in older children is by itself an unreliable diagnostic sign, but remains very important in the follow-up of children with known glaucoma. Older children infrequently present with acute glaucoma inducing nauseating eye pain, headaches, and even colored haloes around lights. This sudden-onset glaucoma may be the result of traumatic hyphema or of angle-closure glaucoma from lens dislocation or cicatricial retinopathy of prematurity. Less frequently, acute glaucoma develops secondary to other processes (Table 12.1).

Loss of vision from childhood glaucoma occurs secondary to pathologic changes in the eye such as corneal opacification and optic nerve damage. Amblyopia is also an important cause of unilateral vision loss, especially in cases where corneal abnormalities and refractive errors are asymmetric.

OCULAR EXAMINATION

The examination of a child with suspected glaucoma includes the components of the complete pediatric eye examination. However, the glaucoma evaluation should address several specific objectives: (a) confirming or excluding the diagnosis of glaucoma, (b) determining the etiology of the glaucoma (if present), and (c) obtaining additional information (including any prior glaucoma treatment) needed to plan for optimal management. If one can confidently exclude the diagnosis of glaucoma, or if an older child with glaucoma is to undergo a trial of medical therapy, examination under anesthesia may *not* be indicated. If indicated, the anesthetized exam allows more detailed gonioscopy and optic nerve head examination, followed by any indicated surgical treatment.

Vision testing techniques vary greatly with the age of the patient. In infants, good fixation and following and the absence of nystagmus are important indicators of good visual function. In children over 3 years of age, visual acuity and eventually visual field testing can also be assessed.

The *external examination* is important to detect evidence of associated abnormalities, inflammation, or lacrimal duct obstruction.

Tonometry should be performed in both the office and operating room settings. Careful measurements of IOP in the office, uninfluenced by general anesthesia, aid in both diagnosing glaucoma and evaluating results of treatment. Among various instruments used to measure IOP in children, the Perkins applanation tonometer (Haag-Streit, Mason, OH) and the Tono-Pen (a hand-held Mackay-Marg-type tonometer, Reichert, Inc, Depew, CA) have been invaluable (5,6), but require the instillation of local anesthetic, which can be anxiety provoking in children. The Icare® rebound tonometer (Finland, Oy), a hand-held tonometer that does not require the use of anesthetic, has demonstrated good clinical correlation when compared with Goldmann applanation among children with glaucoma or suspected glaucoma, and

holds promise as an instrument suitable for home tonometry in selected pediatric glaucoma cases (7,8). In older, cooperative children, the standard slit-lamp-mounted Goldmann applanation instrument is often successful.

IOP measurements are variably lowered by sedatives, narcotics, and inhalation anesthetic agents (9–11), and variably raised by endotracheal intubation and ketamine (3,12). With the possible exception of chloral hydrate conscious sedation (13), most sedative/anesthetic drugs may alter measured IOP but do not usually normalize very high or asymmetrically elevated IOPs. IOP in normal eyes rises from infancy to reach normal adult levels by middle childhood(14). The range of normal IOP in childhood can be considered from 10 to 22 mmHg (3). Newborns with glaucoma may demonstrate a transient postnatal interval of normal IOP, after which the IOP will again rise.

Careful inspection of the anterior segment provides vital information about a childhood glaucoma patient. The cornea is inspected for changes secondary to elevated IOP. The normal horizontal corneal diameter at birth ranges from 9.5 to 10.5 mm (mean 10 mm), enlarging to approximately 11.5 mm by the end of the second year. Under 1 year of age, diameters of 12 to 12.5 mm are suggestive of glaucoma, and a measurement of 13 mm or more at any time in childhood strongly suggests abnormality, as does asymmetry in corneal diameter between the two eyes of a child (3,15–17).

The depth and clarity of the anterior chamber are assessed. The pupil and irides are examined for evidence of primary anomalies or abnormalities secondary to other eye diseases (e.g., aniridia, Axenfeld-Rieger syndrome, and ectropion uveae).

Gonioscopy provides the most important anatomic information about the mechanism of the glaucoma present. Koeppe gonioscopy is a useful technique for this purpose, in both the office and operating room (Figs. 12.11 and 12.12).

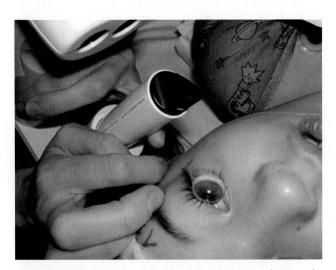

FIGURE 12.11. Operating room gonioscopy using Koeppe lenses and a portable slit lamp provides vital diagnostic information in preparation for glaucoma surgery.

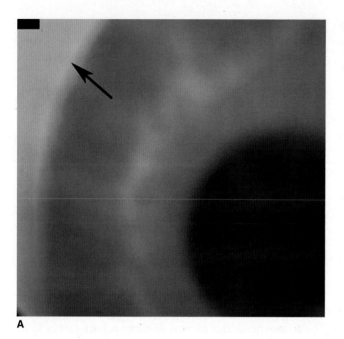

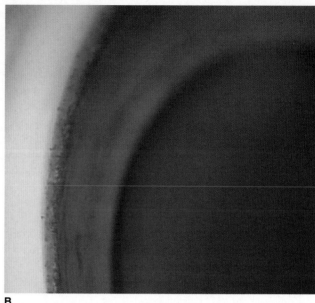

A

B

FIGURE 12.12. Goniophotographs of eyes with congenital glaucoma. **A:** Appearance often seen in lightly pigmented races, showing scalloped border of ciliary body band, no visible scleral spur, and uniform membrane-line appearance of trabecular meshwork band. This eye belongs to the infant shown in Figure 12.1, after initial goniotomy surgery. The cornea is still hazy, and a cleft is visible in the anterior trabecular meshwork at the arrow. **B:** Appearance of angle in a darkly pigmented eye, showing ciliary body band with uveal processes and a narrow trabecular meshwork band, without distinct scleral spur in either A or B.

The iris and angle structures should be inspected carefully and the results recorded. The RetCam® digital imaging system (Clarity Medical Systems, Pleasanton, CA) can also be used in the operating room to photograph angle structures for documentation and future comparison.

The most characteristic feature of the child's anterior chamber angle is the trabecular meshwork, which has the appearance of a smooth, homogeneous membrane, extending from peripheral iris to Schwalbe line, during the first year of life. It becomes coarser and more pigmented with the passing years. In addition, the peripheral iris in the young child tends to be thinner and flatter (18).

The iris in infantile glaucoma often shows a more anterior insertion than that of the normal infant, with altered translucency of the angle face producing an indistinct ciliary body band, trabecular mesh, and scleral spur. This translucent tissue has historically been referred to as "Barkan membrane" (19). The angle may show other characteristics suggestive of the etiology of glaucoma. For example, in glaucoma after cataract surgery, a closed angle with iris bombe suggests pupillary block and the need for peripheral iridectomy/synechiolysis, while an open angle suggests trabecular meshwork dysfunction and the need for a different treatment strategy. An abnormally prominent Schwalbe line and iris adhesions to the angle structures may alternatively suggest Axenfeld-Rieger syndrome (also known as iridocorneal dysgenesis). Juvenile open-angle glaucoma (JOAG) patients

usually demonstrate a normal-appearing open angle, often with a prominent, lacy uveal meshwork.

Taken together with other findings of anterior examination (above), the adequacy of the angle view and its findings are important guides to the appropriate surgical intervention that may be needed.

Funduscopy usually concentrates on a careful assessment of the appearance of the optic nerve head. Other fundus features (e.g., a stalk in persistent fetal vasculature, choroidal hemangioma in Sturge-Weber syndrome) may help confirm the type of glaucoma or help with surgical planning. Large size of the optic nerve cup and asymmetry of cupping between fellow eyes is suggestive but not definite evidence of glaucoma. Illustratively, the cup/disc ratio exceeded 0.3 in 68% of 126 eyes with primary infantile glaucoma examined by Shaffer and Hetherington(20), but in only 2.6% of 936 normal newborn eyes examined by Richardson (21). Marked optic cup asymmetry was noted in only 0.6% of normal eyes in the latter series, contrasted with 89% noted for infants with monocular glaucoma. Indirect ophthalmoscopy using a 28 or 20 diopter condensing lens in the office often underestimates the optic nerve cupping, which more accurately can be assessed by slit-lamp biomicroscopy or with direct ophthalmoscopy through a Koeppe lens in the operating room (Fig. 12.13). In infants and young children, initial findings can be usefully compared with changes seen after control of glaucoma (or failure of control) as a measure of success of

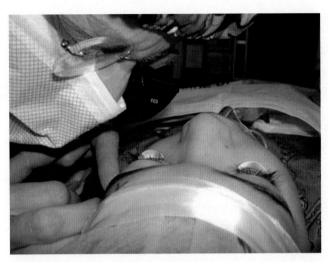

FIGURE 12.13. The appearance of the optic nerve can be well seen through a Koeppe lens. This helps neutralize the changes in size due to refractive error, and facilitates the exam through a fairly small pupil. Drawings of the cupping are helpful, as are photographs that allow future comparisons to be made.

treatment; dramatic reversal of cupping can occur in young eyes after IOP reduction, likely due to an incompletely developed or very flexible lamina cribrosa (22). Drawings (and when possible, photographs) of the optic nerves are valuable for later comparison.

Refraction, Perimetry, Ultrasound, Corneal Pachymetry, and Optical coherence tomography: Determination of refractive errors can be helpful, especially when they are asymmetric in the setting of probable unilateral glaucoma; in this case, relative myopia of the affected eye supports the diagnosis of glaucoma. Visual field testing (using Goldmann kinetic or automated techniques) can be useful in cooperative older children with known glaucoma, allowing assessment of the extent of initial field loss, as well as stability of the remaining visual field over time. Axial length measurement with ultrasound (during examination under anesthesia) can be an adjunct to serial corneal diameter measurements when following infants and young children being treated for glaucoma (17). Ultrasound pachymetry (to measure the central corneal thickness) has proven relevant to evaluation of IOP in cases of adult open-angle glaucoma, especially when the cornea is much thinner or thicker than average; thinner central corneas tend to produce an underestimation of the true IOP by applanation, but also seem to confer additional risk for glaucomatous damage as an independent risk factor in adults (23,24,25). Several studies have reported on central corneal thickness in normal children, as well as in those with glaucoma and ocular diseases associated with childhood glaucoma (26–29). Decreasing target IOP for children's eyes with thinner than average central corneas may be advisable, but the measured IOP should not be "adjusted" downward for eyes with thick corneas, especially in the presence of conditions such as aphakia, where thicker corneas may be acquired rather than congenitally occurring (28).

Optical coherence tomography (OCT) (Carl-Zeiss Meditech, Dublin, CA), a non-contact imaging technology capable of measuring the thickness of the peripapillary retinal nerve fiber layer and the macular area in both adults and children (30–32), correlates with photographic and visual field evidence of glaucomatous optic nerve head damage(33) and may prove valuable to evaluate the thinning of these parameters in children with glaucoma (33,34).

DIFFERENTIAL DIAGNOSIS (TABLE 12.2)

Many conditions of the eye may produce symptoms and ocular signs that suggest possible glaucoma, including simple congenital nasolacrimal duct obstruction, corneal disease, or anterior chamber inflammation, which may variably produce photophobia and tearing. Storage diseases associated with corneal clouding or hereditary corneal dystrophies with opacification of the cornea raise concern for glaucoma in a child, as does isolated corneal enlargement. It is important always to *rule out glaucoma* when any of these signs or symptoms is present, even when initial evidence suggests a more common nonglaucomatous cause. Glaucoma may also complicate inflammation or trauma to the anterior segment, may be found with storage diseases and with primary enlargement of the cornea, and certainly is seen coincidentally with lacrimal duct obstruction (35).

In summary, the signs of glaucoma are shared by other eye diseases and indicate the careful anterior segment examination and tonometry necessary to rule out this abnormality. The identification of some other cause of such signs does not in itself eliminate the risk of glaucoma.

PRIMARY CHILDHOOD GLAUCOMA

Primary Congenital Open-Angle Glaucoma

This disorder is the most common primary pediatric glaucoma, with an estimated incidence of only about one in 10,000 to 20,000 live births in Western countries, but with a higher incidence in Middle East and Slovak Romany populations (1). There is no predilection for race or gender, and most cases (65% to 80%) are bilateral (3). More than 80% of all cases have an onset of disease within the first year of life, with about 25% diagnosed as newborns, and more that 60% presenting by 6 months of age (3,36). Primary congenital (also called primary infantile) glaucoma may present with severe phenotype at birth, or may present with milder signs and symptoms, leading to delay in its diagnosis, sometimes after significant and irreversible optic nerve damage has occurred from chronically elevated IOP. Typically, the corneal abnormalities consisting of progressive edema associated with breaks in Descemet membrane occur during the first year of life. Recognition of glaucoma depends on the sensitivity of caretakers to the significance of these signs and symptoms.

While the majority of primary infantile glaucoma cases are sporadic (no known family history), about 10% are

Table 12.2

DIFFERENTIAL DIAGNOSIS OF FEATURES COMMONLY FOUND IN PEDIATRIC GLAUCOMAS

I. Disorders with "red eye" and/or epiphora and/or photophobia

  A. Congenital nasolacrimal duct obstruction

  B. Conjunctivitis (infectious, non-infectious)

  C. Corneal epithelial defect/abrasion

  D. Keratitis (especially herpes simplex)

  E. Anterior segment inflammation (uveitis, trauma)

II. Disorders with corneal edema or opacification

  A. Forceps-related birth trauma (with Descemet tear)

  B. Congenital malformation/anomaly

    1. Sclerocornea

    2. Peters anomaly

    3. Choristomas (dermoid-like)

    4. Other anterior segment dysgeneses

  C. Corneal dystrophy

    1. Congenital hereditary endothelial dystrophy

    2. Congenital hereditary stromal dystrophy

    3. Posterior polymorphous dystrophy

  D. Keratitis

    1. Herpetic

    2. Rubella[a]

    3. Phlyctenular

  E. Metabolic disease

    1. Mucopolysaccharidoses

    2. Mucolipidoses

    3. Cystinosis

III. Conditions with corneal enlargement

  A. Axial myopia

  B. Megalocornea

  C. Megalophthalmos

IV. Conditions with actual or "pseudo" optic nerve cupping

  A. Physiologically large optic nerve cup

  B. Coloboma or pit of the optic nerve

  C. Atrophic optic nerve (with substance loss)

  D. Hypoplastic optic nerve

  E. Malformation of the optic nerve

Note that some of these conditions may also be associated with glaucoma.

[a]Rare in developed countries.

Adapted from references (3) and (158).

familial, usually transmitted as an autosomal recessive trait, with penetrance varying from 40% to 100% (37,38). Several genetic loci associated with primary congenital glaucoma have been identified in large pedigrees using linkage analysis. Two main causative genes have thus far been reported, the CYP1B1 gene (a cytochrome P450 system enzyme) and the LTB2 gene (39); the MYOC gene has also been implicated in a minority of primary congenital glaucoma cases (40). Mutations in the CYP1B1 gene have been identified in many cases of primary congenital glaucoma worldwide (41–44), but do not seem responsible for many sporadic cases in the United States (unpublished personal data) (45).

The significant inherited defect is confined to the filtration tissues, rendering them less permeable to the passage of aqueous humor. The gonioscopic abnormality typically features decreased transparency of the tissues over the scleral spur and ciliary body band, so that these normal angle landmarks are difficult to define. The width of the trabecular meshwork and ciliary body also may be diminished, giving the impression of an anterior insertion of the iris (see above under *gonioscopy*).

Surgical intervention is the definitive treatment for primary congenital glaucoma, with angle surgery (usually goniotomy or trabeculotomy) successful in the majority of cases, especially those with presentation between 3 and 12 months of age; surgical success drops for those with presentation at birth or after age 1 to 2 years (see below). In cases refractory to angle surgery, filtration surgery (sometimes combined with trabeculotomy) (46–50), glaucoma implant surgery (49,51,54–57), and cycloablation (58) have been used with variable success, depending upon the reported series (see later under Treatment). Visual prognosis is dependent not only upon the timely diagnosis and IOP reduction, but upon the secondary corneal, refractive, and optic nerve changes produced by the initially elevated IOP (3).

Juvenile Open-Angle Glaucoma

In contrast to primary congenital or infantile glaucoma, this rare disease is an autosomal dominant early onset form of primary open-angle glaucoma. JOAG is characterized by acquired and marked bilateral IOP elevation, with usual onset between ages 4 and 35 years, often with a strong family history. Ocular damage, usually in the form of optic nerve cupping and visual field loss, is usually asymptomatic, unless myopia brings the child to eye examination for decreased distance vision. Absent are the corneal stigmata usually present in infant-onset glaucoma. Gonioscopy reveals normal-appearing angle structures. Treatment is difficult, often beginning with medication, and proceeding to filtration or tube implant surgery, although angle surgery may be helpful in some cases (see below).

JOAG was first linked to chromosome 1q21-31 by Sheffield et al. in 1993 (59). Mutations were subsequently reported in the trabecular meshwork glucocorticoid response gene (TIGR, now renamed myocilin) and have

been identified in numerous populations of individuals with JOAG worldwide (60–63).

Primary Pediatric Glaucoma Associated with Systemic Diseases

Primary glaucoma in children may be seen in association with certain systemic diseases in which ocular abnormalities are included in the syndrome complex (see Table 12.1).

Sturge-Weber Syndrome

Glaucoma is present commonly with this disease in association with a facial nevus flammeus of the ipsilateral upper eyelid, and abnormal vasculature of the leptomeninges. Intracranial involvement may be complicated by epilepsy, paralysis, and visual field defects. The glaucoma may be congenital or acquired and is most often unilateral. The onset of glaucoma seems bimodal, with some cases presenting in early infancy, while others occur later in childhood. Inspection of the conjunctiva often shows an abnormal number and tortuosity of blood vessels with elevation of venous pressure. A striking episcleral vascular abnormality is present behind the limbus circumferentially. Gonioscopy reveals minor angle anatomic changes, usually without vascular abnormalities of the angle; blood can often be identified in Schlemm canal. The iris of the involved eye is often more pigmented than that of the fellow eye. Funduscopy generally reveals evidence of a choroidal hemangioma and disc changes secondary to glaucoma. The etiology of glaucoma in Sturge-Weber syndrome is most often considered to be increased episcleral venous pressure secondary to the ipsilateral choroidal hemangioma, although congenitally abnormal angle structures may contribute to infant-onset disease (64,65).

Congenital or infancy-onset glaucoma in Sturge-Weber syndrome usually requires surgical intervention. Although goniosurgery is typically less effective than in cases of primary congenital glaucoma, IOP reduction has been reported with both trabeculotomy and combined trabeculotomy–trabeculectomy for these cases (66,67). Medication is the first-line treatment for glaucoma presenting after infancy, with aqueous suppressants the mainstay of therapy. While guarded trabeculectomy has been performed in these cases, success has also been reported with glaucoma implant surgery (68,69), as well as with careful cycloablation (70). In these eyes with choroidal hemangioma, rapid choroidal expansion and hemorrhage may complicate any intraocular surgery which decompresses the eye, either during or after the procedure; cilioretinal artery occlusion has also been reported after Baerveldt glaucoma implantation (71).

Neurofibromatosis

Neurofibromatosis type 1 (NF-1) is a common systemic disease transmitted by autosomal dominant inheritance. Expression of this disease is variable, as are the tissues affected. Skin involvement with cafe au lait spots is common but may not appear until the end of the first year of life. Lisch nodules appear on the iris in the majority of affected individuals, but often do not appear until puberty. Childhood glaucoma associated with this disease is congenital, rare, usually unilateral, and most often associated with a lid plexiform neuroma (72). Enlargement of the involved eye may be striking, suggesting other causes of accelerated growth in addition to glaucoma. The iris develops an ectropion uveae by the end of the first year of life, and the choroid often appears more densely pigmented than the contralateral structure. The angle shows a circumferential covering by an anterior extension of iris stromal tissue.

Several possible mechanisms of glaucoma in NF-1 have been proposed, including direct effects on the normal angle development, secondary changes to the angle tissue, as well as angle closure by thickened ciliary body and choroid or directly by fibrovascular tissue (73). NF-1 has been linked to the Neurofibromin gene, located on 17q11.2 (OMIM reference #162200) (74). The treatment of glaucoma associated with NF-1 is difficult, with angle surgery unlikely to be successful in glaucoma control. If medical therapy is unsuccessful, reasonable surgical options in the older child include filtration surgery, glaucoma implant surgery, or cycloablation.

Lowe (Oculocerebrorenal) Syndrome

This rare X-linked recessive disease is associated with a high incidence of bilateral glaucoma and cataracts. Affected children usually have associated mental retardation, renal rickets, aminoaciduria, hypotonia, acidemia, and irritability. Additional ophthalmic features of Lowe syndrome include microphthalmia, strabismus, nystagmus, miosis (rendering cataract removal difficult), and iris atrophy. Lowe syndrome has been linked to the locus Xq26.1 [OMIM reference #309000] (74,75). Gonioscopy does not show a characteristic angle anomaly; rather, the angle closely resembles that seen in patients with primary congenital open-angle glaucoma.

Treatment of this glaucoma is difficult, and medical control rarely proves adequate. Goniotomy surgery may be disappointing and is more frequently complicated by serious hemorrhage than when tried in primary congenital open-angle glaucoma (76). Judicious use of glaucoma drainage implant devices and cyclodestructive surgery may also be needed in cases refractory to medications (77–79).

Axenfeld-Rieger Syndrome

This condition represents a type of the anterior chamber cleavage disorder often associated with systemic abnormalities. The collective term Axenfeld-Rieger (A-R) syndrome includes all clinical variations within this spectrum of developmental anomalies (80). Regardless of ocular manifestations, all patients with A-R syndrome share the same general features: (a) a bilateral, developmental disorder of the eyes; (b) a frequent family history of the disorder, with an autosomal dominant mode of inheritance; (c) no sex predilection; (d) frequent systemic developmental defects; and (e) a high incidence of associated glaucoma. The iris may show hypoplasia of the anterior stromal leaf, iridotrabecular and iridocorneal processes, and posterior embryotoxon. Other deformities may occur in the iris, such as corectopia. Glaucoma is a common complication, occurring in more than 50% of cases, often in middle or late childhood. Dental anomalies in the form of oligodontia and anodontia, dysplasias of the skull and skeleton, and umbilical abnormalities are common.

Three chromosomal loci have recently been demonstrated to link to Axenfeld-Rieger syndrome and related phenotypes. These loci are on chromosomes 4q25, 6p25, and 13q14. The genes at chromosomes 4q25 and 6p25 have been identified as PITX2 and FOXC1, respectively (81). Mutations in these genes can cause a wide variety of phenotypes that share features with Axenfeld-Rieger syndrome (82). Genetically, the Axenfield-Rieger syndromes are considered in three types (OMIM#601542, 602482, and 601090) (82). There has been phenotype–genotype correlation between glaucoma severity and underlying genetic defects in Axenfeld-Rieger syndrome, with milder glaucoma in individuals with mutations in FOXC1 vs. more refractory glaucoma in those having either PITX2 defects or FOXC1 duplication (83).

Primary Pediatric Glaucoma Associated with Ocular Anomalies

Primary pediatric glaucomas may also be associated with other ocular anomalies. In some of these well-recognized disorders, systemic abnormalities may also occur.

Aniridia

Aniridia is a bilateral developmental disorder, characterized by the congenital absence of a normal iris; the iris is invariably partially absent, with a rudimentary stump of variable width. Glaucoma occurs in at least 50% of patients with aniridia. Aniridia is associated with multiple ocular defects, which variably manifest from birth to late childhood or teenage years. Some forms of aniridia also have associated systemic abnormalities.

Aniridia is inherited in an autosomal dominant fashion with almost complete penetrance in about two thirds of cases; the remaining cases are sporadic. This disorder has been associated with mutations in the PAX6 gene, located on chromosome 11p13 (locus symbol AN2), telomeric to the Wilms tumor predisposition gene (WT1)(74,82) [(OMIM reference #106210].

It has been reported that approximately 68% of patients with a deletion of chromosome 11 and aniridia will develop Wilms tumor before age 3 years (84).

The congenital ocular anomalies associated with aniridia include a small cornea, hypoplastic iris leaf, cataracts, macular hypoplasia, and filtration angle abnormalities. Progressive dystrophic ocular abnormalities occur in aniridia, causing corneal opacification, increased lens opacification, and glaucoma secondary to increased filtration angle abnormalities. On gonioscopy, progressive trabecular blockage by movement of the residual iris tissue in front of the trabeculum can usually be seen in most aniridia patients with glaucoma (85).

In aniridic infants with a family history of aniridic glaucoma, careful monitoring of the angle by serial gonioscopy is indicated, with consideration of prophylactic goniosurgery to prevent blockage of the trabecular meshwork if progressive abnormalities of the angle occur (86).

If significant glaucoma is present, medical therapy is appropriate. No single form of surgical treatment has been proven to be best for aniridic glaucoma. Goniotomy may be helpful in infantile cases. Trabeculectomy may be successful, but is particularly challenging due to the propensity of these eyes to develop postoperative flat anterior chambers. Glaucoma implant surgery and very careful cycloablation may be needed for particularly refractory cases (87–90).

Anterior Chamber Cleavage Syndrome (Iridocorneal Dysgenesis)

Malformations of the ocular anterior segment involving the cornea, angle, iris, and lens usually show evidence of incomplete formation of the anterior chamber cavity. Although there are variable phenotypes, several of these conditions may actually be allelic with the A-R syndrome. Axenfeld Anomaly, in which the filtration angle is partially obscured from view by attachments between the iris and a prominent Schwalbe line, is better considered as part of the A-R syndrome (see above).

Peters Anomaly

This variation of the so-called anterior chamber cleavage syndrome consists of a posterior defect in Descemet membrane associated with a leukoma in that area with attachment of the iris to much of the periphery of the corneal abnormality. The lens may also be involved, with cataract and/or attachment between the lens and the posterior corneal defect. The angle may also be defective, and glaucoma may develop in about 50% of cases.

Peters anomaly presents at birth, and is usually bilateral and sporadic. Although it typically occurs in the absence of additional abnormalities, associations with a wide range of systemic and other ocular anomalies have been reported (91). Because of the varied genetic and nongenetic patterns and the spectrum of ocular and systemic abnormalities, some consider Peters anomaly to be a morphologic finding rather than a distinct entity (92). Peters anomaly can be caused by mutations in the PAX6 gene, the PITX2 gene, the CYP1B1 gene, or the FOXC1 gene (82) (OMIM reference, #s 607108, 601542, 601771, 601090, respectively) (82).

Management of the glaucoma associated with Peters anomaly is often complicated by the presence of corneal opacity, cataract, and shallow or absent anterior chamber.

In these cases, where angle surgery is not feasible, medical therapy is the first-line treatment, followed by surgical treatment with glaucoma implant surgery and/or cycloablation. Repeated surgeries are often needed, often with an adverse effect on an existing corneal transplant. Phthisis and retinal detachment may result from a variety of mechanisms in these small, complex eyes (93). Corneal transplant should be avoided in favor of optical iridectomy in cases where corneal opacification is only partial, and a visual axis can be obtained without it (94–96). A recent published series of 47 children reported on 144 penetrating keratoplasty procedures; 29% of eyes had visual acuity better than 20/400, while 38% had light perception or no light perception. This series included only 14 eyes with glaucoma (97). While Zaidman reported reasonable visual outcomes after corneal transplant in mild Peters anomaly (lens not involved), his series also noted poorer outcomes in eyes with glaucoma (98) (Fig. 12.14).

Familial Hypoplasia of the Iris

Individuals with this rare cause of childhood glaucoma may have congenital hypoplasia of the iris but lack the anterior chamber abnormalities of the A-R syndrome. This autosomal dominant disorder (also termed iridogoniodysgenesis anomaly, type I), characterized by iris hypoplasia, goniodysgenesis, and juvenile glaucoma, has been mapped to gene locus 6p26 and appears due to mutations in the gene FKHL7. A similar condition has been identified, which includes nonocular features; this has been dubbed iridogoniodysgenesis type 2, maps to 4q25, results from mutations in the gene PITX2, and may be allelic to A-R syndrome (OMIM reference entries #6011631, #137600, respectively) (74). Treatment by goniotomy is sometimes successful in these cases.

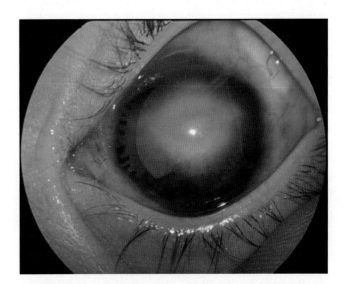

FIGURE 12.14. Left eye of an infant afflicted with severe bilateral Peters anomaly. After lowering of IOP by Ahmed glaucoma implant, an optical iridectomy has been performed, creating an imperfect visual axis in this phakic eye, without resorting to penetrating keratoplasty (which has already failed in the fellow eye). Vision corrects to 20/100.

Posterior Polymorphous Dystrophy

This spectrum of disorders is an autosomal dominant condition that is characteristically responsible for bilateral defects of the cornea at the level of Descemet membrane and usually has little effect on vision. A more severe expression of this disease presents in children from birth or early life, and is characterized by corneal opacification secondary to edema of the stroma and epithelium and opacification at the level of Descemet membrane. These abnormalities may be associated with the acute onset of light sensitivity during the first year of life, with or without complicating glaucoma. In some affected individuals, corneal changes are associated with peripheral iridocorneal adhesions, iris atrophy, and corectopia. Glaucoma occurs in about 15% of patients with posterior polymorphous dystrophy, in both the presence and apparent absence of iridocorneal adhesions. The genetically heterogeneous disorder has been mapped to mutations in the VSX1 gene (chromosome 20p (OMIM reference #605020), in the COL8A2 gene on chromosome 1p34.3 (OMIM #120252), and in the ZEB1 gene on chromosome 10p (OMIM # 189909) (74,82).

SECONDARY CHILDHOOD GLAUCOMA

Pediatric glaucoma may occur secondary to a wide variety of ophthalmic conditions (see Table 12.1). Secondary glaucoma is a complication of another eye disease rather than a primary disorder of the aqueous humor filtration mechanism.

Trauma

The most important glaucoma in children following injury is that caused by an acute or secondary hemorrhage into the anterior chamber (hyphema). This may occur acutely in association with blunt injury, but is more commonly seen 1 to 3 days after the injury in association with a secondary hemorrhage or with a very large initial hyphema. Children with significant trauma to the eye should be examined promptly for evidence of serious injury. The finding of a gross hyphema increases the likelihood of secondary hemorrhage. Such patients are placed at rest and treated with topical steroids and cycloplegics, with avoidance of acetylsalicylic acid. Serial examination including IOP measurement is important, especially in children with sickle cell hemoglobinopathies, where moderate IOP rise may result in significant optic nerve damage (99). There are conflicting reports regarding the use of various agents to reduce the risk of rebleeding, including oral steroids, and antifibrinolytic agents (most notably aminocaproic acid) (100). The occurrence of glaucoma secondary to recurrent hemorrhage can be both painful and damaging. Medical glaucoma treatment and anterior chamber irrigation for persistent glaucoma may be required. IOP usually normalizes after resolution of acute hyphema; however, such eyes need long-term follow-up for the development of angle-recession glaucoma, which may be delayed many years in onset (101).

Neoplasm

The most common cause of glaucoma secondary to neoplasia is retinoblastoma. Its occurrence usually is not associated with the presence of tumor cells in the anterior chamber but rather is secondary to rubeosis iridis and/or angle closure. Such eyes usually show advanced posterior segment tumor growth and require enucleation. Medulloepithelioma, a neoplasm of the ciliary epithelium, can also induce secondary neovascular glaucoma.

Juvenile xanthogranuloma is a rare condition associated with histiocytic infiltration of the iris. Glaucoma may occur secondary to the accumulation of histiocytes in the angle structures or secondary to spontaneous hyphema formation. Treatment is usually medical. Acetazolamide may be necessary for better control of the IOP, and systemic and topical steroids should be used to treat the histiocyte accumulation. Difficult cases may require surgical intervention in the form of glaucoma implant and/or cycloablation (102).

Inflammation

Acute or chronic glaucoma in children may occur secondary to inflammation. When acute, the blockage of aqueous humor outflow is usually secondary to iris bombe formation and angle closure.

Chronic glaucoma secondary to inflammation is more common than the acute form and may be asymptomatic. It is most often seen with chronic anterior uveitis, which may be associated with signs of juvenile rheumatoid arthritis or chronic cyclitis. The possible adverse effect of steroid medication on the glaucoma must also be considered. Treatment of acute glaucoma associated with iris bombe is usually surgical, to produce an iridotomy or iridectomy. Synecholysis may be necessary to open the angle, even after pupillary block is relieved. Both goniotomy and medical treatment of chronic open-angle glaucoma secondary to iritis are helpful for treatment of this condition; tube implant surgery has also been reported quite successful in refractory cases (103–109).

Lens-Induced Glaucoma

Children with ectopia lentis (from a variety of causes, e.g., homocystinuria, Weill-Marchesani, Marfan syndrome) may develop acute glaucoma secondary to forward shifting of the lens into the papillary aperture, with resultant pupillary block and angle closure. This glaucoma is acute, painful, and often associated with vomiting and high IOP. Nonsurgical treatment of this acute glaucoma includes: placing the patient supine, manual displacement of the lens posteriorly in the eye, using a muscle hook (often with a bandage contact lens placed), medication with aqueous suppressants, mydriatics, and analgesics, and post-episode use of miotics.

Iridectomy performed at a later time will prevent the acute glaucoma but may not prevent displacement of the lens into the pupil and the anterior chamber (110). Surgical lensectomy, for repeated cases, is more safely accomplished after IOP has been normalized.

Aphakic Glaucoma (Glaucoma Following Cataract Removal in Childhood)

Glaucoma is quite common after removal of congenital or developmental cataracts (reported incidence from 3% to 41%) and is usually of the open-angle type, although cases of angle-closure glaucoma have also been reported (usually associated with forward movement of the vitreous face, and/or iris bombe from pupil seclusion). Children with cataract removal at an early age, those associated with microphthalmia, and those with persistent fetal vasculature, are at higher risk for glaucoma after lens removal. The onset of open-angle glaucoma after cataract removal is often delayed by many years and may be asymptomatic (111,112). The angle, while open, demonstrates typical abnormalities not present before cataract removal (113). Peripheral iridectomy (with or without vitrectomy) can be curative in angle-closure cases. Medical therapy is the first-line treatment for cases of open-angle glaucoma in aphakia. Angle surgery is not usually successful in these cases (114), but glaucoma implant surgery, and cycloablation may be successful in selected refractory cases (115,116). Primary or secondary intraocular lens implantation does not have an obvious impact, either causative or protective, with regard to associated glaucoma. The mechanism of aphakic glaucoma is not known, although several disparate theories each have their proponents.

Miscellaneous Causes

Secondary glaucoma in children may occur after use of steroid eye drops, and as a complication of retinopathy of prematurity. It may also occur secondary to prenatal infection with rubella virus and manifests as a congenital glaucoma or may occur later in childhood. Other rarer causes have also been noted.

In summary, the causes of secondary childhood glaucoma are extensive, and this possibility must be considered frequently in pediatric ophthalmology. Determining the mechanism of glaucoma in each given case helps the physician to outline the optimal treatment strategy for that particular child.

TREATMENT

As with adult glaucoma, the success of pediatric glaucoma treatment depends on early diagnosis and adequate IOP control. The specific therapy is determined by the type of glaucoma present. Both medical treatment and surgery are often used.

Medical Management

Although surgical management is still the first-line treatment for many children with glaucoma, medical therapy plays an ever-important role in the management of many childhood glaucomas. Hence, surgery is indicated for most cases of primary congenital glaucoma (usually angle surgery), and all angle-closure glaucomas, while medical therapy is the initial first treatment for juvenile and aphakic open-angle glaucoma, as well as most causes of secondary open-angle glaucoma (see above). In the past decade, tremendous advances in pharmacologic therapy of glaucoma have increased the options for medical treatment of childhood glaucoma. However, all currently FDA-approved hypotensive drugs achieved that approval without safety or efficacy testing in the pediatric population. Clinical experience has proven the worth of some drugs, while highlighting the significant dangers of others when used in infants and young children. Besides inadequate IOP reduction, multiple factors conspire against the success of long-term medical therapy of children with glaucoma: The difficulties with long-term compliance, adequate ascertainment of drug-induced side effects, and potential adverse systemic effects of protracted therapy are among the many obstacles to the success of long-term medical therapy.

The glaucoma drugs can be divided into five main categories. The following brief descriptions and comments regarding their use in children will hopefully guide the clinician who uses medications to treat children with glaucoma.

Carbonic Anhydrase Inhibitors

Oral carbonic anhydrase inhibitors, primarily acetazolamide (Diamox), have effectively reduced elevated IOP in infants and children with primary infantile (and other types of) glaucoma for decades, and often reduce IOP in these patients by about 20% to 35 %. Acetazolamide should be given orally with food or milk three times daily, at a dose range of 10 to 20 mg/kg/day. Notable side effects include diarrhea, diminished energy levels, and loss of appetite and weight. Metabolic acidosis may develop in infants, often manifest in infants as tachypnea, and treatable with oral sodium citrate and citric acid oral solution (Bicitra, 1 mEq/kg/day).

Two topical carbonic anhydrase inhibitors are now available—dorzolamide (Trusopt) and brinzolamide (Azopt). These two drugs offer a viable alternative to acetazolamide, with little to no occurrence of systemic side effects. The combination of dorzolamide and oral acetazolamide has been reported, in selected cases, to reduce IOP further than when either drug is used alone (117). Both dorzolamide and brinzolamide should be dosed twice daily (or three times daily for maximal effect), and produce similar IOP reduction, with slightly less ocular stinging reported from brinzolamide (author's personal experience).

The carbonic anhydrase inhibitors are very useful drugs for treating pediatric glaucoma patients, and may be appropriate first- and second-line agents, respectively, in cases where beta blocker use is contraindicated, or inadequate (see Table 12.3).

Table 12.3		
GUIDE TO THE USE OF TOPICAL GLAUCOMA MEDICATIONS IN PEDIATRIC GLAUCOMA		
Medication (*Class*, Name)	**Indications**	**Contraindications/Side Effects**
Beta Blockers Nonselective (timolol) Selective (betaxolol) (possibly safer with asthma)	First line for many, second line for some older children	Systemic effects: bronchospasm, bradycardia; avoid in premature or tiny infants, any history of reactive airways; start with 0.25% in higher risk children
Carbonic Anhydrase Inhibitors Topical (dorzolamide, brinzolamide)	First or second line in young children, add well to other classes	Systemically safe; may wish to avoid or use as later option in children with compromised corneas, especially with corneal transplant
Miotics Echothiophate iodide Pilocarpine	Echothiophate rarely used in aphakia; pilocarpine after angle surgery and some JOAG	Systemic effects (echothiophate): diarrhea (sometimes), interaction with succinyl choline for general anesthesia, possible pro-inflammatory effect; (both) headache; (both) myopic shift

Adrenergic Agonists
 	
Epinephrine compounds
 	
Alpha-2 agonists
 	
  -Apraclonidine (0.5%)
 	
  -Brimonidine (0.1%, 0.15%, 0.2%)
	Not very useful
	
	During/after angle surgery; short term in infants and after corneal transplant
	
	Only in older children!!! Second or third line in JOAG, aphakia, older children with other glaucoma types
		Systemic effects: hypertension, tachycardia
		
		Systemically safe; effect may wear off; rarely local allergy or red eye
		
		DO NOT USE IN INFANTS/SMALL CHILDREN < ~40 pounds (may cause bradycardia, hypotension, hypothermia, hypotonia, apnea (especially if used with beta blocker)

Prostaglandins and similar Latanoprost; travoprost; bimatoprost; unoprostone	First, second, or third line in JOAG; usually second or third line after beta blockers and topical CAIs in others	Systemically safe; grows long, thick, eyelashes; may darken periorbital skin; may cause redness; use with caution or avoid in uveitic glaucoma

Miotics

Miotic drugs (cholinergic stimulators) have largely been supplanted by newer medications, in the treatment of both adults and children with glaucoma. Pilocarpine retains its usefulness to induce and maintain miosis before and after goniotomy or trabeculotomy for congenital glaucoma. Stronger miotics such as echothiophate iodide (Phospholine Iodide) have also been useful in selected cases of aphakic glaucoma.

Beta-Adrenergic Antagonists (Beta Blockers)

Topical beta blockers are effective aqueous suppressants, and play an important role in the treatment of children with glaucoma. Most published studies have examined the effects of timolol, the first topical beta blocker to become available (in 1978). Although beta blockers are well tolerated from an ocular point of view, systemic side effects—most notably bradycardia and respiratory distress due to apnea or asthma exacerbation—have been reported in a minority of children treated with timolol (118). Topical beta blockers should be used with extreme caution (or not at all) in neonates. When used in small children, timolol treatment should always begin with 0.25% drops, excluding those children with a history of asthma or bradycardia; punctal occlusion should be performed when possible (119). Based on experience in adults, betaxolol, as a relatively beta 1-selective agent, may be less prone to precipitating acute asthma attacks (which may present as coughing) than the nonselective beta blockers. A recent randomized prospective study demonstrated that betaxolol and timolol gel-forming solution (0.25% and 0.5%) were all well tolerated and produced modest but statistically significant decreases in IOP in pediatric glaucoma patients younger than 6 years old (120). Beta blockers are usually additive to carbonic anhydrase inhibitors in treating children with glaucoma. Topical beta blockers have an important role in treating children with glaucoma, and are appropriate first-line drugs for many (Table 12.3).

Adrenergic Agonists

Epinephrine compounds—with significant systemic and ocular side effects, coupled with limited effectiveness—have little place in the current treatment of adults and children with glaucoma. Two alpha-2 agonists (apraclonidine and brimonidine) are currently approved for treating adults with glaucoma. Apraclonidine has been safely used for the short-term treatment of children undergoing angle surgery without significant systemic side effects (121). This medication may also have a role in the short-term treatment of infants and small children who cannot tolerate beta blockers, or who have had recent corneal transplantation, and in whom one therefore wishes to avoid topical carbonic anhydrase inhibitors (personal unpublished data).

Brimonidine (currently available as Alphagan P 0.15% and brimonidine 0.2%) can be useful in reducing IOP in older children, but must be used with extreme caution in younger children. Topical brimonidine use has produced life-threatening systemic side effects in infants (bradycardia, hypotension, hypothermia, hypotonia, and apnea), and severe somnolence in toddlers (122). Concurrent use of a topical beta blocker may increase the systemic risk of brimonidine exposure in infants (123). Even older children placed on brimonidine should be warned of its propensity to cause fatigue (124). Brimonidine is rarely an appropriate first-line drug for children, but may be a useful adjunctive therapy in those older children needing additional IOP reduction (Table 12.3).

Prostaglandins

The newest class of drugs for glaucoma treatment are the prostaglandin-like drugs, which lower IOP primarily by enhancing the outflow of aqueous humor through the non-trabecular uveoscleral pathway. In a randomized, double-masked trial of latanoprost and timolol monotherapy in children with pediatric glaucoma, latanoprost was found to be at least as effective as timolol, and both produced clinically significant IOP reduction across glaucoma diagnoses (125). In a retrospective study of latanoprost (Xalatan) use for varied pediatric glaucomas, "responder rates" were highest among children with JOAG (126). Selected cases of juvenile onset glaucoma secondary to Sturge-Weber syndrome have also responded well to latanoprost therapy (127). While no serious systemic side effects have been reported in children, exuberant lengthening and darkening of eyelashes occurs frequently, with increased iris pigmentation and aphakic cystoid macular edema not yet reported (128). Travoprost, in a retrospective study, was found to be well tolerated by children and to reduce IOP in select cases of pediatric glaucoma (primarily eyes that were already

receiving medications) (129). No published series using the other drugs in this group (bimatoprost and unoprostone) have yet been reported to our knowledge. All drugs in this class can produce eye redness, growth of eyelashes, and increased pigmentation around the eyes. They should be used with extreme caution in cases of uveitis, and have produced cystoid macular edema in aphakic/pseudophakic eyes of adults (130). Prostaglandin-like agents may be appropriate first-line agents for older children with glaucoma, especially JOAG, but may not yet be appropriate as first-line treatment for most children (Table 12.3).

Surgical Management

Glaucoma surgery is indicated as primary treatment for primary congenital glaucoma, angle-closure glaucoma, and other cases of childhood glaucoma where medical therapy has failed to adequately control IOP. While the appropriate intervention (angle surgery) is widely agreed upon in the case of primary congenital glaucoma, the optimal surgical algorithm is, in numerous circumstances, open to disagreement, even among experts in the care of these children. The diversity of opinions on the optimal surgical algorithm for pediatric glaucoma undoubtedly relates to the challenges inherent in the surgical management of these children, and in the often suboptimal outcomes of such surgery.

Surgical interventions used for pediatric glaucoma can be broadly divided into these categories: angle surgery (goniotomy or trabeculotomy), filtering surgery (trabeculectomy +/− antifibrotic agents), glaucoma drainage device (seton) surgery, cycloablation (cryotherapy or using laser), and others (such as peripheral iridectomy, combined trabeculotomy/trabeculectomy). Finally, enucleation may be the appropriate procedure for blind, disfigured, and painful eyes. While most surgical procedures used in children with glaucoma are similar to those regularly applied to adult glaucoma patients, angle surgery (goniotomy and trabeculotomy) is used almost exclusively in children, and deserves special mention.

Goniotomy

Goniotomy, a procedure in which the uveal trabecular meshwork is incised under direct visualization, is the surgical procedure of choice in most cases of primary congenital glaucoma. Trabeculotomy ab externo (see below), an alternative and equally effective procedure, is especially useful when corneal clouding prevents an optimal view of the angle structures by gonioscopy. The discovery of the benefit of goniotomy by Barkan (131) represents the most significant advance that has occurred in the surgical management of this condition, and ~70 % of children may be cured by this procedure (Figs. 12.15 and 12.16) (131). Goniotomy also deserves special consideration as a prophylactic procedure in congenital aniridia (132).

Various modifications have been used for performing this simple, but elegant procedure. Common to all of them are: fixation of the globe, magnification and light source

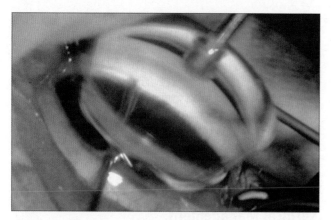

FIGURE 12.15. Goniotomy. Actual surgical photograph of goniotomy surgery. Fixation of the eye is obtained by the assistant grasping the tenon's insertion near the limbus at the 6- and 12-o'clock positions. A Barkan goniotomy lens is shown (modified by addition of a handle), cushioned on healon, and held in place by the surgeon. The cleft is being made with a 25-gauge needle, beginning to the left side of the angle.

(loupes or microscope), operating goniotomy lens, and a sharp instrument for incision (goniotomy knife or disposable needle). The ability to view the angle intended for surgery is critical to the goniotomy surgery. Corneal clearing is promoted by preoperative treatment with aqueous suppressant drugs for several days, and with Apraclonidine 0.5%, Pilocarpine 2%, and sodium chloride 5% drops upon entry to the operating room.

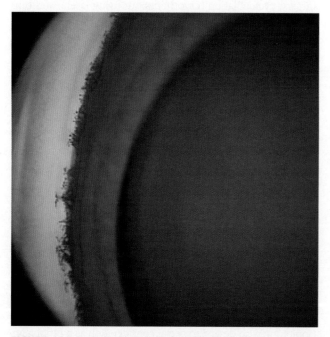

FIGURE 12.16. Goniophotograph showing cleft seen after successful goniotomy surgery in a darkly pigmented eye with primary infantile glaucoma. Note the fine lace-like anterior synechiae bridging the ciliary body band and extending over the cleft in the trabecular meshwork.

One technique involves the use of a modified Barkan goniotomy lens (with a handle), placed onto the cornea on a cushion of Healon. The surgeon sits opposite the angle to be operated (e.g., on the temporal side for nasal goniotomy), using the microscope tilted about 45 degrees from the vertical. The assistant fixates the eye with locking forceps placed on the Tenon's insertion near the limbus at 6- and 12-o'clock for a nasal or temporal goniotomy, and the head is slightly turned away from the surgeon. A 25-gauge disposable needle on a syringe filled with miochol or viscoelastic is used to enter the peripheral clear cornea opposite the intended angle surgery, and the needle is carefully guided over the iris to engage the trabecular meshwork in its anterior one-third. The needle is carefully passed first in one direction, and then in the other, with slight rotation of the eye by the assistant to maximize the incised angle tissue. A cleft should be seen in the wake of the incision, and often the peripheral iris will move slightly posteriorly in the case of congenital glaucoma. The needle is then carefully withdrawn after injection of a small amount of viscoelastic near the entry point, and the entry is closed with a single suture of 10-0 vicryl suture. Approximately 4 to 5 clock hours of angle can be opened in this way. Bleeding, while common, is minimized by refilling the eye to a normal pressure prior to suture closure, with use of a filtered air bubble if the patient is not due to fly in an airplane within 72 hours after surgery. Subconjunctival antibiotic may be used. Postoperatively, antibiotic, steroid, and miotics (except in uveitic glaucoma) are used for various time periods by different surgeons.

Endoscopic goniotomy in children with opaque corneas has shown potential for IOP reduction in a small series, but larger studies are necessary to demonstrate safety and IOP reduction when compared to other surgical alternatives (133,134). There is no clear indication for use of the Trabectome® (NeoMedix Corporation, Tustin, CA) at this time for angle surgery in pediatric eyes (135).

The results of goniotomy surgery are best—reportedly from 70 up to more than 90%—in patients with primary congenital open-angle glaucoma who possess a less severe angle anomaly and who are recognized between 3 and 12 months of age. Newborn patients who are found to have glaucoma because of enlarged and cloudy corneas often possess a more severe angle defect and do significantly less well with goniotomy surgery. Patients found to have primary congenital open-angle glaucoma later in childhood also do less well with goniotomy, possibly as a result of damage to the filtration mechanism caused by the chronic elevation of IOP.

Trabeculotomy Ab Externo

In this procedure, Schlemm canal is identified by radial incision in the bed of a partial-thickness scleral flap, cannulated, and opened from the outside inward, tearing through the poorly functioning trabecular meshwork in that area (136,137) (Fig. 12.17). Standard trabeculotomy uses a stiff

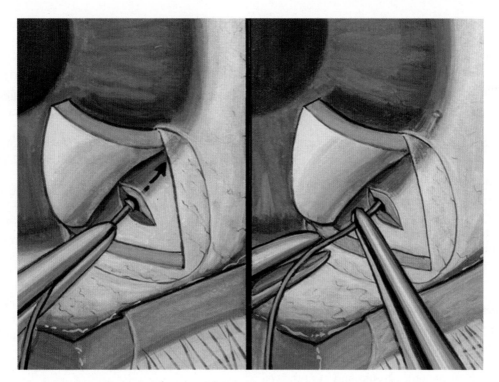

FIGURE 12.17. Suture trabeculotomy, left eye. *Left panel,* A fornix-based flap is made inferotemporal at the limbus. A 3 × 3 mm wide limbus-based scleral flap is made extending one half to two thirds the thickness of the sclera. A radial scratch incision is made in the base of the sclera flap bed, and gradually deepened, until the Schlemm canal is located. A blunted 6-0 prolene suture is shown entering the cut end of Schlemm canal. *Left panel,* The blunted prolene suture is advanced into the canal. If the suture can be advanced for 360 degrees, it can be retrieved from the other cut end of Schlemm canal, and then the two ends pulled to "cheese-wire" an opening for 360-degrees. The same procedure can also be completed by confirming the canal location with the suture, followed by its cannulation using an illuminated catheter (the iScience® microcatheter [iScience Interventional, Menlo Park, CA]). (Modified from medical illustration by Tom Waldrup, from Freedman SF. Medical and surgical treatments for childhood glaucoma, Figure 40.5. In: Rand R, Allingham RR, Damji KF, Freedman SF, Moroi S, Saranov, eds. *Shields textbook of glaucoma,* 6th Ed. Philadelphia, PA: Wolters Kluwer Health/Lippincott Williams & Wilkins, 2011.)

curved metal trabeculotome to tear through the inner wall of Schlemm canal, opening a comparable portion of the angle to goniotomy. A modification, suture trabeculotomy, involves the threading of a flexible 6-0 prolene suture into Schlemm canal for 180- or 360-degrees; when the suture is then pulled taut, the angle is opened up to 360-degrees (Fig. 12.18) (138,139). A recent modification in the trabeculotomy technique involves the use of the iScience® microcatheter (iScience Interventional, Menlo Park, CA) to cannulate Schlemm canal. The illuminated fiber-optic tip is visible through the scleral wall, allowing for visualization of the cannulation process, and theoretically facilitating the success of a 360-degree trabeculotomy (140). While these procedures produce excellent success in uncomplicated cases of primary congenital open-angle glaucoma, they have not been compared against each other, or against goniotomy, in a randomized prospective fashion. Advantages to trabeculotomy include its similarity to trabeculectomy for surgeons comfortable with the prior procedure, the theoretical ability to cannulate the entire angle in one surgery, and the ability

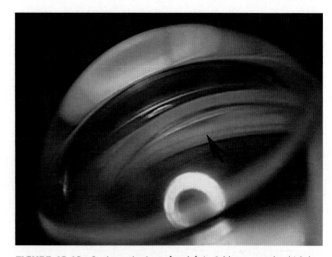

FIGURE 12.18. Gonioscopic view of a cleft in Schlemm canal, which has been created using the 360-degree Trabeculotomy described in Figure 12.17. This is the eye of a 6-year-old boy with pseudophakia and glaucoma developing 4 years after the removal of congenital cataracts in both eyes. The pressure is controlled on one drop, now 2 years post trabeculotomy surgery.

to perform the surgery in the absence of an angle view. Disadvantages include the need to incise conjunctiva and sclera, and the possibility of being unable to locate or cannulate Schlemm canal. Viscocanalostomy has been used for cases of primary congenital glaucoma, with reported short-term success (141).

Combined Trabeculotomy—Trabeculectomy

Some surgeons advocate the combined use of trabeculotomy and trabeculectomy in cases resistant to goniotomy, or in selected populations where birth presentation, severely opaque corneas, and poor prior success with primary trabeculotomy have been reported. These surgeons report excellent success with this technique in selected cases.

Trabeculectomy (Filtering Surgery)

This procedure bypasses the resistance of the angle tissues by excising them under a partial thickness scleral flap, creating a filtering bleb of aqueous fluid, which seeps out through the overlying tenon's capsule and conjunctival layers. This procedure is usually reserved for cases having failed, or likely to fail, angle surgery. As might be expected from the exuberant healing response in young children, simple trabeculectomy has a very low success rate in infants and children in most published series. The use of the antifibrotic agents 5-fluorouracil and mitomycin-C has improved the success of trabeculectomy in adults and in young patients, but at an increased risk of later bleb leak and infection (49,142,143). Variable doses of mitomycin, ranging from 0.2 to 0.5 mg/mL have been applied to the sclera for variable time periods, with little evidence supporting a single dosing strategy. Most pediatric glaucoma surgeons have long used a limbus-based conjunctival incision for trabeculectomy; now several advocate fornix-based incisions (personal communication). Even with the use of mitomycin, infants younger than age 1 to 2 years, and aphakic children do not fare well with trabeculectomy (46,47,144–147). Children with successful filtering blebs must be diligently observed for any signs of bleb leak or infection, as the risk of this occurrence may be cumulative over time. Fibrosis and loss of IOP control can likewise occur years after successful filtration surgery in children. There is no data to support the use of the metal EX-PRESS™ Glaucoma Filtration device (Alcon Laboratories Inc, Fort Worth, TX) in pediatric eyes at this time; indeed, the use of a metal implant to maintain an internal sclerostomy is questionable at best, since the usual site of filtration failure is at the level of the scleral flap or tenon's capsule. There are a few reports of viscocanalostomy and/or deep sclerectomy, some combined with trabeculectomy for refractory pediatric cases, and time will tell whether these modifications are an improvement over current surgical options for these eyes (147). In infants, aphakic eyes, and children at especially high risk for inadequate

infection precautions, alternative surgical strategies may be warranted (see later).

Glaucoma Drainage Device (Seton) Surgery

This surgery involves the placement of a flexible tube into the eye to conduct aqueous humor posteriorly to a plate sewn against the sclera, which becomes encapsulated to form a posterior reservoir, out of which aqueous then percolates into surrounding tissues (Figs. 12.19 and 12.20). While the Molteno (Molteno Ophthalmic Limited, Dunedin, New Zealand) valve implant was used in children for nearly two decades, the Baerveldt (Abbott Medical Optics, Abbott Park, Il) and the Ahmed (New World Medical, Inc. Rancho Cucamonga, CA) glaucoma implants are now more commonly used. Several of the glaucoma drainage devices have undergone modifications in recent years, including the flexible plate Ahmed (FP-7) and the larger Molteno 3 plate). Reported success and complications rates vary widely (52–55,148). Although common problems with the use of drainage implants in children include tube malposition and encapsulation of the reservoir (the latter with elevation of IOP), numerous other complications including fibrovascular ingrowth (Ahmed plates only), motility disturbance, anterior segment and posterior segment complications have been reported, as with this procedure in adult patients. The incidence of endophthalmitis, while non-zero, does seem lower with this procedure than with mitomycin-augmented trabeculectomy in children. However, the final IOP achieved after drainage implant surgery is not as low as after successful filtering surgery, and at least 50% of cases require continued adjunctive medication. Several authors have reviewed moderately large series of refractory pediatric glaucoma patients treated with glaucoma drainage devices; reported success is variable, but 5-year success has been in the range of 60%, with acceptably low rates of visually-devastating complications (56,57,149–151). One series reported both cyclophotocoagulation and a second glaucoma drainage device were both modestly successful (~60% at 24 months) in cases with inadequate IOP control after a single glaucoma drainage device (152). In another reported series, drainage implant surgery appeared more successful at IOP control than did trabeculectomy, for children below the age of 2 years (153).

Cycloablation

In contrast to all the procedures described above, cyclodestructive procedures reduce the rate of aqueous production by injuring the ciliary processes; results are often unpredictable, and complications frequent. Once medical and other surgical means have been exhausted or have proven inadequate to the task, cyclodestruction nonetheless constitutes a valid means of attempting control of otherwise vision-threatening glaucoma in children.

Cyclocryotherapy (freezing the ciliary processes from an external approach) has been used as therapy for difficult childhood glaucomas for many years and is applied

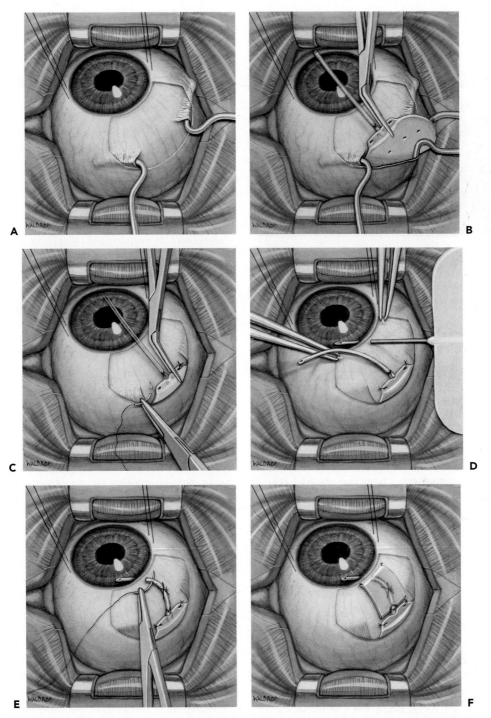

FIGURE 12.19. Technique of glaucoma drainage implant surgery in children. This procedure may also be performed through a fornix incision, without changing any other portion of the procedure. **A:** Surgeon's view of the right eye. A traction suture of 7-0 vicryl has been placed through the limbal tissue/peripheral cornea at the 2- and 8-o'clock positions. A conjunctival peritomy has been made from 9- to 12-o'clock, with a radial wing on each end. A muscle hook has been placed under the superior and lateral rectus muscles to expose the superotemporal quadrant. **B:** Baerveldt glaucoma implant (size 250 mm²) is being placed into the superotemporal quadrant against the sclera. The tubing of the implant has been completely ligated 1 mm from the anterior edge of the reservoir, using a 6-0 vicryl suture. A muscle hook retracts the conjunctiva and tenon's capsule, as the superior wing of the reservoir enters the space just behind the superior rectus insertion. **C:** Final position of the Baerveldt reservoir, being secured into place with 8-0 nylon suture through the anterior positioning holes of the plate, 6 to 8 mm from the limbus. **D:** The eye is stabilized with forceps at the limbus, while a 23-gauge needle enters the anterior chamber parallel to the iris, and almost parallel to the superior limbus. The tube of the Baerveldt implant has been trimmed to its desired length with a bevel up. **E:** The Baerveldt tube has been placed into the anterior chamber through the 23-gauge needle tract, and is secured in place with a figure-of-eight suture of 9-0 nylon. The 9-0 nylon needle is then used to create several "venting slits" in the tubing anterior to its ligature. **F:** A patch graft of donor sclera is fashioned to cover the Baerveldt tubing at its entry site into the eye. Care is taken not to cover the 6-0 vicryl suture around the tubing. The scleral patch graft is secured with 8-0 vicryl suture. (Illustration by Tom Waldrup).

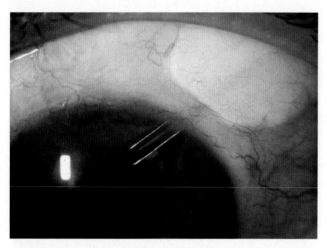

FIGURE 12.20. Right eye of a girl with uveitic glaucoma and pseudophakia, showing tube of Ahmed glaucoma implant (and sclera patch graft) placed 6 years earlier. Note the peaked pupil, which developed slowly over several years, despite good control of intraocular pressure and uveitis.

with a similar technique to that used in adults. Success of this procedure is modest at best, with repeat sessions frequently needed, and with an appreciable incidence of devastating complications such as phthisis and severe visual loss reported in up to 15%. In children, cryotherapy should be applied to a maximum of 180 degrees of the circumference of the eye at one session, using six or seven freezes (30 to 45 seconds each at –80°C) with the anterior edge of a 2.5-mm diameter cryoprobe placed 1 to 1.5 mm from the limbus (in a non-buphthalmic eye) (88,154). This technique is perhaps best reserved for refractory cases where cycloablation is indicated, but where anatomic considerations make laser modalities unlikely to be effective (see below).

Laser Cyclophotocoagulation (Transscleral and Endoscopic). Transscleral laser to the ciliary processes has been performed in children using both the Nd:YAG sapphire probe as well as the diode laser G-probe. These techniques have met with modest success (reported at ~50%, with retreatments in most cases), seem to produce less severe pain and inflammation than cyclocryotherapy, and may have a lower incidence of phthisis and severe complications seen with cyclocryotherapy. Limitations include loss of effect over time, inaccurate placement of the laser energy from an external approach in eyes which often have unusual anterior segment anatomy (155–157). This procedure may be reasonable adjunctive

treatment after a glaucoma drainage device has incompletely controlled the IOP (152).

Endoscopic cyclophotocoagulation has recently been applied in children with refractory glaucoma, using the diode laser and a microendoscopic system with a 20-gauge probe (Microprobe (Endo Optiks, Little Silver, NJ). This procedure allows direct application of laser energy to the intended target of the ciliary processes and may produce less inflammation than either cyclocryotherapy or transscleral cycloablation. However, this procedure has only modest reported success, with retreatment often needed. Hence cumulative success of all procedures at last follow-up was 43% in a reported series of 36 eyes, after a mean cumulative arc of treatment of 260 degrees, with mean follow-up time 19 months. Retinal detachment, hypotony, and visual loss were reported in this series, which included both aphakic and phakic eyes (58). A series of children who underwent endocyclophotocoagulation for aphakic or pseudophakic glaucoma demonstrated a similar success rate of 38% after one treatment (116). This technique may have application as an adjunct after inadequate IOP control in eyes having glaucoma drainage device implantation (personal unpublished data).

Long-Term Follow-Up of Children with Glaucoma

All children with glaucoma require lifetime follow-up. The older child/young adult may suffer asymptomatic loss of IOP control months or even decades after initial successful surgery; progressive changes such as cataract or corneal decompensation may occur many years after initial presentation of glaucoma. Children with functioning filtering surgery or glaucoma drainage devices must be followed for complications specific to these surgeries. The target pressure must be reassessed if progressive optic nerve or visual field changes occur despite previously acceptable levels of IOP control. In addition, young children with glaucoma often face vision-threatening difficulties such as corneal scarring, anisometropia, and resultant amblyopia even after IOP control has been achieved. Children with glaucoma that is controlled without medications should be followed at least every 6 months, and young children, or those whose IOP has been controlled for less than 2 years, should probably be evaluated at least every 3 or 4 months. Despite tremendous advances in the treatment of childhood glaucomas, many children still suffer permanent visual loss from these serious diseases.

REFERENCES

1. Papadopoulos M, Cable N, Rahi J, Khaw PT. The British Infantile and Childhood Glaucoma (BIG) Eye Study. *Invest Ophthalmol Vis Sci* Sep 2007;48(9):4100–4106.
2. Yeung HH, Walton DS. Clinical classification of childhood glaucomas. *Arch Ophthalmol* June 2010;128(6):680–684.
3. DeLuise VP, Anderson DR. Primary infantile glaucoma (Congenital glaucoma). *Surv Ophthalmol* 1983;28:1–18.
4. Chandler PA, Grant WM. *Glaucoma.* Philadelphia, PA: Lea and Febiger, 1980.
5. Van Buskirk EM, Plamer EA. Office assessment of young children for glaucoma. *Ann Ophthalmol* 1979;11:1749.

6. Minckler DS, Baerveldt G, Heuer DK, Quillan-Thomas B, Walonker AF, et al. Clinical evaluation of the Oculab tono-pen. *Amer J Ophthalmol* 1987;104:168–173.

7. Flemmons MS, Hsiao YC, Dzau J, Asrani S, Jones S, Freedman SF. Icare rebound tonometry in children with known and suspected glaucoma. *J AAPOS* Apr 2011;15(2):153–157.

8. Flemmons MS, Hsiao YC, Dzau J, Asrani S, Jones S, Freedman SF. Home tonometry for management of pediatric glaucoma. *Am J Ophthalmol* Sep 2011;152(3):470–478.e2.

9. Watcha MF, Chu FC, Stevens JL, Forestner JE. Effects of halothane on intraocular pressure in anesthetized children. *Anesth Analg* 1990;71:181–184.

10. Murphy DF. Anesthesia and intraocular pressure. *Anesth Analg* 1985;64:520–530.

11. Dominiguez A, Banos MS, Alvare MG, Contra GF, Quintela FB. Intraocular pressure measurement in infants under general anesthesia. *Am J Ophthalmol* 1974;78:110–116.

12. Ausinsch B, Rayburn RL, Munson ES, Levy NS. Ketamine and intraocular pressure in children. *Anesth Analg* 1976;55:773–775.

13. Jaafar MS, Ghulamqadir AK. Effect of oral chloral hydrate sedation on the intraocular pressure measurement. *J Ped Ophthalmol Strabismus* 1993;30:372–376.

14. Pensiero S, DaPozza S, Perissutti P, Cavallini GM, Guerra R. Normal intraocular pressure in children. *J Pediatr Ophthalmol Strabismus* 1992;29:79–84.

15. Sampaolesi R, Caruso R. Ocular echometry in the diagnosis of congenital glaucoma. *Arch Ophthalmol* 1982;100(4):574–577.

16. Becker B, Shaffer RN. *Diagnosis and therapy of the glaucomas.* St. Louis, MO: C.V. Mosby, 1965.

17. Kiskis AA, Markowitz SN, Morin JD. Corneal diameter and axial length in congenital glaucoma. *Can J Opthhalmol* 1985;20:93.

18. Walton DS. Primary congenital open-angle glaucoma. In: Chandler PA, Grant WM, eds. *Glaucoma.* Philadelphia, PA: Lea and Febiger, 1979;329.

19. Barkan O. Pathogenesis of congenital glaucoma: gonioscopic and anatomic observation of the angle of the anterior chamber in the normal eye and in congenital glaucoma. *Am J Ophthalmol* 1955;40:1–11.

20. Shaffer RN, Heatherington J. Glaucomatous disc in infants. A suggested hypothesis for disc cupping. *Trans Am Acad Ophthalmol Otolaryngol* 1969;73:929–935.

21. Richardson KT. Optic cup symmetry in normal newborn infants. *Invest Ophthalmol* 1968;7:137–147.

22. Quigley HA. The pathogenesis of reversible cupping in congenital glaucoma. *Am J Ophthalmol* Sep 1977;84(3):358–370.

23. Argus AA. Ocular hypertension and central corneal thickness. *Ophthalmology* 1995;102:1810–1812.

24. Herndon LW, Choudhri SA, Cox T, Damji KF, Shields MB, Allingham RR. Central corneal thickness in normal, glaucomatous, and ocular hypertensive eyes. *Arch Ophthalmol* 1997;115:1137–1141.

25. Gordon MO, Beiser JA, Brandt JD, et al. The Ocular Hypertension Treatment Study: baseline factors that predict the onset of primary open-angle glaucoma. *Arch Ophthalmol* June 2002;120(6):714–720.

26. Tai TY, Mills MD, Beck AD, et al. Central corneal thickness and corneal diameter in patients with childhood glaucoma. *J Glaucoma* Dec 2006;15(6):524–528.

27. Freedman SF. Central corneal thickness in children—does it help or hinder our evaluation of eyes at risk for glaucoma? *J AAPOS* Feb 2008;12(1):1–2.

28. Lim Z, Muir KW, Duncan L, Freedman SF. Acquired central corneal thickness increase following removal of childhood cataracts. *Am J Ophthalmol* Mar 2011;151(3):434–441.e431.

29. Bradfield YS, Melia BM, Repka MX, et al. Central corneal thickness in children. *Arch Ophthalmol* Sep 2011;129(9): 1132–1138.

30. El-Dairi MA, Asrani SG, Enyedi LB, Freedman SF. Optical coherence tomography in the eyes of normal children. *Arch Ophthalmol* Jan 2009;127(1):50–58.

31. Salchow DJ, Oleynikov YS, Chiang MF, et al. Retinal nerve fiber layer thickness in normal children measured with optical coherence tomography. *Ophthalmology* May 2006;113(5): 786–791.

32. Wang XY, Huynh SC, Burlutsky G, Ip J, Stapleton F, Mitchell P. Reproducibility of and effect of magnification on optical coherence tomography measurements in children. *Am J Ophthalmol* Mar 2007;143(3):484–488.

33. El-Dairi MA, Holgado S, Asrani S, Enyedi L, Freedman S. Correlation between optical coherence tomography and glaucomatous optic nerve head damage in children. *Br J Ophthalmol* 2009;93(10):1325–1330.

34. Hess DB, Asrani SG, Bhide MG, Enyedi LB, Stinnett SS, Freedman SF. Macular and retinal nerve fiber layer analysis of normal and glaucomatous eyes in children using optical coherence tomography. *Am J Ophthalmol* Mar 2005;139(3):509–517.

35. Shaffer RN, Weiss DI. *Congenital and pediatric glaucomas.* St. Louis, MO: C.V. Mosby, 1970.

36. Chandler PA, Grant WM. *Lectures in glaucoma.* Philadelphia, PA: Lea and Febiger, 1965.

37. Phelps DD, Podos SM. *Glaucoma.* Vol Chapter 9. Boston, MA: Little Brown, 1974.

38. Waardenburg PJ, Franceschetti P, Klein D. *Genetics and ophthalmology.* Vol 1. Springfield, IL: Charles C Thomas, 1961.

39. Narooie-Nejad M, Paylakhi SH, Shojaee S, et al. Loss of function mutations in the gene encoding latent transforming growth factor beta binding protein 2, LTBP2, cause primary congenital glaucoma. *Hum Mol Genet* Oct 2009;18(20):3969–3977.

40. Kaur K, Reddy AB, Mukhopadhyay A, et al. Myocilin gene implicated in primary congenital glaucoma. *Clin Genet* Apr 2005;67(4):335–340.

41. Sarfarazi M, Stoilov I, Schenkman JB. Genetics and biochemistry of primary congenital glaucoma. *Ophthalmol Clin North Am* Dec 2003;16(4):543–554, vi.

42. Zenteno JC, Hernandez-Merino E, Mejia-Lopez H, et al. Contribution of CYP1B1 mutations and founder effect to primary congenital glaucoma in Mexico. *J Glaucoma* Apr–May 2008;17(3):189–192.

43. Tanwar M, Dada T, Sihota R, Das TK, Yadav U, Dada R. Mutation spectrum of CYP1B1 in North Indian congenital glaucoma patients. *Mol Vis* 2009;15:1200–1209.

44. Abu-Amero KK, Osman EA, Mousa A, et al. Screening of CYP1B1 and LTBP2 genes in Saudi families with primary congenital glaucoma: genotype-phenotype correlation. *Mol Vis* 2011;17:2911–2919.

45. Messina-Baas OM, Gonzalez-Huerta LM, Chima-Galan C, et al. Molecular analysis of the CYP1B1 gene: identification of novel truncating mutations in patients with primary congenital glaucoma. *Ophthalmic Res* 2007;39(1):17–23.

46. Freedman SF, McCormick K, Cox T. Mitomycin c-augmented trabeculectomy with postoperative wound modulation in pediatric glaucoma. *J AAPOS* 1999;3:117–124.

47. Beck AD, Wilson WR, Lynch MG, Lynn MJ, Noe R. Trabeculectomy with adjunctive Mitomycin c in pediatric glaucoma. *Am J Ophthalmol* 1998;126:648–657.

48. Mandal AK, Prasad K, Naduvilath TJ. Surgical results and complications of mitomycin C-augmented trabeculectomy in refractory developmental glaucoma. *Ophthalmic Surg Lasers* 1999;30(6):473–480.

49. Sidoti PA, Belmonte SJ, Liebmann JM, Ritch R. Trabeculectomy with Mitomycin c in the treatment of pediatric glaucomas. *Ophthalmology* 2000;107:422–429.

50. Mandal AK, Gothwal VK, Nutheti R. Surgical outcome of primary developmental glaucoma: a single surgeon's long-term experience from a tertiary eye care centre in India. *Eye* June 2007;21(6):764–774.

51. Molteno AC, Ancker E, Van Biljon G. Surgical technique for advanced juvenile glaucoma. *Arch Ophthalmol* 1984;102(1):51–57.

52. Englert JA, Freedman SF, Cox TA. The Ahmed valve in refractory pediatric glaucoma. *Am J Ophthalmol* 1999;127:34–42.

53. Fellenbaum PS, Sidoti PA, Heuer DK, Mincker DS, Baerveldt G, Lee PP. Experience with the Baerveldt implant in young patients with complicated glaucomas. *J Glaucoma* 1995;4:91–97.

54. Coleman AL, Smyth RJ, Wilson MR, Tam M. Initial clinical experience with the Ahmed glaucoma valve implant in pediatric patients. *Arch Ophthalmol* 1997;115:186–191.

55. Morad Y, Craig ED, Kim YM, Abdolell M, Levin AV. The Ahmed drainage implant in the treatment of pediatric glaucoma. *Am J Ophthalmol* 2003;135:821–829.

56. O'Malley Schotthoefer E, Yanovitch TL, Freedman SF. Aqueous drainage device surgery in refractory pediatric glaucoma: II. Ocular motility consequences. *J AAPOS* Feb 2008;12(1):40–45.

57. O'Malley Schotthoefer E, Yanovitch TL, Freedman SF. Aqueous drainage device surgery in refractory pediatric glaucomas: I. Long-term outcomes. *J AAPOS* Feb 2008;12(1):33–39.

58. Neely DE, Plager DA. Endocyclophotocoagulation for management of difficult pediatric glaucomas. *J AAPOS* 2001;5(4):221–229.

59. Sheffield VC, Stone EM, Alward WL, et al. Genetic linkage of familial open angle glaucoma to chromosome 1q21-1q31. *Nature Genet* 1993;4:47–50.

60. Stone DL, Fingert JH, Alward WL, al. e. Identification of a gene that causes primary open angle glaucoma. *Science* 1997;275:668–670.

61. Bayat B, Yazdani S, Alavi A, et al. Contributions of MYOC and CYP1B1 mutations to JOAG. *Mol Vis* 2008;14:508–517.

62. Avisar I, Lusky M, Robinson A, et al. The novel Y371D myocilin mutation causes an aggressive form of juvenile open-angle glaucoma in a Caucasian family from the Middle-East. *Mol Vis* 2009;15:1945–1950.

63. Wei YT, Li YQ, Bai YJ, et al. Pro370Leu myocilin mutation in a Chinese pedigree with juvenile-onset open angle glaucoma. *Mol Vis* 2011;17:1449–1456.

64. Phelps CD. The pathogenesis of glaucoma in Sturge-Weber syndrome. *Ophthalmology* 1978;85(3):276–286.

65. Akabane N, Hamanaka T. Histopathological study of a case with glaucoma due to Sturge-Weber syndrome. *Jpn J Ophthalmol* Mar–Apr 2003;47(2):151–157.

66. Mandal AK. Primary combined trabeculotomy-trabeculectomy for early-onset glaucoma in Sturge-Weber syndrome. *Ophthalmology* 1999;106(8):1621–1627.

67. Olsen KE, Huang AS, Wright MM. The efficacy of goniotomy/trabeculotomy in early-onset glaucoma associated with the Sturge-Weber syndrome. *J AAPOS* 1998;2(6):365–368.

68. Budenz DL, Sakamoto D, Eliezer R, Varma R, Heuer DK. Two-staged Baerveldt glaucoma implant for childhood glaucoma associated with Sturge-Weber syndrome. *Ophthalmology* 2000;107(11):2105–2110.

69. Hamush NG, Coleman AL, Wilson MR. Ahmed glaucoma valve implant for management of glaucoma in Sturge-Weber syndrome. *Am J Ophthalmol* 1999;128(6):758–760.

70. van Emelen C, Goethals M, Dralands L, Casteels I. Treatment of glaucoma in children with Sturge-Weber syndrome. *J Pediatr Ophthalmol Strabismus* 2000;37(1):29–34.

71. Chang L, Mruthyunjaya P, Rodriguez-Rosa RE, Freedman SF. Postoperative cilioretinal artery occlusion in Sturge Weber-associated glaucoma. *J AAPOS* Aug 2010;14(4):358–360.

72. Payne MS, Nadell JM, Lacassie Y, Tilton AH. Congenital glaucoma and neurofibromatosis in a monozygotic twin: case report and review of the literature. *J Child Neurol* 2003;18:504–508.

73. Grant WM, Walton DS. Distinctive gonioscopic findings in glaucoma due to neurofibromatosis. *Arch Ophthalmol* 1968;79(2):127–134.

74. *Online Mendelian Inheritance in Man, OMIM (TM)*. World Wide Web URL: http://www.ncbi.nlm.nih.gov/omim/: Johns Hopkins University (Baltimore, MD) and National Center for Biotechnology Information, National Library of Medicine (Bethesda, MD); 2000.

75. Mueller OT, Hartsfield JK Jr, Gallardo LA, et al. Lowe oculocerebrorenal syndrome in a female with a balanced X;20 translocation: mapping of the X chromosome breakpoint. *Am J Hum Genet* 1991;49(4):804–810.

76. Walton DS, Katsavounidou G, Lowe CU. Glaucoma with the oculocerebrorenal syndrome of Lowe. *J Glaucoma* June 2005;14(3):181–185.

77. Walton DS. Congenital glaucoma associated with congenital cataract. In: Epstein DL, ed. *Chandler and Grant's glaucoma*, 3rd Ed. Philadelphia, PA: Lea & Febinger, 1986:515–517.

78. Donahue SP, Keech RV, Munden P, Scott WE. Baerveldt implant surgery in the treatment of advanced childhood glaucoma. *J AAPOS* 1997;1:41–45.

79. Colas-Tomas T, Gutierrez-Diaz E, Tejada-Palacios P, Barcelo-Mendiguchia A, Mencia-Gutierrez E. Management of congenital glaucoma in neurofibromatosis type 1: a report of two cases. *Int Ophthalmol* Apr 2 2009.

80. Shields MB, Buckley EG, Klintworth GK, Thresher R. Axenfeld-Rieger syndrome. A spectrum of developmental disorders. *Surv Ophthalmol* 1985;29:387.

81. Alward WL. Axenfeld-Rieger syndrome in the age of molecular genetics. *Am J Ophthalmol* 2000;130(1):107–115.

82. Online Mendelian Inheritance in Man, OMIM (TM). *An Online Catalog of Human Genes and Genetic Disorders Updated 20 January 2012*. 2011.

83. Strungaru MH, Dinu I, Walter MA. Genotype-phenotype correlations in Axenfeld-Rieger malformation and glaucoma patients with FOXC1 and PITX2 mutations. *Invest Ophthalmol Vis Sci* Jan 2007;48(1):228–237.

84. Turleau C, DeGrouchy J, Tournade M-F, al. e. Del 11p/aniridia complex. Report of three patients and review of 37 observations from the literature. *Clin Genet* 1984;26:356.

85. Grant WM, Walton DS. Progressive changes in the angle in congenital aniridia, with development of glaucoma. *Am J Ophthalmol* 1974;78(5):842–847.

86. Chen TC, Walton DS. Goniosurgery for prevention of aniridic glaucoma. *Arch Ophthalmol* 1999;117:1144–1148.

87. Adachi M, Dickens CJ, Hetherington J Jr, et al. Clinical experience of trabeculotomy for the surgical treatment of aniridic glaucoma. *Ophthalmology* 1997;104(12):2121–2125.

88. Wagle NS, Freedman SF, Buckley EG, Davis JS, Biglan AW. Long-term outcome of cyclocryotherapy for refractory pediatric glaucoma. *Ophthalmology* 1998;105(10):1921–1926; discussion 1926–1927.

89. Wiggins RE, Jr., Tomey KF. The results of glaucoma surgery in aniridia. *Arch Ophthalmol* 1992;110(4):503–505.

90. Arroyave CP, Scott IU, Gedde SJ, Parrish RK 2nd, Feuer WJ. Use of glaucoma drainage devices in the management of glaucoma associated with aniridia. *Am J Ophthalmol* 2003;135(2):155–159.

91. Traboulsi EI, Maumenee IH. Peters' anomaly and associated congenital malformations. *Arch Ophthalmol* 1992;110(12):1739–1742.

92. Kivlin JD, Fineman RM, Crandall AA, Olson RJ. Peters' anomaly as a consequence of genetic and nongenetic syndromes. *Arch Ophthalmol* 1986;104:61.

93. Yang LL, Lambert SR, Lynn MJ, Stulting RD. Surgical management of glaucoma in infants and children with Peters' anomaly: long-term structural and functional outcome. *Ophthalmology* Jan 2004;111(1):112–117.

94. Yang LL, Lambert SR. Peters' anomaly. A synopsis of surgical management and visual outcome. *Ophthalmol Clin North Am* 2001;14(3):467–477.

95. Zaidman GW, Rabinowitz Y, Forstot SL. Optical iridectomy for corneal opacities in Peter's anomaly. *J Cataract Refract Surg* 1998;24(5):719–722.

96. Gollamudi SR, Traboulsi EI, Chamon W, Stark WJ, Maumenee IH. Visual outcome after surgery for Peters' anomaly. *Ophthalmic Genet* 1994;15(1):31–35. 20: Astle WF, et al. Bilateral penetrating keratop…[PMID:8299053]Related Articles, Links.

97. Yang LL, Lambert SR, Drews-Botsch C, Stulting RD. Long-term visual outcome of penetrating keratoplasty in infants and children with Peters anomaly. *J AAPOS* Apr 2009;13(2):175–180.

98. Zaidman GW, Flanagan JK, Furey CC. Long-term visual prognosis in children after corneal transplant surgery for Peters anomaly type I. *Am J Ophthalmol* Jul 2007;144(1):104–108.

99. Goldberg MF. The diagnosis and treatment of secondary glaucoma after hyphema in sickle cell patients. *Am J Ophthalmol* 1979;87:43.

100. Farber MD, Fiscella R, Goldberg MF. Aminocaproic acid versus prednisone for the treatment of traumatic hyphema. A randomized clinical trial. *Ophthalmology* 1991;98:279.

101. Ozer PA, Yalvac IS, Satana B, Eksioglu U, Duman S. Incidence and risk factors in secondary glaucomas after blunt and penetrating ocular trauma. *J Glaucoma* Dec 2007;16(8):685–690.

102. Vendal Z, Walton D, Chen T. Glaucoma in juvenile xanthogranuloma. *Semin Ophthalmol* Jul–Sep 2006;21(3):191–194.

103. Da Mata A, Burk SE, Netland PA, Baltatzis S, Christen W, Foster CS. Management of uveitic glaucoma with Ahmed glaucoma valve implantation. *Ophthalmology* 1999;106(11):2168–2172.

104. Freedman SF, Rodriguez-Rosa RE, Rojas MC, Enyedi LB. Goniotomy for glaucoma secondary to chronic childhood uveitis. *Am J Ophthalmol* 2002;133(5):617–621.

105. Ho CL, Walton DS. Management of childhood glaucoma. *Curr Opin Ophthalmol* Oct 2004;15(5):460–464.

106. Ho CL, Wong EY, Walton DS. Goniosurgery for glaucoma complicating chronic childhood uveitis. *Arch Ophthalmol* June 2004;122(6):838–844.

107. Ho CL, Walton DS. Goniosurgery for glaucoma secondary to chronic anterior uveitis: prognostic factors and surgical technique. *J Glaucoma* Dec 2004;13(6):445–449.

108. Papadaki TG, Zacharopoulos IP, Pasquale LR, Christen WB, Netland PA, Foster CS. Long-term results of Ahmed glaucoma valve implantation for uveitic glaucoma. *Am J Ophthalmol* Jul 2007;144(1):62–69.

109. Bohnsack BL, Freedman SF. (2013) Surgical outcomes in childhood uveitic glaucoma. *Am J Ophthalmol.* 2013 Jan;155(1):134–42. doi: 10.1016/j.ajo.2012.07.008. Epub 2012 Oct 2. PMID: 23036573

110. Harrison DA, Mullaney PB, Mesfer SA, Awad AH, Dhindsa H. Management of ophthalmic complications of homocystinuria. *Ophthalmology* 1998;105(10):1886–1890.

111. Egbert JE, Wright MM, Dahlhauser KF, Keithahn MA, Letson RD, Summers CG. A prospective study of ocular hypertension and glaucoma after pediatric cataract surgery. *Ophthalmology* 1995;102(7):1098–1101.

112. Parks MM, Johnson DA, Reed GW. Long-term visual results and complications in children with aphakia. A function of cataract type. *Ophthalmology* 1993;100(6):826–840; discussion 840–821.

113. Walton DS. Pediatric aphakic glaucoma: a study of 65 patients. *Trans Am Ophthalmol Soc* 1995;93:403–413; discussion 413–420.

114. Beck AD, Lynn MJ, Crandall J, Mobin-Uddin O. Surgical outcomes with 360-degree suture trabeculotomy in poor-prognosis primary congenital glaucoma and glaucoma associated with congenital anomalies or cataract surgery. *J AAPOS* Feb 2011;15(1):54–58.

115. Plager DA, Neely DE. Intermediate-term results of endoscopic diode laser cyclophotocoagulation for pediatric glaucoma. *J AAPOS* 1999;3(3):131–137.

116. Carter BC, Plager DA, Neely DE, Sprunger DT, Sondhi N, Roberts GJ. Endoscopic diode laser cyclophotocoagulation in the management of aphakic and pseudophakic glaucoma in children. *J AAPOS* Feb 2007;11(1):34–40.

117. Sabri K, Levin AV. The additive effect of topical dorzolamide and systemic acetazolamide in pediatric glaucoma. *J AAPOS* Oct 2006;10(5):464–468.

118. Passo MS, Palmer EA, Van Buskirk EM. Plasma timolol in glaucoma patients. *Ophthalmology* 1984;91:1361–1363.

119. Zimmerman TJ, Kooner KS, Morgan KS. Safety and efficacy of timolol in pediatric glaucoma. *Surv Ophthalmol* 1983;28:262–264.

120. Plager DA, Whitson JT, Netland PA, et al. Betaxolol hydrochloride ophthalmic suspension 0.25% and timolol gel-forming solution 0.25% and 0.5% in pediatric glaucoma: a randomized clinical trial. *J AAPOS* Aug 2009;13(4):384–390.

121. Wright TM, Freedman SF. Exposure to topical apraclonidine in children with glaucoma. *J Glaucoma* June–Jul 2009;18(5):395–398.

122. Enyedi LB, Freedman SF. Safety and efficacy of brimonidine in children with glaucoma. *J AAPOS* 2001;5(5):281–284.

123. Mungan NK, Wilson TW, Nischal KK, Koren G, Levin AV. Hypotension and bradycardia in infants after the use of topical brimonidine and beta-blockers. *J AAPOS* Feb 2003;7(1):69–70.

124. Al-Shahwan S, Al-Torbak AA, Turkmani S, Al-Omran M, Al-Jadaan I, Edward DP. Side-effect profile of brimonidine tartrate in children. *Ophthalmology* Dec 2005;112(12):2143.

125. Maeda-Chubachi T, Chi-Burris K, Simons BD, et al. Comparison of latanoprost and timolol in pediatric glaucoma: a phase 3, 12-week, randomized, double-masked multicenter study. *Ophthalmology* Oct 2011;118(10):2014–2021.

126. Black AC, Jones S, Yanovitch TL, Enyedi LB, Stinnett SS, Freedman SF. Latanoprost in pediatric glaucoma—pediatric exposure over a decade. *J AAPOS* Dec 2009;13(6):558–562.

127. Yang CB, Freedman SF, Myers JS, Buckley EG, Herndon LW, Allingham RR. Use of latanoprost in the treatment of glaucoma associated with Sturge-Weber syndrome. *Am J Ophthalmol* 1998;126(4):600–602.

128. Enyedi LB, Freedman SF. Latanoprost for the treatment of pediatric glaucoma. *Surv Ophthalmol* 2002;47(Suppl 1):S129–S132.

129. Yanovitch TL, Enyedi LB, Schotthoeffer EO, Freedman SF. Travoprost in children: adverse effects and intraocular pressure response. *J AAPOS* Feb 2009;13(1):91–93.

130. Moroi SE, Gottfredsdottir MS, Schteingart MT, et al. Cystoid macular edema associated with latanoprost therapy in a case series of patients with glaucoma and ocular hypertension. *Ophthalmology* May 1999;106(5):1024–1029.

131. Barkan O. Operation for congenital glaucoma. *Am J Ophthalmol* 1942;25:552.

132. Chen TC, Walton DS. Goniosurgery for prevention of aniridic glaucoma. *Trans Am Ophthalmol Soc* 1998;96:155–165; discussion 165–159.

133. Kulkarni SV, Damji KF, Fournier AV, Pan I, Hodge WG. Endoscopic goniotomy: early clinical experience in congenital glaucoma. *J Glaucoma* Apr–May 2010;19(4):264–269.

134. Bayraktar S, Koseoglu T. Endoscopic goniotomy with anterior chamber maintainer: surgical technique and one-year results. *Ophthalmic Surg Lasers* 2001;32(6):496–502.

135. Nguyen QH. Trabectome: a novel approach to angle surgery in the treatment of glaucoma. *Int Ophthalmol Clin* Fall 2008;48(4):65–72.

136. Burian HM. A case of Marfan's syndrome with bilateral glaucoma with a description of a new type of operation for developmental glaucoma. *Am J Ophthalmol* 1960;50:1187–1192.

137. Smith R. A new technique for opening the canal of Schlemm. *Brit J Ophthalmol* 1960;44:370–373.

138. Beck AD, Lynch MG. 360 degrees trabeculotomy for primary congenital glaucoma. *Arch Ophthalmol* Sep 1995;113(9):1200–1202.

139. Mendicino ME, Lynch MG, Drack A, et al. Long-term surgical and visual outcomes in primary congenital glaucoma: 360 degrees trabeculotomy versus goniotomy. *J AAPOS* 2000;4(4):205–210.

140. Sarkisian SR, Jr. An illuminated microcatheter for 360-degree trabeculotomy [corrected] in congenital glaucoma: a retrospective case series. *J AAPOS* Oct 2010;14(5):412–416.

141. Noureddin BN, El-Haibi CP, Cheikha A, Bashshur ZF. Viscocanalostomy versus trabeculotomy ab externo in primary congenital glaucoma: 1-year follow-up of a prospective controlled pilot study. *Br J Ophthalmol* Oct 2006;90(10):1281–1285.

142. Waheed S, Ritterband DC, Greenfield DS, Liebmann JM, Sidoti PA, Ritch R. Bleb-related ocular infection in children after trabeculectomy with mitomycin C. *Ophthalmology* 1997;104(12):2117–2120.

143. Giampani J, Jr., Borges-Giampani AS, Carani JC, Oltrogge EW, Susanna R Jr. Efficacy and safety of trabeculectomy with mitomycin C for childhood glaucoma: a study of results with long-term follow-up. *Clinics (Sao Paulo)* Aug 2008;63(4):421–426.

144. Susanna RJ, Oltrogge EW, Carani JCE, Nicolela MT. Mitomycin as adjunct chemotherapy with trabeculectomy in congenital and developmental glaucomas. *J Glaucoma* 1995;4(3):151–157.

145. Mandal AK, Bagga H, Nutheti R, Gothwal VK, Nanda AK. Trabeculectomy with or without mitomycin-C for paediatric glaucoma in aphakia and pseudophakia following congenital cataract surgery. *Eye* Jan 2003;17(1):53–62.

146. Low S, Hamada S, Nischal KK. Antimetabolite and releasable suture augmented filtration surgery in refractory pediatric glaucomas. *J AAPOS* Apr 2008;12(2):166–172.

147. Francis BA, Singh K, Lin SC, et al. Novel glaucoma procedures: a report by the American Academy of Ophthalmology. *Ophthalmology* Jul 2011;118(7):1466–1480.

148. Molteno ACB. Children with advanced glaucoma treated by draining implants. *S Afr Arch Ophthalmol* 1973;1:55–61.

149. Ishida K, Mandal AK, Netland PA. Glaucoma drainage implants in pediatric patients. *Ophthalmol Clin North Am* Sep 2005;18(3):431–442, vii.

150. Tanimoto SA, Brandt JD. Options in pediatric glaucoma after angle surgery has failed. *Curr Opin Ophthalmol* Apr 2006;17(2):132–137.

151. Autrata R, Helmanova I, Oslejskova H, Vondracek P, Rehurek J. Glaucoma drainage implants in the treatment of refractory glaucoma in pediatric patients. *Eur J Ophthalmol* Nov–Dec 2007;17(6):928–937.

152. Sood S, Beck AD. Cyclophotocoagulation versus sequential tube shunt as a secondary intervention following primary tube shunt failure in pediatric glaucoma. *J AAPOS* 2009;13(4):379–383.

153. Beck AD, Freedman S, Kammer J, Jin J. Aqueous shunt devices compared with trabeculectomy with mitomycin-C for children in the first two years of life. *Am J Ophthalmol* 2003;136:994–1000.

154. Al Faran MF, Tomey KF, Al Mutlag FA. Cyclocryotherapy in selected cases of congenital glaucoma. *Ophth Surg* 1990;21:794–798.

155. Kirwan JF, Shah P, Khaw PT. Diode laser cyclophotocoagulation: role in the management of refractory pediatric glaucomas. *Ophthalmology* 2002;109(2):316–323.

156. Bock CJ, Freedman FF, Buckley EG, Shields MB. Transscleral diode laser cyclophotocoagulation for refractory pediatric glaucomas. *J Pediatr Ophthalmol Strabismus* 1997;34:235–239.

157. Phelan MJ, Higginbotham EJ. Contact transscleral Nd:YAG laser cyclophotocoagulation for the treatment of refractory pediatric glaucoma. *Ophthalmic Surg Lasers* 1995;26:401–403.

158. Allingham RR, Damji KF, Freedman SF, Moroi S, Saranov, eds. *Shields textbook of glaucoma*, 6th Ed. Philadelphia, PA: Wolters Kluwer Health/Lippincott Williams & Wilkins, 2011.

13

Pediatric Uveitis

Grace T. Liu • *Alex V. Levin*

INTRODUCTION

Uveitis in the pediatric population is a significant cause of ophthalmic morbidity. Approximately 2% to 14% of patients seen in uveitis clinics are children (1–3). Unique to the pediatric age group in the management and timely diagnosis of uveitis is the threat of amblyopia. In addition, the associated systemic disease profile is much different than that seen in adults. Children more often (71%) have an associated systemic illness than adults (55%) (4). Although juvenile idiopathic arthritis (JIA) is the predominant cause of anterior uveitis in children (5,6), it is important to recognize that uveitis in a child can be due to a wide range of etiologies, including serious life-threatening masquerade syndromes such as retinoblastoma and leukemia. Presenting signs and symptoms are often not recognized until advanced stages, and the disorder may even be entirely asymptomatic until irreversible ocular damage has been sustained (Fig. 13.1). The child may be unable to verbalize his/her symptoms, and can often function normally with visual acuity well below 20/20 for activities of daily living, especially when the disease is unilateral and the child is younger. The approach to pediatric uveitis requires the understanding that early recognition through screening, where appropriate, can be of utmost importance.

Table 13.1 summarizes the diagnostic approach to the child with pediatric uveitis.

EPIDEMIOLOGY

The frequency and etiology of childhood uveitis is in part dependent on geography. Widespread globalization may also affect the current distribution of the disease. A meta-analysis of worldwide studies showed that 7% of patients with uveitis are children. Parasitic anterior uveitis (49.3%) is the most common etiology globally, with idiopathic being the second most common (25.5%) (7). A group from Saudi Arabia reported idiopathic anterior non-granulomatous uveitis as the most common type of uveitis in children (26%) (8). A report from Israel found infectious diseases to be the primary etiology of uveitis in children and adolescents (31.2%) (1).

To the contrary, a study from the US National Eye Institute found that idiopathic uveitis (28.8%) was the leading etiology in the United States, followed by JIA (20.9%), and pars planitis (17.1%). A retrospective study characterizing disease characteristics and visual outcome of 527 children in the United States with uveitis, found that 54% were female; 62% White, 15% Hispanic, 12% Black, 3% Asian, and 2% multiracial (9). The median age at diagnosis was 9.4 years.

CLASSIFICATION

Although consortium-driven classification systems have been proposed, they may be difficult to use in the clinical setting. The Standardization of Uveitis Nomenclature (SUN) criteria were developed for classification and description of uveitis by anatomic location (Table 13.2). Specific grading criteria, such as quantitative grading of inflammation, were also elaborated (10). Morphologic classification, according to cell type, for example granulomatous versus nongranulomatous, may be less useful in children. A broader classification might separate etiologies into exogenous, representing any external injury or invasion of microorganisms from outside the globe, versus endogenous, resulting from factors that originate within the patient.

TREATMENT AND COMPLICATIONS

Topical Medical Therapy

Even with low-grade iritis, the goal is early, aggressive treatment to suppress inflammation maximally, in hopes of preventing the development of vision-threatening complications (11–14). When inflammation is more severe, topical corticosteroids may be indicated as frequently as every 1 to 2 hours. Follow-up within 1 to 2 weeks after initiating treatment is critical to ensure improvement. Perhaps the most common reason for recalcitrant and recurrent uveitis is the too rapid tapering of topical steroids. Although a fairly rapid taper may be appropriate on the first episode, any indication of iritis recurrence during the taper should be met with a change to a slow taper. It may take weeks, months, or even

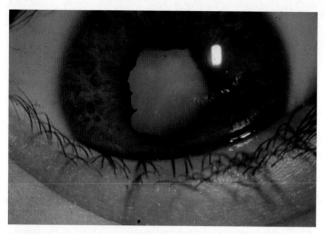

FIGURE 13.1. Child with asymptomatic oligoarticular juvenile idiopathic arthritis who did not present until visual loss was noted by which time she had a dense white cataract, multiple posterior synechiae, and active anterior uveitis. Note the absence of conjunctival inflammation.

years to accomplish a full taper in some children. Although there are certainly risks of steroid-induced cataract or glaucoma, the risk of these complications from inadequately treated uveitis is even greater. Our experience with high dose and chronic topical steroid use actually shows a reduction in such complications and better vision outcomes (15).

Cycloplegic agents are also important, given the increased tendency of children to form synechiae. Many different regimens have been suggested (16). We prefer a minimum of one dose of cyclopentolate 1% at bedtime. It is also important to consider (and treat with glasses if needed) the blur induced by cycloplegia, especially in school-aged children.

A recent study specifically on the use of difluprednate in pediatric uveitis demonstrated its use to be effective for anterior segment inflammation and reduction of cystoid macular edema (CME) when used as an adjuvant to systemic immunomodulatory therapy, but it was not without risks (17). Glaucoma

Table 13.1

EVALUATION AND TESTING FOR PEDIATRIC UVEITIS

History of Present Illness

Medical history:

Systemic illnesses (e.g., sarcoidosis, JIA, AIDS, TB)

Social history:

Sexual history (where appropriate based on age)

Birthplace

Travel (e.g., Ohio River Valley), camping/environment (exposure to ticks)

Review of Systems:

General: fever, weight loss, malaise, night sweats, weight loss, lymphadenopathy

Ear, nose, throat: hearing loss, tinnitus

Cardiac: murmurs (e.g., mitral regurgitation in Kawasaki disease)

Respiratory: shortness of breath, cough, history of "asthma" (e.g., could be sarcoid)

Gastrointestinal: oral ulcers, diarrhea, bloody stools

Genitourinary: dysuria, discharge, ulcers

Musculoskeletal: lower back pain, arthralgias, joint stiffness, myalgia

Dermatologic: rashes, desquamation, alopecia, vitiligo, tick and insect bites

Neurologic: headaches, meningitis, paresthesias

Laboratory Studies:

First line: CBC, ESR, ANA, RF, serum calcium, FTA-ABS, RPR, HLA-B27 (if clinically appropriate based on age and presentation), Lyme titers (if endemic region), urinalysis, tuberculin skin test, chest radiograph

Second line:

Serology: EBV titers, HSV/HZV, toxoplasmosis, toxocara, brucellosis titers, BUN and Cr, serum lysozyme

(continued)

Table 13.1

(continued)

Other radiographic studies, when indicated:

Sacroiliac joint, gastrointestinal series

Ultrasound—joints

Ancillary tests, when indicated:

Fluorescein angiography

Vitreous tap

Lumbar puncture

Renal biopsy

AIDS, acquired immunodeficiency syndrome; ANA, antinuclear antibody; BUN, blood urea nitrogen; CBC, complete blood count; Cr, creatinine; EBV, Epstein-Barr virus; ESR, erythrocyte sedimentation rate; FTA-ABS, fluorescent treponemal antibody absorption; HLA-B27, human leukocyte antigen-B27; HSV, herpes simplex virus; HZV: herpes zoster virus; JIA, juvenile idiopathic arthritis; RF, rheumatoid factor; RPR, rapid plasma reagin; TB, tuberculosis.

and cataract were both observed at significant rates, and the authors recommend close monitoring of pediatric patients on this medication.

Systemic Medical Therapy

Methotrexate is usually the first-line systemic agent if topical therapy fails to control the iritis, or if chronic high frequency dosing of topical steroids is needed. Absorption of oral methotrexate in children can be variable, and subcutaneous injection may be more effective. GI upset is a common side effect of oral administration (18)

Caution should be taken with use of chronic oral corticosteroids in children. The risks of growth retardation, osteoporosis, adrenal suppression, gastrointestinal upset, emotional lability, and susceptibility to infection must be

Table 13.2

THE SUN WORKING GROUP CLASSIFICATION OF UVEITIS (10)

Type	Primary Site of Inflammation	Includes
Anterior uveitis	Anterior chamber	Iritis
		Iridocyclitis
		Anterior cyclitis
Intermediate uveitis	Vitreous	Pars planitis
		Posterior cyclitis
		Hyalitis
Posterior uveitis	Retina or choroid	Focal, multifocal, or diffuse choroiditis
		Chorioretinitis
		Retinochoroiditis
		Retinitis
		Neuroretinitis

Note: panuveitis includes inflammation in anterior chamber, vitreous, and retina or choroid.
SUN, Standardization of Uveitis Nomenclature.

considered. Secondary glaucoma may occur more frequently in children than in adults (19,20). In general, oral corticosteroids are reserved for short course (<14 days) as an acute intervention, to test for steroid responsiveness, or perioperatively. Although nonsteroidal anti-inflammatory medications (NSAIDs) may be a useful adjunct in managing the systemic symptoms of JIA, and there has been some suggestion of ocular benefit, they play a minor role in the management of pediatric uveitis (21).

In recent years, the use of anti-tumor necrosis factor (anti-TNF) and other biologic agents has become the mainstay of second-line systemic therapeutics in uveitis management. These agents, along with methotrexate, may also assist as steroid-sparing interventions to reduce the risks of topical steroids.

Infliximab is approved for many autoimmune diseases, including ankylosing spondylitis, rheumatoid arthritis, psoriatic arthritis, and JIA. It has good efficacy in children with oligo- or polyarthritis from JIA (22). It appears to be superior to etanercept (23). Infliximab should be considered as the first-line anti-TNF agent in treating pediatric uveitis refractive to topical treatment and methotrexate. During infliximab treatment, low dose methotrexate is usually continued. One disadvantage, however, of infliximab in addition to the high cost, is the need for in-hospital infusion and the risk of anaphylaxis.

Adalimumab is a subcutaneous injection approved for polyarticular JIA since 2008 with favorable results in pediatric uveitis (2-year study) (24). Adverse effects include injection site pain, reaction or burning, headache, respiratory or viral infection, trauma, and headache. Although usually given every other week, dosage intervals may be shortened to every week to improve uveitis control.

Etanercept is another TNF inhibitor that has been approved for the treatment of JIA and other autoimmune diseases. It has been studied especially for the treatment of polyarticular JIA (25–28). It is less effective than infliximab (23). It is administered subcutaneously, usually weekly. Compared to the other anti-TNFs in use for pediatric uveitis, etanercept may have lower rates for the development of malignancy (29).

Abatacept, a biologic disease-modifying antirheumatic drug, prevents the costimulatory signal for T cells to fully activate. It gained approval for treatment of polyarticular JIA in 2008 after an international, multicenter trial demonstrated a statistically significant difference in the time period to flare compared to placebo (30,31). There is less data available regarding its efficacy in pediatric uveitis (32).

Other Drugs

In patients who do not respond to the agents above (and switching amongst those agents may also be effective), anakinra, rilonacept (both interleukin-1 inhibitors) and tocilizumab (interleukin-6 inhibitor) have been used.

Mycophenolate mofetil has been studied in children with uveitis. Because of its selective mechanism of action, its side effect profile is more tolerable (33,34). Doycheva and colleagues found a steroid-sparing effect and possible reduced relapse rates. Side effects include, gastrointestinal disturbances, headache, rash, leukopenia, and possible increase in opportunistic infection (35,36).

Surgical Treatment

Band Keratopathy

Band keratopathy (Fig. 13.2) is one of the most common complications associated with chronic anterior chamber inflammation in children (16). Treatment is not required unless visual acuity is compromised, or the patient has symptoms.

Cataract

Cataract can be secondary to the inflammation itself or the chronic use of corticosteroid drops. Most commonly, the opacity begins as a posterior subcapsular cataract, but this can progress, sometimes rapidly, to a total white cataract with or without lens intumescence. In the latter circumstance, phacomorphic or phacolytic glaucoma may rarely ensure.

Though controversy still exists over when and whether to place an intraocular lens (IOL), most physicians agree that a quiescent period is desirable before surgery. Perioperative and postoperative oral steroids are recommended along with intraoperative intravenous steroids. Some authors have recommended intracameral, in addition to the usual subconjunctival steroids at the end of surgery (37). We usually prescribe a 3-day course of oral prednisone at approximately 1 mg/kg/day prior to surgery. This

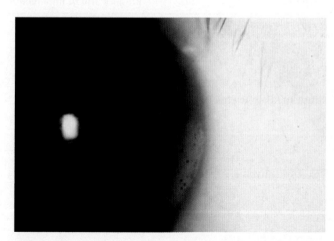

FIGURE 13.2. Typical band keratopathy of chronic pediatric anterior uveitis. Usually starts at medial and temporal limbus and then spreads over interpalpebral cornea.

is continued for 7 to 10 days thereafter, along with a topical regimen of frequent prednisolone acetate (q1-2h) and a cycloplegic agent.

The implantation of an IOL in an eye already predisposed to inflammation is known to potentially complicate the postoperative course. BenEzra and colleagues found that children with JIA-associated uveitis had more postoperative complications after cataract surgery than those with other forms of uveitis (38). Lundvall's study of 10 eyes in children with uveitis who underwent IOL implantation showed that 7 required reoperation (39). There remains no agreement as to whether or not primary posterior capsulotomy is beneficial in these patients (38–40).

Glaucoma

The mechanism of glaucoma in pediatric uveitis may be due to "clogging" of the trabecular meshwork by inflammatory cells and/or fibrin, toxic or immunologic "poisoning" of meshwork cells, peripheral anterior synechiae, or the use of corticosteroids. Given the known complications of intraocular surgery in this population, medical management is recommended for initial therapy. The prostaglandin analogues may be used when maximizing topical therapy, despite reservation about their use in the past because of the propensity to perpetuate inflammation in adults (41). If topical treatment fails, and there are no systemic contraindications, oral acetazolamide may be tried.

Goniotomy has become the first choice in surgical management of uveitic glaucoma, offering a success rate of approximately 70% (42,43). Goniotomy-induced hyphema rates in uveitic children approach 100%, but in our experience, these clear rapidly. Immediate pre- and postoperative topical alpha-2 agonist instillation may be useful in reducing this complication. When goniotomy fails, other standard surgical choices for glaucoma apply. If tube implantation is selected, remember that some "valved" tubes may get clogged by fibrin and other cellular debris from iritis. One study found a higher rate of scleral patch graft erosion over tubes placed in children with uveitis (44). Cyclodestructive procedures can disproportionately induce intraocular inflammation.

Other Complications

Hypotony is usually a late complication of chronic uveitis secondary to ciliary body shutdown after chronic inflammation, or it can be due to cyclitic membrane formation. Topical steroids may improve hypotony secondary to inflammation. Surgery may relieve hypotony due to cyclitic membranes. If hypotony is left untreated, macular and optic nerve edema, and eventually phthisis bulbi, may result. CME is less common in pediatric uveitis but can be associated with pediatric intermediate uveitis (pars-planitis). A retrospective review conducted in Iran reported CME as the second most frequent complication (19.7%) with pars planitis (45).

PEDIATRIC ANTERIOR UVEITIS

Juvenile Idiopathic Arthritis

Table 13.3 provides a differential diagnosis for pediatric anterior uveitis.

This term encompasses all idiopathic childhood arthritis in children younger than 16 years old, persisting for more than 6 weeks, as defined by the International League of Associations of Rheumatology (ILAR) (46). This classification defines seven categories of JIA.

Systemic Juvenile Idiopathic Arthritis

Systemic-onset JIA (sJIA, Still's disease) constitutes 10% to 20% of JIA, yet accounts for approximately two-thirds of mortality associated with JIA (47,48). Morbidity and mortality is often secondary to destructive arthritis, secondary amyloidosis, and other treatment complications, including infection and osteoporosis. sJIA is characterized by arthritis, daily spiking fever, evanescent rash, serositis, and a variety of other extraarticular features (Still GF). Males and females are affected equally. Patients are both antinuclear antibody (ANA) and rheumatoid factor (RF) negative. Because of the infrequency of uveitis,

TABLE 13.3

DIFFERENTIAL DIAGNOSIS OF ANTERIOR UVEITIS IN CHILDREN

Juvenile idiopathic arthritis
Juvenile spondyloarthropathies
Juvenile ankylosing spondylitis
Juvenile psoriatic arthritis
Juvenile reactive arthritis
Sarcoidosis
Blau syndrome
Tubulointerstitial nephritis and uveitis
Kawasaki disease
Inflammatory bowel disease related (ulcerative colitis, Crohn's disease)
Autoinflammatory syndromes: periodic fevers, cryoprin-associated periodic syndromes
Herpes
Syphilis
Trauma
Idiopathic

screening by ophthalmologists is advised only yearly (49,50). Acquired tenosynovitis of the superior oblique tendon (Brown syndrome) has been described (51).

Oligoarthritis

Oligoarthritis, also known as *pauciarticular* arthritis, involves no more than 1 to 4 joints in the first 6 months of disease onset. It is characterized by asymmetric arthritis, early onset (before age 6), female predilection, positive ANA, and high risk of iridocyclitis (52). Oligoarthritis is further subdivided into *persistent*, affecting four joints or less throughout the disease course and *extended*, affecting more than 4 joints after the first 6 months (46). Boys are affected more commonly in the late-onset pauciarticular JIA. These patients are both ANA and RF negative, and approximately 75% of boys with this subtype are HLA-B27 positive.

Chronic iridocyclitis is seen in up to 50% of patients (53). Ophthalmologic screening is recommended every 3 months in this group for a minimum of 5 years after JIA diagnosis (50).

Polyarthritis

Polyarticular JIA affects five or more joints during the first 6 months of disease. It may be characterized by low-grade fever, anemia, and malaise within the first 3 months. Girls are more affected than boys. There are two subtypes: RF positive and RF negative. The former seldom develop uveitis and tend to develop arthritis in late childhood and adolescence. Definitive diagnosis of RF-positive polyarthritis must be confirmed on two separate occasions at least 3 months apart (46). Between 7% and 15% of patients with JIA with uveitis have polyarticular onset (54). Screening is recommended every 6 months (50).

Enthesis-Related Arthritis

Enthesis-related JIA is characterized by chronic arthritis associated with inflammation of muscle and tendon attachment to bone as well as arthritis of one or more joints. Patients are more often HLA-B27–positive boys, usually in the preadolescent to adolescent age group. Uveitis often presents suddenly, and is symptomatic and unilateral. Extraarticular manifestations can occur, such as gastrointestinal, mucosal, and cutaneous manifestations (55–57).

Psoriatic Arthritis

In addition to the presence of psoriasis and arthritis, this diagnosis requires at least two of the following: dactylitis, nail pitting or onycholysis, psoriasis in a first-degree relative. Positive RF is an exclusion criterion (46). Uveitis is usually insidious and chronic anterior, and is seen in 10% of affected children (58).

Undifferentiated Arthritis

This is the last subtype of JIA, which is essentially a diagnosis of exclusion of the other subtypes.

JUVENILE SPONDYLOARTHROPATHIES

The juvenile spondyloarthropathies (JSpA) are an interrelated group of uveitic entities, in children under 16 years old, associated with systemic disease, that are strongly HLA-B27 positive and usually RF negative. They represent the third most common etiology of anterior uveitis in children (59–61).

Juvenile Ankylosing Spondylitis

Over 90% of patients are HLA-B27 positive (62,63). Ocular symptoms are characterized by a recurrent nongranulomatous anterior uveitis. Bilateral uveitis occurs in 80% but usually not simultaneously (64). Severe uveitis can present with hypopyon.

Boys are affected more than girls, and lower extremities are affected, as opposed to lower back involvement in adults. Peripheral arthropathy may present prior to the radiographic finding of sacroiliac joint involvement. Early detection of sacroiliitis may require contrast-enhanced magnetic resonance imaging (65). Stamato et al. reported the occurrence of aortic regurgitation in children with JSpA (66).

Juvenile Psoriatic Arthritis

Girls are affected more frequently. Ocular manifestations include chronic nongranulomatous anterior uveitis. Juvenile psoriatic arthritis (JPsA) is the cause of approximately 3% to 4% of HLA-B27–positive uveitis and accounts for approximately 5% of JIA. Joint disease may be pauciarticular or polyarticular. Systemic features include psoriatic skin changes and nail pitting (46).

Juvenile Reactive Arthritis (Previously Known as Reiter Syndrome)

Reactive arthritis is described as the classic triad of conjunctivitis, arthritis, and urethritis, though more recently, it has been recognized that all three need not necessarily occur simultaneously (67). Conjunctivitis is the most frequent presenting sign in children. Boys are more commonly affected than girls. Ocular involvement includes nongranulomatous anterior uveitis in approximately 3% to 12% of patients (54). Possible etiologies include prior infection with *Salmonella* or *Shigella* enterocolitis.

SARCOIDOSIS

Most reported cases of pediatric sarcoidosis are in the age group 13 to 15 years, but it can present even in infancy (68–71). Definitive diagnosis is made through histopathologic demonstration of a non-caseating epithelioid granuloma along with the correlating clinical and laboratory findings (72,73). Sarcoid eye disease can present with uveitis involving the anterior or posterior segment. Sarcoidosis in

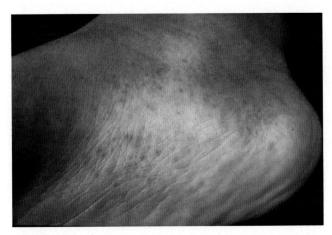

FIGURE 13.3. Characteristic sarcoidosis skin rash of foot.

children can include arthritis, skin rash, lymphadenopathy, pulmonary involvement, and hepatosplenomegaly depending on the age of onset (54). While pulmonary involvement is much more common in adults, it is less likely in children, who tend to have more skin and joint involvement (72,74). There are two distinct categories of pediatric sarcoidosis: early onset sarcoidosis (EOS), which is more similar to JIA in its presentation, and juvenile sarcoidosis (72,73,75). EOS is rarer and is characterized by the triad of rash, arthritis, and uveitis, usually in children less than 5 years old (76–79). The characteristic rash is usually asymptomatic and appears as eczematous or infiltrated plaques or papules (Fig. 13.3). Chest and joint radiographs are usually normal (76). Juvenile sarcoidosis presents in children older than 4 years of age and its manifestations are mainly pulmonary.

BLAU SYNDROME

Blau syndrome is another chronic systemic granulomatous entity that is important to consider when the differential includes sarcoidosis or JIA. The initial and early presentation of this disease is often mistaken for JIA or EOS, and the laboratory findings can be misleading. It is an autosomal dominant disease and can involve multiple organ systems with a classic triad of symmetric arthritis, recurrent uveitis, and granulomatous dermatitis (80). It is not associated with HLA-B27. A mutation in *NOD2/CARD15* on chromosome 16 has been described in families with both Blau syndrome and EOS (81,82). Systemic corticosteroids and/or steroid-sparing agents are required for control of the arthritis, dermatitis, and uveitis. Because of abnormal calcium metabolism, serum calcium and calcium excretion should be closely monitored. Therefore, any patient with this clinical picture and lab reports consistent with hypercalcemia, hypercalciuria, proteinuria, elevated angiotensin-converting enzyme, and in some cases, abnormal liver function tests, should be considered for Blau syndrome (70).

TUBULOINTERSTITIAL NEPHRITIS AND UVEITIS

Tubulointerstitial nephritis and uveitis (TINU) is characterized by bilateral anterior uveitis with renal failure from an eosinophilic interstitial nephritis (83). It has been thought to be related to infection, antibiotic drugs, as well as the coexistence of other autoimmune (84–86). TINU is more prevalent in females (3:1), particularly adolescents and young adults, and can vary in clinical presentation with ocular symptoms preceding renal diagnosis (20%) or following renal diagnosis (65%) (87). Constitutional symptoms such as weight loss, fatigue, arthralgia, and fever may be present (84). Sedimentation rate and serum creatinine are usually elevated. Urinalysis reveals glucosuria, microhematuria, casts, and beta-2 microglobulin. Diagnosis requires renal biopsy. Overall, TINU has a good prognosis, with good response to treatment with oral prednisolone, although recurrence rates can be as high as 56% (84,88).

KAWASAKI DISEASE

Kawasaki disease is an acute multisystem exanthematous vasculitis, affecting small- and medium-sized blood vessels (with propensity for the coronary arteries) which occurs in childhood. It is characterized by fever, mucocutaneous lesions, and cervical lymphadenopathy (89–91).

One of the classic diagnostic findings of Kawasaki disease is bilateral bulbar conjunctival erythema, without exudation, follicles, or papillae, and can be seen in more than 90% of children with the disease (Fig. 13.4) (89,92). Other ocular findings can include superficial punctate keratitis, vitreous opacities, papilledema, and subconjunctival hemorrhage (90). Anterior uveitis is often seen within the first week of systemic illness and can have associated keratic precipitates (KP) (89). The uveitis usually resolves in 2 to 8 weeks

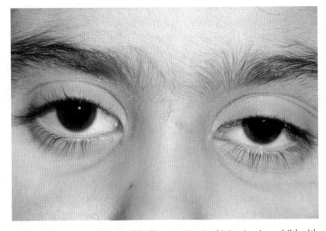

FIGURE 13.4. Mild bilateral bulbar conjunctival injection in a child with Kawasaki disease.

without long-term sequelae. Topical treatment is often not required. When Kawasaki disease is suspected, prompt referral to a pediatric cardiologist is of utmost importance, as sudden death secondary to coronary arteritis is a fatal complication (1% to 2%) (54). Serial echocardiography is a vital part of the workup as surveillance to evaluate for coronary artery aneurysms (93).

Use of systemic steroids has been discouraged as it may increase the risk for coronary aneurysm. A single infusion of high-dose (2 g/kg) γ-globulin (with or without systemic steroids) remains the mainstay of therapy (94,95).

INFLAMMATORY BOWEL DISEASE

Inflammatory bowel disease (IBD) includes multisystem immune-mediated disorders affecting mainly the gastrointestinal tract including Crohn's disease and ulcerative colitis. Common extraintestinal manifestations can include uveitis, ocular surface disease, arthritis, erythema nodosum, and pyoderma gangrenosum. Children with IBD are often asymptomatic when it comes to ocular involvement, which emphasizes the need for ophthalmologic screening exams in this population. One study found the prevalence of asymptomatic uveitis in their pediatric population to be 12.5%. All patients with asymptomatic uveitis were male, and most had Crohn's disease as opposed to ulcerative colitis. Posterior subcapsular cataract was seen in 15.6% (96). Another larger study found that asymptomatic transient uveitis was more prevalent in children with Crohn's disease than ulcerative colitis as well as in those who had experienced extraintestinal manifestations (97). Multiple studies have agreed that there is no relationship between the activity of gastrointestinal disease and the presence of ocular inflammation (97,98).

OTHER AUTOINFLAMMATORY SYNDROMES

There are a few other autoinflammatory syndromes worth addressing when considering the cause of chronic, recurrent, multisystem inflammation with uveitis in pediatrics. They include the *periodic fevers* (familial Mediterranean fever, mevalonate-kinase deficiency, and TNF receptor-associated periodic syndrome), and *cryoprin-associated periodic syndromes or CAPS* (Muckle-Wells syndrome, chronic infantile neurologic cutaneous and articular syndrome, which are cold-induced autoinflammatory syndromes from mutations in CIAS-1 or NLRP3). Given their genetic basis, these syndromes are often seen in specific ethnic groups and show an onset often before the age of 5. They are characterized by recurrent flares of systemic inflammation. Most present with attacks of fever, rash, and arthralgias, along with elevation of acute phase reactants, as well as other multisystem signs of inflammation, such as peritonitis, pleurisy, pericarditis, splenomegaly, and lymphadenopathy (99–101).

INTERMEDIATE UVEITIS

Intermediate uveitis involves the posterior ciliary body, vitreous, and peripheral retina (10). It is the second most common form of pediatric uveitis, after anterior uveitis, with some reports as high as 42% (1,102). Most cases are idiopathic, perhaps as high as 87% (103). The disease may be unilateral or bilateral, and onset is typically in the teenage to young adult years (104). Common complications include cataracts, CME, and band keratopathy Nikkhah (46,103). Pars planitis is characterized by inflammatory clumps (snowballs and snowbanking) usually along the inferior ora serrata, in the absence of systemic disease (Fig. 13.5) (10). It is important to examine the area for neovascularization, which can lead to vitreous hemorrhage. This finding, in addition to inferior peripheral retinoschisis is more often seen in children than in adults (105). In active disease retinal vascular leakage and periphlebitis may occur, and in 50% of children, optic disc edema can be seen as well (106). Macular edema is the leading cause of ocular morbidity (105,107).

Treatment of Intermediate Uveitis

In the setting of CME, choices for treatment include periocular steroid injections and short-term oral steroids, with or without retinal cryopexy. Systemic steroid-sparing agents, including biologic agents are used when inflammation is severe. Giles and Bloom have devised a treatment algorithm for children with intermediate uveitis based on visual acuity and presence or absence of anterior chamber reaction (16). In children who have 20/40 or better visual acuity, the presence of cells in the anterior chamber warrants treatment with topical corticosteroids and cycloplegia. In the absence of anterior chamber cells, no treatment is warranted. For those with less than 20/40 visual acuity and subretinal exudation, optic nerve papillitis, or floaters, weekly injections of periocular steroids are recommended. If there is still no improvement with the maximal dose, including reinjection, retinal cryopexy would be indicated. The authors also

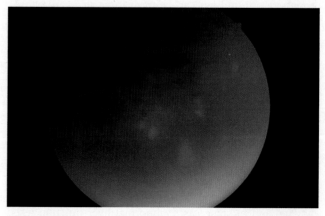

FIGURE 13.5. Vitreous "snowballs" overlying pars plana in pars planitis.

Table 13.4
DIFFERENTIAL DIAGNOSIS OF POSTERIOR UVEITIS AND PANUVEITIS IN CHILDREN
Toxoplasmosis
Toxocariasis
Diffuse unilateral subacute neuroretinitis
Lyme disease
Tuberculosis
Viral: Herpetic, cytomegalovirus, rubella, rubeola, measles, Epstein-Barr virus
Syphilis
Fungal: candidiasis, aspergillosis, leptospirosis
Histoplasmosis
Bartonella
Sarcoidosis
Lyme disease
Vogt-Koyanagi-Harada syndrome
Behçet disease
Idiopathic

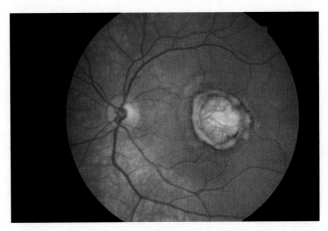

FIGURE 13.6. Macular scar from congenital toxoplasmosis.

reserve immunosuppressive agents such as cyclosporine for bilateral disease or if the above treatment fails (16).

Posterior Uveitis

Posterior uveitis accounts for the majority of uveitis cases in children, and of these, toxoplasmosis is the most common (108,109). Table 13.4 summarizes the common causes of pediatric posterior uveitis.

Toxoplasmosis

The intracellular protozoan *Toxoplasma gondii* can result in a retinochoroiditis. Cats are the definitive and primary host, whereas humans are the intermediate or secondary host, usually after ingestion of the organism in undercooked meat. The majority of human infection is congenital as the result of transplacental transmission by an infected mother.

Congenital disease usually presents bilaterally, with macular scars (Fig. 13.6), whereas acquired disease more often presents as active retinitis without scarring, often in the setting of immunocompromise (54).

If toxoplasmosis is suspected, serologic testing will show the presence of toxoplasma IgG antibody, which confirms prior exposure, but does not necessarily indicate active infection (110). After acute infection, toxoplasma IgM antibodies may continue to persist even for a year (111). Thus, given the high rate of positive anti-toxoplasma serology, which has been found to be anywhere from 10.2% to 21.5% in schoolchildren, a negative test may be a more valuable test result than a positive test to rule out toxoplasma infection (112–114). Because toxoplasmosis has a predilection for neural tissue, the most common findings are in the retina and posterior pole. The classic presentation of focal overlying vitritis from active toxoplasmosis gives a "headlight in the fog" appearance (115,116).

In immunocompetent patients, infection is usually self-limited. When vision is threatened because of optic nerve or macular involvement, or if the individual is immunocompromised, treatment is then indicated. Peripheral retinochoroiditis has been found to be associated with visual impairment in approximately 17% of patients, while 50% of children with posterior pole lesions can be visually impaired. Thus, it is important to monitor lesions closely even when sparing the macula (117). Treatment consists of pyrimethamine, clindamycin, and sulfonamides. Corticosteroids should be used cautiously to help quiet active inflammation but only with concomitant antibiotics. Alternative regimens include sulfamethoxazole with trimethoprim or doxycycline.

Toxocariasis

Ocular toxocariasis secondary to hematogenous spread to the eye is seen after initial tissue invasion from the second-stage larvae of the canine or feline roundworm *Toxocara canis* or *Toxocara cati*. The majority of cases are seen in the pediatric population, who are often in close contact with puppies and kittens.

Ocular toxocariasis can lead to significant morbidity and vision loss. Systemic involvement of the liver, brain, and lungs occurs more often in younger children (approximately 1 to 4 years old) with a history of pica.

The classic presentation of ocular toxocariasis is leukocoria with decreased vision that may be accompanied by pain, photophobia, floaters, or strabismus. Five clinically

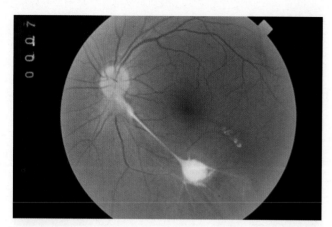

FIGURE 13.7. Posterior pole granuloma in toxocariasis.

distinct forms may occur: peripheral retina and vitreous lesions, posterior pole lesions, endophthalmitis, optic nerve involvement, and anterior segment involvement (118). The most common form of ophthalmic toxocariasis in children 6 to 14 years old is the isolated granuloma (Fig. 13.7) (54). Children with peripheral granuloma usually are older and show traction bands extending from the granuloma to the macula and optic nerve.

The diagnosis made is by clinical history and examination findings. Negative enzyme-linked immunosorbent assay (ELISA) should not rule out the diagnosis, especially when the clinical suspicion is high. There have been several reports of undetectable serum anti-toxocara antibodies. It may be necessary to perform ELISA testing on aqueous or vitreous fluid. Cytology may often reveal eosinophilia. Stool samples are not helpful.

As antihelminthic agents (e.g., albendazole) have been found to potentially worsen inflammation after treatment, oral and periocular steroids are recommended (119). Surgical treatment may be indicated in the presence of retinal detachment, fibrovascular membrane proliferation, and endophthalmitis.

Diffuse Unilateral Subacute Neuroretinitis

Diffuse unilateral subacute neuroretinitis (DUSN) is a progressive inflammatory multietiologic disease that can be caused by several species of nematodes. As raccoons are the definitive host, *Baylisascaris procyonis* (*B. procyonis*) is the most common cause of DUSN in North America (120). Humans are accidental hosts and can be affected variably. The three clinical states of infection are visceral larva migrans, neural larva migrans, and ocular larva migrans. Ophthalmic findings include vitritis, retinitis with migration tracks, retinal vasculitis, optic neuritis, and choroidal infiltrates in the early stages, while late changes may include optic atrophy, retinal vessel attenuation, and retinal pigment epithelium (RPE) degeneration. The clinical picture may be similar to toxocariasis as endophthalmitis, posterior pole granuloma, or retinal detachment (121–125). The definitive

diagnosis involves intraocular identification of the nematode in the subretinal space. Systemic anthelminthic therapy can be considered. Otherwise, laser photocoagulation directed at the nematode followed by a short course of steroids is the definitive treatment.

Lyme Disease

Lyme borreliosis has been described in causes of intermediate uveitis in adults, but it is a rare cause in children (126–128). It is during the late stages of Lyme disease that uveitis (anterior and intermediate) and keratitis have been described. A transient conjunctivitis can be seen in the early stages (126,127). Systemic findings include arthritis, and an annular "bull's-eye" rash called erythema migrans. Recommended treatment is with antibiotics, usually amoxicillin, in children under 8 years of age, and doxycycline in older children (129). Good results have also been reported with intravenous ceftriaxone (130).

Tuberculosis

Tuberculosis (TB) uveitis is a common cause of infectious uveitis in children and was found to be the second most common cause after toxoplasmosis in a global review of the literature (7). Whereas in the past, TB was implicated as a cause for the majority of infectious uveitis cases, currently it is a relatively less frequent cause in developed countries (131,132).

TB uveitis is one of the "great mimickers" in that it can present as an anterior uveitis, intermediate uveitis with vitritis and macular edema, neuroretinitis, choroiditis, endophthalmitis, or panophthalmitis (133–137). Posterior uveitis, consisting of vitritis with serpiginous multifocal lesions involving the posterior pole and periphery, has been described (138).

Intermediate uveitis from TB is the least common manifestation of intraocular TB. More commonly, TB manifests as a posterior uveitis, and the most common intraocular manifestation of TB consists of choroidal tubercles and large solitary tuberculomas (135,139).

Treatment of ocular TB is targeted against the infection as well as the inflammatory reaction, and consists of antituberculous drugs with concomitant systemic corticosteroids (140).

Herpes Simplex

Herpes simplex virus type 2 (HSV-2) accounts for herpetic infections in newborns, with the majority being during the first months of life (141). Neonatal HSV is symptomatic and has a high mortality. Infection is contracted from the maternal birth canal at delivery but can also occur prenatally or through Cesarean section. Neonatal HSV can manifest as isolated mucocutaneous infection, central nervous system disease, or disseminated infection (142). Approximately 45% of cases present with only skin, external eye, or mucosal findings (mucocutaneous HSV), without brain involvement.

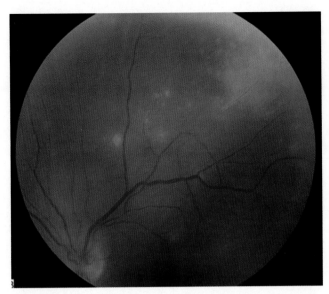

FIGURE 13.8. Acute retinal necrosis in a patient with herpes simplex virus. (Image courtesy of Dr. Sunir J. Garg, Wills Eye institute.)

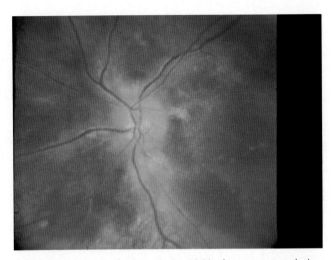

FIGURE 13.9. Hemorrhagic necrotic retinitis due to cytomegalovirus retinitis in a child with severe systemic manifestations of acquired immune deficiency syndrome (AIDS).

Magnetic resonance imaging of the brain and lumbar puncture are recommended for all infants for which HSV infection is considered (142–144).

Ocular manifestations of HSV-2 infection in the newborn can include vitritis and chorioretinitis, and even choroidal hemorrhage (145,146). Acute retinal necrosis is a necrotizing and rapidly progressing chorioretinitis associated with vitritis and an occlusive vasculopathy (Fig. 13.8). Prophylactic laser photocoagulation is often required to prevent retinal detachment. Late ocular manifestations may include atrophy of the RPE and optic disc as well as late retinitis with exudation into vitreous years later (147). All patients should be treated with antivirals (e.g., acyclovir), which has been shown to improve mortality significantly (143).

Congenital Syphilis

The incidence of congenital syphilis has drastically decreased in the United States because of serologic testing at pregnancy and the widespread availability of antibiotic therapy (148). Active congenital disease in infants can manifest systemically with fever, rash, pneumonitis, and hepatosplenomegaly. Ophthalmic findings of congenital syphilis can include the classic funduscopic appearance of the "salt and pepper" or "bone spicule" chorioretinitis. Acquired syphilis can also present with either anterior or posterior inflammation including vitritis, vasculitis, chorioretinitis, papillitis, or optic atrophy. A 10-day course of intravenous penicillin is the recommended treatment (54).

Cytomegalovirus

Cytomegalovirus (CMV) is the most common cause of congenital infection in humans. The birth prevalence of congenital CMV infection is from 0.3% to 2.3% of live births (149).

Approximately 0.7% of all newborns are born with congenital CMV infection annually in the USA, leaving approximately 6,000 children with disabilities such as hearing and vision loss or mental retardation (150). CMV is also seen as an acquired infection in children and the immunosuppressed and can manifest as a necrotic and hemorrhagic chorioretinitis (Fig. 13.9). Retinal tears and detachment may ensue. Compared to adults, CMV retinitis is not as common in the pediatric age group (5% in one series), but should be considered especially in those children who are immunocompromised and with positive CMV laboratory results (151). Congenital infection resulting in a maculitis is usually self-limited (152). Treatment of congenital CMV requires intravenous or intravitreal antivirals (e.g., ganciclovir) (153). Other studies report at least a 3-month course of therapy to control the chorioretinitis (154).

Fungal

Fungal causes of endophthalmitis, such as candidiasis (Fig. 13.10), aspergillosis, or leptospirosis, in children are rare and most often found in the immunocompromised. Chorioretinitis may involve the periphery or posterior pole (155,156). Despite the frequency of candidemia in immunocompromised patients, ocular involvement is highly unusual (157). Treatment involves systemic and intravitreal antifungal agents as well as possible vitrectomy.

Masquerade Syndromes

Masquerade syndromes in the pediatric population can be devastating and should be considered when evaluating a child with uveitis. These can present with anterior or posterior inflammation. Some of these entities include: retinoblastoma (Fig. 13.11), leukemia, and juvenile xanthogranuloma (Table 13.5). Each of these entities can present with leukocoria or strabismus, and findings can

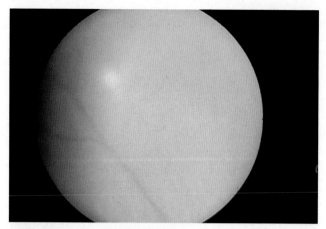

FIGURE 13.10. Candida endophthalmitis with "fungus ball" in posterior vitreous in an immunosuppressed patient.

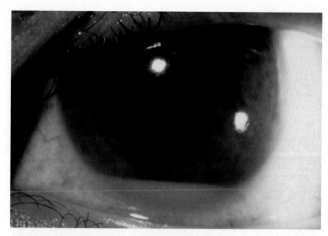

FIGURE 13.12. Relapse of acute lymphoblastic leukemia presenting with pseudohypopyon.

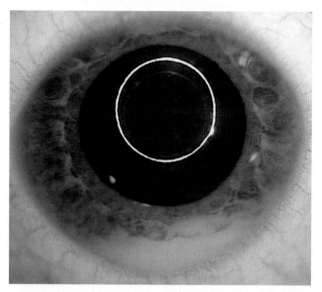

FIGURE 13.11. Child presenting with pseudohypopyon due to retinoblastoma. Note collection of white material in inferior anterior chamber over iris. White rings in pupil are photographic artifact. (Image courtesy of Carol L. Shields, M.D.)

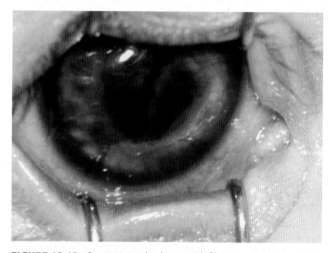

FIGURE 13.13. Spontaneous hyphema with fibrinous uveitis seen in an infant with juvenile xanthogranuloma.

Table 13.5
DIFFERENTIAL DIAGNOSIS OF MASQUERADE SYNDROMES OF PEDIATRIC UVEITIS
Retinoblastoma
Leukemia
Juvenile xanthogranuloma
Metastatic tumors
Malignant melanoma
Intraocular foreign body
Coats disease
Endophthalmitis

include pseudohypopyon and spontaneous hyphema (158–162). As retinoblastoma must be ruled out especially in cases with dense inflammation, B-scan ultrasound should be performed to look for calcification, which is not usually seen in other causes of uveitis. Relapses of acute lymphoblastic leukemia (ALL) can present with ocular findings ranging from anterior chamber and iris involvement to leukemic retinopathy (Fig. 13.12), and these patients require oncologic-targeted treatment of the central nervous system and eye (161,162). Juvenile xanthogranuloma, a rare nonneoplastic, non-Langerhans-cell, histiocytic inflammatory skin disorder, can mimic anterior uveitis or any of the above syndromes, presenting with hyphema (Fig. 13.13), iris heterochromia, or cell and flare. It is a self-limited disease, and treatment is targeted toward lowering inflammation and where indicated, lowering intraocular pressure.

REFERENCES

1. BenEzra D, Cohen E, Maftzir G. Uveitis in children and adolescents. *Br J Ophthalmol* 2005;89:444–448.

2. Azar D, Martin F. Paediatric uveitis: a Sydney clinic experience. *Clin Exp Ophthalmol* 2004;32:468–471.

3. Edelsten C, Reddy MA, Stanford MR, Graham EM. Visual loss associated with pediatric uveitis in English primary and referral centers. *Am J Ophthalmol* 2003;135:676–680.

4. Pivetti-Pezzi P. Uveitis in children. *Eur J Ophthalmol* Jul–Sep 1996;6(3):293–298.

5. de Boer J, Wulffraat N, Rothova A. Visual loss in uveitis of childhood. *Br J Ophthalmol* 2003;87:879–884.

6. Kadayifcilar S, Eldem B, Tumer B. Uveitis in childhood. *J Pediatr Ophthalmol Strabismus* 2003;40:335–340.

7. Rathinam SR, Namperumalsamy P. Global variation and pattern changes in epidemiology of uveitis. *Indian J Ophthalmol* 2007;55:173–183.

8. Hamade IH, Al Shamsi HN, Al Dhibi H, Chacra CB, Abu El-Asrar AM, Tabbara KF. Uveitis survey in children. *Br J Ophthalmol* May 2009;93(5):569–572.

9. Smith JA, Mackensen F, Sen HN, et al. Epidemiology and course of disease in childhood uveitis. *Ophthalmology* 2009;116(8):1544–1551.e1.

10. Jabs DA, Nussenblatt RB, Rosenbaum JT. The Standardization of Uveitis Nomenclature (SUN) Working Group. Standardization of uveitis nomenclature for reporting clinical data. Results of the First International Workshop. *Am J Ophthalmol* 2005;140:509–516.

11. Holland GN, Stiehm ER. Special considerations in the evaluation and management of uveitis in children. *Am J Ophthalmol* June 2003;135(6):867–878.

12. Foster CS, Barrett F. Cataract development and cataract surgery in patients with juvenile rheumatoid arthritis-associated iridocyclitis. *Ophthalmology* 1993;100:809–817.

13. Foster CS, Havrlikova K, Baltatzis S, et al. Secondary glaucoma in patients with juvenile rheumatoid arthritis- associated iridocyclitis. *Acta Ophthalmol Scand* 2000;78:576–579.

14. Tugal-Tutkun I, Havrlikova K, Power WJ, Foster CS. Changing patterns in uveitis of childhood. *Ophthalmology* 1996;103:375–383.

15. Sabri K, Saurenmann RK, Silverman ED, Levin AV. Course, complications and outcome of juvenile arthritis related uveitis. *J AAPOS* 2008;12(6):539–545.

16. Giles CL, Bloom JN. Uveitis in childhood. In: Tasman W, Jaeger EA, eds. *Duane's foundations of clinical ophthalmology*, Vol 4. Philadelphia, PA: Lippincott Williams and Wilkins, 2000:1–21.

17. Slabaugh MA, Herlihy E, Ongchin S, van Gelder RN. Efficacy and potential complications of difluprednate use for pediatric uveitis. *Am J Ophthalmol* May 2012;153(5):932–938.

18. Veld J in't, Wulffraat NM, JF Swart JF. Adverse events of methotrexate treatment in JIA. *Pediatr Rheumatol* 2011; 9(Suppl 1):P203. Poster presentation: Proceedings of 18th Pediatric Rheumatology European Society (PReS) Congress.

19. Kwok AK, Lam DS, Ng JS, et al. Ocular-hypertensive response to topical steroids in children. *Ophthalmology* 1997;104:2112–2116.

20. Ng JS, Fan DS, Young AL, et al. Ocular hypertensive response to topical dexamethasone in children: a dose- dependent phenomenon. *Ophthalmology* 2000;107:2097–2100.

21. Dana MR, Merayo-Lloves J, Schaumberg DA, Foster CS. Visual outcomes prognosticators in juvenile rheumatoid arthritis-associated uveitis. *Ophthalmology* 1997;104:236–244.

22. Saurenmann RK, Levin AV, Feldman BM, Laxer RM, Schneider R, Silverman ED. Risk of new-onset uveitis in patients with juvenile idiopathic arthritis treated with anti-TNFalpha agents. *J Pediatr* Dec 2006;149(6):833–836.

23. Saurenmann RK, Levin AV, Rose JB, et al. Tumour necrosis factor alpha inhibitors in the treatment of childhood uveitis. *Rheumatology* 2006;45:982–989.

24. Lovell DJ, Ruperto N, Goodman S, et al. Adalimumab is safe and effective during long-term treatment of patients with juvenile rheumatoid arthritis: results from a 2-year study. *Arthritis Rheum* 2007;56:S292.

25. Mori M, Takei S, Imagawa T, et al. Safety and efficacy of long-term etanercept in the treatment of methotrexate-refractory polyarticular-course juvenile idiopathic arthritis in Japan. *Mod Rheumatol* Sep 2012;22(5):720–726.

26. Lovell DJ, Reiff A, Jones OY, et al. Pediatric Rheumatology Collaborative Study Group. Long-term safety and efficacy of etanercept in children with polyarticular-course juvenile rheumatoid arthritis. *Arthritis Rheum* June 2006;54(6):1987–1994.

27. Lovell DJ, Reiff A, Ilowite NT, et al. Pediatric Rheumatology Collaborative Study Group. Safety and efficacy of up to eight years of continuous etanercept therapy in patients with juvenile rheumatoid arthritis. *Arthritis Rheum* May 2008;58(5):1496–1504.

28. Bracaglia C, Buonuomo PS, Tozzi AE, et al. Safety and efficacy of etanercept in a cohort of patients with juvenile idiopathic arthritis under 4 years of age. *J Rheumatol* June 2012;39(6):1287–1290.

29. Kerensky TA, Gottlieb AB, Yaniv S, Au SC. Etanercept: efficacy and safety for approved indications. *Expert Opin Drug Saf* Jan 2012;11(1):121–139.

30. Giannini EH, Ruperto N, Prieur AM, et al. Efficacy of abatacept in different sub-populations of juvenile idiopathic arthritis (JIA): results of a randomized withdrawal study. *Arthritis Rheum* 2007;56:S291.

31. Lovell DJ, Ruperto N, Prieur AM, et al. Abatacept treatment of juvenile idiopathic arthritis (JIA): safety report. *Arthritis Rheum* 2007;56:S292.

32. Kenawy N, et al. Abatacept: a potential therapy in refractory cases of juvenile idiopathic arthritis-associated uveitis. *Graefes Arch Clin Exp Ophthalmol* Feb 2011;249(2):297–300.

33. Lipsky JJ. Mycophenolate mofetil. *Lancet* 1996;348:1357–1359.

34. Allison AC, Eugui EM. Immunosuppressive and other effects of mycophenolic acid and an ester prodrug, mycophenolate mofetil. *Immunol Rev* 1993;136:5–28.

35. Dipchand AI, Benson L, McCrindle BW, et al. Mycophenolate mofetil in pediatric heart transplant recipients: a single-center experience. *Pediatr Transplant* 2001;5:112–118.

36. Doycheva D, Deuter C, Stuebiger N, Biester S, Zierhut M. Mycophenolate mofetil in the treatment of uveitis in children. *Br J Ophthalmol* 2007;91:180–184.

37. Li J, Heinz C, Zurek-Imhoff B, Heiligenhaus A. Intraoperative intraocular triamcinolone injection prophylaxis for post-cataract surgery fibrin formation in uveitis associated with juvenile idiopathic arthritis. *J Cataract Refract Surg* Sep 2006;32(9):1535–1539.

38. BenEzra D, Cohen E. Cataract surgery in children with chronic uveitis. *Ophthalmology* 2000;107:1255–1260.

39. Lundvall A, Zetterstrom C. Cataract extraction and intraocular lens implantation in children with uveitis. *Br J Ophthalmol* 2000;84:791–793.

40. Jensen AA, Basti S, Greenwald MJ, Mets MB. When may the posterior capsule be preserved in pediatric intraocular lens surgery? *Ophthalmology* 2002;109:324–327.

41. Ravinet E, Mermoud A, Birgnoli R. Four years later: a clinical update on latanoprost. *Eur J Ophthalmol* 2003;13:162–175.

42. Ho CL, Wong EY, Walton DS. Goniosurgery for glaucoma complicating chronic childhood uveitis. *Arch Ophthalmol* June 2004;122(6):838–844.

43. Freedman SF, Rodriguez-Rosa RE, Rojas MC, Enyedi LB. Goniotomy for glaucoma secondary to chronic childhood uveitis. *Am J Ophthalmol* May 2002;133(5):617–621.

44. Morad Y, Donaldson CE, Kim YM, Abdolell M, Levin AV. The Ahmed seton in the treatment of pediatric glaucoma. *Am J Ophthalmol* 2003;135(6):821–829.

45. Nikkhah H, Ramezani A, Ahmadieh H, et al. Childhood pars planitis; clinical features and outcomes. *J Ophthalmic Vis Res* Oct 2011;6(4):249–254.

46. Petty RE, Southwood TR, Manners P, et al. International League of Associations for Rheumatology classification of juvenile idiopathic arthritis: second revision, Edmonton. *J Rheumatol* 2004;31:390–392.

47. Schneider R, Laxer RM. Systemic onset juvenile rheumatoid arthritis. *Bailliere's Clin Rheumatol* 1998;12(2):245–271.

48. Gurion R, Lehman TJ, Moorthy LN. Systemic arthritis in children: a review of clinical presentation and treatment. *Int J Inflam* 2012:271569.

49. Kanski JJ. Screening for uveitis in juvenile chronic arthritis. *Br J Ophthalmol* Mar 1989;73(3):225–228.

50. Cassidy J, Kivlin J, Lindsley C, Nocton J; Section on Rheumatology; Section on Ophthalmology. Ophthalmologic examinations in children with juvenile rheumatoid arthritis. *Pediatrics* May 2006;117(5):1843–1845.

51. Roifman CM, Lavi S, Moore AT, Morin DJ, Stein LD, Gelfand EW. Tenosynovitis of the superior oblique muscle (Brown syndrome) associated with juvenile rheumatoid arthritis. *J Pediatr* Apr 1985;106(4):617–619.

52. Guillaume S, Prieur AM, Coste J, Job-Deslandre C. Long-term outcome and prognosis in oligoarticular-onset juvenile idiopathic arthritis. *Arthritis Rheum* 2000;43:1858–1865.

53. Jordan A, McDonagh JE. Juvenile idiopathic arthritis: the pediatric perspective. *Pediatr Radiol* 2006;36:734–742.

54. Giles CL, Capone Jr A, Joshi MM. Uveitis in children. In: Nelson LB, Olitsky SE, eds. *Harley's pediatric ophthalmology*, 5th Ed. Philadelphia, PA: Lippincott Williams and Wilkins, 2005:305–327.

55. Burgos-Vargas R. The juvenile-onset spondyloarthritides: rationale for clinical evaluation. *Best Pract Res Clin Rheumatol* 2002;16:551–72.

56. Flato B, Hoffmann-Vold AM, Reiff A, Førre Ø, Lien G, Vinje O. Long-term outcome and prognostic factors in enthesitis-related arthritis. *Arthritis Rheum* 2006;54:3573–3582.

57. Burgos-Vargas R, Vazquez-Mellado J, Cassis N, et al. Genuine ankylosing spondylitis in children: a case-control study of patients with early definite disease according to adult onset criteria. *J Rheumatol* 1996;23:2140–2147.

58. Paiva ES, Macaluso DC, Edwards A, Rosenbaum JT. Characterisation of uveitis in patients with psoriatic arthritis. *Ann Rheum Dis* Jan 2000;59(1):67–70.

59. Patel H, Goldstein D. Pediatric uveitis. *Pediatr Clin North Am* 2003;50:125–136.

60. McCannel CA, Holland GN, Helm CJ et al. Causes of uveitis in the general practice of ophthalmology. UCLA Community based Uveitis Study Group. *Am J Ophthalmol* 1996;121:35–46.

61. Henderly DE, Genstler AJ, Smith RE. Changing patterns of uveitis. *Am J Ophthalmol* 1987:103:131–136.

62. Khan MA, Braun WE, Kushner I, et al. HLA-B27 in ankylosing spondylitis: differences in frequency and relative risk in American blacks and Caucasians. *J Rheumatol Suppl* 1977;3:39–43.

63. Masi AT, Medsger TA Jr. A new look at the epidemiology of ankylosing spondylitis and related syndromes. *Clin Orthop Relat Res* 1979;143:15–20.

64. Burgos-Vargas R, Petty RE. Juvenile ankylosing spondylitis. *Rheum Dis Clin North Am* 1992;18:123–142.

65. Bollow M, Braun J, Biedermann T, et al. Use of contrast-enhanced magnetic resonance (MR) imaging to detect sacroiliitis in children. *Skeletal Radiol* 1998;27:606–616.

66. Stamato T, Laxer RM, de Freitas C, et al. Prevalence of cardiac manifestations of juvenile ankylosing spondylitis. *Am J Cardiol* 1995;75:744–746.

67. Zivony D, Nocton J, Wortmann D, Esterly N. Juvenile Reiter's syndrome: a report of four cases. *J Am Acad Dermatol* 1998;38:32–37.

68. Stanworth SJ, Kennedy CT, Chetcuti PA, Carswell F. Hypercalcaemia and sarcoidosis in infancy. *J R Soc Med* Mar 1992;85(3):177–178.

69. Shetty AK, Gedalia A. Childhood sarcoidosis: a rare but fascinating disorder. *Pediatr Rheumatol Online* 2008;6:6.

70. Pattishall EN, Strope GL, Spinola SM, Denny FW. Childhood sarcoidosis. *J Pediatr* Feb 1986;108(2):169–177.

71. Kendig EL Jr. Sarcoidosis in children: personal observations on age distribution. *Pediatr Pulmonol* 1989;6(2):69–70.

72. Cimaz R, Ansell BM. Sarcoidosis in the pediatric age. *Clin Exp Rheumatol* 2002;20:231–237.

73. Pattishall EN, Kendig EL Jr. Sarcoidosis in children. *Pediatr Pulmonol* 1996;22:195–203.

74. Shetty AK, Gedalia A. Sarcoidosis in children. *Curr Probl Pediatr* 2000;30:153–176.

75. Mallory SB, Paller AS, Ginsburg BC, McCrossin ID, Abernathy R. Sarcoidosis in children: differentiation from juvenile rheumatoid arthritis. *Pediatr Dermatol* 1987;4:313–319.

76. Rasmussen JE. Sarcoidosis in young children. *J Am Acad Dermatol* Nov 1981;5(5):566–570.

77. Fink CW, Cimaz R. Early onset sarcoidosis: not a benign disease. *J Rheumatol* 1997;24:174–177.

78. Hetherington S. Sarcoidosis in young children. *Am J Dis Child* Jan 1982;136(1):13–15.

79. Häfner R, Vogel P. Sarcoidosis of early onset. A challenge for the pediatric rheumatologist. *Clin Exp Rheumatol* Nov–Dec 1993;11(6):685–691.

80. Pastores GM, Michels VV, Stickler GB, Su WP, Nelson AM, Bovenmyer DA. Autosomal dominant granulomatous arthritis, uveitis, skin rash, and synovial cysts. *J Pediatr* Sep 1990;117(3):403–408.

81. Wang X, Kuivaniemi H, Bonavita G, et al. CARD15 mutations in familial granulomatosis syndromes: a study of the original Blau syndrome kindred and other families with large-vessel arteritis and cranial neuropathy. *Arthritis Rheum* Nov 2002;46(11):3041–3045.

82. Miceli-Richard C, Lesage S, Rybojad M, et al. CARD15 mutations in Blau syndrome. *Nat Genet* Sep 2001;29(1):19–20.

83. Dobrin RS, Vernier RL, Fish AL. Acute eosinophilic interstitial nephritis and renal failure with bone marrow lymph node granulomas and anterior uveitis. A new syndrome. *Am J Med* 1975;59:325–333.

84. Mandeville JTH, Levinson RD, Holland GN. The tubulointerstitial nephritis and uveitis syndrome. *Surv Ophthalmol* 2001;46:195–208.

85. Cigni A, Soro G, Faedda R, et al. A case of adult-onset tubulointerstitial nephritis and uveitis ("TINU syndrome") associated with sacroileitis and Epstein-Barr virus infection with good spontaneous outcome. *Am J Kidney Dis* 2003;42:E4–E10.

86. Stupp R, Mihatsch MJ, Matter L, Streuli RA. Acute tubulointerstitial nephritis with uveitis (TINU syndrome) in a patient with serologic evidence for Chlamydia infection. *Klin Wochenschr* 1990;68:971–915.

87. Vohra S, Eddy A, Levin AV, Taylor G, Laxer RM. Tubulointerstitial nephritis and uveitis in children and adolescents: four new cases and a review of the literature. *Pediatr Nephrol* 1999;13(5):321–426.

88. Goda C, Kotake S, Ichiishi A et al. Clinical features in tubulointerstitial nephritis and uveitis (TINU) syndrome. *Am J Ophthalmol* 2005;140:637–641.

89. Burns JC, Joffe L, Sargent RA et al. Anterior uveitis associated with Kawasaki syndrome. *Pediatr Infect Dis* 1985;4:258.

90. Ohno S, Miyajima T, Higuchi M et al. Ocular manifestations of Kawasaki's disease (mucocutaneous lymph node syndrome). *Am J Ophthalmol* 1982;93:713.

91. Puglise JV, Rao NA, Weiss RA et al. Ocular features of Kawasaki's disease. *Arch Ophthalmol* 1982;100:1101.

92. Morens DM, Anderson LJ, Hurwitz ES. National surveillance of Kawasaki disease. *Pediatrics* 1980;65:21.

93. Newburger JW, Takahashi M, Gerber MA, et al. Diagnosis, treatment, and long-term management of Kawasaki disease: a statement for health professionals from the Committee on Rheumatic Fever, Endocarditis and Kawasaki Disease, Council on Cardiovascular Disease in the Young, American Heart Association. *Circulation* Oct 2004;110(17):2747–2771.

94. Newburger JW, Takahashi M, Burns JC, et al. The treatment of Kawasaki syndrome with intravenous gamma globulin. *N Engl J Med* 1986;315:341–347.

95. Newburger JW, Takahashi M, Beiser AS, et al. A single intravenous infusion of gamma globulin as compared with four infusions in the treatment of acute Kawasaki syndrome. *N Engl J Med* 1991;324:1633–1639.

96. Rychwalski PJ, Cruz OA, Alanis-Lambreton G, Foy TM, Kane RE. Asymptomatic uveitis in young people with inflammatory bowel disease. *J AAPOS* June 1997;1(2):111–114.

97. Hofley P, Roarty J, McGinnity G, et al. Asymptomatic uveitis in children with chronic inflammatory bowel diseases. *J Pediatr Gastroenterol Nutr* Nov 1993;17(4):397–400.

98. Daum F, Gould HB, Gold D, et al. Asymptomatic transient uveitis in children with inflammatory bowel disease. *Am J Dis Child* Feb 1979;133(2):170–171.

99. Federici S, Caorsi R, Gattorno M. The autoinflammatory diseases. *Swiss Med Wkly* June 2012;142:w13602.

100. Siegal S. Benign paroxysmal peritonitis. *Ann Intern Med.* 1945;23:1–21.

101. Ben-Chetrit E, Touitou I. Familial Mediterranean fever in the world. *Arthritis Rheum* 2009;61(10):1447–1453.

102. Nagpal A, Leigh JF, Acharya NR. Epidemiology of uveitis in children. *Int Ophthalmol Clin* 2008;48(3):1–7. Medline.

103. Romero R, Peralta J, Sendagorta E, Abelairas J. Pars planitis in children: epidemiologic, clinical, and therapeutic characteristics. *J Pediatr Ophthalmol Strabismus* Sep–Oct 2007;44(5):288–293.

104. Park DW, Folk JC, Whitcup SM, et al. Phakic patients with cystoid macular edema, retinal periphlebitis, and vitreous inflammation. *Arch Ophthalmol.* Aug 1998;116(8):1025–1029.

105. Guest S, Funkhouser E, Lightman S. Pars planitis: a comparison of childhood onset and adult onset disease. *Clin Exp Ophthalmol* 2001;29:81–84.

106. Whitcup SM. Intermediate uveitis. In: Nussenblatt RB, Whitcup SM, ed. *Uveitis: Fundamentals and Clinical Practice.* Philadelphia, PA: Mosby; 2004:269–277.

107. de Boer J, Berendschot TT, van der Does P, Rothova A. Long-term follow-up of intermediate uveitis in children. *Am J Ophthalmol* 2006;141:616–621.

108. Perkins ES. Pattern of uveitis in children. *Br J Ophthalmol* Apr 1966;50(4):169–185.

109. Makley TA Jr, Long J, Suie T et al. Uveitis in children: a follow-up study. *J Pediatr Ophthalmol* 1969;6:136.

110. Hovakimyan A, Cunningham ET Jr. Ocular toxoplasmosis. *Ophthalmol Clin North Am* 2002;15:327–332.

111. Holland GH, O'Connor GR, Belfort R Jr, et al. Toxoplasmosis. In: Pepose JS, Holland GH, Wilhelmus KR, eds. *Ocular infection and immunity.* St Louis, MO: Mosby-Year Book, 1996:1183–1223.

112. Fan CK, Hung CC, Su KE, et al. Seroprevalence of Toxoplasma gondii infection among pre-schoolchildren aged 1–5 years in the Democratic Republic of Sao Tome and Principe, Western Africa. *Trans R Soc Trop Med Hyg* May 2006;100(5):446–449.

113. Taylor MR, Lennon B, Holland CV, Cafferkey M. Community study of toxoplasma antibodies in urban and rural schoolchildren aged 4 to 18 years. *Arch Dis Child* Nov 1997;77(5):406–409.

114. Huldt G, Lagercrantz R, Sheehe PR. On the epidemiology of human toxoplasmosis in Scandinavia especially in children. *Acta Paediatr Scand* 1979;68:745–749.

115. Couvreur, Desmonts G. Congenital and maternal toxoplasmosis. A review of 300 congenital cases. *Dev Med Child Neurol* Oct 1962;4:519–530.

116. Wilson CB, Remington JS, Stagno S, Reynolds DW. Development of adverse sequelae in children born with subclinical congenital Toxoplasma infection. *Pediatrics* Nov 1980;66(5):767–774.

117. Tan HK, Schmidt D, Stanford M, Tear-Fahnehjelm, Ferret N, Salt A, Gilbert R. European multicenter study on congenital toxoplasmosis (emscot). Risk of Visual Impairment in Children with Congenital Toxoplasmic Retinochoroiditis. *Am J Ophthalmol* 2007;144:648–653.

118. Hagler WH, Pollard ZF, Jarret WH, et al. Result for surgery for ocular Toxocara canis. *Ophthalmology* 1981;88:1081–1086.

119. Barisant-Asenbaker T, Maca SM, Hauff W. Treatment of ocular toxocariasis with albendazole. *J Ocul Pharmacol Ther* 2001;17:287–294.

120. Kuchle M, Knorr HL, Medenblik-Frysch, Weber SA, Bauer C, Naumann, GO. Diffuse unilateral subacute neuroretinitis syndrome in a German most likely caused by the raccoon roundworm, Baylisascaris procyonis. *Graefes Arch Clin Exp Ophthalmol* 1993;231:48–51.

121. Barbazetto IA, Lesser RL, Tom D, Freund KB. Diffuse unilateral subacute neuroretinitis masquerading as a white-dot syndrome. *Br J Ophthalmol* 2009;93:574–576, 655.

122. Gass JD, Braunstein RA. Further observations concerning the diffuse unilateral subacute neuroretinitis syndrome. *Arch Ophthalmol* 1983;101:1689–1697

123. Gass JD, Scelfo R. Diffuse unilateral subacute neuroretinitis. *J R Soc Med.* 1978;71:95–111.

124. Kazacos KR. Baylisascaris procyonis and related species. In: Samuel WM, Pybus MJ, Kocan AA, eds. *Parasitic diseases of wild mammals*, 2nd Ed. Ames, IA: Iowa State University Press, 2001:301–341.

125. Mets MB, Noble AG, Basti S, et al. Eye findings of diffuse unilateral subacute neuroretinitis and multiple choroidal infiltrates associated with neural larva migrans due to Baylisascaris procyonis. *Am J Ophthalmol* 2003;135: 888–890.

126. Zaidman GW. The ocular manifestations of Lyme disease. *Int Ophthalmol Clin* 1997;37:13–28.

127. Berglöff J, Gasser R, Feigl B. Ophthalmic manifestations in Lyme borreliosis. *J Neuro-ophthalmol* 1994;14:15–20.

128. Karma A, Seppälä I, Mikkilä H, et al. Diagnosis and clinical characteristics of ocular Lyme borreliosis. *Am J Ophthalmol* 1995;119:127–135.

129. Wormser GP, Dattwyler RJ, Shapiro ED, et al. The clinical assessment, treatment, and prevention of Lyme disease, human granulocytic anaplasmosis, and babesiosis: clinical practice guidelines by the Infectious Diseases Society of America. *Clin Infect Dis* Nov 2006;43(9):1089–1134. Epub 2006 Oct 2. Erratum in: *Clin Infect Dis* Oct 2007;45(7):941.

130. Suttorp-Schulten MSA, Kuiper H, Kijlstra A, et al. Long-term effects of ceftriaxone treatment on intraocular Lyme borreliosis. *Am J Ophthalmol* 1993;116:571–575.

131. Woods AC. Modern concepts of the etiology of uveitis. *Am J Ophthalmol* 1960;50:1170–1187.

132. Wakabayashi T, Morimura Y, Miyamoto Y, Okada AA. Changing pattern of intraocular inflammatory disease in Japan. *Ocul Immunol Inflamm* 2003;11:277–286.

133. Rosen PH, Spalton DJ, Graham EM. Intraocular tuberculosis. *Eye* 1990;4:486–492.

134. Helm CJ, Holland GN. Ocular tuberculosis. *Surv Ophthalmol* 1993;38:229–256.

135. Biswas J, Madhavan HN, Gopal L, Badrinath SS. Intraocular tuberculosis: clinocopathologic study of five cases. *Retina* 1995;15:461–468.

136. Gupta A, Gupta V, Arora S, Dogra MR, Bambery P. PCR-positive tubercular retinal vasculitis: clinical characteristics and management. *Retina* 2001;21:435–444.

137. Demirci H, Shields CL, Shields JA, Eagle RC Jr. Ocular tuberculosis masquerading as ocular tumors. *Surv Ophthalmol* 2004;49:78–89.

138. Vasconcelos-Santos DV, Rao PK, Davies JB, Sohn EH, Rao NA. Clinical features of tuberculous serpiginous like choroiditis in contrast to classic serpiginous choroiditis. *Arch Ophthalmol* Jul 2010;128(7):853–858.

139. Gupta V, Gupta A, Rao NA. Intraocular tuberculosis: an update. *Surv Ophthalmol* 2007;52:561–587.

140. Bodaghi B, LeHoang P. Review ocular tuberculosis. *Curr Opin Ophthalmol* Dec 2000;11(6):443–448.

141. Hutchison DS, Smith RE., Haughton PB. Congenital herpetic keratitis. *Arch Ophthalmol* 1975;93:70–73.

142. Corey L, Wald A. Maternal and neonatal herpes simplex virus infections. *N Engl J Med* 2009;361:1376–1385.

143. Meehan WP, Bachur RG. Predictors of cerebrospinal fluid pleocytosis in febrile infants aged 0 to 90 days. *Pediatr Emerg Care* 2008;24(5):287–293.

144. Kimberlin D, Lin C-Y, Jacobs RF, et al. Natural history of neonatal herpes simplex virus infections in the Acyclovir era. *Pediatrics* 2001;108:223–229.

145. Hagler WS, Walters DV, Nahmias, AJ. Ocular involvement in neonatal herpes simplex virus infection. *Arch Ophthalmol* 1969;82:169–176.

146. Nahmias AJ, Hagler WS. Ocular manifestations of herpes simplex in the newborn (neonatal herpes simplex). *Int Ophthalmol Clin* 1972;12,191–213.

147. Tarkkanen A, Laatikainen L. Late ocular manifestations in neonatal herpes simplex infection. *Br J Ophthalmol* Sep 1977; 61(9):608–616.

148. Wilhemus KR. Syphilis. In: Insler MS, ed. *AIDS and other sexually transmitted diseases and the eye*, Orlando, FL: Grune & Stratton, 1987:73–104.

149. Kenneson A, Cannon MJ. Review and meta-analysis of the epidemiology of congenital cytomegalovirus (CMV) infection. *Rev Med Virol* 2007;17:253–276.

150. Cannon MJ. Congenital cytomegalovirus (CMV) epidemiology and awareness. *J Clin Virol* 2009;46(Suppl):S6–S10.

151. Baumal CR, Levin AV, Kavalec CC, Petric M, Khan H, Read SE. Screening for pediatric cytomegalovirus retinitis. *Arch Pediatr Adolesc Med* 1996;150(11):1186–1192.

152. Baumal CR, Levin AV, Read SE. Cytomegalovirus retinitis in immunosuppressed children. *Am J Ophthalmol* 1999;127:550–558.

153. Kimberlin DW, Lin CY, Sanchez PJ, et al. Effect of ganciclovir therapy on hearing in symptomatic congenital cytomegalovirus disease involving the central nervous system: a randomized, controlled trial. *J Pediatr* 2003;143:16–25

154. Nigro G, Scholz H, Bartmann U. Ganciclovir therapy for symptomatic congenital cytomegalovirus infection in infants: a two-regimen experience. *J Pediatr* 1994;124:318–322.

155. Feigin RD, Anderson DC. Human leptospirosis. *CRC Crit Rev Clin Lab Sci* 1975;5:413–467.

156. Maalouf T, Schmitt C, Crance J, George J, Angioi K. [Endogenous aspergillus endophthalmitis: a case report]. *J Fr Ophtalmol* Feb 2000;23(2):170–173.

157. Donahue SP, Hein E, Sinatra RB. Ocular involvement in children with candidemia. *Am J Ophthalmol* June 2003;135(6): 886–887.

158. Materin MA, Shields CL, Shields JA, Eagle RC Jr. Diffuse infiltrating retinoblastoma simulating uveitis in a 7-year-old boy. *Arch Ophthalmol* Mar 2000;118(3):442–443.

159. Shields JA, Shields CL, Eagle RC, Blair CJ. Spontaneous pseudohypopyon secondary to diffuse infiltrating retinoblastoma. *Arch Ophthalmol* 1998;106:1301–1302.

160. Foster BS, Mukai S. Intraocular retinoblastoma presenting as ocular and orbital inflammation. *Int Ophthalmol Clin* 1996;36:153–160.

161. Decker EB, Burnstine RA. Leukemic relapse presenting as acute unilateral hypopyon in acute lymphocytic leukemia. *Ann Ophthalmol* 1993;25:346–349.

162. Yi DH, Rashid S, Cibas ES, Arrigg PG, Dana MR. Acute unilateral leukemic hypopyon in an adult with relapsing acute lymphoblastic leukemia. *Am J Ophthalmol* 2005;139: 719–721

14

Diseases of the Retina and Vitreous

Eric D. Weichel • James F. Vander • William Tasman • William E. Benson

X-LINKED RECESSIVE RETINOSCHISIS

X-linked recessive retinoschisis is an inherited ocular disorder that occurs in males (1). It is characterized by degeneration of the vitreous and splitting of the retina at the level of the nerve fiber layer. The most common finding involves the macula and consists of a petaloid configuration. Usually there are numerous folds that radiate in a spoke-wheel configuration (Fig. 14.1). This may give the clinical appearance of cystoid macular edema, but the macula does not stain with fluorescein. When seen in a young boy, this sign should alert the observer to the possibility of the peripheral changes seen in X-linked retinoschisis. Peripheral retinoschisis, seen 50% of the time, is more common in the inferotemporal quadrant. The schisis is always bilateral but may be asymmetric. The anterior limit of the retinoschisis seldom extends to the ora serrata, and the posterior limit may extend to the optic disc. Nerve fiber layer breaks are common and appear as large round or oval holes (Fig. 14.2). In some eyes the nerve fiber layer breaks are so large that only remnants of the nerve fiber layer remain. Often, bridging retinal blood vessels are present, and there is hemorrhage into the vitreous. When vitreous hemorrhaging occurs, some patients develop dragging of the retina. Most recently, ocular coherence tomography (OCT) has demonstrated a characteristic finding of a wide hyporeflective space between the thin reflective outer layer and the thicker, more reflective inner retinal layers (Fig. 14.3) (2).

Vitreous veils and strands may also be present. The electroretinogram (ERG) often shows a subnormal b-wave in conjunction with a normal a-wave. Color vision abnormalities parallel the degree of foveal involvement. The results of electrooculogram (EOG) and dark adaptation tests are usually normal. Most commonly, patients are first seen because of decreased vision. The visual acuity on presentation is usually between 20/70 and 20/100 mmHg. This often (but not always) deteriorates up until age 20 years, reaching the 20/200 range. Other presenting symptoms are vitreous hemorrhage, retinal detachment, and strabismus.

The natural history of retinoschisis is that of a stationary or slowly progressive disease. The most important complications are vitreous hemorrhage and retinal detachment. It is important to realize that progression of X-linked retinoschisis may be followed by spontaneous partial regression, and that fluctuations in the appearance of the fundus are common during the first few years of life.

Differential diagnoses include retinal detachment, persistent fetal vasculature (PFV), Goldmann-Favre disease, retinitis pigmentosa (RP), Norrie disease, Stickler's syndrome, and (because of occasional dragged retinas) retinopathy of prematurity (ROP) and familial exudative vitreoretinopathy (FEVR).

Retinal detachment in a child may be differentiated from X-linked retinoschisis because the latter is always bilateral. In addition, retinal detachment, unlike X-linked retinoschisis, usually extends to the ora serrata.

In some cases of PFV, extensive hyaloid remnants that are adherent to the disc and inferior retina may contract and cause an inferior retinal detachment, with or without visible retinal breaks. This condition is generally unilateral and associated with microphthalmos, and is neither familial nor hereditary.

Goldmann-Favre vitreoretinal degeneration is transmitted as an autosomal recessive trait. Although peripheral retinoschisis is often present, the disease is also characterized by night blindness and fundus changes resembling those of RP.

Stickler's syndrome is transmitted as an autosomal dominant trait. Elevation of the retina is attributable to rhegmatogenous retinal detachment rather than retinoschisis. Additional ophthalmologic and systemic features help to distinguish this entity from X-linked retinoschisis.

Although dragging of the retina may occur in ROP and FEVR, the additional fundus features of these two entities are distinct and rarely confused with X-linked retinoschisis. In addition, ROP and FEVR can usually be identified because of a history of prematurity in the case of ROP and autosomal dominant inheritance with respect to FEVR.

As long as X-linked retinoschisis is not accompanied by rhegmatogenous retinal detachment, no treatment is indicated. Recurrent vitreous hemorrhages are usually best treated conservatively, but vitrectomy occasionally becomes necessary because of the presence of organized vitreous membranes leading to retinal detachment.

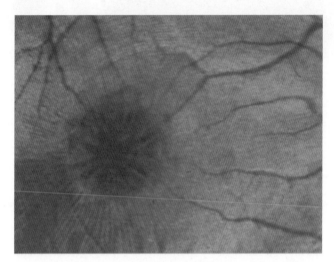

FIGURE 14.1. Foveoschisis with typical retinal cysts in a petaloid configuration and radial striae in X-linked retinoschisis.

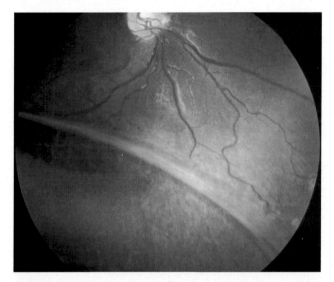

FIGURE 14.2. Peripheral nerve fiber layer dehiscence in X-linked retinoschisis.

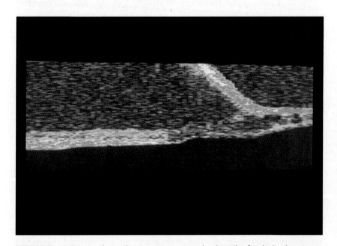

FIGURE 14.3. Ocular coherence tomography (OCT) of X-linked retinoschisis showing schisis of nerve fiber layer.

X-linked retinoschisis has a prevalence ranging from 1:5,000 to 1:25,000. Female carriers of X-linked retinoschisis generally do not show any ocular abnormalities, although peripheral retinal alterations similar to those found in affected males have been reported (3). The X-linked retinoschisis gene (XLRS1) is located on the distal short arm of the X chromosome (Xp22) (4). DNA analysis can reveal evidence of the carrier state and is of use when performing genetic counseling.

HEREDITARY VITREORETINOPATHY WITH SYSTEMIC FINDINGS

Stickler's Syndrome

Stickler and associates (5) described an autosomal dominant, progressive arthro-ophthalmopathy associated with high myopia, optically empty vitreous, and retinal detachment. Stickler's syndrome is the most common disorder associated with high myopia and retinal detachment. Systemic findings include midfacial flattening (Fig. 14.4), cleft palate, micrognathia, glossoptosis, hearing loss, and skeletal dysplasia. The ocular findings include an optically empty vitreous with bands. Myopia is common. Lattice degeneration is present and often radial and perivascular (Fig. 14.5). There is a high

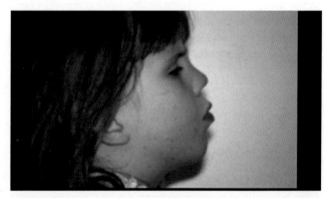

FIGURE 14.4. Flattened facies in a young patient with Stickler's syndrome.

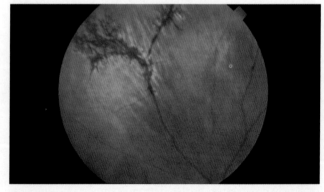

FIGURE 14.5. Radially oriented lattice degeneration in a patient with Stickler's syndrome.

incidence of retinal breaks, which may be multiple or giant retinal tears. Cataracts and glaucoma are often present.

Treatment of retinal detachment in Stickler's syndrome is difficult because of posterior retinal breaks and a high incidence of proliferative vitreoretinopathy. Prophylactic laser treatment to areas of lattice degeneration and retinal breaks may reduce the risk of detachment.

Stickler's syndrome has been linked to mutations in the type II procollagen (*COL2A1*) gene. A polymerase chain reaction assay is available to assist in genetic counseling (6).

HEREDITARY VITREORETINOPATHY WITHOUT SYSTEMIC FINDINGS

Wagner's Syndrome

Wagner's syndrome (Wagner's hereditary vitreoretinal degeneration) (7) is similar to Stickler's syndrome but without any systemic abnormalities. These patients have myopia, an optically empty vitreous cavity, preretinal avascular membranes, perivascular pigmentation, retinal degeneration, and progressive chorioretinal atrophy. They also develop lenticular changes between the ages of 20 and 40 years. Wagner's syndrome is autosomal dominant and has been localized to chromosome 5q13–q14 (8). Patients with Wagner's syndrome infrequently develop retinal detachment compared with a much higher incidence of retinal detachments in patients with Stickler's syndrome.

Goldmann-Favre Disease

Goldmann-Favre disease (9) is inherited in an autosomal recessive manner. It is characterized by night blindness with absent or diminished ERG response, foveal and peripheral retinoschisis, pigment changes resembling RP, and progressive decreased visual function (Fig. 14.6) (6). As in Stickler's syndrome, the vitreous is liquefied with vitreous strands and veils. Retinal detachments and cataract formation are common in this condition. Retinal detachments have a guarded prognosis for successful repair; therefore, asymptomatic

breaks should be treated prophylactically before detachment. The enhanced S cone syndrome is a variant of Goldmann-Favre disease with night blindness and foveal cystic changes without the vitreous abnormalities.

STARGARDT'S DISEASE (FUNDUS FLAVIMACULATUS)

Stargardt's disease is most often an autosomal recessive condition that usually appears between 8 and 14 years of age. It is bilateral, slowly progressive, and sometimes associated with macular degeneration (10). Characteristically, the foveal reflex is absent or grayish in color. Pigmentary spots sometimes develop in the macular area and may accumulate irregularly. Yellowish-white pisciform flecks may be visible in the deep retina or retinal pigment epithelium (RPE) (Fig. 14.7). They are typically seen in the posterior pole but can extend out to the equator. Eventually, in some cases, a circular area of depigmentation and chorioretinal atrophy of the macula follow (Figs. 14.8 and 14.9). In the early stages of the disease, the loss of central vision may be out of proportion to the appearance of the fundus. Fluorescein angiography may reveal abnormalities, particularly a dark fundus (the so-called silent choroid) (11) before any fundus abnormalities become apparent. Fluorescein angiography of the flecks may reveal hypofluorescence, presumably because of blockage. Later, some areas may hyperfluoresce because of damage to the RPE. Sometimes, the entire choroid may show blockage on fluorescein angiography.

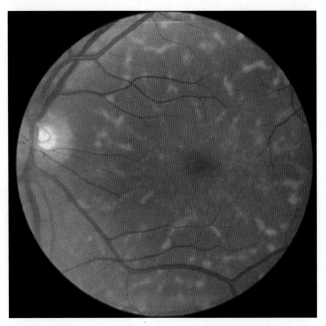

FIGURE 14.7. Typical pisciform lesion of fundus flavimaculatus. The dark fundus and pisciform lesions are the result of excessive amounts of lipofuscin in the pigment epithelium.

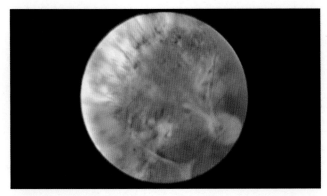

FIGURE 14.6. Preretinal membranes and retinal pigmentary changes in a 34-year-old woman with Goldmann-Favre disease.

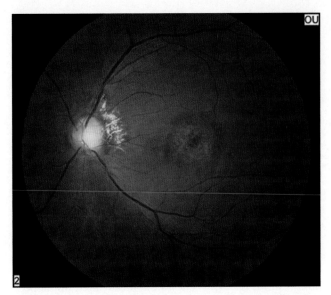

FIGURE 14.8. Typical retinal pigment epithelium (RPE) atrophy in a bull's-eye pattern in a patient with Stargardt's disease.

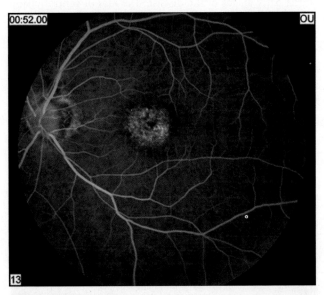

FIGURE 14.9. Corresponding fluorescein angiography with central hyperfluorescence.

The evolution is slow, symmetric, and progressive, and the disease is usually well established by age 30 years, with vision in the 20/200 range. Late in life, large areas of chorioretinal atrophy may develop (12).

The disease was first described by Stargardt in 1909. Fundus flavimaculatus was described independently as a separate entity. Today, however, Stargardt's disease and fundus flavimaculatus are thought to have a common cause and to represent different parts on the spectrum of a single disease. Stargardt's disease is caused by a mutation of the ABCR gene located on the short arm of chromosome 1 (13). Other sites have been identified in patients with

the autosomal dominant form. The mechanism of photoreceptor death has been postulated (14) with histopathology revealing the accumulation of lipofuscin within the RPE. Stargardt's disease refers to predominantly macular involvement, and fundus flavimaculatus refers to more peripheral involvement. In fundus flavimaculatus, the vision is near normal unless macular involvement develops.

BEST'S VITELLIFORM DEGENERATION

In 1905, Best reported eight members of one family with an interesting macular dystrophy, now called Best's vitelliform degeneration (15). The transmission in this disease is autosomal dominant, but there may be variable expressivity. Vitelliform macular degeneration has a distinctive appearance characterized by a sharply defined discoid formation in, or immediately adjacent to, the macula (Fig. 14.10). The disc is usually yellow-orange or pinkish yellow and varies in size from 0.5 to 4 disc diameters. The abnormality is subretinal and resembles the yolk of a poached egg (16). It is usually diagnosed between 5 and 15 years of age and is bilateral, although unilateral cases have been reported. Multiple vitelliform lesions in the same eye have also been described. The condition is very slowly progressive. The vision is usually normal or mildly reduced at this stage. Gradually the homogeneous contents of the vitelliform disc may "scramble," giving an irregular yellow lesion, eventually leaving abnormal pigmentation and chorioretinal atrophy (Fig. 14.11). The appearance at that point is often indistinguishable from that associated with other types of macular degeneration. Vision loss develops from these atrophic changes or, in some cases, a choroidal neovascular membrane. These macular changes can also be assessed with the OCT (17).

Best's dystrophy of the macula is present at birth and if no change is visible postnatally, the clinical signs will not develop later.

ERG results are normal, as are the peripheral visual fields. Central scotomata cannot be elicited in eyes with normal visual acuity but are present late in the disease. Dark adaptation is normal. The EOG, however, is always

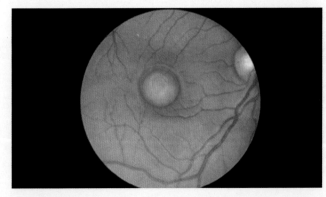

FIGURE 14.10. Fried-egg appearance of a typical vitelliform macular degeneration.

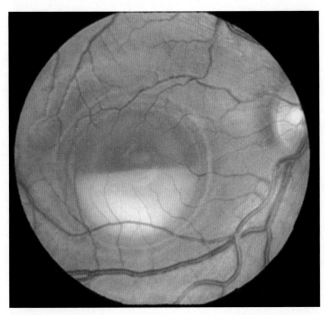

FIGURE 14.11. Pseudohypopyon stage of Best's disease resulting from a fluid level within a cystic space.

abnormal in patients with vitelliform macular degeneration, even in those who do not express the disease clinically. Thus, EOG testing is helpful diagnostically and in genetic counseling, because unaffected carriers have a 50% chance of passing the condition to their offspring. Carriers who have a normal ophthalmologic examination will have a subnormal EOG (18).

The pathogenesis of vitelliform degeneration is uncertain. The gene causing Best's disease has been localized to 11q13 with an identified encoded protein called bestrophin, which has an unknown function (19).

STATIONARY FORMS OF CONGENITAL NIGHT BLINDNESS

The stationary forms of congenital night blindness are congenital stationary night blindness, Oguchi's disease, and fundus albipunctatus. These diseases should be considered in the differential diagnosis of early-onset night blindness that is not progressive. All of the former differ from the progressive disorders, such as RP, Goldmann-Favre disease, and gyrate atrophy.

Congenital Stationary Night Blindness

Congenital stationary night blindness exhibits three modes of inheritance: (a) X-linked (most common), (b) autosomal dominant, and (c) autosomal recessive. Molecular genetic testing has found numerous mutations in genes encoding proteins of photoreceptors or the RPE (20). Color vision and visual fields characteristically are normal. Visual acuity is normal or mildly reduced. The fundi are entirely

normal. Histopathologically the retina is normal. Dark adaptation reveals a reduced retinal sensitivity, and ERG shows a decreased scotopic response with a normal photopic response. The defect is caused from a failure of communication between the proximal end of the photoreceptor and the bipolar cell. No Purkinje shift in relative luminosity curves is seen. Initially, the disease can be confused with early-onset RP, but the lack of progression with the former serves to distinguish these two entities.

Oguchi's Disease

Oguchi's disease, another stationary form of congenital night blindness, is usually diagnosed by a combination of two readily observable phenomena. First is the unusual color of the fundus, which has been described as various shades of gray-white to yellow. The abnormal color may be limited to a small section of the mid-periphery or extend throughout the entire fundus in a discontinuous or homogeneous pattern. The second unique characteristic of Oguchi's disease is the Mizuo phenomenon (21), which is a change in the color of the fundus in the dark-adapted state (Fig. 14.12). When light is prevented from entering the eye, the color of the fundus changes from the light shade, seen initially, to a reddish, more normal appearance. The time needed to elicit this change varies among patients. Dark adaptation testing reveals a prolonged dark adaptation time and normal retinal sensitivities. ERG testing reveals a decreased scotopic response, which may revert to normal during prolonged dark adaptation. The genetic defect has been localized to the arrestin gene, which is responsible for terminating the signaling that triggers cellular response in the rod phototransduction cascade (22). These patients have a good prognosis, with near-normal vision that remains stable (23).

Fundus Albipunctatus

Fundus albipunctatus is another stationary form of night blindness. Patients present with nyctalopia and have essentially normal visual acuity, color vision, and visual fields. This presentation is identical to that of congenital stationary

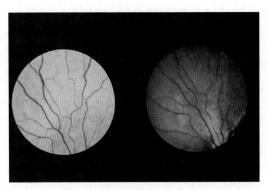

FIGURE 14.12. Oguchi disease and light-adapted retina (*left*) and dark-adapted retina exhibiting the Mizuo phenomenon (*right*).

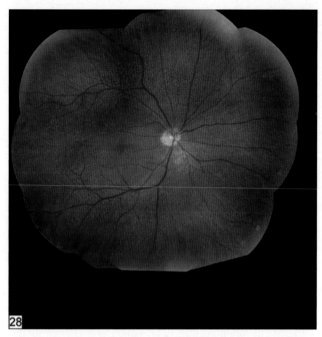

FIGURE 14.13. Patient with fundus albipunctatus with punctate white spots at the level of the RPE throughout the posterior pole, sparing the macula. Note that the disc and retinal vessels are normal.

night blindness and Oguchi's disease, but fundus albipunctatus is easily differentiated by the presence of multiple white dots scattered throughout the fundus (24) (Fig. 14.13), most likely at the level of the RPE. Patients with fundus albipunctatus have normal-appearing vessels and discs. These patients have a good prognosis, because the vision usually remains normal; however, macular degeneration may develop.

This condition is ophthalmoscopically similar to retinitis punctata albescens. However, retinitis punctata albescens is a form of night blindness with progressive retinal degeneration. The discrete uniform white dots in this condition involve the mid-peripheral retina and spare the macula. The autosomal dominant form is associated with a mutation in the human peripherin/RDS gene (25), and the autosomal recessive form is associated with a mutation in the retinaldehyde binding protein gene (RLBP1) (26).

CONGENITAL DEVELOPMENTAL ABNORMALITIES

Aplasia and Hypoplasia of the Macula

Aplasia of the macula is a rare disorder often associated with gross ocular deformities such as microphthalmos, aniridia, coloboma of the optic nerve, monocular myopia, albinism, and medullated nerve fibers. *Hypoplasia of the macula,* another rare entity, has been suggested as a possible cause of certain forms of amblyopia. In this condition, the central retina does not differentiate completely and is usually arrested at a stage equivalent to 6 to 8 months of intrauterine development. Clinically, this is detected by the lack of the

normal perifoveal capillary network, lack of a foveal reflex, absence of the macula lutea pigment, and decreased pigmentation in the foveal pigment epithelium. Visual loss is variable. The cause is uncertain.

Persistent Fetal Vasculature

The most constant feature in PFV, previously known as persistent hyperplastic primary vitreous (PHPV) (27), is a dense, white vitreous band that usually extends from the disc to the fundus periphery or to the lens (Fig. 14.14). It may occur in any meridian but is most common nasally. Limited retinal detachments or other evidence of vitreoretinal traction, such as traction folds, macular pigmentary degeneration, or pigmented demarcation lines, are often associated findings. Prominent uveal processes (Fig. 14.15) and relative microphthalmos are also characteristic of PFV.

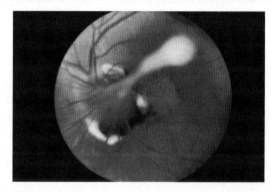

FIGURE 14.14. Persistent hyperplastic vitreous emanating from the disc.

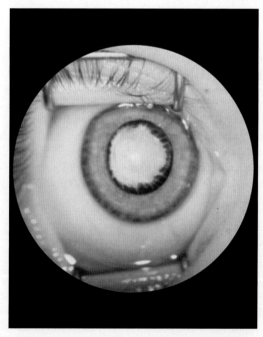

FIGURE 14.15. Elongated ciliary processes and white pupil, characteristic of persistent fetal vasculature (PFV).

As in other anomalous vascular systems, PFV can vary in degree. The spectrum includes Bergmeister's papilla, vitreoretinal veils around the disc and macula, vitreous stalks and hyaloid remnants, and retinal folds. Each is related to the other and to congenital abnormalities of the anterior primary vitreous.

The prognosis in PFV is variable depending largely on the severity of the microphthalmia and retinal detachment, if present. Removal of the vitreous opacification and cataract may yield significant visual improvement in selected cases. Aggressive amblyopia therapy is usually necessary.

Myelinated Nerve Fibers

Myelinated nerve fibers occur because of extension of myelination anterior to the lamina cribrosa where it does not belong. The cause is unknown. Myelinated nerve fibers appear during the first year of life, rarely affect visual acuity, and occur predominantly among males; although bilateral cases occur, unilaterality is the rule. The medullated fibers have a feather-like appearance and are usually adjacent to the disc. Sometimes the myelination process is located away from the optic nerve, but unless the macula is affected, vision is preserved (Fig. 14.16). If it is inherited, the mode of transmission is usually autosomal dominant.

Coats' Disease

Coats' disease is a nonhereditary abnormality of the retinal vasculature, first described by Coats in 1908 (28). Peripheral retinal telangiectasia, sometimes with a "light bulb" appearance, and secondary exudation are the characteristic findings (Fig. 14.17). In advanced cases, serous detachment of the sensory retina may occur. Discrete dilated vessels and telangiectasia are noted early on fluorescein angiography with

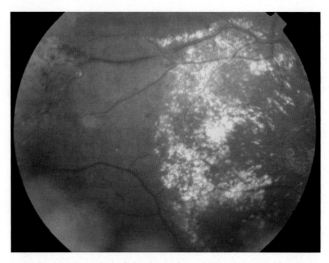

FIGURE 14.17. Light bulb lesions with exudation in Coats' disease.

marked late leakage. In addition, extensive capillary dropout in areas of peripheral retinal telangiectasia is common. In certain cases, telangiectasia and microaneurysms can occur in the posterior pole and may be associated with exudation posterior to the equator. Macular exudate may also develop in eyes in which the retinal vascular leakage is limited to the periphery. Although the vitreous is usually clear in mild cases, retinal neovascularization and vitreous hemorrhage may occur in advanced cases. Optic nerve involvement in Coats' disease is rare. In the end stages of Coats' disease, neovascular glaucoma and phthisis bulbi may develop.

Coats' disease is much more common in males than in females but does affect both sexes. It is unilateral in 90% of cases and tends to occur in childhood. A similar, although usually less severe, condition occurs in adulthood. It is uncertain whether this represents the same underlying disease as the classic form of Coats' disease.

Treatment is directed at elimination of the abnormal vessels. Cryotherapy is an effective means of eliminating the vessels and can be used from the equator to the ora serrata. Indirect laser photocoagulation may be possible if there is no subretinal fluid and the exudate is not too marked. In patients with vascular abnormalities posterior to the equator, photocoagulation is preferable. Usually, two to three treatment sessions are necessary at 4- to 6-week intervals to eliminate the abnormal vasculature.

Patients with marked Coats' disease may develop serous detachment of the sensory retina. In these individuals, scleral buckling with drainage of subretinal fluid followed by cryotherapy to the anomalous vessels can lead to reattachment of the retina.

With elimination of the anomalous vessels, subretinal exudate begins to clear. This is a slow process that may take as long as 1 year until all the exudation has absorbed. With macular involvement, a subretinal organized nodule may remain permanently in the fovea. The prognosis for recovery of macular function is poor if foveal exudation is present.

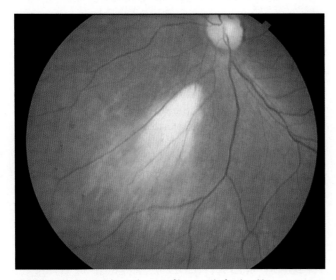

FIGURE 14.16. Myelinated nerve fibers with feather-like appearance away from the optic nerve.

Even in patients who have been successfully treated, recurrences have been noted up to 5 years later. It is therefore recommended that patients be followed at 6-month intervals, so further treatment can be given if necessary before the process becomes too extensive.

The differential diagnosis of Coats' disease includes angiomatosis of the retina, retinoblastoma, FEVR, ROP, PFV, nematode infestation, and astrocytoma of the retina.

PRIMARY AND SECONDARY RETINAL DEGENERATION

Retinitis Pigmentosa

Although given the name "retinitis pigmentosa" by Donders in 1855, this condition probably is more accurately called "retinal pigmentary dystrophy." It is often hereditary and is characterized by progressive deterioration of the visual cells, pigment epithelium, and choroid. Typical clinical findings are thinning of the retinal vessels, waxy pallor of the optic disc, and appearance of "bone-corpuscle" pigment, initially at the equator. The pigmentary changes typically become visible during the first decade of life and may begin as fine dots that gradually assume the spidery bone-corpuscle appearance (Fig. 14.18). As the disease progresses, the equatorial girdle widens and a ring scotoma is produced in the visual field.

The ring scotoma is the characteristic field defect. The defect usually begins inferotemporally and enlarges to form the ring scotoma. In more advanced stages, the scotoma may progress so only inferotemporal field and central vision are preserved.

Almost all patients with RP have night blindness, and this is reflected initially by abnormalities in dark adaptation. The adaptation curve initially shows an increased rod

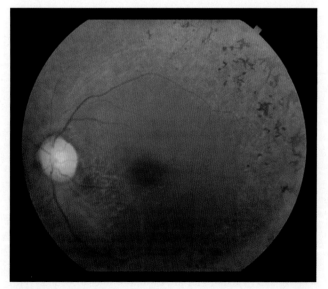

FIGURE 14.18. Attenuation of retinal vessels, waxy pallor of the optic disc, and peripheral "bone-corpuscle" pigmentation in a patient with retinitis pigmentosa (RP).

threshold with a normal cone response. As the disease progresses, the rods and the cones become involved, the curve being monophasic.

Of equal importance in the diagnosis is the ERG. In primary pigmentary degeneration of the retina, the ERG response is subnormal or absent, a change that appears before the subjective visual deterioration or ophthalmoscopically visible changes.

Histologic study reveals a general disappearance of the neuroepithelial elements, a proliferation of glial cells, changes in the pigment epithelium, and an obliterative sclerosis of the retinal vessels. First to be affected are the rods, as opposed to the ganglion cells and nerve fiber layer, which may remain unaffected even when the eye is blind. The migration of pigment into the retina, aided by macrophages, follows the degeneration.

Previously, classification of the photoreceptor degeneration depended largely on the clinical manifestations and the modes of inheritance: autosomal recessive, autosomal dominant, and X-linked. Recent advances in genetic analysis have shown that one gene may be responsible for several different clinical entities (phenotypes) and that several different genes may be responsible for one phenotype. Mutations affecting multiple loci of the rhodopsin and peripherin genes are among the many described (29). Although the advent of genetic analysis is dramatically altering the classification and genetic counseling of RP, some general statements concerning inheritance are still worth noting. The most common form is autosomal recessive, followed by autosomal dominant and X-linked recessive. The autosomal dominant type is the most benign form, and X-linked is the most severe form (30). Of greater importance, however, is that the severity and rate of progression are similar within a family; this can be helpful in individual patient counseling.

Other significant ocular findings include posterior subcapsular cataract, vitreous opacities, glaucoma, myopia, and keratoconus. Macular changes occur as cystoid macular edema and retinal pigment epithelial atrophy.

Numerous systemic associations with RP have been described (Table 14.1). Well-established extraocular manifestations include deafness, diencephalic and endocrine anomalies, oligophrenia, ophthalmoplegia, and lipidoses.

Perhaps the best known condition in the differential diagnosis of RP is the Laurence-Moon–Biedl-Bardet syndrome, which is characterized by mental retardation, hypogenitalism, retinal changes, polydactyly, obesity, and a recessive inheritance pattern (31). It occurs predominantly among males, and the retinal changes may simulate typical RP or be characterized by macular degeneration.

Other disorders associated with an atypical RP pattern are Refsum syndrome and Bassen-Kornzweig disease. In Refsum syndrome, phytanic acid accumulates in swollen RPE because of a deficiency of the enzyme phytanoyl-CoA hydroxylase. The sensory retina is affected (32), and there are changes in the RPE. Systemic findings include cerebellar ataxia, polyneuritis, and anosmia.

Table 14.1

RETINITIS PIGMENTOSA AND ASSOCIATED SYSTEMIC DISORDERS

1. Lipidoses

   a. Gaucher disease

   b. Neuronal ceroid lipofuscinosis

   A constant finding in the juvenile form (Batten-Mayou disease, Spielmeyer-Vogt disease), but a variable finding in the late infantile form (Jansky-Bielschowsky disease), in which ocular signs may vary between the infantile and juvenile forms

2. Late form of Pelizaeus-Merzbacher disease (a form of sudanophilic cerebral sclerosis)

3. Progressive familial myoclonic epilepsy

4. Spinopontocerebellar degeneration

   a. Marie ataxia

   b. Friedreich ataxia

   c. Unclassified spastic paraplegias

   d. Charcot-Marie-Tooth disease

   e. Progressive pallidal degeneration with retinitis pigmentosa

   f. Hereditary muscular atrophy, ataxia, and diabetes mellitus

5. Specific syndromes with progressive external ophthalmoplegia and retinitis pigmentosa

   a. Progressive external ophthalmoplegia (progressive nuclear ophthalmoplegia ocular myopathy)

   b. Retinitis pigmentosa, external ophthalmoplegia, and heart block

   c. Retinitis pigmentosa, ophthalmoplegia, and spastic quadriplegia

   d. Abetalipoproteinemia (Bassen-Kornzweig syndrome, acanthocytosis)

   e. Refsum syndrome

6. Generalized muscular dystrophy

7. Myotonic dystrophy (Steinert disease)

8. Syndromes in which a hearing loss is a prominent finding

   a. Hallgren syndrome

   b. Refsum syndrome

   c. Usher syndrome

   d. Retinitis pigmentosa with deafness of varying severity

   e. Cockayne disease (Cockayne-Neill disease, Neill-Dingwall syndrome)

   f. Alstrom syndrome (retinitis pigmentosa, deafness, obesity, and diabetes)

9. Syndromes with renal disease as a prominent feature

   a. Familial juvenile nephrophthisis (Fanconi nephrophthisis)

   b. Hereditary nephritis, retinitis pigmentosa, and chromosomal abnormalities

   c. Cystinuria

   d. Cystinosis (Fanconi syndrome I)

   e. Oxalosis

(continued)

Table 14.1

(continued)

10. Syndromes in which bone disease is a prominent feature

   a. Paget disease

   b. Osteogenesis imperfecta (Lobstein syndrome)

   c. Marfan syndrome

   d. Osteopetrosis "familiaris" (marble bone, osteosclerosis fragilis generalisata, Albers-Schonberg disease)

11. Syndromes with skin disease

   a. Werner disease

   b. Psoriasis

12. Laurence-Moon–Biedl-Bardet syndrome

13. Dresbach syndrome (elliptocytosis, ovalocytosis)

14. Klinefelter syndrome

15. Mucopolysaccharidoses: retinal degeneration has now been reported in types I, II, III, and V

16. Hooft disease (hypolipidemia syndrome)

Adapted from Krill AE. Retinitis pigmentosa: a review. *Sight Sav Rev* 1972;42:26, with permission.

In Bassen-Kornzweig disease, an absence of serum 3-lipoprotein leads to malabsorption and subsequent vitamin A deficiency. Systemic findings include steatorrhea, acanthocytosis, ataxic neuropathy, and growth retardation (33).

In addition to these two syndromes, any vitamin A or zinc deficiency can cause symptoms of nyctalopia. It is important to recognize Refsum syndrome and Bassen-Kornzweig disease, because treatment is often possible. The differential diagnosis also includes syphilis, rubella, trauma, and drug-induced retinopathies.

Leber's Congenital Amaurosis

Leber's congenital amaurosis is an autosomal recessive congenital retinal dystrophy that has a broad spectrum of fundal presentations, ocular findings, and systemic associations. Mutations have been found on four known genes for this condition. Clinically, patients present with decreased vision during the first year of life. The ophthalmoscopic appearance is variable, ranging from normal to an RP-like picture. Other findings in the fundus are macular colobomas, salt-and-pepper changes, a marbleized pattern and a nummular pigmentary pattern (Fig. 14.19) (34). Other ocular signs include eye rubbing "oculodigital sign," high hyperopia, pendular nystagmus, poorly reactive pupils, cataracts, keratoconus, and strabismus.

The ERG is essential to a correct diagnosis because of the varied clinical presentation. The photopic and scotopic ERG response is extinguished in Leber's congenital amaurosis.

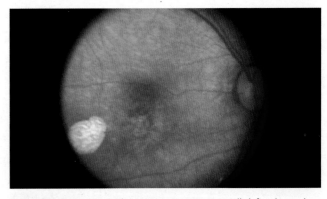

FIGURE 14.19. Nummular pigmentary pattern; well-defined round-to-oval pigmented lesions in a patient with Leber's congenital amaurosis.

Leber's congenital amaurosis has been associated with many systemic abnormalities and neurologic disorders. Systemic associations include polycystic kidney disease, osteopetrosis, cleft palate, and skeletal anomalies. Neurologic associations include mental retardation, seizures, and hydrocephalus.

There is much controversy concerning these associations as well as over the classification of Leber's congenital amaurosis. It is important to realize that this is not a single disease state but a constellation of eye findings associated with several diseases.

Treatable metabolic disorders confused with Leber's congenital amaurosis include abetalipoproteinemia

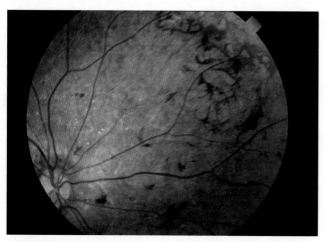

FIGURE 14.20. Bietti's crystalline retinopathy with crystals in retinal layers associated with bone spicules.

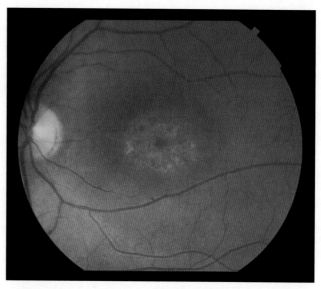

FIGURE 14.21. Cone dystrophy with pigmentary changes and areas of chorioretinal atrophy involving the macula.

(Bassen-Kornzweig syndrome), infantile phytanic acid storage disease (Refsum disease), and infantile Batten disease (ceroid lipofuscinosis) (35).

Bietti's Crystalline Dystrophy

This retinal degeneration was first described by Bietti in 1937 (36) characterized by crystalline deposits in all retinal layers with associated choriocapillaris and RPE loss (Fig. 14.20). Some cases also have limbal corneal crystals. This condition is inherited in an autosomal recessive pattern, and the genetic defect has been mapped to 4q35 (37).

Patients complain of progressive decrease in night vision, which correlates with a decrease in the ERG. The fluorescein angiogram typically demonstrates focal areas of choriocapillaris atrophy in the posterior pole.

Cone Dystrophy

Cone degeneration is characterized by loss of central vision, photophobia, abnormalities of color vision, and an abnormal photopic ERG. Most patients present in the first or second decade of life. There is usually no family history, because most patients have an autosomal recessive inheritance pattern, although autosomal dominant pedigrees have been described. An acquired nystagmus is occasionally a presenting sign. Ophthalmoscopically, the patient may be normal, exhibit the classic "bull's-eye" lesion, have diffuse pigmentary changes, or have regions of chorioretinal atrophy involving the macula (Fig. 14.21). Optic atrophy has also been described. The diagnosis is confirmed, however, by the presence of an abnormally low ERG response to a 25-Hz flickering light, an abnormal photopic ERG, and a normal scotopic ERG. Color vision testing shows severe abnormalities early in the course of the disease. The prognosis is usually poor, most patients progressing to a vision of 20/200 or worse.

Another rare cone disorder is achromatopsia or rod monochromatism. This disorder presents in the first year of life with a pendular nystagmus, photopia, and decreased vision. The fundus appears normal on examination. The inheritance is typically autosomal recessive, and the diagnosis is confirmed by the presence of an abnormal response to a flicker stimulus, an abnormal photopic ERG, and a normal scotopic ERG. Vision usually is in the 20/200 to 20/400 range and remains unchanged throughout life.

Choroideremia

Choroideremia is a progressive retinal degeneration that can be confused with RP first described by Mauthner in 1871 (38). Patients present with progressive nyctalopia and visual field loss secondary to a progressive degeneration of the RPE, retina, and choroid. The choroideremia gene has been cloned from chromosome Xq13–q22 (39).

The condition is inherited as an X-linked trait, and affected males show loss of the RPE and choriocapillaris (Fig. 14.22). This loss begins in the mid-periphery and progresses both anteriorly and posteriorly. An island of normal macula is retained until late in the disease. The patient therefore can have good central vision with poor peripheral fields. The disease is seen in the first two decades, and loss of central vision appears by the fifth decade. Female carriers usually display mild abnormalities involving the RPE. This disorder should be differentiated from RP and gyrate atrophy, which can usually be identified by a careful examination of the fundus. The X-linked pattern of inheritance and examination of the female carriers, who often demonstrate irregular pigment clumping, also provide useful clues.

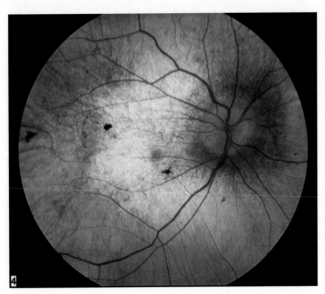

FIGURE 14.22. Extensive atrophy of the choroid and RPE in a patient with choroideremia, with preservation of some of the RPE centrally.

Gyrate Atrophy

Gyrate atrophy is an autosomal recessive disorder with a typical onset in the late teens to mid-40s (40). The disease gene for gyrate atrophy, ornithine aminotransferase has been linked to chromosome 10q26 and has been cloned (41) with application of cryotherapy at threshold disease. It can also present as early as 10 years of age with symptoms of nyctalopia and loss of visual field. The initial changes are first seen in the mid-periphery as "scalloped," well-circumscribed atrophic areas in the RPE and choriocapillaris. The fundi are more pigmented than in choroideremia. High myopia and cataracts are associated ocular findings. The disease generally progresses slowly, with patients maintaining central vision into the fourth decade. As new areas of atrophy appear and the older areas coalesce, the peripheral vision worsens.

The disorder is believed to be the result of a deficiency of the mitochondrial enzyme ornithine aminotransferase. This deficiency leads to elevated levels of ornithine, which is believed to be toxic to the RPE. The elevated levels of ornithine can be detected in the blood and help in establishing the diagnosis. The diagnosis can also be confirmed by determining enzyme levels in cultures of skin fibroblasts. Levels are reduced or absent in affected individuals and reduced in carriers. Treatment with pyridoxine and restriction of arginine in the diet can reduce serum ornithine levels by 27% or more, but whether this slows or halts progression of the disease is unproved.

Albinism

The term "albinism" refers to decreased pigmentation. True albinism is often divided into oculocutaneous and ocular varieties, depending on whether the skin is involved or not. In ocular albinism (X-linked disease), only the eyes are affected and there is a decrease in the number of melanosomes, but each melanosome is often fully pigmented—a so-called macromelanosome (42). Female carriers may show partial iris transillumination defects or fundus hypopigmentation. In oculocutaneous albinism (autosomal recessive disease), both the skin and the eyes are involved, and there is a decreased amount of melanin deposited in each melanosome (43). Oculocutaneous albinism is further subdivided on the basis of tyrosinase test results. Tyrosinase-negative albinos lack any pigment in the eyes, skin, or hair.

The eye findings are similar in all true cases of albinism, regardless of type. Patients present with decreased vision and pendular nystagmus secondary to foveal hypoplasia. OCT has been used to demonstrate a widespread thickening of the retina throughout the fovea (44). These patients are sometimes photophobic, display iris transillumination defects, and have decreased pigmentation in the RPE and choroid (Figs. 14.23 and 14.24). Abnormal retinogeniculostriate projections have been found in true albinos, in whom many of the temporal nerve fibers decussate rather than project to the ipsilateral geniculate body.

Two important forms of albinism for the clinician to be aware of are the Hermansky-Pudlak and the Chediak-Higashi

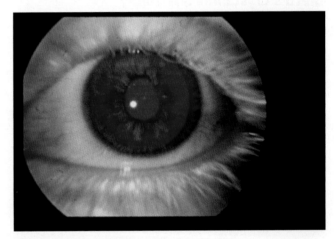

FIGURE 14.23. Iris transillumination defects secondary to ocular albinism.

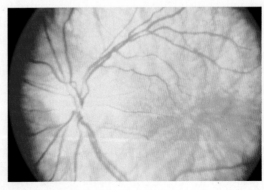

FIGURE 14.24. Decreased pigmentation in the retinal pigment epithelium with choroids associated with albinism.

syndromes. In the former, petechiae and ecchymoses are present because of a platelet defect; these patients are susceptible to bleeding. In the latter, patients are susceptible to recurrent infections because of a leukocyte defect.

Retinopathy of Prematurity

ROP is a peripheral proliferative retinal vascular disorder affecting primarily, markedly premature infants and leading, in severe cases, to complex retinal detachment and profoundly abnormal vision. Fortunately, with the timely application of treatment this devastating result can often be avoided.

ROP was first described by Terry in 1942. In the 1950s, Campbell and, later, Patz implicated high levels of inspired oxygen in the development of ROP. Although hyperoxia shortly after birth is a definite risk factor for ROP, even with modern oxygen monitoring techniques and avoidance of high oxygen levels, ROP continues to develop. The most important risk factor for the development of ROP is low birth weight. Infants with a birth weight of 1,250 g have a 47% risk of developing ROP, whereas infants weighing only 750 g have a 90% risk. The signs of ROP usually are first apparent 32 to 34 weeks after conception, regardless of the gestational age at birth.

The International Classification of Retinopathy of Prematurity describes the various features of ROP and is widely accepted (45,46). Funduscopic variables include the anteroposterior location ("zone"), circumferential extent ("clock hours" or "sectors"), severity ("stage") of disease, and presence or absence of "plus disease" (Figs. 14.25 and 14.26). Plus disease is an extremely important prognostic variable and is defined as dilation and tortuosity of vessels in the posterior pole. The features of the International Classification are defined in Table 14.2.

Although the fundamental reason for failure of normal peripheral retinal vascularization to develop in the extrauterine environment of the premature infant is unknown, the

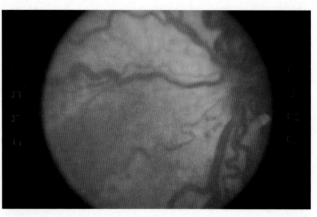

FIGURE 14.26. Tortuous and dilated retinal vasculature in plus disease.

Table 14.2

STAGES OF RETINOPATHY OF PREMATURITY

Stage No.	Characteristic
1	Demarcation line
2	Ridge
3	Ridge with extraretinal fibrovascular proliferation
4	Subtotal retinal detachment
A	Extrafoveal
B	Retinal detachment including fovea
5	Total retinal detachment
Funnel	
	Anterior
	Open
	Narrow
	Posterior
	Open
	Narrow

clinical progression through the stages of ROP is well documented and shares many features with other retinal vascular disorders such as diabetes and venous occlusions. Initially, shunting of blood through dilated vascular channels occurs at the border of vascularized and nonvascularized retina. Peripheral retinal nonperfusion presumably alters the balance of growth and inhibitory factors within the eye, leading to the development of neovascularization. Progressive traction leads to the end-stage sequelae of ROP, including retinal detachment, retinal fold, and vitreous hemorrhage.

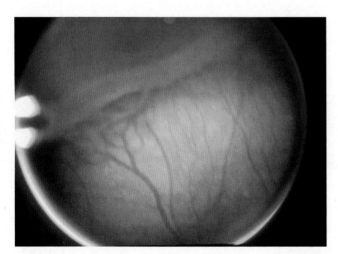

FIGURE 14.25. Stage 3 ROP ridge with extraretinal fibrovascular proliferation.

The most severe expression of the acute phase of ROP usually occurs by 40 to 42 weeks postconceptional age. Regression is the most common outcome of ROP. In general, the more severe the acute changes, the more advanced the fundus changes during regression. The first sign of regression is usually growth of normal-appearing retinal vessels across the ridge into the anterior, avascular retina. Regression may take several months and in some cases, the retinal vessels fail to advance fully to the ora serrata. Associated with the International Classification is a list of common long-term sequelae of ROP (Table 14.3).

One of the most common findings associated with regressed ROP is myopia. Myopia occurs in more than 80% of children with regressed ROP and is usually more than

---

Table 14.3

LONG-TERM SEQUELAE OF RETINOPATHY OF PREMATURITY

Peripheral Changes

Vascular

1. Failure to vascularize peripheral retina

2. Abnormal, nondichotomous branching of retinal vessels

3. Vascular arcades with circumferential interconnection

4. Telangiectatic vessels

Retinal

1. Pigmentary changes

2. Vitreoretinal interface changes

3. Thin retina

4. Peripheral folds

5. Vitreous membranes with or without attachment to retina

6. Lattice-like degeneration

7. Retinal breaks

8. Traction/rhegmatogenous retinal detachment

Posterior Changes

Vascular

1. Vascular tortuosity

2. Straightening of blood vessels in temporal arcade

3. Decrease in angle of insertion of major temporal arcade

Retinal

1. Pigmentary changes

2. Distortion and ectopia of macula

3. Stretching and folding of retina in macular region leading to periphery

4. Vitreoretinal interface changes

5. Vitreous membrane

6. Dragging of retina over disc

7. Traction/rhegmatogenous retinal detachment

6 diopters. The condition may be noted within the first 2 months of life and may progress during the first 6 years. There appears to be a significant relationship between the degree of myopia and the severity of ROP. The myopia is most likely caused by forward displacement of the lens iris diaphragm rather than by increased axial length.

Retinal pigmentation alterations are common in regressed ROP and may be found in the posterior pole and the fundus periphery. Pigment clumping similar to that seen in hyperplasia of the pigment epithelium may occur, as well as discrete patches characterized by loss of the pigment epithelium and outer sensory retinal layers.

In mild regressed ROP, peripheral vitreous membranes develop anterior to the equator, especially on the temporal side. These may be present when there are no alterations in the posterior pole. However, the converse is not true. If posterior pole changes (e.g., dragging of the retina) are detected, peripheral changes will almost invariably be present.

Equatorial retinal folds usually occur between the equator and the ora serrata and may be the sole retinal finding consistent with regressed ROP. They are found at the location of the vascular demarcation line that was present during the active phase of ROP and are often associated with areas of retinal pigmentation. The retinal vessels cross the folds and travel anteriorly toward the ora serrata (Fig. 14.27).

Dragging of the retina is a hallmark of regressed ROP. In 80% of the cases, dragging or displacement is to the temporal side (Fig. 14.28). The macular displacement causes pseudoheterotopia.

Lattice-like degeneration occurs in 15% of patients with regressed ROP. This is considerably higher than the 6% to 7% incidence reported in the general population.

Retinal breaks associated with ROP tend to be primarily on the temporal side. Usually they are round or oval in shape and equatorial in location. They may occur in association with lattice degeneration. Marked equatorial folds indicative of severe vitreous traction are common just anterior to the

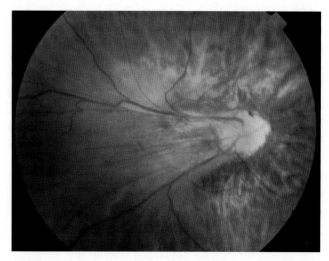

FIGURE 14.28. Dragging of the retina in a patient with cicatricial ROP.

breaks. Retinal breaks and detachment secondary to ROP may occur many years after regression, even in adulthood. Thus, ROP is truly a lifelong disease and requires periodic fundus examination.

Treatment for ROP consists primarily of ablative therapy to the peripheral retina once funduscopic evidence of early proliferative changes develops. The Cryotherapy for Retinopathy of Prematurity (CRYO-ROP) study (47) assessed patients with at least 5 contiguous or 8 cumulative clock hours of extraretinal fibrovascular proliferation in stage 3 ROP, zone I or II disease, and the presence of plus disease. Cryotherapy was then used to treat the entire anterior avascular retina back to the ridge. An unfavorable result was defined as a macular fold, retinal detachment, or retrolental tissue.

The CRYO-ROP study revealed that an unfavorable outcome was significantly less common (48). Early anatomic results have been correlated with long-term visual results.

Indirect laser photocoagulation has produced comparable results in several reports and has gained favor, especially for the treatment of zone I ROP. Although a few reports of cataract after laser therapy have appeared, the advantages of laser therapy, including ease of application, less physical stress to small infants, and less postoperative swelling, have led to its widespread use.

Most recently, the Early Treatment for Retinopathy of Prematurity Randomized Trial (ETROP) demonstrated a reduction of unfavorable outcomes in treatment of high-risk pre-threshold ROP compared with conventional treatment. (48).

The ETROP defined two groups of high-risk pre-threshold ROP. Type 1 ROP was defined as (a) zone 1, any stage ROP with plus disease; (b) zone 1, stage 3 ROP with or without plus disease; and (c) zone 2, stage 2 or 3 ROP with plus disease. Type 2 ROP was defined as (a) zone 1, stage 1 or 2 ROP without plus disease, and (b) zone 2, stage 3 ROP without plus disease.

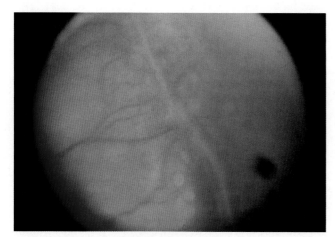

FIGURE 14.27. Regressing ROP showing retinal vessels growing past the vascular demarcation line toward the ora serrata.

The ETROP treated all type 1 ROP with peripheral retinal ablation and observed type 2 ROP for regression of ROP or progression to type 1 ROP. The results showed a reduction in both functional and structural unfavorable outcomes with ablation of the avascular retina in Type 1 eyes compared with conventional treatment. Unfavorable visual acuity outcomes were reduced from 19.5% to 14.5%," and unfavorable structural outcomes were reduced from 15.6% to 9.1%. Clinical judgment will continue to assist in determining the ideal time for intervention.

The use of an intravitreal injection of an anti-VEGF agent (bevacizumab) has been recently described (49). Rapid resolution of plus disease and neovascularization will occur. Long-term efficacy and safety remain uncertain, however, and the role of this therapy as either primary treatment or rescue for severe posterior disease is unknown.

In cases with an unfavorable outcome, surgical intervention may be considered. Cases with a macular fold or retrolental tissue are not good candidates for surgery. Scleral buckling and/or vitrectomy, with or without lens removal often successfully repair stage 4 retinal detachments and shallow, "open funnel" stage 5 detachments. Unfortunately, long-term follow-up reveals that useful vision frequently fails to develop even in eyes with a successful anatomic result. Therefore, prevention with prompt treatment for those eyes at risk for developing severe anatomic changes is critical.

Familial Exudative Vitreoretinopathy

Criswick and Schepens (50) described a hereditary disease of the vitreous and retina that they termed "familial exudative vitreoretinopathy." The striking feature on ophthalmoscopic examination is peripheral retinal exudation, which is subretinal and intraretinal and, unlike peripheral uveitis, occurs posterior to the ora serrata, most commonly on the temporal side. Occasionally, however, exudation is not present. Peripheral retinal nonperfusion, often with retinal neovascularization, is present. Unlike in ROP, no discrete ridge is present in FEVR. Typically, neovascularization appears as isolated tufts at a brush border between vascular and avascular retina. FEVR may be diagnosed shortly after birth but may not produce symptoms until early adulthood. Although evidence of the condition is invariably present bilaterally, marked asymmetry may be noted. In advanced cases, the vitreous cavity features organized membranes in all quadrants, both peripherally and centrally, that appear to be intimately bound to the retina. Localized retinal detachment, often forming a broad fold, usually extends temporally from the disc (Fig. 14.29). The ocular changes are slowly progressive and tend to run a downhill course, with increasing proliferation of blood vessels, increasing exudation, membrane formation, and retinal detachment.

FEVR usually has an autosomal dominant mode of inheritance with incomplete penetrance. A family history is

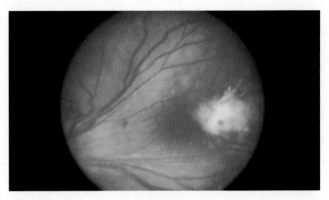

FIGURE 14.29. Dragging of the retina in a 6-year-old girl with familial exudative vitreoretinopathy (FEVR). This condition may simulate ROP (see Fig. 14.28).

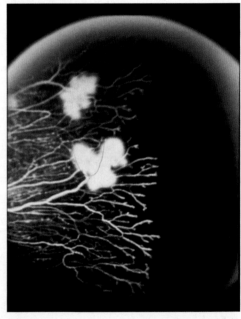

FIGURE 14.30. Avascular zone and retinal periphery of an asymptomatic man with FEVR.

often not present, however. The condition may occur subclinically in relatives of symptomatic patients. In a review of three separate families with FEVR, 85% of those with the disorder were asymptomatic. In asymptomatic persons with the condition, the retina often has an avascular peripheral zone (Fig. 14.30). In some pedigrees, an X-linked inheritance pattern is suspected, and in some cases there is no family involvement and a new mutation is suspected as the source for the disease. The frizzled 4 (FZD4) gene mutation has been found in both autosomal and sporadic cases of FEVR (51). The mutant allele of FZD4 encodes a truncated protein that is retained in the endoplasmic reticulum and is linked to FEVR (52).

The role of treatment with laser or cryotherapy during the proliferative phase of the disease has not been proven in a clinical trial. Some studies have shown a benefit of performing vitrectomy surgery for retinal detachments or vitreous hemorrhage (53,54).

The features of FEVR resemble those seen in ROP. It differs from ROP in that it is hereditary and there is no history of prematurity or oxygen therapy. The disorder may also resemble ROP, Norrie's disease, incontinentia pigmenti, Coats' disease, PFV, retinoblastoma, nematode endophthalmitis, and peripheral uveitis.

Norrie's Disease

Norrie's disease is a bilateral X-linked recessive syndrome associated with degeneration of the ocular structures with auditory and mental impairment. The condition was first described by Norrie in 1935; Norrie's disease only affects males, and females are silent carriers. The penetrance is complete, which prevents unaffected males from passing this genetic defect to their offspring. The Norrie's disease gene has been localized to Xp11.3 and encodes a protein called norrin with unknown function (55). The gene for Norrie's disease has also been associated with the FEVR gene (56). Most cases demonstrate bilateral blindness observed at birth secondary to retinal detachments, PFV, vitreous hemorrhage, iris atrophy, or corneal opacities. Eventually, these eyes progress to phthisis bulbi.

The systemic findings include mental retardation (60%) and hearing impairment (30%). The mental retardation is variable in progression. Sensorineural hearing loss appears in the second to fifth decade of life. The life span is of normal duration. Treatment of the retinal detachment has not been successful in long-term retinal attachment rates or functional success. Prenatal testing has been used to exclude Norrie's disease in the male fetus of a high-risk carrier (57).

Incontinentia Pigmenti

Incontinentia pigmenti (Bloch-Sulzberger syndrome) is inherited as an X-linked dominant trait at gene locus Xq28. The NEMO gene, an NF-κB pathway gene deletion, accounts for 90% of new mutations (58). It is lethal in males. Peripheral retinal nonperfusion and neovascularization are the typical fundus features, similar to FEVR and ROP. The diagnosis is generally made by the associated findings, which include: (a) skin vesicles in infancy on the trunk and extremities with later form areas of skin depigmentation (Figs. 14.31 and 14.32); (b) central nervous system defects such as cortical blindness, developmental delay, mental retardation, and spastic paralysis; (c) alopecia; and (d) incomplete dentition or pegged teeth (Fig. 14.33). Other ophthalmologic features are strabismus, cataract, microphthalmia, optic nerve atrophy, iris hypoplasia, nystagmus, corneal opacities, retinal folds, and macular ischemia (59,60).

The differential diagnosis of incontinentia pigmenti includes ROP, Norrie's disease, FEVR, Coats' disease, and PFV. The management includes laser or cryotherapy for neovascularization and vitrectomy for retinal detachment.

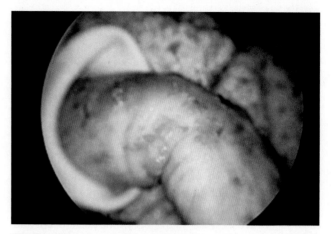

FIGURE 14.31. Incontinentia pigmenti skin vesicles on the arm of an infant.

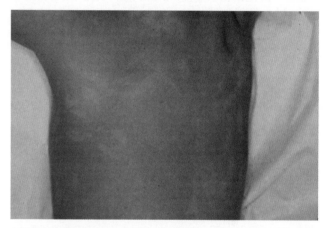

FIGURE 14.32. "Whorls" of skin depigmentation of the trunk of an incontinentia pigmenti patient.

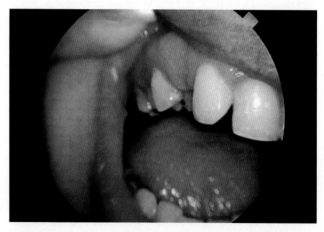

FIGURE 14.33. Peg-shaped tooth in a patient with incontinentia pigmenti.

Retinal Detachment

Primary rhegmatogenous retinal detachment is rare in children. Risk factors for retinal detachment include congenital or developmental structural ocular abnormalities, trauma, previous ophthalmic surgery, and preceding uveitis (61).

Traumatic retinal detachment occurs more often in males than in females. Blunt trauma and penetrating injuries can both cause detachment. However, in the case of blunt trauma there may be a latent period of months or even years between the injury and the diagnosis of detachment. This is understandable for two reasons: first, children are often reluctant to report an injury or symptom, and second, many traumatic detachments start inferiorly and do not cause a subjective awareness until the macula is threatened.

Because traumatic retinal detachments may initially be asymptomatic, one or more demarcation lines are often present. When found, these confirm a duration of at least several months. A multiplicity of demarcation lines indicates successive increases in the size of the detachment and is evidence that chorioretinal adhesions cannot be counted on to wall off a detachment. The detachments are seldom bullous but tend to be smooth and flat. Fixed star folds are rare, although they may occur, and intraretinal cysts may be present if the detachment is old. These disappear spontaneously in a few days if the retina reattaches after surgery.

Retinal detachment often results from a retinal dialysis, which tends to occur primarily in the inferotemporal and superonasal quadrants (Fig. 14.34). Sometimes the retina tears along both the anterior and posterior borders of the vitreous base; the base itself is avulsed and may hang like a pigmented loop in the vitreous cavity with its underlying

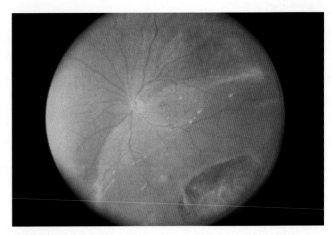

FIGURE 14.34. Inferior temporal retinal dialysis in a young patient who had a retinal detachment in the fellow eye from dialysis.

strip of attached retina. Superonasal avulsion of the vitreous base is pathognomonic of traumatic retinal detachment.

Another form of traumatic peripheral retinal damage is extensive detachment of the ora serrata, with retinal breaks in the nonpigmented epithelium of the pars plana ciliaris along the anterior border of the vitreous base. Pars plana breaks appear as small or large dialyses and cannot usually be seen without scleral depression. Traumatic retinal detachments with dialyses have a favorable surgical prognosis.

REFERENCES

1. Ewing CC, Ives EJ. Juvenile hereditary retinoschisis. *Trans Ophthalmol Soc UK* 1970;89:29–39.
2. Ozdemir H, Karacorlu S, Karacorlu M. Optical coherence tomography findings in familial foveal retinoschisis. *Am J Ophthalmol* 2004;137(1):179–181.
3. Kaplan J, Pelet A, Hentati H, et al. Contribution to carrier detection and genetic counseling in X linked retinoschisis. *J Med Genet* 1991;28(6):383–388.
4. Sauer CG, Gehrig A, Warneke-Wittstock R, et al. Positional cloning of the gene associated with X-linked juvenile retinoschisis. *Nat Genet* 1997;17(2):164–170.
5. Stickler GB, Belau PG, Farrell FJ, et al. Hereditary progressive arthro-ophthalmopathy. *Mayo Clin Proc* 1965;40:433–455.
6. Ahmad NN, McDonald-McGinn DM, Dixon P, et al. PCR assay confirms diagnosis in syndrome with variably expressed phenotype: mutation detection in Stickler syndrome. *J Med Genet* 1996;33(8):678–681.
7. Wagner H. Ein Bisher unbekanntes Erbleiden des Auges (degeneratio hyaloideo-retinalis hereditaria) beobachtet im Kanton Zurich. *Klin Monatsbl Augenheilkd* 1938;100:840.
8. Zech JC, Morle L, Vincent P, et al. Wagner vitreoretinal degeneration with genetic linkage refinement on chromosome 5q13–q14. *Graefes Arch Clin Exp Ophthalmol* 1999;237(5):387–393.
9. Favre M. [Two cases of hyaloid-retinal degeneration.] *Ophthalmologica* 1958;135(5–6):604–609.
10. Franceschetti A. A special form of tapetoretinal degeneration: fundus flavimaculatus. *Trans Am Acad Ophthalmol Otolaryngol* 1965;69(6):1048–1053.
11. Fish G, Grey R, Sehmi KS, et al. The dark choroid in posterior retinal dystrophies. *Br J Ophthalmol* 1981;65(5):359–363.
12. Fishman GA, Farber M, Patel BS, et al. Visual acuity loss in patients with Stargardt's macular dystrophy. *Ophthalmology* 1987;94(7):809–814.
13. Allikmets R, Singh N, Sun H, et al. A photoreceptor cell-specific ATP-binding transporter gene (ABCR) is mutated in recessive Stargardt macular dystrophy. *Nat Genet* 1997;15(3):236–246.
14. Glazer LC, Dryja TP. Understanding the etiology of Stargardt's disease. *Ophthalmol Clin North Am* 2002;15(1):93–100, viii.
15. Best F. Uber eine hereditare Macullaffektoin: Beitrage zur Vererbungslere. *Z Augenheilkd* 1905;13:199.
16. Cavender JC. Best's macular dystrophy. *Arch Ophthalmol* 1982;100(7):1067.
17. Pierro L, Tremolada G, Introini U, et al. Optical coherence tomography findings in adult-onset foveomacular vitelliform dystrophy. *Am J Ophthalmol* 2002;134(5):675–680.
18. Deutman AF. Electro-oculography in families with vitelliform dystrophy of the fovea. Detection of the carrier state. *Arch Ophthalmol* 1969;81(3):305–316.
19. Bakall B, Marknell T, Ingvast S, et al. The mutation spectrum of the bestrophin protein—functional implications. *Hum Genet* 1999;104(5):383–389.
20. Dryja TP. Molecular genetics of Oguchi disease, fundus albipunctatus, and other forms of stationary night blindness: LVII Edward Jackson Memorial Lecture. *Am J Ophthalmol* 2000;130(5):547–563.
21. Mizuo A. On new discovery in dark adaptation in Oguchi's disease. *Acta Soc Ophthalmol Jpn* 1913;17:1148.

22. Nakazawa M, Wada Y, Fuchs S, et al. Oguchi disease: phenotypic characteristics of patients with the frequent 1147delA mutation in the arrestin gene. *Retina* 1997;17(1):17–22.

23. Oguchi C. Über die eigenartige Hemeralopie mit diffuser weissgraulicher Verfarbung des Augenhintergrundes. *Albrecht von Graefes Arch Ophthalmol* 1912(81):109.

24. Carr RE, Margolis S, Siegel IM. Fluorescein angiography and vitamin A and oxalate levels in fundus albipunctatus. *Am J Ophthalmol* 1976;82(4):549–558.

25. Kajiwara K, Sandberg MA, Berson EL, et al. A null mutation in the human peripherin/RDS gene in a family with autosomal dominant retinitis punctata albescens. *Nat Genet* 1993;3(3):208–212.

26. Burstedt MS, Sandgren O, Holmgren G, et al. Bothnia dystrophy caused by mutations in the cellular retinaldehyde-binding protein gene (RLBP1) on chromosome 15q26. *Invest Ophthalmol Vis Sci* 1999;40(5):995–1000.

27. Goldberg MF. Persistent fetal vasculature (PFV): an integrated interpretation of signs and symptoms associated with persistent hyperplastic primary vitreous (PHPV). LIV Edward Jackson Memorial Lecture. *Am J Ophthalmol* 1997;124(5):587–626.

28. Coats G. Forms of retinal disease with massive exudation. *R Lond Ophthalmol Hosp Rep* 1908;17:440–525.

29. Bird AC. Retinal photoreceptor dystrophies LI. Edward Jackson Memorial Lecture. *Am J Ophthalmol* 1995;119(5):543–562.

30. Bird AC. X-linked retinitis pigmentosa. *Br J Ophthalmol* 1975;59(4):177–199.

31. Blumel J, Kniker WT. Laurence-Moon-Bardet-Biedl syndrome: review of the literature and a report of five cases including a family group with three affected males. *Tex Rep Biol Med* 1959;17:391–410.

32. Refsum S. Heredopathia atactica polyneuritiformis phytanic acid storage disease (Refsum's disease) with particular reference to ophthalmological disturbances. *Metab Ophthalmol* 1977;1:73.

33. Bassen FA, Kornzweig AL. Malformation of the erythrocytes in a case of atypical retinitis pigmentosa. *Blood* 1950;5:381.

34. Schroeder R, Mets MB, Maumenee IH. Leber's congenital amaurosis. Retrospective review of 43 cases and a new fundus finding in two cases. *Arch Ophthalmol* 1987;105(3):356–359.

35. Batten FE. Cerebral degeneration with symmetrical changes in the maculae in two members of a family. *Trans Ophthalmol Soc U K* 1903;23:386.

36. Bietti G. Uber familiärs Vorkommen von "Retinitis punctata albescens" (verbunden mit "Dystrophia marginalis cristallinea corneae"). Glitzern des Glaskörpers und anderen degeneration Augenveränderungen. *Klin Monatsbl Augenheilkd* 1937;99:737–756.

37. Jiao X, Munier FL, Iwata F, et al. Genetic linkage of Bietti crystallin corneoretinal dystrophy to chromosome 4q35. *Am J Hum Genet* 2000;67(5):1309–1313.

38. Mauthner L. Ein Fall von Choroideremia. *Berd Naturw Med Ver Innsbruch* 1871;2:191.

39. van Bokhoven H, van den Hurk JA, Bogerd L, et al. Cloning and characterization of the human choroideremia gene. *Hum Mol Genet* 1994;3(7):1041–1046.

40. McCulloch C, Marliss EB. Gyrate atrophy of the choroid and retina: clinical, ophthalmologic, and biochemical considerations. *Trans Am Ophthalmol Soc* 1975;73:153–171.

41. Mitchell GA, Looney JE, Brody LC, et al. Human ornithine-deltaaminotransferase. cDNA cloning and analysis of the structural gene. *J Biol Chem* 1988;263(28):14288–14295.

42. Garner A, Jay BS. Macromelanosomes in X-linked ocular albinism. *Histopathology* 1980;4(3):243–254.

43. Fulton AB, Albert DM, Craft JL. Human albinism. Light and electron microscopy study. *Arch Ophthalmol* 1978;96(2):305–310.

44. Meyer CH, Lapolice DJ, Freedman SF. Foveal hypoplasia in oculocutaneous albinism demonstrated by optical coherence tomography. *Am J Ophthalmol* 2002;133(3):409–410.

45. An international classification of retinopathy of prematurity. The Committee for the Classification of Retinopathy of Prematurity. *Arch Ophthalmol* 1984;102(8):1130–1134.

46. An international classification of retinopathy of prematurity. II. The classification of retinal detachment. The International Committee for the Classification of the Late Stages of Retinopathy of Prematurity. *Arch Ophthalmol* 1987;105(7):906–912.

47. Multicenter trial of cryotherapy for retinopathy of prematurity. Preliminary results. Cryotherapy for Retinopathy of Prematurity Cooperative Group. *Arch Ophthalmol* 1988;106(4):471–479.

48. Early Treatment for Retinopathy of Prematurity Cooperative Group. Revised indications for the treatment of retinopathy of prematurity: results of the early treatment for retinopathy of prematurity randomized trial. *Arch Ophthalmol* 2003;121(12):1684–1694.

49. Mintz-Hittner HA, Kennedy KA, Chuang AZ for the BEAT-ROP Cooperative Group. Efficacy of intravitreal bevacizumab for Stage 3+ retinopathy of prematurity. *N Engl J Med* 2011;364:603–615.

50. Criswick VG, Schepens CL. Familial exudative vitreoretinopathy. *Am J Ophthalmol* 1969;68(4):578–594.

51. Kondo H, Hayashi H, Oshima K, et al. Frizzled 4 gene (FZD4) mutations in patients with familial exudative vitreoretinopathy with variable expressivity. *Br J Ophthalmol* 2003;87(10):1291–1295.

52. Kaykas A, Yang-Snyder J, Heroux M, et al. Mutant frizzled 4 associated with vitreoretinopathy traps wild-type frizzled in the endoplasmic reticulum by oligomerization. *Nat Cell Biol* 2004;6(1):52–58. Epub 2003 Dec 14.

53. Pendergast SD, Trese MT. Familial exudative vitreoretinopathy. Results of surgical management. *Ophthalmology* 1998;105(6):1015–1023.

54. Ikeda T, Fujikado T, Tano Y, et al. Vitrectomy for rhegmatogenous or tractional retinal detachment with familial exudative vitreoretinopathy. *Ophthalmology* 1999;106(6):1081–1085.

55. Berger W, Meindl A, van de Pol T, et al. Isolation of a candidate gene for Norrie disease b positional cloning. *Nat Genet* 1992;(1):199–203.

56. Chen Z, Battinelli EM, Hendriks RW. Norrie disease gene: characterization of deletions and possible function. *Genomics* 1993;16:533–535.

57. Redmond RM, Graham CA, Kelly ED, et al. Prenatal exclusion of Norrie's disease. *Br J Ophthalmol* 1992;76(8):491–493.

58. Aradhya S, Woffendin H, Jakins T, et al. A recurrent deletion in the ubiquitously expressed NEMO (IKK-gamma) gene accounts for the vast majority of incontinentia pigmenti mutations. *Hum Mol Genet* 2001;10(19):2171–2179.

59. Goldberg MF. The blinding mechanisms of incontinentia pigmenti. *Trans Am Ophthalmol Soc* 1994;92:167–176; discussion 176–179.

60. Holmstrom G, Thoren K. Ocular manifestations of incontinentia pigmenti. *Acta Ophthalmol Scand* 2000;78(3):348–353.

61. Weinberg DV, Lyon AT, Greenwald MJ, et al. Rhegmatogenous retinal detachments in children: risk factors and surgical outcomes. *Ophthalmology* 2003;110(9):1708–1713.

15

Congenital Abnormalities of the Optic Disk

Gary C. Brown • *Melissa M. Brown*

VASCULAR ANOMALIES OF THE OPTIC DISK

Prepapillary Vascular Loops

First described by Liebrich in 1871 (1), prepapillary vascular loops were originally thought to be remnants of an incompletely regressed hyaloid system. Most evidence now suggests they occur as a separate entity (2–4). Despite the fact these anomalies appear dark, thus venous, approximately 95% of prepapillary loops are arterial (3).

Clinically, the vessels appear as loops that extend from the optic disk into the vitreous cavity and then back to the disk (Fig. 15.1). In contrast to a single hyaloid artery, each prepapillary loop has at least one ascending and one descending branch. Loops can assume a spiral or corkscrew shape, a figure-of-eight appearance, or manifest with a simple hairpin turn configuration (3). Spontaneous movement, coincident with the heartbeat, is seen in approximately half of cases, whereas approximately 30% are encased by a white, glial-appearing sheath (Fig. 15.2).

Arterial prepapillary loops average approximately 1.5 mm in height and project in the vitreous cavity into Cloquet's canal, rather than into the vitreous gel (3). In contrast to a persistent hyaloid artery, arterial prepapillary loops achieve a maximum height of approximately 5 mm and do not extend anteriorly to the posterior capsule of the lens.

Bilaterality is present in 9% to 17% of cases (2), and cilioretinal arteries have been noted in up to 75% of affected eyes. Systemic associations have not been routinely noted.

Histopathologically, a prepapillary arterial loop has been shown to contain intima, but not an internal elastic lamina (Fig. 15.3) (5). The vessel lies beneath a loose connective tissue sheath continuous with the internal limiting membrane of the retina.

Mann (4) has suggested that prepapillary arterial loops arise at approximately the 100 mm stage (3.5 to 4 months) of gestation. At this time, mesenchymal cells, the precursors of retinal capillary endothelial cells, and retinal vessels, inadvertently grow anteriorly into the supporting tissue of

Bergmeister's papilla overlying the optic nerve head. They then proceed back down onto the disk and on their course into the developing retina. Bergmeister's papilla subsequently regresses, leaving the vascular abnormality within Cloquet's canal.

The major complication associated with prepapillary arterial loops is retinal artery obstruction in the distribution of the area supplied by the loop (Fig. 15.4) (2). Reported in approximately 10% of cases of prepapillary loops described in the literature, the obstruction has been hypothesized to occur secondary to turbulent flow, which predisposes to endothelial damage and thrombus formation. Vitreous hemorrhage and hyphema also have been noted (3).

Congenital prepapillary venous loops are usually single vessels that extend 0.5 mm or less into the vitreous cavity (Fig. 15.5). Acquired prepapillary venous loops are more common and often multiple, typically seen in adults, and found in conjunction with retinal venous obstruction or diseases associated with retinal venous obstruction, such as glaucoma, meningioma, or increased intracranial pressure (Fig. 15.6).

Persistent Hyaloid Artery

A persistent hyaloid artery presents clinically as a single vessel traveling from the optic disk—through Cloquet's canal—anteriorly to the posterior capsule of the lens (Fig. 15.7) (2). The point of attachment to the posterior capsule, most often located inferonasal to the visual axis, is known as Mittendorf's dot.

Hyaloid artery remnants are seen in the eyes of premature infants in up to 95% of cases, but are observed in only 3% of full-term infants (6). The incidence in children and adults is lower, but exact figures are lacking. Most commonly, a persistent hyaloid artery in a child is bloodless, but in rare instances it can contain blood and be associated with vitreous hemorrhage (7). Ocular associations reported with persistent hyaloid artery include persistent hyperplastic primary vitreous, coloboma of the optic disk, optic nerve hypoplasia, and posterior vitreous cysts (2).

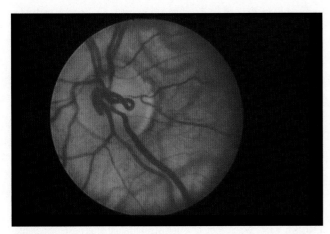

FIGURE 15.1. Congenital prepapillary arterial loop with a figure-of-eight configuration.

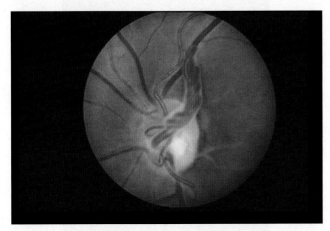

FIGURE 15.2. White, fibroglial sheath (*arrow*) surrounding a prepapillary arterial loop extending into Cloquet's canal. The cilioretinal artery at the 3:30 o'clock position off the optic disk is sheathed and shows temporal pallor, both occurred secondary toxemia of pregnancy 15 years previously.

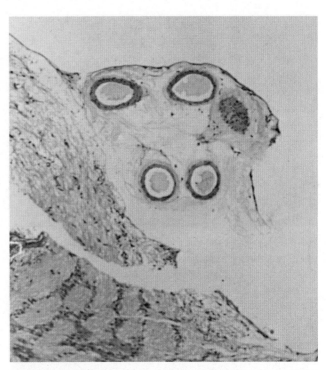

FIGURE 15.3. Histopathology of prepapillary arterial loop. The vessel is located with amorphous connective tissue beneath the internal limiting membrane of Elschnig.

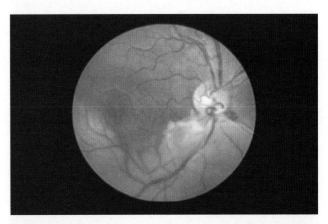

FIGURE 15.4. Inferior branch retinal artery obstruction in the right eye of an 18-year-old youth with a prepapillary arterial loop. (Reprinted from Brown GC, Magargal LE, Augsburger JJ, et al. Preretinal arterial loops and retinal arterial occlusion. *Am J Ophthalmol* 1978;87:646–651, with permission of Ophthalmic Publishing Company.)

Persistent Bergmeister's Papilla

Although not a vascular abnormality in the strictest sense, Bergmeister's papilla develops around the posterior aspect of the fetal hyaloid artery. It is therefore included herein.

Between the first and second months of gestation, neuroectodermal cells within the optic cup at the superior end of the embryonic fissure differentiate into the primitive epithelial papilla (8). This primitive epithelial papilla becomes the optic nerve head when axons traveling from retinal ganglion cells to the respective lateral geniculate nuclei within the thalamus of the brain pass through it.

At the end of the fourth month of gestation, neuroectodermal glial cells on the surface of the optic disk multiply and form a sheath around the hyaloid artery that extends anteriorly for approximately one-third the length of the vessel (Fig. 15.8). The sheath is maximally developed at approximately 5.5 months of gestation, after which atrophy occurs. The degree of regression determines, in part, the physiologic cupping of the optic disk.

Incomplete regression of Bergmeister's papilla causes a persistent Bergmeister's papilla, also known as *epipapillary veil*. Clinically, the entity appears as a tuft of glial tissue most commonly located on the nasal aspect of the nerve head (Fig. 15.9). Absence of physiologic cupping can also be seen in affected eyes. The visual acuity is unaffected by the abnormality, and systemic associations are generally lacking.

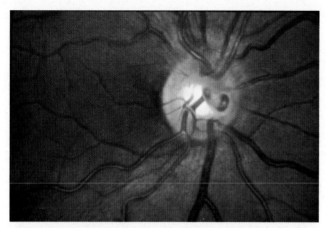

FIGURE 15.5. Single congenital prepapillary venous loop in the right eye on the nasal side of this right optic disk. The white fibroglial tissue overlying the loop has the clinical appearance of a Bergmeister's papilla. (Reprinted with permission from Brown GC, Tasman WS. *Congenital anomalies of the optic disc.* New York: Grune & Stratton, 1983:53.)

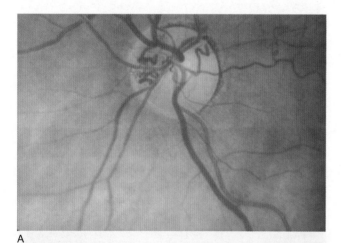

A

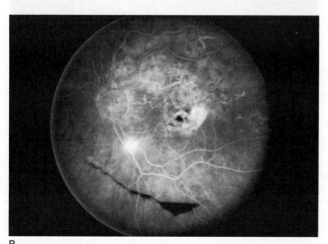

B

FIGURE 15.6. A: Multiple acquired prepapillary venous loops. **B:** Fluorescein angiogram corresponding to **(A)** reveals evidence of a previous superotemporal retinal branch vein obstruction. (Reprinted with permission from Brown GC, Tasman WS. *Congenital anomalies of the optic disc.* New York: Grune & Stratton, 1983:54–55.)

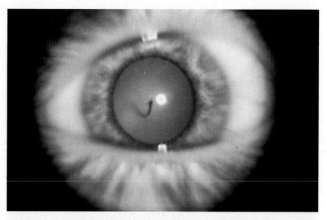

FIGURE 15.7. Single loop of a persistent hyaloid artery extending anteriorly within Cloquet's canal to insert on the posterior capsule of the lens.

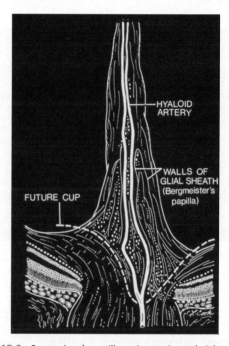

FIGURE 15.8. Bergmeister's papilla at its maximum height during the fifth month of gestation. It usually regresses by birth. The *dotted white line* shows the future cup of the optic disk.

Enlarged Vessels

Causes of enlarged vessels on the optic disk in children include arteriovenous (AV) malformations, retinal capillary hemangiomas (von Hippel tumors), and retinoblastoma. Because the latter two conditions are most appropriately classified as tumors, they will not be addressed in this section. Choroidal melanoma also has been noted to cause enlarged vessels on the optic disk (9), but the tumor is generally not seen in children.

AV malformations in the retina can be mild, moderate, or severe, and thus have been correspondingly classified by Archer and associates (10) as grades I, II, and III abnormalities. A grade I AV communication, the mildest variant, has also been called a *congenital retinal macrovessel* by Brown et al.

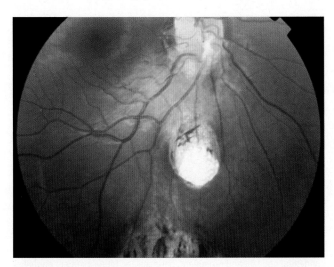

FIGURE 15.9. Yellowish, persistent Bergmeister's papilla (*star*) overlying the inferonasal optic disk. Incomplete retinochoroidal colobomatous lesions are present inferior to the optic disk.

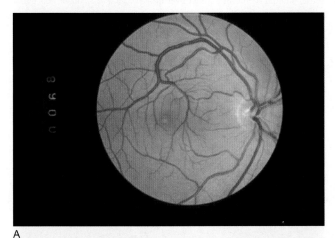

A

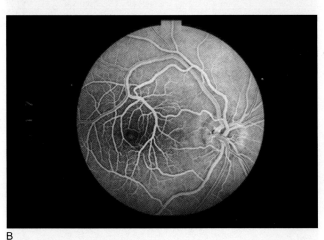

B

FIGURE 15.10. A: Congenital retinal macrovessel. Enlarged vein drains the retina, both superior and inferior to the horizontal raphe. Visual acuity in the eye was 20/20, despite the presence of a yellow foveolar cyst. **B:** Fluorescein angiogram of the central macula seen in **(A)**. The small circular area of central hyperfluorescence in the foveal avascular zone corresponds to the retinal cyst. Vessel forming the superior border of the foveal avascular zone is an arteriovenous (AV) communication.

(11). A congenital macrovessel is a single enlarged retinal vessel, usually a vein, that traverses both sides of the horizontal raphe (Fig. 15.10). Some of these vessels are associated with readily apparent AV communications, whereas others are not. Transient cysts in the central fovea have been seen in association with congenital retinal macrovessels, but appear to affect the visual acuity minimally.

Grade II and III AV communications have also been called racemose angiomas or racemose hemangiomas. The grade II variant is moderate and is usually associated with normal vision (Fig. 15.11), whereas with grade III AV communications the vision can be severely reduced due of replacement of optic nerve tissue by enlarged vascular elements (Fig. 15.12) (12,13). Both grade II and III AV communications can be associated with AV communications in the face, scalp, mandible, and central nervous system. The eponym Wyburn-Mason syndrome has been applied to retinal AV communications associated with systemic AV

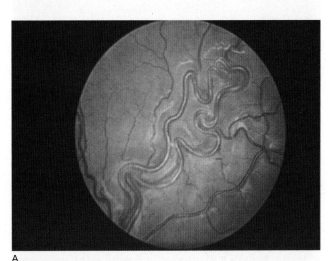

A

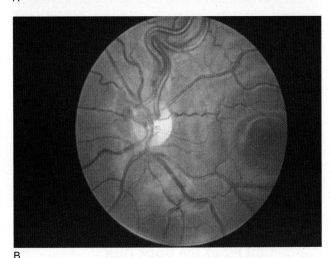

B

FIGURE 15.11. Grade II arteriovenous (AV) communication in a 12-year-old boy. Visual acuity in the eye was 20/20. (Reprinted with permission from Brown GC, Tasman WS. *Congenital anomalies of the optic disc.* New York: Grune & Stratton, 1983:75.)

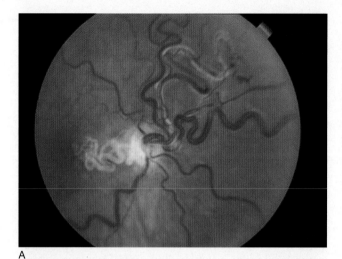

A

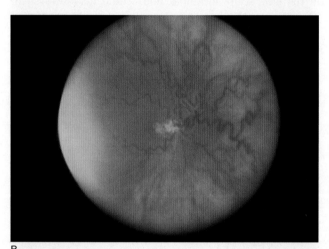

B

FIGURE 15.12. A: Grade III arteriovenous (AV) communication. Visual acuity in the eye was no light perception, presumably because of the replacement of the normal optic nerve tissue by vessel (courtesy of Dr. Jerry A. Shields). **B:** Grade III AV communication shown in **(A)** with equator-plus photography. Multiple AV communications are present. The patient also had a maxillary AV communication that caused severe bleeding after tooth extraction. The yellow illuminating light is at the left of the photograph (courtesy of Dr. Jerry A. Shields).

communications (14). Rundles and Falls (15) found that, among 34 cases of congenital retinal AV malformations reported through 1951, 18 (53%) had associated central nervous system and/or dermatologic involvement.

COLOBOMATOUS AND OTHER EXCAVATED DEFECTS

Congenital Pit of the Optic Disk

Found in approximately 1 per 11,000 patients (16), a congenital pit of the optic nerve head appears as a localized depression that can be yellow-white (Fig. 15.13), gray (Fig. 15.14), black (Fig. 15.15), or other variants in color.

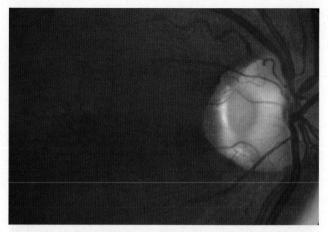

FIGURE 15.13. Right eye of a patient with a yellow/white, temporal congenital optic pit and prominent, peripapillary, retinal pigment epithelial changes adjacent to the pit. A serous detachment of the sensory retina involves the macular, and a lamellar macular hole is present with the internal limiting membrane intact over it. (Reprinted with permission from Brown GC, Tasman WS. *Congenital anomalies of the optic disc.* New York: Grune & Stratton, 1983:107.)

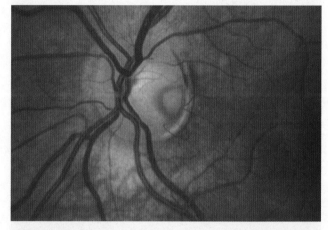

FIGURE 15.14. Gray congenital pit of the optic nerve head with peripapillary atrophy.

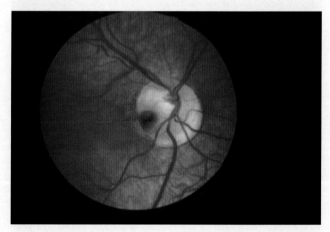

FIGURE 15.15. Black congenital pit of the optic nerve head with an adjacent macular retinal detachment. The background choroidal vessels are more obscured in the region of the retinal detachment.

The defects generally range in size from 0.25 to 0.40 disk diameters. More than 50% are located on the temporal aspect of optic disk, versus inferiorly, nasally, or centrally (Fig. 15.16). Although found anywhere on the optic disk, they occasionally have a peripapillary location.

Peripapillary retinal pigment epithelial disturbances are present in 95% of eyes with optic pits that are not centrally located (see Fig. 15.13) (17). Peripapillary choroidal neovascularization has been seen rarely in these cases (18). In unilateral cases, the nerve head with the pit is larger than a normal contralateral nerve head in 85% of patients. Most pits are single, but approximately 5% of affected eyes have more than one defect on the disk. Cilioretinal arteries are frequently associated.

Approximately 40% of eyes with a congenital optic pit have an associated or previous serous detachment of the sensory retina and/or posterior retinoschisis (see Fig. 15.13) (17,19,20). Retinal detachment is more commonly seen with larger, temporally located pits and usually involves the macula. Posterior splitting of the retinal layers, or macular retinoschisis, can be seen in eyes with congenital optic pits in association with, or not associated with, retinal detachment (21). We are unaware that centrally located pits (see Fig. 15.16) have been associated with retinal detachment. The subretinal fluid rarely extends beyond the posterior pole and, in the great majority of cases, can be seen extending to the optic disk in the vicinity of the pit. Cystic changes within the detached retina are found in two-thirds of cases, and an outer macular hole develops in approximately 25%. In contrast with most lamellar macular holes, in which absence of the inner retinal layers is observed, the macular holes seen in conjunction with congenital optic pits tend to involve the outer retina, giving the appearance the internal limiting membrane is intact.

The age of onset of the retinal detachment is variable, with the mean of approximately 30 years (17). Nevertheless, retinal detachment has been seen within the first decade of life.

Uncertainty exists as to the origin of the subretinal/intraretinal fluid seen in conjunction with congenital optic pits. Although evidence in the collie dog model suggests it originates from the vitreous cavity (19), other possible sources in the human include cerebrospinal fluid from the subarachnoid space, leakage from choroidal vessels, and leakage from small vessels located at the base of the pit (17).

Evidence indicates that, in many instances, the presence of an associated retinal detachment of the posterior pole is visually disabling. Although the fluid can wax and wane spontaneously, Brown et al. (20) found that among 20 such untreated eyes followed for at least 1 year the visual acuity was 20/100 or worse in 55%. When the vision is decreased because of serous macular retinal detachment, laser treatment has been advocated in the peripapillary region to induce reattachment of the retina to the underlying retinal pigment epithelium and subsequent reabsorption of the subretinal fluid (Fig. 15.17). The treatment does not have to be sufficiently heavy to involve the nerve fiber layer. With cases of macular retinal detachment that do not respond to laser therapy after 1 to 2 months, repeat laser therapy, possibly in conjunction with pars plana vitrectomy and/or a gas/fluid exchange, can be considered (22,23). Unless a macular hole develops within the detached macular retina, the retina can remain detached for months without negating the possibility of good visual return with therapy.

Fluorescein angiography typically reveals early hypofluorescence of the pit, with progression to late hyperfluorescence. Associated visual field defects, excluding the enlarged blind spots from larger disks (85%) and central scotomas from macular retinal detachments (40%), mimic those found with glaucoma and are seen in 60% of eyes (Fig. 15.18) (20). Included among these are arcuate scotomas (26%), localized constrictions (12%), nasal and/or temporal steps (10%), paracentral scotomas (8%), and generalized constrictions (6%).

In general, systemic abnormalities have not been linked with congenital optic pits. Nevertheless, the association of a basal encephalocele with agenesis of the corpus callosum has been reported (24). A hereditary pattern is not usually present, although autosomal dominant inheritance has been noted (25). The defect is thought to arise, in most cases, from abnormal differentiation of the primitive epithelial papilla (26).

Optic Nerve Coloboma

Occurring in approximately 1 per 12,000 patients (20), an optic nerve coloboma has several identifying features (Fig. 15.19). Included are (a) enlargement of the papillary area; (b) partial or total excavation of the disk, more so inferiorly; (c) a glistening white surface; and (d) retinal blood vessels entering and exiting the nerve head from the border of the defect. Depths are variable and may range up to 50 D (27).

The abnormality can be unilateral or bilateral. Visual acuity is variable and has been noted to range from normal to

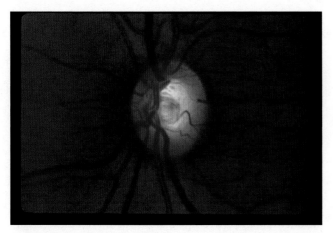

FIGURE 15.16. Central gray/brown congenital pit of the optic nerve head.

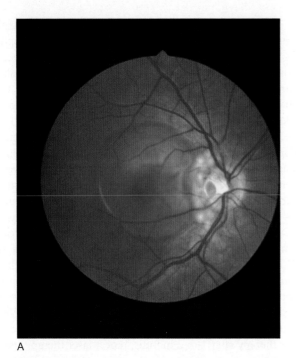

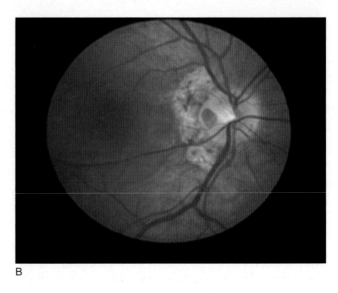

FIGURE 15.17. A: Peripapillary laser treatment with 200 μm burns in the right eye of a 15-year-old girl with a congenital optic pit and serous retinal detachment involving the macula. Visual acuity in the eye was 20/200. **B:** Subretinal fluid reabsorbed within 1 month after treatment of the fundus shown in **(A)**. Visual acuity improved to 20/25.

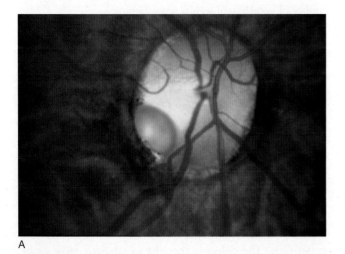

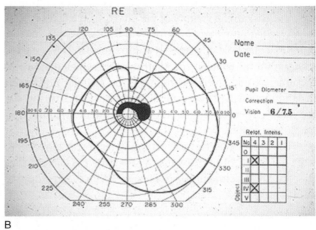

FIGURE 15.18. A: Inferotemporal congenital optic pit. **B:** Superior arcuate scotoma associated with the congenital optic pit shown in **(A)**.

no light perception (28). Concomitant retinochoroidal and/or iris colobomatous defects can also be present (Fig. 15.20). The anomaly is believed to occur secondary to incomplete closure of the embryonic fissure during the second month of gestation (28).

Non-rhegmatogenous retinal detachment can be seen in association with optic nerve colobomas (Fig. 15.21) (28). The detachment most often occurs in the second or third decade of life and usually extends outward from the optic disk (25). Peripapillary laser therapy in association with pars plana vitrectomy and air–gas/fluid exchange has been used successfully in our institution to flatten the retina (22).

The source of the subretinal fluid is uncertain. If a retinochoroidal colobomatous component is also present, a hole within the intercalcary membrane, the thin dysplastic retina overlying the defect, can be causative. In such instances, the retina at the edges of the colobomatous defect may have to be treated with laser photocoagulation in conjunction with vitrectomy and a gas–fluid exchange.

Numerous systemic abnormalities have been reported in conjunction with colobomatous defects in the eye (20). Included among these are diseases of the cardiovascular, central nervous, dermatologic, gastrointestinal, genitourinary, nasopharyngeal, and musculoskeletal systems. Of

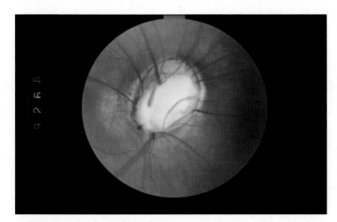

FIGURE 15.19. Coloboma of the optic disk. There is a large inferior excavated defect, the disk is enlarged, and the retinal vessels exit and enter from the margins of the colobomatous disk.

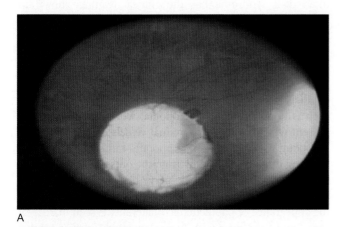

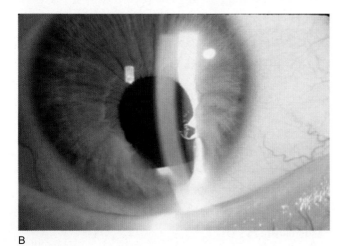

FIGURE 15.20. A: Retinochoroidal coloboma extending superiorly to involve the optic nerve head on equator-plus fundus photography. The optic nerve head is located within the superior aspect of the large, yellow retinochoroidal coloboma. Note the peripheral fundus inferiorly appears normal, indicating that the embryonic fissure partially closed during gestation. Closure typically begins in the region of the peripheral fundus, then extends anteriorly and posteriorly. The yellow illuminating light is at the right of the photograph (courtesy of Dr. Jerry A. Shields). **B:** Iris coloboma associated with the retinochoroidal coloboma shown in **(A)** (courtesy of Dr. Jerry A. Shields).

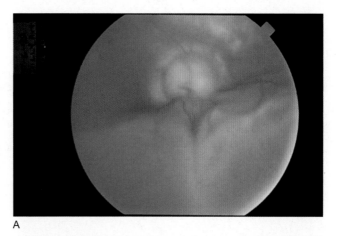

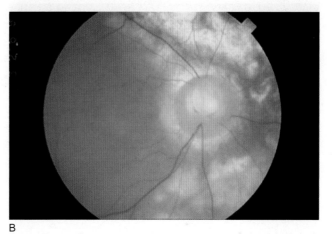

FIGURE 15.21. A: Coloboma of the optic disk associated with a bullous retinal detachment. **B:** Resolution of the retinal detachment shown in **(A)** after a pars plana vitrectomy with gas–fluid exchange.

particular note is the CHARGE syndrome (*c*oloboma, *h*eart disease, *a*tresia choanae, *r*etarded growth, *g*enital hypoplasia, and *e*ar anomalies and/or deafness) (29).

Morning Glory Disk Anomaly

In 1970, Kindler (30) reported on 10 patients with a unilateral, congenital optic nerve head anomaly that resembled the morning glory flower. Among the features of the morning glory optic disk are (a) enlargement and excavation, (b) a central core of white tissue, (c) a peripapillary annulus of variably pigmented subretinal tissue, and (d) retinal vessels that enter and exit from the borders of the defect (Fig. 15.22). The retinal vessels are frequently straightened and sheathed.

In approximately 30% of eyes, a non-rhegmatogenous retinal detachment develops (30,31). It can involve just the posterior pole, or progress to total retinal detachment. As is the case with an optic nerve coloboma, the origin of the subretinal fluid is uncertain. Peripapillary laser therapy in conjunction with vitrectomy and gas–fluid exchange can be of benefit for flattening the retina in some cases (22).

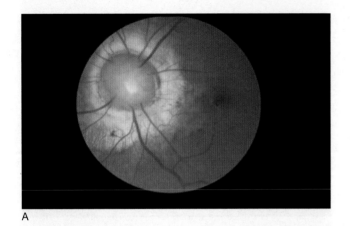

A

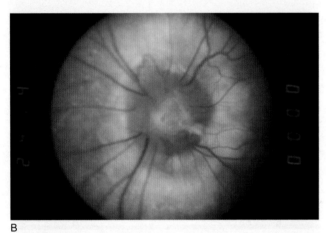

B

FIGURE 15.22. **A:** Morning glory optic disk anomaly. The enlarged disk is excavated centrally and has a central tuft of glial tissue, a surrounding annulus of subretinal, peripapillary fibroglial tissue, and straightened retinal arteries. **B:** Morning glory optic disk anomaly with a central tuft of glial tissue and surrounding annulus of subretinal fibrosis. The yellow peripapillary region off the 3 o'clock position on the optic disk represents xanthophyll pigment in the outer retina of the central macula. (Reprinted with permission from Brown GC, Tasman WS. *Congenital anomalies of the optic disc.* New York: Grune & Stratton, 1983:162.)

The visual acuity in eyes with the morning glory optic disk anomaly and no retinal detachment can range from near normal to hand-motion recognition (20). Strabismus may be associated. In unilateral cases, the possibility of associated amblyopia should be considered, particularly because the visual loss in affected eyes in bilateral cases does not seem to be as severe as the visual loss in unilateral affected eyes (32).

Basal encephalocele has been noted in conjunction with the morning glory disk anomaly (33). Other congenital optic disk abnormalities reported with basal encephalocele include congenital optic pit, optic nerve coloboma, and megalopapilla (20). Intracranial vascular anomalies can also be seen in patients with morning glory disc anomaly. These anomalies may include carotid artery stenosis with moyamoya disease. For this reason magnetic resonance imaging and magnetic resonance angiography may be indicated in these patients (34).

Peripapillary Staphyloma

The peripapillary staphyloma is an excavated defect surrounding a relatively normal appearing optic disk. Mild cases, especially in myopes, are relatively common, though severe cases are rare. Atrophic changes of the choroid and retinal pigment epithelium are usually seen within the walls of the defect. Although the depth of the optic disk can range from 1 to 20 D (20), the macula is usually within 1 to 2 D of emmetropia. The visual acuity can be normal in mild cases, but severe visual loss is generally seen with pronounced defects (20). Contractions of the walls of larger peripapillary staphylomas have been reported (35).

Tilted Disk Syndrome

Present in approximately 1% to 2% of the population, the tilted disk syndrome has the clinical features shown in Table 15.1 (Figs. 15.23 and 15.24) (36,37). It has a number of alternative nomenclatures (20), including the nasal fundus ectasia syndrome, inverse myopia, inversion of the optic disk, and dysversion of the optic disk. The entity may be a variant of colobomatous defects (20). The inferior peripapillary area without choroid and retinal pigment epithelium is known as Fuchs coloboma, while situs inversus is present when the temporal retinal vessels on the optic disk first point nasally and then temporally, rather than normally pointing directly temporally from the outset.

The margins of the optic nerve head are often elevated superiorly because of the tilting effect, at times mimicking the appearance of papilledema. Bilaterality is seen in 75% of cases, and most eyes with hypopigmented, inferior fundus

TABLE 15.1

TILTED DISK SYNDROME

	Percent of eyes
Inferonasal disk tilting	65
Inferonasal or inferior crescent	88
Situs inversus of the retinal vessels	80
Myopia (>1 D)	85–90
Astigmatism (>1 D)	71
Hypopigmented, inferior fundus ectasia of 1–4 D	72–90
Vision of 20/25 to 20/50	75
	Percent of cases
Bilateral	75
Percent of general population	1–2

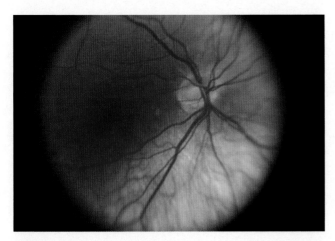

FIGURE 15.23. Tilted disk syndrome. The optic nerve is tilted inferiorly, the superior disk margin is blurred due to anterior tilting, and an inferonasal conus, or Fuchs coloboma (*star*) is present. Mild situs inversus can be seen. A pronounced region of ectatic, lightened fundus is present inferiorly.

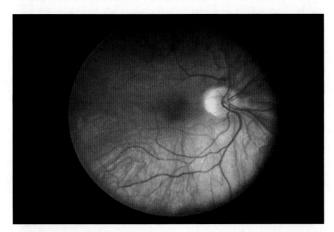

FIGURE 15.24. Tilted disk syndrome in another eye shows lightening of the inferior ectatic fundus and pronounced situs inversus. Absence of an inferior Fuchs coloboma demonstrates that all features of the tilted disk syndrome need not be present to make the diagnosis.

ectasia have associated superotemporal visual field defects. Bilateral disk swelling, decreased vision, and field defects in persons with the tilted disk syndrome have led to the misdiagnosis of a pituitary tumor in the past. Unlike the field abnormalities associated with optic chiasmal lesions, which respect the vertical midline, those seen in the tilted disk syndrome are often relative and cross the vertical midline (Fig. 15.25) (36,37).

In 75% of eyes with the tilted disk syndrome, the visual acuity is reduced to the 20/25 to 20/50 range. Despite decreased visual acuity, these patients do not relate a history of visual loss. It is uncertain why the vision is decreased, but the possibility that obliquely oriented macular cones account for the loss has been proposed (37). This syndrome has considerable clinical relevance, since its prevalence is 1% to 2% in the general population and it is associated with

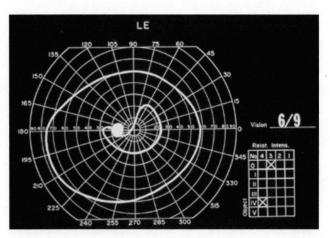

FIGURE 15.25. Superotemporal visual field defect associated with the region of inferior lightened ectasia in an eye with the tilted disk syndrome. The defect crosses the vertical midline, unlike those encountered with pituitary tumors compressing the optic chiasm, which typically respect the vertical midline.

vision loss. It often explains why select astigmatic myopes with the same refractive error as others do not see as well as their comparators.

SIZE ABNORMALITIES

Optic Nerve Hypoplasia

Variants of this entity range from almost imperceptible hypoplasia to severe involvement of the optic disk. The typical funduscopic appearance is that of a small disk in which the retinal vessels enter and exit centrally (Fig. 15.26A), in contrast with their usual more nasal location on the normal optic nerve head. The central location of the entrance and exit of the retinal vessels on the optic disk is key to the diagnosis, especially in more subtle cases with good vision. The retinal vessels are generally normal in caliber, though they may appear relatively large since the disk is small. A "double ring" sign may be present for 360 degrees, but commonly is incomplete. The outer ring has been shown histopathologically to correlate with the juncture of the sclera and lamina cribrosa (Fig. 15.26B). It corresponds with the size of the normal disk (38). The inner ring is formed by the border of the central optic nerve head tissue with the retina and retinal pigment epithelium, which extend further posteriorly over the surface of the disk than in a normal eye.

Optic nerve hypoplasia is believed to occur secondary to failure of development of the ganglion cell layer of the retina (39), although retrograde degeneration caused by congenital lesions of the cerebral hemispheres has also been reported (40). An autosomal dominant hereditary pattern has been rarely noted (41). Pharmacologic insults that have been associated prenatally in mothers of children with optic nerve hypoplasia include the use of phenytoin (42), quinine (43), lysergic acid diethylamide, meperidine, diuretics, and corticosteroids (44). As is the case with pharmacologic agents,

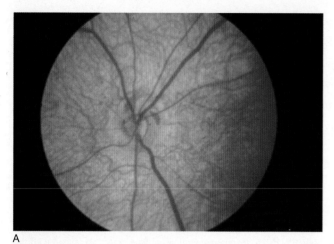

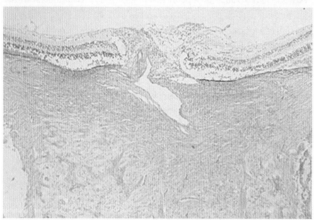

FIGURE 15.26. **A:** Hypoplastic optic disk with a double ring sign. The retinal vessels are normal in size and enter and exit centrally on the disk. The inner ring is formed by the juncture of the remaining nerve tissue and the retina and retinal pigment epithelium extending abnormally posteriorly over the nerve. The outer ring, representing the size of a normal optic nerve, is created by the juncture of the lamina cribrosa and the sclera (Courtesy of Dr. W. Richard Green). **B:** Hypoplastic optic disk histopathology corresponding to **(A)**. The inner ring is formed by the juncture of the remaining nerve tissue (*star*) and the retina and retinal pigment epithelium extending abnormally posteriorly over the nerve. The outer ring, representing the size of a normal optic nerve, is created by the juncture of the lamina cribrosa and the sclera (*ovals*) (Courtesy of Dr. W. Richard Green).

the role of maternal infections during pregnancy in causing optic nerve hypoplasia in the child is uncertain. The entity has been seen in conjunction with congenital cytomegalovirus, as well as maternal syphilis and rubella (44,45). Diabetes mellitus in the mother has also been associated in a number of cases (44,46).

Unilateral and bilateral cases seem to occur with almost equal frequency. The visual acuity is variable and can range from normal to no light perception. Visual field abnormalities can be seen, including altitudinal defects, localized and generalized constriction, centrocecal scotomas, bitemporal hemianopsias, and binasal hemianopsias (20). Concomitant

nystagmus and strabismus may be present, particularly in more severe cases.

Optic nerve hypoplasia has been associated with a number of systemic abnormalities. Approximately 13% of affected patients have pituitary dysfunction, including anterior pituitary defects with growth hormone insufficiency, posterior pituitary dysfunction (diabetes insipidus), hypoglycemia, and panhypopituitarism (47). In such instances, an "empty sella" can be seen. This can occur in unilateral or bilateral cases. Partial or complete absence of the septum pellucidum has been seen in approximately one-fourth of patients. Absence or thinning of the corpus callosum may also be present. Agenesis of the septum pellucidum in conjunction with optic nerve hypoplasia is known as DeMosier's syndrome (48).

Optic Nerve Aplasia

With optic nerve hypoplasia, the retinal blood vessels and optic disk are present. In contrast, with true optic nerve aplasia, both the disk and retinal vessels are absent (Fig. 15.27), as are the retinal ganglion cells (49). Fortunately, the entity is usually unilateral. Some early reported cases of optic nerve aplasia were probably variants of optic nerve hypoplasia.

The visual acuity with optic nerve aplasia is no light perception. Fluorescein angiography discloses only a choroidal flush, whereas electroretinography is subnormal, but a-waves and b-waves can be present (49). Concurrent microphthalmos and retinochoroidal coloboma have been reported (49).

Optic nerve aplasia can occur as an isolated finding, but it has been associated with cyclopia, partial agenesis of the central nervous system, and a Hallermann-Streiff-like syndrome (49). Causative associations are lacking.

Megalopapilla

Abnormalities that have been associated with an enlarged optic disk include coloboma of the optic disk, congenital optic pit, morning glory disk anomaly, high myopia, and

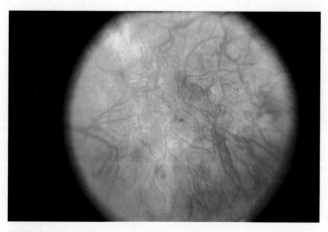

FIGURE 15.27. Optic nerve aplasia. The nerve head and retinal vessels are absent (Courtesy of Dr. Leonard Nelson, Wills Eye Hospital).

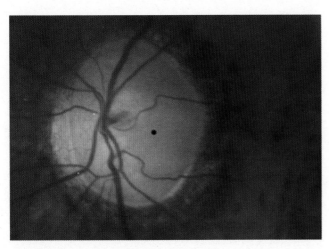

FIGURE 15.28. Megalopapilla. Central fovea (*arrow*). The retinal vessels are normal in caliber but appear small because of the enlarged size of the optic disk. Peripapillary atrophy can be seen.

megalopapilla. Clinically, megalopapilla manifests as an enlarged, but otherwise usually normal appearing, optic disk (Fig. 15.28). A mild peripapillary, retinal pigment epithelial disturbance is frequently observed, but other intraocular abnormalities have not been consistently associated.

First described by Franceschetti and Bock in 1950 (50), megalopapilla is generally not associated with decreased visual acuity, although mild-to-moderate visual loss has been noted (51). By strict definition, the entity includes optic disks with averaged horizontal and vertical diameters that measure approximately 2.1 mm or greater. The embryologic derivation is uncertain, but it is thought to arise from abnormal development of the primitive epithelial papilla (52).

An enlarged blind spot is present on visual field examination, but partial superotemporal quadrantanopsia has also been noted (53). Systemic abnormalities that have been described in conjunction with megalopapilla include basal encephalocele, cleft palate, and mandibulofacial dysostosis (50–54).

REFERENCES

1. Liebrich R. Demonstration of diseases of the eye. Persistent hyaloid artery and vein. *Trans Pathol Soc Lond* 1871;22:221–224.
2. Brown G, Tasman W. *Congenital anomalies of the optic disc.* New York: Grune & Stratton, 1983a:31–93;1983b:95–215.
3. Degenhart W, Brown GC, Augsburger JJ, et al. Prepapillary vascular loops: a clinical and fluorescein angiographic study. *Ophthalmology* 1981;88:1126–1131.
4. Mann I. *Developmental abnormalities of the eye,* 2nd Ed. Philadelphia, PA: JB Lippincott Co., 1957:133–136.
5. Shakin EP, Shields JA, Augsburger JJ, et al. Clinicopathologic correlation of a prepapillary vascular loop. *Retina* 1988;8:55–58.
6. Jones HE. Hyaloid remnants in the eyes of premature babies. *Br J Ophthalmol* 1963;47:37–44.
7. Delaney WW. Prepapillary hemorrhage and persistent hyaloid artery. *Am J Ophthalmol* 1980;90:419–421.
8. Mann IC. *Development of the human eye,* 3rd Ed. New York: Grune & Stratton, 1969:27–28, 228–231.
9. Shields JA, Joffe L, Guibor P. Choroidal melanoma clinically simulating a retinal angioma. *Am J Ophthalmol* 1978;85:67–81.
10. Archer DB, Deutman A, Ernest JT, et al. Arteriovenous communications in the retina. *Am J Ophthalmol* 1973;75:224–241.
11. Brown GC, Donnoso LA, Magargal LE, et al. Congenital retinal macrovessels. *Arch Ophthalmol* 1982;100:1430–1436.
12. Augsburger JJ, Goldberg. RE, Shields JA, et al. Changing appearance of retinal arterial malformation. *Albrecht von Graefes Arch Klin Exp Ophthalmol* 1980;215:65–70.
13. Cameron ME, Greer CH. Congenital arteriovenous aneurysm of the retina. *Br J Ophthalmol* 1968;52:768–772.
14. Wyburn-Mason R. Arteriovenous aneurysm of midbrain and retina, optic nerve, chiasm and brain. *Brain* 1943;66:165–203.
15. Rundles WZ, Falls HF. Congenital arteriovenous (racemose) aneurysm of the retina. *Arch Ophthalmol* 1951;46:408–418.
16. Kranenburg EW. Crater-like holes in the optic disc and central serous retinopathy. *Arch Ophthalmol* 1960;64:912–928.
17. Brown GC, Shields JA, Goldberg RE. Congenital pits of the optic nerve head. II. Clinical studies in humans. *Ophthalmology* 1980;87:51–65.

18. Borodic GE, Gragoudas ES, Edward WO, et al. Peripapillary subretinal neovascularization and serous macular detachment. Association with congenital optic nerve pits. *Arch Ophthalmol* 1984;102(2):229–231.
19. Brown GC, Shields JA, Patty BE, et al. Congenital pit of the optic nerve head. I. Experimental studies in collie dogs. *Arch Ophthalmol* 1979;97:1341–1344.
20. Brown G, Tasman W. *Congenital abnormalities of the optic disc.* New York: Grune and Stratton, 1983b:92–215.
21. Lincoff H, Lopez R, Kreissig I, et al. Retinoschisis associated with optic pits. *Arch Ophthalmol* 1988;106:61–67.
22. Brown GC, Brown MM. Treatment of retinal detachment associated with congenital excavated defects of the optic disc. *Ophthalmic Surg* 1995;26:11–15.
23. Cox MS, Witherspoon CD, Morris RE, et al. Evolving techniques in the treatment of macular detachment caused by optic nerve pits. *Ophthalmology* 1988;95:889–896.
24. Van Nouhuys JM, Bruyn GW. Nasopharyngeal transsphenoidal encephalocele, craterlike hold in the optic disc and agenesis of the corpus callosum; pneumoencephalographic visualisation in a case. *Psychiatr Neurol Neurochir* 1964;67:243–258.
25. Babel PJ, Farpour E. L'origene genetique des fossettes colobomateuses des nerf optique. *J Genet Hum* 1967;16:187–198.
26. Vossias A. Beitrag zur lehre von den angeborenen conis. *Klin Monatsbal Augenheilkd* 1885;23:137–157.
27. Lyle DJ. Coloboma of the optic nerve. *Am J Ophthalmol* 1932;15:347–349.
28. Savell J, Cook JR. Optic nerve colobomas of autosomal-dominant heredity. *Arch Ophthalmol* 1976;94:395–400.
29. Pagan RA, Graham JM, Zonana J, et al. Coloboma, congenital heart disease, and choanal atresia with multiple anomalies: CHARGE association. *J Pediatr* 1981;99:223–227.
30. Kindler P. Morning glory syndrome: unusual congenital optic disc anomaly. *Am J Ophthalmol* 1970;69:376–384.
31. Steinkuller PG. The morning glory disc anomaly: case report and literature review. *J Pediatr Ophthalmol* 1980;17:81–87.
32. Beyer WB, Quencer RM, Osher RH. Morning glory syndrome: a functional analysis including fluorescein angiography,

ultrasonography, and computerized tomography. *Ophthalmology* 1982;100:1361–1367.

33. Pollock JA, Newton TH, Hoyt WF. Transsphenoidal and transethmoidal encephaloceles. *Radiology* 1968;90:442–453.

34. Lenhart PD, Lambert SR, Newman NJ, Biousse V, Atkinson DS Jr, Traboulsi EI, Hutchinson AK. Intracranial vascular anomalies in patients with morning glory disk anomaly. *Am J Ophthalmol* 2006;142(4):644–650.

35. Wise JB, MacLean JL, Gass JDM. Contractile peripapillary staphyloma. *Arch Ophthalmol* 1966;75:626–630.

36. Riise D. Visual field defects in optic disc malformation with ectasia of the fundus. *Acta Ophthalmol* 1966;44:906–918.

37. Riise D. The nasal fundus ectasia. *Acta Ophthalmol* 1975;126 (Suppl):5–108.

38. Mosier MA, Lieberman MF, Green WR, et al. Hypoplasia of the optic nerve. *Arch Ophthalmol* 1978;96:1437–1442.

39. Jerome B, Forster HW. Congenital hypoplasia (partial aplasia) of the optic nerve. *Arch Ophthalmol* 1948;34:669–672.

40. Ellenberger C, Runyan TE. Holoprosencephaly with hypoplasia of the optic nerves, dwarfism and agenesis of the septum pellucidum. *Am J Ophthalmol* 1970;70:960–967.

41. Hackenbruch Y, Meerhoff E, Besio R, et al. Familial bilateral optic nerve hypoplasia. *Am J Ophthalmol* 1975;79:314–320.

42. Hoyt CS, Billson FA. Maternal anticonvulsants and optic nerve hypoplasia. *Br J Ophthalmol* 1978;62:3–6.

43. McKinna AJ. Quinine induced hypoplasia of the optic nerve. *Can J Ophthalmol* 1966;1:261–266.

44. Hotchkiss ML, Green WR. Optic nerve aplasia and hypoplasia. *J Pediatr Ophthalmol* 1979;16:225–240.

45. Hittner HM, Desmond MM, Montgomery JR. Optic nerve manifestations of human congenital cytomegalovirus. *Am J Ophthalmol* 1976;81:661–665.

46. Petersen RA, Walter DS. Optic nerve hypoplasia with good visual acuity and visual field defects. *Arch Ophthalmol* 1977;95:254–258.

47. Acers TE. Optic nerve hypoplasia: septo-optic pituitary dysplasia syndrome. *Trans Am Ophthalmol Soc* 1981;79.425–457.

48. DeMosier G. Agenesie du septum lucidum avec malformation du tractus optique: la dysplasie septo-optique. *Schweiz Arch Neurol Neurochir Psychiatr* 1956;77:267–292.

49. Little LE, Whitmore PU, Wells TU. Aplasia of the optic nerve. *J Pediatr Ophthalmol* 1976;13:84–88.

50. Franceschetti A, Bock RH. Megalopapilla: a new congenital anomaly. *Am J Ophthalmol* 1950;33:227–235.

51. Strieff B. Uber megalopapillae. *Klin Monatsbl Augenheilkd* 1961;139:824–827.

52. Badtke G. Ober die grossenanomalien der papilla nervi optici, unter besonderer: berucksichtigung der schwarzen megalopapille. *Klin Monatsbl Augenheilkd* 1959;135:502–510.

53. Merin S, Harwood-Nash DC, Crawford JS. Axial tomography of optic nerve defects. *Am J Ophthalmol* 1971;72:1122–1129.

54. Malbran JL, Roveda JM. Megalopapilla. *Arch Oftalmol B Aires* 1951;26:331–335.

16

Disorders of the Lacrimal Apparatus in Infancy and Childhood

Donald P. Sauberan

EMBRYOLOGY

The lacrimal gland arises from the ectoderm of the superior conjunctival fornix at the 22 to 24 mm length of the embryo. Condensation of the surrounding mesenchyme leads to the development of the glandular stroma starting about the ninth week of development. This mesenchymal tissue is felt to arise from neural crest cells.

The lacrimal collection system is formed when the lateral nasal prominence and the maxillary prominence fuse at the 10 mm stage of embryonic development. At about the 15 mm stage, a double layer of epithelium is trapped within the space. It extends laterally to form the canalicular system and inferiorly to form the nasolacrimal duct. This epithelial cord is originally horizontal, but as the midface enlarges, it assumes the mature vertical orientation. Cavitation of this system begins to occur at about the third gestational month and continues until about the seventh gestational month. The last part of the nasolacrimal collection system to canalize is the very distal portion where the nasolacrimal duct empties into the inferior meatus in the nasal cavity (valve of Hasner). The valve of Hasner is often still closed at birth, but will spontaneously open during the first few months of life in the majority of cases.

LACRIMAL ANATOMY

There are two main tear-producing structures. The main lacrimal gland secretes reflexive tears in response to peripheral sensory, retinal, or psychogenic stimulation, such as those that occur with crying or reaction to an ocular irritant. The accessory glands of Krause and Wolfring are responsible for non-reflex basal tear secretion, which keeps the corneal surface lubricated. Tears are composed of three layers: an outer oily layer (secreted by the meibomian glands), a central aqueous layer (secreted by the lacrimal glands), and an inner mucinous layer (secreted by the conjunctival goblet cells). Once thought to be three distinct layers, it is now believed that there is mixing of the layers within the tear film.

The main lacrimal gland is located in the superotemporal orbit within the lacrimal gland fossa. It is divided into a larger orbital lobe and a smaller palpebral lobe by the lateral horn of the levator aponeurosis. The ducts of the lacrimal gland empty into the superior cul-de-sac approximately 5 mm above the lateral border of the tarsal plate. The ducts from the orbital lobe pass into the palpebral lobe, so any damage to the palpebral lobe can drastically reduce the outflow of tears from the lacrimal gland onto the corneal surface. The innervation of the lacrimal gland is complex. The afferent system is served by the lacrimal nerve, which is a branch off of the ophthalmic division of the trigeminal nerve (V1). The efferent secretory pathway begins in the lacrimal (salivatory) nucleus within the pons. Parasympathetic presynaptic fibers join the facial nerve that passes through the geniculate ganglion without synapsing. It leaves the facial nerve via the greater superficial petrosal nerve and joins the deep petrosal nerve to form the vidian nerve. This nerve travels to synapse in the pterygopalatine ganglion. Post-synaptic fibers are distributed to the lacrimal gland through the zygomatic branch of the maxillary branch of the trigeminal nerve (V3). They reach the lacrimal gland via an anastomosis between the zygomaticotemporal nerve and the lacrimal nerve. Sympathetic nerve fibers innervate the lacrimal gland as well, but appear to have no impact on secretion.

The accessory lacrimal glands of Krause and Wolfring are located near the conjunctival fornix and at the edge of the tarsal plate, respectively. There are 20 to 40 glands of Krause within the superior conjunctival fornix, and 2 to 8 within the inferior conjunctival fornix. There are 3 to 20 glands of Wolfring located at the upper border of the superior tarsal plate, and 1 to 4 at the lower border of the inferior tarsal plate. There may also be an accessory lacrimal gland within the caruncle or plica semilunaris. As mentioned previously, the accessory lacrimal glands are responsible for basal tear production that is necessary for adequate lubrication of the globe.

Evaporation plays a small role in the removal of tears from the ocular surface, but most tears are drained through a series of collection channels and into the nose. The beginning of the tear drainage system is the lacrimal punctum (plural: punctae). The punctae are openings into the eyelid that sit on an elevation known as the lacrimal papillae. Each punctum lies approximately 6 mm lateral to the medial canthus; however, when the eyelids are open, the upper punctum lies about 0.5 mm nasal to the lower punctum. Normally, the punctae face inward within the tear lake. Each punctual opening is about 0.2 to 0.3 mm in diameter and open into the canalicular system. The ampulla is a 2 mm vertical section extending distally from the punctum perpendicular to the eyelid margin. The horizontal canaliculus then extends from the base of the ampulla toward the medial canthus curving with the eyelid and located just inferior to the eyelid margin. The 8 to 10 mm segment has a diameter slightly less than 1 mm, although elastic tissue surrounding the canalicular system allows for dilation to several times its width. In 90% of patients, the upper and lower canaliculi will join to form a common canaliculus that enters the lateral wall of the lacrimal sac. There are numerous infoldings at the junction of the canaliculus and lacrimal sac which creates a valve-like structure termed the valve of Rosenmuller. This structure helps prevent reflux of material from the sac into the canalicular system.

The lacrimal sac is located within the lacrimal fossa, formed by the frontal process of the maxilla and the lacrimal bone. The fossa and sac lay anterior to the orbital septum and are thus preorbital (not orbital) structures. The sac lies between the anterior of posterior crura of the medial canthal tendon. It is divided into a 3 to 5 mm portion above the canalicular opening known as the fundus, and the remaining distal portion (approximately 10 mm in length) known as the body. Because the majority of the sac is located inferior to the medial canthal tendon, conditions that affect the lacrimal sac (such as dacryoceles or dacryocystitis) are typically found inferior to the medial canthal tendon. Any process that involves the region superior to the medial canthal tendon should be met with suspicion, and an alternate diagnosis to a nasolacrimal disorder should be entertained. The nasolacrimal duct extends from the distal end of the lacrimal sac through the lateral wall of the nose to empty into the inferior meatus of the nose. The duct is approximately 12 mm long, and courses in inferior, lateral, and slightly posterior directions. The valve of Hasner is a fold of tissue that is present at the very distal end of the duct. This valve often does not "open" in infants, and is a common cause of infantile nasolacrimal duct obstruction. The nasolacrimal collecting system is lined with pseudostratified ciliated columnar epithelium, similar to that found in the upper respiratory system. Mucous-producing goblet cells are also present.

Most of the tear lake is actively pumped away from the eye by the actions of the orbicularis muscle. Jones (1) proposed that during eye closure the superficial and deep heads of the pretarsal orbicularis muscle compress the ampullae and shorten the horizontal canaliculus. At the same time the deep heads of the preseptal orbicularis, which are attached to the lacrimal sac fascia, contract, which expands the sac and creates negative pressure. This draws the tears from the canalicular system into the sac. When the eye opens, the orbicularis muscles relax and the resilience of the lacrimal sac fascia collapses the tear sac, forcing tears through the duct and into the nose. As the eyelids open and the puncta move laterally, the tears of the tear lake once again fill the ampullae and canaliculi. An alternative theory (Rosengren-Doane) suggests that the contraction of the orbicularis creates a positive pressure in the tear sac, which forces the tears into the nose, and as the eye opens the negative pressure created from re-expansion of the sac draws tears into the canaliculi when the puncta separate.

LACRIMAL TESTS

Dye Disappearance Test

The dye disappearance test (DDT) can be performed on nearly all children in the clinic. A drop of fluorescein (or a fluorescein strip wet with topical anesthetic) is placed into each conjunctival fornix and the patient is rechecked after 5 minutes. In a normal patient, there should be minimal (if any) fluorescein remaining. Fluorescein visualized after 5 minutes demonstrates obstruction, but does not localize the condition. The DDT is a physiologic test, as it involves no external means of forcing the tears into the collection system. Jones testing, which involves inserting a cotton-tipped applicator under the inferior meatus to collect fluorescein dye, is extremely difficult, if not impossible to perform on pediatric patients. In addition, diagnostic irrigation of the tear system will be resisted by children and can only be performed in more cooperative older patients.

Dacryocystography

Dacryocystography (DCG) is a radiographic test for evaluating the quality (not quantity) of tear outflow. It is particularly useful in the detection of lacrimal fistulae, neoplasms, and lacrimal stones. A radiopaque dye is injected into the lower canaliculus and serial films are taken at 15 and 30 minutes post-injection. This test has a limited use in the pediatric population. First, this test must be undertaken under general anesthetic in the majority of children. Second, the patient is exposed to a fair amount of radiation during the procedure (estimated at 3,000 mrad). Lastly, the majority of conditions that this test is most useful for are rare in the pediatric population.

Dacryoscintigraphy

Dacryoscintigraphy (DSG) is another radiographic test that provides a qualitative view of the lacrimal outflow. Ten microliters containing 100 microcuries of technetium-99m pertechnetate is dropped into each eye. Images are then taken four times per minute for 20 minutes. This test can often be performed while awake, and radiation exposure is much less than with DCG (around 4 to 14 mrad). One can also investigate an anatomic blockage from a functional delay by having the patient perform various maneuvers during the test (such as forceful blinking).

CONGENITAL ANOMALIES OF LACRIMAL SECRETORY APPARATUS

Absence of the lacrimal gland is a rare condition that may present as chronic irritation of the conjunctiva and cornea from dryness, and is treated as such. Computed tomography shows no discernible lacrimal gland (2). Alacrima may also occur in association with conditions of other developmental anomalies, such as anophthalmos or cryptophthalmos, or may be inherited as an autosomal dominant or recessive trait.

"Crocodile tears," or paradoxic gustolacrimal reflex, is unilateral tearing with mastication. This can be seen as a congenital defect, usually associated with an ipsilateral Duane syndrome or lateral rectus palsy. It is more commonly seen as an acquired condition, after a paralysis of the facial nerve, from trauma, or surgery.

Prolapse of the palpebral lobe of the lacrimal gland may occur, and the palpebral lobe can often be identified under the conjunctiva in the lateral aspect of the superior fornix. This should be recognized as normal tissue and left undisturbed, because surgical excision would transect the ducts from the orbital portion and could produce a dry eye.

Aberrant lacrimal tissue may be located elsewhere on the surface of the eye, under the conjunctiva. It may appear similar to a dermoid, except that it is not usually in the lower outer quadrant typical of dermoids. Aberrant lacrimal tissue appears as a slightly raised, well-vascularized, multicystic mass, and histopathologically it is often described as a choristomatous malformation containing a lacrimal gland, among other elements. Usually there are no symptoms, but excision may be performed for diagnosis or cosmesis. Aberrant lacrimal gland tissue may also occur within the sclera or in the eye.

Lacrimal secretory ducts may be absent or become obstructed, leading to distention and cystic development (dacryops) of the lacrimal gland. Rarely, a portion of the tears from the lacrimal gland may exist in the eyelid above the tarsus from a fistula. The opening is typically surrounded by hair, and excision with closure in layers should correct the condition.

Punctal agenesis can range from a simple veil overlying the punctual opening to a complete absence of the punctum (and often the surrounding canalicular system). The presence of appropriate lacrimal papillae will often indicate whether there is an actual opening underneath. Often a punctal opening can be made by inserting a sharp object (such as a safety pin) through the tissue overlying the punctum. This can be followed by a punctal dilator to expand the opening. Punctae may also be anomalous in position or number.

The canalicular system can have any multitude of congenital anomalies. Canalicular atresia can be proximal (adjacent to the punctum), midcanalicular, or distal (adjacent to or involving the opening into the lacrimal sac). The more significant the obstruction, the more significant surgical correction must be entertained.

A lacrimal sac diverticulum is a rare condition that presents as a mass below the medial palpebral ligament and may be uninfected or infected. When the lacrimal system is drained, however, a palpable or visible mass remains. Treatment consists of surgical excision of the diverticulum, suturing the closed wall of the lacrimal sac where the diverticulum originated. It can often mimic a dacryocystocele.

Congenital lacrimal sac fistula is a rare entity, occurring in approximately 1 in 2,000 births (3). They are often asymptomatic, and only become visualized should the child have concurrent nasolacrimal duct obstruction (leading to tearing through the fistula) or the development of an infection. The fistula is a connection lined with stratified squamous epithelium typically located inferonasal to the medial canthus, usually connecting the skin to the common canaliculus or lacrimal sac. The dimple located on the skin is visible, though not always noted if not actively discharging material. Often these patients will have concurrent nasolacrimal duct obstruction, and present with epiphora. Sometimes, the fistula will terminate prior to the nasolacrimal system, and no tears will be present. The fistula can be visualized using fluorescein dye as used to irrigate to check for patency during nasolacrimal duct probing. The fluorescein will be visualized on the skin surface following irrigation. The treatment for symptomatic lacrimal sac fistula is surgical. Cauterization of the external opening has been attempted in the past, but does not appear to be successful (4). Complete closure and excision of the fistula is necessary. Silicone tubes may be placed at the same time should distal nasolacrimal duct obstruction be present.

DACRYOCELE

The presentation of a dacryocele (sometimes called amniotocele, lacrimal sac mucocele, or dacryocystocele) is usually at or near birth. A bluish mass is noted inferior to the medial canthal angle (Fig. 16.1). A dacryocele is formed when the nasolacrimal duct is obstructed at both the proximal and terminal ends, both at the valve of Rosenmuller (at the level of the common canaliculus entering into the nasolacrimal sac) and the valve of Hasner (at the level of the nasolacrimal duct entering the inferior meatus in the nose). The blockage of both the inlet and the outlet of the duct leads to sequestration of mucus which can become secondarily infected. In the case of infection, the skin overlying the lacrimal sac can be erythematous. Schnall and Christian (5) found that 4 out of 21 (19.0%) dacryoceles had evidence of infection, with 3 occurring at the time of presentation. Becker (6) found a much higher percentage of

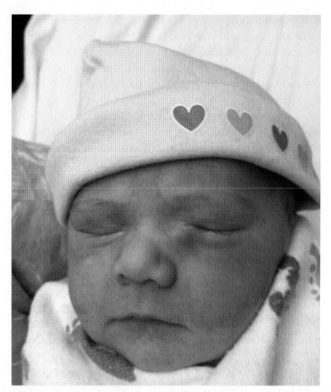

FIGURE 16.1. A dacryocele (sometimes called amniotocele, lacrimal sac mucocele, or dacryocystocele) is usually at or near birth. A bluish mass is noted inferior to the medial canthal angle.

secondary infection, with 21 out of 29 (72.4%) developing dacryocystitis and/or cellulitis. A dacryocystocele may also exhibit intranasal extension causing respiratory distress in the newborn. Paysse et al. (7) found a concurrent intranasal mucocele in 23 out of 30 (77%) dacryoceles, with respiratory distress present in 7 patients. The diagnosis of a dacryocele is usually clinical. As noted above, it is usually a bluish elevation occurring below the medial canthal tendon. The differential diagnosis for such a lesion includes meningoencephalocele (which are normally located superior to the medial canthal tendon), dermoid cyst, or hemangioma. Imaging is not normally necessary. MRI can be performed to assess the area should an atypical lesion be present (8). Suggestions of an atypical presentation include an elevation occurring above the medial canthal tendon, hypertelorism, pulsation, and known CNS abnormality (7). Prenatal diagnosis of dacryocele has also occurred using ultrasound (9). Nasal examination using a nasal speculum or endoscope can be performed to evaluate for the presence of an intranasal mucocele. They often will present with dacryocystitis and/or cellulitis. Wong and Vanderveen (10) found that 30 out of 46 (65%) dacryoceles presented with dacryocystitis or cellulitis. There are differing opinions regarding the treatment of dacryocystoceles. Current conservative measures include digital massage of the lacrimal sac in an attempt to hydrostatically decompress the lacrimal sac. Infrequently, the

dacryocele can decompress through the canalicular system, but the nasolacrimal duct can remain blocked distally at the valve of Hasner (6). Schnall and Christian (5), in a prospective study, found that 16 of 21 (76%) patients resolved with conservative treatment consisting of antibiotics (topical and/or systemic based on presence of infection), digital massage, and warm compresses. In addition, all four dacryoceles that were infected at presentation or became infected after presentation resolved with conservative therapy. All dacryoceles resolved within 1 week, thus he recommended that 1 week of conservative therapy is indicated in these patients prior to nasolacrimal duct probing. Becker (6), however, found that all 7 (100%) patients who had a nasolacrimal duct probing prior to a secondary infection developing had resolution, whereas only 10 out of 19 (53%) with dacryocystitis or cellulitis had resolution following a nasolacrimal duct probing. He advocated early probing in an attempt to open the system prior to the development of thickened cyst wall and turbid purulent fluid which can lead to early closure. Wong and Vanderveen (10) showed that 78% of dacryoceles required surgical intervention, while only 10 out of 46 eyes (22%) resolved with conservative nonsurgical measures. Probing may occur in either the office or in the operating room. Wong and Vanderveen (10) found a 100% success rate in both office probing and operating room probing in cases not complicated by a nasal cyst. Probing should be delayed in the event of an infectious dacryocystitis to minimize the risk of creating a false passage. Systemic antibiotics given at this time may also allow the dacryocele to resolve. Should initial probing fail, repeat probing with or without silicone tube intubation, balloon dacryoplasty; or marsupialization of the intranasal cyst can be undertaken (6).

EVALUATION AND MANAGEMENT OF THE TEARING CHILD

In the evaluation of the tearing child, other causes of tearing such as corneal disease, congenital glaucoma, or infection must be ruled out. Distinction may be made between tearing alone, tearing with discharge, or intermittent tearing and discharge. Office evaluation includes inspection of the eyelid margins for the presence and apparent patency of puncta, as well as an anterior segment examination to look for other causes of tearing. Inspection of the medial canthal region for associated defects, such as medial encephalocele, dacryocele, or fistulae, is important. Digital pressure over the lacrimal sac should be performed to look for reflux. Dye disappearance testing may be performed, and delayed or asymmetric drainage after 5 minutes may provide evidence of partial obstruction. The Jones dye tests are difficult to perform accurately in pediatric patients in the office, because insertion of a cotton applicator into the nose will be resisted by the patient, and irrigation of the lacrimal sac generally cannot be safely performed in young patients.

CONGENITAL NASOLACRIMAL DUCT OBSTRUCTION

Approximately 6% of all neonates have nasolacrimal duct obstruction (11). The number is as high as 75% when fetal autopsies are performed. Most infants present with tearing and/or mattering of the involved eye. Depending on the level of obstruction, the symptoms may be more tearing than mattering or vice versa. Mucopurulent discharge can sometimes be expressed from the lacrimal sac through the punctum with digital massage. Symptoms are often worse in the cold, wind, or when the child has an upper respiratory tract infection. The presentation may be unilateral or bilateral. There is usually no concurrent conjunctival injection, which differentiates it from more typical conjunctivitis. The most common etiology is the failure of the valve of Hasner to open. Premature infants have much higher rates of nasolacrimal duct obstruction. However, because tear production is not occurring until near term, these infants often do not exhibit the symptoms of epiphora. The diagnosis of nasolacrimal duct obstruction is a clinical one. One must be diligent in looking for other, less common causes of tearing. The most important diagnosis on the differential is infantile glaucoma. Increased intraocular pressure can lead to corneal epithelial edema and breakdown, resulting in tearing. Other signs and symptoms consistent with infantile glaucoma include increased corneal diameter, optic nerve cupping, photophobia, and increased axial length resulting in myopia. The combination of epiphora with any of these other signs or symptoms should lead one to consider the diagnosis of infantile glaucoma. Other causes of infantile epiphora include keratitis, foreign body, or agenesis of the lacrimal puncta. The treatment of nasolacrimal duct obstruction is, at first, conservative. Peterson and Robb (12) evaluated the natural history of nasolacrimal duct obstruction, and found that 44 of 50 (88%) patients resolved spontaneously using conservative treatment. A recent study by the Pediatric Eye Disease Investigator Group found spontaneous resolution in 66% of patients aged 6 to <10 months. Conservative treatment usually consists of some mixture of nasolacrimal massage, warm compresses, and antibiotics if needed for secondary infection. Crigler in 1923 (13) described massage of the lacrimal sac in an attempt to open the distal nasolacrimal duct by creating an increase in hydrostatic pressure within the sac to break open the distal membrane. This is still the method of choice for nasolacrimal massage. Surgical intervention consists of the introduction of a flexible metallic probe into the nasolacrimal duct to open it. While classically the obstruction is located at the valve of Hasner, the location of obstruction may be anywhere along the route. Probes of increasing size are placed into the nasolacrimal duct to increase the opening to minimize failure. The nasolacrimal system can also be irrigated to assess patency following probing. This can be done by using fluorescein-stained balanced salt solution to irrigate with nasal suction to collect the fluid. One must remember, however, that this test does not mimic physiologic tear drainage, and that an open system to irrigation may not stay patent. Various opinions remain as to the most beneficial timing to pursue surgical intervention. Some argue that early intervention will have a higher success rate and allow for probing in the office, eliminating the need for general anesthesia. Others state that the procedure should be delayed as long as possible to allow for maximum spontaneous resolution. Classically, it is thought that the older a patient is at the time of the probing, the less successful the probing will be. Katowitz and Welsh (14) found a decreasing level of success after the first year of life. This led to use 1 year of age as an ideal time to perform the initial surgical procedure. Various studies show a success rate between 90% and 95% after initial probing. Should the initial probe fail, one must decide whether to perform a secondary probing or an ancillary procedure. The two main secondary procedures include balloon dacryoplasty and silicone tube intubation. Balloon dacryoplasty involves the insertion of a balloon catheter on a flexible guide wire into the nasolacrimal duct, and the inflation of the catheter to a predetermined pressure for a predetermined time. Success rates for balloon dacryoplasty as a primary procedure have been quoted as high as 94% (15); however, the extra cost associated with its usage may preclude its use for common nasolacrimal duct obstructions. It may be useful in the recalcitrant cases where other modalities have failed. Silicone intubation of the nasolacrimal duct can be used as a secondary or primary procedure. Silicone tubes can be bicanalicular or monocanalicular. Bicanalicular silicone tubes consist of the silicone tube with a flexible metal probe on each end. Each separate end is introduced into the upper or lower punctum and then retrieved from the nose. The tube endings are tied in knots to prevent premature removal, and are often secured into the nasal vestibule via a suture. The tubes are kept in for a varying amount of time (surgeon preference), and then removed under general anesthesia. The disadvantages to this system include the possibility of punctual/canalicular tearing secondary to a tight tube and the injury to the nasal mucosa while removing the tube from inferior meatus. The other type of tube is the monocanalicular stent. This is a single silicone tube with a special footplate at the proximal end to allow for seating in the punctum once located in the duct. The advantage of the monocanalicular stent is that there is no risk for canalicular damage secondary to tight tubing, and the tube may be removed in the office, as it is not secured in the nose. This alleviates the need for a secondary procedure under general anesthesia. There is also much less trauma involved in the insertion of the monocanalicular stent. The two main disadvantages to this system include early unplanned removal of the tube and corneal abrasion. In a large study by Engel et al. (16), 116 of 685 (14.9%) cases had premature tube removal. However, of these patients who had premature tube removal, there was no difference in the recurrence rate compared with those who had the tube removed in the office. There was also a 2% incidence of corneal abrasion. This is believed to be secondary to the footplate rubbing against the cornea. Engel et al. (16) looked at primary monocanalicular stent placement for nasolacrimal duct obstruction and found a success rate of 97.3% in patients of age between 12 and 18 months, and a success rate of 97.5% in patients of age between 18 and 24 months. This suggests that delay of initial treatment could be extended to as late as 24 months if combined with an initial monocanalicular stent placement. The ideal length of time to leave silicone tubes in is unknown. Many surgeons leave them in for about 3 to 6 months. The difficulty in comparing any of these secondary procedures is that they intrinsically all contain a nasolacrimal duct probe in addition to their other steps. When these procedures fail, dacryocystorhinostomy (DCR) may be required. Endoscopic DCR has had a high success rate even in children (17) and avoids an external scar. This involves identification of the site for a nasal ostium using a 20-gauge light pipe and nasal endoscopy to create a new ostium or enlarge the existing ostium, followed by placement of silicone tubing. Endoscopic DCR is less successful for revisions. External DCR remains the gold standard and involves creating an incision nasal to the medial canthus to expose the lacrimal sac and directly making a connection from the lacrimal sac into the nose. Conjunctival DCR may be needed if the puncta and canaliculi are congenitally absent. Jones's technique uses placement of a Pyrex tube in the medial canthal area, which extends through the lacrimal fossa into the nose through a DCR-type incision. Once the passageway becomes epithelialized, a polyethylene tube can be exchanged for the glass tube. Practically speaking, however, the care and preservation of this system in a young child are difficult.

ACQUIRED NASOLACRIMAL SYSTEM OBSTRUCTION

The nasolacrimal collection system is often divided into an upper system (consisting of the punctum and canalicular system) and a lower system (the nasolacrimal duct). In the pediatric population, acquired conditions of the upper nasolacrimal system are much less common than congenital abnormalities. However, acquired abnormalities can occur. Most common, punctual stenosis can develop from infectious etiologies such as Herpes simplex and Varicella zoster. Allergic rhinitis can cause intermittent obstruction of the nasolacrimal system through local edema and inflammation during acute episodes. Malignancies of the nasolacrimal sac are extremely rare in the pediatric population, but may present with a functional obstruction along with blood-tinged tears. The most common cause of an acquired lower system obstruction is trauma, possibly involving midface LeFort fractures.

DECREASED TEAR PRODUCTION

Although not nearly as common as epiphora, some children experience of lack of tearing. Basal tear secretion is nearly always present at birth, whereas reflex tear secretion can occur anywhere from birth to several months of age (11). Often, parents simply notice the lack of tears during crying, and suspect a problem. Children can present with irritation, foreign body sensation, conjunctival injection, photophobia, or corneal scarring.

Absence of reflex tearing may be reported by parents as no tears in one eye or both eyes when the infant is crying. Usually such children do show normal basal tearing, but examination of the ocular surface should be performed to ensure that adequate lubrication exists. There should be no sign of ocular irritation with absent reflex tearing because the basal secretion from accessory lacrimal glands provides a sufficient tear film. No investigation or treatment is necessary.

Congenital or early-onset lack of tear production can be the result of systemic conditions such as Riley-Day syndrome (familial dysautonomia) and Allgrove syndrome (triad consisting of alacrima, achalasia, and adrenocorticoid insufficiency) (18). Medications can cause a decrease in tear production. Antihistamines, useful in the treatment of allergic rhinitis, are a common cause in the pediatric population secondary to the anticholinergic side effect that reduces tear production. Isotretinoin is a common cause in the adolescent population. Examination of the corneal surface is vital when presented with a child with the complaint of absence of tearing. Fluorescein staining can help assess the status of the cornea. Punctate epithelial erosions, frank epithelial defects, or corneal scarring can all be present. The tear lake is diminished. The eyelid margin may have evidence of blepharitis, with eyelid margin erythema, telangiectasia, or debris. Sjogren's syndrome, either primary or secondary to other rheumatologic conditions such as sysemic lupus erythematous (SLE), is rare. Absence of the main lacrimal gland is very uncommon (19).

Treatment is aimed at maintaining the integrity of the cornea epithelium. Copious use of tear substitutes, in liquid, gel, or ointment form, allow for adequate protection. Should the use of artificial tears fail, temporary or permanent punctual occlusion may be necessary. Immunomodulatory medication, such as cyclosporine 0.05%, may be useful in extreme cases. Blepharitis, if present, should be treated with warm compresses, eyelid scrubs, and antibiotics as necessary. Oral antibiotics such as erythromycin or tetracycline may be useful in the treatment of chronic blepharitis. Tetracycline and its derivatives should be avoided in children under age 8 to eliminate the risk of tooth discoloration. Patients with Riley-Day syndrome will also have decreased corneal sensation, which can lead to devastating ocular complications. Tarsorrhaphy should be utilized in these cases of decreased tear production associated with poor corneal sensation.

REFERENCES

1. Jones LT. An anatomical approach to problems of the eyelids and lacrimal apparatus. *Arch Ophthalmol* 1961;66:111–124.
2. Keith CG, Boldt DW. Congenital absence of the lacrimal gland. *Am J Ophthalmol* 1986;102(6):800–801.
3. Tien AM, Tien DR. Bilateral congenital lacrimal sac fistulae in a patient with ectrodactyly-ectodermal dysplasia-clefting syndrome. *J AAPOS* 2006;10(6):577–578.
4. Birchansky LD, Nerad JA, Kersten RC, Kulwin DR. Management of congenital lacrimal sac fistula. *Arch Ophthalmol* 1990; 108(3):388–390.
5. Schnall BM, Christian CJ. Conservative treatment of congenital dacryocele. *J Pediatr Ophthalmol Strabismus* 1996;33(5): 219–222.
6. Becker BB. The treatment of congenital dacryocystocele. *Am J Ophthalmol* 2006;142(5):835–838.
7. Paysse EA, Coats DK, Bernstein JM, Go C, De jong AL. Management and complications of congenital dacryocele with concurrent intranasal mucocele. *J AAPOS* 2000;4(1):46–53.
8. Farrer RS, Mohammed TL, Hahn FJ. MRI of childhood dacryocystocele. *Neuroradiology* 2003;45(4):259–261.
9. D'addario V, Pinto V, Anfossi A, Del bianco A, Cantatore F. Antenatal sonographic diagnosis of dacryocystocele. *Acta Ophthalmol Scand* 2001;79(3):330–331.
10. Wong RK, Vanderveen DK. Presentation and management of congenital dacryocystocele. *Pediatrics* 2008;122(5): e1108–e1112.
11. Robb R. Tearing abnormalities. In: Isenberg S, ed. *The eye in infancy*, 2nd Ed. St. Louis, MO: Mosby, 1994:248–253.
12. Petersen RA, Robb RM. The natural course of congenital obstruction of the nasolacrimal duct. *J Pediatr Ophthalmol Strabismus* 15(4):246–250.
13. Crigler LW. The treatment of congenital dacryocystitis. JAMA 1923;81(1):23–24. doi:10.1001/jama.1923.02650010027009
14. Katowitz JA, Welsh MG. Timing of initial probing and irrigation in congenital nasolacrimal duct obstruction. *Ophthalmology* 1987;94(6):698–705.
15. Becker BB, Berry FD, Koller H. Balloon catheter dilatation for treatment of congenital nasolacrimal duct obstruction. *Am J Ophthalmol* 1996;121(3):304–309.
16. Engel JM, Hichie-Schmidt C, Khammar A, Ostfeld BM, Vyas A, Ticho BH. Monocanalicular silastic intubation for the initial correction of congenital nasolacrimal duct obstruction. *J AAPOS* 2007;11(2):183–186.
17. VanderVeen DK, Jones DT, Tan H, et al. Endoscopic dacryocystorhinostomy in children. *J AAPOS* 2001;5(3)143–147.
18. Brooks BP, Kleta R, Caruso RC, Stuart C, Ludlow J, Stratakis CA. Triple-A syndrome with prominent ophthalmic features and a novel mutation in the AAAS gene: a case report. *BMC Ophthalmol* 2004;4:7.
19. Kim SH, Hwang S, Kweon S, Kim TK, Oh J. Two cases of lacrimal gland agenesis in the same family—clinicoradiologic findings and management. *Can J Ophthalmol* 2005;40(4): 502–505.

17

Pediatric Eyelid Disorders

Forrest J. Ellis

EYELID DEVELOPMENT

Eyelid development is intimately associated with the development of the eye (1). During the fourth week of gestation, the optical vesicle forms as a projection from the side of the forebrain. The optical vesicle invaginates, forming the optic cup. The overlying ectoderm forms the lens placode, which separates and migrates internally to form the lens of the eye. The ectodermal surface overlying the optic cup develops into the cornea. Further development during week 6 results in small folds of the surface ectoderm with its underlying mesenchyme. These two folds become the upper and lower eyelids. These folds grow toward each other and ultimately result in fusion of the upper and lower eyelids between weeks 8 and 10 of gestation. The eyelids remain fused until approximately the sixth month of gestation, at which time separation of the eyelids occurs. In addition to primary eyelid developmental abnormalities, eyelid and ocular development may be affected by abnormalities or defects in facial development. Abnormalities in orbital development can also cause secondary abnormalities in eyelid development.

ANATOMY OF THE EYELIDS

Upper Eyelid

The upper eyelid margin forms a curved arch from the medial canthus to the lateral canthus and overlies the superior 1 to 2 mm of the cornea. The peak of this curve is approximately 1 mm nasal to the center of the cornea. The upper eyelid crease is formed by the attachment of strands of the external levator aponeurosis to the skin (2). An absent upper eyelid crease can be seen in conditions of abnormal levator development such as congenital ptosis. However, the normal Asian eyelid has a low set and less developed eyelid crease. In addition, dehiscence of the levator aponeurosis can result in an abnormally elevated eyelid crease.

The upper eyelid tarsus is approximately 10 mm in its vertical height in the adult and proportionately shorter in children. It is formed of dense fibrous tissue. Medially and laterally the tarsus is attached firmly to the orbital rims by the canthal tendons. The medial canthal tendon attaches to the anterior and posterior lacrimal crests and the fascia of the lacrimal sac. The lateral canthal tendon attaches to the lateral border of the tarsus and to the Whitnall tubercle inside the lateral orbital rim. The lateral canthus is normally even with or just slightly above the medial canthal tendon in the horizontal plane. Externally an extra fold of skin can be seen in the medial canthal area overlying and potentially obscuring the medial canthal tendon. This extra fold of skin is referred to an epicanthal fold.

The anatomy of the upper eyelid overlying the tarsal plate consists of eyelid skin covering the orbicularis oculi muscle. This pretarsal orbicularis is adherent to the underlying tarsal plate. Conjunctiva is also firmly adhered to the tarsus posteriorly. Superior to the tarsus, the skin covers the preseptal orbicularis muscle. Beneath the preseptal muscle is the orbital septum, which defines the anterior boundary of the orbit and overlies orbital fat. The orbital septum is important in eyelid anatomy. In Caucasian upper eyelids, the orbital septum and levator aponeurosis fuse at approximately the superior tarsal boarder 10 mm above the eyelid margin. However, in Asian eyelids, the septum inserts much lower into the levator aponeurosis, resulting in inferior displacement of orbital fat and a lower eyelid crease (3). Posterior to the levator aponeurosis is the underlying Müller muscle.

Lower Eyelid

The lower eyelid margin usually crosses the inferior corneoscleral limbus. Lower eyelid anatomy has similar features to upper eyelid anatomy (4). However, the lower eyelid tarsus is only 5 mm in its greatest vertical height. Arising from the area of inferior rectus muscle is the capsulopalpebral fascia. In a similar, but less well-developed fashion to the levator aponeurosis, this fascia inserts into the lower eyelid tarsus where it retracts and stabilizes the lower eyelid. The orbital septum of the lower eyelid inserts directly onto the tarsus.

Levator Palpebrae Superioris and Müller Muscle

The levator muscle has its origin at the lesser wing of the sphenoid. It runs posterior to anterior in the superior aspect of the orbit. Just inside the superior orbital rim, the levator muscle crosses and fuses with the Whitnall ligament. This attachment provides support to the levator muscle and aponeurosis. At this point, the levator muscle turns in an inferior direction while becoming more fibrous. The levator aponeurosis spreads out horizontally to form a fan-shaped structure with attachments medially and laterally, the medial and lateral horns, which insert in the periosteum. The levator aponeurosis inserts broadly across the anterior surface of the upper eyelid tarsus. Small strands of the levator aponeurosis also project anteriorly, inserting into the eyelid skin and forming the eyelid crease.

The Müller muscle complex arises from the posterior aspect of the levator muscle, lies along the posterior surface of the levator aponeurosis, and inserts into the superior border of the tarsus.

Eyelid Innervation

Cranial nerve VII (the facial nerve), which divides into six branches, innervates the facial musculature. The temporal branch of the facial nerve provides innervation to the orbicularis oculi, frontalis, pars ciliaris, and corrugator muscles. However, the superior division of cranial nerve III innervates the levator palpebrae superioris muscle. The Müller muscle is innervated by the sympathetic nervous system. Interruption of ocular sympathetic supply causes ptosis, miosis, and anhydrosis. This triad of signs is known as Horner syndrome (5).

Vascular Supply to the Eyelids

The vascular supply to the eyelids is rich with many collaterals. The supraorbital, supratrochlear, lacrimal, and dorsal nasal branches of the ophthalmic artery supply the eyelids, forehead, and orbit. An anastomosis between the dorsal nasal and lacrimal arteries in the upper eyelid forms the marginal arcade, which lies 2 mm above the eyelid margin between the tarsus and orbicularis oculi muscles. A peripheral arcade is located at the superior border of the tarsus between the levator aponeurosis and Müller muscle. The lower eyelid has a similar anatomic configuration of the arterial arcades. A rich venous drainage network exists throughout the eyelids. Because of the rich vascular supply, ischemic necrosis of the eyelids is rare.

EYELID DISORDERS

Anophthalmos and Microphthalmos

True anophthalmos is an extremely rare condition and results from an absence of the development of the optic vesicle. Most cases of clinical anophthalmos likely represent severe microphthalmos when careful histology is obtained from serial orbital sections. Microphthalmos represents a range of ocular developmental abnormalities from near complete absence of

identifiable ocular structures to a small normally formed eye, a condition referred to as nanophthalmos. Approximately 25% of patients with anophthalmos/microophthalmos have a diagnosable genetic syndrome (6,7). Because eyelid and orbital development are dependent on the underlying ocular development, microphthalmos often is associated with abnormal or reduced orbital bony size. Eyelid deformities that result include shortened horizontal palpebral fissure lengths. The mainstay of treatment involves serial prosthetic conformers to enlarge the cul-de-sacs. In more severe cases, the orbital volume can be expanded using dermis fat grafts, orbital implants, and orbital expanders (8). Soft tissue growth will parallel bone growth. Using these various techniques, an acceptable cosmetic appearance is often achieved.

Cryptophthalmos

Cryptophthalmos is an extremely rare condition in which there is complete failure of development of the eyelid folds. One of the most distinct features of cryptophthalmos is failure of the brow to develop normally, resulting in fusion of the hairline and brow. This is distinct from an abnormal separation of the eyelid folds. Without development of the normal eyelid folds, the underlying cornea and conjunctiva do not normally form. The anterior segment of the globe is severely malformed, and the posterior segment of the globe is sometimes disorganized. If attempts are made to separate the eyelids, then the globe will often require corneal transplantation to close the anterior segment defect and mucous membrane grafting to form conjunctival cul-de-sacs (9). Preoperative evaluation with an electroretinogram, visual evoked potentials, imaging studies, and ultrasound may provide preoperative insight into the structure and function of the underlying globe. While reconstructive surgery may allow for an improved cosmetic result, useful vision is occasionally achieved. When associated cutaneous syndactyly, malformations of the larynx and genitourinary tract, craniofacial dysmorphism, orofacial clefting, mental retardation, and musculoskeletal anomalies occur, Fraser syndrome should be considered (10).

Congenital Eyelid Coloboma

A congenital defect involving the absence of a portion of the eyelid margin is an eyelid coloboma (Fig. 17.1). Coloboma may affect either the upper or lower eyelids and may vary in size from a small eyelid marginal defect to a near complete absence of the eyelids. Coloboma more typically occur in the nasal aspect of the upper eyelid, and large eyelid coloboma can result in corneal exposure and ulceration.

The etiology of colobomas is varied. Abnormal migration patterns of ectoderm and mesoderm may cause abnormal development of the eyelid margin. Colobomas may also result from a mechanical disruption of eyelid development such as amniotic bands or facial clefts (Fig. 17.2). Eyelid colobomas can be seen in association with other abnormalities

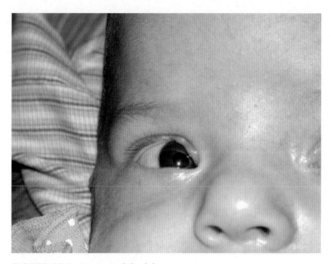

FIGURE 17.1. Upper eyelid coloboma.

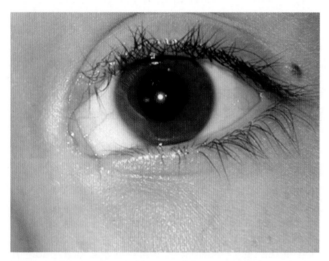

FIGURE 17.2. Small medial lower eyelid congenital cleft, resulting in canalicular atresia.

including dermoids, cleft lip, microphthalmia, and ocular colobomata. Coloboma of the upper eyelids occur commonly in Goldenhar syndrome.

Treatment of upper eyelid coloboma should be directed at maintaining lubrication and protection for the ocular surface. Surgical correction is not emergent as long as the corneal surface is being protected. A larger coloboma may require more aggressive lubrication and perhaps occlusive dressing prior to surgical closure. For smaller colobomas, surgical repair during the latter half of the first year of life is preferable to allow for tissue growth. For defects less than 25% of the horizontal eyelid width, direct closure after excision of the defect is all that is required. The edges of the defect are excised to form a pentagonal defect and then the tarsus is closed with three interrupted absorbable sutures. The eyelid margin is closed with sutures anterior to, through, and posterior to the gray line. The skin is reapproximated with interrupted sutures. Larger defects up to 40% of the

eyelid margin can be closed by a lateral canthotomy and cantholysis with medial rotation of the eyelid. Larger eyelid defects often require a free tarsal conjunctival graft. Eyelid-sharing procedures (e.g., Hughes procedure), which occlude the line of sight, should be avoided in children as they will induce occlusion amblyopia. Because most eyelid colobomas causing corneal exposure are in the upper eyelid, a lateral canthotomy usually can be performed and the eyelid defect closed nasally as described above. If necessary, a temporal tarsal conjunctival sharing procedure can then be performed, taking care not to occlude the visual axis.

Pseudocoloboma

More commonly, pseudocoloboma of the lower eyelid are seen in craniofacial synostosis (Treacher Collins syndrome) (Figs. 17.3 and 17.4). With these pseudocolobomas, the eyelid margin is intact but there is a facial cleft laterally, which results in an inferior and lateral displacement of the lower eyelid. Treacher Collins syndrome is caused by a first brachial arch abnormality. Ophthalmic findings include microphthalmos, iris coloboma, and absence of the puncta. Hypoplasia of the maxilla and zygoma are common with an antimongoloid slant to the palpebral fissures. Deformations of the external ear and hearing loss are associated with this syndrome. Simple soft tissue tightening and elevation of the lateral canthal tendon is frequently ineffective in correcting the lateral dystopia of the eyelid because there is often an absence of vertical and horizontal eyelid tissue. For this reason, transposition flaps from the upper to lower eyelids are useful in addition to resuspension of the lateral canthal tendon.

Ankyloblepharon

Ankyloblepharon is caused by failure of eyelid separation or from an abnormality in the migration of the mesodermal elements of the eyelid. Ankyloblepharon filiforme adnatum may

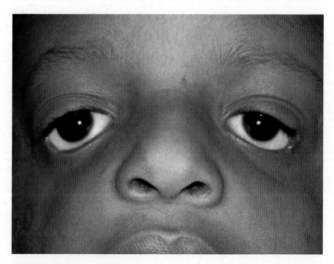

FIGURE 17.3. Pseudocolobomata of the lower eyelids associated with Treacher Collins syndrome.

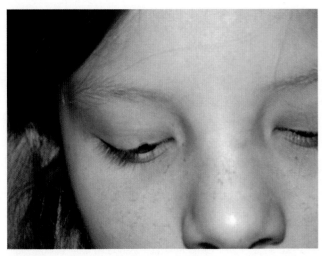

FIGURE 17.4. Small partial coloboma of the upper eyelid.

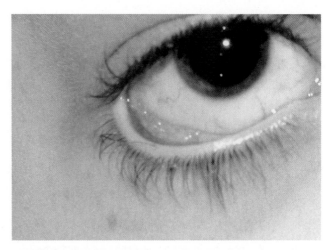

FIGURE 17.6. Acquired distichiasis. Eyelash in association with a meibomian gland orifice.

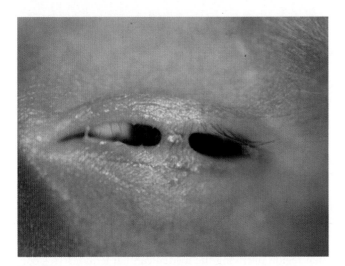

FIGURE 17.5. Ankyloblepharon in a newborn.

be isolated, demonstrating fine bands of tissue between the upper and lower eyelids, or it may be seen with trisomy 18 or other chromosomal abnormalities (11,12). In addition, ankyloblepharon may be part of the Hay-Wells syndrome, which is characterized by congenital ectodermal dysplasia, alopecia, scalp infections, dystrophic nails, hypodontia, ankyloblepharon, and cleft lip and/or cleft palate (13). The treatment of ankyloblepharon is entirely surgical. The bands of the eyelid are separated, and the eyelid margins are reformed as necessary. Figure 17.5 shows ankyloblepharon in a newborn.

Distichiasis

Distichiasis occurs when a developmental abnormality results in cilia formation in association with metaplastic meibomian glands. This condition is often asymptomatic although these lashes may cause superficial corneal irritation and abrasion. In an acquired form, distichiasis may occur with chronic eyelid inflammation such as blepharitis, trachoma, and Stevens-Johnson syndrome (Fig. 17.6).

Trichiasis

Trichiasis refers to an acquired eyelash abnormality resulting from normally located but misdirected cilia. Chronic eyelid inflammation is the most common cause for trichiasis.

Treatment of eyelash abnormalities is not required in the absence of any abnormality of the corneal surface. Electrolysis or split thickness eyelid resections can be used to remove the lash follicles (14). In addition, direct excision of the lash follicles is possible.

Congenital Ectropion

Congenital ectropion is rarely found in isolation. When the lower eyelid is involved, it is often part of the blepharophimosis syndrome or Treacher Collins syndrome. Also, congenital eyelid ectropion may be seen in patients with neonatal erythroderma (collodion baby) (15). When secondary to an insufficiency in the vertical extent of the skin and orbicularis layers, a full-thickness skin graft or transfer flap is usually required in addition to a lateral tightening of the eyelid.

Congenital Entropion and Epiblepharon

Epiblepharon results from an extra fold of pretarsal lower eyelid skin and orbicularis, which rotates the lower eyelid cilia and margin inward (Fig. 17.7). Epiblepharon is more common in Asian eyelids. With downward pressure over the excess skin, the eyelid margin assumes a normal appearance. This condition is typically self-limited and resolves with facial growth. Most children are relatively asymptomatic without corneal injury. If corneal surface changes occur with persistent corneal irritation, a small ellipse of subciliary skin and orbicularis muscle can be removed. Since lower eyelid retraction can result from excessive skin excision, only a minimal amount of skin is removed.

Congenital lower eyelid entropion is caused when preseptal orbicularis overrides the pretarsal orbicularis (Fig. 17.8). In

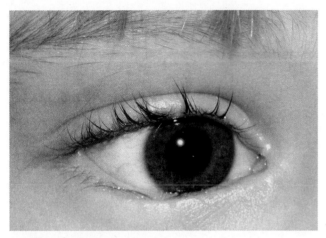

FIGURE 17.7. Epiblepharon, which typically resolves spontaneously.

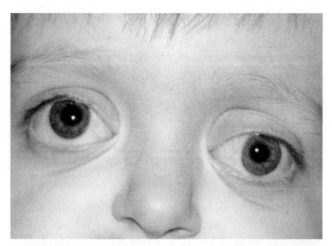

FIGURE 17.9. Lower eyelid retraction associated with shallow orbits and relative proptosis in a patient with Pfeiffer syndrome.

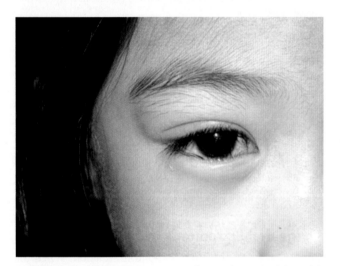

FIGURE 17.8. Lower eyelid entropion with inward rotation of the eyelid, necessitating surgical correction.

addition, there is laxity of the lower eyelid retractors, allowing a true inward rotation of the lower eyelid. Correction requires reattachment of the lower eyelid retractors to the lower border of the tarsus, elimination of horizontal eyelid laxity when present, and resection of overriding skin and orbicularis.

Congenital horizontal tarsal kink results in entropion of the upper eyelid and may be associated with congenital levator aponeurotic disinsertion. More important, corneal ulceration occurs in 50% of cases (16).

Congenital Eyelid Retraction

Congenital eyelid retraction, especially of the lower eyelid, may occur in isolation or secondary to structural anomalies, resulting in very shallow orbits and proptosis (Fig. 17.9). While some infants will have transient upper eyelid retraction, persistent superior scleral show in the absence of a structural cause warrants a medical evaluation for thyroid or neurologic disease. Options to correct eyelid retraction are müllerectomy and levator recession. Spacer grafts are occasionally necessary.

Euryblepharon

Euryblepharon is a condition characterized by increased vertical separation of the temporal aspect of the palpebral opening such that the palpebral conjunctiva is not in apposition with the eye. The lateral canthus is usually displaced inferiorly. This condition is characterized by a lack of vertical skin height, and treatment requires a lateral canthoplasty as well as possible skin graft into the lower eyelid to provide additional vertical height.

Epicanthus

The epicanthus consists of a fold of skin in the medial canthal region overlying the medial canthal tendon. This condition can occur in isolation or it can be associated with multiple genetic disorders such as trisomy 21 and blepharophimosis syndrome. Epicanthal folds are generally classified as being one of the four types: epicanthus supraciliaris, epicanthus inversus, epicanthus palpebralis, and epicanthus tarsalis.

Epicanthus tarsalis is the normal medial canthal structure seen in many Asian eyelids (Fig. 17.10). The eyelid fold arises in the region of the upper tarsal plate and extends to the skin of the medial canthus. Epicanthus inversus is seen in isolation and in patients with blepharophimosis syndrome. This occurs when the fold of skin begins in the lower eyelid tarsal region and extends up through the medial canthal region toward the brow. Epicanthus palpebralis occurs when a fold runs from the upper eyelid tarsal region to the lower border of the orbit. Epicanthus supraciliaris occurs when the fold arises in the brow and terminates in the area of the lacrimal sac.

Epicanthal folds can be corrected with a variety of techniques, including a YV plasty most simply (Fig. 17.11). In addition, the Mustarde (17) and Roveda techniques have been described.

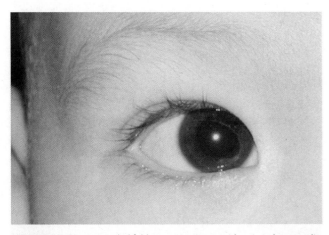

FIGURE 17.10. Epicanthal fold, most consistent with epicanthus tarsalis.

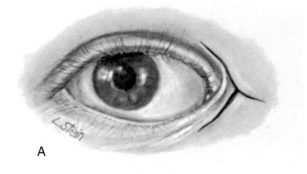

A

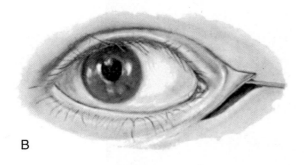

B

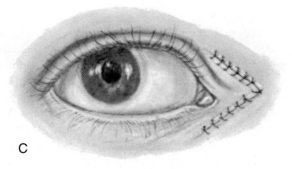

C

FIGURE 17.11. Surgery for epicanthus. **A:** Incision for preparing the skin flap. **B:** Undermining of skin to allow for movement of the tip. **C:** Skin sutures in a V-shape, flattening the epicanthal fold. The skin at the junction of the Y flap is rotated medially to the apex of the V, thus flattening the epicanthus.

Telecanthus

Telecanthus refers to a wide intercanthal distance, differentiated from hypertelorism, which describes an increased interorbital bony separation. Telecanthus is often associated with epicanthus and blepharophimosis. When associated with epicanthal folds, telecanthus may be corrected using the same procedures that are used to treat epicanthus. However, medial canthoplasty and/or transnasal wiring may be necessary in more severe cases.

Blepharoptosis

Ptosis of the child's upper eyelid is most often congenital. It is occasionally due to congenital myasthenia, congenital fibrosis of the extraocular muscles, syndromic associations, or acquired abnormalities such as loss of innervation to Müller or levator muscle. In addition, mechanical factors can contribute to ptosis, such as relative enophthalmos following an orbital fracture, tumor, or traumatic injury. Congenital ptosis of the upper eyelid is typically seen in association with abnormal development of the levator palpebral complex (Fig. 17.12). Although typically sporadic, familial ptosis has been linked to chromosome 1p (18). Perhaps abnormal neurologic innervation during development of the levator muscle results in abnormal development of the muscle complex, similar to what occurs in congenital fibrosis syndrome (19). Congenital ptosis occurs either unilaterally or bilaterally. Superior rectus muscle weakness can occur in association with congenital ptosis.

Myogenic ptosis is also a potential cause of acquired ptosis in children. This is due to conditions such as muscular dystrophy and myasthenia gravis. Another unique type of congenital ptosis occurs in the Marcus Gunn jaw-winking phenomenon (Fig. 17.13). This is a result of aberrant innervation of the levator muscle with nerves normally directed to the muscles of mastication. Usually with contralateral jaw movement, the ptotic eye elevates. This is often noticed in infancy during feeding as the child seems to "wink" when nursing or taking a bottle.

Evaluation

Careful history should be taken as to the variability of the ptosis. Most patients with congenital ptosis will have a history of slight worsening with fatigue; however, they should not have large variability in the ptosis. Certainly alternating ptosis or a history of a normal eyelid position following sleep followed by significant ptosis when the patient is fatigued should raise a concern for myasthenia gravis. Evaluation of a patient with ptosis should include observation for signs of fatigue of the levator muscles. In a young child with poor cooperation, prolonged eyelid elevation to assess fatigability may not be possible. Tests which can be performed to establish the diagnosis of myasthenia gravis include the ice, rest, tensilon, and neostigmine tests. Tests for acetylcholine receptor antibodies are rarely positive in isolated ocular

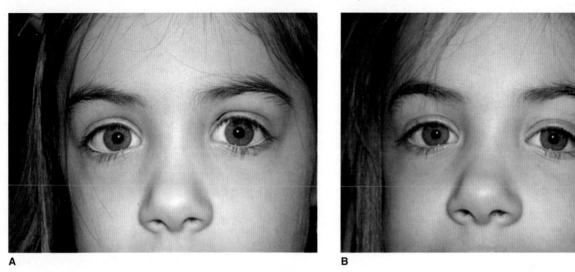

FIGURE 17.12. Congenital ptosis of the left upper eyelid. **A:** Immediate postoperative appearance with desired overcorrection. **B:** Three months post surgical repair.

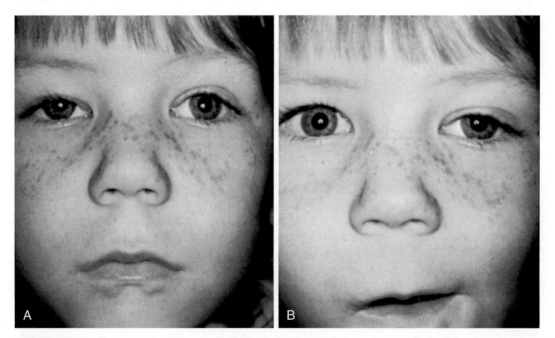

FIGURE 17.13. Right Marcus Gunn phenomenon demonstrated with jaw movement to the left. **A:** After jaw movement. **B:** Before jaw movement.

myasthenia gravis, especially in childhood; however, positive tests are strongly indicative of the presence of myasthenia gravis (20). A positive tensilon test, abnormal single-fiber electromyographic recordings, and therapeutic responses to anticholinesterase medicines or corticosteroids establish this diagnosis. If myasthenia is strongly suspected, then a trial of pyridostigmine bromide or corticosteroids is indicated.

Treatment of uncomplicated congenital ptosis requires measurement of the absolute amount of ptosis present in the primary position. Care should be taken to fix the brow as patients with unilateral or bilateral ptosis often use their frontalis muscle to elevate the eyelids. The eyelid margin–reflex distance (MRD) should be measured. The MRD is the distance from a corneal light reflex to the upper eyelid margin with the patient's eyes in primary gaze. The amount of levator excursion also should be measured. This can be difficult in younger children and infants. In congenital ptosis, the amount of ptosis inversely correlates with the amount of levator function. Repeat examination at separate visits helps the surgeon obtain reliable measurements of the true amount of ptosis and levator function. Levator excursion is measured by first firmly fixing the brow to immobilize the frontalis muscle. The amount of eyelid margin movement from full downgaze to full upgaze is then determined. A full examination of the extraocular muscles should be undertaken. In addition to specific examination of the superior rectus muscle, one should also check the Bell phenomenon (upward deviation of the eye during forced eyelid closure). A normal (present) Bell phenomenon is important because, after repair of congenital ptosis, lagophthalmos is common. A normal Bell phenomenon and normal superior rectus muscle function allow for protection of the cornea postoperatively (21). When superior rectus muscle function is reduced, a surgeon should be more conservative in the amount of surgery performed to correct the ptosis. In a younger child, reliable Schirmer testing is difficult. Examination of the tear film and careful evaluation of the cornea for any signs of exposure both pre- and postoperatively are necessary. In addition to evaluating the tear film, care should be taken to determine the corneal sensitivity. Certainly, patients with diminished corneal sensitivity due to innervational abnormalities are at increased risk of exposure to keratopathy following surgery for correction of congenital ptosis. Corneal sensation can easily be determined using a simple wisp of cotton at the tip of a cotton-tip applicator applied to the corneal surface. Abnormal corneal sensitivity cautions the surgeon to avoid surgery or reduce the amount of ptosis correction.

In patients with Marcus Gunn jaw-winking ptosis, the amount of eyelid retraction with movement of the jaw should be evaluated. In those patients with mild retraction, ptosis repair should be undertaken using standard amounts of surgery dependent on the degree of ptosis. An external levator resection is the usual procedure. If significant retraction is present, extirpation of the involved levator muscle combined with a frontalis suspension should be performed. Failure to extirpate the involved levator muscle will result in persistent wink.

In addition to measuring levator function, the eyelid should be assessed with its response to phenylephrine. One drop of 2.5% is instilled into the lower cul-de-sac in younger children and infants. The MRD is remeasured after approximately 5 minutes; if the eyelid elevates to a near-normal position, tightening or resecting the Müller muscle could be considered for ptosis repair.

All patients with congenital ptosis require repeated visual acuity testing with determinations of refractive error. Amblyopia frequently occurs secondary to strabismus, induced astigmatism, and less commonly, occlusion of the line of sight (22). The presence of a chin elevation may allow for peripheral fusion but does not exclude the presence of amblyopia (23).

Timing of Surgical Intervention

In most situations, congenital ptosis is repaired when the child is 4 to 5 years old. Severe ptosis causing a significant chin-up position or occlusion amblyopia may be surgically repaired when recognized. Nevertheless, most ptosis-associated amblyopia is caused by induced astigmatism. If a significant astigmatism develops, spectacle and amblyopia therapy should be instituted.

Surgical Procedures

There are several options for the surgical management of congenital ptosis. The main forms of treatment are external levator resection and frontalis suspension procedures. The Müller muscle procedures (Fasanella Servat and müllerectomy) may be used for correction in mild ptosis, particularly neurogenic ptosis associated with Horner syndrome.

Levator Muscle Procedures

Levator aponeurosis/muscle-shortening procedures are performed in cases of mild-to-moderate ptosis (Fig. 17.14). Although classic levator dehiscence can be encountered in the pediatric population, more commonly decreased levator excursion and levator muscle dysgenesis are encountered. Although a 1 mm resection generally elevates the eyelid 1 mm in adults, this is not true in most pediatric ptosis patients. A more generous resection is required in children and is dependent on the amount of levator function measured (Table 17.1).

The surgical approach is through the eyelid crease. Dissection is made initially through the skin, followed by the orbital septum. The underlying levator aponeurosis is exposed beneath the preaponeurotic fat. The levator aponeurosis is separated from the tarsal plate, and dissection in the plane between the Müller muscle and levator aponeurosis is carried out superiorly to expose and separate the levator tendon. In cases in which a large resection is anticipated, the lateral and medial horns of the aponeurosis are cut. Three partial thickness permanent sutures are placed in the anterior tarsal surface 3 to 4 mm below the superior border of the tarsus. These sutures are then placed through the levator aponeurosis. Because the patient is usually under general anesthesia, the amount of resection needs to be determined prior to surgery. Sutures are tied with a single-throw knot on the anterior surface of the aponeurosis and are replaced and retied until the surgeon is satisfied with the eyelid height and contour. Square knots are then tied, and levator tendon distal to the sutures is resected. The eyelid crease may be formed with separate sutures between the levator tendon and eyelid skin by incorporating bites of the levator tendon into the skin closure, or the existing sutures securing the levator tendon may be brought through skin edges and retied on the skin surface.

Frontalis Suspension

Frontalis suspension procedures are used in unilateral or bilateral cases of severe ptosis with extremely poor levator function (Fig. 17.15) (24). Autogenous fascia lata can be obtained from the leg of the child; typically, children are 3 to 4 years of age before an adequate length of fascia lata is obtainable. Banked irradiated fascia lata is available, but autogenous fascia lata has a lower rate of recurrent ptosis. Newer nonresorbable materials are available. These include Mersilene mesh, Supramid suture, and expanded

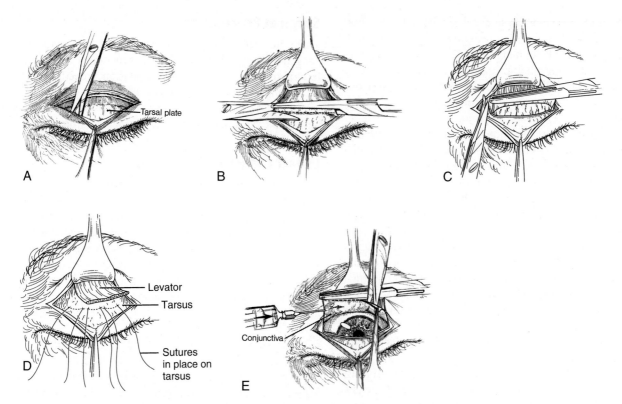

FIGURE 17.14. External levator procedure. **A:** The orbital septum has been opened, exposing the tarsus and levator tendon. **B:** Levator tendon dissected off the tarsus. **C:** The levator tendon is dissected off the Müller muscle. **D:** Reattachment of the tendon to the tarsus. **E:** After the final suture placement, the distal levator tendon is resected.

TABLE 17.1

PTOSIS REPAIR BASED ON LEVATOR MUSCLE FUNCTION AND AMOUNT OF PTOSIS

A. Poor levator muscle function (4 mm) with severe ptosis (4 mm)
 —Frontalis suspension procedure

B. Moderate levator muscle function (5–7 mm) with moderate ptosis (3 mm)
 —External levator resection 17–20 mm

C. Moderate levator muscle function (5–7 mm) with mild ptosis (2 mm)
 —External levator resection 12–15 mm

D. Moderate levator muscle function (8–10 mm) with mild ptosis (2 mm)
 —External levator resection 10–12 mm

E. Good levator muscle function (10–13 mm) with mild ptosis (2 mm)
 —External levator resection 6–9 mm

---

polytetrafluoroethylene (ePTFE). Synthetic Supramid suture can be used for temporary elevation of the eyelid but may result in recurrent ptosis within 18 months (25). ePTFE is now available in strips specifically designed for use in ptosis repair (Fig. 17.15). A higher incidence of infection with similar material has been reported (26). Such infections are unusual if the eyelid skin incisions are closed with sutures and if patients are treated with antibiotics at the time of surgery and postoperatively.

In cases of severe unilateral ptosis, bilateral frontalis suspensions have been performed to provide a symmetric eyelid appearance, particularly in downgaze when lagophthalmos is most notable. However, if unilateral frontalis suspension is performed and postoperative asymmetry is an issue, the fellow normal eyelid can be subsequently operated. In cases of asymmetric bilateral ptosis requiring a frontalis suspension procedure on the more severely affected side, bilateral frontalis suspension will likely result in the best cosmetic result.

The double rhomboid technique provides excellent results (Fig. 17.16). The brow of the child is the most mobile section of the forehead and allows for both adequate elevation of the eyelid as well as good closure of the eyelid. Some surgeons prefer a central knot higher on the forehead. While this provides excellent contour and suspension to the upper eyelid, the more fixed superior forehead does not allow as much dynamic eyelid movement.

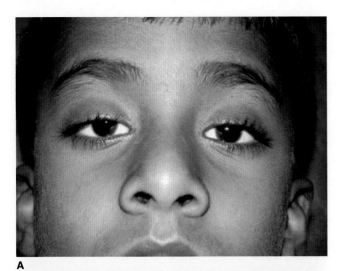

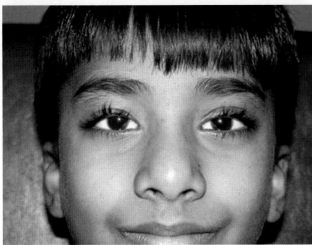

FIGURE 17.15. A: Preoperative bilateral congenital ptosis. **B:** Postoperative appearance after bilateral frontalis suspension with expanded polytetrafluoroethylene (ePTFE).

Tarsal Müller Muscle Procedures

Tarsal Müller muscle procedures result in good outcomes in those patients with excellent levator function and mild ptosis. A positive preoperative phenylephrine test suggests that a Müller muscle procedure will adequately elevate the eyelid. These procedures work particularly well for patients who have ptosis associated with congenital or acquired Horner syndrome.

Complications of Ptosis Surgery

The primary complications of ptosis surgery are undercorrections, overcorrections, and corneal exposure problems. Other complications include abnormal eyelid crease, ectropion, entropion, conjunctival prolapse, infection, and bleeding. Blindness is a rare but devastating complication. Undercorrection is common in congenital ptosis, while overcorrection is unusual. Exposure keratopathy can be serious and should be investigated at all postoperative examinations. Lubrication with ointments and artificial tears should

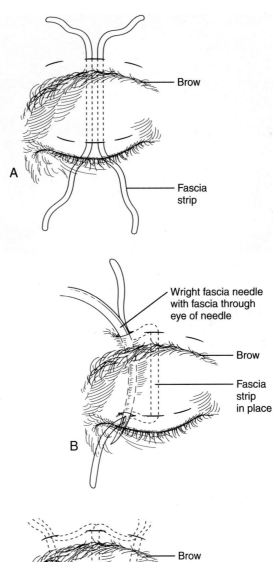

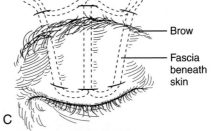

FIGURE 17.16. A–C: Double rhomboid technique for the frontalis suspension.

be used in all patients postoperatively until the corneal examination is stable.

Blepharophimosis Syndrome

Blepharophimosis syndrome is an autosomal dominant condition with characteristic features including ptosis, epicanthus inversus, telecanthus, blepharophimosis (a short horizontal palpebral fissure length), and variable lower eyelid ectropion (Fig. 17.17). Each of the individual abnormalities is addressed surgically, either simultaneously or during separate sessions.

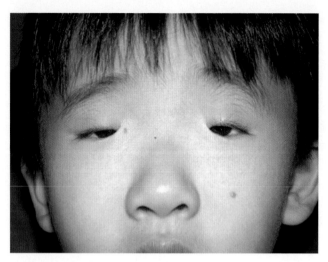

FIGURE 17.17. Blepharophimosis syndrome.

EYELID TUMORS

Benign Lesions
Capillary Hemangiomata

Capillary hemangiomata are the most common eyelid and orbital tumors in infants. They are composed of abnormal capillaries with proliferation of endothelial cells. Clinically, capillary hemangiomata present as superficial or deep lesions. Superficial lesions have a bright red appearance during the rapid growth phase and will blanche with compression, and deeper hemangiomata may give a reddish to purple hue to the overlying skin (Fig. 17.18). Capillary hemangiomata rapidly enlarge during the first several months of life and may continue to enlarge until 18 months of age; this rapid enlargement may lead to areas of necrosis or ulceration as the lesions outgrow their blood supply. These tumors are soft and compressible. Clinically, these lesions are more common in females and in those children born prematurely.

Most hemangiomas regress completely without residua. Involution typically occurs slowly and is complete by 3 to 7 years of age. During the involutional stage, the reddish lesion will slowly change to gray, and the surface epithelium slowly changes to a more normal skin appearance. However, the skin may be thin with fine wrinkles. Hemangiomata on the eyelids can result in deformational abnormalities for the position and contour of the eyelid (Fig. 17.19).

While larger tumors can cause occlusion amblyopia by blocking the visual axis, refractive amblyopia from induced astigmatism is more common. As little as 1.5 D of astigmatism increases the risk of amblyopia (27). Spectacle correction is frequently required along with amblyopia therapy.

Evaluation

For larger lesions and lesions involving the orbit or when the hemangioma appearance is not typical, computed tomography (CT) or magnetic resonance imaging (MRI) are valuable imaging techniques. CT scanning demonstrates an enhancing soft tissue lesion with irregular borders. MRI is often better at differentiating capillary hemangiomata from lymphangiomata. MRI scanning may show the chocolate cysts of lymphangiomata that are not typical of capillary hemangiomata. An MRI of capillary hemangiomata shows characteristic flow voids.

Management

There are a number of management options for capillary hemangiomata. Most commonly, observation alone is all that is required as these lesions typically involute spontaneously. Periocular capillary hemangiomata are more problematic as they have a higher incidence of amblyopia and eyelid deformities. As mentioned above, correction of any refractive error and appropriate amblyopia therapy are important in the management of the patient with periocular hemangiomata.

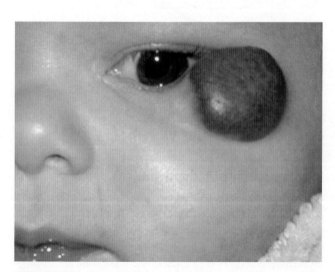

FIGURE 17.18. Large periocular capillary hemangioma. The most superficial components are bright red.

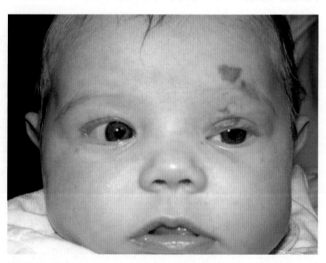

FIGURE 17.19. Hemangioma with upper eyelid inducing ptosis and astigmatism.

In cases of occlusion amblyopia from large periocular hemangiomata, more aggressive intervention needs to be considered. Options to slow the growth or decrease the size of a periocular capillary hemangioma include oral propranolol (29,29), topical propranolol (30), intralesional corticosteroids, oral corticosteroids, topical corticosteroids, superficial laser ablation, surgical excision, and systemic interferon-alpha. In general, oral propranolol has replaced corticosteroid therapy as the primary modality used in the medical treatment of hemangiomata. This is primarily due to lower complications and side effects of propranolol compared to steroids. However, bradycardia, hypotension, bronchospasm, hypoglycemia, and electrolyte disturbances from systemic propranolol treatment of infantile hemangioma have been reported (30). Typically, the dosage is 1 to 2 mg/kg/day in divided doses and tapered slowly once sufficient regression is recognized. Many practitioners obtain a pretreatment electrocardiogram. Topical propranolol preparations have been used for more superficial hemangiomas (30).

Intralesional corticosteroid injections for periocular capillary hemangiomata were first described by Kushner (31). When necessary, a combination of long- and short-acting corticosteroids is injected in one or multiple sites into the lesion. The total steroid dosage per injection should be in the range of 3 to 5 mg/kg (32). Following injection with both long- and short-acting steroid agents, a repeat injection may be required in 4 to 6 weeks. If short-acting agents are used in isolation, then subsequent injections, if necessary, may be repeated at 2- to 4-week intervals. Complications of steroid injection include eyelid necrosis, subcutaneous fat atrophy, and very rarely, central retinal artery occlusion (32,33). The potential complication of retinal artery occlusion is extremely rare and might be minimized by injecting under low pressure, reducing the chance of retrograde flow of particulate steroid material. In addition, immediately before injection, the plunger of the syringe should be retracted to avoid direct intravascular injection. Additional complications that have been described include adrenal suppression (34). Children, pediatricians, and parents should be warned of this potential complication. Consideration should be given to measurement of circulating glucocorticoids. Despite these concerns, Addisonian crisis has not been reported following steroid injection for capillary hemangioma. Oral corticosteroids are sometimes used as either primarily or as secondary modality when other treatments have not been effective. Oral corticosteroids are administered at 1 to 4 mg/kg/day. The length of treatment depends on the size and response of the tumor. In general, it may last for 6 to 12 weeks with a tapering of the steroid dosage.

Alternatives include topical "betasol propionate," although this treatment modality may not be as successful as oral or intralesional steroids (35). In more systemic life-threatening hemangiomata, interferon-alpha has been used. However, significant side effects, including neutropenia and neurologic toxicity, have been reported.

Finally, surgical excision of hemangiomata has been advocated for select cases (36). This may be better for small isolated lesions rather than large diffuse lesions. Excision is particularly useful for those lesions which are very anterior and well circumscribed. Since hemangiomata interdigitate with normal eyelid structures, surgical excision must be done with particular attention to the anatomy to avoid the creation of secondary problems such as ptosis. More commonly, surgery is used once total or near-total regression of the hemangioma has occurred. Surgery may involve correction of eyelid crease abnormalities or ptosis, correction of eyelid contour abnormalities, or removal of excessive skin.

Lymphangioma

Lymphangioma is a tumor that presents in a fashion similar to capillary hemangioma. However, it typically does not show spontaneous involution. While more commonly involving the orbit, it can present as a mass of the eyelid or conjunctiva. Lymphangiomata are composed of endothelial-lined channels, collections of lymphocytes, and occasional blood-filled cysts. These lesions may increase in size with upper respiratory tract infections. More dramatic enlargement occurs with hemorrhage into a cyst. Management is challenging as complete surgical resection is rarely possible. Use of the carbon dioxide laser facilitates surgical excision of these lesions. Unlike capillary hemangiomata, proparanolol and corticosteroids are ineffective in the management of lymphangiomata.

Periocular Dermoid Cysts

Dermoid cysts occur most commonly in the periocular region overlying the frontozygomatic suture, frontolacrimal, or frontomaxillary sutures (Fig. 17.20). These cysts are firm, smooth, nontender subcutaneous masses present from birth. The skin overlying the cysts is freely mobile, and the cyst is usually affixed to bone. Enlargement is typically slow. Rupture secondary to trauma can expose the cystic contents to the subcutaneous tissue and result in significant inflammation and permanent scarring. CT scans demonstrate the dermoid cyst to be a characteristically well-demarcated lesion. The surrounding bone frequently shows some molding around the cyst. Occasionally, a lateral dermoid cyst may have a barbell appearance with an intraorbital and extraorbital component. CT scans are not necessary unless an internal cystic component is suspected.

Treatment of dermoid cysts is surgical excision performed at about 1 year of age. As children become more mobile, the risk of rupture from trauma increases. Care should be taken to avoid rupture of the dermoid cyst during surgery if possible. If rupture does occur, the surgeon needs to ascertain that complete removal of the contents of the cyst as well as the cyst capsule has been accomplished. Remnants of the dermoid can cause significant inflammatory reaction with fibrosis and scarring. Excision may be

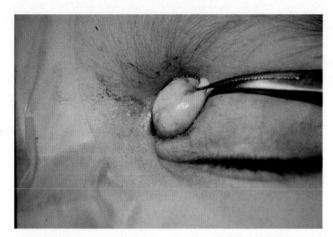

FIGURE 17.20. Typical appearance of a periocular dermoid cyst.

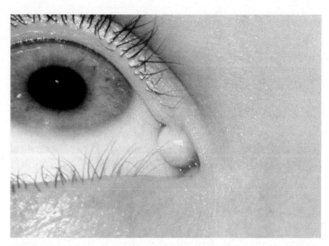

FIGURE 17.21. Pathologically confirmed congenital nevus of the medial upper eyelid.

approached through either the eyelid crease incision or a sub- or suprabrow incision.

Plexiform Neuroma

Plexiform neuroma is most often seen in the setting of type 1 neurofibromatosis. The typical plexiform neuroma causes an S-shaped deformity of the upper eyelid. The eyelid may have a "bag of worms" sensation to palpation, resulting from the underlying nodular plexiform neuroma. A plexiform neuroma interdigitates with normal tissues and grows with age. Surrounding bone may show abnormalities, particularly absence or hypoplasia of the greater wing of the sphenoid. This tumor frequently causes mechanical ptosis with resultant astigmatism and amblyopia (37). If significant ptosis or induced astigmatism is present, surgical debulking of the eyelid components of the tumor may be necessary. However, recurrence is expected over time.

Nevi

The nevus develops as a benign proliferation of the epidermal melanocytes. In children, these can be congenital or acquired. Due to the fusion of the eyelids during fetal development, a nevus may be present on corresponding areas of both the upper and lower eyelids (kissing nevus). Nevi tend to be variable in color and size, but are typically tan colored with focal areas of increased pigmentation (Fig. 17.21). Surgical excision for cosmesis or because of a concern for malignant transformation may be considered. Larger lesions may require skin grafts, flaps, and occasionally multiple-staged surgical procedures. Acquired nevi tend to occur after 6 months of age; these typically have pigmented spots within the lesion (Fig. 17.22).

One form of congenital pigmentation is that of oculodermal melanocytosis (nevus of Ota). The skin, as well as the ocular surface and conjunctiva, have a slate-gray pigmentation. The uvea of the affected eye may also have increased pigmentation. While more common in Asians, when seen in Caucasians, there is an increased risk of uveal melanoma.

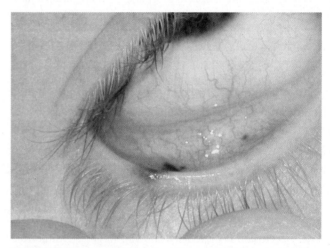

FIGURE 17.22. Acquired nevus in a 12-year-old white male. Pathology confirmed benign melanocytes.

Giant Hairy Nevi

Giant nevi are congenital, hairy, and deeply pigmented melanocytic nevi. A 5% risk of malignant transformation into malignant melanoma is reported (38). Therefore, prophylactic excision of these nevi is performed.

Pilomatrixoma

Pilomatrixoma is a benign proliferation of hair matrix cells. These lesions tend to occur in children and have the appearance of a solid subcutaneous nodule.

Juvenile Xanthogranuloma

Juvenile xanthogranuloma is a proliferation of non-Langerhans cell histiocytes (Fig. 17.23). These lesions in the skin are yellow-red, rounded papules and nodules. When they occur on the iris, they may be associated with spontaneous (atraumatic) hyphema. Since spontaneous resolution

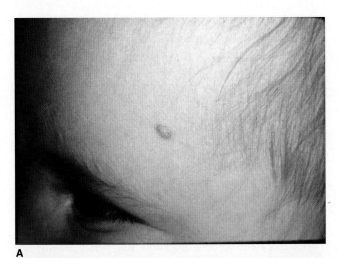

A

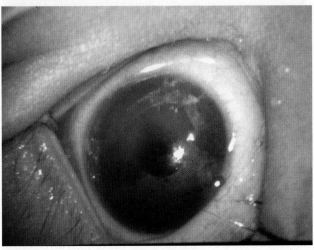

B

FIGURE 17.23. A: Juvenile xanthogranuloma (JXG) skin lesion. **B:** Spontaneous hyphema associated with JXG lesion of the iris.

does occur, surgical excision of skin lesions is rarely necessary. Needle biopsy or anterior chamber aspiration have been used for iris lesions when the diagnosis is uncertain. Low-dose radiation has been used for recalcitrant iris lesions but seldom is necessary.

Chalazion

Chalazia are common lesions of the pediatric eyelid. A chalazion results when obstruction of a meibomian gland occurs, resulting in rupture of the oil gland into the surrounding soft tissue and formation of a pseudocyst. The inflammatory reaction creates an erythematous nodule in the eyelid. Typical treatment includes warm compresses and eyelid hygiene. Topical antibiotic ointment may be used in combination with topical corticosteroids to reduce the inflammatory component of the chalazion. Intralesional corticosteroids are sometimes used. Care should be taken to avoid steroid injection into darkly pigmented skin as this may cause a focal area of hypopigmentation. For persistent chalazia, in which the inflammatory process is quiescent, incision and drainage

may be necessary. For younger children, this is usually done under general anesthesia. A chalazion clamp is used and placed over the involved portion of the eyelid and the eyelid inverted. A number 11 or 15 Bard-Parker blade is used to vertically incise the tarsus from the palpebral conjunctival surface. Care is taken to avoid extending the incision to the eyelid margin as this could result in notching of the eyelid margin. A pseudocyst will typically extrude a gelatinous material when incised. A curette is used to remove the entire contents of the cyst. In larger lesions, excision of the pseudocyst wall is performed.

Milia

Milia are cystic accumulations of keratin within the pilosebaceous units. These are extremely common in neonates and usually regress in the first 3 to 4 weeks of life. No treatment is required.

Pyogenic Granuloma

Pyogenic granulomas are bright red papules or nodules. They are common in children and can occur on any cutaneous or mucosal surface. These lesions are usually rapidly growing and bleed easily from minor trauma. When they occur in the periocular region, they are nearly always associated with a prior ocular injury, surgery, trauma, or with a chalazion. Larger lesions are simply excised and the base cauterized. Smaller lesions may respond to topical corticosteroids.

Syringoma

Syringomas are benign tumors of the eccrine duct structures. They are 1 to 3 mm translucent papules most commonly seen on the lower eyelid. The incidence is increased in Down syndrome.

Xanthelasma

Xanthelasma are typically yellow-colored papules and plaques seen on the upper eyelids near the medial canthus. While rare in the pediatric age group, any child with xanthelasma deserves an evaluation for disorders of lipid metabolism.

Malignant Lesions

Malignant lesions are rare in the childhood eyelid. However, they may occur under certain circumstances. Basal cell carcinoma has been reported on the eyelids of children, but usually in association with nevus sebaceous, xeroderma pigmentosa, or basal cell nevus syndrome. Basal cell carcinomas have smooth pearly edges with telangiectases. The central area may necrose, leaving a raised rim.

Basal cell nevus syndrome is an autosomal dominant disorder. In addition to basal cell carcinoma, jaw cyst, rib and vertebral abnormalities, calcification of the falx cerebri, agenesis of corpus callosum, palmer and plantar pits, ovarian fibromata, cardiac fibromata, and medulloblastomata occur. Additional ocular findings include cataracts, glaucoma, coloboma, microphthalmia, and strabismus.

Squamous cell carcinoma is rare in children and is most typically seen in patients with xeroderma pigmentosa. Unlike basal cell carcinoma, squamous cell carcinoma can metastasize. Xeroderma pigmentosa is an autosomal recessive disorder characterized by defective DNA repair under conditions of UV exposure.

INFECTIOUS EYELID DISORDERS

Preseptal Cellulitis

A common infectious eyelid disorder in children is preseptal cellulitis, an infectious process limited to the skin and subcutaneous tissues anterior to the orbital septum. While the outcome is typically good in preseptal cellulitis, systemic sepsis and meningitis can occur. Preseptal cellulitis may be secondary to upper respiratory tract infections, sinusitis, or trauma. Occasionally, preseptal cellulitis results from an infection of a chalazion or spread from dacryocystitis. Abscess formation requiring surgical drainage can occur. Additionally, orbital and intracranial spread of the infection may occur. Patients with proptosis, pupillary changes, and limited extraocular motility should be evaluated for orbital cellulitis as these findings are not seen in patients with isolated preseptal cellulitis. Treatment of preseptal cellulitis includes antibiotics and surgical drainage of abscesses. Younger children and neonates should be admitted for intravenous antibiotics and monitoring. Older children with milder infections may be managed with oral antibiotics with close follow-up care. Common pathogens found in children with preseptal cellulitis include *Staphylococcus aureus*, *Streptococcus pneumoniae*, *Haemophilus influenza*, and *Streptococcus epidermitis*. If a foreign body is suspected, then surgical removal of the foreign body is necessary for the infection to clear.

Necrotizing fasciitis is an infection caused by aerobic or anaerobic microorganisms, which spreads rapidly through soft tissues. This condition has a high mortality rate. Typically, these patients have signs of systemic toxicity with sepsis, organ failure, and respiratory failure. In the setting of necrotizing fasciitis, aggressive surgical debridement and broad-spectrum antibiotics are necessary.

Blepharitis

Chronic blepharitis is common in children and may result in chronic blepharoconjunctivitis, recurrent chalazia, loss of lashes (madarosis), and thickening of the eyelid margins. Secondary corneal vascularization and scarring can result. Inflammation of the glands of the eyelid margin occurs with collarettes and crusting on the cilia. Treatment consists of warm compresses, tarsal massage, eyelid hygiene with baby shampoo scrubs, and topical erythromycin ointment three or four times daily. Treatment is continued for several weeks. Blepharitis may be chronic in children despite treatment. Oral erythromycin has been effective in children with severe blepharokeratitis (39). Oral tetracycline, minocycline, and doxycycline, while effective in adult blepharitis, are avoided in children due to the risk of dental enamel discoloration.

Herpes Simplex

When primary herpes simplex infection occurs in children, it is usually asymptomatic. Periocular involvement in primary herpes simplex infection usually manifests as vesicles on the eyelid margin. This infection is self-limited, but topical antibiotics may be used to prevent secondary bacterial infection. Latent herpetic infection may persist throughout life and be activated by many nonspecific stimuli. The most common ocular manifestation involves the cornea, but the eyelids may be involved in a recurrent infection. Herpetic blepharitis is characterized by the formation of vesicles that subsequently break down and ulcerate to form a yellow crusted surface. Systemic administration of the antiviral agent acyclovir is beneficial.

Herpes Zoster

Herpes zoster ophthalmicus is unusual in childhood, but the upper or lower eyelids may be involved if the first or second division of the trigeminal nerve is affected. Vesicles occur at the inner half of the upper eyelid when the supratrochlear branch of the first division is involved, and along the side and tip of the nose if the nasociliary branch is involved. In the latter instance, severe keratitis and uveitis may occur. Systemic treatment with acyclovir is used along with antibiotic ointments to prevent secondary bacterial skin infections.

Molluscum Contagiosum

Molluscum contagiosum is a disorder caused by a poxvirus. The lesions are 2- to 4 mm papules, and they may be isolated or multiple. In children, these lesions typically occur on the face, trunk, and extremities, including the eyelids. When present on the eyelids, they can be associated with chronic follicular conjunctivitis. Infection with this agent is self-limited and usually resolves in 6 to 18 months. When conjunctivitis is associated with molluscum contagiosum, the molluscum lesions near the eyelid margins should be excised or curetted. Asymptomatic children do not necessarily need treatment. However, if treatment is undertaken, simple excision or curettage of the surface of the lesions is all that is required.

Fungal Eyelid Infections

Eyelid infections due to fungi are unusual but may occur in immunocompromised individuals. Diagnosis requires a strong index of suspicion, proper culture with Sabouraud medium, and wet smears cleared with 10% potassium hydroxide. Pathogens include *Actinomyces*, *Nocardia*, *Candida*, and *Blastomyces*.

Pediculosis

Louse infections of the eyelids cause severe itching and irritation. The pubic louse has an affinity for the eyelids. Diagnosis is made easily on slit-lamp examination when the ova and adult crab louse are observed. Treatment consists of improving the patient's personal hygiene and application of a bland antibiotic ointment that suffocates the louse. Head and body antilouse shampoos are used along with home hygiene measures. It should be remembered that pediculosis is a sexually transmitted disease. A child presenting with pediculosis should prompt an evaluation for possible abuse.

Contact Dermatitis

The skin of the eyelids may resemble crepe paper, but it becomes markedly swollen after contact with inciting agents. The skin of the eyelids is red, itchy, and irritated. Common irritants include topical medications (e.g., atropine), cosmetics, nail polish, soaps, poison ivy, and sumac. Treatment consists of removal of the inciting substance. Symptomatic relief may be obtained by using systemic antihistamines and local corticosteroid preparations.

EYELID TRAUMA

The spectrum and management of periocular trauma is extensive. However, some common management issues should be considered. In any child who has sustained a periocular injury, the nature and history of the trauma should be elicited to the fullest extent possible. Blunt trauma with periocular ecchymosis will require careful evaluation of the eye and orbital structures. Even seemingly minor periocular trauma may be associated with orbital fractures and muscle entrapment in children (40). Therefore, ocular motility should be assessed and appropriate imaging studies performed when necessary (41). A thorough eye examination including a retinal examination should be included in the evaluation, as the history of the injury may be inconsistent with the physical findings.

Simple eyelid skin lacerations where a foreign body is not present and which do not involve the eyelid margin should be closed directly. Only the skin is closed, and care is taken to avoid vertical eyelid skin tension that can create eyelid retraction and abnormal eyelid contour. The orbital septum need not be closed for the same reason. Even in severe injuries, such as seen with dog bites, it is rare to have missing eyelid skin. When repairing complex skin lacerations where the anatomic relationships may at first not be obvious, start by suturing the skin where anatomic arrangement is recognized (Fig. 17.24). Closure of these areas will

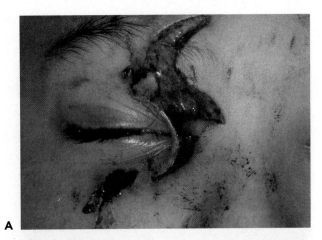

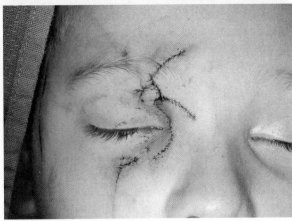

FIGURE 17.24. A: Complex medial canthal eyelid laceration. **B:** By first approximating the areas where the anatomic relationship is easily identified (i.e., the brow cilia area and inferior laceration up to the medial canthal skin), the remaining anatomic relationships can be identified. The canaliculus and lacrimal sac were not involved.

lead to a gradual recognition of the position of the remaining skin tissue so that proper reapproximation of the eyelid skin can be undertaken.

In cases in which the eyelid margin has been violated, the tarsus is closed primarily, followed by skin closure (Fig. 17.25). In full-thickness eyelid lacerations, the tarsus is closed with three interrupted 6-0 absorbable sutures. These are preplaced and positioned such that a slight eversion of the eyelid margin occurs when the sutures are securely tied. Closure of the eyelid margin is performed with interrupted sutures. 7-0 chromic sutures with the tails cut close to the knots are usually used in younger children. These sutures resorb quickly and do not require general anesthesia to remove them. While the risk of corneal abrasion from the sutures at the margin is possible, scheduled application of antibiotic ointment seems preventative. In older children for whom in-office suture removal is possible, 8-0 black silk marginal sutures with the tails cut close to the knots work well without causing corneal surface irritation. Alternatively, the tails can be left long and draped over the anterior surface of the eyelid and then tied beneath superficial skin sutures.

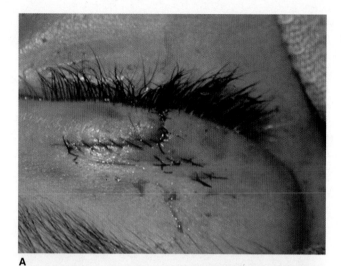

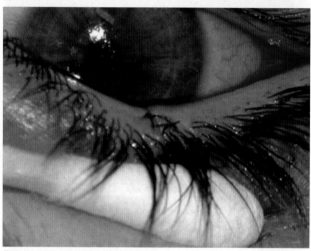

FIGURE 17.25. Repair of eyelid laceration. **A:** Tarsus is closed with interrupted vicryl sutures and the skin is closed with 8-0 silk. **B:** Eyelid margin closed with silk sutures aligning the eyelid margin.

The skin can be closed with the surgeon's choice of absorbable or nonabsorbable suture depending on the child's age.

Trauma involving the lateral canthus will often require reapproximation of the lateral canthus with permanent sutures secured to the periorbita of the lateral orbital rim. Medial canthal reconstruction with canalicular reconstruction can be managed with a Silastic intubation of the canalicular system. If the canaliculus is lacerated, careful inspection utilizing cotton-tipped applicators to retract the injured tissues will typically reveal the medial portion of the lacerated canaliculus, recognized by the glistening epithelium. Typically, this is located more medially and more posteriorly than one might initially suspect. Avoid grasping the lacerated medial canthal area with toothed forceps when searching for the torn edge of the canaliculus. Sharp forceps create bleeding, shred tissues, and make location of the canaliculus more difficult. Once the canaliculus is located, Silastic intubation of the torn canaliculus is performed. The Ritleng introducer with Monoka monocanalicular stents or bicanalicular tubes easily facilitates intubation. Once the tube is in place, the epithelium of the canaliculus is closed with at least two 6-0 Vicryl sutures. These sutures are preplaced and then, with firm traction of the distal tube coming from the nares, the sutures are securely tied. The skin is then closed with either absorbable or nonabsorbable suture, depending on the child's age. Monocanalicular tubes self-seat in the punctum and do not require intranasal suture fixation. Similarly, a bicanalicular tube can be secured to itself within the lacrimal sac, thus avoiding intranasal fixation. Usually, these tubes are removed in the office after 4 to 6 months.

Burn Injuries

Burns may result from caustic chemical exposure or materials from thermal injuries. Lye burns are more serious than acid burns. While base (alkali) penetrates deeply by causing protein dissolution, acid burns cause protein coagulation, which limits the depth of acid penetration. When caustic material comes into contact with the eyelids, the immediate treatment consists of a very thorough lavage with water. The cul-de-sacs should be included in the irrigation and all particulate matter should be removed. Scarring may lead to lagophthalmos, entropion, or ectropion. If scarring and contracture are severe, surgical lysis of the adhesions, excision of the scar tissue, and full-thickness skin grafting may be necessary.

REFERENCES

1. Piest KL. Embryology and anatomy of the developing face. In: Katowitz JA, ed. *Pediatric oculoplastic surgery.* New York: Springer-Verlag, 2002:11–30.
2. Dortzbach RK, Sutula FC. Involutional blepharoptosis. A histopathological study. *Arch Ophthalmol* 1980;98:2045–2049.
3. Jeong S, Lemke BN, Dortzbach RK, et al. The Asian upper eyelid: an anatomical study with comparison to the Caucasian eyelid. *Arch Ophthalmol* 1999;117:907–912.
4. Hawes MJ, Dortzbach RK. The microscopic anatomy of the lower eyelid retractors. *Arch Ophthalmol* 1982;100:1313–1318.
5. Jeffery AR, Ellis FJ, Repka MX, et al. Pediatric Horner syndrome. *J AAPOS* 1998;2:159–167.
6. Slavotinek AM. Eye development genes and known syndromes. *Mol Genet Metab* 2011 Dec;104(4):448–456.
7. Bardakjian TM, Schneider A. The genetics of anophthalmia and microphthalmia. *Curr Opin Ophthalmol* Sep 2011;22(5): 309–313.
8. Gossman MD, Mohay J, Roberts DM. Expansion of the human microphthalmic orbit. *Ophthalmology* 1999;106:2005–2009.
9. Saleh GM, Hussain B, Verity DH, Collin JR. A surgical strategy for the correction of Fraser syndrome cryptophthalmos. *Ophthalmology* Sep 2009;116(9):1707–1712.
10. Slavotinek AM, Tifft CJ. Fraser syndrome and cryptophthalmos: review of the diagnostic criteria and evidence for phenotypic modules in complex malformation syndromes. *J Med Genet* 2002;39:623–633.

11. Weiss AH, Riscile G, Kousseff BG. Ankyloblepharon filiforme adnatum. *Am J Med Genet* 1992;42:369–373.

12. Tuysuz B, Ilikkan B, Vural M, et al. Ankyloblepharon filiforme adnatum (AFA) associated with trisomy 18. *TurkJ Pediatr* 2002;44:360–362.

13. McGrath JA, Duijf PH, Doetsch V, et al. Hay-Wells syndrome is caused by heterozygous missense mutations in the SAM domain of p63. *Hum Mol Genet* 2001;10:221–229.

14. Vaughn GL, Dortzbach RK, Sires BS, et al. Eyelid splitting with excision or microhyfrecation for distichiasis. *Arch Ophthalmol* 1997;115:282–284.

15. Niemi KM, Kanerva L, Kuokkanen K, et al. Clinical, light and electron microscopic features of recessive congenital ichthyosis type I. *Br J Dermatol* 1994;130:626–633.

16. Sires BS. Congenital horizontal tarsal kink: clinical characteristics from a large series. *Ophthal Plast Reconstr Surg* 1999;15:355–359.

17. Mustarde JC. The treatment of ptosis and epicanthal folds. *Br J Plast Surg* 1959;12:252–258.

18. Engle EC, Castro AE, Macy ME, et al. A gene for isolated congenital ptosis maps to a 3-cM region within 1p32–p34.1. *Am J Hum Genet* 1997;60:1150–1157.

19. Engle EC. The molecular basis of the congenital fibrosis syndromes. *Strabismus* 2002;10:125–128.

20. Anlar B. Juvenile myasthenia: diagnosis and treatment. *Paediatr Drugs* 2000;2:161–169.

21. Carter SR, Meecham WJ, Seiff SR. Silicone frontalis slings for the correction of blepharoptosis: indications and efficacy. *Ophthalmology* 1996;103:623–630.

22. Harrad RA, Graham CM, Collin JR. Amblyopia and strabismus in congenital ptosis. *Eye* 1988;2:625–627.

23. McCulloch DL, Wright KW. Unilateral congenital ptosis: compensatory head posturing and amblyopia. *Ophthal Plast Reconstr Surg* 1993;9:196–200.

24. Crawford JS. Repair of ptosis using frontalis muscle and fascia lata. *Trans Am Acad Ophthalmol Otolaryngol* 1956;60:672–678.

25. Liu D. Blepharoptosis correction with frontalis suspension using a supramid sling: duration of effect. *Am J Ophthalmol* 1999;128:772–773.

26. Wasserman BN, Sprunger DT, Helveston EM. Comparison of materials used in frontalis suspension. *Arch Ophthalmol* 2001;119:687–691.

27. Weakley DR Jr. The association between nonstrabismic anisometropia, amblyopia, and subnormal binocularity. *Ophthalmology* 2001;108:163–171.

28. Léauté-Labrèze C, Dumas de la Roque E, Hubiche T, Boralevi F, Thambo JB, Taïeb A. Propranolol for severe hemangiomas of infancy. *N Engl J Med* June 2008;358(24):2649–2651

29. Haider KM, Plager DA, Neely DE, Eikenberry J, Haggstrom A. Outpatient treatment of periocular infantile hemangiomas with oral propranolol. *J AAPOS* June 2010;14(3):251–256.

30. Ni N, Guo S, Langer P. Current concepts in the management of periocular infantile (capillary) hemangioma. *Curr Opin Ophthalmol* Sep 2011;22(5):419–425.

31. Kushner BJ. The treatment of periorbital infantile hemangioma with intralesional corticosteroid. *Plast Reconstr Surg* 1985;76:517–526.

32. Drolet BA, Esterly NB, Frieden IJ. Hemangiomas in children. *N Engl J Med* 1999;341:173–181.

33. Kushner BJ. Hemangiomas in children. *N Engl J Med* 1999;341:2018.

34. Goyal G, Watts P, Lane CM, et al. Adrenal suppression and failure to thrive after steroid injections for periocular hemangioma. *Ophthalmology* 2004;111:389–395.

35. Cruz OA, Zarnegar SR, Myers SE. Treatment of periocular capillary hemangioma with topical clobetasol propionate. *Ophthalmology* 1995;102:2012–2015.

36. Plager DA, Snyder SK. Resolution of astigmatism after surgical resection of capillary hemangiomas in infants. *Ophthalmology* 1997;104:1102–1106.

37. Avery RA, Dombi E, Hutcheson KA, et al. Visual outcomes in children with neurofibromatosis type 1 and orbitotemporal plexiform neurofibromas. *Am J Ophthalmol*;2013; Epub 2013 Feb 26.

38. Lorentzen M, Pers M, Bretteville-Jensen G. The incidence of malignant transformation in giant pigmented nevi. *Scand J Plast Reconstr Surg* 1977;11:163–167.

39. Meisler DM, Raizman MB, Traboulsi EI. Oral erythromycin treatment for childhood blepharokeratitis. *J AAPOS* 2000;4:379–380.

40. Jordan DR, Allen LH, White J, et al. Intervention within days for some orbital floor fractures: the white-eyed blowout. *Ophthal Plast Reconstr Surg* 1998;14:379–390.

41. Criden MR, Ellis FJ. Linear nondisplaced orbital fractures with muscle entrapment. *J AAPOS* Apr 2007;11(2):142–147.

18

Disorders of the Orbit

David B. Lyon

PEDIATRIC ORBITAL DISORDERS have a diverse and complex spectrum and must be approached in an organized and disciplined manner to arrive at the best plan of evaluation, diagnosis, and treatment. The common orbital diseases in childhood overlap little with those found in adults. An initial differential diagnosis should be formulated based on the history and physical examination, and it is helpful to classify the disease process based on features of inflammation, infiltration, mass effect, or vascular changes. Clues about the dynamics and location of the disease process may come from evaluation of the motor and sensory nerve effects and the presence or absence of pain. Pain is caused by a rapid increase of mass or pressure effect such as that seen with infection, inflammation or hemorrhage, or from bone or nerve involvement. Neoplasms rarely cause pain until late in their course.

The time progression of the disease process is also important to establish since some processes occur in minutes (hemorrhage), hours to days (rhabdomyosarcoma, thyroid eye disease [TED], neuroblastoma, granulocytic sarcoma, inflammation, or infection), weeks to months (chronic inflammatory conditions, benign neoplasm, or lymphoma), or months to years (dermoid, neurogenic tumors, fibrous dysplasia). Sometimes it is difficult for the patient or family to remember the exact onset of symptoms, and old photos can be helpful in establishing the time of onset and progression of the disease process. Any past ocular, medical, and family history should be obtained. Systemic investigation may be important in the assessment of the patient since endocrinologic, infectious, immunologic, vascular, and neoplastic diseases may have orbital involvement. Imaging techniques may be employed to best define the lesion as to location, composition, contour, vascularity, and effect on the adjacent orbital structures such as compression and infiltration. Many patients will require an orbitotomy for a diagnostic biopsy or removal of the lesion.

ORBITAL ANATOMY

The orbit is delineated by portions of seven of the bones of the face and skull; is surrounded by the brain, paranasal sinuses, and soft tissues of the face; and contains the globe, optic nerve, motor and sensory nerves, extraocular muscles, connective tissue, fat, glandular structures, and blood vessels. Any of these anatomic structures may be involved in a disease process or give rise to a primary orbital neoplasm.

In adults, the orbit is pyramidal in shape with a total volume of 30 mL. The orbital roof is triangular and composed of the frontal bone and lesser wing of the sphenoid and contains the optic canal. The lateral wall, which is at a 45-degree angle to the medial wall, is composed of the greater wing of the sphenoid and the zygomatic bones. The thinner medial wall is composed of the maxillary, lacrimal, ethmoid, and lesser wings of the sphenoid bones. Finally, the orbital floor, which is also triangular in shape, is made up of the maxillary, zygomatic, and palatine bones. The growth of the orbit is complete sometime between 7 years of age and puberty. Loss of an eye before this time may retard orbital bony development.

The optic canal and superior orbital fissure are in the orbital apex and transmit the optic nerve and ophthalmic artery, and cranial nerves III, IV, V-1, and VI. From their origin in the orbital apex at the annulus of Zinn, the extraocular muscles course anteriorly to insert on the globe in the anterior orbit, except the inferior oblique which has its origin at the medial anterior orbital floor. From the posterior sclera, the orbital portion of the optic nerve resides inside the muscle cone and exits the orbit via the optic canal. For descriptive purposes, the retrobulbar orbital is separated into intraconal and extraconal spaces. The lacrimal gland resides in the superotemporal anterior orbit and the lacrimal drainage apparatus is in the medial anterior orbit.

Paraorbital structures include the anterior cranial fossa superiorly and the paranasal sinuses. The ethmoid sinuses are located medially and are present at birth. Superior to the anterior orbit is the frontal sinus that is rarely well developed before 9 years of age. The maxillary sinus lies inferior to the orbit and expands during childhood with a resulting change in the orbital floor configuration.

ORBITAL EXAMINATION

Evaluation of orbital disease in children should include a complete ocular examination with special attention to inspection, palpation, and documentation of eyelid and globe position. Optic nerve function should be evaluated and followed with best-corrected visual acuity, color vision, pupillary function, visual fields, and optic disk appearance. The status and function of the cranial nerves, corneal and facial sensation, and facial tone and symmetry should be evaluated. Photographic documentation of all abnormalities is helpful at baseline and follow-up exams to evaluate for interval changes of the disease process. Photos should also be taken preoperatively on surgical cases.

Proptosis, or axial globe displacement, is one of the main indicators of orbital disease. Thus, all patients need Hertel exophthalmometer readings to determine if proptosis is present and to quantitate the globe position relative to the lateral orbital rim. The orbit is surrounded by bone, except anteriorly, so that any increase in volume from a mass, infection, or inflammation may result in the displacement of the globe anteriorly, with asymmetry measuring more than 2 mm being significant. Evaluation of globe dystopia vertically or horizontally also helps determine the location of the mass within the orbit. An orbital mass not centered within the orbit will displace the globe off its axis in a direction away from the mass. Intraconal processes usually cause axial proptosis, as seen with optic nerve glioma or TED. Inferomedial displacement can result from superotemporal lesions such as dermoid cysts and lacrimal gland tumors. Lateral displacement can result from medial subperiosteal abscesses (SPAs).

The orbital rims and quadrants should be palpated for masses. If a mass is noted, document its location, size, shape, tenderness, consistency, discreteness, and mobility. Resistance to retropulsion of the globe, compared with the fellow side, may indicate a posterior or apex process that is not palpable. The preauricular and submandibular lymph nodes should also be evaluated with palpation.

Orbital processes can affect ocular motility, either by direct involvement of the muscles or their motor nerves, or by deviation of the axis of the eye. Inflammatory processes often cause pain with eye movements, especially when the muscles or nerves are directly involved.

Pulsation may be secondary to a vascular malformation in the orbit or the absence of orbital bone that allows the transmission of brain pulsation to the orbit as sometimes seen with an encephalocele, surgical removal of the orbital roof, or with absence of the sphenoid wing in some cases of neurofibromatosis. If the flow through an orbital vascular lesion is high, you may hear a bruit or feel a thrill, as with carotid cavernous fistulae, larger dural arteriovenous fistulae, and orbital arteriovenous malformations. Venous lesions of the orbit do not pulsate, but may enlarge with the valsalva maneuver or with the head held in a dependent position.

Evaluation of the visual pathways includes examination of best-corrected visual acuity, color vision, red desaturation, visual fields, and pupillary reactions. All these factors can assist in the detection of visual loss due to an orbital process. Loss of color vision and an afferent pupillary defect are often the first signs of early visual loss. Changes in the size of the pupil can be seen with tumors that invade or compress the parasympathetic (third cranial nerve and ciliary ganglion) or sympathetic fibers that innervate the pupillary muscles. Optic nerve head edema or atrophy helps to determine the duration of the process. Retinal or choroidal striae or folds may be seen from a mass pressing on the globe.

ORBITAL IMAGING

Orbital imaging provides diagnostic information with increased specificity as to the location, character, and size of an orbital lesion. Computed tomography (CT) and magnetic resonance imaging (MRI) are the most commonly used modalities.

CT is utilized in the evaluation of orbital trauma, orbital cellulitis, screening for mass-occupying lesions, and for processes that may involve bone. Spiral CT produces higher quality images with good spatial resolution, faster scanning times (a few minutes per patient), and less expense than MRI scans. The addition of contrast material gives further information regarding the lesion and enhances vascular structures. However, concern of cancer induction from radiation exposure in children is real, and adherence to the as low as reasonably achievable policy of the US Food and Drug Administration is recommended (1).

MRI yields an excellent view of the optic nerve and visual pathways, orbital apex, orbitocranial junction, brain, organic foreign bodies, vascular tumors, or heterogeneous tumors. Fat suppression with gadolinium can be used to enhance orbital structures or processes. With this technique, the normally bright orbital fat will appear dark, allowing visualization of orbital structures and processes such as vascular tumors or inflammation. The advantages of MRI over CT scanning include no radiation exposure, no need for contrast material to visualize vascular structures, and better contrast resolution of soft tissues. The disadvantages of MRI include long acquisition time, sensitivity to motion artifact, possible need for sedation and anesthesia support, higher cost, and decreased spatial resolution. MRI is contraindicated in patients with metallic foreign bodies, metallic clips, or any ferromagnetic material in the area being examined.

Ultrasonography has a complementary role in pediatric orbital disease. Its advantages are no radiation exposure, no contrast needed, readily available, noninvasive, and no sedation required. Useful information regarding the location, size, shape, tissue characteristics, and vascular features of orbital lesions can be obtained. Color Doppler echography will quantitate flow velocity of vascular lesions. Poor resolution around the bone at the orbital apex makes this form of testing less useful. However, it is particularly helpful in identifying lesions adjacent to and involving the globe, such as scleritis and vascular and cystic lesions (2).

Rarely, arteriography is used to study arterial lesions such as aneurysms and arteriovenous malformations. Selective injection, magnification, and subtraction techniques increase visualization of the lesion. CT angiography and magnetic resonance angiography allow noninvasive visualization of large- and medium-sized vessels of the arterial system, but do not provide the fine detail possible with direct angiography.

CONGENITAL ABNORMALITIES OF THE ORBIT

Anophthalmos and Microphthalmos

Anophthalmia and microphthalmia refer to the absence of an eye and the presence of a small eye within the orbit, respectively, and represent a spectrum of maldevelopment resulting from failure of the primary optic vesicle to fully develop during the fourth week of embryologic development. Both anophthalmia and microphthalmia are usually bilateral and occur as part of genetic syndromes in 75% of cases with variable phenotype. The remaining cases are usually due to maternal viral infections or ingestions of teratogens. Isolated nonsyndromic heritable unilateral cases are very rare (3).

In true anophthalmos, the orbits and eyelids are usually normally formed, but small. The conjunctival fornices are decreased in size, and the eye cannot be seen or felt in the orbit on palpation. Histologically, no ocular tissue is present. Extraocular muscles may be present and well developed. Infants with true bilateral anophthalmos show an absence of the chiasm, small geniculate bodies, and small optic foramina. Clinical anophthalmos refers to the condition of no visible or palpable globe without radiographic or histopathologic confirmation of true anophthalmos.

Isolated microphthalmos is usually a unilateral condition that occurs sporadically. The size of the eye is variable and there is sometimes functional vision if it is not too severe. If a coloboma exists, due to failure of closure of the embryonic fissure, microphthalmos may be associated with an orbital cyst that consists of an inner layer of primitive neuroretinal tissue that may contain retinal structures, photoreceptor differentiation, or rosette formation, and an outer layer continuous with the sclera with vascularized connective tissue and occasional cartilage. The size of the cyst varies and often is beneficial for stimulating normal growth of the orbital bone and eyelids. B-scan ultrasonography, CT, or MRI establish the diagnosis, demonstrating a round or irregular cystic lesion adjacent to the microphthalmic globe (Fig. 18.1). Occasionally, the cyst can enlarge greatly, obscuring the microphthalmic globe and expanding the orbit. Management is individualized and may include observation, cyst aspiration or excision, cyst excision with enucleation, and prosthesis fitting with or without surgery (4).

Since both anophthalmos and microphthalmos may be associated with hypoplastic orbits and small eyelids, the goal of treatment is expansion of the eyelids, socket, and bony orbit. Progressively enlarging conformers, fit by an ocularist, are used to expand the eyelids and conjunctival fornices. Clear conformers may be utilized if

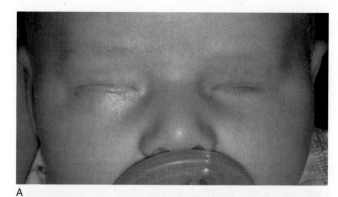

A

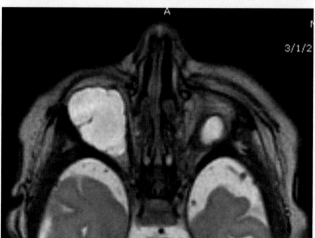

B

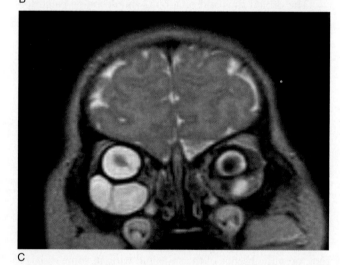

C

FIGURE 18.1. Bilateral microphthalmos with cyst in a newborn. **A:** External photo shows normally formed eyelids, no visible globes, and fullness of the right lower lid with mild ectropion from the cyst. **B** and **C:** Axial and coronal T2 MRI images show the microphthalmos, left eye smaller than right, with cyst inferior to the globes, right larger than left.

a microphthalmic eye may have visual potential. When satisfactory expansion has occurred, an ocular prosthesis can be fabricated. Tissue expanders can be placed in the orbit and progressively expanded to enlarge the hypoplastic orbit to then allow for orbital implant placement for volume augmentation (5). Dermis–fat grafting is another option for volume enhancement with the added advantages of expanding the socket conjunctival surface area and potential for growth with the child.

Cryptophthalmos

Cryptophthalmos is a rare congenital anomaly, usually bilateral, in which the eyelids are fused to the globe. It may be divided into several grades with and without upper eyelid coloboma (6). In complete cryptophthalmos, the eyelids are absent and the globe is entirely covered by skin extending from the brow to the cheek. In partial cryptophthalmos, the medial eyelid is replaced with a layer of skin fused to the globe, but the lateral portion of the eyelid is normal in structure and function. There is partial or complete absence of the eyebrow, eyelids, eyelashes, and conjunctiva with continuation of the forehead skin to the cheek over the eyes. The hidden eye is usually abnormal, with a wide variety of ocular defects. The partially developed adnexa are fused to the anterior segment of the globe. These defects are thought to result from failure of the eyelid fold formation, which normally occurs in the seventh week of gestation. This condition is often associated with multiple congenital deformities such as cleft palate, syndactyly, dental malformations, nasal deformities, urogenital deformities, and hypoplasia of the facial and orbital bones. Histologically, the eyelids are abnormal with absent conjunctiva and diminished or absent orbicularis and levator muscles, tarsal plate, and meibomian glands, making attempts at reconstruction difficult.

ORBITAL INFECTIONS

Orbital infections range from preseptal cellulitis to orbital abscesses. It is extremely important to know the features of these infections and their proper treatment to avoid visual loss or spread of infection to the cavernous sinus or intracranial structures. Infections occur from three primary sources: direct spread from an adjacent sinus (most common); direct inoculation from trauma, surgical or nonsurgical, or skin infection; and hematogenous spread from a distant focus.

Preseptal Cellulitis

Preseptal cellulitis is an infection of the periorbital soft tissues anterior to the orbital septum and thus is not a true orbital infection. However, it may be difficult to distinguish from orbital cellulitis or may spread to involve the postseptal orbital tissues. It is more common than orbital cellulitis in children and is characterized by eyelid erythema and edema, generally more pronounced in the upper eyelid. If the cellulitis is severe, some chemosis may also be present. Staphylococcal and streptococcal organisms are the main pathogens for which antibiotic coverage is required today, including methicillin-resistant strains of *Staphylococcus aureus* (MRSA). Children with preseptal cellulitis often have a history of antecedent upper respiratory tract infections, recent eyelid trauma, insect bites, or infections. Oral antibiotics and close observation are the treatment of choice.

Clinical evaluation, sometimes supplemented with CT scanning, is the best method to distinguish preseptal from orbital cellulitis. Proptosis and decreased motility herald orbital cellulitis. Chemosis is a less specific finding. On CT scan, preseptal cellulitis shows soft-tissue edema or abscess formation anterior to the orbital septum, whereas orbital cellulitis shows involvement of the postseptal orbital tissues. This differentiation, however, is usually made clinically. Rapid progression of preseptal cellulitis to orbital cellulitis can occur, and therefore, patients should be followed closely, and admitted for intravenous antibiotics and imaging if the clinical picture deteriorates.

Orbital Cellulitis

Orbital cellulitis requires prompt identification and treatment to prevent visual or life-threatening complications. It is more common in children than in adults, but it is usually related to sinusitis in both. Orbital extension from the ethmoid sinus is most likely, but any or all of the sinuses may be involved. Upper respiratory tract infections interfere with clearance of secretions by the respiratory cilia, causing poor sinus drainage and predisposing children to sinusitis. The bones separating the orbit and sinuses are thin, allowing spread of the infection. The foramina, especially the ethmoid foramina, and the valveless interconnecting venous system of the orbit and sinuses represent other routes for possible spread of infection from the sinuses to the orbit. Other causes of orbital cellulitis are traumatic and surgical wounds, foreign bodies, or spread from odontogenic infections, dacryoadenitis, panophthalmitis, dacryocystitis, or endogenous septicemia. Immunosuppressed children can develop fungal orbital cellulitis, which is often fatal, and present with fever and neutropenia and mild symptoms (7).

Signs of orbital cellulitis include eyelid edema, pain, decreased motility, proptosis, chemosis, decreased vision, orbital tension, and headache (Fig. 18.2A). Decreased vision, an afferent pupillary defect, or dilated pupil indicate involvement of the orbital apex and require aggressive treatment. Delayed treatment may result in an orbital apex syndrome, cavernous sinus thrombosis, possible blindness due to apical optic nerve compression, cranial nerve palsies, brain abscess, and even death. Permanent visual loss can also result from direct optic neuritis or vasculitis. Spread via the vascular emissaries to the cavernous sinus can lead to cavernous sinus thrombosis, and spread through the diploic vessels to the intracranial cavity can lead to subdural empyema or intracranial abscesses. The recent medical history is usually positive for an upper respiratory tract infection, but the symptoms may be mild. The child is sick, lethargic, tired, and often febrile, which helps to differentiate this from orbital inflammatory disease. CT or MRI scans show orbital

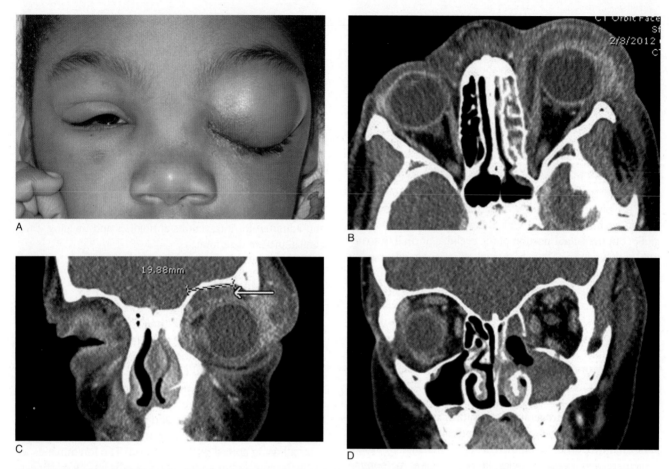

FIGURE 18.2. Orbital cellulitis and subperiosteal abscess (SPA) in a 7-year-old girl. She underwent an endoscopic left maxillary antrostomy with debridement, left anterior ethmoidectomy with lamina papyracea opening, and drainage of a medial SPA 2 days prior to photo. **A:** Clinical appearance with marked left and mild right periorbital edema at the time of ophthalmic consultation. She had extensive left superior chemosis and motility limitation with normal vision. **B:** Axial; **C** and **D:** Coronal CT scan showing left periorbital edema, superior orbital SPA (*arrow* in **C**), left maxillary and ethmoidal opacification, maxillary antrostomy, and bony defect in the lamina papyracea from the prior surgery. An upper eyelid crease approach to the superior orbit was used to culture and drain the superior SPA. There was no growth from the cultures taken at both procedures and rapid improvement following the superior orbital drainage.

involvement by soft-tissue edema, proptosis, fat stranding, phlegmon, and possible intraorbital abscess which may vary in location and extent. They also reveal the accompanying sinus infection, which helps to secure the diagnosis of infection in most cases (Fig. 18.2B–D).

In contrast to adults, the pathogens in orbital cellulitis in young children tend to be single aerobic organisms, including streptococcal and staphylococcal species. Other gram-positive and gram-negative organisms are possible causes. If foul smelling, anaerobic infections should be considered, especially if the wound has been contaminated by soil and bites. Before the introduction of the HiB vaccine in 1985, *Haemophilus influenzae* was the most common pathogen isolated in patients with orbital cellulitis. Antibiotic treatment should be targeted to cover the most likely infecting organisms, again including MRSA. Since the disease process can threaten vision and life, high-dose intravenous antibiotics and nasal decongestants must be used.

Due to the delay in development of the sinuses in children, the most frequent locus of the disease is the ethmoidal sinus. Since the sinuses are the primary site of infection, and the orbit is a bystander, surgical sinus drainage by otolaryngology is often indicated. Close monitoring of vision, pupillary reaction, extraocular motility, and central nervous system (CNS) function must be carried out during the first 24 to 48 hours. If there is no evidence of improvement or if the condition worsens, an orbital or subperiosteal abscess should be considered and looked for with repeat imaging. Abscesses within the orbital soft tissues can extend posteriorly, resulting in life-threatening consequences such as cavernous sinus thrombosis, meningitis, and intracranial abscesses. Third, fourth, fifth (V-1), and sixth cranial nerve dysfunction may occur in septic cavernous sinus thrombosis. Systemic signs of toxicity are present, including sepsis, nausea, vomiting, meningeal signs, and altered levels of consciousness. When an abscess of the orbit or brain is identified, it requires immediate drainage to prevent serious complications.

Subperiosteal Abscess

An SPA or infiltrate occurs when purulent material elevates the periorbita away from the bony walls of the orbit adjacent to an infected sinus. On CT scan, the periorbita is tethered at the orbital suture lines so the abscess creates a smooth, dome-shaped elevation of the periorbita with either a homogeneous or heterogeneous collection (Fig. 18.2C). The signs are similar to those of orbital cellulitis, but may also include nonaxial displacement and deformation of the globe. Initial treatment is with broad-spectrum intravenous antibiotics, based on the age of the child, to obtain adequate drug levels in the relatively avascular subperiosteal space. Garcia and Harris outlined the criteria for initial nonsurgical management based on the absence of the following surgical indicators: age of patient, 9 years or older; presence of frontal sinusitis; nonmedial location of SPA; large SPA; suspicion of anaerobic subperiosteal infection (e.g., presence of gas within the abscess space as visualized on CT scan); recurrence of SPA after previous drainage; evidence of chronic sinusitis (e.g., nasal polyps); acute optic nerve or retinal compromise; infection of dental origin, because the presence of anaerobes would be anticipated (8). These criteria are built on an earlier microbiologic study that found negative or single aerobic organisms on cultures of drained material in children less than 9 years old, more severe infections in those 10 to 14 years old, and positive cultures at drainage, even after 3 days of usually appropriate antibiotics, which were often polymicrobial including anaerobes in those 15 and older (9).

Although these guidelines are helpful, each child has to be individually managed in conjunction with otolaryngology. If there is a poor response to antibiotics after 24 to 48 hours, or if there is a threat to the optic nerve, retinal function, suspicion of anaerobic infection, or very tense orbit with significant pain, drainage and culture is indicated either via orbitotomy or endoscopic sinus surgery with orbital drainage. If sinus surgery is being performed, despite the lack of clear criteria for SPA drainage, it is wise to include its drainage if feasible. Large SPAs, now defined as 2 cm or larger in greatest dimension or greater than 1,250 mm³, or that extend along the orbital roof or floor from the ethmoid, or those associated with frontal sinusitis or intracranial complications should be drained promptly (10,11). Sinus infections of dental origin also constitute an indication for surgical intervention because the presence of anaerobes is anticipated. Decisions should be based on the clinical course as improvement on serial CT scans may lag. The use of intravenous corticosteroids may also be beneficial for treatment of the sinusitis and SPA (12).

Dacryoadenitis

Dacryoadenitis, or lacrimal gland inflammation, may be infectious. It is most often viral in nature, occasionally bacterial, and very rare in children. It presents with an inflamed, tender lacrimal gland that is palpable through an edematous upper eyelid. The child may have adenopathy, fever, malaise, and leukocytosis. Since the orbital lobe of the gland is postseptal, infectious dacryoadenitis is a localized form of orbital cellulitis. CT scan shows diffuse lacrimal gland swelling without bony defects. It usually improves spontaneously, and since there is generally no bacterial involvement, antibiotics are rarely indicated. Systemic steroids frequently help accelerate resolution of the process and keep the patient more comfortable. Infectious dacryoadenitis may be difficult to distinguish from the more common idiopathic lacrimal gland inflammation. The presence of preauricular adenopathy makes a diagnosis of viral dacryoadenitis more likely. Other infectious causes include mononucleosis, herpes zoster, mumps, trachoma, syphilis, and tuberculosis.

ORBITAL INFLAMMATION

Thyroid Eye Disease

TED is an inflammatory orbital disorder associated with autoimmune thyroid dysfunction, most commonly Graves' disease. It is the most common cause of orbital inflammation in adults with manifestations that vary from mild to severe and may cause significant pain and disfigurement, visual disability, and blindness. Pediatric TED is uncommon, but occurs in up to 30% of children with Graves' disease, especially in teenagers when the incidence of primary and second-hand smoke exposure increases. Like in adults, there is a female predominance. Antithyroid medications are usually the first line of treatment in pediatric Graves' disease and thyroidectomy is uncommon. Available studies suggest that childhood TED is less severe than in adults, with eyelid retraction and proptosis as the predominant eye changes (Fig. 18.3), whereas the more severe manifestations of restrictive myopathy and optic dysfunction almost never occur in children (13–15). Most children require no treatment or supportive treatment of exposure keratitis only with ocular lubricants. Severe inflammation is rare, and thus oral corticosteroids are

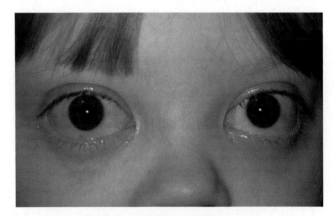

FIGURE 18.3. Thyroid eye disease in a 6-year-old girl. She has bilateral proptosis and upper and lower eyelid retraction. Lubricating ointment residue is visible on the eyelids.

seldom used. Orbital decompression, extraocular muscle, and eyelid surgery are very infrequently needed.

Idiopathic Orbital Inflammation

Idiopathic orbital inflammation (IOI) is described histologically as a pleomorphic inflammatory cellular response and fibrovascular tissue reaction without known cause. IOI is rare in children and is a diagnosis of exclusion, accepted after ruling out other known causes of orbital inflammation such as orbital cellulitis, Langerhans cell histiocytosis (LCH), sarcoidosis, TED, Wegener's granulomatosis, or lymphoproliferative disorders. The character of presentation and temporal sequence help to form the essential diagnostic framework for orbital inflammation. Classically, IOI presents acutely or subacutely with signs of inflammation (pain, swelling, and redness), whereas chronic inflammation from granulomatous disease often presents with a mass effect or chronic bony destruction.

IOI is a multifaceted disease with a wide spectrum of clinical, radiologic, and histopathologic presentations. Many classification schemes have been applied based on location of the inflammatory process, histopathologic characteristics, and stage of inflammation. However, the most useful classification is by the anatomic site of involvement: dacryoadenitis, myositis, sclerotenonitis, diffuse anterior inflammation, perioptic neuritis, or the superior orbital fissure and cavernous sinus syndrome of Tolosa-Hunt.

The inflammatory process is typically characterized by an abrupt onset of pain, proptosis, and inflammatory signs and symptoms, such as swelling and erythema, depending on the location and degree of inflammation, fibrosis, and mass effect. Pediatric IOI differs from the adult presentation by an increased incidence of bilateral involvement and may have associated headache, fever, vomiting, abdominal pain, lethargy, and eosinophilia. The IOI syndromes are initially managed with systemic corticosteroids, with biopsy reserved for cases that are atypical, poorly responsive to treatment, or steroid dependent.

Anterior involvement presents with visual loss, pain, proptosis, ptosis, eyelid swelling, chemosis, and decreased ocular motility. Associated findings may include uveitis, scleritis, papillitis, and even exudative retinal detachments. This syndrome is more common in children and young adults. Systemic evaluation in the younger age group may show an increased sedimentation rate and cerebrospinal fluid pleocytosis. Characteristically, the CT scan shows diffuse anterior orbital infiltration, producing scleral and choroidal thickening, as well as some optic nerve sheath thickening. Ultrasonography shows thickening of the sclera, with accentuation of tenon's space and doubling of the optic nerve shadow (the T-sign). Differential diagnosis must include orbital cellulitis, ruptured dermoid cyst, hemorrhage within a vascular lesion, acute hemorrhage, rhabdomyosarcoma, metastatic neuroblastoma, collagen vascular diseases, and leukemic infiltrates. Histopathologically, the infiltration is characterized by a pleomorphic cellular infiltrate of lymphocytes, plasma cells, and eosinophils with variable degrees of reactive fibrosis. The fibrosis is more prominent as the process becomes more chronic. Treatment consists of oral prednisone, 1 to 2 mg/kg daily, which generally results in a dramatic improvement of symptoms, especially pain, and complete resolution may be expected over several weeks with slow tapering of the systemic corticosteroids. Recurrences occur more frequently in younger patients and require reinstitution of the corticosteroids and may require nonsteroidal anti-inflammatory medications or rarely, immunosuppressive medications. Topical corticosteroid eye drops may help to decrease the superficial inflammatory and anterior chamber reactions. Lesions that do not respond promptly to treatment necessitate orbital biopsy to determine the diagnosis. If the biopsy confirms the diagnosis, treatment should be coordinated by rheumatology and may include antimetabolites, alkylating agents such as methotrexate and cyclophosphamide, or biologics to control the disease process.

Diffuse inflammation is similar to anterior inflammation, but the signs and symptoms are more severe, including limitation of ocular motility, papillitis, and exudative retinal detachment. CT and MRI scans show soft-tissue infiltration involving the entire orbit from the apex to the posterior globe. Again, treatment with corticosteroids is indicated, and a rapid response is usually seen; however, it is more difficult to taper the corticosteroids, and recurrences are more frequently seen than with anterior involvement.

Orbital myositis presents with pain on eye movement, retrobulbar pain, diplopia, swelling of the eyelids, localized injection and/or chemosis over the affected muscle insertions, and occasionally proptosis. Eye movement is often limited in the direction of the affected muscle, and movement in its field of action, or when it is stretched in the field of its antagonist, may exacerbate pain. CT scan shows enlargement of the affected muscle(s) with irregular margins. The superior muscle complex is most commonly involved, followed by the medial rectus. The extraocular muscle insertion may be thickened in up to 50% of patients, in contrast with thyroid orbitopathy, in which the muscle tendon insertions are spared. The condition may be bilateral and can recur with recurrences usually involving different muscles. Treatment is initiated with oral prednisone 1 to 2 mg/kg daily. A good response is usually noted within several days in most patients. If they fail to respond adequately, biopsy should be performed (Fig. 18.4). Patients with bilateral or multiple muscle involvement are more prone to recurrences and should be followed closely and evaluated for associated systemic disease.

Apical orbital inflammation presents with pain, minimal proptosis, decreased vision, limitation of eye movements and diplopia, often with minimal external inflammatory signs. CT scan shows irregular infiltration of the apex of the orbit, with possible extension along the muscles and nerves. This process should rarely be treated nonspecifically without a very rigorous systemic evaluation, since a variety of disorders can present in this fashion. Lymphoma, secondary tumors from adjacent sinuses, sclerosing inflammation, fungal infections, metastases, Wegener's granulomatosis, meningioma,

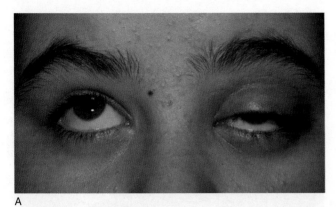

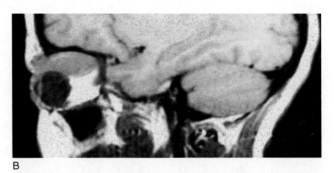

FIGURE 18.4. Idiopathic orbital inflammation (IOI) in a 13-year-old girl with previous indeterminate biopsy and no response to oral steroids. **A:** Clinical photo in upgaze shows mild left upper eyelid erythema, ptosis with reduced lid excursion, upgaze limitation, and a sub-brow scar from the previous biopsy. **B:** Sagittal MRI shows an extensive soft-tissue mass in the superior orbit engulfing the levator-superior rectus complex. Repeat biopsy of the levator muscle confirmed IOI and she responded well to high-dose intravenous steroids.

mucormycosis, and Tolosa-Hunt syndrome should be ruled out. This process often requires a longer course of high-dose corticosteroids, usually 6 to 8 weeks, for complete resolution.

Lacrimal gland inflammation, or dacryoadenitis, can result from a multitude of causes, including infections, lymphoma, sarcoidosis, Sjogren's syndrome, hematopoietic malignancy, Wegener's granulomatosis, and myriad of auto-immune disorders. It is the most common form of child-hood orbital inflammation and may be bilateral (16). The patient presents with pain, tenderness, and injection of the lateral upper eyelid and conjunctiva. The upper eyelid often demonstrates an S-shaped deformity with mild-to-moder-ate inferomedial displacement of the globe. CT scan shows infiltration confined to the superior lateral orbit, with an enlarged lacrimal gland with irregular margins that enhance with contrast, and often inferior and medial displacement of the globe. Since lacrimal gland inflammation is frequently related to systemic syndromes and has multiple causes, inci-sional biopsy through a percutaneous route is indicated if the lesion does not respond promptly to steroid treatment. Idiopathic inflammation shows a polymorphous cellular infiltration with edema, vascular dilatation, and minimal destruction of the lacrimal gland. If there is destruction of the gland, then a rigorous evaluation for organ-specific immune disorders should definitely be performed.

ORBITAL TUMORS

Orbital tumors can be classified based on the tissue of ori-gin or by the route of orbital involvement. Primary lesions originate within the orbit; secondary lesions invade the orbit from contiguous structures; and metastatic tumors spread from distant sites.

The most common primary orbital tumors in children include benign developmental cysts, vascular lesions, and neural tumors. Congenital hamartomas, anomalous growth

of tissue consisting only of mature cells normally found at the involved site (hemangioma, neurofibroma, and glioma), and choristomas, normal tissue in an abnormal anatomic location' (dermoid cyst, epidermoid cyst, lipodermoid, and teratoma), are the most common. Malignant orbital tumors are in the minority and represent a variable percentage in several large series based on referral and geographic biases (17–19). Rhabdomyosarcoma must be considered in any child presenting with a rapidly enlarging mass or progres-sive proptosis and it is the most common primary malignant orbital tumor in children. Fibro-osseous lesions arise within the orbital walls and impinge on orbital structures. Lacrimal gland tumors in children are rare. Secondary orbital tumors arise due to extension from the sinuses, intracranial fossa, eyelids, or globe. Metastatic neoplasms include neuroblas-toma, leukemia, and Ewing's sarcoma.

Dermoid Cysts and Lipodermoids

Epidermal dermoid cysts, or dermoids, are lined with nor-mal keratinizing stratified squamous epithelium with various adnexal structures in the wall, including sebaceous glands, hair follicles, and eccrine sweat glands, and the contents of the cyst include keratin, sebaceous secretions, and hair. These choristomas are formed when a piece of surface ectoderm is pinched off in a bony suture line where the tissue will gradu-ally form a cyst. They are frequently attached to the bone at the frontozygomatic (Fig. 18.5) or frontonasal suture lines. Such cysts are firm, smooth, painless, oval masses on palpa-tion that may transilluminate and may cause some bony ero-sion at the site of attachment. They may be freely mobile or may be fixed to the periosteum at the underlying suture. The more superficial cysts usually become clinically symptomatic in childhood, but the deeper orbital cysts may not become clinically symptomatic until adulthood. On CT scan, they are well-circumscribed oval masses with a low-density lumen

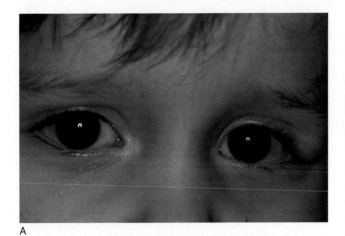
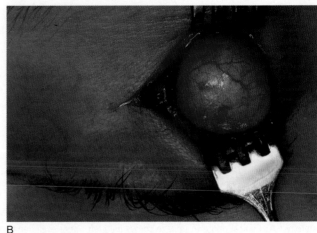

FIGURE 18.5. Dermoid cyst in a 2-year-old boy. **A:** Left superotemporal dermoid adjacent to the frontozygomatic suture. **B:** Intraoperative appearance at time of excision via a lateral lid crease incision.

and can exhibit bony expansion and erosion (Fig. 18.6). Some may occur partly in the orbit and partly in the temporal fossa, connected through a defect in the zygomatic or frontal bone, the so-called dumbbell dermoid.

Most anteriorly situated dermoid cysts can be excised easily through a lid crease incision that hides the scar nicely. Every effort should be made to remove the tumor in one piece, employing meticulous dissection, since the contents of the dermoid cyst are irritating and may result in lipogranulomatous inflammation of orbital tissues or lead to recurrences. If the dermoid cyst is accidentally ruptured or leaks during removal, copious irrigation and removal of the entire cyst should be performed. Deep orbital dermoid cysts, such as those originating from the sphenozygomatic suture and extending along the orbital roof, may require a lateral orbitotomy or occasionally a transcranial approach to assist removal. These deeper cysts generally present in young adults as a slowly progressive, painless proptosis, and inferior globe dystopia.

Lipodermoids are solid tumors that present subconjunctivally on the lateral bulbar surface over the lateral rectus muscle and may have deep extensions (Fig. 18.7). Occasionally, they also present in a medial location. Only the anterior portion of these tumors should be excised, preserving the overlying conjunctiva if at all possible. Postoperative complications include problems of motility, ptosis, and keratitis sicca secondary to damage to the lacrimal ducts.

Teratoma

Teratomas are composed of tissue elements derived from two or more of the three primary embryonic cell layers (ectoderm, endoderm, and mesoderm) and are thought to arise from pluripotent embryonic tissue. They most commonly occur in the testes, ovaries, and retroperitoneum. Orbital teratomas are rare and typically grow rapidly after birth, causing proptosis and exposure keratitis. Most are benign and localized to the

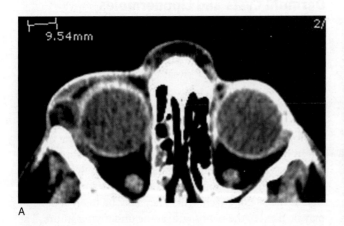
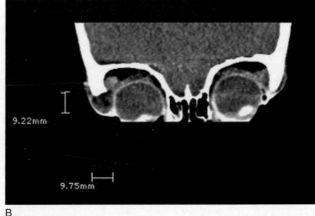

FIGURE 18.6. Dermoid cyst in a 3½-year-old boy. **A:** Axial and **B:** Coronal CT scan showing an oval cystic mass at the right superolateral orbital rim with adjacent bony remodeling. Imaging was performed because the lesion could not be distinguished from the supraorbital rim by palpation and its posterior extent could not be determined clinically.

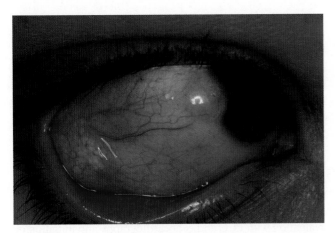

FIGURE 18.7. Lateral bulbar lipodermoid and limbal dermoid of the right eye in a 6-year-old girl.

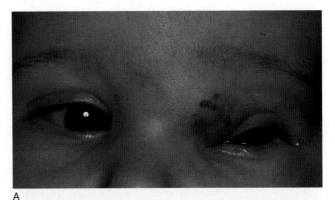

A

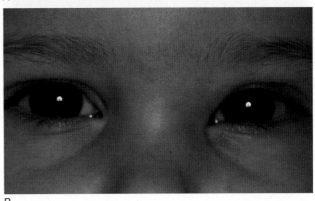

B

FIGURE 18.8. Infantile hemangioma in an 8-month-old girl. **A:** External photo shows a left superomedial orbital and upper eyelid lesion with both superficial and deeper components causing ptosis, globe dystopia, and visual axis obstruction. **B:** Appearance 4 months after intralesional steroid injection with minimal residual disease.

orbit, but rarely they can be highly malignant. They may be sharply circumscribed and, if posterior to the globe, can cause substantial deformity and remodeling of the bone orbit. They are usually heterogeneous masses with calcification, adipose tissue, and occasional bone formation. Orbital teratomas are usually multiloculated, cystic masses with solid areas. The affected eye may be dwarfed by the extent of the tumor mass. The tumor is a choristoma and consists of skin, hair, sebaceous glands, cartilage, connective tissue, and epithelium. All three layers may be represented: ectoderm, with keratinizing squamous epithelium and adnexal glandular structures; endoderm, with gastrointestinal mucosal and glandular tissues; mesoderm, with fibrous tissue, cartilage, fat, muscle, and/or bone; and neuroectoderm by mature brain. Some may be associated with brain and/or periorbital involvement and may be extensions of a primary teratoma from these sites. CT scan reveals large heterogeneous lesions with many cystic cavities and possible intracranial involvement. Treatment consists of surgical excision, perhaps with a combined neurosurgical and orbital approach, with preservation of the globe whenever possible. Occasionally, aspiration of the fluid from a large cyst may facilitate complete removal. Teratomas in other locations of the body have been known to undergo malignant transformation; those confined to the orbit are generally benign.

Infantile Hemangioma

Infantile hemangiomas (IHs) arise in infancy and are the most common benign orbital tumor of childhood. They usually appear in the first few weeks of life with increasing growth over the first 6 to 12 months of age, with an infiltrative growth pattern that may involve any portion of the orbit. The lesions may be multiple and primarily involve the head and neck regions. The clinical appearance depends on the depth of the tumor under the skin. Most have both cutaneous and subcutaneous components. When the tumor involves the skin, it is commonly called a strawberry nevus because of the reddish coloration and irregularly dimpled surface. The subcutaneous portion can extend into the orbit

causing ptosis, globe displacement, proptosis, strabismus, or astigmatism; therefore, it is important to monitor these patients for amblyopia (Fig. 18.8). IHs are soft and blanch on gentle pressure. Although benign, these tumors are unencapsulated and are hypercellular invasive lesions.

When the orbit is involved, there may be a bluish discoloration or no skin changes, and they may present as a progressively enlarging mass. The rapid growth may suggest a rhabdomyosarcoma, but the diagnosis may be differentiated by the presence of a soft mass that increases in size and assumes a blue or purplish discoloration when the child cries or strains due to vascular engorgement. Multiple large visceral capillary hemangiomas can lead to sequestration of thrombocytes and red blood cells, causing a thrombocytopenia and bleeding diathesis, the Kasabach-Merritt syndrome.

IHs have an initial growth phase, usually for up to 6 to 12 months, a stable phase, and then a spontaneous involution phase, usually after 1 year up until age of 8. They often increase remarkably in size during the first 6 months of life and then gradually diminish. The majority of the vessels disappear, but the larger veins persist. In rapidly proliferating lesions, ulceration, necrosis, bleeding, and infection can occur. As the lesion becomes smaller, the reddish color fades to a light gray and the mass is less compressible.

CT and MRI scans of these lesions demonstrate the margins to vary from moderately well defined to infiltrating masses. They may involve any compartment, both intraconal and extraconal, preseptal and postseptal. Intravenous contrast causes a moderate to intense enhancement, which can be homogeneous or nonhomogeneous. On T1-weighted MRI, capillary hemangiomas have a low signal intensity compared to fat, and a high signal intensity compared to the extraocular muscles. On T2-weighted MRI, they have high signal intensity with respect to fat and extraocular muscles, and there may be areas of flow void.

Conservative treatment is usually best since there is a strong tendency for these lesions to spontaneously regress. However, treatment must be considered when visual complications develop such as deprivational amblyopia from ptosis, anisometropia from induced astigmatism, or strabismus. A variety of therapeutic options, depending on location, depth, and patient age are available for lesions that require treatment. Historically, the primary treatment was systemic, topical, and/or intralesional corticosteroids, managed in conjunction with the pediatrician who monitored for systemic side effects. The mechanism of action of steroids is not fully understood, but they probably stimulate vasoconstriction by making the tumor more sensitive to circulating catecholamines.

Intralesional corticosteroids are helpful, especially for IH of the upper eyelid causing amblyopia. A combination of a long-acting steroid (e.g., triamcinolone, 40 mg/mL) and short-acting steroid (e.g., betamethasone, 6 mg/mL) is injected directly into the lesion with a 23-gauge needle (20). The needle is placed into a few areas of the lesion, withdrawn first, and then injected. There is a small risk of embolization of the depot material into a vessel, which could result in a central retinal artery occlusion. Most lesions will involute with one injection, but occasionally a second injection may be required if the response is not adequate.

For large hemangiomas, or deep orbital lesions, oral corticosteroids (e.g., prednisone 1 to 2 mg/kg/day) may be required. Systemic corticosteroids should be administered under the guidance of a pediatrician while monitoring for side effects. The response is often complete in 6 weeks, but the lesion may increase in size as the dose is tapered. The side effects of corticosteroids, both local and systemic, are many and include eyelid necrosis, linear subcutaneous fat atrophy, local fat atrophy, retrobulbar hemorrhage, ocular penetration, central retinal and/or choroidal embolization, gastritis, Cushing syndrome, adrenal suppression, and failure to thrive.

Lasers and surgical procedures have limited application as primary treatments. However, cutaneous laser therapy is helpful in reducing remaining vessels that do not involute completely. In rare instances of circumscribed lesions, excision may be indicated. There is no capsule surrounding these lesions, but a safe excision can be performed with the appropriate use of cautery. The surgeon should be aware that IHs in and around the orbit usually have a high blood flow, derived from multiple fine feeder arterial vessels from the internal and/or external carotid artery, and are capable of bleeding profusely if surgical excision is undertaken.

Currently, the primary treatment for periocular IH is oral propranolol based on the incidental discovery of its efficacy (21). Since this initial report in severe refractory hemangiomas, the efficacy and safety of oral and even topical beta-blockers has been reported in several retrospective series (22–25). The usual dosage is 0.5 mg/kg/day, divided into three doses, for the first week and increasing to 1 to 2 mg/kg/day provided the children have no cardiac or pulmonary disease and are not premature infants. The studies varied in the need for pretreatment pediatric cardiology evaluation with ECG and echocardiography and initiation of treatment on an inpatient or outpatient basis. Home pulse and blood pressure monitoring is recommended. Treatment is discontinued when the response plateaus and side effects such as bradycardia, hypotension, hypoglycemia, and sleep disturbances are generally mild.

The three potential explanations for the therapeutic effects of propranolol on IHs are induction of vasoconstriction, reducing expression of basic fibroblast growth factor and vascular endothelial growth factor, and triggering apoptosis of capillary endothelial cells. Propranolol is not always successful and prospective randomized trial data on its use are needed.

Lymphangioma

Lymphangiomas are typically diffuse unencapsulated choristomatous primitive vascular tumors that infiltrate the normal tissues of the eyelid and orbit and usually become clinically apparent in the first decade of life. They are generally multilobular and easily compressible and may involve the conjunctiva, eyelids, orbit, scalp, oropharynx, and sinuses, and rarely spread intracranially. The natural progression is variable and unpredictable. Some are small, localized, and slowly progressive and others may diffusely infiltrate the orbital structures and enlarge relentlessly. They may be exacerbated by viral upper respiratory tract infection due to an activation of the lymphoid follicles located in the interstitium. The female-to-male ratio is approximately 3:1 and the tumors show a predilection for the superior and inferior nasal aspects of the orbit.

The histogenesis remains unclear, but they are thought to represent a combined vascular malformation with both venous and lymphatic components. Lymphangiomas are characterized by slow, indolent growth, with acute exacerbations occurring over minutes to a few hours secondary to spontaneous or traumatic hemorrhage. The thin walls of the lymphatic channels may rupture spontaneously or with minor trauma, creating blood-filled cysts (chocolate cysts), which contain old, dark blood. Patients have pain due to the rapid distention of the orbital tissues. There is no connection with the lymphatic or vascular system, so no pulsation is present. Patients may also have induced ptosis, proptosis

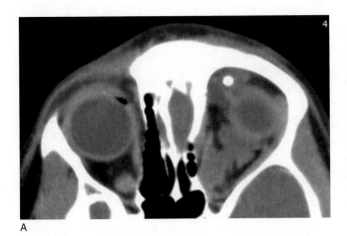
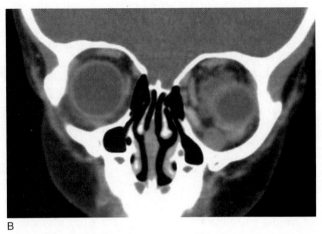

FIGURE 18.9. Lymphangioma in a 5-year-old girl. She presented to the ER with left eye pain and swelling with associated nausea and vomiting. There was no history of trauma. **A:** Axial CT scan with both intraconal and extraconal homogeneous soft-tissue disease of the left orbit and with a calcified phlebolith superonasally that suggested the diagnosis. **B:** Coronal CT scan showing a multilobular left orbital soft-tissue mass in the medial, inferior, and retrobulbar areas.

or globe dystopia, glaucoma, optic nerve compression, and strabismus. Induced astigmatism may develop because of pressure on the globe and this may precipitate anisometropia and amblyopia.

CT and MRI scans demonstrate an unencapsulated infiltrative lesion that extends across the orbital spaces into many tissues, with variable densities, creating a heterogeneous mass (Figs. 18.9 and 18.10). Cystic spaces containing blood, plasma, or lymphatic tissue may be present. This combination of solid and cystic components in a pediatric tumor is typical of lymphangioma. Noncontiguous intracranial vascular malformations have been reported in up to 25% of patients (Fig. 18.10), and therefore MRI imaging of the brain should be performed to detect asymptomatic CNS lesions that may subsequently bleed.

Histologically, lymphangiomas are composed of irregularly sized and shaped dilated, serum-filled, thin-walled vascular channels lined with flattened endothelium in a loose fibrous stroma that contains bundles of smooth muscle and collections of lymphocytes. The endothelial spaces have no pericytes or smooth muscle in their walls. Scattered follicles of lymphoid tissues are located in the interstitium. The stroma has a variable amount of connective tissue that may exhibit evidence of scarring, hemosiderin deposition, and cholesterol clefts from previous hemorrhagic episodes. Thrombosis and calcification (see Fig. 18.9) may be present. The tumors have an infiltrative growth pattern and are not encapsulated. The vascular channels are partially filled with proteinaceous and homogeneous eosinophilic fluid material.

These tumors are often progressive from early childhood until mid-adolescence. Older patients tend to stabilize and have fewer of the acute manifestations commonly observed in children. However, the tumors do not regress like IHs.

Complete surgical excision is usually not possible due to the infiltrative intertwining pattern of growth and a conservative approach is generally recommended. Surgical debulking of the tumor or aspiration of blood cysts may

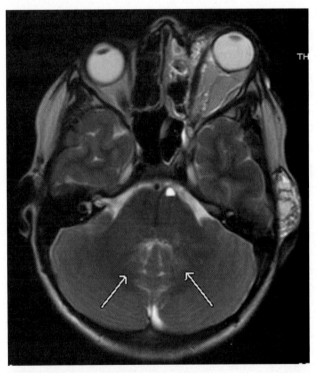

FIGURE 18.10. Lymphangioma in a 12-year-old boy with a long history and several prior drainage procedures and partial excisions. He presented with acute hemorrhage, deep orbital pain and nausea, and bradycardia from the oculocardiac (vasovagal) reflex. Axial T2 MRI reveals extensive orbital cysts in the intraconal space extending to the orbital apex and cavernous sinus. Bilateral developmental venous anomalies in the cerebellum and cerebrum, most predominantly seen in the deep white matter of the cerebellum (*arrows*), are also present. Another lymphangioma deposit is present in the left periauricular scalp.

be considered when acute orbital hemorrhage compromises the globe or optic nerve, for marked proptosis and exposure complications, or for intractable vasovagal symptoms. Bleeding may result from minimal trauma with rupture of a component vessel, or possibly spontaneous hemorrhage from fragile neovascular tufts. After a hemorrhage occurs, excision of the blood cyst is possible, but spontaneous regression is common. There is a high incidence of recurrent hemorrhage. The orbital tissues may become fibrotic and infiltrated with the malformation, making differentiation of normal and abnormal tissues difficult during surgery. Since the lesions do not respect tissue planes, portions of the tumor may be left to avoid damage to important normal structures.

Systemic corticosteroids have been used with some success for symptomatic relief of pain, loss of vision, and motility dysfunction during acute exacerbations, presumably by decreasing inflammation and edema (26). They may cause a reduction of lymphoid hypertrophy, stabilizing the vasculature to decrease hemorrhage and fluid osmosis into the tissues and causing the channels to involute. Corticosteroid use in children seems to have a better effect on proptosis and mass effect than in adults.

Recently, percutaneous aspiration and intralesional sclerosing therapy has added another promising treatment modality for lymphangiomas (27,28). It is hypothesized that this therapy targets the endothelial cells of the abnormal membranes that make up the cystic spaces leading to fibrous adhesion and obliteration while sparing the normal orbital tissues. These retrospective studies showed sclerosing agents to be safe with limited adverse outcomes, but larger prospective studies are needed.

Rhabdomyosarcoma

Rhabdomyosarcoma is the most common primary orbital malignant tumor in children, with an average age of onset of 8 to 10 years. The orbit is considered a prognostically favorable site. It arises from undifferentiated pluripotent mesenchymal cells of the orbit with histologic features of striated muscle in various stages of embryogenesis. This mesenchymal tumor can originate from many different areas of the body, including the orbit (10%), head and neck (25%), genitourinary tract (23%), and extremities (17%). It also originates in smaller percentages from the trunk, retroperitoneum, chest, perineum, and gastrointestinal tract. Histologic subtypes include embryonal, alveolar, botryoid, and pleomorphic. More than 70% will occur in the first decade of life, but this tumor may present from birth to the seventh decade.

Embryonal rhabdomyosarcoma is the most common histologic type, present in more than 80% of cases, and consists of loose fascicles of undifferentiated spindle cells with eosinophilic cytoplasm. It characteristically develops in the superior nasal orbit, displacing the eye down and outward, and is associated with a survival rate of 94% (29). The tumor may involve any part of the orbit and rarely arises from the conjunctiva.

The most malignant form is alveolar, accounting for 9% of orbital rhabdomyosarcoma, with a predilection for the inferior orbit. It consists of rhabdomyoblasts arranged in an alveolar pattern with necrotic cells sloughing into the center.

The pleomorphic, which is the least common and most differentiated form, occurs in older persons and has the best prognosis of 97% survival. The botryoid is a rare variant, appears grapelike, and is not a primary tumor of the orbit, but invades the orbit from the paranasal sinuses or conjunctiva.

Any child presenting with the rapid onset of painless proptosis, over a period of several days to a few weeks, should be considered to have a rhabdomyosarcoma until proven otherwise (Figs. 18.11 and 18.12). There is often discoloration and edema of the eyelids and frequently there is a vague history of unrelated trauma. Imaging should be performed promptly and CT scan typically reveals a well-circumscribed mass of homogeneous density, which is isodense in relation to normal muscle with moderate to marked contrast enhancement, and may have areas of bone destruction. On MRI scan, they appear isointense or slightly hypointense compared to brain on T1-weighted images, and hyperintense on T2-weighted imaging.

If rhabdomyosarcoma is still suspected after imaging, evaluation should proceed rapidly in conjunction with a pediatric oncologist. Biopsy of the tumor by an anterior orbitotomy approach should be performed as soon as possible. If possible, an attempt to remove the entire lesion should be made, provided this does not risk visual loss, and frequently the pseudocapsule allows complete resection. If not, larger lesions should be debulked as extensively as possible, as the staging is partially dependent on the extent of disease and the smaller the volume of residual tumor, the more effective the subsequent treatment (30).

Preauricular, submandibular, and cervical lymph nodes should be palpated to detect regional metastasis and a chest CT scan, bone marrow aspirate and biopsy, and lumbar puncture are performed to evaluate for distant metastasis. The brain and lungs are primary sites for metastases. The tumor can also erode into the sinuses, causing nasal stuffiness and nosebleeds.

Statistics from the Intergroup Rhabdomyosarcoma Study reveal a 3-year survival rate of 93% for children with localized orbital rhabdomyosarcoma (29). Chemotherapy appears to be of greatest value when disease is limited to the orbit. Completely resected tumors with negative margins may not require radiation, whereas patients with microscopic residual orbital disease and/or lymph node metastases receive both chemotherapy and radiation. The Intergroup Rhabdomyosarcoma Studies I–IV delivered a total dose of local radiation, from 4,500 to 6,000 cGy, over a 6-week period and systemic chemotherapy to eliminate microscopic cellular metastases with a survival rate of more than 90% if the tumor was confined to the orbit, compared with only a 25% to 35% survival rate in 1970. There is a worse prognosis if tumor spreads into the paranasal sinuses or meninges. Disfiguring orbital exenteration is reserved for the rare radio-resistant or multidrug-resistant tumor.

With a longer survival rate for patients with rhabdomyosarcoma treated with chemotherapy and radiation, ocular and orbital complications are common including visual

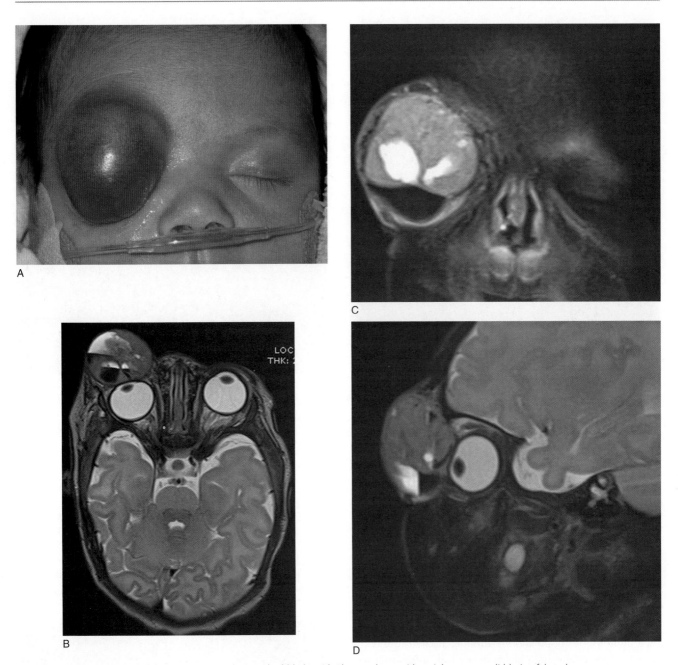

FIGURE 18.11. Possible rhabdomyosarcoma in a 2-week-old baby girl. She was born with a right upper eyelid lesion felt to be vascular, most likely an infantile hemangioma. **A:** Clinical photo of the rapidly enlarging right superoanterior orbital mass that precluded a view of the globe. **B:** Axial T2 MRI; **C:** Coronal T2 MRI; and **D:** Sagittal T2 MRI show a large relatively encapsulated mass anterior to the right globe with cystic areas containing fluid levels compatible with hemorrhage and solid portions with homogeneous enhancement, most consistent with rhabdomyosarcoma. Anterior orbitotomy via an upper eyelid crease incision showed a partially necrotic mass with hemorrhagic cysts that was nearly totally excised with frozen section pathology revealing a small round blue cell neoplasm. After extensive review of histologic, immunophenotypic, and cytogenetic findings, and outside pathologic consultation, the final diagnosis was undifferentiated round cell sarcoma with biphenotypic mesenchymal and epithelial features.

impairment, cataracts, dry eye, radiation retinopathy, ptosis, enophthalmos, and orbital hypoplasia (31). After finishing treatment, children need to be followed closely every few months with a comprehensive ocular examination to monitor for these complications. Also, the incidence of second malignant neoplasms is increasing and includes acute nonlymphoblastic leukemia, leiomyosarcoma, adrenocortical carcinoma, epidermoid carcinoma, malignant melanoma, fibrillary astrocytomas, and osteogenic sarcoma. Any bone in the radiation field may be involved. Thus, these patients require lifelong follow-up with craniofacial and systemic evaluations.

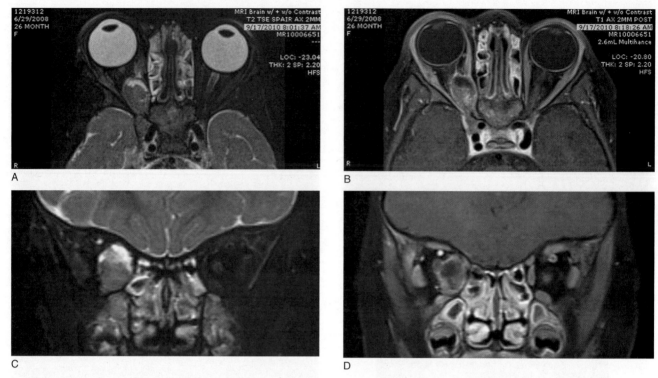

FIGURE 18.12. Malignant rhabdoid tumor in a 2-year-old girl who presented with right-sided proptosis and third cranial nerve palsy that developed over a 2-week period. **A:** Axial T2 MRI; **B:** Axial T1 fat sat postcontrast MRI; **C:** Coronal T2 MRI; **D:** Coronal T1 fat sat postcontrast MRI images show a right orbital apex mass extending into the superior orbital fissure and cavernous sinus. It has mixed cystic and solid contrast-enhancing components. A swinging lower eyelid inferior fornix transconjunctival anterior orbitotomy approach was used for biopsy and revealed a small round blue cell tumor (SRBCT) on frozen section that subsequently was diagnosed as a malignant rhabdoid tumor.

Small Round Blue Cell Tumors

When an orbital biopsy is performed in a child with possible rhabdomyosarcoma, the frozen section report from the pathologist is usually interpreted as a small round blue cell tumor (SRBCT), final diagnosis pending (Figs. 18.11 and 18.12). This group of malignant neoplasms is characterized by a monotonous population of undifferentiated round cell tumors that require immunohistochemical, ultrastructural, cytogenetic, and molecular techniques to accurately diagnose. The differential diagnosis of SRBCTs in children varies according to the site of presentation and age, but includes alveolar rhabdomyosarcoma, Ewing's sarcoma/primitive neuroectodermal tumor (EWS/PNET), neuroblastoma, malignant rhabdoid tumor (Fig. 18.12), and lymphoblastic lymphoma for the orbit. Achieving the correct diagnosis by representative biopsy is important so that the oncologist can select the proper treatment protocol.

Neurofibroma

Neurofibromas are slow-growing congenital tumors of the peripheral nerves, composed of proliferating Schwann cells within the nerve sheaths, with axons, endoneural fibroblasts, and mucin. Large plexiform neurofibromas may produce a

slowly progressive proptosis and may also involve the eyelids (Fig. 18.13). Neurofibroma of the orbit may occur as an isolated lesion, where it may be excised without recurrence, or it may be part of the generalized disease neurofibromatosis. Due

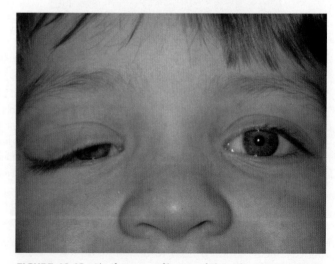

FIGURE 18.13. Plexiform neurofibroma of the right orbit in a 5-year-old boy. He has an S-shaped lid deformity, ptosis, and an expanded and elongated upper eyelid from the orbitopalpebral tumor.

to the variable expression of the mutations and the fact that the disease manifests in multiple tissues and organs, the NIH in 1990 established guidelines for the diagnoses of neurofibromatosis type 1 (NF1) and neurofibromatosis type 2 (NF2). NF1 includes any two of the following: six or more café au lait spots, two or more neurofibromas or one plexiform neurofibroma, axillary or inguinal freckling, optic glioma, osseous lesions, Lisch nodules, or a first-degree relative with NF1. NF2 includes either bilateral acoustic neuromas or a first-degree relative with NF2, in addition to either a unilateral eighth nerve palsy or two other lesions: neurofibroma, meningioma, glioma, schwannoma, or juvenile posterior subcapsular lenticular opacity. A negative family history does not exclude the disease as half of all new cases of NF1 and even a greater proportion of NF2 cases present as new, sporadic mutations.

NF1 is inherited as an autosomal dominant disorder with irregular penetrance, variable expressivity, and a high spontaneous mutation rate, with the defect localized to the long arm of chromosome 17. It is classified as a phakomatosis since the hamartomas involves the skin, eye, CNS, and viscera. It has multiple manifestations including Lisch nodules, café au lait spots, prominent corneal nerves, perilimbal neurofibromas, neurofibromas, glaucoma, megaloglobus, pigmentary hamartomas of the uveal tract, optic nerve and CNS tumors, and occasionally tumors of the spinal cord, sympathetic nerves, and adrenals. About one-third of patients that present with optic nerve glioma have NF1.

NF2 is ten times more rare than NF1 and has CNS meningiomas, acoustic neuromas, and presenile lens opacities. The defect is localized to the long arm of chromosome 22. Many of the typical characteristics are absent during infancy and develop only later in childhood and adolescence, and signs and symptoms often worsen during periods of high hormonal activity such as pregnancy.

Palpation of an orbitopalpebral plexiform neurofibroma reveals a typical "bag of worms" feeling and it may cause an S-shaped deformity of the upper eyelid (Fig. 18.13). These tortuous, fibrous cords infiltrate normal tissues, making excision of the tumor difficult and often incomplete. The globe itself, including sclera, iris, ciliary body, cornea, and choroid, can be infiltrated, resulting in glaucoma and buphthalmos. Pulsation of the eye may occur due to a partial absence of the sphenoid bone. On CT imaging, neurofibromas are contrast enhancing, irregular soft-tissue infiltrations. On MRI scans, they are heterogeneous and hypointense on T1-weighted images and have high signal intensity on T2-weighted images with respect to orbital fat. They have variable enhancement with gadolinium and are best visualized with fat suppression.

The management of plexiform neurofibromas is difficult and frustrating for the patient and family, as well as the ophthalmologist. The cosmetic results are often inadequate and temporary. The surgical management is repeated debulking with eyelid reconstruction and ptosis repair. The management of these lesions differs in adults and children. Rapid growth of neurofibromas typically occurs in children and adolescents, and they should be followed with close observation to allow timely intervention with appropriate surgical procedures. If there is normal development of the visual system, major surgical procedures should be delayed until the disease process has slowed, at which time a more permanent and definitive procedure may be performed. Radiotherapy is ineffective for neurofibromas.

Optic Nerve Glioma

Optic nerve glioma, also known as juvenile pilocytic astrocytoma, is cytologically benign and is the most common pediatric optic nerve tumor. They may occur anywhere along the optic pathway or hypothalamus and may be isolated or may occur with NF1. Thus, NF1 patients should be monitored for early detection of optic pathway glioma, examining for signs such as visual loss, afferent pupillary defects, and optic atrophy. Annual routine follow-up should be continued until the patient is at least 17 years old. In asymptomatic NF1 patients, routine imaging has little benefit (32). However, if symptomatic, MRI should be performed which shows fusiform enlargement of the optic nerve, often with chiasmal involvement, confirming the diagnosis, and biopsy is not warranted. The behavior of optic nerve glioma can be quite variable, but in the absence of progressive visual loss or extreme proptosis, observation is indicated. Little correlation exists between visual function and tumor size. Surgical excision of the optic nerve may be indicated if there is progression intracranially through the optic canal, to protect the optic chiasm, or for reduction of extreme proptosis with exposure keratitis in nonsighted eyes. Radiation and chemotherapy have also been utilized for selected cases, but the decision to initiate treatment is complicated by reports of spontaneous regression.

Lymphoma

Orbital lymphoma is rare in childhood, except for Burkitt lymphoma (BL) and, more recently, acquired immunodeficiency syndrome-associated lymphoma. BL is a mature B-cell non-Hodgkin lymphoma that has three major variants: the endemic (African) form; the sporadic form; and the immunodeficiency-associated form (33). The endemic form occurs in equatorial Africa, where it commonly involves the mandible or maxilla, and secondarily the orbit. It has also been reported to occur in association with Epstein–Barr virus (EBV) infection and as a manifestation of HIV infection and AIDS. The sporadic form of the disease occurs in nonendemic areas around the world where it typically manifests as an abdominal tumor with bone marrow involvement, but rarely occurs with orbital involvement. A recent review of orbital BL in immunocompetent patients found children to be most frequently effected, usually presenting with proptosis without a palpable mass and often with adjacent sinus involvement and eventual systemic disease with a guarded prognosis (33). If a biopsy specimen confirms the presence of a malignant lymphoma, a careful systemic examination of the child is necessary to reveal the exact stage of the disease process.

There is a wide spectrum of lymphoproliferative diseases from benign lymphoid hyperplasia to malignant lymphoma. These lymphoid proliferations may present a diagnostic challenge because the biopsies are generally small and neither cytologic nor architectural findings may be sufficient to distinguish between reactive and malignant processes. An open biopsy is preferred and an experienced pathologist, using immunophenotyping and flow cytometric analysis in conjunction with clinical and histologic findings, is required to arrive at the correct diagnosis. Chemotherapy is the treatment of choice for lymphoma with the specific regimen depending on the histology and extent of the disease.

Neuroblastoma

Neuroblastoma arises from the adrenal medulla of infants and young children or from any cells of neural crest origin in the autonomic chain of the postganglionic sympathetic nervous system. Neuroblastoma originates in the abdomen in the majority of cases. It is the most common solid tumor in children, accounting for about 10% of pediatric cancers. Most present before the age of 3 years and 90% occur in children younger than 5 years of age, but they can occur any time in the first two decades of life. Orbital involvement occurs as metastatic disease and neuroblastoma is second to rhabdomyosarcoma as the most frequent orbital malignancy of childhood. When it metastasizes to the orbital bones, usually to the lateral wall, it produces periorbital ecchymosis and marked proptosis. Almost all orbital involvement in

neuroblastoma represents advanced, widely metastatic disease (stage IV) with poor survival (34).

CT imaging, as well as bone scan and bone marrow biopsy, should be performed to find the primary lesion and metastatic deposits. If CT scan of the orbits demonstrates a mass with bony destruction, metastatic neuroblastoma must be considered in the differential diagnosis (Fig. 18.14). Urinary excretion of catecholamines is increased in 90% of neuroblastoma patients. Treatment of neuroblastoma includes surgical excision of the primary lesion, radiation therapy with or without total body irradiation, autologous bone marrow rescue, and aggressive combination chemotherapy for disseminated disease.

Leukemia

Leukemic infiltration of one or both orbits in the pediatric age group occurs most commonly with acute myelogenous leukemia, but may also occur with chronic myelogenous and acute and chronic lymphocytic disease (35). Granulocytic sarcoma (chloroma) is soft-tissue infiltration by myelogenous leukemia. The term chloroma comes from the greenish hue of the fresh specimen due to the presence of myeloperoxidase. Orbital involvement may develop before, during, or after the diagnosis of systemic leukemia. It presents as a rapidly expanding tumor causing proptosis, which is often bilateral, with a mean age of onset of 7 to 9 years. The CT scan appearance is as homogeneous masses that mold to orbital bone, most commonly the lateral wall. In the absence of any hematologic evidence of disease, orbital biopsy is needed. The primary treatment is multi-agent chemotherapy. If the lesion is large, or if there is compressive optic neuropathy;

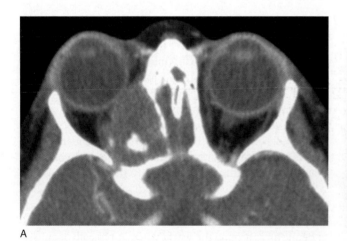

A

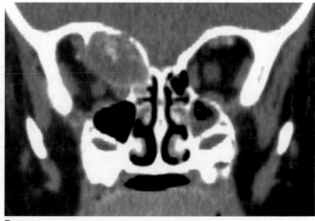

B

FIGURE 18.14. Myofibroma in a 14-month-old boy who presented with right proptosis that developed over 1 week. **A:** Axial and **B:** Coronal CT scans show an expansile bony destructive mass, partially calcified, within the posterior medial wall of the right orbit, most consistent with neuroblastoma or Langerhans cell histiocytosis. Biopsy via an upper eyelid crease anterior orbitotomy showed a cytologically bland spindle cell proliferation with collagenous stroma consistent with myofibromatosis. **C:** Two-week postoperative photo shows a healing right upper eyelid crease scar with residual inferior dystopia of the right eye. **D:** Axial T2 MRI; **E:** Axial T1 fat sat post-contrast MRI; **F:** Coronal T2 MRI images done after biopsy as a baseline showing T2 isointense mass with diffuse homogeneous enhancement.

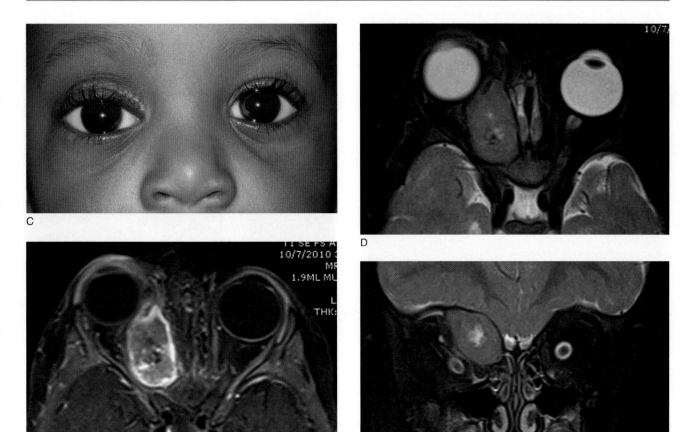

FIGURE 18.14. (*continued*)

radiotherapy can be efficacious. The prognosis is improving with intensive chemotherapy and bone marrow transplantation when in remission (35).

BONY DISEASES OF THE ORBIT

Fibrous Dysplasia of Bone

Fibrous dysplasia of bone manifests as a replacement of the normal bone medullary cavity with immature bone, fibrous hyperplasia, and osteoid, which distorts the medullary bone. The lack of osteoblasts prevents normal bone formation. It is a benign developmental disorder of the bone that can be mono- or polyostotic. Most orbital lesions involve multiple skull bones, not respecting the suture lines, and all bones may be involved. When the orbital bones are affected, the volume of the orbit is reduced resulting in proptosis and globe displacement. CT scan confirms the diagnosis by showing a sclerotic bony lesion with ground-glass appearance (Fig. 18.15). Histopathologic examination reveals bony trabeculae composed of woven bone within a fibrous stroma. These lesions often grow rapidly during early life and then stabilize after puberty, but occasionally they may progress into adulthood. The association of polyostotic fibrous bony

lesions with cutaneous pigmentation and endocrine disorders is known as McCune-Albright syndrome, which occurs largely in females and is also associated with sexual precocity and a postzygotic mutation in the G-protein. The etiology of fibrous dysplasia is unknown, and malignant transformation is very rare and usually associated with prior irradiation.

The major clinical signs and symptoms vary according to the site and extent of bone involvement. Facial asymmetry, proptosis, and globe displacement are the most common presentations. A slowly progressive visual loss may occur from compression of the optic nerve in the optic canal or at the optic chiasm. Although rare, there can be rapid progression, increased pain, and infiltrative features, and one must rule out malignant transformation to osteosarcoma, fibrosarcoma, chondrosarcoma, and giant cell sarcoma.

Treatment is generally conservative with diagnostic imaging and regular observation, with intervention for gross deformity, functional deficits, pain, or sarcomatous transformation. If the lesion is well localized, resection, curettage with bone grafting, or contouring may be performed. Recently, a more aggressive and earlier intervention, using a multidisciplinary craniofacial approach, has been reported with removal of as much affected bone as possible and reconstruction as a one-stage procedure (36).

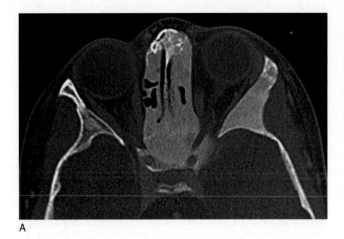
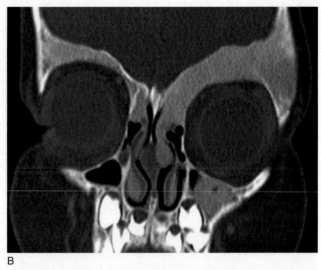

FIGURE 18.15. Fibrous dysplasia in a 7-year-old girl evaluated for facial asymmetry and left hypoglobus. **A:** Axial and **B:** Coronal CT showing osseous expansion of the diploic space with ground-glass density involving the frontal, ethmoid, and sphenoid bones bilaterally, left greater than right, and left zygomatic bone.

Langerhans Cell Histiocytosis

LCH includes a broad spectrum of disorders including acute disseminated LCH (e.g., Letterer-Siwe disease), multifocal LCH (e.g., Hand-Schüller-Christian syndrome), and unifocal LCH (e.g., eosinophilic granuloma) (37). Orbital involvement by LCH most often represents unifocal disease. The condition is uncommon and orbital disease usually involves the superior temporal quadrant, associated with an osteolytic defect of the orbital roof caused by proliferating Langerhans cells in the bone marrow (Fig. 18.16). There is a male predominance, with onset in the first or second decade of life. Symptoms include rapidly progressive upper eyelid edema and erythema, bone pain, and tenderness that

is often initially misdiagnosed as periorbital or orbital cellulitis (Fig. 18.16). CT scan shows extensive destruction of the frontal bone which suggests LCH, or possibly metastatic malignancy, and anterior orbitotomy with incisional biopsy is required to confirm the diagnosis. If frozen section pathology supports the diagnosis, curettage or intralesional steroid injection may be performed.

The lesion's cellular components include pathologic Langerhans cells, chronic inflammatory cells, and eosinophils. Once pathologically confirmed, systemic evaluation by a pediatric oncologist is undertaken including a thorough physical exam, skeletal survey, and bone scan. Although controversial, pediatric oncologists consider the

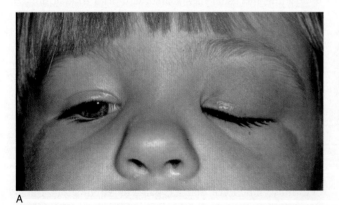
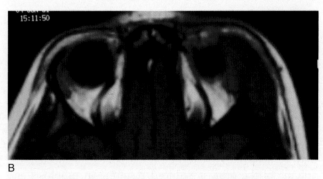

FIGURE 18.16. Langerhans cell histiocytosis in a 2-year-old girl. She had been treated with oral antibiotics for 2 weeks for presumed left preseptal cellulitis with no response. **A:** Presenting appearance on downgaze with left upper eyelid erythema, edema, and ptosis. There was a mass palpable along the lateral supraorbital rim. **B:** Axial T1 and **C:** Coronal T1 MRI show a left superolateral orbital mass that extends through the bone into the anterior cranial fossa. **D:** Appearance 6 weeks after anterior orbitotomy with biopsy, curettage, and intralesional steroid injection.

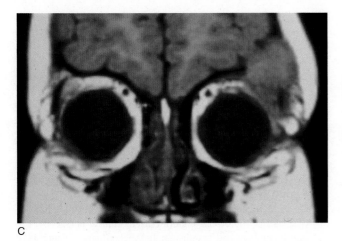

C

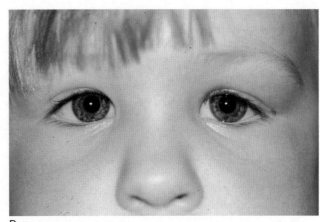

D

FIGURE 18.16. (*continued*)

orbit a risk site for CNS involvement, and for development of diabetes insipidus, and often recommend chemotherapy, even with unifocal orbital disease (38). Patients should be

followed to confirm resolution of the orbital disease with timely reossification and to monitor for progression to multifocal disease (39).

REFERENCES

1. Mills DM, Tsai S, Meyer DR, Belden C. Perspective: pediatric ophthalmic computed tomographic scanning and associated cancer risk. *Am J Ophthalmol* 2006;142:1046–1053.
2. Neudorfer M, Leibovitch I, Stolovitch C, et al. Intraorbital and periorbital tumors in children-value of ultrasound and color doppler imaging in the differential diagnosis. *Am J Ophthalmol* 2004;137:1065–1072.
3. Griepentrog GJ, Lucarelli MJ. Heritable unilateral clinical anophthalmia. *Ophthal Plast Reconstr Surg* 2004;20:166–168.
4. Chaudhry IA, Arat YO, Shamsi FA, Boniuk M. Congenital microphthalmos with orbital cysts: distinct diagnostic features and management. *Ophthal Plast Reconstr Surg* 2004;20:452–457.
5. Tse DT, Abdulhafez M, Orozco MA, et al. Evaluation of an integrated orbital tissue expander in congenital anophthalmos: report of preliminary clinical experience. *Am J Ophthalmol* 2011;151:470–482.
6. Nouby G. Congenital upper eyelid coloboma and cryptophthalmos. *Ophthal Plast Reconstr Surg* 2002;18:373–377.
7. McCarty ML, Wilson MW, Fleming JC, et al. Manifestations of fungal cellulitis of the orbit in children with neutropenia and fever. *Ophthal Plast Reconstr Surg* 2004;20:217–223.
8. Garcia GH, Harris GJ. Criteria for nonsurgical management of subperiosteal abscess of the orbit. Analysis of outcomes 1988–1998. *Ophthalmology* 2000;107:1454–1458.
9. Harris GJ. Subperiosteal abscess of the orbit: age as a factor in the bacteriology and response to treatment. *Ophthalmology* 1994;101:585–595.
10. Todman MS, Enzer YR. Medical management versus surgical intervention of pediatric orbital cellulitis: the importance of subperiosteal abscess volume as a new criterion. *Ophthal Plast Reconstr Surg* 2011;27:255–259.
11. Dewan MA, Meyer DR, Wladis EJ. Orbital cellulitis with subperiosteal abscess: demographics and management outcomes. *Ophthal Plast Reconstr Surg* 2011;27:330–332.

12. Yen MT, Yen KG. Effect of corticosteroids in the acute management of pediatric orbital cellulitis with subperiosteal abscess. *Ophthal Plast Reconstr Surg* 2005;21:363–367.
13. Krassas GE, Segni M, Wiersinga WM. Childhood Graves' ophthalmopathy: results of a European questionnaire study. *Eur J Endocrinol* 2005;153:515–520.
14. Durairaj VD, Bartley GB, Garrity JA. Clinical features and treatment of Graves ophthalmopathy in pediatric patients. *Ophthal Plast Reconstr Surg* 2006;22:7–12.
15. Goldstein SM, Katowitz WR, Moshang T, Katowitz JA. Pediatric thyroid–associated orbitopathy: the children's hospital of Philadelphia experience and literature review. *Thyroid* 2008;18:997–999.
16. Belanger C, Zhang KS, Reddy AK, Yen MT, Yen KG. Inflammatory disorders of the orbit in childhood: a case series. *Am J Ophthalmol* 2010;150:460–463.
17. Bullock JD, Goldberg SH, Rakes SM. Orbital tumors in children. *Ophthal Plast Reconstr Surg* 1989;5:13–16.
18. Shields JA, Bakewell B, Augsburger JJ, et al. Space-occupying orbital masses in children: a review of 250 consecutive biopsies. *Ophthalmology* 1986;93:379–384.
19. Kodsi SR, Shetlar DJ, Campbell RJ, et al. A review of 340 orbital tumors in children during a 60-year period. *Am J Ophthalmol* 1994;117:177–182.
20. Kushner BJ. Intralesional corticosteroid injection for infantile adnexal hemangioma. *Am J Ophthalmol* 1982;93:496–506.
21. Léauté-Labrèze C, Dumas de la Roque E, Hubiche T, Boralevi F, Thambo JB, Taïeb A. Propranolol for severe hemangiomas of infancy. *N Engl J Med* 2008;358(24):2649–2651.
22. Missoi TG, Lueder GT, Gilbertson K, Bayliss SJ. Oral propranolol for treatment of periocular infantile hemangiomas. *Arch Ophthalmol* 2011;129:899–903.
23. Dhaybi RA, Superstein R, Milet A, Powell J, et al. Treatment of periocular infantile hemangiomas with propranolol: case series of 18 children. *Ophthalmology* 2011;118:1184–1188.

24. Fridman G, Grieser E, Hill R, Khussus N, Bersani T, Slonim C. Propranolol for the treatment of orbital infantile hemangiomas. *Ophthal Plast Reconstr Surg* 2011;27:190–194.

25. Guo S, Ni N. Topical treatment for capillary hemangioma of the eyelid using beta-blocker solution. *Arch Ophthalmol* 2010;128:255–256.

26. Sires BS, Goins CR, Anderson RL, et al. Systemic corticosteroid use in orbital lymphangioma. *Ophthal Plast Reconstr Surg* 2001;17:85–90.

27. Schwarcz RM, Ben Simon GJ, Cook T, Goldberg RA. Sclerosing therapy as first line treatment for low flow vascular lesions of the orbit. *Am J Ophthalmol* 2006;141:333–339.

28. Hill III RH, Shiels II WE, Foster JA, et al. Percutaneous drainage and ablation as first line therapy for macrocystic and microcystic orbital lymphatic malformations. *Ophthal Plast Reconstr Surg* 2012;28:119–125.

29. Wharam M, Beltangady M, Hays D, et al. Localized orbital rhabdomyosarcoma. *Ophthalmology* 1987;94:251–254.

30. Browning MB, Camitta BM. The surgeon's role in pediatric orbital malignancies: an oncologist's perspective. *Ophthal Plast Reconstr Surg* 2003;19:340–344.

31. Raney RB, Anderson JR, Kollath J, et al. Late effects of therapy in 94 patients with localized rhabdomyosarcoma of the orbit: report from the intergroup rhabdomyosarcoma study (IRS)-III, 1984–1991. *Med Pediatr Oncol* 2000;34:413–420.

32. Thiagalingam S, Flaherty M, Dillson F, et al. Neurofibromatosis type 1 and optic pathway gliomas. *Ophthalmology* 2004;111: 568–577.

33. Baker PS, Gold KG, Lane KA, Bilyk JR, Katowitz JA. Orbital Burkitt lymphoma in immunocompetent patients: a report of 3 cases and a review of the literature. *Ophthal Plast Reconstr Surg* 2009;25:464–468.

34. Smith SJ, Diehl NN, Smith BD, Mohney BG. Incidence, ocular manifestations, and survival in children with neuroblastoma: a population-based study. *Am J Ophthalmol* 2010;149:677–682.

35. Bidar M, Wilson MW, Laquis SJ, et al. Clinical and imaging characteristics of orbital leukemic tumors. *Ophthal Plast Reconstr Surg* 2007;23:87–93.

36. Goisis M, Biglioli F, Guareschi M, Frigerio A, Mortini P. Fibrous dysplasia of the orbital region: current clinical perspectives in ophthalmology and cranio-maxillofacial surgery. *Ophthal Plast Reconstr Surg* 2006;22:383–387.

37. Woo KI, Harris GJ. Eosinophilic granuloma of the orbit: understanding the paradox of aggressive destruction responsive to minimal intervention. *Ophthal Plast Reconstr Surg* 2003;19:429–439.

38. Harris GJ. Langerhans cell histiocytosis of the orbit: a need for interdisciplinary dialogue. *Am J Ophthalmol* 2006;141:374–378.

39. Vosoghi H, Rodriguez-Galindo C, Wilson MW. Orbital Involvement in langerhans cell histiocytosis. *Ophthal Plast Reconstr Surg* 2009;25:430–433.

19

Ocular Tumors of Childhood

Carol L. Shields • *Jerry A. Shields*

OVERVIEW

There are several benign and malignant ocular tumors that can occur in childhood. Tumors in the ocular region can lead to loss of vision, loss of the eye and, in the case of malignant neoplasms, loss of life. Therefore, it is important for the clinician to recognize childhood ocular tumors and to refer affected patients for further diagnostic studies and appropriate management. Based on our extensive clinical experience with ocular tumors over the past 50 years, we review general concepts of childhood eye tumors and discuss the clinical manifestations of specific tumors of the eyelid, conjunctiva, intraocular structures, and orbit in children (1–5).

Clinical Signs of Childhood Ocular Tumors

The clinical characteristics of childhood ocular tumors vary with its location: whether the tumor is located in the eyelids, conjunctiva, intraocular tissues, or the orbit. Each location imparts different signs and symptoms.

Eyelids and Conjunctiva

Eyelid and conjunctival tumors are generally more evident than intraocular or orbital tumors, prompting an early visit to a physician. Most tumors in the eyelid or conjunctival region have characteristic features, so an accurate diagnosis can generally be made with inspection. However, additional diagnostic studies of optical coherence tomography (OCT) or magnetic resonance imaging (MRI) can be helpful.

Intraocular Tumors

Intraocular tumors are often hidden until the patient is visually symptomatic. Young children often do not complain of visual loss and visual acuity can be difficult to assess due to cooperation. However, several features should alert the pediatrician to consider the possibility of an intraocular tumor and prompt a timely referral, particularly the presence of leukocoria (white pupil), strabismus (crossed eye), or lack of visual response.

Leukocoria There are several causes of leukocoria in children (2,4–7) (Fig. 19.1). The more common causes include congenital cataract, retinal detachment from retinopathy of prematurity, persistent fetal vasculature (persistent hyperplastic primary vitreous), and Coats's disease. Retinoblastoma is likely the most serious condition to cause leukocoria in children. Any child with leukocoria should be referred promptly to an ocular oncologist for diagnostic evaluation and management.

Strabismus Most children with strabismus do not have an intraocular tumor. However, about 30% of patients with retinoblastoma present initially with either esotropia or exotropia, due to the tumor location in the macular area which disrupts central fixation. It is important that a complete retinal examination with indirect ophthalmoscopy be performed to exclude an underlying tumor in these cases.

Visual Impairment An older child with an intraocular tumor might complain of visual impairment or could be found to have decreased vision on visual screening in school. This can occur from reduction of central retinal function by a tumor or by the presence of vitreous hemorrhage, hyphema, or secondary cataract formation.

Orbital Tumors

Unlike tumors of the eyelid and conjunctiva, orbital tumors are not directly visualized by the physician. Therefore, these tumors can attain a large size before becoming clinically evident. These patients generally present with proptosis or displacement of the eye (3). Pain, diplopia, and conjunctival edema can also be early clinical features of an orbital tumor. Computed tomography (CT) and MRI have revolutionized the diagnosis and treatment of orbital tumors (8). Caution is issued for use of CT in children to reduce radiation exposure (9).

Diagnostic Approaches

Although some atypical tumors can defy clinical diagnosis, most ophthalmic tumors in children can be accurately diagnosed by a competent ophthalmologist or ocular oncologist.

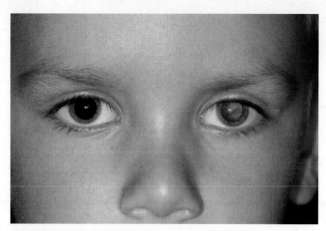

FIGURE 19.1. Leukocoria secondary to retinoblastoma.

Eyelid and Conjunctiva

Most eyelid and conjunctival tumors are recognized by their classic clinical features. Diagnostic studies can provide additional help. Smaller suspicious tumors can be removed by excisional biopsy and larger tumors are best diagnosed by incisional biopsy and definitive treatment withheld until a definite diagnosis is established.

Intraocular Tumors

Concerning intraocular tumors, lesions of the iris can often be recognized with external ocular examination or slit-lamp biomicroscopy. Tumors of the retina and choroid can be visualized with ophthalmoscopy, which can reveal typical features depending on the type of tumor. Many small tumors are difficult to visualize and may only be detected by an experienced ophthalmologist using binocular indirect ophthalmoscopy. Ancillary studies such as fundus photography, autofluorescence, OCT, fluorescein angiography, indocyanine green angiography, ocular ultrasonography, and occasionally CT or MRI are of supplemental value in establishing the diagnosis. OCT is a relatively newer fundus scanning method using a rapid, noncontact, comfortable technique providing cross-sectional imaging of the retina to 4 to 5 μm resolution in a few minutes. Children comfortably tolerate this technique (10). OCT can provide in vivo, high-resolution information of the retina to the 10 μm level. Fine needle aspiration biopsy under general anesthesia has recently been employed in selected intraocular tumors of children (11).

Orbital Tumors

Some orbital tumors occur in an anterior location and can be recognized by their extension into the conjunctiva and eyelid area. This is particularly true of childhood vascular tumors such as capillary hemangioma and lymphangioma. Other tumors reside in the deeper orbital tissues and are less accessible. Orbital ultrasonography can be performed in the office, but often more formal imaging with CT or MRI is necessary.

Therapeutic Approaches

The treatment of an ocular tumor in a child depends on the type of tumor as well as the location and size of the lesion, and the general health of the patient.

Eyelid and Conjunctiva

Neoplasms of the eyelid and conjunctiva can be removed surgically by a qualified ophthalmologist or ocular oncologist. Inflammatory lesions that simulate neoplasia can be managed by antibiotics or corticosteroids, depending on the diagnosis. Some malignant neoplasms such as leukemias and lymphomas are best managed with a limited diagnostic biopsy followed by irradiation and/or chemotherapy.

Intraocular Tumors

The management of intraocular tumors is more complex. Certain benign intraocular tumors that are asymptomatic are usually managed by serial observation. Some symptomatic benign tumors can be treated with laser or cryotherapy, depending on the mechanism of visual impairment. Malignant tumors, such as retinoblastoma, are managed with chemotherapy (intravenous chemotherapy, intra-arterial chemotherapy [IAC], sub-Tenon chemotherapy, or intravitreal chemotherapy approaches), radiotherapy (external beam or plaque radiotherapy), laser photocoagulation, thermotherapy, cryotherapy, or enucleation of the eye (2,4,12,13). More recently, there is a strong trend toward using methods of chemotherapy for retinoblastoma control (13,14).

Orbital Tumors

The treatment of an orbital tumor varies greatly with the clinical signs of histopathologic diagnosis. Benign vascular tumors, such as capillary hemangioma and lymphangioma, can be managed by serial observation or amblyopia patching of the opposite eye to decrease the severity of associated amblyopia. Circumscribed tumors in the anterior orbit may be managed by excisional biopsy. Many malignant tumors, such as rhabdomyosarcoma and orbital leukemia, require limited biopsy to establish the diagnosis, followed by irradiation or chemotherapy (3,5).

EYELID TUMORS

There are several pediatric cutaneous tumors that affect the skin of the eyelids (3,14).

Capillary Hemangioma

The capillary hemangioma or strawberry hemangioma can occur on skin in 10% of infants and is recognized to be

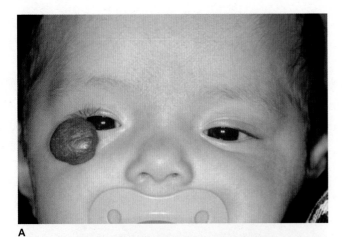

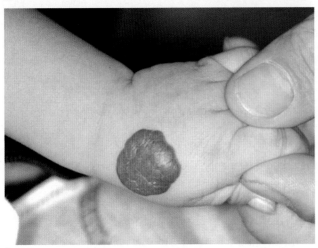

FIGURE 19.2. Capillary hemangioma of the eyelid. **A:** Eyelid hemangioma in an infant twin #1 managed with observation as it did not obstruct visual acuity. **B:** Cutaneous hemangioma in twin #2 on the hand.

more common in premature infants and twins. Capillary hemangioma of the eyelids can be a reddish, diffuse, or circumscribed mass (15) (Fig. 19.2). It usually has clinical onset at birth, or shortly thereafter, tends to enlarge for a few months, and then slowly regress. The main complications of this benign tumor are strabismus and amblyopia. In the recent years, the most frequently used treatment has been refraction, glasses for refractive error, patching of the opposite eye, and close follow-up. More recently, there has been a trend toward oral propranolol or complete surgical excision of those lesions that are relatively small and localized (16). Propranolol can hasten tumor regression with little side effect. Corticosteroids or radiotherapy are reserved for lesions that do not respond to standard measures.

Facial Nevus Flammeus

Facial nevus flammeus is a congenital cutaneous vascular lesion that occurs in the distribution of the fifth cranial nerve

(Fig. 19.3). It may be an isolated entity or it may occur with variations of the Sturge-Weber syndrome. Infants with this lesion have a higher incidence of ipsilateral glaucoma, diffuse choroidal hemangioma, and secondary retinal detachment. Affected infants should be referred to an ophthalmologist as early as possible in order to diagnose and treat these serious ocular conditions. Management of the cutaneous lesion includes observation, cosmetic make-up, or tunable-dye laser treatment delivered at infancy.

Kaposi Sarcoma

Opportunistic neoplasms such as Kaposi sarcoma can be found in immunosuppressed children, particularly those with acquired immunodeficiency syndrome. Although the affected patient can display red cutaneous lesions elsewhere, the eyelid can occasionally be the initial site of involvement. The lesion appears as a reddish-blue subcutaneous mass near the eyelid margin. This tumor is managed by improvement of immunosuppression. In children with human immunodeficiency virus (HIV) infection, treatment with highly active anti-retroviral therapy is employed.

Basal Cell Carcinoma

Although basal cell carcinoma is primarily a disease of adults, it is occasionally seen in younger patients, particularly if there is a family history of the basal cell carcinoma (nevus) syndrome. It generally occurs on the lower eyelid as a slowly progressive mass that can develop a central ulcer (rodent ulcer) and loss of eyelashes. Treatment generally involves local excision, frozen section margin control, and eyelid reconstruction.

Taylor and coauthors reviewed 39 patients with basal cell carcinoma (nevus) syndrome (Gorlin-Goltz syndrome) and found the age of presentation between 5 and 72 years (17). The presenting clinical features included odontogenic

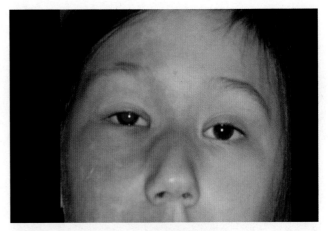

FIGURE 19.3. Nevus flammeus of the face in a child with Sturge-Weber syndrome.

keratocyst (*n* = 17 patients), basal cell carcinoma (*n* = 13), and congenital malformations (*n* = 2). Family history of the syndrome was present in 17 of 39 patients. Basal cell carcinoma developed in 18 of 28 (64%) patients before the age of 30 years. Newer treatment with systemic hedgehog inhibition has been a breakthrough in the control of this disease (18).

Melanocytic Nevus

Melanocytic nevus can occur on the eyelid as a variably pigmented well-circumscribed lesion, similar to those that occur elsewhere on the skin. Nevus does not usually cause loss of cilia. In some instances, the nevus is congenital and large and involves both the upper and lower eyelids and is termed "kissing nevus" or "divided nevus" (Fig. 19.4). There is some evidence that early intervention with curettage of the lesion within the first 3 to 4 weeks after birth can successfully remove the lesion without the need for extensive grafting. At infancy, the nevus is superficial and can be scraped off the skin whereas later it deepens into the subcutaneous tissue, making surgical removal difficult. Following curettage, topical antibiotic ointment is applied and the skin heals by granulation.

The blue nevus is often apparent at birth, whereas the junctional or compound nevus may not become clinically apparent until puberty. Transformation into malignant melanoma is rare and usually occurs later in life. Although most eyelid nevi in children can be safely observed, they are occasionally excised because of cosmetic considerations or because of fear of malignant transformation.

Neurofibroma

Neurofibroma can occur on the eyelid as a diffuse or plexiform lesion that is often associated with von Recklinghausen's neurofibromatosis. In the earliest stages, the lesion produces a characteristic S-shaped curve to the upper eyelid. Larger lesions produce thickening of the eyelid with secondary blepharoptosis (Fig. 19.5). Since these diffuse tumors are often difficult or impossible to completely excise,

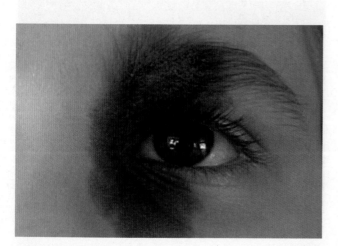

FIGURE 19.4. Eyelid margin kissing nevus.

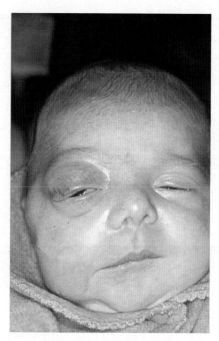

FIGURE 19.5. Neurofibroma of the eyelid and orbit in an infant.

they should be managed by periodic observation or surgical debulking if they cause a major cosmetic problem.

Neurilemoma (Schwannoma)

Neurilemoma is a benign peripheral nerve sheath tumor that is composed purely of Schwann cells of peripheral nerves. It can appear in the orbit or on the eyelid and is managed by surgical resection. This tumor may or may not be associated with neurofibromatosis.

CONJUNCTIVAL TUMORS

Introduction

Tumors of the conjunctiva and epibulbar tissues involve a large spectrum of conditions ranging from benign lesions such as limbal dermoid, myxoma, and scleral melanocytosis to aggressive, life-threatening malignancies such as melanoma, Kaposi sarcoma, and sebaceous carcinoma (1,3,19–22). The clinical differentiation of the various tumors is based primarily on the clinical features of the tumor as well as the patient history. The clinical features as well as the management of each tumor are discussed, based on the authors' personal experience with approximately 2,000 patients with conjunctival tumors over a 40-year period (22). Herein, we review and illustrate the features of conjunctival tumors in children.

Spectrum of Tumors in Children

Several previously published surveys (20–22) have reported on the incidence of conjunctival lesions in adults. However, the epidemiologic features, anatomic characteristics, and malignant potential of such lesions differ in the pediatric age group. There have been only three large series of conjunctival tumors in children (1,23,24). Elsas and Green, and Cunha and coworkers evaluated the incidence of these lesions from a pathology laboratory standpoint, whereas Shields and associates presented their data from a clinical standpoint (1,23,24) (Tables 19.1 and 19.2).

In a clinical series of 262 children referred to an Oncology Service with a conjunctival tumor, Shields and coworkers found that the most common lesions were of melanocytic (67%), choristomatous (10%), vascular (9%), and benign epithelial (2%) origin (1) (Table 19.1). They noted that 10% of cases were non-neoplastic lesions simulating a tumor such as epithelial inclusion cyst, nonspecific inflammation/infection, episcleritis, scleritis, and foreign body.

Specific Tumors

The following tumors are classified based on tissues of origin, including choristomatous, epithelial, melanocytic, vascular, fibrous, xanthomatous, and lymphoid/leukemic origin.

TABLE 19.1

CLINICAL DIAGNOSTIC CATEGORIES OF CONJUNCTIVAL TUMORS IN 262 CHILDREN (1)

Classification of Tumors	Number of Patients (%)
Choristomatous	26 (10%)
Benign epithelial	5 (2%)
Premalignant and malignant epithelial	1 (<1%)
Melanocytic	175 (67%)
Vascular	23 (9%)
Fibrous	2 (<1%)
Neural	0 (0%)
Xanthomatous	1 (<1%)
Myxomatous	0 (0%)
Lipomatous	0 (0%)
Lacrimal gland	0 (0%)
Lymphoid	4 (1.5%)
Leukemic	0 (0%)
Metastatic	0 (0%)
Secondary	0 (0%)
Non-neoplastic lesions simulating a tumor	25 (9.5%)

Data from the Oncology Service at Wills Eye Institute.

Choristomatous Conjunctival Tumors

A variety of tumors can be present at birth or become clinically apparent shortly after birth. Most of the lesions are choristomas, consisting of displaced tissue elements normally not found in these areas. A simple choristoma is comprised of one tissue element such as epithelium, whereas a complex choristoma represents variable combinations of ectopic tissues like bone, cartilage, and lacrimal gland.

Dermoid Conjunctival dermoid is a congenital well-circumscribed yellow-white solid mass that involves the bulbar or limbal conjunctiva (25,26). It characteristically occurs inferotemporally and often this tumor has fine white hairs (Fig. 19.6). In rare cases, it can extend to the central cornea or be located in other quadrants on the bulbar surface. Most often dermoid straddles the limbus, but in rare cases it can be extensive and involves the full-thickness cornea, anterior chamber, and iris stroma. The more severe dermoids occur earlier in embryogenesis.

The conjunctival dermoid can occur as a solitary lesion or can be associated with Goldenhar's syndrome. The patient should be evaluated for ipsilateral or bilateral preauricular skin appendages, hearing loss, eyelid coloboma, orbitoconjunctival dermolipoma, and cervical vertebral anomalies. Histopathologically, the conjunctival dermoid is a simple choristomatous malformation that consists of dense fibrous tissue lined by conjunctival epithelium with deeper dermal elements including hair follicles and sebaceous glands.

The management of an epibulbar dermoid includes observation if the lesion is small and visually asymptomatic. Anterior segment OCT can assist in judging depth of involvement. It is possible to excise the lesion for cosmetic reasons, but the remaining corneal scar can be cosmetically unacceptable. Larger or symptomatic dermoids can produce visual loss from astigmatism. These can be approached by lamellar keratosclerectomy with primary closure of overlying tissue if the defect is superficial, or closure using corneal graft if the defect is deep or of full thickness. The cosmetic appearance might improve, but the refractive and astigmatic error and visual acuity might not change. When the lesion involves the central cornea, a lamellar or penetrating keratoplasty is necessary and long-term amblyopia should be anticipated.

Dermolipoma Dermolipoma is believed to be congenital, but it classically remains asymptomatic for years and might not be detected until adulthood. This tumor tends to occur in the conjunctival fornix superotemporally and appears as a yellow, soft, fluctuant mass with fine white hairs on its surface (Fig. 19.7). It can extend into the orbital fat and onto the bulbar conjunctiva, sometimes reaching the limbus.

Dermolipoma has features similar to orbital fat on CT and MRI scans. Histopathologically, it is lined by conjunctival epithelium on its surface and the subepithelial tissue has variable quantities of collagenous connective tissue and adipose tissue. Pilosebaceous units and lacrimal gland tissue might be

TABLE 19.2

COMPARISON OF DATA FROM THREE SERIES OF CONJUNCTIVAL LESIONS IN YOUNG PATIENTS

Classification of Tumors	% Tumors	% Tumors	% Tumors
Data source	Clinical series (1)	Pathology series (24)	Pathology series (23)
	(n = 262)	(n = 282)	(n = 302)
Choristomatous	10	22	33
Benign epithelial (papilloma)	2	10	7
Premalignant and malignant epithelial	<1	0	1
Melanocytic	67	23	29
Vascular	9	6	2
Fibrous	<1	na	<1
Neural	0	1	na
Xanthomatous	<1	na	na
Myxomatous	0	na	na
Lipomatous	0	4	2
Lacrimal gland	0	na	na
Lymphoid	1.5	3	na
Leukemic	0	na	na
Metastatic	0	na	na
Secondary	0	na	na
Non-neoplastic lesions simulating a tumor[a]	9.5	30	23

[a]Includes epithelial inclusion cyst, inflammatory lesions, vernal conjunctivitis, pyogenic granuloma, nonspecific granuloma, foreign body, scar tissue, keloid, and others.

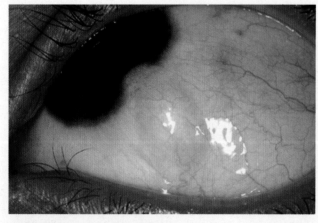

FIGURE 19.6. Conjunctival dermoid.

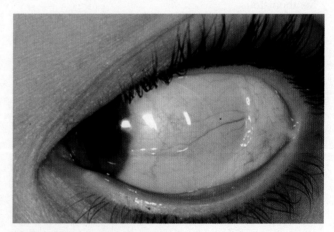

FIGURE 19.7. Conjunctival dermolipoma.

present. The majority of dermolipomas require no treatment, but larger ones or those that are cosmetically unappealing can be managed by excision of the entire orbitoconjunctival lesion through a conjunctival forniceal approach or by removing the anterior portion of the lesion in a manner similar to that used to remove prolapsed orbital fat. Amniotic membrane graft might be necessary to repair the defect.

Epibulbar Osseous Choristoma Epibulbar osseous choristoma is a tumor comprised of mature bone, usually located in the bulbar conjunctiva superotemporally (3,27) (Fig. 19.8). It is believed to be congenital and typically remains undetected until palpated by the older patient. On ultrasonography or CT scanning, the mass demonstrates calcium. This tumor is usually managed by observation. Occasionally, a foreign body sensation necessitates excision of the mass using a conjunctival forniceal incision followed by dissection of the tumor to bare sclera.

Lacrimal Gland Choristoma Lacrimal gland choristoma is a congenital lesion, discovered in young children as an asymptomatic pink stromal mass, typically in the superotemporal or temporal portion of the conjunctiva. It is speculated that this lesion represents small sequestrations of the embryonic evagination of the lacrimal gland from the conjunctiva. The lacrimal gland choristoma can masquerade as a focus of inflammation due to its pink color. Rarely, this mass can be cystic due to ongoing secretions if there is no connection to the conjunctival surface. Excisional biopsy is usually performed to confirm the diagnosis.

Complex Choristoma The conjunctival dermoid and epibulbar osseous choristoma are simple choristomas as they contain one tissue type such as skin or bone. A complex choristoma contains a greater variety of tissue derived from two germ layers such as lacrimal tissue and cartilage. It is variable in its clinical appearance and can cover much of the epibulbar surface, or it may form a circumferential growth pattern around the limbus.

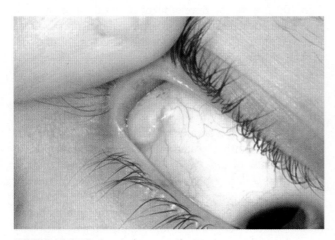

FIGURE 19.8. Conjunctival osseous choristoma.

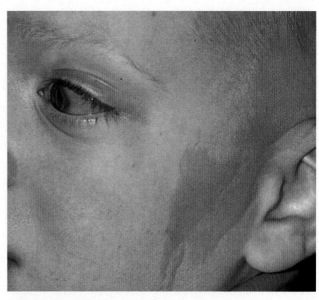

FIGURE 19.9. Complex conjunctival choristoma in a child with nevus sebaceous of Jadassohn and organoid nevus syndrome.

The complex choristoma has an association with the linear nevus sebaceous of Jadassohn (26) (Fig. 19.9). The nevus sebaceous of Jadassohn includes cutaneous features with sebaceous nevus in the facial region and neurologic features including seizures, mental retardation, arachnoidal cyst, and cerebral atrophy. The ophthalmic features of this syndrome include epibulbar complex choristoma and posterior scleral cartilage. The management of complex choristoma depends upon the extent of the lesion. Observation or wide local excision followed by mucous membrane graft reconstruction are options.

Epithelial Conjunctival Tumors

There are several benign and malignant tumors that can arise from the squamous epithelium of the conjunctiva.

Papilloma Squamous papilloma is a benign tumor, documented to be associated with human papillomavirus infection of the conjunctiva (28,29). This tumor can occur in both children and adults. It is speculated that the virus is acquired through transfer from the mother's vagina to the newborn's conjunctiva as the child passes through the mother's birth canal. Papillomas appear as a pink fibrovascular frond of tissue arranged in a sessile or pedunculated configuration (Fig. 19.10). The numerous fine vascular channels ramify through the stroma beneath the epithelial surface of the lesion. In children, the lesion is usually small, multiple, and located in the inferior fornix. Histopathologically, the lesion shows numerous vascularized papillary fronds lined by acanthotic epithelium.

There are several treatment options for small sessile papillomas. Sometimes observation allows for slow spontaneous resolution of this tumor. Larger or more pedunculated

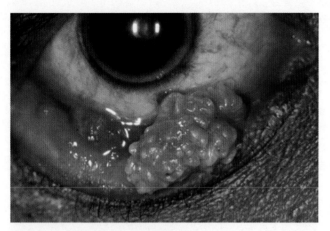

FIGURE 19.10. Conjunctival papilloma.

tumors can lead to foreign body sensation, chronic mucous production, hemorrhagic tears, incomplete eyelid closure, and poor cosmetic appearance, requiring therapeutic intervention. Complete removal of the mass without direction manipulation of the tumor (no touch technique) is advisable to avoid spreading of the virus (30). Double freeze–thaw cryotherapy is applied to the remaining conjunctiva around the excised lesion in order to prevent tumor recurrence. In some instances, the pedunculated tumor is frozen alone and then excised while frozen. Topical or injection interferon and Mitomycin C have been employed for resistant or multiply recurrent conjunctival papillomas (31,32). For difficult recurrent lesions, oral cimetidine for several months following surgical resection can minimize recurrence by boosting the patient's immune system and suppressing the virally stimulated mass (33).

Hereditary Benign Intraepithelial Dyskeratosis

Hereditary benign intraepithelial dyskeratosis (HBID) is a rare, benign condition seen in an inbred isolate of Caucasian, African American, and Native Americans (Haliwa Indians), initially identified in North Carolina. It is an autosomal dominant disorder characterized by bilateral elevated fleshy plaques on the nasal or temporal perilimbal conjunctiva and on the buccal mucosa. It can remain asymptomatic or can cause redness and foreign body sensation. It is characterized histopathologically by acanthosis, dyskeratosis on the epithelial surface and deep within the epithelium, and prominent chronic inflammatory cells. HBID does not usually require aggressive treatment. Smaller, less-symptomatic lesions can be treated with ocular lubricants and topical corticosteroids. Larger symptomatic lesions can be managed by local resection with mucous membrane grafting if necessary.

Squamous Cell Carcinoma/Conjunctival Intraepithelial Neoplasia

Squamous cell carcinoma and conjunctival intraepithelial neoplasia (CIN) are malignancies of the surface epithelial cells. Intraepithelial neoplasia displays anaplastic cells within the epithelium, whereas squamous cell carcinoma displays extension of anaplastic cells through the basement membrane into the conjunctival stroma. Clinically, invasive squamous cell carcinoma is usually larger and more elevated than CIN. Leukoplakia can be seen with either condition.

Patients who are medically immunosuppressed from organ transplantation, those with HIV, or those with underlying DNA repair abnormalities like xeroderma pigmentosum are at particular risk to develop conjunctival squamous cell carcinoma and malignant melanoma (34). In these cases, the risk for life-threatening metastatic disease is greater.

The management of conjunctival squamous cell carcinoma varies with the extent of the lesion. Tumors in the limbal area require alcohol epitheliectomy for the corneal component and partial lamellar scleroconjunctivectomy with wide margins for the conjunctival component followed by freeze–thaw cryotherapy to the remaining adjacent bulbar conjunctiva. Extensive tumors or those tumors that are recurrent, especially with extensive corneal component, are treated with adjuvant topical Interferon, Mitomycin C, or 5-Fluorouracil (31,32,34,35).

Melanocytic Conjunctival Tumors

There are several lesions that arise from the melanocytes of the conjunctiva and episclera. The most important ones include nevus, racial melanosis, primary acquired melanosis (PAM), and malignant melanoma (Table 19.3). Ocular melanocytosis should be included in this section as its scleral pigmentation can masquerade as conjunctival pigmentation.

Ocular Melanocytosis Ocular melanocytosis is a congenital pigmentary condition of the periocular skin, sclera, orbit, meninges, and soft palate. Typically, there is no conjunctival pigment. However, this condition is clinically confused with PAM (Table 19.3). In ocular melanocytosis, flat, gray-brown pigment scattered posterior to the limbus on the sclera is visualized through the thin overlying conjunctival tissue (Fig. 19.11). Partial or entire uvea can be affected by similar increased pigment (36,37). This condition imparts a 1 in 400 risk for the development of uveal melanoma and not conjunctival melanoma (36). Affected patients should be followed once or twice yearly for the development of uveal, orbital, or meningeal melanoma.

Nevus The conjunctival nevus is the most common melanocytic tumor. It becomes clinically apparent in the first or second decade of life as a discrete, variably pigmented, slightly elevated lesion that contains fine clear cysts in 65% of cases (38,39). Conjunctival nevus can manifest as a darkly pigmented (65%), lightly pigmented (19%), or completely nonpigmented (16%) mass (39) (Fig. 19.12). It is typically located in the interpalpebral bulbar conjunctiva near the limbus and remains stationary throughout life with <1% risk for transformation into malignant melanoma. Over time, nevus can become more

Table 19.3

DIFFERENTIAL DIAGNOSIS OF PIGMENTED EPIBULBAR LESIONS (1)

Condition	Anatomic Location	Color	Depth	Margins	Laterality	Other Features	Progression
Nevus	Inter-palpebral limbus usually	Brown or yellow	Stroma	Well defined	Unilateral	Cysts	<1% progress to conjunctival melanoma
Racial melanosis	Limbus > bulbar > palpebral conjunctiva	Brown	Epithelium	Ill defined	Bilateral	Flat, no cysts	Very rare progression to conjunctival melanoma
Ocular melano-cytosis	Bulbar conjunctiva	Gray	Episclera	Ill defined	Unilateral more so than bilateral	Congenital, usually 2 mm from limbus, often with periocular skin pigmentation	<1% progress to uveal melanoma
Primary acquired melanosis	Anywhere, but usually bulbar conjunctiva	Brown	Epithelium	Ill defined	Unilateral	Flat, no cysts	Progresses to conjunctival melanoma in nearly 50% cases that show cellular atypia
Malignant melanoma	Anywhere	Brown or pink	Stroma	Well defined	Unilateral	Vascular nodule, dilated feeder vessels, may be nonpigmented	32% develop metastasis by 15 y

or less pigmented in about 5% of cases (38). Rarely, giant nevus can be found, often with numerous cysts (40).

Histopathologically, the conjunctival nevus is composed of nests of benign melanocytes in the stroma near the basal layers of the epithelium. Like cutaneous nevus, it can be junctional, compound, or deep. The management is periodic observation with photographic comparison. If growth is documented, then local excision of the lesion

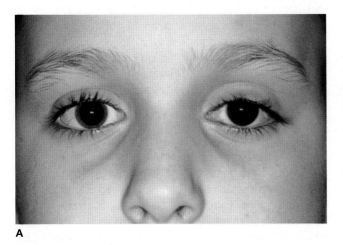
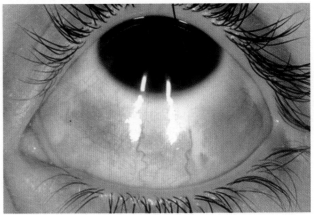

FIGURE 19.11. Ocular melanocytosis. **A:** Heterochromia with light brown right iris and dark brown left iris. **B:** Episcleral melanocytosis.

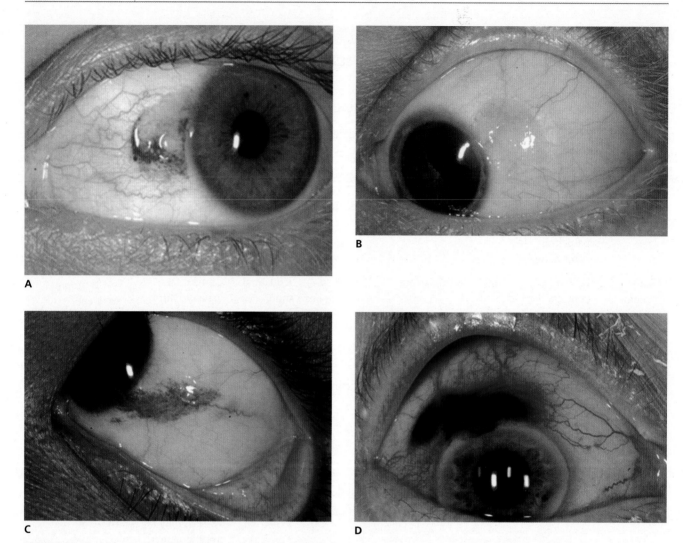

FIGURE 19.12. Melanocytic conjunctival lesions. **A:** Partially pigmented conjunctival nevus with cysts. **B:** Nonpigmented conjunctival nevus. **C:** Primary acquired melanosis (PAM). **D:** Conjunctival melanoma.

should be considered. In some cases, excision for cosmetic reasons is desired. At the time of excision, the entire mass is removed using the no touch technique and if it is adherent to the globe, then a thin lamella of underlying sclera is removed intact with the tumor. Standard double freeze–thaw cryotherapy is applied to the remaining conjunctival margins. These precautions are employed to prevent recurrence of the nevus and also to prevent recurrence should the lesion prove to be a melanoma.

Racial Melanosis Racial melanosis is an acquired pigmentation of the conjunctiva usually detected in darkly pigmented individuals and occasionally in children. This pigment is most often present at the limbus and less on the limbal cornea and bulbar conjunctiva. This pigmentation is often patchy and rarely evolves into melanoma. Histopathologically, the pigmented cells are benign melanocytes located in the basal layer of the epithelium. The recommended management is observation.

Primary Acquired Melanosis Primary acquired melanosis (PAM) is an important benign conjunctival pigmentary condition that can give rise to conjunctival melanoma. In contrast to conjunctival nevus, it is acquired in middle age and rarely in children. It appears diffuse, patchy, flat, and noncystic. In contrast to ocular melanocytosis, the pigment is acquired, located within the conjunctiva, and appears brown, not gray, in color (41) (Fig. 19.12). In contrast to racial melanosis, PAM generally is found in fair-skinned individuals as a unilateral patchy condition.

Histopathologically, PAM is characterized by the presence of abnormal melanocytes near the basal layer of the epithelium. Pathologists should attempt to classify the melanocytes as having atypia or no atypia based on nuclear features and growth pattern. PAM with atypia carries 13% to 46% risk for ultimate evolution into malignant melanoma, whereas PAM without atypia carries nearly 0% risk for melanoma development (41).

The management of PAM depends on the extent of involvement and the association with melanoma. If PAM is minor, occupying less than 2 clock hours of the conjunctiva, then periodic observation or complete excisional biopsy and cryotherapy are options. If the PAM occupies more than 2 or 3 clock hours, then incisional map biopsy of all four quadrants is warranted, followed by double freeze–thaw cryotherapy to all affected pigmented sites. If the patient has a history of melanoma or if there are areas of nodularity or vascularity suspicious for melanoma, then a more aggressive approach is warranted with complete excisional biopsy of the suspicious areas using the no touch technique. Topical Mitomycin C can also be beneficial, especially if there is recurrent corneal PAM. This medication should be used with extreme caution in children due to its toxicities.

Malignant Melanoma Malignant melanoma of the conjunctiva most often arises from PAM, but can also arise from a preexisting nevus or de novo (42–44). Melanoma typically arises in middle-aged to older adults, but rare cases in children have been recognized (Fig. 19.12). In our practice, 1% of all conjunctival melanoma occur in children. Conjunctival melanoma shows considerable clinical variability as it can be pigmented or nonpigmented; pink, yellow, or brown in color; and involve the limbal, bulbar, forniceal, or palpebral conjunctiva.

Vascular Conjunctival Tumors

There are several vascular tumors of the conjunctiva, including capillary hemangioma, lymphangioma, pyogenic granuloma, cavernous hemangioma, racemose hemangioma, varix, hemangiopericytoma, and Kaposi sarcoma. We discuss the first three conditions as they are typically found in children or young adults.

Capillary Hemangioma Capillary hemangioma of the conjunctiva is generally presented in infancy, several weeks following birth, as a red stromal mass, sometimes associated with cutaneous or orbital component. Similar to its cutaneous counterpart, the conjunctival mass might enlarge over several months and then spontaneously involute. Management includes observation most commonly, but surgical resection or oral propranolol can be employed.

Lymphangioma Conjunctival lymphangioma can occur as an isolated conjunctival lesion or it can represent a superficial component of a deeper diffuse orbital lymphangioma. It usually becomes clinically apparent in the first decade of life and appears as a multliloculated mass containing variable-sized clear dilated cystic channels. In most instances, blood is visible in many of the cystic spaces. These have been called "chocolate cysts." The treatment of conjunctival lymphangioma is often difficult because surgical resection or radiotherapy cannot completely eradicate the mass.

Pyogenic Granuloma Pyogenic granuloma is a proliferative fibrovascular response to prior tissue insult by inflammation, surgery, or nonsurgical trauma. It is sometimes classified as a polypoid form of acquired capillary hemangioma. It appears clinically as an elevated red mass, often with a prominent blood supply. Microscopically, it is composed of granulation tissue with chronic inflammatory cells and numerous small caliber blood vessels. The term "pyogenic granuloma" is a misnomer as this lesion is not pyogenic, nor does it display granuloma. Pyogenic granuloma will sometimes respond to topical corticosteroids but many cases ultimately require surgical excision.

Xanthomatous Conjunctival Tumors

Xanthomatous conjunctival tumors include juvenile xanthogranuloma, found in children, and xanthoma and reticulohistiocytoma, typically found in adults.

Juvenile Xanthogranuloma Juvenile xanthogranuloma is a cutaneous condition that presents as painless, pink skin papules with spontaneous resolution, generally in children under the age of 2 years. Rarely, conjunctival, orbital, and intraocular involvement is noted. In the conjunctiva, the mass appears as an orange-pink stromal mass, typically in teenagers or young adults. If the classic skin lesions are noted, the diagnosis is established clinically and treatment with observation or topical steroid ointment is provided. Otherwise, biopsy is suggested and recognition of the typical histopathologic features of histiocytes admixed with Touton giant cells confirms the diagnosis.

Lymphoid/Leukemic Conjunctival Tumors

Lymphoid and leukemic tumors of the conjunctiva can both appear as an orange-pink stromal mass. Systemic evaluation for underlying malignancy is important.

Lymphoid Tumors Lymphoid tumors can occur in the conjunctiva as isolated lesions or they can be a manifestation of systemic lymphoma (45–47). This condition is most often found in older adults and rarely in children. Clinically, the lesion appears as a diffuse, slightly elevated pink mass located in the stroma or deep to Tenon's fascia, most commonly in the forniceal region. This appearance is similar to that of smoked salmon; hence it is termed the "salmon patch." It is not possible to differentiate clinically between a benign and malignant lymphoid tumor. Therefore, biopsy is necessary to establish the diagnosis and a systemic evaluation should be done in affected patients to exclude the presence of systemic lymphoma. The lymphoid tumors found in children are most often hyperplasia and not lymphoma and generally not associated with systemic lymphoma. Treatment of the conjunctival lesion should include chemotherapy or rituximab if the patient has systemic lymphoma, or external beam irradiation (2,000 to 4,000 cGy) if the lesion is localized to the conjunctiva. Other options include excisional biopsy and cryotherapy, local interferon injections, or observation. There is new information that some lymphoid tumors are related to *Helicobacter pylori* or *Chlamydia psittici* infection and treatment with appropriate antibiotics could be beneficial.

Leukemia Leukemia generally manifests in the ocular region as hemorrhages from associated anemia and thrombocytopenia rather than leukemic infiltration. In the rare instance of leukemic infiltration of the conjunctiva, the mass appears pink and smooth within the conjunctival stroma either at the limbus or the fornix, similar to a lymphoid tumor. Biopsy reveals sheets of large leukemic cells. Treatment of the systemic condition is advised with secondary resolution of the conjunctival infiltration.

Non-neoplastic Lesions That Simulate Conjunctival Tumors

A number of non-neoplastic conditions can simulate neoplasms. These include epithelial inclusion cyst, inflammatory lesions, vernal conjunctivitis, pyogenic granuloma, nonspecific granuloma, foreign body, scar tissue, keloid, and others. In most instances, the history and clinical findings should allow for the diagnosis, however, excision of the mass might be necessary in order to exclude a neoplasm.

Conclusion

Most conjunctival tumors in children are benign. The most common conjunctival tumor in children is the nevus. Conjunctival nevus rarely evolve into melanoma (<1%). Episcleral melanocytosis is a sign of possible uveal melanocytosis and affected eyes should be dilated once or twice a year as there is a risk for uveal melanoma. Conjunctival papillomas can be treated with observation, cryotherapy, topical chemotherapy or interferon, and oral cimetidine.

INTRAOCULAR TUMORS

Retinoblastoma

Retinoblastoma represents approximately 4% of all pediatric malignancies and is the most common intraocular malignancy in children (2,4,14,48). It is estimated that 250 to 300 new cases of retinoblastoma are diagnosed in the United States each year and 7,000 to 8,000 cases are found worldwide (49). Asia estimates over 4,000 and Africa estimates approximately 2,000 new cases of retinoblastoma per year (49). Most (>97%) children with retinoblastoma in the United States and other medically developed nations survive their malignancy, whereas approximately 50% survive worldwide. The reason for the poor survival in undeveloped nations relates to late detection of advanced retinoblastoma, often presenting with orbital invasion or metastatic disease.

Systemic Concerns with Retinoblastoma

Retinoblastoma can be grouped in four different ways: sporadic or familial, unilateral or bilateral, nonheritable or heritable, and somatic or germline mutation. About two-thirds of all cases are unilateral and one-third of cases are bilateral. Genetically, it is simpler to discuss retinoblastoma with the latter classification of somatic or germline mutation. Germline mutation implies that the mutation is present in all cells of the body, whereas somatic mutation means that only the tissue of concern, the retinoblastoma, has the mutation. All patients are offered genetic testing for retinoblastoma. The testing is performed on the tumor specimen (when available) and a blood sample. Mutations for retinoblastoma have been found predominantly on chromosome 13 long arm (50).

Patients with germline mutation have mutation in both the tumor and the peripheral blood, whereas those with somatic mutation show only mutation in the tumor and not the blood. This implies that all cells might be affected with the mutation in germline cases so these patients could be at risk for other cancers (second cancers and pinealoblastoma). Patients with bilateral and familial retinoblastoma have presumed germline mutation because they have multifocal or heritable disease. Patients with unilateral sporadic retinoblastoma usually carry somatic mutation, but approximately 7% to 15% of these patients will show a germline mutation. Nichols and coworkers performed sensitive multistep clinical molecular screening of 180 unrelated individuals with retinoblastoma and found germline *RB1* mutations in 77 out of 85 bilateral retinoblastoma patients (91%), 7 out of 10 familial unilateral patients (70%), and 6 out of 85 unilateral sporadic patients (7%). Mutations included 36 novel alterations spanning the entire *RB1* gene (50). Thus, it is important to have children with retinoblastoma tested for genetic mutations, particularly those with unilateral sporadic retinoblastoma.

Children with retinoblastoma are at risk for three important, life-threatening problems including metastasis from retinoblastoma, intracranial neuroblastic malignancy (trilateral retinoblastoma/pinealoblastoma), and second primary cancers.

Retinoblastoma metastasis typically develops within 1 year of the diagnosis of the intraocular tumor. Those at greatest risk (high risk) for metastasis show histopathologic features of retinoblastoma invasion beyond the lamina cribrosa in the optic nerve, in the choroid, sclera, orbit, or anterior chamber (51–53). It is critical that a qualified ophthalmic pathologist examines the eye for the high-risk features. High-risk retinoblastoma has been found in 24% of group E and 14% of group D eyes, so this feature is not uncommon and could be life-threatening to the patient (53). Patients with postlaminar optic nerve invasion or gross (>3 mm) choroidal invasion or a combination of any optic nerve or choroidal invasion should be treated with chemotherapy. Chemotherapy with vincristine, etoposide, and carboplatin for 4 to 6 months is highly effective in preventing metastatic disease (52).

Pinealoblastoma or related brain tumors typically occur in the first 5 years of life, most often within 1 year of diagnosis of the retinoblastoma (54,55). This has been termed "trilateral" retinoblastoma and overall is found in about 3% of all children with retinoblastoma, but those with germline mutation manifest this tumor in up to 10% of cases. Unfortunately, pinealoblastoma is usually fatal with only few survivors. Systemic chemotherapy, particularly the chemoreduction protocol currently used for retinoblastoma can prevent trilateral retinoblastoma (56). Longer follow-up in our series of over 500 children with retinoblastoma treated with chemoreduction continue to show the same trend with very few cases of pinealoblastoma. It should be noted that benign pineal cyst can simulate pinealoblastoma and can best be differentiated using high-resolution MRI (57). With MRI, the benign cyst shows gadolinium enhancement of the wall but not the center cavity, whereas pinealoblastoma are typically larger than cysts and show full enhancement. Pineal cysts require no treatment.

Second cancers occur in survivors of bilateral or heritable (germline mutation) retinoblastoma (58–60). Patients with hereditary retinoblastoma have approximately a 4% chance of developing a second cancer during the first 10 years of follow-up, 18% during the first 20 years, and 26% within 30 years (58). Second cancers most often include osteogenic sarcoma, spindle cell sarcoma, chondrosarcoma, rhabdomyosarcoma, neuroblastoma, glioma, leukemia, sebaceous cell carcinoma, squamous cell carcinoma, and malignant melanoma. Therapeutic radiotherapy previously delivered for the retinoblastoma can further increase the rate of second cancers. Hereditary retinoblastoma patients who received ocular radiation carried a 29% chance for periocular second cancer compared with only 6% risk in hereditary retinoblastoma patients treated without radiotherapy (58). Abramson and colleagues have shown that less than 50% of patients survive their second cancer and they are at risk to develop a third nonocular cancer (22% by 10 years) at a mean interval of 6 years (60). Survivors continue to be at risk for fourth and fifth nonocular cancers. There is some concern that patients treated with chemoreduction, particularly etoposide, might be at risk for secondary acute myelogenous leukemia (61).

Ophthalmic Diagnosis and Management of Retinoblastoma

The clinical manifestations of retinoblastoma vary with the stage of the disease (2,4,12,48). A small retinoblastoma, <2 mm in diameter, appears transparent or slightly translucent in the sensory retina. Larger tumors stimulate dilated retinal blood vessels feeding the tumor, foci of intrinsic calcification, and can produce subretinal fluid (exophytic pattern), subretinal seeding, and vitreous seeding (endophytic pattern) (Fig. 19.13). Retinoblastoma of any size can produce leukocoria, but this is most often seen with large tumors (Fig. 19.1). Diffuse retinoblastoma is an advanced form of endophytic retinoblastoma and often occurs silently in older children (61).

A number of ocular disorders in infants and children can resemble retinoblastoma. The most common pseudoretinoblastomas includes Coats's disease, persistent hyperplastic primary vitreous (also known as persistent fetal vasculature), ocular inflammation such as toxocariasis, and familial exudative vitreoretinopathy (62). Any child with retinal detachment, vitreous hemorrhage, or intraocular mass should be evaluated for retinoblastoma. Keep in mind that approximately 25% of children referred with the presumed diagnosis of retinoblastoma actually have a simulating, often benign condition (pseudoretinoblastoma) (62).

Several classifications of retinoblastoma have been developed including the Reese Ellsworth classification and the more recent International Classification of Retinoblastoma (ICRB) (48,63) (Tables 19.4 to 19.6). The ICRB is simple to remember and is useful for prediction of chemoreduction success (64).

Management of retinoblastoma is tailored to each individual case and is based on the overall situation, including the threat of metastatic disease, risks for second cancers, systemic status, laterality of the disease, size and location of the tumor(s), and estimated visual prognosis. The currently available treatment methods include chemotherapy using intravenous (chemoreduction, CRD), IAC, sub-Tenon, or intravitreal routes; thermotherapy; cryotherapy; laser photocoagulation; plaque radiotherapy; external beam radiotherapy; and enucleation (12,13,65) (Table 19.5). Based on the ICRB, chemoreduction success is achieved in 100% of group A, 93% of group B, 90% of group C, and 47% of group D eyes (64) (Fig. 19.13) (Table 19.6).

For unilateral retinoblastoma, focal treatment with laser photocoagulation or cryotherapy is used if the disease is minor and plaque radiotherapy is used for larger tumors. IAC now plays an important role for unilateral groups C and D eyes, with high control (65–69) (Fig. 19.13). Enucleation is used for group E eyes in which there is little chance for useful vision. For bilateral retinoblastoma, CRD plus thermotherapy or cryotherapy is necessary in most cases and IAC is used as salvage for recurrent disease. Enucleation of one eye still plays an important role in the management of retinoblastoma. Enucleation of both eyes is only necessary in <1% of cases in the United States.

With over two decades of experience with CRD, we have witnessed excellent retinoblastoma control (70–72). The tumor reduces by approximately 35% in base and nearly 50% in thickness. Retinal detachment completely resolves in nearly every eye. In spite of these successes, vitreous and subretinal seeds pose the greatest problem with potential for recurrence, often remote from the main tumor. In a report on 158 eyes with retinoblastoma treated using vincristine, etoposide, and carboplatin for six cycles, all retinoblastomas, subretinal seeds, and vitreous seeds showed initial regression (70). However, approximately 50% of the

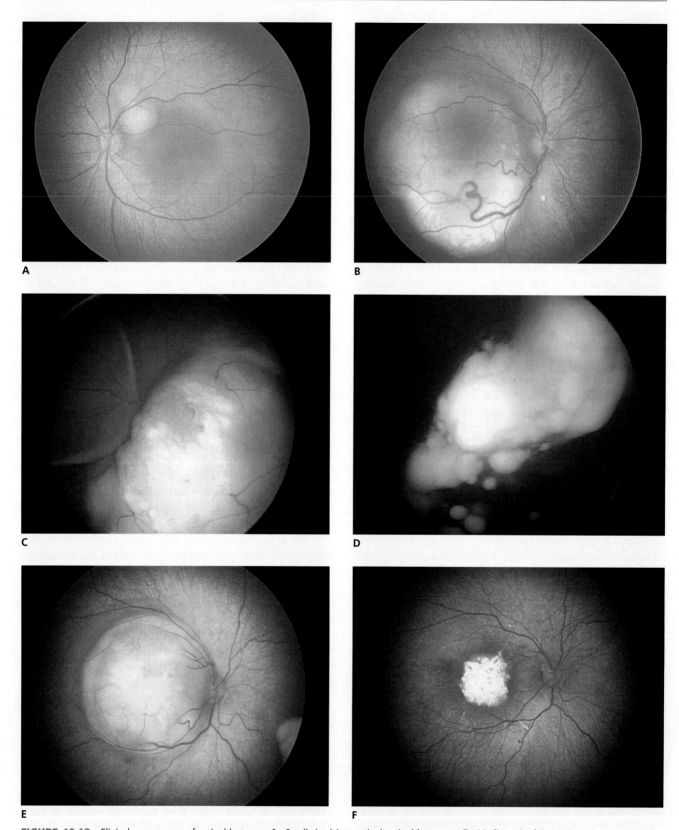

FIGURE 19.13. Clinical appearance of retinoblastoma. **A:** Small-sized intraretinal retinoblastomas. **B:** Medium-sized intraretinal retinoblastoma with surrounding subretinal fluid. **C:** Large-sized exophytic retinoblastoma with subretinal fluid. **D:** Endophytic retinoblastoma. **E:** Macular retinoblastoma before chemoreduction. **F:** Macular retinoblastoma (same as in Fig. 19.13E) following chemoreduction and thermotherapy. **G:** Advanced retinoblastoma before intra-arterial chemotherapy (IAC). **H:** Following IAC (patient 13G), the tumor has completely regressed. **I:** Large retinoblastoma managed with enucleation.

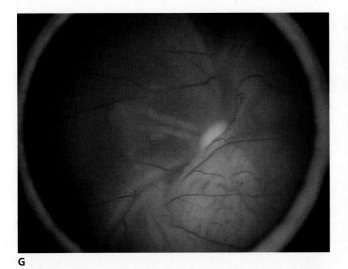

G

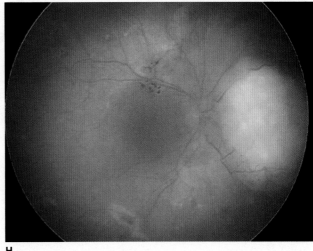

H

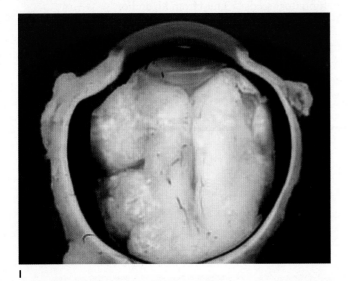

I

FIGURE 19.13. (*continued*)

eyes with vitreous seeds showed at least one vitreous seed recurrence at 5 years, and 62% of the eyes with subretinal seeds showed at least one subretinal seed recurrence at 5 years (70). Of the 158 eyes, recurrence of at least one retinal tumor per eye was found in 51% eyes by 5 years. A more recent analysis of 457 consecutive retinoblastomas showed those treated with chemoreduction alone had recurrence in 45% by 7 years follow-up, whereas those treated with chemoreduction plus thermotherapy, cryotherapy, or both showed recurrence in 18% by 7 years (71).

Plaque radiotherapy is a method of brachytherapy in which a radioactive implant is placed on the sclera over the base of a retinoblastoma to irradiate the tumor transclerally. It is limited to tumors less than 16 mm in base and 8 mm in thickness and complete treatment can be achieved in approximately 4 days. Plaque radiotherapy provides long-term tumor control in 90% of eyes when used as a primary treatment (2,4,72). In those eyes that need plaque radiotherapy for tumor recurrence after chemoreduction, complete control of the tumor is achieved in 96% of cases.

Plaque radiotherapy can be used for recurrent subretinal seeds or vitreous seeds but there is a higher failure rate. In such eyes, IAC is used for tumor control.

Enucleation is an important and powerful method for managing retinoblastoma (2,4). Enucleation is employed for advanced tumor with no hope for useful vision in the affected eye or if there is a concern for invasion of the tumor into the optic nerve, choroid, or orbit. Eyes with unilateral groups E are usually managed with primary enucleation. Eyes with bilateral groups D or E often require enucleation of one eye for tumor control.

Retinal Capillary Hemangioma

Retinal capillary hemangioma is a reddish-pink retinal mass that can occur in the peripheral fundus or adjacent to the optic disk (73). The tumor often has prominent dilated retinal blood vessels that supply and drain the lesion (Fig. 19.14). Untreated lesions can cause intraretinal exudation and retinal detachment. Fluorescein angiography shows rapid filling

Table 19.4

INTERNATIONAL CLASSIFICATION OF RETINOBLASTOMA (ICRB) (48)

Group	Quick Reference	Specific Features
A	Small tumor	Rb $\leq$ 3 mm[a]
B	Larger tumor Macula Juxtapapillary Subretinal fluid	Rb > 3 mm[a] or • macular Rb location ($\leq$ 3 mm to foveola) • juxtapapillary Rb location ($\leq$ 1.5 mm to disk) • Rb with subretinal fluid
C	Focal seeds	Rb with • subretinal seeds $\leq$ 3 mm from Rb and/or • vitreous seeds $\leq$ 3 mm from Rb
D	Diffuse seeds	Rb with • subretinal seeds > 3 mm from Rb and/or • vitreous seeds > 3 mm from Rb
E	Extensive Rb	Extensive Rb nearly filling globe or • Neovascular glaucoma • Opaque media from intraocular hemorrhage • Invasion into optic nerve, choroid, sclera, orbit, anterior chamber

Rb, retinoblastoma.
[a]Three millimeters in basal dimension or thickness.

Table 19.5

TREATMENT STRATEGY BASED ON LATERALITY AND RETINOBLASTOMA GROUPING

International Classification of Retinoblastoma	Unilateral	Bilateral[a]
A	Laser or cryotherapy	Laser or cryotherapy
B	IAC, VEC, or plaque	VEC
C	IAC, VEC, or plaque	VEC
D	IAC, VEC, or enucleation	VEC + STC Reserve IAC, if recurrence
E	Enucleation	VEC + STC Reserve IAC, if recurrence Reserve EBRT, if recurrence in only remaining eye Reserve IVC, if recurrent vitreous seeds

EBRT, external beam radiotherapy; IAC, Intra-arterial chemotherapy; IVC, Intravitreal chemotherapy; Laser, laser photocoagulation; Plaque, plaque radiotherapy; STC, Sub-Tenon chemotherapy; VEC, vincristine, etoposide, carboplatin plus thermotherapy or cryotherapy.
[a]Treatment in bilateral cases is usually based on the most advanced eye.

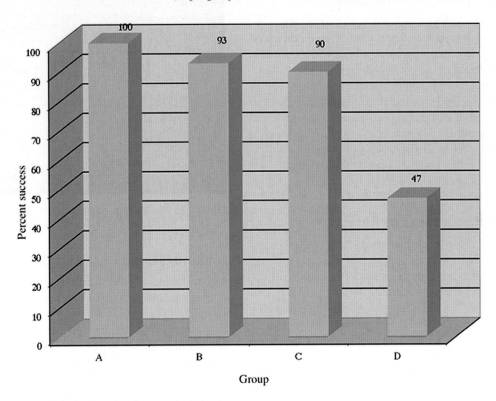

Table 19.6

CHEMOREDUCTION SUCCESS BASED ON INTERNATIONAL CLASSIFICATION OF RETINOBLASTOMA (64)

Success of chemoreduction using the International Classification of Retinoblastoma (major groups) in 249 consecutive cases

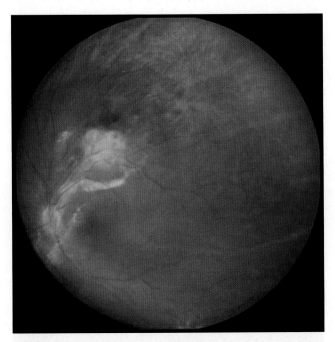

of the tumor with dye and intense late staining of the mass. Patients with retinal capillary hemangioma should be evaluated for the von Hippel-Lindau syndrome, an autosomal dominant condition characterized by cerebellar hemangioblastoma, pheochromocytoma, hypernephroma, and other visceral tumors and cysts. If the tumor produces macular exudation of retinal detachment, it can be treated with methods of laser photocoagulation, cryotherapy, photodynamic therapy (PDT), plaque radiotherapy, or external beam radiotherapy. The gene responsible for this syndrome has been localized to the short arm of chromosome 3.

Retinal Cavernous Hemangioma

The retinal cavernous hemangioma typically appears as a globular or sessile intraretinal lesion that is composed of multiple vascular channels that have a reddish-blue color (2,4). This tumor can show patches of gray-white fibrous tissue on the surface from previous preretinal hemorrhage. Cavernous hemangioma is a congenital retinal vascular hamartoma that is probably present at birth. This tumor can be associated with similar intracranial and cutaneous vascular hamartomas. In general, retinal cavernous hemangioma

FIGURE 19.14. Retinal capillary hemangioma with subretinal fluid and exudation in a child with von Hippel-Lindau syndrome.

requires no active treatment. If vitreous hemorrhage should occur, plaque radiotherapy to the tumor can be performed to induce sclerosis. If vitreous blood does not resolve, removal by vitrectomy may be necessary.

Retinal Racemose Hemangioma

The retinal racemose hemangioma is not a true neoplasm but rather a simple or complex arteriovenous communication (2,4). It is characterized by a large dilated tortuous retinal artery that passes from the optic disk for a variable distance into the fundus where it then communicates directly with a similarly dilated retinal vein which passes back to the optic disk (Fig. 19.15). It can occur as a solitary unilateral lesion or it can be part of the Wyburn-Mason syndrome which is characterized by other similar lesions in the midbrain and sometimes the orbit, mandible, and maxilla. It does not appear to have a hereditary tendency.

Astrocytic Hamartoma of Retina

Astrocytic hamartoma of the retina is a yellow-white intraretinal lesion that can also occur in the peripheral fundus or in the optic disk region. The lesion can be homogeneous or it may contain glistening foci of calcification (Fig. 19.16). Unlike retinal capillary hemangioma, it does not generally produce significant exudation or retinal detachment. Patients with astrocytic hamartoma of the retina should be evaluated for tuberous sclerosis, characterized by intracranial astrocytoma, cardiac rhabdomyoma, renal angiomyolipoma, pleural cysts, and other tumors and cysts. Growing astrocytic hamartoma can be treated with PDT.

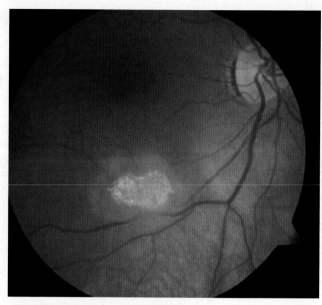

FIGURE 19.16. Retinal astrocytic hamartoma with glistening calcification.

Melanocytoma of the Optic Nerve

Melanocytoma of the optic nerve is a deeply pigmented congenital tumor that overlies a portion of the optic disk (Fig. 19.17) (2,74). Unlike uveal melanoma that occurs predominantly in whites, melanocytoma occurs with equal frequency in all races. It must be differentiated from malignant melanoma.

Intraocular Medulloepithelioma

Medulloepithelioma is an embryonal tumor that arises from the primitive medullary epithelium or the inner layer of the optic cup (75,76). It generally becomes clinically apparent in the first decade of life and appears as a fleshy, often cystic mass in the ciliary body (Fig. 19.18). Cataract and secondary

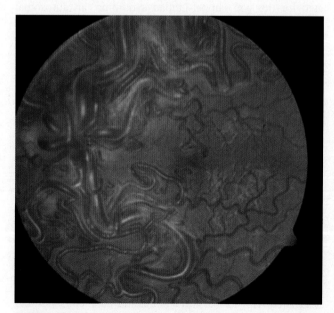

FIGURE 19.15. Retinal racemose hemangioma.

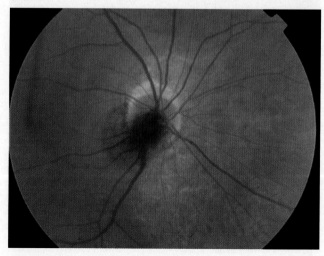

FIGURE 19.17. Optic disk melanocytoma with choroidal component.

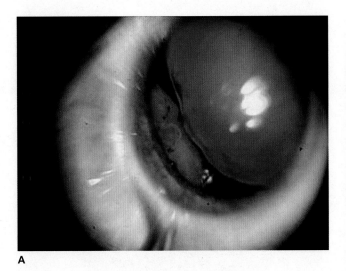

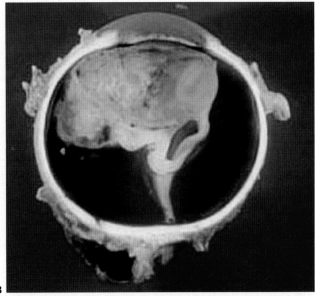

FIGURE 19.18. Medulloepithelioma of the ciliary body. **A:** Mass is visible peripheral to the lens on scleral depression. **B:** Following enucleation in another case, the mass is seen in the ciliary body with total retinal detachment.

glaucoma are frequent complications. Although approximately 60% to 90% are cytologically malignant, intraocular medulloepithelioma tends to be only locally invasive and distant metastasis is exceedingly rare. Larger tumors generally require enucleation of the affected eye. It is possible that some smaller tumors can be resected locally without enucleation.

Choroidal Hemangioma

Choroidal hemangioma is a benign vascular tumor that can occur as a circumscribed lesion in adults or as a diffuse tumor in children (77). The diffuse choroidal hemangioma usually occurs in association with ipsilateral facial nevus flammeus or variations of the Sturge-Weber syndrome. Ipsilateral congenital glaucoma is a frequent association. Secondary retinal detachment frequently occurs. Affected children often develop amblyopia in the involved eye. If vision loss from retinal detachment is found, then treatment of circumscribed hemangioma involves PDT (78), whereas diffuse hemangioma is treated with PDT, plaque radiotherapy, or external beam radiotherapy.

Choroidal Osteoma

Choroidal osteoma is a benign choroidal tumor, more common in females, and is probably congenital. Although it has been recognized in infancy, it may not be diagnosed clinically until young adulthood (79,80). This tumor consists of a plaque of mature bone that generally occurs adjacent to the optic disk (Fig. 19.19). Slow enlargement and choroidal neovascularization with subretinal hemorrhage and visual loss is a frequent complication. The pathogenesis is unknown and serum calcium and phosphorus levels are normal. Treatment with intravitreal anti-vascular endothelial growth factors is warranted.

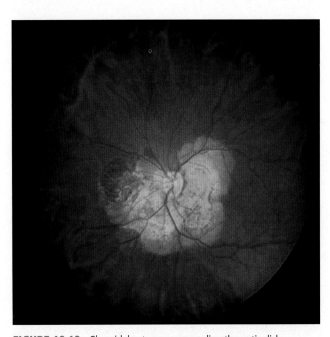

FIGURE 19.19. Choroidal osteoma surrounding the optic disk.

Uveal Nevus

Uveal nevus is a flat or minimally elevated variably pigmented tumor that may occur in the iris (Fig. 19.19) or in the choroid (81–83) (Figs. 19.20 and 19.21). With age, choroidal nevus shows increasing thickness, multifocality, and overlying drusen (82). Most nevi are stationary and nonprogressive but malignant transformation into melanoma can occur in approximately 1 in 8,000 cases. Factors that predict risks for transformation of iris nevus into melanoma and factors for choroidal nevus into melanoma are listed in Table 19.7.

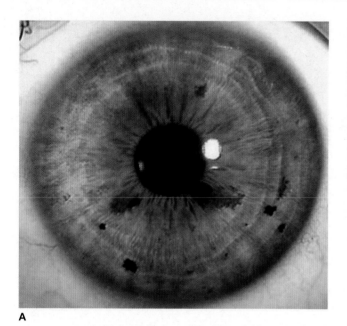

A

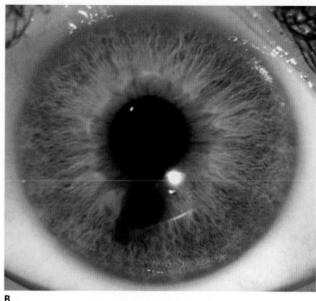

B

FIGURE 19.20. Iris freckles and nevi. **A:** Flat iris freckles on iris surface. **B:** Slightly thickened iris nevus distorting the iris stroma and causing corectopia.

Uveal Melanoma

Although uveal melanoma is generally a disease of adulthood, it is occasionally diagnosed in children (84,85) (Fig. 19.22). This malignancy can metastasize liver, lung, and other distant sites, and factors important in metastatic disease rely on tumor chromosomal typing as well as tumor size. Younger patient age at diagnosis is a factor for improved survival (85). Plaque radiotherapy or local tumor resection can be employed for most tumors and enucleation for large tumors.

Congenital Hypertrophy of Retinal Pigment Epithelium

Congenital hypertrophy of the retinal pigment epithelium (RPE) is a well-circumscribed, flat, pigmented tumor that occurs most often in the periphery of the fundus (86). It often shows depigmented lacunae within the lesion and a surrounding pale halo. It can occur as a solitary lesion or it can be multiple as part of congenital grouped pigmentation (Fig. 19.23). This condition is not a marker for familial adenomatous polyposis or Gardner's syndrome. A similar appearing but unrelated RPE lesion with irregular configuration is the marker.

Leukemia

Childhood leukemias can occasionally exhibit tumor infiltration in the retina, optic disk, and uveal tract. It is characterized by a swollen optic disk and thickening of the retina and choroid, often with hemorrhage and secondary retinal detachment. Intraocular leukemic infiltrates are generally responsive to irradiation and chemotherapy, but generally portend a poor systemic prognosis.

ORBITAL TUMORS

A variety of neoplasms and related space-occupying lesions can affect the orbit (87,88). Orbital cellulitis secondary to sinusitis and inflammatory pseudotumors are more common than true neoplasms. Only about 5% of orbital lesions in children that come to biopsy prove to be malignant. Cystic lesions are the most common group and vascular lesions are the second most common. This section covers orbital tumors and cysts but does not discuss orbital inflammatory or infectious conditions.

Dermoid Cyst

Dermoid cyst is the most common noninflammatory space-occupying orbital mass in children (89). This mass usually appears in the first decade of life as a fairly firm, fixed, subcutaneous mass at the superotemporal orbital rim near the zygomaticofrontal suture (Fig. 19.24). Occasionally, a dermoid cyst may occur deeper in the orbit unattached to the bone. This tumor can slowly enlarge or rupture, inciting an intense inflammatory reaction. Management is either observation or surgical removal of the mass.

Teratoma

A teratoma is a cystic mass that contains elements of all three embryonic germ layers (3,5). An orbital teratoma causes proptosis that is generally quite apparent at birth. The diagnosis should be suspected by imaging studies. Larger orbital teratomas can destroy the eye. Smaller teratomas can be removed intact without sacrificing the eye, but larger ones that have caused blindness may require orbital exenteration.

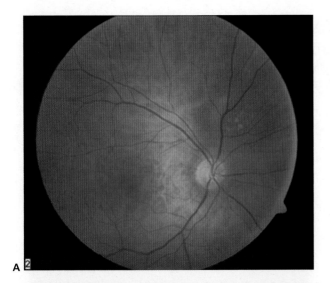

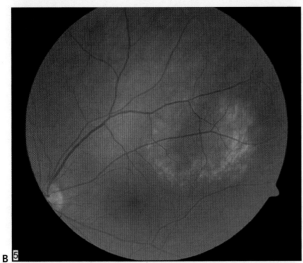

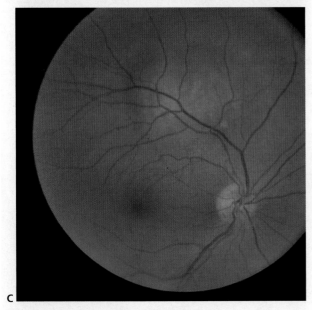

FIGURE 19.21. Choroidal nevus. **A:** Choroidal nevus with drusen. **B:** Choroidal nevus with halo. **C:** Suspicious choroidal nevus versus small melanoma with orange pigment and subretinal fluid.

Capillary Hemangioma

Capillary hemangioma is the most common orbital vascular tumor of childhood. It usually is clinically apparent at birth or within the first few weeks after birth and shows progressive enlargement with proptosis during the first few months of life. Thereafter, this mass slowly involutes. Orbital imaging studies show a diffuse, poorly circumscribed, orbital mass that enhances with contrast material. Management includes refraction, treatment of induced amblyopia with patching of the opposite eye, and consideration of oral propranolol. Occasionally, surgical resection for circumscribed tumors is performed.

Lymphangioma

Lymphangioma is an important vascular tumor of the orbit in children. This tends to become clinically apparent during the first decade of life (89). It can cause abrupt proptosis following orbital trauma, secondary to hemorrhage into the lymphatic channels within the lesion (Fig. 19.25). Such spontaneous hemorrhages, called chocolate cysts, can require aspiration or surgical evacuation to prevent visual loss from compression of the eye. Occasionally, surgical resection or debulking of the mass is necessary. More recently, aspiration of large cysts followed by injection of tissue glue has been performed and allowed avoidance of major surgery.

Juvenile Pilocytic Astrocytoma

Juvenile pilocytic astrocytoma (optic nerve glioma) is the most common orbital neural tumor of childhood (3,5). It is a cytological benign hamartoma that is generally stationary or very slowly progressive. The affected child develops ipsilateral visual loss and slowly progressive axial proptosis (Fig. 19.26). Orbital imaging studies show an elongated or oval-shaped mass that is well circumscribed because of the overlying dura mater. There is a greater incidence of this tumor in patients with neurofibromatosis. Since surgical excision necessitates blindness, the best management is periodic observation and surgical removal if there is blindness and cosmetically unacceptable proptosis. In cases that extend to the optic chiasm and are surgically unresectable, chemotherapy or radiotherapy may be necessary.

Rhabdomyosarcoma

Rhabdomyosarcoma is the most common primary orbital malignant tumor of childhood (90,91). This tumor most often occurs in the first decade of life with a mean age of 8 years at the time of diagnosis. It causes rapid proptosis and displacement of the globe over weeks, usually without pain or major inflammatory signs (Fig. 19.27). Imaging studies show an irregular but fairly well-circumscribed mass usually

Table 19.7
CLINICAL FEATURES PREDICTIVE OF TRANSFORMATION OF IRIS NEVUS (81) AND CHOROIDAL NEVUS (83) INTO MELANOMA
ABCDEF Guide Risk factors for transformation of iris nevus into melanoma
A, age ≤ 40 y
B, blood (hyphema)
C, clock hour inferiorly
D, diffuse configuration
E, ectropion
F, feathery margins
TFSOM-UHHD Risk factors for transformation of choroidal nevus (≤3 mm thickness) into melanoma (Mnemomic: *To Find Small Ocular Melanoma—Using Helpful Hints Daily*)
T, thickness >2 mm
F, fluid subretinal
S, symptoms
O, orange pigment
M, margin within 3 mm of optic disk
UH, ultrasound hollow
H, halo absent
D, drusen absent

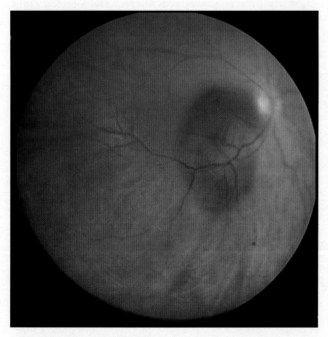

FIGURE 19.22. Choroidal melanoma in a 16-year-old boy.

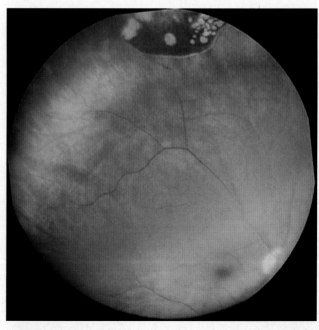

FIGURE 19.23. Congenital hypertrophy of the retinal pigment epithelium (RPE), solitary type.

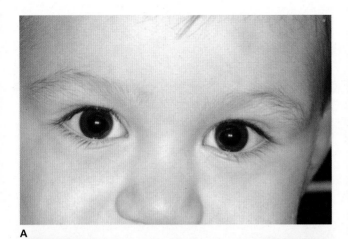

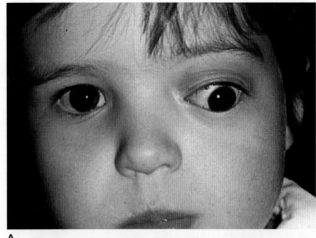

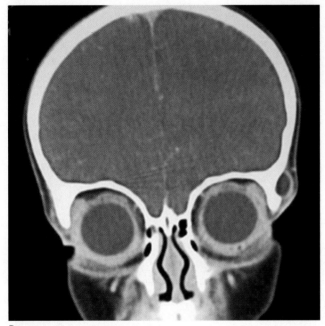

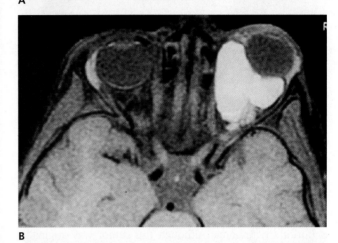

FIGURE 19.24. Dermoid cyst near the lateral orbital rim, barely visible clinically. **A:** Slight elevation of lateral orbital skin is shown. **B:** Coronal CT showing the cystic mass.

in the extraconal anterior orbit. The best approach is to obtain a generous biopsy to confirm the diagnosis and treat with combined chemotherapy and radiotherapy, depending on the staging of the disease.

Granulocytic Sarcoma (Chloroma)

Granulocytic sarcoma is the soft tissue infiltration by myelogenous leukemia. Although leukemia usually appears first in the blood and bone marrow, the orbit soft tissues may be the initial site to become clinically apparent. The child presents with a fairly rapid onset of proptosis and displacement of the globe. Confirmation of the orbital lesion can be made

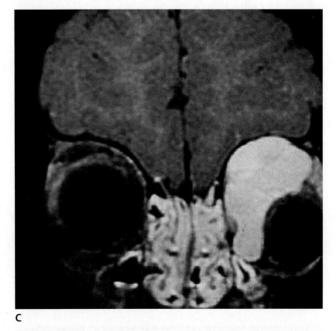

FIGURE 19.25. Orbital lymphangioma producing rapid proptosis in a young child. **A:** Downward displacement of the globe is shown. **B:** Axial MRI showing bright signal in the blood-filled cyst. **C:** Coronal MRI showing the mass displacing the globe.

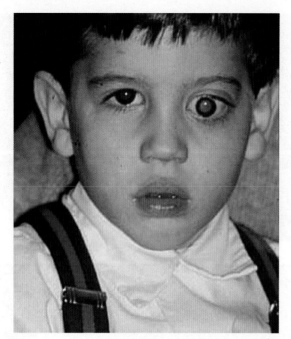

FIGURE 19.26. Juvenile pilocytic astrocytoma of optic nerve causing proptosis.

by biopsy and the condition is treated by chemotherapy or low-dose irradiation.

Lymphoma

The most important lymphoma to affect the orbit of children is Burkitt's lymphoma. Although this tumor was originally recognized exclusively in African tribes, it is recognized in otherwise normal children from the United States who are HIV positive (3,5).

Langerhan's Cell Histiocytosis

Eosinophilic granuloma can affect the orbital bones as an intraosseous bone-destructive inflammatory lesion (3,5). Although it can occur anywhere in the orbit, it most often occurs in the anterior portion of the frontal and zygomatic bones. Ultrastructural studies have suggested the stem cell in eosinophilic granuloma is the Langerhans cell. Hence, the term "Langerhans cell histiocytosis" is becoming preferable.

Metastatic Neuroblastoma

Although orbital metastasis in children can occur secondary to Wilm's and Ewing's tumors, metastatic neuroblastoma is the most common metastatic orbital tumor of childhood (3,5). The majority of children with orbital metastasis from

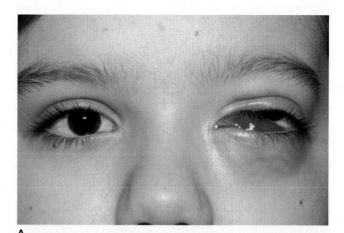

A

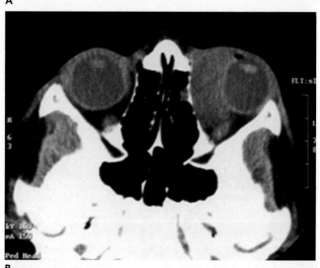

B

FIGURE 19.27. Orbital rhabdomyosarcoma. **A:** Proptosis and tumor involving the inferior fornix is shown. **B:** Axial CT scan showing mass in medial orbit.

neuroblastoma have a previously diagnosed primary neoplasm in the adrenal gland. However, the orbital metastasis can be diagnosed before the adrenal primary in about 3% of cases.

ACKNOWLEDGMENT

This work was supported by the Eye Tumor Research Foundation, Inc., Philadelphia, PA; the Lucille Wiedman Fund for Pediatric Eye Cancer Research, Philadelphia, PA; and the Carlos G. Bianciotto Retinoblastoma Research Fund, Philadelphia, PA.

REFERENCES

1. Shields CL, Shields JA. Conjunctival tumors in children. *Curr Opin Ophthalmol* 2007;18:351–360.

2. Shields JA, Shields CL. *Intraocular tumors. A text and atlas.* Philadelphia, PA: W.B. Saunders, 1992.

3. Shields JA, Shields CL. *Eyelid, conjunctival, and orbital tumors. An atlas and textbook*, 2nd Ed. Philadelphia, PA: Lippincott Williams and Wilkins, 2008.

4. Shields JA, Shields CL. *Intraocular tumors. An atlas and textbook*, 2nd Ed. Philadelphia, PA: Lippincott Williams and Wilkins, 2008.

5. Shields JA. *Diagnosis and management of orbital tumors.* Philadelphia, PA: W.B. Saunders, 1989.

6. Shields JA, Parsons HM, Shields CL, Shah P. Lesions simulating retinoblastoma. *J Ped Ophthalmol Strabism* 1991;28:338–340.

7. Shields JA, Shields CL. Review: coats disease. The 2001 LuEsther Mertz Lecture. *Retina* 2002;22:80–91.

8. De Potter P, Shields JA, Shields CL. *MRI of the eye and orbit.* Philadelphia, PA: JB Lippincott, 1994.

9. Mills DM, Tsai S, Meyer DR, Belden C. Pediatric ophthalmic computed tomographic scanning and associated cancer risk. *Am J Ophthalmol* 2006;142:1046–1053.

10. Shields CL, Mashayekhi A, Luo CK, Materin MA, Shields JA. Optical coherence tomography in children. Analysis of 44 eyes with intraocular tumors and simulating conditions. *J Ped Ophthalmol Strabism* 2004;41:338–344.

11. O,Hara BJ, Ehya H, Shields JA, Augsburger JJ, Shields CL, Eagle RC Jr. Fine needle aspiration biopsy in pediatric ophthalmic tumors and pseudotumors. *Acta Cytologica* 1993;37:125–130.

12. Shields CL. Forget-me-nots in the care of children with retinoblastoma. *Seminars in Ophthalmol* Sep–Oct 2008;23(5):324–334.

13. Epstein J, Shields CL, Shields JA. Trends in the management of retinoblastoma; Evaluation of 1,196 consecutive eyes during 1974–2001. *J Ped Ophthalmol Strabismus* 2003;40:196–203.

14. Ramasubramanian A, Shields CL, eds. *Retinoblastoma.* New Delhi, India: Jaypee Brothers Medical Publishers, 2012.

15. Haik BG, Karcioglu ZA, Gordon RA, Pechous BP. Capillary hemangioma (infantile periocular hemangioma). Review. *Surv Ophthalmol* 1994;38:399–426.

16. Schupp CJ, Kleber JB, Günther P, Holland-Cunz S. Propranolol therapy in 55 infants with infantile hemangioma: dosage, duration, adverse effects, and outcome. *Pediatr Dermatol* 2011;28:640–644.

17. Taylor SF, Cook AE, Leatherbarrow B. Review of patients with basal cell nevus syndrome. *Ophthal Plast Reconstr Surg* 2006;22:259–265.

18. Tang JY, Mackay-Wiggan JM, Aszterbaum M, et al. Inhibiting the Hedgehog pathway in patients with the Basal-Cell Nevus syndrome. *NEJM* 2012;366:2180–2188.

19. Shields CL, Shields JA. Tumors of the conjunctiva and cornea. *Surv Ophthalmol* 2004;49:3–24.

20. Grossniklaus HE, Green WR, Luckenbach M, Chan CC. Conjunctival lesions in adults. A clinical and histopathologic review. *Cornea* 1987; 6;78–116.

21. Shields CL, Shields JA, White D, Augsburger JJ. Types and frequency of lesions of the caruncle. *Am J Ophthalmol* 1986;102:771–778.

22. Shields CL, Demirci H, Karatza EC, Shields JA. Clinical Survey of 1,643 melanocytic and nonmelanocytic conjunctival tumors. *Ophthalmology* 2004;111:1747–1754.

23. Elsas FJ, Green WR. Epibulbar tumors in childhood. *Am J Ophthalmol* 1975;79:1001–1007.

24. Cunha RP, Cunha MC, Shields JA. Epibulbar tumors in children: a survey of 282 biopsies. *J Pediatr Ophthalmol Strabismus* 1987;24:249–254.

25. Scott JA, Tan DT. Therapeutic lamellar keratoplasty for limbal dermoids. *Ophthalmology* 2001;108:1858–1867.

26. Shields JA, Shields CL, Eagle RC Jr, Arevalo F, DePotter P. Ophthalmic features of the organoid nevus syndrome. *Ophthalmology* 1997;104:549–557.

27. Shields CL, Qureshi A, Eagle RC Jr, Lally SE, Shields JA. Epibulbar osseous choristoma in 8 patients. *Cornea* 2012;31:756–770.

28. Kaliki S, Arepalli S, Shields CL, Klein K, Sun H, Hysenj E, Lally SE, Shields JA. Conjunctival papilloma. Features and outcomes based on age at presentation. *JAMA Ophthalmol* 2013; 28:1–9.

29. Sjo NC, Heegaard S, Prause JU, von Buchwald C, Lindeberg H. Human papillomavirus in conjunctival papilloma. *Br J Ophthalmol* 2001;85:785–787.

30. Shields JA, Shields CL, De Potter P. Surgical management of conjunctival tumors. The 1994 Lynn B. McMahan Lecture. *Arch Ophthalmol* 1997;115:808–815.

31. Karp CL, Moore JK, Rosa RH Jr. Treatment of conjunctival and corneal intraepithelial neoplasia with topical interferon alpha-2b. *Ophthalmology* 2001;108:1093–1098.

32. Shields CL. Kaliki S, Kim HJ, et al. Interferon for ocular surface squamous neoplasia in 81 cases: Outcomes based on American Joint Committee on Cancer Classification. *Cornea* 2012; May 10. [Epub ahead of print] PMID: 22580436.

33. Shields CL, Lally MR, Singh AD, Shields JA, Nowinski T. Oral cimetidine (Tagamet) for recalcitrant, diffuse conjunctival papillomatosis. *Am J Ophthalmol* 1999;128:362–364.

34. Shields CL, Ramasubramanian A, Mellen P, Shields JA. Conjunctival squamous cell carcinoma arising in immunosuppressed patients (organ transplant, human immunodeficiency virus infection). *Ophthalmology* 2011;118:2133–2137.

35. Shields CL, Naseripour M, Shields JA. Topical Mitomycin C for extensive, recurrent conjunctival squamous cell carcinoma. *Am J Ophthalmol* 2002;133:601–606.

36. Singh AD, DePotter P, Fijal BA, Shields CL, Shields JA, Elston RC. Lifetime prevalence of uveal melanoma in white patients with oculo(dermal) melanocytosis. *Ophthalmology* 1998;105:195–198.

37. Shields CL, Qureshi A, Mashayekhi A, et al. Sector (partial) oculo(dermal) melanocytosis in 89 eyes. *Ophthalmology* 2011;118:2474.

38. Gerner N, Norregaard JC, Jensen OA, Prause JU. Conjunctival naevi in Denmark 1960–1980. A 21-year follow-up study. *Acta Ophthalmol Scand* 1996;74:334–337.

39. Shields CL, Fasiudden A, Mashayekhi A, Shields JA. Conjunctival nevi: clinical features and natural course in 410 consecutive patients. *Arch Ophthalmol* 2004;122:167–175.

40. Shields CL, Regillo A, Mellen PL, Kaliki S, Lally SE, Shields JA. Giant conjunctival nevus: Clinical features and natural course in 32 cases. *JAMA Ophthalmol* 2013; in press.

41. Shields JA, Shields CL, Mashayekhi A, Marr BP, Eagle RC Jr, Shields CL. Primary acquired melanosis of the conjunctiva. Risks for progression to melanoma in 311 eyes. The 2006 Lorenz E. Zimmerman lecture. *Ophthalmology* 2007; Epub 2007 Sep 18.

42. Shields CL, Shields JA, Gunduz K, et al. Conjunctival melanoma: risk factors for recurrence, exenteration, metastasis, and death in 150 consecutive patients. *Arch Ophthalmol* 2000;118:1497–1507.

43. Strempel I, Kroll P. Conjunctival malignant melanoma in children. *Ophthalmologica* 1999;213:129–132.

44. Shields CL, Markowitz JS, Belinsky I, et al. Conjunctival melanoma. Outcomes based on tumor origin in 382 consecutive cases. *Ophthalmology* 2011;118:389–395.

45. Knowles DM II, Jakobiec FA. Ocular adnexal lymphoid neoplasms: clinical, histopathologic, electron microscopic, and immunologic characteristics. *Hum Pathol* 1982;123:148–162.

46. McKelvie PA, McNab A, Francis IC, Fox R, O'Day J. Ocular adnexal lymphoproliferative disease: a series of 73 cases. *Clin Experiment Ophthalmol* 2001;29:387–393.

47. Shields CL, Shields JA, Carvalho C, Rundle P, Smith AF. Conjunctival lymphoid tumors: clinical analysis of 117 cases and relationship to systemic lymphoma. *Ophthalmology* 2001;108:979–984.

48. Shields CL, Shields JA. Basic understanding of current classification and management of retinoblastoma. *Curr Opin Ophthalmol* 2006;17:228–234.

49. Kivela T. The epidemiological challenge of the most frequent eye cancer: retinoblastoma, an issue of birth and death. *Br J Ophthalmol* 2009;93:1129–1131.

50. Nichols KE, Houseknecht MD, Godmilow L, et al. Sensitive multistep clinical molecular screening of 180 unrelated individuals with retinoblastoma detects 36 novel mutations in the RB1 gene. *Hum Mutat* 2005;25:566–574.

51. Honavar SG, Singh AD, Shields CL, et al. Postenucleation adjuvant therapy in high-risk retinoblastoma. *Arch Ophthalmol* 2002;120:923–931.

52. Kaliki S, Shields CL Shah SU, Eagle RC Jr, Shields JA, Leahey A. Postenucleation adjuvant chemotherapy with vincristine, etoposide, and carboplatin for the treatment of high-risk retinoblastoma. *Arch Ophthalmol* 2011;129:1422–1427.

53. Kaliki S, Shields CL, Rojanaporn, Al-Dahmash S, McLaughlin J, Shields JA, Eagle RC. High-risk retinoblastoma based on International Classification of Retinoblastoma. Analysis of 519 enucleated eyes. *Ophthalmology* 2013; Feb 8. pii: S0161-6420(12)01063-9. doi: 10.1016/j.ophtha.2012.10.044. [Epub ahead of print]

54. Kivela T. Trilateral retinoblastoma: A meta-analysis of hereditary retinoblastoma associated with primary ectopic intracranial retinoblastoma. *J Clin Oncol* 1999;17:1829–1837.

55. De Potter P, Shields CL, Shields JA. Clinical variations of trilateral retinoblastoma: a report of 13 cases. *J Pediatr Ophthalmol Strabismus* 1994;31:26–31.

56. Shields CL, Meadows AT, Shields JA, Carvalho C, Smith AF. Chemoreduction for retinoblastoma may prevent intracranial neuroblastic malignancy (trilateral retinoblastoma). *Arch Ophthalmol* 2001;119:1269–1272.

57. Karatza E, Shields CL, Flanders AE, Gonzalez ME, Shields JA. Pineal cyst simulating pinealoblastoma in 11 children with retinoblastoma. *Arch Ophthalmol* 2006;124:595–597.

58. Roarty JD, McLean IW, Zimmerman LE. Incidence of second neoplasms in patients with bilateral retinoblastoma. *Ophthalmology* 1988;95:1583–1587.

59. Wong FL, Boice JD Jr, Abramson DH, et al. Cancer incidence after retinoblastoma. Radiation dose and sarcoma risk. *JAMA* 1997;278:1262–1267.

60. Abramson DH, Melson MR, Dunkel IJ, Frank CM. Third (fourth and fifth) nonocular tumors in survivors of retinoblastoma. *Ophthalmology* 2001;108:1868–1876.

61. Shields CL, Ghassemi F, Tuncer S, Thangappan A, Shields JA. Clinical spectrum of diffuse infiltrating retinoblastoma in 34 consecutive eyes. *Ophthalmology* 2008;115:2253–2258.

62. Shields CL, Schoenfeld E, Kocher K, Shukla SY, Kaliki S, Shields JA. Lesions simulating retinoblastoma (pseudoretinoblastoma) in 604 cases. *Ophthalmology* 2012; Oct 27. doi:pii: S0161-6420 (12)00721-X. 10.1016/j.ophtha.2012.07.067. [Epub ahead of print] PMID: 23107579.

63. Murphree AL. Intraocular retinoblastoma: the case for a new group classification. *Ophthalmol Clin North Am* 2000;18:41–53, viii.

64. Shields CL, Mashayekhi A, Au AK, et al. The International Classification of Retinoblastoma predicts chemoreduction success. *Ophthalmology* 2006;113:2276–2280.

65. Shields CL, Fulco E, Kaliki S, et al. Retinoblastoma frontiers with intravenous, intra-arterial, periocular and intravitreal chemotherapy. *Eye* 2013. doi:10.1038/eye.2012.175

66. Shields CL, Kaliki S, Shah SU, et al. Minimal exposure (one or two cycles) intra-arterial chemotherapy in the management of retinoblastoma. *Ophthalmology* 2012;119:188–192.

67. Shields CL, Kaliki S, Rojanaporn D, Al-Dahmash S, Bianciotto C, Shields JA. Intravenous and intra-arterial chemotherapy for retinoblastoma: What have we learned. *Curr Opin Ophthalmol* 2012;23:202–209.

68. Shields CL, Bianciotto CG, Ramasubramanian A, et al. Intra-arterial chemotherapy for retinoblastoma. Report #1: Control of tumor, subretinal seeds, and vitreous seeds. *Arch Ophthalmol* 2011;129:1399–1406. [published online June 13, 2011]

69. Shields CL, Bianciotto CG, Jabbour P, et al. Intra-arterial chemotherapy for retinoblastoma. Report #2: Treatment complications. *Arch Ophthalmol* 2011;129:1407–1415. [published online June 13, 2011]

70. Shields CL, Honavar SG, Shields JA, Demirci H, Meadows AT, Naduvilath TJ. Factors predictive of recurrence of retinal tumor, vitreous seeds and subretinal seeds following chemoreduction for retinoblastoma. *Arch Ophthalmol* 2002;120:460–464

71. Shields CL, Mashayekhi A, Cater J, Shelil A, Meadows AT, Shields JA. Chemoreduction for retinoblastoma Analysis of tumor control and risks for recurrence in 457 tumors. *Am J Ophthalmol* 2004;138:329–337.

72. Shields CL, Mashayekhi A, Sun H, et al. Iodine 125 plaque radiotherapy as salvage treatment for retinoblastoma recurrence after chemoreduction in 84 tumors. *Ophthalmology* 2006;113:2087–2092.

73. Singh AD, Shields CL, Shields JA. Major review: Von Hippel-Lindau disease. *Surv Ophthalmol* 2001;46:117–142.

74. Shields JA, Demirci H, Mashayekhi A, Shields CL. Melanocytoma of the optic disc in 115 cases. The 2004 Samuel Johnson Memorial Lecture. *Ophthalmology* 2004;111:1739–1746.

75. Shields JA, Eagle RC Jr, Shields CL, De Potter P. Congenital neoplasms of the nonpigmented ciliary epithelium. (medulloepithelioma). *Ophthalmology* 1996;103:1998–2006

76. Kaliki S, Shields CL, Eagle RC Jr, et al. Ciliary body medulloepithelioma: analysis of 41 cases. 2013; in press.

77. Shields CL, Honavar SG, Shields JA, Cater J, Demirci H. Circumscribed choroidal hemangioma. Clinical manifestations and factors predictive of visual outcome in 200 consecutive cases. *Ophthalmology* 2001;108:2237–2348.

78. Blasi MA, Tiberti AC, Scupola A, et al. Photodynamic therapy with verteporfin for symptomatic circumscribed choroidal hemangioma: five-year outcomes. *Ophthalmology* 2010;117:1630–1637.

79. Shields CL, Shields JA, Augsburger JJ. Review: choroidal osteoma. *Surv Ophthalmol* 1988;33:17–27.

80. Shields CL, Sun H, Demirci H, Shields JA. Factors predictive of tumor growth, tumor decalcification, choroidal neovascularization and visual outcome in 74 eyes with choroidal osteoma. *Arch Ophthalmol* 2005;123:658–666.

81. Shields CL, Kaliki S, Hutchinson A, Nickerson S, Patel J, Kancherla S, Peshtani A, Nakhoda S, Kocher K, Kolbus E, Jacobs E, Garoon R, Walker B, Rogers B, Shields JA. Iris nevus

growth into melanoma: Analysis of 1611 consecutive eyes. The ABCDEF guide. *Ophthalmology* 2013;120:766–72.

82. Shields CL, Furuta M, Mashayekhi A, et al. Clinical spectrum of choroidal nevi based on age at presentation in 3422 consecutive eyes. *Ophthalmology* 2008;115(3):546–552.

83. Shields CL, Cater JC, Shields JA, Singh AD, Santos MCM, Carvalho C. Combination of clinical factors predictive of growth of small choroidal melanocytic tumors. *Arch Ophthalmol* 2000;118:360–364.

84. Shields CL, Kaliki S, Shah S, Luo W, Furuta M, Shields JA. Iris melanoma features and prognosis in children and adults in 317 patients. The 2011 Leonard Apt Lecture. *J AAPOS* 2012;16: 10–16.

85. Shields CL, Kaliki S, Furuta M, Mashayekhi A, Shields JA. Clinical spectrum and prognosis of uveal melanoma based on age at presentation in 8033 cases. *Retina* 2012;32: 1363–1372.

86. Shields CL, Mashayekhi A, Ho T, Cater J, Shields JA. Solitary congenital hypertrophy of the retinal pigment epithelium:

clinical features and frequency of enlargement in 330 patients. *Ophthalmology* 2003;110:1968–1976.

87. Shields, JA, Shields CL, Scartozzi R. Survey of 1264 orbital tumors and pseudotumors. The 2002 Montgomery Lecture. Part 1. *Ophthalmology* 2004;111:997–1008.

88. Shields JA, Bakewell B, Augsberger JJ, Bernardino V. Space-occupying orbital masses in children: A review of 250 consecutive biopsies. *Ophthalmology* 1988;93:379–384.

89. Shields JA, Kaden IH, Eagle RC Jr, Shields CL. Orbital dermoid cysts. Clinicopathologic correlations, classification, and management. The 1997 Josephine E. Schueler Levture. *Ophthal Plast Reconstr Surg* 1997;13:265–276.

90. Wright JE, Sullivan TJ, Garner A, Wulc AE, Moseley IF. Orbital venous anomalies. *Ophthalmology* 1997;104:905–913.

91. Shields CL, Shields JA, Honavar SG, Demerci H. The clinical spectrum of primary ophthalmic rhabdomyosarcoma. *Ophthalmology* 2001;108:2284–2292

92. Shields JA, Shields CL. Rhabdomyosarcoma: review for the ophthalmologist. *Surv Ophthalmol* 2003;48:39–57.

20

Systemic Hamartomatoses ("Phakomatoses")

Carol L. Shields • *Jerry A. Shields*

THE SYSTEMIC HAMARTOMATOSES (phakomatoses) comprise a group of syndromes with variable clinical manifestations that primarily affect the ocular region, central nervous system (CNS), skin, and occasionally, the viscera (1–7). The recognition of singular ocular or cutaneous features should prompt a referral to specialists familiar with the variety of manifestations of these conditions for diagnostic purposes and to provide patient management. In this chapter, we review the hamartomatoses, otherwise termed phakomatoses or oculoneurocutaneous syndromes. We emphasize the clinical spectrum of findings and illustrate the salient features.

GENERAL CONSIDERATIONS

Historical Aspects

The term "phakoma" was coined by Van der Hoeve in 1932 to indicate a mother spot or birthmark, a characteristic finding in many of these conditions (1). At that time, retinal and cerebellar hemangiomatosis (von Hippel-Lindau syndrome), neurofibromatosis (von Recklinghausen syndrome), and tuberous sclerosis (Bourneville syndrome) were grouped under this heading. Later, encephalofacial hemangiomatosis (EFH; Sturge-Weber syndrome), racemose hemangiomatosis (Wyburn-Mason syndrome), and cavernous hemangioma of the retina with cutaneous and CNS involvement were grouped with these other conditions.

Terminology

To better understand these syndromes, the clinician should be familiar with certain terms such as hamartia, hamartoma, chorista, and choristoma.

Hamartia and hamartoma are terms that refer to malformations that are composed of tissues that are ordinarily present at the location where they occur. A hamartia is a nontumorous anomaly composed of tissues that are normally present at the involved site, while a hamartoma is a tumorous malformation composed of tissues that are normally present at the involved site. Most of the entities discussed in this chapter are characterized by the presence of hamartomas. The term systemic hamartomatosis is used to designate multiple-organ involvement. Examples of hamartomas include the vascular tumors that occur in patients with either retinocerebellar hemangiomatosis or EFH, and the glial and peripheral nerve tumors are those that occur with tuberous sclerosis or neurofibromatosis. These tumors develop in areas where vascular and neural tissues are normally present.

Chorista and choristoma, on the other hand, are terms that refer to malformations composed of elements that are not ordinarily present at the location where they occur. A chorista is a nontumorous anomaly composed of tissues which are not normally present at the involved site. The microscopic rests of ectopic lacrimal gland tissue that sometimes occur in the anterior chamber and deep orbit are examples of choristas. A choristoma is a tumorous malformation composed of tissues that are not normally present at the involved site. The classic example of a choristoma is the limbal dermoid, a tumor composed of dermal elements that are not normally present in the bulbar conjunctiva or cornea.

A particular lesion can be classified as either a hamartoma or a choristoma depending on the organ involved. For example, a 5 mm nodule of mature bone would be classified as a hamartoma if it occurred on the superior orbital rim, but a similar mass of osseous tissue in the liver would be classified as a choristoma.

Heredity

Most of the hamartomatoses have an autosomal dominant mode of inheritance, often with incomplete penetrance. Specific chromosomal abnormalities have been recognized in association with these entities. Notable exceptions are EFH (Sturge-Weber syndrome) and racemose hemangiomatosis (Wyburn-Mason syndrome) in which heredity does not appear to play a role and genetic abnormalities are not yet delineated. In Sturge-Weber syndrome, there is some evidence that the condition is a mosaic mutation with only segmental involvement. Those that receive the full mutation die in utero. Although these conditions are generally hereditary, many do not become clinically apparent until the teenage years or young adulthood.

Benign and Malignant Tumors

In general, the tumors that develop in these syndromes are benign. They differ from true neoplasms by virtue of the fact that they are anomalies of tissue formation, rather than tumors that arise from fully developed tissues. Furthermore, they are usually stationary or slowly progressive lesions that generally lack the capacity for the limitless proliferation seen with malignant neoplasms (5,6). Some of these syndromes, however, can be associated with malignant neoplasms. For example, there is an increased incidence of malignant schwannomas of the peripheral nerves in patients with neurofibromatosis. Hypernephroma occurs with greater frequency in patients with retinal capillary hemangiomatosis.

Formes Frustes and Combined Phakomatoses

It is common for patients with systemic hamartomatoses to only manifest some of the clinical features of a particular syndrome. This lack of complete expressivity is referred to as a forme fruste. Furthermore, patients can occasionally exhibit certain lesions characteristic of one entity and other lesions characteristic of another. For example, the café au lait spots seen in patients with neurofibromatosis can occasionally be seen in patients with tuberous sclerosis. Some patients with features of Sturge-Weber syndrome also manifest oculodermal melanocytosis, a condition termed phakomatosis pigmentovascularis. This coincidence of two conditions has been attributed to a genetic phenomenon of twin spotting (8–10).

TUBEROUS SCLEROSIS COMPLEX (BOURNEVILLE SYNDROME)

Definition, Incidence, and Genetics

Tuberous sclerosis complex (TSC) is a syndrome characterized by retinal astrocytic hamartomas cutaneous abnormalities, CNS astrocytomas, and internal tumors such as cardiac rhabdomyoma, renal angiomyolipoma, and other tumors (11–14). It is best known to produce a triad of adenoma sebaceum, epilepsy, and mental deficiency. The term "epiloia" (which implies epilepsy and "mindlessness") has often been used to describe this condition, but the names TSC has become more widely accepted.

TSC is an autosomal dominant condition and displays two genetic loci including 9q34 (TSC1) and 16p13 (TSC2).

These two sites control products of hamartin (TSC1) and tuberin (TSC2) that act synergistically to regulate cellular growth and differentiation (15,16). Deregulation of these products leads to hamartomatous tumor development.

The major and minor diagnostic criteria for TSC were established by the Tuberous Sclerosis Consensus Conference in 1998 (15,16) (Table 20.1). The major features include facial angiofibromas, ungual or periungual fibromas, hypomelanotic (ash leaf) macules (≥3), shagreen patch, retinal nodular (astrocytic) hamartomas, cortical tuber, subependymal nodule, subependymal giant cell astrocytoma, cardiac rhabdomyoma, lymphangiomyomatosis, and renal angiomyolipoma. The minor features include dental enamel pits, rectal hamartomatous polyps, bone cysts, cerebral white matter migration lines, gingival fibromas, nonrenal hamartoma, retinal achromatic patch, confetti skin lesions, and multiple renal cysts. A definite diagnosis of TSC is established by the presence of two major or one major plus two minor features. Probable TSC requires one major and one minor feature and possible TSC requires either one major or two or more minor features.

The incidence of TSC is about 1 in 10,000. Although TSC is usually diagnosed during the first few years of life, it has occasionally been recognized in patients as young as 1 month or as old as 50 years. This syndrome has been identified in all races, and there is no sex predilection.

Ophthalmologic Features

The retinal astrocytic hamartoma is the characteristic fundus lesion of TSC (17–21). The smaller noncalcified tumor can be extremely subtle and appear only as ill-defined translucent thickening of the nerve fiber layer. A slightly larger tumor is more opaque and appears as a sessile white lesion at the level of the nerve fiber layer of the retina (Fig. 20.1). It may contain characteristic dense yellow, refractile foci of calcification that resemble fish eggs or tapioca (Fig. 20.2). In some cases, this tumor can develop a central cavity and occasionally, there can be localized overlying vitreous seeds (22,23). The retinal astrocytic hamartoma is generally stable but can rarely enlarge and produce retinal detachment and neovascular glaucoma.

A fairly common but often overlooked fundus feature of TSC is the retinal pigment epithelial (RPE) depigmented (punched out) lesion (19,20). This finding can be tiny at only 50 to 100 μm diameter or it can be obvious at 3 to 4 mm diameter. Multiple RPE depigmented lesions should be suggestive of TSC.

Ancillary studies, such as fluorescein angiography, ultrasonography, and optical coherence tomography, can assist in the diagnosis (24). Fine-needle aspiration has been used to make a diagnosis in atypical cases.

The retinal astrocytic hamartoma shows rather typical pathologic features. It is located in the nerve fiber layer of the retina and is composed of fibrillary astrocytes. Foci of dystrophic calcification, sometimes resembling psammoma

Table 20.1

DIAGNOSTIC CRITERIA (REVISED) FOR ESTABLISHING THE DIAGNOSIS OF TUBEROUS SCLEROSIS COMPLEX (TSC)

Category	Feature
Major features	• Facial angiofibromas or forehead plaque • Ungual or periungual fibroma • Hypomelanotic macules (>3) (ash leaf macule) • Shagreen patch (connective tissue nevus) • Multiple retinal nodular hamartomas • Cortical tuber • Subependymal nodule • Subependymal giant cell astrocytoma • Cardiac rhabdomyoma • Lymphangiomyomatosis • Renal angiomyolipoma
Minor features	• Multiple pits in dental enamel • Hamartomatous rectal polyps • Bone cysts • Cerebral white matter migration lines • Gingival fibromas • Non-renal hamartoma • Retinal achromic patch • Confetti skin lesions • Multiple renal cysts
Classification	• Definite TSC: Either 2 major or 1 major with two minor features • Probable TSC: 1 major and 1 minor features • Possible TSC: Either 1 major or ≥2 minor features

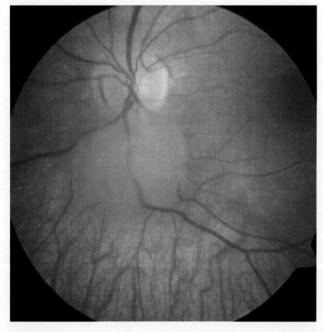

FIGURE 20.1. Tuberous sclerosis complex: non-calcified retinal astrocytic hamartoma.

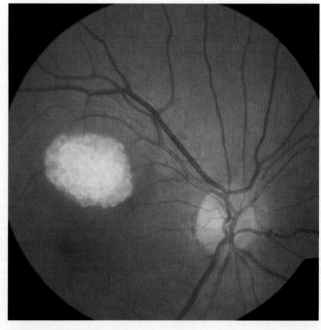

FIGURE 20.2. Tuberous sclerosis complex: calcified retinal astrocytic hamartoma.

bodies, are frequently present in the tumor. The uveal tract is rarely affected in tuberous sclerosis. A depigmented iris sector, seen in some affected patients, is believed to be the equivalent of depigmented cutaneous lesions.

Dermatologic Features

The main cutaneous manifestations of TSC include adenoma sebaceum, depigmented macules, and café au lait spots. Adenoma sebaceum is characterized clinically by multiple slightly elevated, rubbery, yellow-red papules. They are most often found on the face, frequently in a butterfly-shaped distribution (Fig. 20.3). They are composed microscopically of a benign proliferation of fibrous tissue and blood vessels. In reality, these tumors are angiofibromas, and the sebaceous gland hyperplasia appears to be a secondary change and is not part of the primary process. Consequently, the term "sebaceous adenoma" is a misnomer. Similar angiofibromas can occur beneath or adjacent to the fingernails or toenails in patients with tuberous sclerosis. These subungual fibromas, when present, are highly suggestive of tuberous sclerosis.

Depigmented macules resembling vitiligo are commonly present on the skin of patients with TSC (25). Because these patches frequently assume a configuration of a leaf from the mountain ash tree, the characteristic lesion is often referred to as the ash leaf sign (Fig. 20.4). These lesions are considered to be highly characteristic or even pathognomonic of tuberous sclerosis.

Other Features

The characteristic brain findings in patients with TSC include subependymal and cortical astrocytomas, sometimes with giant tumor cells (13,14,26) (Fig. 20.5). Both can demonstrate cystic and calcific changes, which account for the name tuberous sclerosis (potato-like masses). These lesions

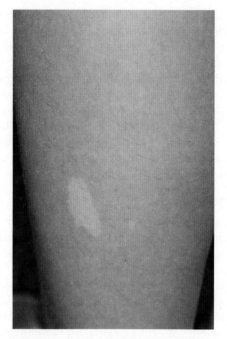

FIGURE 20.4. Tuberous sclerosis complex: ash leaf sign.

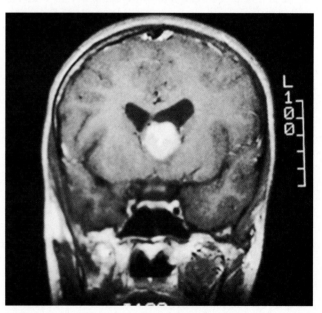

FIGURE 20.5. Tuberous sclerosis complex: brain astrocytoma.

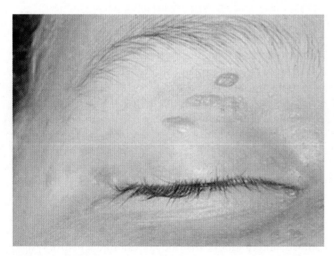

FIGURE 20.3. Tuberous sclerosis complex: adenoma sebaceum in the periocular region.

contribute to the seizures and mental deficiency. Contrary to early reports, mental deficiency is not necessarily a part of this syndrome. Many of the early reported patients were recruited from mental institutions where individuals with mental derangement were hospitalized. It is now recognized that many patients have only mild symptoms and signs and are of normal or near-normal intelligence.

The renal lesions commonly predispose the patient to recurrent nephritis and elevated blood urea nitrogen. They have been shown histologically to be benign angiomyolipomas, with no tendency to undergo malignant transformation or to metastasize (26). The cardiac lesions have been shown to be rhabdomyomas, composed of large spider cells with prominent vacuoles containing glycogen. Some patients with tuberous sclerosis develop slowly progressive subpleural cysts that result from anomalous development of pulmonary tissue. These cysts can rupture, leading to spontaneous pneumothorax. Irregular cortical thickenings of bones, particularly the metatarsals and metacarpals, as well as hamartomas of the liver, thyroid, pancreas, testes, and other organs, have been reported.

Management

The retinal astrocytic hamartoma and RPE depigmented lesions are typically asymptomatic, nonprogressive, and do not require treatment. Ocular examination should be performed yearly, and the patient followed for other manifestations of tuberous sclerosis. If there should be an associated retinal detachment that extends into the foveal area, then laser photocoagulation, photodynamic therapy, or plaque radiotherapy can be employed to bring about resolution of the subretinal fluid. The astrocytic hamartoma of the retina has an extremely low tendency to undergo malignant change and has no tendency to metastasize. The visual prognosis is also excellent, except in the rare instances in which exudation, retinal detachment, or vitreous hemorrhage occur.

Most of the cutaneous lesions of TSC require no treatment. Larger facial angiofibromas may require surgical excision for cosmetic purposes. In recent years, the brain lesions have been treated with mTOR inhibitors (27).

NEUROFIBROMATOSIS (VON RECKLINGHAUSEN SYNDROME)

Definition, Incidence, and Genetics

Neurofibromatosis is an oculoneurocutaneous syndrome characterized by multisystem involvement that can lead to a wide variety of clinical symptoms and signs. Although a number of isolated reports during the 19th century described many of the clinical features of this syndrome, von Recklinghausen published a classic monograph in 1882 that provided a better understanding of this condition (28). The condition is now known as von Recklinghausen syndrome. The National Institute of Health Consensus Development Conference established criteria for the diagnosis of neurofibromatosis.

Neurofibromatosis is categorized into types 1 and 2. Type 1 is called peripheral neurofibromatosis or von Recklinghausen syndrome, whereas type 2 is called central or bilateral acoustic neurofibromatosis. Type 1 neurofibromatosis is characterized by peripheral and cutaneous manifestations and is related to an abnormality on chromosome 17. Type 2 is characterized by CNS tumors and early onset of posterior subcapsular cataract. Type 2 neurofibromatosis is related to an abnormality on chromosome 22.

Neurofibromatosis Type 1
General Considerations

Neurofibromatosis type 1 occurs at a rate of 1 in 3,000 persons, but it is estimated that the frequency could be higher as some individuals manifest only mild features. Approximately one-half of affected patients represent a new mutation. This condition is caused by an autosomal dominant mutation in the *NF1* gene that leads to decreased production of the protein neurofibromin, which has a tumor suppressor function. Only one deleted is necessary to manifest this condition. The *NF1* gene is chromosome 17q. There have been more than 250 mutations identified. Complete gene deletion leads to severe phenotype. This highly penetrant phenotype has a wide variety of manifestations and can vary within families. Another locus, the *SPRED1* gene, has been found in patients with "mild neurofibromatosis" and this represents Legius syndrome.

The criteria for diagnosis of neurofibromatosis type 1 are listed in Table 20.2 (29,30). This condition more often affects patients of the Caucasian race and equally in boys and girls. Scoliosis can be a prominent feature.

Ophthalmologic Features

Neurofibromatosis has the most diversified ocular findings among the phakomatoses. This condition can involve the eyelid, conjunctiva, aqueous outflow channels, uveal tract, retina, orbit, and optic nerve (31,32).

Eyelid involvement is characterized by nodular or plexiform neurofibroma. Nodular neurofibroma appears as a solitary or multifocal painless, smooth-surfaced and well-defined mass, often the size of a pea, and without color change. Plexiform neurofibroma presents as a diffuse thickening of the eyelid that can produce the typical S-shaped curvature to the eyelid, a finding highly characteristic of neurofibromatosis. The conjunctiva can be involved by diffuse or localized neurofibromas. Patients with neurofibromatosis have an increased incidence of congenital glaucoma, which can be secondary to several mechanisms. There is a high association of neurofibromatosis type 1 with optic nerve glioma.

Iris Lisch nodules are the most common ophthalmic abnormality of neurofibromatosis type 1. These characteristically orange-tan nodules appear in early childhood (usually by age of 5 to 6 years) as discrete, multiple, bilateral tumors of the anterior border layer of the iris, classically measuring less than 1 mm diameter, and best detected by slit lamp biomicroscopy (Fig. 20.6). Histopathologically, iris Lisch nodules are hamartomas composed of aggregates of melanocytes on the anterior border layer of the iris.

The choroidal findings in patients with neurofibromatosis type 1 include unifocal or multifocal choroidal nevus, diffuse plexiform neurofibroma, neurilemoma, and melanoma. Multiple bilateral, choroidal nevi are highly suggestive of neurofibromatosis type 1. They are usually small, ill-defined, and randomly distributed. Choroidal neurofibroma usually appears a diffuse thickening of the uveal tract from an increased number of neurofibromatous and melanocytic

Table 20.2	
DIAGNOSTIC CRITERIA FOR NEUROFIBROMATOSIS TYPE 1 (NF1)	
Feature	**Number**
Café au lait	≥6 café au lait spots larger than 5 mm in diameter in prepubertal children (<10 y) or ≥6 café au lait spots larger than 15 mm in diameter in postpubertal individuals (adults)
Freckles in axilla or inguinal region	Crowe sign
Skin neurofibroma	≥2 typical neurofibroma or ≥1 plexiform neurofibroma
Optic nerve glioma	—
Iris Lisch nodules	≥2 lesions
Osseous lesion	Sphenoid dysplasia or long bone abnormalities (cortex thinning or pseudoarthrosis)
Relative (first degree) with NF1 by above criteria	Parent, sibling, or offspring

At least two of the seven criteria should be present for diagnosis. Some manifestations do not appear until later life, delaying diagnosis. Adapted from: Stumpf DA, Alksne JF, Annegers JF. Neurofibromatosis. Conference Statement. National Institute of Health Consensus Development Conference. *Arch Neurol* 1988;45:575–578; Gutmann DH, Aylsworth A, Carey JC, et al. The diagnostic evaluation and multidisciplinary management of neurofibromatosis 1 and neurofibromatosis 2. *JAMA* 1997;278:51–57.

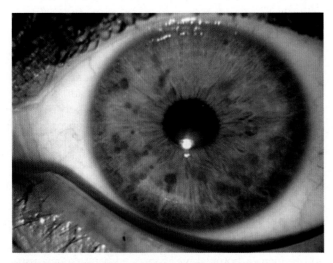

FIGURE 20.6. Neurofibromatosis type 1: Iris Lisch nodules.

elements. There appears to be a higher incidence of uveal melanoma in patients with neurofibromatosis.

Several retinal and optic disk lesions can occur with neurofibromatosis type 1. Retinal astrocytic hamartoma is a manifestation of neurofibromatosis, but is more often found with TSC. Retinal vasoproliferative tumor can occur with neurofibromatosis, leading to exudative retinopathy and risk for blindness (33). Congenital hypertrophy of the RPE is believed to be more common in patients with neurofibromatosis type 1. Fundus changes can occur secondary to optic nerve glioma including optic disk edema, optic atrophy, opticociliary shunt vessels, and central retinal vein obstruction.

Dermatologic Features

The most important cutaneous manifestations of neurofibromatosis include café au lait spots (pigmented macules), freckles in the axillary or inguinal region, and urticarial pigmentosa (Fig. 20.7). Café au lait spots are found in 95% of patients with neurofibromatosis type 1, but they can be seen in patients with other conditions such as McCune-Albright syndrome, TSC, and Fanconi anemia. Café au lait spots are also found in persons without neurofibromatosis type 1. They can become more noticeable over time with sun exposure.

Subcutaneous or cutaneous benign neurofibromas are an important finding but typically appear in older children or later. Deep neurofibromas might not be visible and are only detected by palpation. Puberty and pregnancy can increase number and growth of neurofibromas. Plexiform neurofibromas can be invasive and ill defined, occasionally associated with pain. Rapid growth of neurofibroma is suggestive of malignant degeneration.

Central Nervous System Features

The most important CNS feature of neurofibromatosis type 1 is the optic nerve glioma (juvenile pilocytic astrocytoma). Optic nerve glioma can present with painless proptosis

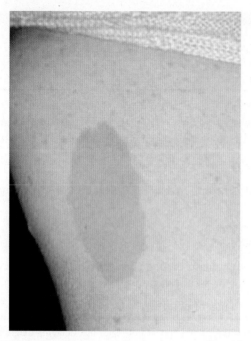

FIGURE 20.7. Neurofibromatosis type 1: cutaneous café au lait spot.

or subtle features of color or visual acuity abnormalities (Figs. 20.8 and 20. 9). Magnetic resonance imaging shows enlargement of the optic nerve, often so large that it develops a fold (kink) within its substance to accommodate the orbit, leading to down-and-out proptosis. This mass shows enhancement on T1-weighted, gadolinium contrast images, particularly notable in the axial and coronal views. It is important to differentiate this tumor from optic nerve sheath meningioma as the systemic implications and therapy differ. This is best determined using gadolinium-enhanced, orbital fat suppressed, T1-weighted coronal views. With glioma, the central substance of the nerve enhances, whereas with meningioma the peripheral encircling arachnoid sheath enhances.

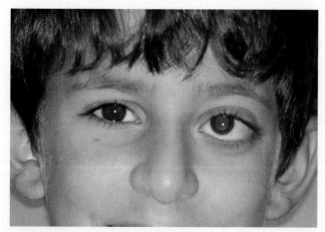

FIGURE 20.8. Neurofibromatosis type 1: mild proptosis from optic nerve glioma.

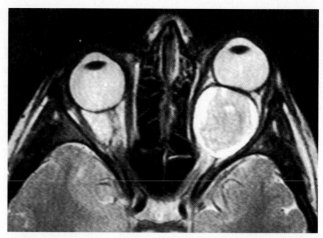

FIGURE 20.9. Neurofibromatosis type 1: magnetic resonance image of optic nerve glioma.

Glioma is more often associated with neurofibromatosis type 1, whereas meningioma with neurofibromatosis type 2.

Other Features

There are several orthopedic problems in patients with neurofibromatosis type 1: sphenoid wing dysplasia, congenital pseudoarthrosis with tibial or forearm bowing, thoracic cage asymmetry with inferior rib prominence, and scoliosis/kyphosis. Scoliosis at a young age (under 10 years) can progress. Other findings include macrocephaly and hypertension.

A number of other benign and malignant systemic tumors have been associated with neurofibromatosis. Sarcomas can arise from the peripheral nerve sheath, either de novo or from preexisting benign cutaneous nerve sheath tumors. Malignant peripheral nerve sheath tumors can occur in over 20% of patients. There seems to be an increased incidence of breast, genitourinary, and gastrointestinal tumors, as well as cutaneous melanoma.

Management

The management of neurofibromatosis varies with the location and the extent of the disease. Most fundus lesions require no treatment. Choroidal melanoma and neurilemoma usually required plaque radiotherapy, resection, or enucleation. Iris Lisch nodules, congenital hypertrophy of the RPE, and retinal astrocytic hamartoma are observed. Retinal vasoproliferative tumors often require cryotherapy, laser photocoagulation, photodynamic therapy, or plaque radiotherapy to control exudative findings.

Neurofibromatosis Type 2
General Considerations

Neurofibromatosis type 2 is a multisystem disorder with prominent features of CNS tumors including bilateral vesibular schwannomas (acoustic neuromas), spinal cord schwannomas, meningiomas, gliomas, and juvenile posterior subcapsular cataract. This condition is also referred to as MISME syndrome, a mnemonic referring to related tumors of MIS—multiple inherited schwannomas, M—meningiomas, and E—ependymomas (34). Cutaneous features are less often seen with this form of neurofibromatosis. The criteria for diagnosis of neurofibromatosis type 2 are listed in Table 20.3.

Neurofibromatosis type 2 can be associated with reduced life span secondary to CNS tumors, particularly if they are present at a young age and are multiple. The average age at symptom onset is approximately 20 years but can be delayed. Early age at symptoms and the presence of intracranial meningioma at diagnosis are two signs of higher risk for disease severity and mortality. In an analysis of 150 affected patients in 1992, more than 40% were expected to die by 50 years (35). Recent advances in treatment has extended life prognosis.

The incidence of neurofibromatosis type 2 is 1 in 25,000 live births and has nearly 100% penetrance by 60 years of age (36). It is estimated that this condition has a diagnostic prevalence of 1 in 100,000 people in 2005. Neurofibromatosis type 2 is related to a mutation in the *NF2* gene at chromosome 22q12.2. This gene produces merlin (also called neurofibromin-2), a tumor suppressor.

When mutated, decreased function of merlin leads to the uncontrolled development of tumors, particularly in the CNS. One-half of affected patients have a de novo mutation.

Ophthalmologic Features

Neurofibromatosis type 2 displays three important ophthalmologic findings, notably posterior subcapsular cataract in childhood, combined hamartoma of the retina and RPE, and epiretinal membranes (37–40) (Fig. 20.10). The juvenile posterior subcapsular cataract (<50 years) is a criterion for diagnosis of this condition. Other lens opacities in the capsular or cortical region of young patients are believed to be related to neurofibromatosis type 2. Lisch nodules are not a feature of neurofibromatosis type 2.

Epiretinal membranes and combined hamartoma of the retina and RPE can have overlapping clinical phenotype and can be multifocal. Of those with severe clinical features of neurofibromatosis type 2, 80% display epiretinal membranes (38). The hamartomas are along the inner retina but lead to prominent retinal dragging, corkscrew retinal vessels, gray-green appearance, and tumor formation (40).

Table 20.3
DIAGNOSTIC CRITERIA FOR NEUROFIBROMATOSIS TYPE 2 (NF2)

Feature
Bilateral eighth cranial nerve tumors confirmed on magnetic resonance imaging or computed tomography
Unilateral eighth cranial nerve tumor
Plus
Relative (first degree) with NF2
Two of the following:
• Meningioma
• Glioma
• Schwannoma
• Juvenile posterior subcapsular lens opacity
Plus
Relative (first degree) with NF2

Diagnosis is established with at least one of the three situations listed above.
Adapted from: Stumpf DA, Alksne JF, Annegers JF. Neurofibromatosis. Conference statement. National Institute of Health Consensus Development Conference. *Arch Neurol* 1988;45:575–578; Gutmann DH, Aylsworth A, Carey JC, et al. The diagnostic evaluation and multidisciplinary management of neurofibromatosis 1 and neurofibromatosis 2. *JAMA* 1997;278:51–57.

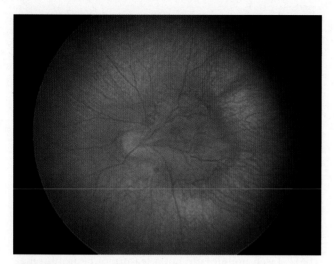

FIGURE 20.10. Neurofibromatosis type 2: epiretinal membrane (combined hamartoma retina and retinal pigment epithelium, RPE).

Dermatologic Features

The cutaneous features of neurofibromatosis type 2 are different than those in type 1. Occasionally, overlap of the two conditions can be seen. Café au lait spots are occasionally found. Axillary or inguinal freckling is not often found with neurofibromatosis type 2. Subcutaneous schwannomas or neurofibromas can be found. Neurofibromatosis type 2 displays skin plaques, represented by well-circumscribed, roughened areas less than 2 cm² and often with slight hyperpigmentation and hypertrichosis.

Central Nervous System Features

Neurofibromatosis type 2 is also called CNS neurofibromatosis because of the importance of these related tumors. The CNS tumors represent the majority of findings in neurofibromatosis type 2 and vary with the size and extent of the associated tumors. Acoustic neuromas (vestibular schwannomas) are the most common and well-recognized feature. If bilateral, they are considered pathognomonic of neurofibromatosis type 2. Patients present with symptoms of tinnitus, gradual hearing loss, and later growth of the tumor produce brainstem compression, hydrocephalus, and facial palsy.

Spinal cord schwannomas, particularly dumbbell shaped, are common. Spinal cord ependymomas, astrocytomas, and meningiomas can occur less frequently. Intracranial meningiomas are frequent and can manifest with or without symptoms. Nonvestibular schwannomas, particularly of cranial nerves 3 and 5, are diagnosed at a fairly early age, but can be indolent and slow growing.

Other Features

Sensory motor polyneuropathy can be found, particularly in those with schwannomas.

Management

Patients with neurofibromatosis type 2 should have annual ophthalmic, neurologic, dermatologic, and auditory examinations. This requires a multidisciplinary team. Surgical resection of symptomatic neurologic tumors is performed, but radiotherapy or chemotherapy can be used, particularly for ependymomas. Erlotinib has been used for unresectable progressive vestibular schwannomas and this medication is under trial. Additionally, bevacizumab and Gleevac have been investigated for treatment of schwannomas. Regarding ophthalmic care, cataract surgery can be beneficial. Additionally, monitoring of epiretinal membrane with clinical examination and optical coherence tomography, with surgical removal if progressive, can be considered.

RETINOCEREBELLAR HEMANGIOMATOSIS (VON HIPPEL-LINDAU SYNDROME)

Definition, Incidence, and Genetics

In 1895, von Hippel reported the clinical findings of so-called retinal angiomatosis (41) and in 1926 Lindau studied cerebellar lesions and pointed out their relationship to the retinal tumors previously described by von Hippel (42). Consequently, the combination of retinal and cerebellar involvement has been called von Hippel-Lindau (VHL) syndrome. The definition of VHL syndrome has now been expanded to include all of the clinical manifestations of this intriguing condition (43,44) (Table 20.4).

Table 20.4

DIAGNOSTIC CRITERIA FOR THE DIAGNOSIS OF VON HIPPEL LINDAU DISEASE

Family history	Feature
Positive	Any one of the following: • Retinal hemangioblastoma • Brain hemangioblastoma • Visceral lesion
Negative	Any one of the following: • Two or more retinal hemangioblastomas • Two or more brain hemangioblastomas • Single retinal or brain hemangioblastoma with a visceral lesion

Family history of retinal or brain hemangioma or visceral lesion. Visceral lesions include renal cysts, renal carcinoma, pheochromocytoma, pancreatic cysts, islet cell tumors, epididymal cystadenoma, endolymphatic sac tumor, and adnexal papillary cystadenoma of probable meonephirc origin.

VHL syndrome is recognized to be a hereditary disorder, with an autosomal dominant mode of inheritance and incomplete penetrance. Many cases occur as spontaneous mutations with no apparent family history. About 20% of cases have a positive family history (35). The exact frequency of familial occurrence is not known because many cases are lowly penetrant and express only subtle subclinical features of the syndrome. The condition is related to a partial deletion of chromosome 3p (45,46).

Ophthalmologic Features

The most common ocular manifestation of VHL syndrome is the retinal or optic disk capillary hemangioma, currently termed "hemangioblastoma." Multiple and bilateral retinal hemangioblastoma are diagnostic of VHL. The diagnosis of the ocular lesions is usually made in the second or third decade of life.

The ophthalmoscopic appearance of a retinal hemangioblastoma varies with the location of the lesion in the fundus (Figs. 20.11 and 20.12). In the earliest stages, a tumor in the peripheral retina can be subtle and difficult to recognize ophthalmoscopically. As the tumor enlarges, it appears as a distinct red nodule with a dilated tortuous afferent artery and efferent vein. The dilated blood vessels extend from the optic disk to the tumor. The capillary hemangioblastoma of the optic disk does manifest the well-defined feeding and draining blood vessels. A retinal capillary hemangioblastoma can assume either an exudative form or vitreoretinal form.

Histopathologically, the capillary hemangioblastoma consists of a proliferation of retinal capillaries that usually

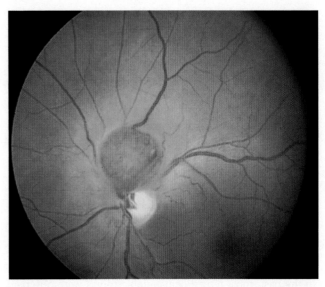

FIGURE 20.12. von Hippel-Lindau disease: retinal hemangioblastoma at optic disk.

replace the full thickness of the sensory retina. With light microscopy, there appears to be a benign proliferation of both endothelial cells and pericytes. It has recently been demonstrated that the clear "stromal cell" which characterizes the capillary hemangioma is the cell of origin for the neoplasm, but the exact nature of these cells is still not known (46). In the end stages, total retinal detachment can ensue with massive gliosis of the retina, cataract, and phthisis bulbi.

Fluorescein angiography is the most helpful ancillary study in confirming the diagnosis. In the arterial phase, the tumor fills rapidly by way of the feeding retinal artery and shows numerous fine capillaries within the tumor. In the venous phase, the lesion shows marked hyperfluorescence as the dye leaks from the capillaries. In the late phase, fluorescein leaks from the tumor into the overlying vitreous (6).

Dermatologic Features

In contrast to the other systemic hamartomatoses, VHL syndrome usually has no major cutaneous involvement. Congenital cutaneous hemangiomas have been observed on rare occasions.

Other Features

The cerebellar hemangioblastoma is the classic CNS lesion in VHL syndrome. It can be small and asymptomatic, but it usually enlarges slowly and can eventually produce profound cerebellar signs and symptoms. The cerebellar symptoms usually occur in the fourth decade of life, and patients with known ocular disease should have periodic neurologic evaluation to detect early onset. Identical lesions can occasionally occur in the medulla oblongata and spinal cord.

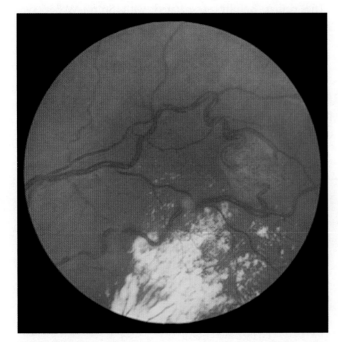

FIGURE 20.11. von Hippel-Lindau disease: retinal hemangioblastoma in periphery with subretinal and intraretinal exudation.

The cerebellar hemangioblastoma is best diagnosed with magnetic resonance imaging. Like retinal hemangioblastoma, it characteristically has large blood vessels that supply and drain the lesion. The vascular tumor frequently occurs within a cerebellar cyst. Histologically, the tumor is a hemangioblastoma with features similar to the vascular tumor that occurs in the retina.

Various systemic hamartomas can occur in patients with VHL syndrome. These include hypernephroma, pheochromocytoma, renal cyst, and pancreatic and epididymal cysts. A detailed medical and family history should be taken on all patients with retinal capillary hemangioma and, if indicated, appropriate studies be undertaken to detect any of the systemic components of VHL syndrome.

Management

In the past, most retinal hemangioblastomas were observed until leakage discovered and treatment was provided. Currently, our philosophy is to treat most lesions promptly, especially small peripheral retinal hemangioblastomas. The only exception is the macular and peripapillary lesions that we often wait for leakage to justify treatment as treatment complications could be detrimental to visual acuity in those cases.

The patient should be examined periodically, perhaps on a 3- to 4-month basis. Treatment should be delivered to prevent or resolve exudation or subretinal fluid. Several methods have been advocated, including laser photocoagulation, photodynamic therapy, cryotherapy, or plaque radiotherapy. Occasionally, systemic corticosteroids can be of benefit. Pars plana vitrectomy and/or scleral buckling procedure may be necessary to treat vitreous fibrosis and retinal detachment. Anti-vascular endothelial growth factors can be of help to manage related macular edema (47).

ENCEPHALOFACIAL HEMANGIOMATOSIS (STURGE-WEBER SYNDROME)

Definition, Incidence, and Genetics

EFH is frequently referred to as Sturge-Weber syndrome. In 1879, Sturge described a syndrome composed of a facial hemangioma with ipsilateral buphthalmos and contralateral seizures (48). He speculated that an associated intracranial angioma may have been present. In 1884, Milles established the association of a choroidal hemangioma with this condition (49). Later, Weber studied the clinical manifestations in greater detail, and the fully expressed entity became to known as Sturge-Weber syndrome (50). Sturge-Weber syndrome is now recognized to consist of a facial hemangioma, buphthalmos, seizures, and radiographic evidence of intracranial calcification (51). Some patients display a forme fruste, or partial expression, rather than the entire syndrome. In contrast to the other systemic hamartomatoses, there is no recognizable hereditary pattern associated with Sturge-Weber syndrome. There is no predisposition for sex or race.

This condition affects 1 per 50,000 persons. Roach has designed a classification for Sturge-Weber syndrome (52) (Table 20.5).

In 1987, Happle proposed that Sturge-Weber syndrome was an example of somatic mosaicism of a genetic trait (53). In 2003, Comi and associates supported this theory but demonstrating abnormality in the gene expression of fibronectin in fibroblasts from the region of the port-wine stain compared to normal skin (54).

Ophthalmologic Features

The ocular findings associated with Sturge-Weber syndrome include eyelid involvement with nevus flammeus, prominent epibulbar blood vessels, glaucoma, retinal

Table 20.5		
ROACH DIAGNOSTIC SCALE FOR THE CLASSIFICATION OF ENCEPHALOTRIGEMINAL ANGIOMATOSIS (STURGE-WEBER SYNDROME)		
Type	**Title**	**Involvement of skin, eye, and brain**
Type I	Classic Sturge-Weber syndrome	Leptomenimgeal angioma present. Cutaneous facial angioma present. Glaucoma likely present.
Type II	Sturge-Weber syndrome	Leptomeningeal angioma absent. Cutaneous facial angioma present. Glaucoma possibly present.
Type III	Sturge-Weber syndrome (forme fruste)	Leptomeningeal angioma present. Cutaneous facial angioma absent. Glaucoma absent.

Adapted from: Roach ES. Neurocutaneous syndromes. *Pedatr Clin North Am* 1992;39:591–620.

vascular tortuosity, and diffuse choroidal hemangioma (55) (Figs. 20.13 and 20.14).

The nevus flammeus can involve the eyelids. Although it is usually unilateral, bilateral involvement can occur. Involvement of the upper eyelid has a high association with ipsilateral glaucoma. Prominent tortuous epibulbar blood vessels, in both the conjunctiva and episclera, are common findings. Glaucoma is more common in patients with Sturge-Weber syndrome than it is in the other systemic hamartomatoses.

The main abnormality of the uveal tract in patients with Sturge-Weber syndrome is the diffuse choroidal hemangioma. Patients with this tumor usually have a bright-red

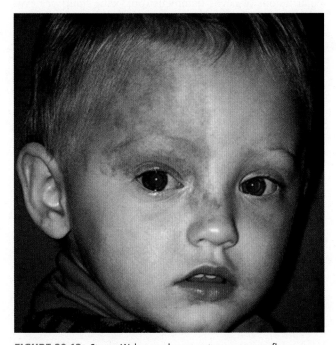

FIGURE 20.13. Sturge-Weber syndrome: cutaneous nevus flammeus.

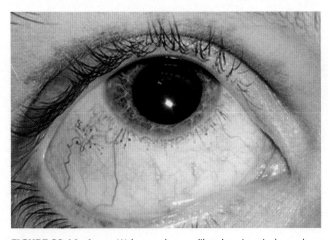

FIGURE 20.14. Sturge-Weber syndrome: dilated conjunctival vessels.

pupillary reflex in the involved eye as compared with the normal contralateral eye. This phenomenon, which is due to the light reflex from the highly vascularized tumor in the posterior pole, has been called the "tomato catsup" fundus. The choroidal hemangioma can be unilateral or bilateral. The diffuse tumor is usually diagnosed when the affected patient is young (median age 8 years) because either the associated facial hemangioma prompts a fundus examination or visual impairment occurs from hyperopic amblyopia or from a secondary retinal detachment. The diffuse choroidal hemangioma can produce total retinal detachment and neovascular glaucoma. Histopathologically, the lesion is a diffuse thickening of the choroid consisting of variable sized venous channels (56).

The precise incidence of the diffuse choroidal hemangioma in patients with facial nevus flammeus syndrome has not been determined. The incidence of choroidal hemangioma appears to be higher in patients who have both facial nevus flammeus and leptomeningeal hemangiomatosis.

Dermatologic Features

The classic skin lesion of Sturge-Weber syndrome is the nevus flammeus or port-wine stain (3,4). Although it classically occurs in the cutaneous distribution of the fifth cranial nerve, it can have many variations, ranging from minor involvement of the first division of the nerve to massive involvement of all three divisions. It sometimes crosses the midline in an irregular pattern and is occasionally bilateral.

Other Features

The typical CNS change associated with Sturge-Weber syndrome is a diffuse leptomeningeal hemangioma that is ipsilateral to the facial hemangioma and classically in the occipital region. The adjacent cerebral cortex can show secondary calcification that appears on computed tomography (CT) as a radiopaque double line, called the "railroad track" sign. The calcific process progresses during the first 20 years of life and then stabilizes. Seizures can be localized to the side contralateral to the CNS involvement.

Management

The management of diffuse choroidal hemangioma can be difficult (57). Asymptomatic tumors with no subretinal fluid require refraction as tumor-induced hyperopia can occur, leading to amblyopia in the small child. If secondary retinal detachment is detected, treatment with photodynamic therapy, external beam radiotherapy, plaque radiotherapy, or propranolol can be effective. Radiotherapy is remarkably effective for management of this condition.

The nevus flammeus of Sturge-Weber syndrome should be managed by dermatologic consultation for tunable dye laser early in life. Cover-up cosmetics can also be employed.

PHAKOMATOSIS PIGMENTOVASCULARIS

Definition, Incidence, and Genetics

Phakomatosis pigmentovascularis is a condition that shows combination of pigmentary cutaneous lesion (ocular melanocytosis, nevus of Ota) with nevus flammeus (Sturge-Weber syndrome) (8–10,58–60).

Since the first report on this condition by Ota in 1947, there have been few reports, mostly in the dermatologic literature. In 2005, Happle proposed reclassification (8) (Table 20.6). There is a relationship of the Nevus of Ota component with uveal melanoma and the Sturge-Weber component with choroidal hemangioma (10).

According to Happle, phakomatosis pigmentovascularis is divided into three types including phakomatosis cesioflammea, phakomatosis spilorosea, and phakomatosis cesiomarmorata (Table 20.6). Phakomatosis cesioflammea is characterized by coexistence of a dermal melanocytosis (blue spot) and nevus flammeus (port-wine stain). "Caesius" is the Latin term for "bluish-gray" and "flammea" for "flame" or "fire." The other two types have less relationship to the eye.

The association of dermal melanocytosis with cutaneous nevus flammeus is believed to be due to "twin spotting" phenomenon, which is the association of two genetically different clones of cells within a region of normal cells. This involves sporadic somatic recombination and a mosaic distribution of lesions. Moutray and associates describe monozygotic twins discordant for phacomatosis cesioflammea, supporting post-zygotic twin spotting theory (9).

Ophthalmologic Features

The ophthalmologic features of phakomatosis pigmentovascularis include a spectrum of findings with unilateral or bilateral periocular facial nevus flammeus (port-wine stain), ocular or oculodermal melanocytosis, secondary glaucoma, and risk for uveal or conjunctival melanoma (Fig. 20.15). There are only few reports in the ophthalmic literature.

Dermatologic Features

The cutaneous manifestations included mostly pigmented lesions of nevus of Ota (melanocytosis), Mongolian spot, or café au lait spot, nonpigmentation of vitiligo, as well as vascular lesions of nevus flammeus (port-wine stain) or nevus anemicus. These cutaneous findings tended to be patchy without midline separation and scattered over the surface of the body.

Central Nervous System Features

Neurologic features of phakomatosis pigmentovascularis include seizures, cortical atrophy, Arnold Chiari type 1, bilateral deafness, idiopathic facial paralysis, hydrocephalus, diabetes insipidus, plexiform neurofibroma, psychomotor developmental delay, and electroencephalogram alterations.

Other Features

Miscellaneous features include scoliosis, extremity length asymmetry, syndactyly, macrocephaly, renal agenesis, renal angiomatosis, hepatosplenomegaly, cavernous

---

Table 20.6		
CLASSIFICATION OF PHAKOMATOSIS PIGMENTOVASCULARIS (PPV)		
New classification	**Findings**	**Old classification**
Phakomatosis cesioflammea	Nevus cesius (blue spot) or melanocytosis with nevus flammeus	PPV II a/b
Phakomatosis spilorosea	Nevus spilus (speckled lentiginous nevus) with pale pink telangiectatic nevus	PPV II a/b
Phakomatosis cesiomarmorata	Nevus cesius (blue spot) with cutis marmorata	PPV V a/b
Phakomatosis pigmentovascularis unclassifiable	Various pigmentary and vascular nevi	PPV IV a/b and no name

Note: Phakomatosis and phacomatosis are both terms used in publications.

Adapted from: Happle R. Phacomatosis pigmentovascularis revisited and reclassified. *Arch Dermatol* 2005;141:385–388.

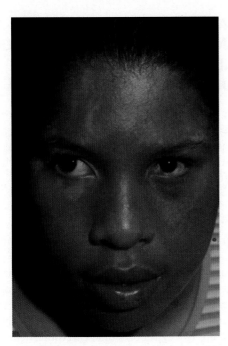

FIGURE 20.15. Phakomatosis pigmentovascularis: cutaneous nevus flammeus and oculodermal melanocytosis.

hemangioma, umbilical hernia, hypoplasia of leg veins, IgA deficit, hyper-IgE syndrome, eczema, and premature eruption of teeth.

Management

The cutaneous features should be managed by a dermatologist. Often the port-wine stain responds to tunable dye laser therapy. The ophthalmologist should follow the patient lifelong for the development of glaucoma and melanoma. Monitoring of neurologic status should also be performed.

RACEMOSE HEMANGIOMATOSIS (WYBURN-MASON SYNDROME)

Definition, Incidence, and Genetics

Racemose hemangioma of the midbrain and ipsilateral retina is called Wyburn-Mason syndrome (61). In contrast to the other oculoneurocutaneous syndromes, there are few skin abnormalities except for occasional small facial hemangiomas. The ocular and CNS changes, however, can be quite striking. Wyburn-Mason first recognized this relationship in 1943 (61). He estimated that intracranial aneurysms were present in 81% of known cases of retinal arteriovenous aneurysms. Conversely, he estimated that retinal arteriovenous aneurysms occurred in about 70% of cases of midbrain arteriovenous aneurysms. This congenital condition does not appear to be familial and does not exhibit a hereditary pattern. The characteristic arteriovenous communications can range from very subtle asymptomatic lesions to more extensive ones which form tumor-like masses, often referred to as racemose or cirsoid hemangiomata.

Ophthalmologic Features

The classic ocular finding is the racemose hemangioma of the retina (50–52). Similar vascular malformations can occur in the orbit and adjacent structures. These retinal arteriovenous communications have been divided into three groups according to the Archer classification (62,63) (Table 20.7). Group I is characterized by interposition of an abnormal capillary plexus between the major vessels. It is not a true tumor and the affected patient is generally asymptomatic. Group II is typified by a direct arteriovenous communication without interposition of capillary or arteriolar elements (Fig. 20.16). The dilated blood vessels in this group can superficially resemble a retinal hemangioblastoma, but no tumor is found. In general,

Table 20.7		
ARCHER CLASSIFICATION FOR WYBURN-MASON SYNDROME		
Group	**Feature**	**Comments**
I	Abnormal capillary plexus between the major vessels of the arteriovenous malformations.	Such lesions tend to be small, patients asymptomatic, and intracranial involvement uncommon.
II	Arteriovenous malformations lack any intervening capillary bed between the artery and vein.	Risk of retinal decompensation resulting in retina edema, hemorrhage, and vision loss. Low risk for intracranial arteriovenous malformations.
III	Extensive arteriovenous malformations with dilated and tortuous vessels and no distinction between artery and vein.	High risk for visual loss due to retinal decompensation or retinal compression of nerve fiber layer, optic nerve, or other vessels. High risk for intracranial arteriovenous malformations.

Adapted from: Archer DM, Deutman A, Ernest JT, Krill AE. Arteriovenous communications of the retina. *Am J Ophthalmol* 1973;75:224–241.

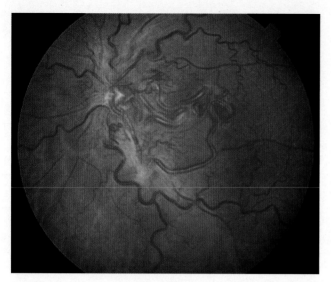

FIGURE 20.16. Wyburn-Mason syndrome: retinal racemose hemangioma.

these patients have few visual symptoms, but they may have associated cerebral arteriovenous malformations. Group III is characterized by a more extensive and complex arteriovenous communication which is often associated with visual loss. The fundus changes in this group are similar to those described by Wyburn-Mason (49) and the affected patient has a high incidence of CNS lesions. There is characteristically no exudation or retinal detachment. Although these lesions are believed to remain stationary indefinitely, remarkable changes have been observed in the distribution of the blood vessels over several years.

Dermatologic Features

There are no related cutaneous changes with racemose hemangiomatosis, except for the rare occurrence of small facial angiomas.

Other Features

The seizures that occur with Wyburn-Mason syndrome are probably related to the CNS vascular malformations. Spontaneous intracranial hemorrhages, secondary to the vascular anomaly in the midbrain, can lead to a variety of neurologic symptoms and signs. Intracranial hemorrhage occurs more frequently than intraocular hemorrhage. The bones of the skull can frequently be involved with the vascular malformation. When the mandible or maxilla are involved, abnormal bleeding can follow dental work.

Management

In general, treatment is not necessary for retinal racemose hemangiomatosis. If the hemangioma produces persistent vitreous hemorrhage, then the blood can be removed by vitrectomy. Panretinal photocoagulation may be necessary for neovascular complications of retinal vein obstruction.

RETINAL CAVERNOUS HEMANGIOMATOSIS WITH CUTANEOUS AND CENTRAL NERVOUS SYSTEM VASCULAR MALFORMATIONS

Although not historically grouped with the phakomatoses, cavernous hemangioma of the retina has been recognized to be frequently associated with skin and CNS changes and should perhaps be considered one of the systemic hamartomatoses (64–67).

Definition, Incidence, and Genetics

The syndrome of cavernous hemangiomas of the retina, CNS, and skin can be diagnosed at any age and seems to be more common in women than in men. The retinal and skin tumors are frequently asymptomatic, but the CNS hamartomas can sometimes produce dramatic clinical symptoms. In many instances, there is an autosomal dominant mode of inheritance.

There are two types of retinal cavernous hemangioma, including those that occur sporadically/independently and those associated with the syndrome of cutaneous and CNS vascular malformations. The latter is associated with a highly penetrant autosomal dominant mutation and is a part of the phakomatoses. Genetic abnormalities have been found on chromosomes 3q, 7p, and 7q.

Ophthalmologic Features

Ophthalmoscopically, this tumor appears as a dark grape-like cluster of venous intraretinal aneurysms either at the optic disk, macula, or in the peripheral retina (63–65). There is no obvious feeding artery and the lesion is typically centered along the course of a vein (Fig. 20.17). This lesion

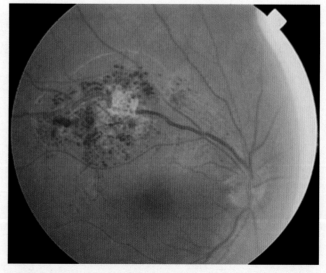

FIGURE 20.17. Retinal cavernous hemangiomatosis with cutaneous and central nervous system vascular malformations: retinal cavernous hemangioma.

produces no exudation or subretinal fluid, likely due to the fact that the thin-walled channels are lined by nonfenestrated endothelium. Repetitive vitreous hemorrhages (often mild and subclinical) can lead to white fibroglial tissue on the surface. This nonprogressive thin-walled, aneurysmal retinal tumor can remain hidden in the fundus for decades until dilation is performed or the patient develops vitreous hemorrhage.

The most important diagnostic test for retinal cavernous hemangioma is fluorescein angiography, which produces highly characteristic, if not pathognomonic, features of hypofluorescence persistent into the late frames with slow nonleaking filling of the aneurysms. Fluorescein is contained within the venous aneurysms of the lesion and pools in the plasma in the superior portion of each vascular space, whereas the blood elements collect in the inferior portion. This produces the typical fluorescein–blood interface in the late angiograms that characterizes retinal cavernous hemangioma. Rarely related iris cavernous hemangiomatosis with repetitive hyphema can be found (66).

Dermatologic Features

The hemangiomas of the skin in this syndrome are quite variable in their appearance and distribution on the body. The lesions occur most commonly on the back of the neck. Involvement of the eyelids is rare.

Other Features

This condition can lead to seizures from the CNS vascular involvement. Atypical symptoms of diplopia or neurological symptoms have been observed.

Management
Dermatologic Disease

The cutaneous hemangiomas seen are generally small and asymptomatic and require no treatment.

Ophthalmologic Disease

Most retinal cavernous hemangiomas are asymptomatic and require no treatment. They can produce visual loss from vitreous hemorrhage and could require pars plana vitrectomy. For direct tumor control, low-energy plaque radiotherapy can be employed.

ORGANOID NEVUS SYNDROME

Definition, Incidence, and Genetics

Organoid nevus syndrome (ONS) is an oculoneurocutaneous condition characterized by the sebaceous nevus of Jadassohn, cerebral atrophy, epibulbar complex choristoma, posterior scleral cartilage, and occasionally other features

(67,68). Although the sebaceous nevus of Jadassohn is a well-known dermatologic entity, the complete syndrome is uncommon and the exact incidence is unknown. It is generally a sporadic condition with familial occurrence being extremely rare. This condition was originally described by Jadassohn with the term "organoid nevus" to emphasize the prominence of the cutaneous component. Later, terms such as "nevus sebaceous of Jadassohn" and "Solomon syndrome" were applied to this condition.

Ophthalmologic Features

Although there are several ophthalmic features of ONS, the two most important ones are the epibulbar complex choristoma and posterior scleral cartilage. The epibulbar complex choristoma is a fleshy lesion of the conjunctiva that often extends onto the cornea (Figs. 20.18 and 20.19). It is composed, histopathologically, of a dermolipoma that contains variable combinations of ectopic lacrimal gland and hyaline cartilage. The posterior scleral cartilage produces a peculiar yellow-white discoloration of the fundus in the area of involvement. Since the cartilage produces a pattern similar to bone with ultrasonography and CT, it has sometimes been misinterpreted as a choroidal osteoma.

Dermatologic Features

The main dermatologic feature of ONS is the sebaceous nevus of Jadassohn. It appears as a geographic yellow-brown lesion that often involves the preauricular region and extends onto the scalp where it is associated with alopecia.

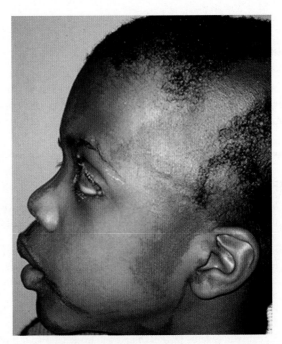

FIGURE 20.18. Organoid nevus syndrome: nevus sebaceous of Jadassohn with alopecia.

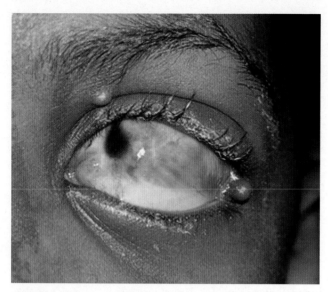

FIGURE 20.19. Organoid nevus syndrome: conjunctival complex choristoma.

Other Features

Patients with the ONS can develop seizures, due mainly to enlarging subarachnoid cysts in the CNS, and mental retardation. Imaging studies have shown arachnoidal cysts, leptomeningeal hemangiomas, hamartomas, cerebral cortical atrophy, and the MEAN tumor (meningoencephaloangioneuronomatosis). Rarely, ONS can have cardiac and renal abnormalities including patent ductus arteriosus, ventricular septal defect, coarctation of the aorta, nephroblastomatosis, and horseshoe kidney. Other rare relationships include vitamin D–resistant rickets and liver cysts.

Management

The epibulbar choristoma remains fairly stationary and can be safely observed if small. Larger or progressive lesions, however, may require surgical excision. Amblyopia can ensue. There is no treatment of the fundus lesion. The sebaceous nevus requires close follow-up and surgical resection when possible, since basal cell carcinoma or other adnexal tumors can develop in about 20% of cases.

OTHER CONDITIONS RELATED TO PHAKOMATOSES

Other oculoneurocutaneous conditions that are sometimes loosely classified with the phakomatoses include ataxia telangiectasia (Louis-Bar syndrome), oculodermal melanocytosis (68,69), Klippel-Trenaunay-Weber syndrome, and diffuse neonatal hemangiomatosis. These associations are discussed in the literature but are beyond the scope of this discussion.

SUMMARY

The systemic hamartomatoses, or phakomatoses, are characterized by hamartias and hamartomas, which can involve the eye, skin, CNS, and occasionally viscera. Although these syndromes all represent congenital abnormalities of tissue formation, the lesions may not become clinically apparent until later in life. The conditions which are presently included in this classification are tuberous sclerosis (Bourneville syndrome); neurofibromatosis type 1 (von Recklinghausen syndrome); neurofibromatosis type 2 (MISME syndrome); retinocerebellar capillary hemangiomatosis (VHL syndrome); encephalofacial cavernous hemangiomatosis (Sturge-Weber syndrome); phakomatosis pigmentovascularis; racemose hemangiomatosis (Wyburn-Mason syndrome); retinal, cutaneous, and CNS cavernous hemangiomatosis; and ONS. Several other syndromes are occasionally included under this category as well.

ACKNOWLEDGMENTS

This work was supported by the Eye Tumor Research Foundation, Inc., Philadelphia, PA.

REFERENCES

1. Van der Hoeve J. The Doyne memorial lecture. Eye symptoms in phakomatoses. *Trans Ophthalmol Soc UK* 1932;52: 380–401.
2. Shields JA, Shields CL. Systemic hamartomatoses ("phakomatoses"). In: Shields JA, Shields CL, eds. *Intraocular tumors. A text and atlas*. Philadelphia, PA: WB Saunders Co., 1992:513–39.
3. Shields CL, Shields JA. Phakomatoses. Chapter 132. In: Ryan SJ, ed. *Retina*, 5th Ed. St. Louis, MO: Elsevier Inc, 2013;2170–2183.
4. Shields CL, Shields JA. Phakomatoses. In: Regillo CD, Brown GC, Flynn HW Jr, eds. *Vitreoretinal disease. The essentials*. New York: Thieme Medical Publishers, Inc, 1999;377–390.
5. Shields JA, Shields CL. Eyelid, *Conjunctival, and orbital tumors. An atlas and textbook*, 2nd Ed. Philadelphia, PA: Lippincott Williams and Wilkins, 2008.
6. Shields JA, Shields CL. *Intraocular tumors. An atlas and textbook*. 2nd Ed. Philadelphia, PA: Lippincott Williams and Wilkins, 2008.
7. Ebert EM, Albert DM. The phakomatoses. In: Albert DM, Jakobiec FA, eds. *Principles and practice of ophthalmology*. Philadelphia, PA: WB Saunders Co., 2000:5120–46.
8. Happle R. Phacomatosis pigmentovascularis revisited and reclassified. *Arch Dermatol* 2005;141:385–388.
9. Moutray T, Napier M, Shafiq A, et al. Monozygotic twins discordant for phacomatosis pigmentovascularis: evidence

for the concept of twin spotting. *Am J Med Genet* 2010;152: 718–720.

10. Shields CL, Kligman BE, Suriano M, et al. Phacomatosis Pigmentovascularis of Cesioflammea Type in 7 Cases. Combination of ocular pigmentation (melanocytosis, melanosis) and nevus flammeus with risk for melanoma. *Ophthalmology* 2011;129:746–750.

11. Bourneville D. Sclereuse tubereuse des circonvolution cerebrales. Idiote et epilepsie hemiphlegique. *Arch Neurol (Paris)* 1880;1:81–91.

12. Kwiatkowski DJ, Short MP. Tuberous sclerosis. *Arch Dermatol* 1994;130:348–354.

13. Roach ES, DiMario FJ, Kandt RS, Northrup H. Tuberous Sclerosis Consensus Conference: recommendations for diagnostic evaluation. National Tuberous Sclerosis Association. *J Child Neurol* 1999;14:401–407.

14. Roach ES, Gomez MR, Northrup H. Tuberous sclerosis complex consensus conference: revised clinical diagnostic criteria. *J Child Neurol* 1998;13:624–628.

15. Astrinidis A, Senapedis W, Henske EP. Hamartin, the tuberous sclerosis complex 1 gene product, interacts with polo-like kinase 1 in a phosphorylation-dependent manner. *Hum Mol Genet* 2006;15:287–297.

16. Povey S, Burley MW, Attwood J, et al. Two loci for tuberous sclerosis: one on 9q34 and one on 16p13. *Ann Hum Genet* 1994;58:107–127.

17. Lucchese NJ, Goldberg MF. Iris and fundus pigmentary changes in tuberous sclerosis. *J Pediatr Ophthalmol Strabismus* 1981;18:45–46.

18. Nyboer JH, Robertson DM, Gomez MR. Retinal lesions in tuberous sclerosis. *Arch Ophthalmol* 1976;94:1277–1280.

19. Rowley SA, O'Callaghan FJ, Osborne JP. Ophthalmic manifestations of tuberous sclerosis: a population based study. *Br J Ophthalmol* 2001;85:420–423.

20. Shields CL, Reichstein DA, Bianciotto CG, Shields JA. Retinal pigment epithelial depigmented lesions associated with tuberous sclerosis complex. *Arch Ophthalmol* 2012; 130:387–390.

21. Aronow ME, Nakagawa JA, Gupta A, et al. Tuberous sclerosis complex: genotype'phenotype correlation of retinal findings. *Ophthalmology* Sep 2012;119(9):1917–1923.

22. Veronese C, Pichi F, Guidelli Guidi SG, et al. Cystoid changes within astrocytic hamartomas of the retina in tuberous sclerosis. *Retin Cases Brief Rep* 2011;5:113–116.

23. Cohen V, Shields CL, Furuta M, Shields JA. Vitreous seeding from retinal astrocytoma in three cases. *Retina* 2008;28:884–888.

24. Shields CL, Benavides R, Materin MA, Shields JA. Optical coherence tomography of retinal astrocytic hamartoma in 15 cases. *Ophthalmology* 2006;113:1553–1557.

25. Gold AP, Freeman JM. Depigmented nevi; the earliest sign of tuberous sclerosis. *Pediatrics* 1965;35:1003–1005.

26. Reed WB, Nickel WR, Campion G. Internal manifestations of tuberous sclerosis. *Arch Dermatol* 1963;87:715–728.

27. Franz DN, Belousova E, Sparagana S, et al. Efficacy and safety of everolimus for subependymal giant cell astrocytomas associated with tuberous sclerosis complex (EXIST-1): a multicenter, randomized placebo-controlled phase 3 trial. *Lancet* Nov 2012. doi:pii:S0140-6736(12)61134-9. 10.1016/S0140-6736(12)61134-9.

28. von Recklinghausen FD. Uber die multiplen fibrome der haut und ihre beziehungen zu den neurrommen. Festschr Feier fundfund-zwanzigjahrigen Best Path Inst. Berlin, 1882, A Hirschwald.

29. Stumpf DA, Alksne JF, Annegers JF. Neurofibromatosis. Conference Statement. National Institute of Health Consensus Development Conference. *Arch Neurol* 1988;45:575–578.

30. Gutmann DH, Aylsworth A, Carey JC, et al. The diagnostic evaluation and multidiscipliniary management of neurofibromatosis 1 and neurofibromatosis 2. *JAMA* 1997; 278:51–57.

31. Lewis RA, Riccardi VM. von Recklinghausen neurofibromatosis. Incidence of iris hamartoma. *Ophthalmology* 1981;88: 348–354.

32. Lewis RA, Gerson LP, Axelson KA, et al. Von Recklinghausen neurofibromatosis II. Incidence of optic gliomata. *Ophthalmology* 1984;91:929–935.

33. Shields CL, Kaliki S, Al-Daamash S, et al. Retinal vasoproliferative tumors. Comparative clinical features of primary versus secondary tumors in 334 cases. *JAMA Ophthalmol* 2013;131:328–334.

34. Evans DG. Neurofibromatosis 2 (Bilateral acoustic neurofibromatosis, central neurofibromatosis, NF2, neurofibromatosis type II). *Genet Med* 2009;11:599–610.

35. Evans DGR, Huson SM, Donnai D, et al. A clinical study of type 2 neurofibromatosis. *Q J Med* 1992;84:603–618.

36. Asthagiri AR, Butman JA, Kim HJ, et al. Neurofibromatosis type 2. *Lancet* 2009;373:1974–1986.

37. Kaiser-Kupfer MI, Freidlin V, Dariles MB, et al. The association of posterior capsular lens opacities with bilateral acoustic neuromas in patients with neurofibromatosis type 2. *Arch Ophthalmol* 1989;107:541–544.

38. Meyers SM, Gutman FA, Kaye LD, et al. Retinal changes associated with neurofibromatosis 2. *Trans Am Ophthalmol Soc* 1995;93:245–257.

39. Shields CL, Mashayekhi A, Dai VV, et al. Optical coherence tomography findings of combined hamartoma of the retina and retinal pigment epithelium in 11 patients. *Arch Ophthalmol* 2005;123:1746–1750.

40. Shields CL, Thangappan A, Hartzell K, et al. Combined hamartoma of the retina and retinal pigment epithelium in 77 consecutive patients. Visual outcome based on macular versus extramacular tumor location. *Ophthalmology* 2008;115: 2246–2252.

41. von Hippel E Jr. Vorstellung eines patienten mit einem sehr ungewohnlichen aderhautleiden. *Ber Versamml Ophthalmol Gesellsch* 1895;24:269.

42. Lindau A. Studien uber kleinhirncystein. Bau, pathogenese und beziehungen zur angiomatose retinae. *Acta Pathol Microbiol Scand* 1926;3(suppl 1):1–28.

43. Singh AD, Shields CL, Shields JA. Major review: Von Hippel-Lindau disease. *Surv Ophthalmol* 2001;46:117–142.

44. Hardwig P, Robertson DM. Von Hippel-Lindau disease: a familial, often lethal, multi-system phakomatosis. *Ophthalmology* 1984;91:263–270.

45. Latif F, Tory K, Gnarrra J, et al. Identification of the von Hippel-Lindau tumor suppressor gene. *Science* 1993;260:1317–1320.

46. Chan CC, Vortmeyer AO, Chew EY, et al. VHL gene deletion and enhanced VEGF gene expression detected in the stromal cells of retinal angioma. *Arch Ophthalmol* 1999;117:625–630.

47. Dahr SS, Cusick M, Rodriguez-Coleman H, et al. Intravitreal anti-vascular endothelial growth factor therapy with pegaptanib for advanced von Hippel-Lindau disease of the retina. *Retina* Feb 2007;27(2):150–158.

48. Sturge WA. A case of partial epilepsy apparently due to a lesion of one of the vasomotor centers of the brain. *Trans Clin Soc Lond* 1879;12:162–167.

49. Milles WJ. Naevus of the right temporal and orbital region; naevus of the choroid and detachment of the retina in the right eye. *Trans Ophthalmol Soc UK* 1884;4:168–171.

50. Weber FP. Right-sided hemihypertrophy resulting from right-sided congenital spastic hemiplegia with a morbid condition of the left side of the brain revealed by radiogram. *J Neurol Psychopathol (London)* 1922;37:301–311.

51. Alexander GL, Norman RM, eds. *The Sturge-Weber syndrome.* Bristol, England: J Wright, 1960.

52. Roach ES. Neurocutaneous syndromes. *Pedatri Clin North Am* 1992;39:591–620.

53. Happle R. Lethal genes surviving by mosaicism: a possible explanation for sporadic birth defects involving the skin. *J Am Acad Serm* 1987;16:899–906.

54. Comi AM, Hunt P, Vawter MP, et al. Increased fibronectin expression in Sturge-Weber syndrome fibroblasts and brain tissue. *Pediatr Res* 2003;53:762–79.

55. Sullivan TJ, Clarke MP, Morin JD. The ocular manifestations of the Sturge-Weber syndrome. *J Pediatr Ophthalmol Strabismus* 1992;29:349–356.

56. Witschel H, Font RL. Hemangioma of the choroid. A clinicopathologic study of 71 cases and a review of the literature. *Surv Ophthalmol* 1976;20:415–431.

57. Ramasubramanian A, Shields CL. Current management of choroidal hemangioma. *Retina Today* November/December 2010:52–55.

58. Ota M, Kawamura T, Ito N. Phakomatosis pigmentovascularis [In Japanese]. *Jpn J Dermatol* 1947;52:1–3.

59. Tran HV, Zografos L. Primary choroidal melanoma in phacomatosis pigmentovascularis IIa. *Ophthalmology* 2005;112:1232–1235.

60. Fernandez-Guarino M. Boixeda P, de las Heras B, et al. Phacomatosis pigmentovascularis: Clinical findings in 15 patients and review of the literature. *J Am Acad Dermatol* 2008;58:88–93.

61. Wyburn-Mason R. Arteriovenous aneurysm of midbrain and retina, facial naevi and mental changes. *Brain* 1943;66:163–203.

62. Archer DM, Deutman A, Ernest JT, et al. Arteriovenous communications of the retina. *Am J Ophthalmol* 1973;75:224–241.

63. Materin MA, Shields CL, Marr BP, et al. Retinal racemose hemangioma. *Retina* 2005;25:936–937.

63. Gass JDM. Cavernous hemangioma of the retina. A neuro-oculocutaneous syndrome. *Am J Ophthalmol* 1971;71:799–814.

64. Goldberg RE, Pheasant TR, Shields JA. Cavernous hemangioma of the retina. A four generation pedigree with neurocutaneous involvement. *Arch Ophthalmol* 1979;97:2321–2324.

65. Lewis RA, Cohen MH, Wise GN. Cavernous hemangioma of the retina. A report of three cases and a review of the literature. *Br J Ophthalmol* 1975;59:422–434.

66. Thangappan A, Shields CL, Gerontis CC, et al. Iris cavernous hemangioma associated with multiple cavernous hemangiomas in the brain, kidney, and skin. *Cornea* 2007;26:481–483.

67. Shields JA, Shields CL, Eagle RC Jr, et al. Ophthalmic features of the organoid nevus syndrome. *Ophthalmology* 1997;104:549–557.

68. Kraus JN, Ramasubramanian A, Shields CL, Shields JA. Ocular features of the organoid nevus syndrome. *Retin Cases Brief Rep* 2010;4:385–386.

68. Singh AD, De Potter P, Fijal BA, et al. Lifetime prevalence of uveal melanoma in Caucasian patients with ocular (dermal) melanocytosis. *Ophthalmology* 1998;105:195–198.

69. Shields CL, Qureshi A, Mashayekhi A, et al. Sector (partial) oculo(dermal) melanocytosis in 89 eyes. *Ophthalmology* 2011;118:2474–2479.

21

Ocular Abnormalities in Childhood Metabolic Disorders

Avery H. Weiss

DISORDERS OF AMINO ACID METABOLISM

Albinism

Albinism represents a group of inherited disorders characterized by a congenital reduction of melanin pigment in the developing eye. Specific changes in the eye and visual system result from this pigmentary defect and are common to all types of albinism. Although the reduction in melanin synthesis can be localized to the eye (ocular albinism [OA]), it is much more likely to involve the skin, hair, and eye (oculocutaneous albinism [OCA]) (Fig. 21.1). Affected individuals show hypopigmentation of skin and hair with characteristic eye involvement. Therefore, the diagnosis is usually made on the basis of the clinical findings (1).

Melanin is exclusively produced by a relatively small population of melanocytes with two embryonic origins. Melanocytes deriving from the neural crest migrate to and settle in the skin, hair, and eye (choroid and iris). Melanocytes in the retinal pigment epithelium (RPE) originate from the outer layer of neuroectoderm that makes up the optic vesicle. Production of melanin occurs in specialized intracytoplasmic organelles known as melanosomes. These membrane-bound organelles contain the enzymes needed to convert tyrosine to melanin. Hydroxylation of tyrosine to dihydroxyphenylalanine is mediated by tyrosinase. Then additional enzymes, including tyrosinase-related proteins 1 and 2, regulate subsequent oxidative steps in the pathway, resulting in the synthesis of eumelanin and pheomelanin, the two major forms of melanin (1).

Proteins other than the family of tyrosine enzymes are involved in melanogenesis. The OCA2 locus in humans (pink eye dilution gene in mice) encodes for a transmembrane protein important for the synthesis of melanin (2). Mutations within this locus are associated with OCA2 and a subset of patients with Prader-Willi syndrome (PWS) and Angelman syndrome (AS). This locus has been mapped to chromosome 15q. The genes associated with Chédiak-Higashi (*CHS1*) and Hermansky-Pudlak (*HPS1-8*) syndromes encode for proteins involved in the biogenesis and trafficking of melanosomes and other lysosomal-related organelles. Combined abnormalities of melanosomes, along with lysosomal and other lysosomal-related organelles (platelet-dense granules, basophil granules, major histocompatibility complex class 2 compartments), in these genetic disorders demonstrate the shared properties of these organelles (3).

Congenital nystagmus with an abrupt onset during the first 3 months of life is usually the presenting clinical sign. The nystagmus has a pendular or jerk waveform or can evolve from a pendular to jerk waveform. Nystagmus severity can be invariant or vary with horizontal gaze position. Patients with gaze position differences will often adopt a compensatory head turn to align the target at this eccentric gaze position where retinal slip is minimized and visual acuity is optimized. Unstable fixation and immature tracking in infancy can lead to vision concerns. Despite delays in acuity development, final visual acuities range from 20/40 to 20/200.

Iris hypopigmentation is an important diagnostic finding observed in most but not all albinism patients. Incident light reflected from within the eye can penetrate the iris in albinism, owing to reduced melanin in its posterior pigmented layer. Diffuse iris defects can be grossly detected by transscleral illumination using a light source placed on the bulbar conjunctiva, but punctate defects are subtle and best appreciated at slit-lamp examination (4) (Fig. 21.2A).

Fundus pigmentation is typically commensurate with skin pigmentation; in albinism, the fundus is hypopigmented. Loss of melanin pigmentation within the RPE allows for direct visualization of the underlying and prominent choroidal vessels (Fig. 21.2). The macula, unlike the peripheral retina, contains luteal (carotenoid) pigments. Since the luteal pigments are intact in albinism, the hypopigmentation is more conspicuous in the peripheral retina than the macula. Functionally, the RPE is intact, and the full-field electroretinogram (ERG) is normal.

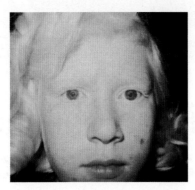

FIGURE 21.1. Oculocutaneous albinism (OCA). The skin, hair, and irides of this black child are hypopigmented.

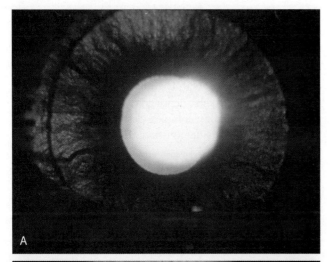

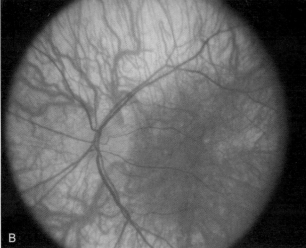

FIGURE 21.2. Ocular fundus in albinism. Pertinent findings include absence of macular reflex and blonde fundus. In **(A)** and **(B)**, the choroidal vessels are abnormally prominent because overlying pigment epithelium is hypopigmented. **A:** Slit-lamp photograph shows diffuse iris transilluminations. **B:** Fundus in albinism showing absence of retinal pigmentation and hypoplastic macula.

The hallmark of albinism is macular hypoplasia (Fig. 21.2B). The normal eye is characterized ophthalmoscopically by the presence of a concave depression in the region of the macula, owing to the lateral displacement of the inner retinal layers. In albinism, the macula is coplanar with the surrounding retina, causing loss of the macular and foveal light reflexes, and blood vessels may course through this normally avascular structure. As a result of the loss of ganglion cells originating from the fovea, the optic disk contains fewer axons and its diameter tends to be smaller but within the normal range. The anatomic abnormalities of the macula especially the blunted macula reflex, due to abnormal persistence of the inner retinal layers, and reduced density of cone photoreceptors are best characterized with optical coherence tomography (OCT) (5).

The visual pathways are abnormal in albinism. Melanin plays an important developmental role in the routing of optic nerve axons. Normally, the ratio of fibers that project to the contralateral hemisphere versus those that project to the ipsilateral hemisphere is 53:47. In albinism, the ratio is increased because axons from the temporal retina are routed contralaterally rather than ipsilaterally. This leads to altered binocular representation of the visual scene in which spatial correspondence in the retina is not maintained in the visual cortex. If the two retinal images are not in precise cortical registration, then binocular interactions cannot develop normally, and stereopsis is severely reduced or absent. Because stereopsis provides a feedback signal that helps to establish and maintain eye alignment, albinos frequently have strabismus. Misrouting of optic axons can be demonstrated in albinism using a lateralizing visually evoked potential (VEP) (4). The response to a pattern-onset stimulus presented monocularly is recorded with electrodes offset to the right and left of the midline. Asymmetric amplitudes between the two hemispheres are indirect evidence of abnormal decussations. Because the various types of albinism share overlapping clinical features, albinism is most reliably classified by the underlying molecular defect (Table 21.1). In OCA1A, there is a complete lack of tyrosinase activity. Individuals with OCA1A are usually diagnosed at birth on the basis of having white scalp hair, white skin, and blue irides, especially in dark-complexioned families. Nystagmus, reduced acuity, and strabismus may be the initial manifestations in light-complexioned families in whom pigmentary differences are less conspicuous. The skin and hair remain white throughout life, visual acuity ranges from 20/100 to 20/400, and no melanin pigmentation develops within the iris or retina.

In OCA1B, tyrosinase activity is reduced or temperature dependent (6). Although affected individuals have white or light yellow hair and white skin at birth, the skin, hair, and eyes acquire pigmentation by the age of 1 to 3 years. At slit-lamp examination, peripapillary clumps or radial spokes of pigmentation become evident, along with fine granular pigmentation of the retina. Despite these pigmentary changes, there is typically no improvement in visual acuity.

Table 21.1

CLASSIFICATION OF ALBINISM

Clinical Condition	Molecular Defect
Oculocutaneous albinism type 1 (OCA1)	
OCA1A	No tyrosinase activity
OCA1B	Reduced tyrosinase activity
Yellow OCA	Reduced tyrosinase activity
Minimal pigment OCA	Reduced tyrosinase activity
Temperature-sensitive OCA	Temperature-sensitive tyrosinase
Oculocutaneous albinism type 2 (OCA2)	
OCA2	*P* gene mutation
Brown OCA	*P* gene mutation
Oculocutaneous albinism type 3 (OCA3)	
OCA3	Tyrosinase-related protein 1
Oculocutaneous albinism type 4 (OCA4)	
OCA4	Membrane-associated transporter gene
Ocular albinism type 1 (OA1)	
OA1	G-protein coupled membrane receptor (GPCR)
OA1 with sensorineural deafness	GPCR + contiguous gene

Individuals with OCA2 have a defective P protein with normal tyrosinase activity (2). The *OCA2* gene encodes for the P protein, which is an integral component of the melanosomal membrane. These individuals produce some melanin but predominantly yellow pheomelanin rather than black-brown eumelanin. The phenotype is determined by the relative amounts of pigmentation of skin, hair, and eyes, which can range from minimal to near normal. In general, the pigmentary deficiency is less severe than that observed in OCA1A but can overlap with that in OCA1B. Scalp hair and skin coloration vary from off-white to blond to brown. The ocular findings are identical except for the increased amounts of iris and retinal pigmentation. Visual acuity ranges from 20/30 to 20/400 but is usually near the 20/200 level (1).

PWS and AS have hemizygous deletions within chromosomal locus 15q where the *OCA2* gene colocalizes (1,7). Individuals with PWS and AS can have hypopigmented skin and hair, but the ocular features of albinism are usually lacking. When the ocular findings of albinism are found, affected individuals are reported to have an *OCA2* gene mutation of the nondeleted chromosome (8). PWS is characterized by hypotonia, obesity, mental retardation, hypogonadism, short stature, and small hands and feet. The diagnosis of AS should

be suspected in any albino with microcephaly, developmental delay, inappropriate laughter, and seizures. Craniofacial stigmata include flat occiput, thin upper lip, prominent jaw, and widely spaced teeth.

OA has an X-linked inheritance pattern and is less prevalent than OCA. Affected males have normal skin and hair pigment along with ocular features of albinism. Despite normal skin appearance, light and electron microscopy demonstrate aggregates of abnormal melanosomes within keratinocytes and melanocytes in affected males and carrier females. The ocular findings include congenital nystagmus, reduced visual acuity (20/40 to 20/200), hypopigmentation of the iris and retina, and foveal hypoplasia. In individuals with dark complexions, the iris and retinal pigmentary changes can be subtle or absent, and there is less severity of foveal hypoplasia and reductions in visual acuity. The *OA1* gene encodes a G-protein-coupled membrane receptor that localizes to melanosome membranes (9). The obligate ligand for the putative OA1 receptor has not been identified but is likely important to melanosome function.

OA is rarely associated with sensorineural deafness and vestibular dysfunction. Inheritance is autosomal dominant. The presence of heterochromia iridis and a prominent white forelock in some patients suggests overlap with Waardenburg syndrome. Therefore, a digenic interaction between microphthalmia-associated transcription factor (MITF), a transcription factor linked to Waardenburg syndrome, and OA has been proposed (10). OA is associated with late-onset deafness and X-linked inheritance. This phenotype is attributed to a variant of a G-protein-coupled receptor or contiguous gene defect (11).

OCA can appear as part of a multisystem disease in which the melanocyte and other intracellular organelles are affected. The classic example is Hermansky-Pudlak syndrome (HPS), which includes a group of genetic disorders resulting from defects in membrane trafficking. Membrane and secretory proteins are synthesized in the endoplasmic reticulum, then move on to the Golgi complex where they undergo posttranslational modifications. These proteins are then shuttled to the plasma membrane, secretory granules or vesicles, and to organelles of the endocytic pathway. To date, eight genotypes have been identified, HPS1-8 (12–14). The gene for type 2 HPS encodes for the β3A subunit of adaptor complex 3 is known to assist in the transport of tyrosinase into melanosomes and lytic granules into NK cells and cytotoxic lymphocytes (15). The remaining HPS proteins are involved in the assembly of additional lysosomal-related organelles. Progressive accumulation of ceroid lipofuscin leads to interstitial fibrosis and granulomatous colitis. A bleeding diathesis can occur as a result of a deficiency of platelet storage granules or dense bodies. Reduction or absence of these granules, which contain serotonin, adenine nucleotides, and calcium, results in defective platelet aggregation. Easy bruisability, of soft tissues especially, and prolonged bleeding time in individuals of Puerto Rican descent are characteristic features.

Chédiak-Higashi is another multisystem disease associated with albinism. Patients with this disorder have the typical features of albinism, and skin biopsy reveals the presence of abnormally large melanosomes. In addition, they have an associated immune defect, increased susceptibility to lymphoproliferative disorders, and presence of larger intracytoplasmic granules in leukocytes and other tissues. Defective chemotaxis and decreased bactericidal activity predisposes these children to bacterial infections. The diagnosis is usually suspected on the basis of the clinical findings and presence of abnormal granules in their leukocytes. Most patients die by the second decade of life from an overwhelming infection or malignancy.

Alkaptonuria

Alkaptonuria is a rare autosomal recessive disease resulting from a deficiency of the enzyme that degrades homogentisic acid (HGA), an intermediary product in the metabolism of phenylalanine and tyrosine. The gene encoding for this enzyme, homogentisate 1, 2-dioxygenase, is mutated (16). Accumulation of HGA and its metabolites in cartilage and other connective tissues (ochronosis) leads to arthritis, joint destruction, and cardiac-valve calcification. The

earliest pigmentation changes involve the eyes and ears, but not until patients reach their twenties. Patches of pigmentation are usually found in the sclera in front of the extraocular muscles but can be detected in the conjunctiva or cornea (17). Ochronotic pigmentation of many internal areas of the body (cartilage, tendons, and ligaments) can be quite striking. Arthritis is a long-standing complication of alkaptonuria and is the major cause of disability. Clinically, it resembles ankylosing spondylitis involving the spine and large joints, leading to lumbosacral ankylosis with limitation of motion and need for joint replacement (18). Nitisinone, an inhibitor of the second enzyme in the catabolic pathway of tyrosine, has been shown to reduce the plasma and urine levels of HGA over 3 years (19). Early treatment can potentially prevent the development of the disabling arthritis.

Cystinosis

Cystinosis is an autosomal recessive disorder with an estimated incidence of 1 case per 150,000 live births. It is a lysosomal storage disorder resulting from defective transport of cystine across lysosomal membranes (20). Cystine is the homodimer of the amino acid cysteine, which is generated by protein catabolism. Cystinosin, a selective transmembrane protein, transports cystine out of the lysosome. Mutations in the gene encoding for cystinosin (CTNS) impair cystine transport, resulting in accumulation at levels of 5 to 500 times normal—levels that initiate crystallization and cell damage (21). The most common mutation is a 57,257 bp deletion that can be detected by polymerase chain reaction (22). The kidney is particularly susceptible to cystine toxicity, resulting in kidney damage beginning in the first year of life. By comparison, central nervous system (CNS) damage does not become evident before the patient's third decade of life (23).

The term cystinosis includes infantile and late-onset nephropathic forms and a benign nonnephropathic form. The most common and clinically important type is the infantile nephropathic form. Infants with cystinosis are typically normal at birth. Beginning at about 6 months of age, development slows, linear growth falls, and the child suffers from isolated or repeated episodes of acidosis and dehydration. Urinalysis reveals excessive losses of glucose, amino acids, phosphate, calcium, bicarbonate, and other small molecules (Fanconi syndrome). Progressive glomerular damage usually leads to renal failure in untreated patients by 10 years of age (29). Phosphaturia can lead to hypophosphatemic rickets. Accumulation of cystine crystals in other tissues causes hypothyroidism, diabetes mellitus, and delayed onset of puberty. Patients with treated nephropathic cystinosis can develop late complications such as distal myopathy, swallowing difficulties, hepatomegaly, and cortical atrophy and calcifications evidenced by computed tomography (CT) (23).

Late-onset cystinosis is clinically similar to the infantile form except for the delayed onset and slower progression of the disease. Patients may have preserved renal function into the third decade of life, and growth delay is mild. Accumulation of corneal crystals is slower. Patients with nonnephropathic disease have isolated ocular involvement. Molecular testing reveals the presence of mutations with residual activity of the cystine transporter (24).

The eye, like the kidney, is predisposed to cystine-related damage. Although they are not present at birth, cystine crystals can be found in the cornea of patients with nephropathic cystinosis by 1 year of age (Table 21.2). Slit-lamp detection of corneal crystals is an easy way to help confirm the diagnosis and should be done in all patients with Fanconi syndrome or renal failure of uncertain etiology. These refractile crystals first appear in the epithelium and anterior stroma of the cornea, but with increasing age, they occupy its entire thickness and become densely packed (Fig. 21.3). With continued buildup of cystine crystals, the cornea becomes opacified, resulting in decreased vision and the need for corneal transplantation in some patients. Cystine crystals are abundant on the conjunctiva, but there are relatively fewer on the surface of the iris, lens capsule, and trabecular meshwork.

Photophobia and secondary blepharospasm are significant problems for most patients with cystinosis and can be disabling in some patients. Symptomatic children often wear heavily tinted sunglasses and brimmed hats to avoid undue levels of light

Table 21.2

CORNEAL OPACITIES AS AN IMPORTANT OCULAR FINDING

Age at Onset	Disorder	Major Systemic Signs
3–12 mo	Tyrosinosis type II	Keratitis, Eratitis, photophobia, hyperkeratosis (palms/soles)
	Cystinosis	Renal Fanconi syndrome, failure to thrive
		Storage symptoms
	Hurler (MPS type I-H)	Coarse facies
	Scheie (MPS type I-S)	Hepatosplenomegaly
	α-mannosidosis (infantile)	Bone changes
	Maroteaux-Lamy syndrome	Cardiomyopathy
	I-cell disease	Inguinal hernias
	Steroid sulfatase deficiency	X-linked ichthyosis
1–6 y	Morquio syndrome (MPS type IV)	Bone changes, dwarfism
	Mucolipidosis type IV	Psychomotor retardation, retinal degeneration
	α-mannosidosis	Mental deterioration, cataract
	Tangier disease	Yellow tonsil, hypocholesterolemia
	LCAT deficiency	Hemolytic anemia, lipoprotein abnormalities
Late childhood, adolescence to adulthood	Fabry disease	Abdominal pain, painful neuropathy, angiokeratoma
	Galactosialidosis	Cherry-red spot, angiokeratoma, neurologic deterioration
	Wilson disease	Kayser-Fleischer ring, hepatic dysfunction, extrapyramidal signs

LCAT, lecithin-cholesterol acyltransferase; MPS, mucopolysaccharidosis.
Modified from Saudubray JM, Charpentier C. Clinical phenotypes: diagnosis/algorithms. In: Scriver CR, Beaudet AL, Sly WC, et al., eds. *The metabolic and molecular basis of inherited disease,* 8th Ed. New York: McGraw-Hill, 2001:1374, with permission.

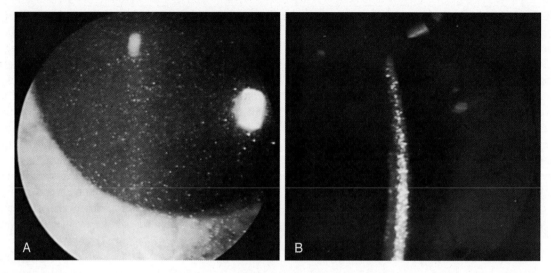

FIGURE 21.3. A: Cornea of an 8-year-old girl with cystinosis, seen in direct illumination. The crystals are too small to see with the naked eye but are readily visible with proper magnification. **B:** Slit-beam view of the cornea shown in **(A)**. The refractile, iridescent crystals are scattered throughout the stroma but are most dense in the anterior two-thirds.

exposure. The severity of photophobia seems to be correlated with the density of cystine crystals rather than the loss of the corneal epithelium. Possible reasons for the photophobia include a tear deficiency, subtle corneal inflammation, and glare (25).

Increased long-term survival of patients with cystinosis has led to the emergence of late ocular sequelae (26). The most important sequelae are due to progressive cystine accumulation in the retina (27). Decreases in visual acuity, color vision loss, and pigmentary disturbances of the macula and peripheral retina have been described (Table 21.3). Visual testing shows elevation of dark-adaptation thresholds, visual field constriction and variable reduction in the rod- and cone-mediated ERGs. Severe visual loss and even blindness can occur in patients who go untreated for years. Progressively increasing deposits of cystine crystal can be detected in most ocular tissues, including extraocular muscles and the optic nerve.

Replacement of electrolytes, calcium, carnitine, and glucose due to renal losses, kidney transplantation, and oral cysteamine are the mainstays of systemic treatment. Several studies have documented the ability of cysteamine to preserve renal function and to prevent growth retardation (28,29). However, cystine crystals continue to accumulate in the cornea, indicating that the drug does not achieve adequate levels in this avascular tissue. To overcome this delivery problem, topical cysteamine was formulated and found to be highly successful in removing cystine crystals from the cornea. Cysteamine eye drops (0.5%) administered as often as hourly are well tolerated and dramatically reduce the intense photophobia and blepharospasm that accompany cystine accumulation (30).

Table 21.3
PIGMENTARY DISTURBANCE OF THE RETINA AS AN IMPORTANT MANIFESTATION
Abetalipoproteinemia
Carbohydrate glycoprotein deficiency syndrome
Cystinosis
Hyperornithinemia
Refsum disease
Mitochondrial disorders
Long-chain 3-hydroxyacyl-CoA dehydrogenase deficiency
Mucopolysaccharidosis (types I, IV, VI, VIII)
Peroxisomal disorders
Primary hyperoxaluria (PH1)
Zellweger syndrome
Infantile phytanic acid storage
Neonatal adrenoleukodystrophy
Acyl-CoA oxidase deficiency
Primary hyperoxaluria (PH2)

Hyperornithinemia (Gyrate Atrophy of the Choroid and Retina)

Gyrate atrophy of the choroid and retina is a retinal degeneration related to a deficiency of ornithine aminotransferase (OAT). As a result, 10- to 20-fold elevations of ornithine accumulate in plasma, cerebrospinal fluid (CSF), and aqueous humor. More than 50 different mutations of the gene encoding for OAT have been identified to date (31). The functional gene has been mapped to chromosome 10q26. Gyrate atrophy occurs worldwide, but its prevalence is much higher in the Finnish population.

Clinically, the disease begins with myopia, night blindness, and contracted visual fields in the first decade of life (32). Examination of the fundus reveals punctate or circular patches of chorioretinal atrophy in the retinal periphery (see Table 21.3). With increasing age, the lesions become larger and more numerous, gradually coalescing and forming confluent areas of chorioretinal atrophy with scalloped margins posteriorly (Fig. 21.4). Near puberty, increased pigment appears at the back edge of the chorioretinal lesions and in the posterior pole. Posterior subcapsular cataracts are present in patients by the end of their second decade. Visual loss parallels the fundus changes, showing slowly progressive contraction of the visual field until blindness occurs in the third to seventh decades of life. Likewise, the ERG progressively deteriorates until the response to light becomes extinguished.

Various therapies have been tried to prevent or delay the onset of blindness. Initially pharmacologic doses of vitamin B6, a cofactor for OAT activity, were given in an attempt to stimulate the enzyme. This strategy failed in all but a small percentage of patients (33,34). A second strategy involved creatine supplementation based on the fact that ornithine is a potent inhibitor of creatine biosynthesis. Creatine supplementation appeared to have no beneficial effect (35).

Another strategy called for an arginine-restricted diet with the intent of lowering plasma ornithine levels. The effect of long-term reduction of ornithine accumulation is still controversial. Some authors report slowed progression of the retinal degeneration, while others observe continued progression (36–38).

Primary Hyperoxaluria

Primary hyperoxaluria (PH) is a rare autosomal recessive disorder characterized by increased synthesis and toxic accumulation of oxalic acid. Failure of either of two enzymes to detoxify glyoxalate, an oxidation product of glycine, leads to its increased conversion to oxalate. PH type 1 (PH1), which is the most common type, is due to a deficiency of the liver-specific peroxisomal enzyme alanineglyoxylate aminotransferase (39). PH type 2 (PH2) is caused by a defect in the more widespread cytosolic enzyme D-glycerate dehydrogenase/glyoxylate reductase (40). Because oxalate cannot be metabolized further, elevated levels accumulate in the urine, leading to the formation of stones and resulting in nephrocalcinosis in the kidney, and eventually renal failure. In PH1, oxalate crystals can accumulate in extrarenal tissues including bone, heart, nerves, joint, and teeth (oxalosis). In general, PH2 is a milder disease, and there is no evidence of systemic oxalosis.

Retinopathy is the major clinical finding in the eye, but histopathologically oxalate crystals are deposited throughout the ocular tissues (41,42). Initially, multiple crystalline deposits (100 to 200 μm) with a vascular distribution are found in the posterior pole out to the equator. Later, ringlets of pigmentation may surround the crystals and coalesce in the macula, forming a black geographic lesion (see Table 21.3). Visual acuity is relatively good when the optic disk is normal but reduced when there is optic atrophy (42). Fluorescein angiography initially shows multiple areas of hypofluorescent centers (oxalate crystal) surrounded by hyperfluorescent rings (atrophic RPE). Later, angiography can show small-vessel occlusion and localized subretinal neovascularization.

The diagnosis is usually based on the presence of increased urinary excretion of oxalate and glyoxylate in PH1, and of oxalate and glycerate in PH2. Enzyme assay of biopsied tissue or molecular testing is necessary to confirm the diagnosis. Treatment is directed at reducing exogenous oxalate intake, administration of pharmacologic doses of pyridoxine (essential cofactor for aminotransferases), or enzyme replacement by liver transplantation. The associated renal failure is managed in the short term with renal dialysis and in the long term with kidney transplantation (43).

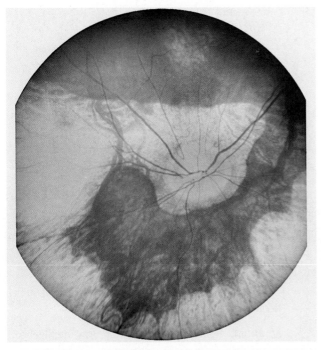

FIGURE 21.4. Peripheral fundus in gyrate atrophy of the retina and choroid. Areas of pigment epithelial atrophy enlarge and coalesce with time.

Galactosemia

The galactosemias are a group of three inherited disorders characterized by an inability to metabolize galactose. The main source of galactose is milk, which contains lactose, a disaccharide composed of glucose and galactose. Galactose is primarily converted to glucose by sequential enzymatic activity of galactokinase, galactose-1-phosphate uridyl transferase (Gal-1-UDP transferase), and uridine diphosphate (UDP)-galactose-4-epimerase. Decreased activity of any one of these enzymes is a cause of galactosemia. The gene for each galactose enzyme has been characterized, and numerous mutations have been identified (44–46).

Patients with Gal-1-UDP transferase deficiency, the most common form of galactosemia, typically present in infancy with failure to thrive. Vomiting and diarrhea begin with milk ingestion. Jaundice and unconjugated hyperbilirubinemia are the earliest signs of hepatic dysfunction, followed by hepatomegaly and abnormal liver function tests. Untreated, the liver disease can progress to cirrhosis. Aminoaciduria and proteinuria are evidence of renal tubular dysfunction, and there is a higher incidence of *Escherichia coli* sepsis. A minority of patients present with developmental delay, hepatomegaly, and cataracts later in life (47).

Cataract is the major ocular complication (Table 21.4). The cause of the cataract is most likely related to the

Table 21.4

CATARACT AS AN IMPORTANT MANIFESTATION OF METABOLIC DISEASE

Age at Onset	Disorder	Major Important Features
Congenital (at birth)	Lowe syndrome	Hypotonia, renal disease
	Zellweger syndrome and variants	Dysmorphia, hypotonia, seizures
	Rhizomelic chondrodysplasia punctata	Dwarfism, bone changes
Newborn (1–4 wk)	Galactosemias	Liver disease, failure to thrive, *Escherichia coli* sepsis
	Gal-1-UDP transferase deficiency	
	Epimerase deficiency	
Infancy (1 mo to 1 y)	Galactosemia	Isolated
	Galactokinase deficiency	
	Oligosaccharidoses	Coarse facies, hepatosplenomegaly
	Sialidosis	
	α-mannosidosis	
	Nonketotic hypoglycemia	Seizures, developmental delay
Childhood (1–15 y)	Hypoparathyroidism and pseudohypoparathyroidism	Bone changes, hypocalcemia
	Diabetes mellitus	Hyperglycemia
	Wilson disease	Chronic hepatitis, neurologic involvement
	Neutral lipid storage disease (OMIM 275630)	Ichthyosis, hepatosplenomegaly, myopathy
	Sjogren-Larson	Ichthyosis, mental retardation, spastic paraplegia
Adulthood (>15 y)	Galactosemia (heterozygotes)	Isolated
	Hyperornithinemia	Myopia, night blindness, chorioretinal atrophy
	Fabry disease	Renal failure, angiokeratoma
	Cerebrotendinous xanthomatosis	Xanthoma, neurologic dysfunction, low intelligence

Gal-1-UDP transferase, galactose-1-phosphate uridyltransferase.

Modified from Endres W, Shin YS. Cataract and metabolic disease. *J Inherit Metab Dis* 1990;13:509–516, with permission from Kluwer Academic Publishers.

accumulation of galactitol in the lens. In the presence of lenticular aldose reductase, galactose is reduced to galactitol, which is impermeable to cellular membranes, leading to its intracellular accumulation. Increased intracellular levels of galactitol create an osmotic gradient causing the lens to imbibe water, which in turn leads to hydropic degeneration of lens fiber cells. The earliest observable lens change is an increased refractive power of the fetal lens nucleus, giving the appearance of an "oil drop." This is usually followed by development of a zonular or nuclear cataract (48).

The mainstay of treatment is elimination of galactose-rich foods from the diet. Long-term studies indicate that dietary elimination of galactose can reverse or delay the development of cataracts and liver disease, but it has no ameliorative effect on the damage to the CNS and ovaries (49). Children with galactosemia are often delayed in acquisition of language skills, mildly retarded, and girls suffer from ovarian failure.

Patients with galactokinase deficiency have cataracts but there is no evidence of hepatic or renal disease, or mental retardation (50). Because cataracts may be the first and only abnormality, it is important to routinely screen for galactosemia in infants and children who develop cataracts (51). Homozygous deficiency of galactokinase is associated with the zonular cataracts that typically develop in the first year of life. By comparison, the causal relationship between partial galactokinase deficiency and cataracts is less clear. Individuals with reduced galactokinase activity seem to have a higher prevalence of cataracts than those with normal galactokinase activity. Cataracts that develop later in life can be nuclear or subcapsular. Rarely pseudotumor cerebri has been reported.

There are two forms of the UDP-galactose-4-epimerase deficiency. In the benign form, the child is normal and the epimerase deficiency is limited to red blood cells and leukocytes. With generalized loss of epimerase activity, the clinical presentation resembles transferase deficiency with vomiting, weight loss, hepatomegaly, hypotonia, aminoaciduria, and galactosuria. Cataracts have not been noted in either form of this rare disorder (49,52).

DISORDERS OF LIPID METABOLISM: FAMILIAL HYPERCHOLESTEROLEMIA

Familial hypercholesterolemia (FH) is one of the most common metabolic diseases and a frequent cause of coronary arteriosclerosis. The amount of low-density lipoprotein (LDL), the major cholesterol-carrying lipoprotein in human plasma, is the major determinant of cholesterol levels. This spherical particle consists of an inner core of cholesterol esters surrounded by an outer layer of phospholipids and apolipoprotein B (apoB) (53). LDL is the obligate ligand for the LDL receptor (LDLR), which is located on cell surface of hepatocytes. After binding to the receptor, LDL is internalized and then degraded in lysosomes, releasing free cholesterol into the intracellular cholesterol pool. The intracellular

concentration of cholesterol provides the feedback signal that controls transcription of LDLR. When the intracellular cholesterol level is low, transcription of LDLR is upregulated; when levels are high, transcription is downregulated (53). Hepatic stores of cholesterol are influenced by intestinal absorption and reexcretion of dietary cholesterol, and excretion into bile. Recent studies indicate that intestinal absorption is mediated by ATP binding cassette transporter G5 (ABCG5), and excretion is mediated by another ABC transporter, ABCG8 (54,55).

Four monogenic disorders that cause LDL to accumulate in plasma are known, and their underlying molecular defects have been characterized. Each of these disorders is characterized by hypercholesterolemia with cholesterol deposits in skin and tendons, premature atherosclerosis, and coronary heart disease. The most common is FH. Heterozygous patients exhibit hypercholesterolemia in the first decade of life, corneal arcus and tendon xanthoma in their teens, and generalized atherosclerosis by their thirties (53). Homozygotes develop all of these complications in early childhood and can die from a myocardial infarction in childhood. The second disorder is familial ligand-defective apoB-100. The clinical manifestations are similar but not as severe as those seen in heterozygous FH (56). The third disorder is sitosterolemia in which there is increased absorption of dietary cholesterol and plant phytol, and reduced excretion of these sterols into bile. Mutations of the ABC transporters (ABCG5 and ABCG8) have been identified in this disorder (54,55). The fourth disorder is autosomal recessive hypercholesterolemia (ARH), in which intracellular processing of the LDL–LDLR complex is altered (57). Children and young adults with ARH, like homozygotes with FH, have severe hypercholesterolemia, coronary heart disease, and cholesterol-laden skin deposits.

The major ocular manifestations of FH are palpebral xanthomata (xanthelasmata) and corneal arcus (58). Xanthelasmata appear as orange-yellow plaques within the eyelid skin. Corneal arcus is caused by cholesterol deposits in the periphery of the stroma where it is separated from the limbus by a narrow zone of clear cornea (Fig. 21.5). The presence of

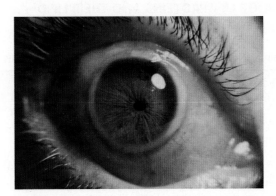

FIGURE 21.5. Arcus senilis. The severe degree of corneal arcus seen here is uncommon even in the elderly. When observed in those under 40 years of age, arcus may be a sign of hypercholesterolemia.

xanthelasmata or corneal arcus in a young person is associated with a higher incidence of hypercholesterolemia, but they can be found in normal individuals (59). The diagnosis is suspected on finding an elevated plasma cholesterol and normal triglycerides, and confirmed by molecular testing.

DISORDERS OF LIPOPROTEIN METABOLISM

Cholesterol, triglycerides, and other lipids are transported in body fluids by lipoproteins classified according to increasing density (Table 21.5). A lipoprotein is a particle consisting of a central core of hydrophobic lipids surrounded by a shell of polar lipids and apolipoproteins. The apolipoproteins are synthesized and secreted by the liver and intestine. They have two roles: solubilizing hydrophobic lipids and serving as shuttles and sinks for lipids moving to and from specific cells and tissues.

Tangier Disease

Tangier disease is characterized by a deficiency of high-density lipoproteins (HDL) and accumulation of cholesterol esters in the reticuloendothelial system and other tissues. HDL transport cholesterol and phospholipids from peripheral tissues to the liver (reverse cholesterol transport). Extracellular lipid efflux is initially dependent upon shuttling of cholesterol from endocytotic vesicles to the cellular surface by ABC1 (60). In Tangier disease, the *ABC1* gene is mutated, and intracellular lipids cannot be exported (61,62). Deficiency of HDL leads to reduced total serum cholesterol, usually below 125 mg/dL, whereas plasma triglycerides are normal or elevated. These findings together with lipoprotein electrophoresis showing absence of HDL are pathognomonic of Tangier disease.

The classic findings of Tangier disease include yellow-colored tonsils, hepatosplenomegaly, peripheral neuropathy,

and orange-brown spots of the rectal mucosa (63). Corneal opacities are noted in 25% to 50% of patients. A diffuse or dot-like haze of the central cornea develops with advancing age, owing to the continued accumulation of cholesterol esters. Conjunctival biopsies reveal intracellular lipid droplets outside of lysosomes, which helps to distinguish Tangier disease from Niemann-Pick and other lysosomal diseases. Additional ocular findings include orbicularis oculi weakness and secondary ectropion (64,65).

Familial Lipoprotein Lipase Deficiency

Familial lipoprotein lipase deficiency is a rare autosomal recessive disorder in which there is defective clearance of chylomicrons from plasma and a corresponding increase in triglyceride levels. Lipoprotein lipase is responsible for the hydrolysis of chylomicrons and very low density lipoprotein (VLDL) triglyceride release of fatty acids to tissues for energy. The diagnosis is usually based on a history of failure to thrive, recurrent abdominal pain or pancreatitis, and detection of elevated triglycerides after overnight fasting. Hepatomegaly and eruptive xanthomata are evidence of extravascular phagocytosis of chylomicrons by hepatic and skin macrophages. Ocular manifestations are limited to the retinal vessels, which take on a pink color known as "lipemia retinalis" when triglyceride levels are above 2,000 mg/dL (Fig. 21.6). The color changes reflect altered scattering of light owing to the massive presence of chylomicrons. Visual acuity is normal, and the retinal vascular changes are reversible. Treatment is restriction of dietary fat.

Abetalipoproteinemia

Abetalipoproteinemia is a rare autosomal recessive disorder characterized by a defect in the assembly or secretion of plasma lipoproteins that contain apoB. This results in the failure to form chylomicrons in the intestine and VLDL in the liver. Critical to the assembly of apoB is microsomal

---

Table 21.5

MAJOR LIPOPROTEINS AND THEIR LIPID AND PROTEIN COMPONENTS

Lipoprotein	Major Core Lipid	Apoproteins
Chylomicron	Dietary triacylglycerols	ApoE, CII, B-48
Very low density lipoprotein	Endogenous triacylglycerides	ApoE, CII, B-100
Low-density lipoprotein	Endogenous cholesterol esters	ApoE, B-100
High-density lipoprotein	Endogenous cholesterol esters	ApoI, AII

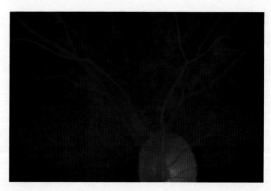

FIGURE 21.6. Lipemia retinalis. The marked fundus changes in this 23-year-old black man with fat-induced hyperlipemia (type 1 hyperlipoproteinemia) cleared within several days after ingestion of fat was stringently limited.

triglyceride transfer protein (MTP), which facilitates the transport of triglyceride, cholesterol ester, and phospholipid between membranes. Individuals with abetalipoproteinemia lack MTP activity and have mutations in the *MTP* gene (66,67). Because these lipoproteins transport cholesterol and triglycerides, plasma levels of both lipids are greatly reduced. The inability to form chylomicrons leads to the abnormal accumulation of triglycerides in the intestinal mucosa and malabsorption of fat and fat-soluble vitamins.

Chronic diarrhea owing to fat malabsorption is the initial clinical manifestation in infancy and early childhood. The presence of "star-shaped" erythrocytes (acanthocytes) in the peripheral blood is highly characteristic. This peculiar shape of red blood cells is related to the abnormal lipid composition of their membranes. Severe anemia can result from the secondary deficiency of iron and folate. Neurologic disease begins during the teenage years with decreased deep tendon reflexes and loss of vibratory and proprioceptive senses, followed by ataxic gait. Progressive spinocerebellar degeneration peripheral neuropathy, along with myopathic changes, can lead to generalized weakness and confinement to a wheelchair by the third decade of life (66,67).

Retinal degeneration is considered one of the cardinal manifestations of abetalipoproteinemia (Fig. 21.9). In the original reports, progressive visual loss, especially night blindness; pigmentary disturbances of the retina; and reductions in the ERG were noted (Fig. 21.7). More recently, it has become generally accepted that the neurologic disease and degenerative pigmentary retinopathy are secondary to a deficiency of vitamin E and therefore preventable. Presumably the high levels of polyunsaturated fatty acids in the outer retina and inadequate levels of vitamin E predispose the retina

to oxidative damage. Several studies have shown that the retinal degeneration and neurologic disease is preventable with administration of large oral doses of vitamin E (68,69). Long-standing studies of patients on oral vitamin E reveal normal vision, subtle pigmentary disturbances limited to the retinal equator and/or macula, and normal ERGs. Angioid streaks are a rare manifestation of abetalipoproteinemia, predisposing affected individuals to the development of subretinal neovascular membranes and sudden visual loss (70).

Horizontal ophthalmoplegia occurs in approximately one-third of affected patients. It is characterized by an acquired exotropia, with progressive medial rectus paresis, decreased saccadic velocities, and dissociated nystagmus of the adducting eye (71). One reported patient had ptosis with eyelid synkinesis and anisocoria, findings consistent with aberrant regeneration and peripheral involvement of the oculomotor nerve (72). However, reduced saccadic velocities implicate the brainstem burst generator, and histopathology shows myopathic changes.

Lecithin-Cholesterol Acyltransferase Deficiency and Fish-Eye Disease

Lecithin-cholesterol acyltransferase (LCAT) is a plasma enzyme that transfers a fatty acid from lecithin to cholesterol. Esterified cholesterol can then be used in the synthesis of cell membranes and other cellular components. It normally circulates in the plasma bound to HDL and LDL. Deficiencies of LCAT limit the available pool of cholesterol esters and lysolecithin required for membranogenesis and other synthetic pathways. Consequently, elevated levels of free cholesterol and lecithin accumulate in serum and various tissues. Serum levels of total cholesterol and triglycerides can be normal or high (73).

The major findings of LCAT deficiency are anemia, proteinuria, renal failure, early-onset atherosclerotic changes, and corneal opacities (73). The corneal changes are found in all patients from early childhood (see Table 21.2). They appear centrally as numerous, minute gray dots distributed throughout the corneal stroma. Along the peripheral cornea, the opacities are more confluent, forming a ring of opacification resembling a corneal arcus. Slit-beam views of the cornea can reveal a sawtooth configuration to the anterior and posterior corneal surfaces (crocodile shagreen) attributed to degenerative changes of stromal collagen. Histopathologic studies reveal the presence of vacuoles containing electron-dense particles within the Bowman layer and stroma (74). Heterozygotes appear to have a higher incidence of arcus-like corneal lesions.

Fish-eye disease is a rare autosomal recessive disease with main clinical manifestations of corneal opacifications (the eye resembling the eye of a boiled fish) and hypertriglyceridemia. It is caused by a selective functional loss of LCAT activity associated with HDL but not LDL. Serum levels of HDL are 10% of normal, whereas levels of LDL and VLDL are elevated. Furthermore, their lipid composition

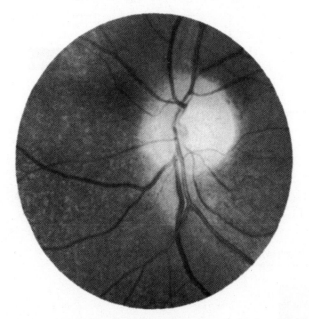

FIGURE 21.7. Granular mottling of retinal pigment epithelium (RPE) in abetalipoproteinemia. Electroretinography reveals diminished or absent signals in such eyes.

is abnormal: HDL contains relatively high amounts of free cholesterol, whereas LDL and VLDL contain relatively high amounts of cholesterol esters. Interestingly, neither patients with fish-eye disease nor familial LCAT deficiency in whom HDL levels are severely reduced show an increased incidence of atherosclerotic heart disease (73).

Patients with fish-eye disease have pronounced corneal opacities but no renal or hematologic abnormalities, unlike those with familial LCAT deficiency. These opacities can cause progressive visual loss, for which corneal transplantation is sometimes required (73–75).

Sphingolipidoses

The sphingolipidoses are a group of inherited disorders caused by defects in the degradation of various sphingolipids resulting in their excessive intralysosomal accumulation (Fig. 21.8). Sphingolipids are found in cellular membranes of all tissues but are enriched in membranes of brain and nervous tissue. Beginning with sphingosine as the basic backbone, the various kinds of sphingolipids are formed by the sequential addition of a fatty acid (ceramide), one or more sugar residues (cerebroside), and sialic acid (ganglioside). Because the sphingolipid composition differs across tissues, the clinical phenotype can vary widely, depending on the nature and severity of the enzyme defect.

G$_{M2}$ Gangliosidoses (Tay-Sachs Disease and Sandhoff Disease)

Lysosomal degradation of G$_{M2}$ gangliosides requires three genetically distinct proteins: hexosaminidase A (HexA), hexosaminidase B (HexB), and G$_{M2}$ activator. Hexosaminidase is a dimeric enzyme composed of alpha and beta chains encoded by the genes *HexA* and *HexB*, respectively. Mutations of these genes cause Tay-Sachs disease and Sandhoff disease. Clinical phenotypes associated with deficiency of HexA and HexB vary widely, ranging from infantile onset with rapidly progressive neurologic deterioration and death to adult-onset slowly progressive neurologic disease compatible with prolonged survival. However, Tay-Sachs and Sandhoff diseases are clinically indistinguishable and therefore considered together. Defective activity of the G$_{M2}$ activator is rarely diagnosed and clinically is indistinguishable from both infantile Tay-Sachs and Sandhoff diseases (76).

Infants with acute G$_{M2}$ gangliosides due to HexA deficiency (Tay-Sachs disease) or HexB deficiency (Sandhoff disease) are normal at birth. At 3 to 5 months of age, motor

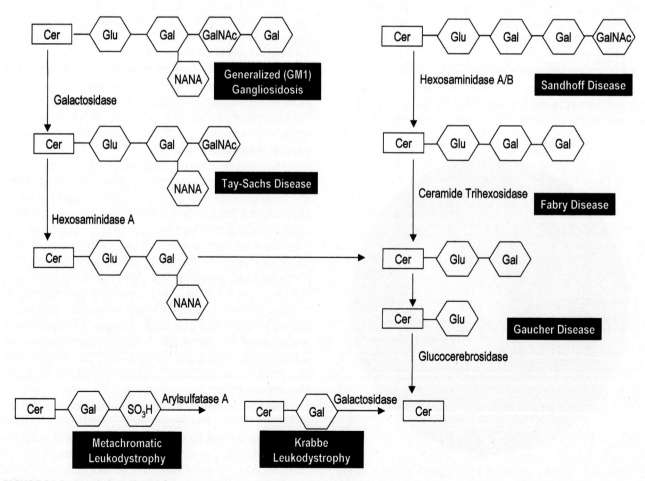

FIGURE 21.8. Metabolic pathways for sphingolipid metabolism. Cer, ceramide; Glu, glucose; Gal, galactose; Glc Nac, N-acetyl-glucosaminyl; NANA, N-acetyl neuraminic acid.

weakness is detected, and the startle reaction to sudden sounds is exaggerated. Between 6 and 10 months of age, the failure to achieve, or loss of, gross motor skills becomes more obvious. After 10 months of age, there is rapid neurologic deterioration associated with severe visual loss and increasing seizures. Death caused by aspiration or bronchopneumonia ensues between 2 and 4 years of age (76).

The earliest and most important ocular finding from a diagnostic viewpoint is the cherry-red spot (Table 21.6). Ophthalmoscopically, the normal-appearing fovea stands out against the background of the peripheral retina in which the ganglion cells are swollen with sphingolipids (Fig. 21.9). Progressive lipid accumulation leads to ganglion cell damage, resulting in severe visual loss, optic atrophy, and extinguished VEP (76,77). Abnormalities of eye movements have been noted long after blindness occurred (78).

Subacute G_{M2} gangliosidosis is characterized by the progressive loss of motor and cognitive skills between 2 and 10 years of age. Seizures, increasing spasticity, and generalized neurologic deterioration predominate between 10 and 15 years of age until death occurs from intercurrent infection. Typically, a macular cherry-red spot is not found, but visual loss from optic atrophy or retinal degeneration can develop late in the disease.

Chronic G_{M2} gangliosidosis has its onset in adolescence or adulthood during which there is an insidious onset of progressive dystonia, spinocerebellar degeneration, dysarthria, and psychoses. Visual acuity is normal, and the fundi

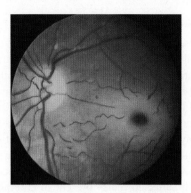

FIGURE 21.9. Cherry-red spot seen in the fundus of an infant with Tay-Sachs disease. There is optic atrophy, indicating that the disease is in its late stages.

are unaffected. Eye movement studies show hypometric saccades with premature termination of saccades, decreased smooth pursuit, and slow phase OKN gains (79).

G_{M1} Gangliosidosis

G_{M1} gangliosidosis is a rare storage disease with autosomal recessive inheritance caused by β-galactosidase deficiency. This enzyme deficiency leads to the accumulation of G_{M1} ganglioside within the brain and complex carbohydrates within soft tissues, bone, and viscera. On the basis of age of onset, it can be classified clinically into infantile, late infantile/juvenile, and chronic/adult types (80).

The infantile type is the most common and is usually recognized because of the combined presence of neurologic abnormalities, coarse facial features, and hepatomegaly. Psychomotor delay is present at birth or develops within 3 to 6 months of age. Neurologic deterioration is rapid, leading to seizures, blindness, spastic rigidity, and death before 2 years of age. Generalized skeletal dysplasia is often present. Visual loss develops early, and macular cherry-red spots are found in at least 50% of patients. Subtle corneal clouding may occur owing to the stromal accumulation of keratan sulfate. Strabismus, nystagmus, and optic atrophy have been noted. Peripheral blood smear shows vacuolated lymphocytes, and foamy histiocytes are found in the bone marrow, liver, spleen, and lymph nodes (80).

In juvenile G_{M1} gangliosidosis, neurologic deterioration begins in the first or second year of life with gait disturbance, progressive stiffness, and mental regression. Seizures are common, and patients expire between 3 and 10 years of age. Many patients have skeletal dysplasia, but facial dysmorphism and visceromegaly are not present. Visual acuity is appropriate for age, and the fundi are normal (80).

Adult G_{M1} gangliosidosis is a chronic disease with onset between 3 and 30 years of age that is mainly found in Japan. Initial clinical manifestations are gait or speech disturbance with progressive dystonic posturing. Mental deterioration is mild, and there are pyramidal signs. Facial dysmorphism is mild, and there is no visceromegaly. Cherry-red spots are not observed, but corneal opacities can occur (80).

Table 21.6	
METABOLIC DISORDERS WITH MACULAR CHERRY-RED SPOTS	
Disorder	**Frequency of Occurrence**
G_{M2} gangliosidosis	
Tay-Sachs disease	All cases
Sandhoff disease	Most cases
G_{M1} gangliosidosis	50%
Niemann-Pick disease (type A)	50%
Metachromatic leukodystrophy	Occasional cases
Farber disease	Variable
Sialidosis (type 1)	All cases
Sialidosis (type 2)	Variable
Galactosialidosis	Variable
Disorders with macular halos	
Niemann-Pick disease (type B)	10% of cases

Fabry Disease

Fabry disease is a lysosomal storage disorder caused by a deficiency of the enzyme α-galactosidase A. As a result, the substrate ceramide trihexoside accumulates within vascular endothelial cells, leading to ischemia and infarction, especially of the kidney, heart, and brain (Fig. 21.10). Parenchymal deposition of ceramide in podocytes causes proteinuria, and cardiomyopathy and conduction abnormalities in cardiomyocytes. Inheritance is X-linked. The encoding gene, which maps to the X chromosome, has been fully characterized (81).

Typically, affected males present in childhood or adolescence with painful extremities (acral paresthesias); fever lasting a few minutes to a few days; heat, cold, and exercise intolerance; and gastrointestinal problems. Examination of the skin reveals angiokeratomata (Fig. 21.11), which are red or blue-black nodules and are found between the umbilicus and knees. In adulthood, cardiac disease becomes problematic owing to angina, myocardial infarction, and arrhythmias. Proteinuria is found early, but there is progressive renal impairment with onset of renal failure between the third and fourth decades of life. Patients are also at risk for cerebrovascular events including thrombosis, transient ischemic attacks, and focal neurologic deficits (diplopia, hearing loss, and vestibular hypofunction). As further evidence of their cardiovascular risk, Fabry disease was identified in 0.5% of a large cohort of stroke patients of age 18 to 55 years (82). Female carriers may be asymptomatic or present with full-blown systemic disease. The diagnosis is established by demonstration of deficient α-galactosidase A activity in serum, white cells, or even tears (83). In the past, premature demise usually resulted from renal failure or widespread small-vessel occlusive disease of the heart or brain (82). Ocular involvement is present early in life and helps in making the diagnosis. Slit-lamp examination reveals characteristic changes of the cornea and lens. Yellowish deposits extend from a central vortex to the periphery, giving the corneal epithelium a whorl-like appearance (Fig. 21.12). The opacities may be the only clinical finding in asymptomatic female carriers (77). Similar deposits are found in patients on long-term chloroquine or amiodarone. Inspection of the lens reveals granular opacities within the inferior portion of the anterior capsule or on the posterior capsule (Fig. 21.13). The granular deposits align linearly and radiate from a central region of the posterior capsule, giving rise to a characteristic spoke-like opacity in about 50% of affected males and a smaller percentage of carrier females (84). The vessels of the conjunctiva and retina, like vessels elsewhere, are often dilated and tortuous (Fig. 21.14). Along with superimposed renal failure and hypertension, retinal vascular complications, including central retinal artery occlusions, can occur even in young patients (85,86).

Treatment with enzyme replacement (recombinant α-galactosidase A) is now available for patients with Fabry

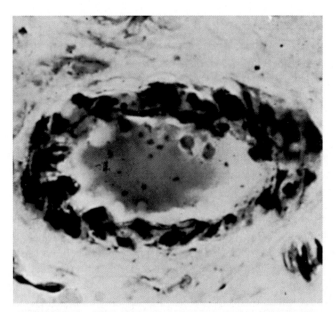

FIGURE 21.10. Sudan black-stained conjunctival tissue demonstrates the glycolipid material present in the media of small blood vessels in Fabry disease (×1,000).

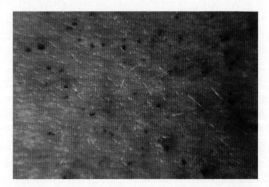

FIGURE 21.11. Skin lesions, the "angiokeratomata" of Fabry disease, most prominent in the bathing suit area.

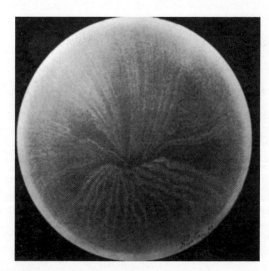

FIGURE 21.12. Cornea of a female carrier of Fabry disease, showing the whorl-like changes in the epithelium.

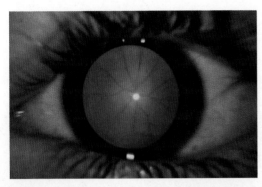

FIGURE 21.13. Cataract noted in the posterior capsular area of the lens in about 50% of patients with Fabry disease. Carriers may also show this capacity, which is best seen by retroillumination.

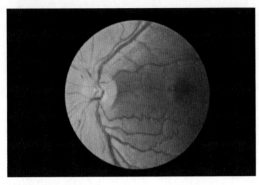

FIGURE 21.14. Characteristic retinal vessel tortuosity of a 22-year-old man with Fabry disease.

disease. Two recent clinical trials have conclusively shown that with therapy the deposits of ceramide trihexoside in the kidney, heart, and skin, and neuropathic pain are reduced, and there is improved renal function and cardiac conduction (87,88).

Metachromatic Leukodystrophy

Metachromatic leukodystrophy (MLD) is an autosomal recessive disorder caused by a deficiency of arylsulfatase. This lysosomal enzyme removes the sulfate moiety from cerebroside sulfate, a glycolipid that is mainly found in myelin sheaths of the nervous system. Levels of arylsulfatase A activity are correlated with symptomatic disease, age of onset, and rapidity of neurologic deterioration (89). Approximately 0.5% to 2.0% of the population have arylsulfatase A activities of 5% to 15 % but are asymptomatic. Molecular testing reveals loss of a polyadenylation signal that encodes for a glycosyl subunit, resulting in a smaller, less-efficient enzyme. Mutations associated with no enzyme activity (type I) are associated with early-onset and rapidly progressive disease. In comparison, mutations with residual arylsulfatase A are associated with late onset of milder disease (90). Histologic studies of the central and peripheral nervous systems show demyelination and loss of white matter and the presence of metachromatic material in macrophages.

Three clinical forms of MLD can be distinguished according to age at onset: infantile (1 to 2 years), juvenile (3 to 16 years), and adult (older than 16 years). Affected infants initially present with loss of acquired motor skills, hypotonia, and depressed deep tendon reflexes that progress to hypertonia with exaggerated reflexes, along with ataxia, truncal titubations, nystagmus, and optic atrophy (90). Prior to cellular death, swelling and opacification of the ganglion cells filled with cerebroside can lead to a cherry-red spot or grayness of the macula (91,92). Within a few years, the blind unresponsive quadriplegic infant with decerebrate or decorticate rigidity dies, usually from pneumonia. Bone marrow transplantation has limited success in the treatment of late infantile disease (93).

Patients with late-onset MLD present with cognitive and behavioral disturbances, and peripheral neuropathy including optic atrophy. Brain magnetic resonance imaging (MRI) scans show loss of white matter, especially periventricular white matter. Protein levels are elevated in the CSF. The diagnosis is confirmed by the demonstration of metachromatic lipids in tissue specimens (including conjunctiva), reduced arylsulfatase activity (including tears), or a mutated arylsulfatase A allele.

Multiple sulfatase deficiency is an extended form of MLD in which there is a deficiency of arylsulfatase, steroid sulfatase, and various sulfatases that degrade glycosaminoglycans. In addition to the neurologic manifestations of infantile MLD, these children have coarse facial features, hepatosplenomegaly, skeletal anomalies, and ichthyosis. Besides optic atrophy, cherry-red spot, or grayness of the macula, the eye findings may include retinal degeneration, corneal opacities, and equatorial lens opacities (94).

Krabbe Disease (Globoid Cell Leukodystrophy)

Krabbe disease is an autosomal recessive disorder caused by a deficiency of galactocerebrosidase, the lysosomal enzyme that cleaves galactose from ceramide. The onset is usually between 3 and 6 months of age, although later onset in childhood and adulthood is reported. The infantile onset form accounts for 85% to 90% of cases. Early signs include irritability, hypersensitivity to sensory stimuli, spasticity, and seizures, followed by regression of psychomotor development and generalized neurologic deterioration (95). Optic atrophy and blindness are prominent early signs (88). Macular cherry-red spots have been noted in one patient. CSF protein is elevated. Neuroimaging studies show diffuse cerebral atrophy, hypodensity of white matter, and abnormal signal intensity of white matter on T2-weighted images. Histologically, there is extensive loss of myelin and the presence of globoid cells, which are macrophages distended with galactocerebroside (96). Disease progression is rapid and patients rarely survive beyond 2 years of age.

The late-onset forms have a more insidious onset, progress over a period of years, and account for 10% to

15% of cases. Children may present with decreased visual acuity due to optic atrophy along with spastic or ataxic gait disturbance, loss of fine motor skills, and deterioration in school performance (95). Allogeneic bone marrow transplantation can slow disease progression and reverse the central nervous manifestations, especially in patients with presymptomatic infantile-onset disease or late-onset disease (97).

Gaucher Disease

Gaucher disease is the most common sphingolipidosis having an estimated prevalence of 1 in 4,000 among the general population and 1 in 850 among Ashkenazic Jews. It is caused by a deficiency of glucocerebrosidase and results in the accumulation of glucocerebroside in liver, spleen, bone, brain, and sometimes other tissues (90). Clinically, three types have been delineated: nonneuropathic (type 1), acute neuropathic (type 2), and subacute neuropathic (type 3).

Type 1 is the most common and represents the mildest form of the disease. It is characterized by progressive hepatosplenomegaly and structural skeletal changes. Splenic sequestration and displacement of the bone marrow often lead to anemia and coagulation abnormalities. Bone involvement can be mild or severely debilitating. Radiographic findings include the Erlenmeyer flask deformity of the distal femur, aseptic necrosis, and pathologic fractures. Although the splenomegaly and bone complications may appear in early life, the course of the disease is slowly progressive and patients survive into adulthood. Infants with type 2 disease develop marked hepatosplenomegaly by 6 months of age, show progressive neurologic deterioration, and usually die before 2 years of age. In type 3 disease, the severity of involvement is between that for types 1 and 2, and patients can survive beyond their second decade (98).

Ocular manifestations are usually related to the accumulation of lipid within macrophages and neuronal tissues. White deposits, presumably filled with undigested glucocerebroside, have been noted on the surface of the cornea, trabecular meshwork, iris, and retina and within the vitreous (99,100). The retinal spots are usually seen in type 3 disease but have been reported in severe type 1 disease (Fig. 21.15). Fundus abnormalities include perimacular grayness, but the typical cherry-red spot of the macula is not found. Premature onset of pingueculae on the conjunctiva has been reported, but histologic studies have revealed elastic degeneration rather than lipid-laden macrophages. Neuroophthalmic manifestations are sequelae of CNS involvement in type 2 and type 3 diseases. Abnormalities of eye movements can be a prominent neurologic finding and, in conjunction with the visceromegaly, should bring Gaucher disease to mind. Decreased saccadic velocity detected by eye movement recording is often the first sign of neurologic involvement, followed by a horizontal gaze palsy (101). These findings indicate that there is early involvement of the saccadic burst neurons, abducens motoneurons, and parapontine reticular formation. The diagnosis

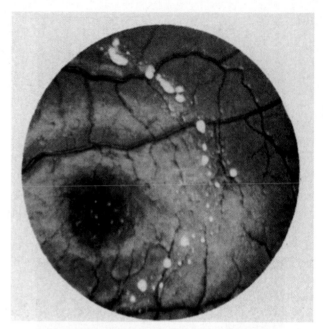

FIGURE 21.15. Characteristic white spots in or on the retina in a patient with juvenile neuronopathic Gaucher disease.

of Gaucher disease is usually made on the basis of the clinical findings, demonstration of Gaucher cells in the bone marrow, and is confirmed by enzymatic or molecular testing. In the past, the only therapy was symptomatic correction of the hematologic or skeletal complication. Enzyme replacement is now recommended for children with type 1 Gaucher disease (102–104). Treatment reduces the amount of storage material in liver and spleen, improves the red blood cell and platelet counts, and increases bone mineralization and remodeling.

Niemann-Pick Disease

Niemann-Pick disease (NPD) includes a heterogeneous group of disorders separable on the basis of clinical phenotype and genetic defect into types A, B, C1, and C2. Each of these variants is an autosomal recessive disorder characterized by variable involvement of the CNS and visceromegaly. NPA and NPB are due to a deficiency of acid sphingomyelinase (ASM). NPC1 and NPC2 result from a defect in intracellular transport of cholesterol from the lysosome to plasma membrane.

ASM cleaves sphingomyelin into ceramide and phosphocholine. As a result of the ASM deficiency in NPA and NPB, sphingomyelin accumulates in macrophages in the spleen, liver, lymph nodes, and lung. Histopathology reveals cells having a foamy cytoplasm representing storage material that stains for lipid. Wright stain gives the cytoplasm a striking blue appearance referred to as the sea-blue histiocyte (105).

Niemann-Pick type A (NPA) is the most common subtype of NPD and, like Tay-Sachs disease, has a higher prevalence among Ashkenazic Jews. Typically, newborns are normal, but during the first few months of life, feeding problems, hepatosplenomegaly, and failure to thrive become evident. By 6 months of age, the infant loses motor and cognitive skills and thereafter, the emaciated appearance with protuberant abdomen and spastic rigidity dominates the clinical picture. Although respiratory symptoms are minimal, chest radiographs show alveolar infiltrates. Death usually occurs by 3 years of age. The major ocular finding in NPA is the macular cherry-red spot, present in 50% of affected infants (77). The cherry-red spot in NPD is related to sphingomyelin accumulation in the lysosomes of retinal ganglion cells (see Fig. 23.14). Vision is retained until optic atrophy develops late in the disease. Walton and coworkers (106) have reported subtle lens opacities and peculiar corneal opacification that can progress in some cases.

Niemann-Pick type B (NPB) is a milder disease because there may be no neurologic deficits or only mild ataxia (105). However, storage material accumulates in the brain. Although residual ASM activity of 2% to 10% of normal is reported in some individuals, it is not significantly correlated with disease severity. Affected patients are found to have splenomegaly, pancytopenia secondary to hypersplenism, or pulmonary disease related to lipid-laden histiocytes filling the alveoli. Longevity usually depends on the severity of lung involvement. A distinctive macular halo is thought to be pathognomonic of NPB, but it is found in only 10% of cases (107). It is variably described as a concentric ring of gray deposits or crystalloid opacities centered on the foveola. Intraretinal localization of the opacities is uncertain, but the preservation of good visual acuities for as long as 20 years is consistent with sparing of the photoreceptors.

Niemann-Pick C1 (NPC1) is characterized by the accumulation of cholesterol within lysosomes, resulting from its defective transport from the lysosome to plasma membrane. Two proteins encoded by different genes are responsible for this intracellular movement of cholesterol (108–110). Mutations of NPC1 account for 95% of NPC cases, and mutations of NPC2 for the remaining 5%. The clinical phenotype is somewhat correlated with the specific gene mutation.

The clinical phenotype is highly variable in terms of age of onset and disease progression. Some patients have an acute onset in infancy with early demise, and others do not become symptomatic until adolescence or adulthood. Most patients are normal until 1 to 2 years of age after which they develop progressive neurologic signs (111). Neither cherry-red spots nor macular halos are observed. The hallmark of type C disease is a vertical ophthalmoplegia in conjunction with ataxia/athetosis and foam cells in the bone marrow—a triad known as the DAF syndrome. Vertical saccades are slow and hypometric, whereas horizontal saccades are normal initially but a total ophthalmoplegia develops with disease progression (112). Reductions of cerebellar grey and white matter are correlated with decreased saccade gains and severity of ataxia (113).

Treatment is currently limited to symptomatic relief and liver transplantation in individual patients. Enzyme replacement with recombinant sphingomyelinase for NPA and NPB and hematopoietic stem cell transplantation (HSCT) hold great promise based on preliminary evidence in mouse models of NPD. Enzyme replacement shows limited effectiveness in stabilizing neurologic function in juvenile-onset NPC.

Farber Disease

Farber disease (disseminated lipogranulomatosis) is an autosomal recessive disorder caused by a deficiency of lysosomal acid ceramidase (114). As a result, ceramide accumulates in macrophages within various tissues. The clinical triad of subcutaneous nodules around joints and over pressure points, progressive arthropathy, and laryngeal hoarseness is virtually diagnostic of this disease (Fig. 21.16). The lungs, liver, heart, and lymph nodes may also be involved. Motor impairment and mental deterioration may result when ceramide accumulates in neurons. There are several phenotypes having variable involvement of the CNS. In the classic type, there is progressive neurologic deterioration, and death occurs within the first few years of life. Without CNS involvement, there is still progressive joint deformity, but longevity is significantly prolonged. Although few patients have been treated, HSCT causes regression of the granuloma and dramatically increases joint mobility (115).

The major ocular finding is a macular cherry-red spot owing to subtle opacification of the surrounding retina. Histopathologic studies of the retina have shown the presence of intracytoplasmic lipid vacuoles containing curvilinear tubular structures known as "Farber bodies" (116). Granulomatous nodules on the eyelid, skin, and conjunctiva can be prominent in some patients. Nodular opacities in the cornea and lens are less-frequent findings.

Mucopolysaccharidosis

The mucopolysaccharidoses (MPS) are caused by deficiency of enzymes catalyzing the stepwise degradation of glycosaminoglycans (mucopolysaccharides). Specifically, the catabolism of dermatan sulfate, keratan sulfate, heparan sulfate, or chondroitin sulfate is involved individually or in combination. There are six types of mucopolysaccharidoses distinguished on the basis of clinical features and specific

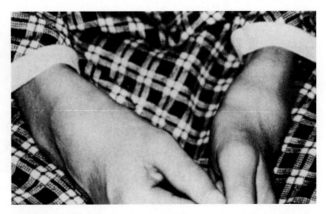

FIGURE 21.16. Nodular thickening of the wrists in a patient with Farber lipogranulomatosis.

enzyme deficiency (107). Ocular findings are common in MPS-I, MPS-IV, MPS-VI, and MPS-VII.

Mucopolysaccharidosis (MPS) type I includes three clinical phenotypes linked by a common deficiency of α-L-iduronidase. At the severe end of the spectrum is Hurler syndrome (MPS-IH), with onset between 6 and 24 months of age and characterized by the development of coarse facial features, enlarged tongue, hepatosplenomegaly, stiff joints, and cardiac disease (coronary artery disease, endocardial fibroelastosis). Developmental delay and progressive deterioration become obvious after 2 years of age. Affected children seldom live to 10 years of age. Bone X-ray studies show a constellation of findings referred to as dysostosis multiplex (Fig. 21.17). At the mild end of the spectrum is Scheie syndrome (MPS-IS) in which coarse facies, joint stiffness, and aortic valve disease predominate, but stature and intelligence are normal. In Hurler/Scheie syndrome, the clinical phenotype is intermediate between MPS-IH and MPS-IS (117).

Detection of corneal opacities is the main reason that the ophthalmologist is asked to evaluate patients with MPS. Functionally, the opacifications are consistent with normal vision or only mild reductions until corneal clouding becomes severe (Fig. 21.18). Additional ophthalmic involvement is mostly related to the abnormal accumulation of glycosaminoglycans within various parts of the eye (Fig. 21.19). Excessive accumulation in the trabecular meshwork is associated with glaucoma (118) and the retina with progressive degeneration (119), both of which can lead to blindness (see Table 21.3). Another potentially blinding complication is indirectly related to increased intracranial pressure presumably due to infiltration of the meninges and defective resorption of CSF (120). Sustained increases in intracranial pressure are frequently associated with ventricular enlargement and progressive optic atrophy.

Morquio syndrome is caused by an individual's inability to degrade keratan sulfate, resulting from either a deficiency of

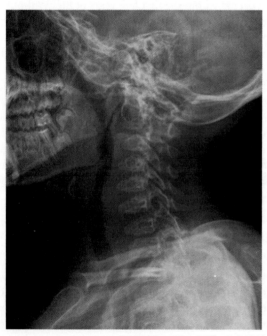

FIGURE 21.17. X-ray of cervical spine in patient with mucopolysaccharidosis showing platyspondyly and anterior breaking of the cervical vertebrae.

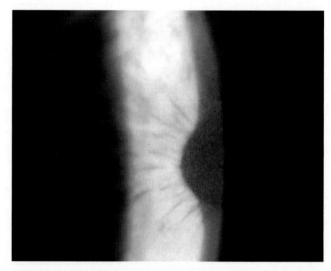

FIGURE 21.18. Slit-lamp photograph of the cornea in a 50-year-old patient with Hurler/Scheie syndrome showing diffuse stromal opacities.

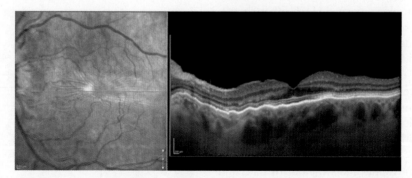

FIGURE 21.19. Optical coherence tomography (OCT) of globe in a patient with Hurler/Scheie syndrome having discrete accumulation of mucopolysaccharides, a choroidal effusion due to obstruction of uveal-scleral outflow and degeneration of the outer nuclear layer. Note the large low reflective areas in the choroid and retinal striae.

N-acetylgalactosamine 6-sulfatase (MPS-IVA) or β-galactosidase (MPS-IVB). Both types are characterized by short trunk dwarfism, skeletal deformities, normal intelligence, and fine corneal deposits that progress with advancing age (117).

Maroteaux-Lamy syndrome is characterized by defective degradation of dermatan sulfate resulting from a deficiency of arylsulfatase B. The clinical phenotype resembles that of Hurler syndrome except that mental development is normal. Corneal opacities are obvious and can interfere with vision (121).

Mucopolysaccharidosis (MPS) type VII (Sly syndrome) exhibits a wide clinical spectrum and is caused by a deficiency of β-glucuronidase. Patients with early-onset disease present with hepatosplenomegaly, dysostosis multiplex, and developmental delay. Corneal opacities are variably present. Children with onset after 4 years of age have milder disease with normal intelligence and clear corneas (117).

Enzyme replacement with alpha-L-iduronidase is one treatment option for Hurler syndrome (122). Weekly administration reduces hepatic storage, increases degradation of glycosaminoglycans, and ameliorates some aspects of clinical disease. HSCT provides an attractive alternative because it delivers enzyme inside and outside the blood compartment. HSCT has been shown to increase longevity and improve systemic health in patients with various types of MPS (123,124). A recent consensus long-term ophthalmologic follow-up indicates stabilization of ocular involvement in some patients but progressive corneal opacification, optic atrophy, and deterioration of ERGs in others (125–127).

DISORDERS OF GLYCOPROTEIN

Glycoproteins are ubiquitous proteins to which oligosaccharide chains are covalently linked through the hydroxyl groups of serine or threonine or through the free amino group of asparagine. Degradation of glycoproteins is accomplished by a series of lysosomal enzymes. Deficiency or faulty intracellular trafficking of any one of these enzymes results in the abnormal accumulation of storage material and specific clinical manifestations. Each of these disorders has an autosomal recessive mode of inheritance. Affected patients have a Hurler-like phenotype with coarse facial features, visceromegaly, and dysostosis multiplex, but increased amounts of oligosaccharides are found in the urine. The most relevant clinical features of each of these disorders are outlined in Table 21.7.

Sialidosis

Sialidosis is a rare lysosomal storage disease due to an inherited deficiency of sialidase, the enzyme that cleaves sialic acid residues from oligosaccharides. As a result, there is tissue accumulation and increased urinary excretion of sialylated oligosaccharides and glycoproteins (128). Two clinical variants are distinguished on the basis of age of onset and disease severity. Type I sialidosis is a late-onset mild form characterized by normal facies, cherry-red spot

with decreased visual acuity, and myoclonus or gait disturbance (129,130). Visual loss is progressive and likely related to progressive optic nerve disease. As ganglion cells atrophy, the cherry-red spot may fade. The myoclonus initially involves the limbs but can become generalized and disabling with disease progression.

Type II sialidosis is the dysmorphic form in which early onset and disease severity are correlated with lower levels of residual sialidase activity. Congenital sialidosis type II patients present at birth with hydrops fetalis, ascites, hepatosplenomegaly, stippled epiphyses, and early demise. Individuals with infantile or childhood-onset have coarse facial features, visceromegaly, dysostosis multiplex, and developmental delay. Cherry-red spots, punctate lens opacities, myoclonus, and ataxia are observed in older children who survive into the second decade of life. Vacuolated lymphocytes and foam cells in the bone marrow are found in type II but not in type I (128).

The diagnosis is confirmed by the detection of sialylated oligosaccharides in the urine and reduced activity of lysosomal sialidase. The gene coding for sialidase was cloned, and mutations have been identified in individuals with sialidosis (131). Some of these mutations may affect active site residues, but others affect surface sites that are likely important for interaction with other lysosomal enzymes. Recent evidence indicates sialidase is part of a multienzyme complex including cathepsin A (protective protein), β-galactosidase (132), and others.

Galactosialidosis

Galactosialidosis is associated with a combined deficiency of neuraminidase and β-galactosidase secondary to a deficiency of cathepsin A (133). The conformational structure of this lysosomal protein is important for the protection and maintenance of the catalytic activity of both of the other enzymes (134). All patients have a Hurler-like phenotype, and three clinical phenotypes are recognized on the basis of age of onset.

The early infantile form is associated with nonimmune fetal hydrops, coarse facial features, hepatosplenomegaly, proteinuria that progresses to renal failure, cardiomegaly with heart failure, and early death. The late infantile form has features similar to those of the early infantile form except that heart involvement is characterized by thickening of aortic and mitral valves, and longevity is longer. Approximately 60% of reported patients, mostly Japanese, have the juvenile/adult form. Unlike the infantile forms, neurologic involvement is common and includes generalized seizures, myoclonus, ataxia, and mental retardation with progressive deterioration. Skeletal changes are mild, and there is no visceromegaly (133). Ocular findings are common to all three forms and include cherry-red spots with progressive acuity loss, corneal clouding, and punctate lens opacities (133,135). Histopathologic studies reveal intracytoplasmic inclusions within retinal ganglion and amacrine cells that

Table 21.7

CLINICAL FEATURES OF MANNOSIDOSIS, FUCOSIDOSIS, AND SIALIDOSIS[a]

Disorder	Age of Onset	Facies	Dysostosis Multiplex	Neurologic	Hepatosplenomegaly	Eye Findings
α-mannosidosis						
Type I	3–12 mo	Coarse	+++	Mental retardation	+++	Cataracts, corneal opacities
Type II	1–4 y	Coarse	++	Mental retardation	++	Cataracts, corneal opacities
β-mannosidosis	<1–6 y	Some dysmorphism	±	Mental retardation	–	–
Fucosidosis						
Type I	3–18 mo	Mild coarsening	++	Mental retardation, seizures	++	Infrequent
Type II	1–2 y	Mild coarsening	++	Mental retardation	++	Tortuous conjunctival vessels
Sialidosis						
Type I and type II	8–25 y	Normal	–	Myoclonus, seizures, neuropathy	–	Blindness, cherry-red spot
Congenital	In utero	Coarse	+++	Mental retardation	++	
Infantile	0–12 mo	Coarse	+++	Mental retardation	±	Cherry-red spots
Juvenile	2–20 y	Mild coarsening	++	Myoclonus, mental retardation	–	Reduced acuity, cherry-red spots
Aspartylglycosaminuria	1–5 y	Coarse, sagging skin	+	Mental retardation	–	Lens opacities

±, borderline; +, mild; ++, moderate; +++, severe.
[a]Other important findings include the presence of vacuolated lymphocytes and angiokeratoma.
Modified from Thomas GH. Disorders of glycoprotein degradation: α-mannosidosis, β mannosidosis, fucosidosis, and sialidosis. In: Scriver CR, Beaudet AL, Sly WS, et al., eds. *The metabolic and molecular basis of inherited disease*, 8th Ed. New York: McGraw-Hill, 2001:3507–3534, with permission.

lead to severe loss of these cell types. The cherry-red spot may fade as the ganglion cells atrophy. In support of the anatomic changes, pattern VEPs show severely reduced amplitudes, and full-field ERGs demonstrate a reduction in the b-wave (136).

Mannosidosis

Mannosidosis is a lysosomal disorder caused by a deficiency of α-mannosidase, the enzyme that cleaves mannose from the oligosaccharide chain of glycoproteins. Consequently, mannose-rich oligosaccharides accumulate in numerous tissues. In soft tissues, this leads to coarse features, macroglossia, hypertrophic gums, and hernias. Abnormal storage in the CNS results in mental deterioration and hearing loss. Hepatosplenomegaly is common. Dysostosis multiplex and thickened calvarium are the predominant skeletal changes. Vacuolated lymphocytes are found in the peripheral blood and foam cells in the bone marrow. The severity of disease varies with age at onset. In infantile onset (type I), clinical signs appear rapidly, and death often occurs between 3 and 10 years of age. The milder juvenile form (type II) is characterized by normal early development with appearance of mental deterioration and hearing loss in childhood or later (137). Ocular manifestations are most apparent in the lens where mannose-rich glycoproteins have been found. In type I, a spoke-like opacity of the posterior cortex is highly characteristic (137). In type II, punctate opacities are scattered throughout the lens (138). Occasionally, anteriorly located opacities have been noted in the lens and cornea. Electron microscopy of skin and conjunctiva shows membrane-bound vacuoles in fibroblasts, suggestive of lysosomal storage disease.

I-Cell Disease (Mucolipidosis II)

I-cell disease was initially named after the abundant intracytoplasmic inclusions noted on microscopy. Although cells are filled with storage material in mucolipidosis II and III, lysosomal enzymes are paradoxically present at elevated levels in serum and other body fluids (139). To better understand this paradox, it is necessary to briefly review intracellular sorting and trafficking of proteins. Lysosomal enzymes, like many other proteins, are synthesized in ribosomes and then translocated to the endoplasmic reticulum, where mannose side chains are added. These glycoproteins are then transferred to the Golgi apparatus, where the terminal mannose is phosphorylated, a reaction catalyzed by *N*-acetyl-glucosaminyl (Glc Nac) phosphotransferase. A second enzyme, phosphodiesterase, then cleaves off the *N*-acetylglucosamine, leaving mannose-6-phosphate. Exposure of the mannose-6-phosphate marker allows the protein to be recognized by specific receptors and translocated to lysosomes. The lack of this obligate marker results in these proteins being diverted from lysosomes to the plasma membrane for extracellular secretion. The activity of Glc Nac phosphotransferase activity is absent in mucolipidosis II and reduced in mucolipidosis III. Cell types dependent on the mannose-6-phosphate marker are therefore deficient in multiple lysosomal enzymes. Although all cells are deficient in phosphotransferase activity, certain cell types still accumulate lysosomal enzymes, suggesting there are alternative targeting pathways (139).

I-cell disease is characterized by the early onset of coarse facial features, dysostosis multiplex, psychomotor retardation, and reduced linear growth. Deficiency of lysosomal enzymes leads to the progressive accumulation of mucopolysaccharides in bones and soft tissues, especially skin, ears, and gingiva. With advancing age, joint immo-

bility, cognitive deficits, cardiomegaly progress, and respiratory infections become more frequent. Most children die of cardiorespiratory complications before 8 years of age (139). Corneal clouding is a late manifestation, in contrast to Hurler syndrome (140).

Mucolipidosis III/Pseudo-Hurler Polydystrophy

Mucolipidosis III is a much milder disease than mucolipidosis II owing to residual phosphotransferase activity. Onset of involvement is between 2 and 4 years of age. Stiffness of the hands and shoulders is a common manifestation. By 6 years of age, claw-hand deformity, scoliosis, and short stature are apparent, and there is mild mental retardation. Coarsening of facial features, skin thickening, and corneal clouding become evident with increasing age. Carpel tunnel syndrome and progressive destruction of the joints, especially the hip joint, are disabling. Milder disease with slower progression allows survival into adulthood (139). Ophthalmologic manifestations are due to the accumulation of storage material causing axial hyperopia (increased scleral thickness), puffiness of the eyelids, and fine discrete opacities of the corneal stroma that progress but do not compromise vision. Optic nerve head swelling can result from mechanical compression due to accumulation of storage material within the scleral canal or meninges. Nonspecific tortuosity of retinal vessels and surface wrinkling maculopathy are reported, but ERGs are normal (140).

The diagnosis of mucolipidosis II and III is based on demonstration of increased levels of hexosaminidase B, iduronate sulfatase, and arylsulfatase A in the serum and deficient levels of these enzymes in the lysosomes of cultured fibroblasts. Alternatively, the level of phosphotransferase activity can be directly measured. To date, molecular testing is limited to the detection of mutations in the phosphotransferase gamma subunit (141).

Mucolipidosis IV

Mucolipidosis IV is an autosomal recessive neurodegenerative disease characterized by ophthalmologic and neurologic abnormalities. On the basis of electron microscopic evidence of membrane-bound storage material, it was first considered to be a mucolipidosis. Recent evidence indicates that type IV is caused by mutations in the mucolipin gene, which encodes a novel transient receptor potential (TRP) channel (142,143). The TRP channel proteins are implicated in a variety of cellular functions, including calcium entry into epithelial cells, stabilization of membranes, and transport of lipids to lysosomes.

Affected individuals typically present in infancy with hypotonia, developmental delay, and corneal epithelial haze. More than 80% are Ashkenazi Jews. Brain MRI scans show a dysplastic corpus callosum and white matter demyelination early, and cerebellar atrophy later. All patients have constitutive achlorhydria with elevated serum gastrin levels. Delay in establishing the diagnosis is related to the nonspecificity of the clinical findings (144–146). A subset of developmentally normal patients can present with an isolated retinal degeneration (147).

Bilateral corneal clouding and strabismus often bring these children to an ophthalmologist in the first year of life. Fundus examination reveals optic nerve pallor, retinal vascular attenuation, and retinal pigmentary abnormalities that progress with increasing age (148,149). Pradhan and colleagues (150) documented progressive amplitude reduction for the photopic and scotopic ERG, suggesting a rod-cone dystrophy. The scotopic ERG is electronegative at the highest stimulus intensity. Progressive corneal opacification can contribute to visual loss. Keratoplasty fails to correct the problem as the corneal opacification recurs when the epithelium of the donor graft is replaced by host stem cells. Nystagmus and cataract (posterior subcapsular and nuclear) have been noted in a minority of patients. Histopathologic studies of conjunctiva obtained by biopsy or topical swab show characteristic lysosomal inclusions on microscopy.

Congenital Disorders of Glycosylation

The carbohydrate-deficient glycoprotein syndromes include a heterogeneous group of multisystem genetic disorders characterized by defective addition of oligosaccharides to the asparagine moiety of glycoproteins. These N-linked glycoconjugates are an important feature of various serum transport proteins (apolipoprotein B, transferrin), hormones (thyroid-stimulating hormone), lysosomal enzymes, and circulating proteins (immunoglobulin G). As a result of the large number of potentially defective proteins, affected individuals have multisystem disease, and there are multiple phenotypes (151). Based on the pattern of isoelectric focusing of transferrin, patients are diagnosed with CDG-1 or CDG-2.

CDG-1a, due to a deficiency of phosphomannomutase, is the most common form (152). Infants typically present with microcephaly, seizures, axial hypotonia, hyporeflexia, and abnormal eye movements, probably related to cerebellar and/ or vermis hypoplasia (153,154). Later, psychomotor retardation, stroke, microcephaly, retinal dystrophy, and stroke-like episodes become more apparent. Although pigmentary retinopathy is found only in some patients, full-field ERG demonstrates abnormalities in all patients (155). The cone response is characterized by broad a-waves of normal amplitude followed by sharply defined narrow b-waves. Photopic prolonged on–off ERGs show a well-defined off-response but the photopic on-response b-wave is absent. The scotopic a-wave falls within the normal range but the scotopic b-wave falls below the 5th percentile, giving a reduced a:b ratio. The ERG findings indicate a selective defect of on-bipolar cells (156). Older children can present with ataxia, mental retardation, and skeletal deformities. Additional signs are unusual distribution of subcutaneous fat, inverted nipples, and growth delay.

The recent discovery of additional defects in novel glycosylation pathways has led to a new classification based on the corresponding gene defect of which there are 12 to date (157). For example, ATP6VOA2-CDG is the most common form of CDG-2. Typical clinical findings of this genotype include microcephaly, neonatal seizures, axial and peripheral hypotonia with cutis laxa, strabismus, and nystagmus. This subtype comes to medical attention with a congenital myasthenia-like syndrome as glycosylation of acetylcholine receptors is critical to their assembly and surface localization. Treatment of all types is primarily supportive.

DISORDERS OF PEROXISOMES

Peroxisomes are membrane-bound organelles that are found in virtually all eukaryotic cells and catalyze a variety of anabolic and catabolic functions. These functions include the biosynthesis of plasmalogens and bile acids, and α- and β-oxidation of long-chain fatty acids and related compounds. Disorders of peroxisomes are divided into defects of peroxisomal biogenesis that are associated with multiple enzyme deficiencies (or defects of single enzymes) (158). Recent studies have identified more than 30 matrix and membrane peroxin proteins that are involved in the biogenesis of peroxisomes. To date, mutations in 11 different PEX genes have been characterized in humans (159). Defects in the importation of peroxisomal proteins lead to metabolic disturbances and excessive accumulation of substrates that are responsible for the clinical manifestations. A mutation in PEX1 is found in 65% of patients with peroxisomal biogenesis disorders (PBD) (160). Inheritance is autosomal recessive. Despite their genotypic diversity, PBDs share the following clinical characteristics: facial dysmorphism (large fontanel, shallow orbits, low or broad nasal bridge, anteverted nostrils), psychomotor retardation, hypotonia, hearing loss, and retinal degeneration (Fig. 21.20).

Cerebrohepatorenal Syndrome of Zellweger

Zellweger syndrome is the most severe phenotype, characterized by facial dysmorphism, severe hypotonia, neonatal seizures, neuronal migration defects, and hepatomegaly. Brain MRI scans demonstrate cortical dysplasia, neuronal heterotopia, and dysmyelination with early loss of cerebellar white matter. Skeletal CT often reveals highly characteristic stippling of the epiphyses (Fig. 21.21). Most infants die before 1 year of age. Histopathology reveals the absence of peroxisomes, along with the presence of small (microgyria) and thickened (pachygyria) cerebral convolutions and multiple renal cysts. Biochemical abnormalities include reduced levels of plasmalogens, defective oxidation, accumulation of very long chain fatty acids (VLCFA) and phytanic acid, and accumulation of bile and its intermediates (158).

Ocular involvement is common (161,162). Abnormalities of the anterior segment include corneal clouding, cataract, congenital glaucoma, and Brushfield spots (Fig. 21.22). In the posterior segment, there can be a dysplastic or

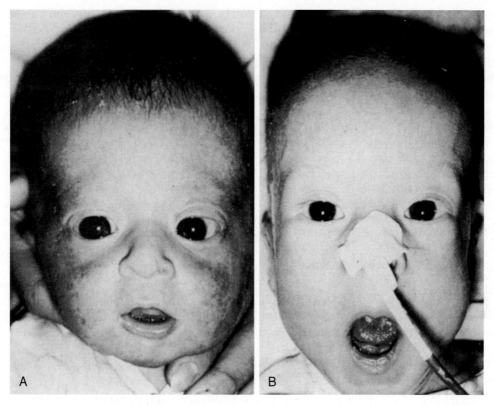

FIGURE 21.20. A, B: Two infants with Zellweger cerebrohepatorenal syndrome, showing characteristic high forehead, shallow orbits, and broad nasal bridge.

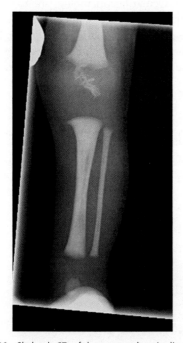

FIGURE 21.21. Skeletal CT of knee reveals stippling of the distal femoral epiphysis.

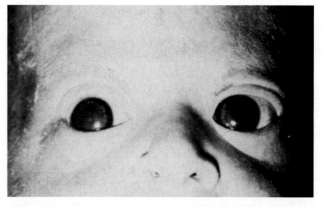

FIGURE 21.22. Infant with Zellweger syndrome and bilateral congenital cataracts. A full surgical iridectomy is present superiorly in the left eye.

Treatment with docosahexaenoic acid (DHA) ethyl ester has been shown to stabilize visual acuity and retinal function indexed by ERG in DHA-deficient patients with peroxisome biogenesis disorders (164).

Infantile Phytanic Acid Storage Disease

Infantile phytanic acid storage disease is the mildest phenotype among the PBD. The concurrence of sensorineural deafness, pigmentary degeneration of the retina, and elevated phytanic acid are the hallmarks of this disorder (165,166). It is distinguished from adult Refsum disease by the presence of

atrophic optic disk and disturbance of retinal pigmentation (163). The ERG is extinguished, but the striking clinical features distinguish Zellweger syndrome from Leber congenital amaurosis and other early-onset retinal dystrophies.

facial dysmorphism, mental retardation, hepatomegaly, and severe reduction of peroxisomes. The levels of phytanic acid and VLCFA are increased, and other peroxisomal metabolites are elevated. All patients develop retinal degeneration. The fundus can be normal or with early-onset involvement, there can be visual loss, congenital nystagmus, pigmentary mottling of the macula, and optic disk pallor. The ERG demonstrates severe reduction of the rod- and cone-mediated responses. Because of the relatively mild systemic involvement, the ophthalmologist plays a central role in making the diagnosis. Successful treatment with a low phytol, low phytanic acid diet, and plasma exchange has been reported (167,168).

Adrenoleukodystrophy

The term adrenoleukodystrophy is used to describe two genetically distinct diseases characterized by CNS demyelination, adrenal insufficiency, and abnormally high levels of VLCFA in tissues and body fluids (169,170). The X-linked type has normal-appearing peroxisomes, but there is impaired function of VLCFA coenzyme A (CoA) ligase. This protein is a member of the ABC transmembrane transporter protein superfamily and possibly transports VLCFA into peroxisomes (171). Clinically, there are three distinct phenotypes: cerebral (35% to 40%), adrenomyeloneuropathy (30% to 35%), and isolated Addison disease.

The cerebral form of X-linked adrenoleukodystrophy has its onset between 4 and 8 years of age. Early development is normal, and behavioral changes and difficulties performing in school are the most common initial symptoms. Then there is progressive neurologic deterioration leading to a vegetative state within 6 months to 10 years. More than 90% of patients have clinical or biochemical evidence of adrenal insufficiency. Brain CT or MRI scans demonstrate progressive demyelination of the periventricular white matter in the posterior parietal, occipital, and frontal regions. The diagnosis is confirmed by the detection of abnormally high levels of VLCFA in plasma, red cells, and fibroblasts (169). Treatment consists of adrenal hormone replacement, HSCT for early-onset disease, and Lorenzo's oil (glyceryl trioleate-trierucate) (172).

Ocular abnormalities become evident 6 months to 6 years after the onset of systemic involvement (173). Visual acuity may initially be 20/20 but can rapidly deteriorate to no light perception. Although the fundi are frequently normal in appearance, most patients develop optic atrophy, and some show pigmentary mottling of the macula and midperipheral retina (Fig. 21.23). Ocular histopathology showed marked degeneration of photoreceptor cells, including the macula in severe neonatal onset disease (174). Visual field defects vary with the severity of optic nerve and posterior visual pathway involvement. Strabismus is common, and acquired pendular nystagmus can occur (175). Progressive visual acuity loss is correlated with onset of disease before 10 years, severity of brain MRI scoring, parieto-occipital involvement and performance IQ (176).

The second type of adrenoleukodystrophy is one of the PBD in which the number and size of peroxisomes are diminished, the function of multiple peroxisomal enzymes is impaired, and inheritance is autosomal recessive. Affected individuals present in infancy with hypotonia, failure to thrive, and seizures. Dysmorphic facial features may or may not be present. Later psychomotor delay and blindness, secondary to progressive optic atrophy, become evident. Additional ocular findings include focal pigmentary disturbances in the peripheral retina and visible clumps of macrophages in the vitreous. Ocular histopathology shows marked degeneration of photoreceptor cells, including the macula. The clinical course varies from early death to survival into the midteens. The diagnosis is confirmed by showing absence of hepatic peroxisomes, reduced plasmalogen levels, and increased plasma levels of VLCFA and other peroxisomal metabolites.

Refsum Disease

Refsum disease is a rare autosomal recessive disorder caused by a defect in the α-oxidation of phytanic acid (177). Most

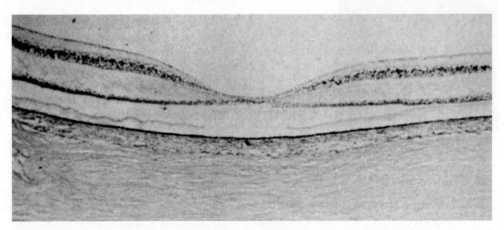

FIGURE 21.23. Section of the retinal fovea in a patient with childhood adrenoleukodystrophy, showing loss of ganglion cells; the bipolar and photoreceptor layers are intact (×60).

patients have a mutation of phytanoyl-CoA hydroxylase, a peroxisomal protein catalyzing the first step in α-oxidation (178). A subset of patients has mutations in PEX7, which is required for targeting to the peroxisome (178). In homozygotes, phytanic acid accumulates to high levels accounting for 5% to 30% of the total plasma lipids, compared with 0.3% in normal individuals. Heterozygotes have intermediate levels and are largely asymptomatic. It is believed that accumulation of phytanic acid leads to its incorporation into lipid membranes, displacing normal straight-chain fatty acids. Incorporation of this multiple-branched molecule may distort membrane structure and impair cellular function. Clinically, there are four cardinal features—retinitis pigmentosa, peripheral neuropathy, cerebellar ataxia, and elevated CSF protein. Brain MRI shows abnormal T2 signal intensity in the dentate nuclei and corticospinal tracts in the brainstem and within the periventricular and cerebral white matter (Fig. 21.24). Additional systemic manifestations can include deafness, ichthyosis, epiphyseal dysplasia, and cardiomyopathy. Although the onset of disease may occur between the first and fifth decade of life, most patients have symptoms by 20 years of age (179).

All patients have retinitis pigmentosa with visual field loss that begins in the midperiphery and marches centrally and peripherally, leaving a central island of intact vision (177,178). Nystagmus, secondary to cerebellar involvement, can develop in Refsum disease, unlike patients with typical retinitis pigmentosa. Ophthalmoscopy reveals a diffuse pigmentary retinopathy and attenuation of retinal vessel

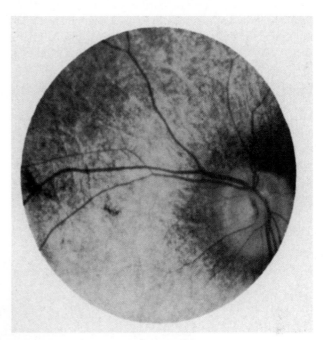

FIGURE 21.25. Pigmentary retinopathy in a patient with Refsum disease. Note the narrow retinal vessels.

caliber early in the disease and secondary optic atrophy in later stages (Fig. 21.25). The ERG shows predominant loss of rod function. Pupillary miosis and poor pupillary dilation have been repeatedly noted (178). Cataracts, typically posterior subcapsular, develop in midlife. Treatment is elimination of phytanic acid and its precursor, phytol, from the diet (158,160,179,180). The basis for this successful therapy is that phytanic acid is exclusively of exogenous origin (dairy products) and not endogenously synthesized. Dietary compliance can prevent progressive visual loss but does not restore visual deficits already incurred.

DISORDERS OF COPPER METABOLISM

Wilson Disease

Wilson disease is an autosomal recessive disorder caused by a genetic defect of the copper ATP transporter (ATP7B), which plays a role in copper distribution in the liver, brain, and kidney (181). Recent evidence indicates that a copper chaperone (Atox1) first transfers copper from the cytosol to ATP7B through protein–protein interactions. Then the copper-transport protein delivers the metal to the secretory pathway for incorporation into copper-dependent enzymes or to the membrane for exportation from the cell. Mutations of the protein lead to a deficiency of copper-dependent enzymes, like ceruloplasmin, and to excretion into bile (1,182,183). Copper accumulates to toxic levels in liver, brain, and other tissues, where it presumably stimulates the production of reactive oxygen species and disrupts cell metabolism.

Patients with Wilson disease present with liver disease, neurologic signs, or both (184). Liver involvement may develop

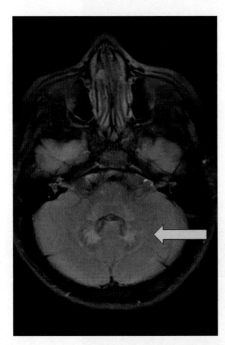

FIGURE 21.24. Head CT scan demonstrates characteristic signal enhancement within the dentate nuclei bilaterally (*yellow arrow*). Similar signal enhancement was noted in Globus pallidus, substantia nigra, and corticospinal tracts.

at any age beyond 6 years and can be mild or fulminant, rapidly progressing to hepatic failure and death. Of particular importance, Wilson disease is the most common cause of chronic or recurrent liver disease in childhood. Neurologic signs are unusual before 12 years of age. Dysarthria, incoordination of voluntary movements, tremor, and choreoathetosis are early extrapyramidal signs of neurologic involvement. Deterioration in intellectual function and behavioral disturbances are usually late manifestations. Brain MRI scans reveal cortical and subcortical signal abnormalities, especially in the basal ganglia. Additional extrahepatic manifestations include hemolytic anemia, joint disease, and defects of renal tubular acidification.

The Kayser-Fleischer ring is the most important ophthalmologic sign in Wilson disease (184). It is a green-to-brown granular deposit located within the Descemet membrane at the corneal periphery (Fig. 21.26). It first appears at the superior and inferior limbus but then progresses to involve the entire circumference of the cornea. In advanced cases, the ring can be seen on gross inspection but is best seen with slit-lamp examination in its early stage. The Kayser-Fleischer ring is present in nearly 100% of patients with neurologic disease and in 70% to 95% of patients with liver disease. Although the Kayser-Fleischer ring is considered to be pathognomonic of Wilson disease, it occurs in primary biliary cirrhosis and other chronic liver diseases.

Cataract is another ocular manifestation of Wilson disease (184). Copper accumulates in a spoke-like pattern on the anterior lens capsule, in a pattern resembling a sunflower (Fig. 21.27). The sunflower cataract is present in only 10%

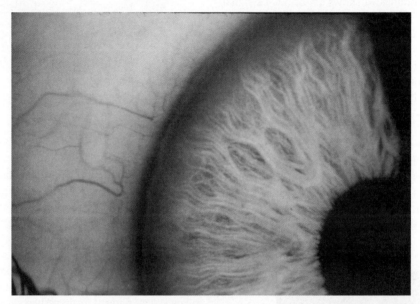

FIGURE 21.26. Slit-lamp photograph of the cornea reveals prominent Kayser-Fleischer ring in a patient with Wilson disease.

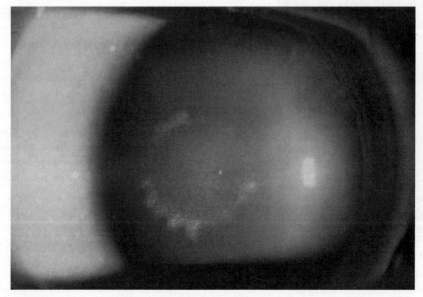

FIGURE 21.27. Slit-lamp photograph shows a "sunflower cataract" in Wilson disease.

to 20% of patients with Wilson disease and does not affect vision.

Neurologic involvement in Wilson disease largely spares the ocular motor system. Versions are normal and pathologic nystagmus is not observed. Electrooculographic recordings have demonstrated slow saccades and pursuits with reduced gain more so for vertical than horizontal eye movements (185–187). Additionally, loss of accommodation and accommodative convergence interferes with near vision and can be very problematic (188). Neuronal degeneration has been reported but the evidence is limited to marginal decreases in the nerve fiber layer by OCT and delays of the VEP (189). MRI scans demonstrate abnormalities in the midbrain, where the neural centers for accommodation and convergence are located (190).

Laboratory studies are necessary to confirm the diagnosis. Serum copper and ceruloplasmin levels are low, whereas urinary copper excretion is high. The observed levels, however, are variable, especially in younger patients with hepatic disease. Therefore, liver biopsy is the most reliable method for documenting increased copper accumulation.

Treatment is directed at reducing tissue stores of copper using copper chelators. Penicillamine has been the copper chelator of choice, but long-term follow-up shows neurologic deterioration in 50% of patients. Preliminary evidence indicates that tetrathiomolybdate, an alternative copper chelator, is associated with a lower incidence of neurologic deterioration (191). Liver transplant is well tolerated in patients with end-stage liver disease (184).

REFERENCES

1. King RA, Hearing VJ, Creel DJ, et al. Albinism. In: Scriver Beaudet AL, Sly WS, et al., eds. *The metabolic and molecular bases of inherited disease*, 8th Ed. New York: McGraw-Hill, 2001:5587–5627.

2. Rinchik EM, Bultman SJ, Horsthemke B, et al. A gene for the mouse pink-eyed dilution locus and for human type II oculocutaneous albinism. *Nature* 1993;361:72–76.

3. Huizing M, Gahl WA. Disorders of vesicles of lysosomal lineage: the Hermansky-Pudlak syndromes. *Curr Mol Med* 2002; 2:451–467.

4. Creel DJ, Summers CG, King RA. Visual anomalies associated with albinism. *Ophthalmic Pediatric Genet* 1990;11: 193–200.

5. McAllister JT, Dubis AM, Tait DM, et al. Arrested development: high-resolution imaging of foveal morphology in albinism. *Vision Res* Apr 2010;50(8):810–817.

6. King RA, Townsend D, Oetting W, et al. Temperature-sensitive tyrosinase associated with peripheral pigmentation in oculocutaneous albinism. *J Clin Invest* 1991;87:1046–1053.

7. King RA, Wiesner GL, Townsend D, et al. Hypopigmentation in Angelman syndrome. *Am J Med Genet* 1993;46:40–44.

8. Horsthemke B, Dittrich B, Buiting K. Imprinting mutations on human chromosome 15. *Hum Mutat* 1997;10:329–337.

9. Schiaffino MV, d'Addio M, Alloni A, et al. Ocular albinism: evidence for a defect in an intracellular signal transduction system. *Nat Genet* 1999;23:108–112.

10. Morell R, Spritz RA, Ho L, et al. Apparent digenic inheritance of Waardenburg syndrome type 2 (WS2) and autosomal recessive ocular albinism (AROA). *Hum Mol Genet* 1997;6:659–664.

11. Bassi MT, Ramesar RS, Caciotti B, et al. X-linked late-onset sensorineural deafness caused by a deletion involving OA1 and a novel gene containing WD-40 repeats. *Am J Hum Genet* Jun 1999;64(6):1604–1616

12. Gahl WA, Brantly M, Kaiser-Kupfer MI, et al. Genetic defects and clinical characteristics of patients with a form of oculocutaneous albinism (Hermansky-Pudlak syndrome). *N Engl J Med* 1998;338:1258–1264.

13. Anderson PD, Huizing M, Claassen DA, et al. Hermansky-Pudlak syndrome type 4 (HPS-4): clinical and molecular characteristics. *Hum Genet* 2003;113:10–17.

14. Wei ML. Hermansky-Pudlak syndrome: a disease of protein trafficking and organelle function. *Pigment Cell Res* Feb 2006;19(1): 19–42. Review.

15. Bonifacino JS, Gahl WA. A new variant of Hermansky-Pudlak syndrome due to mutations in a gene responsible for vesicle formation. *Am J Med* 2000;108:423–427.

16. Fernandez-Canon JM, Granadino B, Beltran-Valero de Bernabe D, et al. The molecular basis of alkaptonuria. *Nat Genet* 1996;14:19–24.

17. Kampik A, Sani JN, Green WR. Ocular ochronosis: clinicopathological, histochemical and ultrastructural studies. *Arch Ophthalmol* 1980;98:1441–1447.

18. Phornphutkul C, Introne WJ, Perry MB, et al. Natural history of alkaptonuria. *N Engl J Med* 2002;347:2111–2121.

19. Suwannarat P, O'Brien K, Perry MB, et al. Use of nitisinone in patients with alkaptonuria. *Metabolism* June 2005;54(6):719–728.

20. Gahl WA, Thoene JG, Schneider JA. Cystinosis: a disorder of lysosomal membrane transport. In: Scriver CR, Beaudet AL, Sly WS, et al., eds. *The metabolic and molecular basis of inherited disease*, 8th Ed. New York: McGraw-Hill, 2001:5085–5108.

21. Town M, Jean G, Cherqui S, et al. A novel gene encoding an integral membrane protein is mutated in nephropathic cystinosis. *Nat Genet* 1998;18:319–324.

22. Forestier L, Jean G, Attard M, et al. Molecular characterization of CTNS deletions in nephropathic cystinosis: development of a PCR-based detection assay. *Am J Hum Genet* 1999;65: 353–359.

23. Theodoropoulos DS, Krasnewich D, Kaiser-Kupfer MI, et al. Classic nephropathic cystinosis as an adult disease. *JAMA* 1993;270:2200–2204.

24. Gahl WA, Thoene JG, Schneider JA. Cystinosis. *N Engl J Med* 2002;347:111–121.

25. Katz B, Melles RB, Schneider JA. Corneal sensitivity in nephropathic cystinosis. *Am J Ophthalmol* 1987;104:413–416.

26. Kaiser-Kupfer MI, Caruso RC, Minkler DS, et al. Long-term ocular manifestations in nephropathic cystinosis. *Arch Ophthalmol* 1986;104:706–711.

27. DaSilva VA, Zurbrugg RP, Lavanchy B, et al. Long-term treatment of infantile nephropathic cystinosis with cysteamine. *N Engl J Med* 1985;313:1460–1464.

28. Gahl WA, Reed GF, Thoene JG, et al. Cysteamine therapy for children with nephropathic cystinosis. *N Engl J Med* 1987;316:971–977.

29. Kaiser-Kupfer MI, Fujikawa L, Kuwabara T, et al. Removal of corneal crystals by topical cysteamine in nephropathic cystinosis. *N Engl J Med* 1987;316:775–779.

30. Tsilou ET, Rubin BI, Reed G, et al. Therapy. *Ophthalmology* June 2006;113(6):1002–1009.

31. Valle D, Simell O. The hyperornithinemias. In: Scriver CR, Beaudet AL, Sly WS, et al., eds. *The metabolic and molecular basis of inherited disease*, 7th Ed. New York: McGraw-Hill, 1995:1147–1185.

32. Kaiser-Kupfer M, Ludwig D, DeMonasterio R, et al. Gyrate atrophy of the choroid and retina: early findings. *Ophthalmology* 1985;92:394–401.

33. Weleber R, Kennaway N. Clinical trial of vitamin B, for gyrate atrophy of the choroid and retina. *Ophthalmology* 1981;88:316–324.

34. Hayasaka S, Saito T, Nakagima H, et al. Clinical trials of vitamin B, and protein supplementation for gyrate atrophy of the choroid and retina. *Br J Ophthalmol* 1985;69:283–290.

35. Vannas-Sulonen K, Sipila I, Vannas A, et al. Gyrate atrophy of the choroid and retina. A five-year follow-up of creatine supplementation. *Ophthalmology* 1985;92:1719–1727.

36. Kaiser-Kupfer M, Caruso R, Valle D. Gyrate atrophy of the choroid and retina: chronic reduction of ornithine slows retinal degeneration. *Arch Ophthalmol* 1991;109:1539–1548.

37. Valle D, Walser M, Brusilow S, et al. Gyrate atrophy of the choroid and retina: amino acid metabolism and correction of hyperornithinemia with an arginine-restricted diet. *J Clin Invest* 1980;65:371–378.

38. Vannas-Sulonen K, Simell O, Spilia I. Gyrate atrophy of the choroid and retina: the ocular disease progresses in juvenile patients despite normal or near normal plasma ornithine concentration. *Ophthalmology* 1987;94:1428–1433.

39. Purdue PE, Lumb MJ, Fox M, et al. Characterization and chromosomal mapping of a genomic clone encoding human alanine: glyoxylate aminotransferase. *Genomics* 1991;10:34–42.

40. Cramer SD, Ferree PM, Lin K, et al. The gene encoding hydroxypyruvate reductase (GRHPR) is mutated in patients with primary hyperoxaluria type II. *Hum Mol Genet* 1999;8:2063–2069.

41. Meredith TA, Wright JD, Gammon JA, et al. Ocular involvement in primary hyperoxaluria. *Arch Ophthalmol* 1984;102:584–587.

42. Small KW, Letson R, Scheinman J. Ocular findings in primary hyperoxaluria. *Arch Ophthalmol* 1990;108:89–93.

43. Hoppe B, Langman CB. A United States survey on diagnosis, treatment, and outcome of primary hyperoxaluria. *Pediatr Nephrol* 2003;18:986–991.

44. Stambolian D, Ai Y, Sidjanin D, et al. Cloning of the galactokinase cDNA and identification of mutations in two families with cataracts. *Nat Genet* 1995;10:307–312.

45. Maceratesi P, Daude N, Dallapiccola B, et al. Human UDP-galactose 4' epimerase (GALE) gene and identification of five missense mutations in patients with epimerase-deficiency galactosemia. *Mol Genet Metab* 1998;63:26–30.

46. Tyfield L, Reichardt J, Fridovich-Keil J, et al. Classical galactosemia and mutations at the galactose-1-phosphate uridyl transferase (GALT) gene. *Hum Mutat* 1999;13:417–430.

47. Holton JB, Walter JH, Tyfield LA. Galactosemia. In: Scriver CR, Beaudet AL, Sly WS, et al, eds. *The metabolic and molecular basis of inherited disease*, 8th Ed. New York: McGraw-Hill, 2001:1553–1588.

48. Stambolian D. Galactose and cataract. *Surv Ophthalmol* 1988;32:333–349.

49. Waggoner DD, Buist NBM, Donnell GV. Long-term prognosis in galactosemia: results of a survey of 350 cases. *J Inherit Metab Dis* 1990;13:802–815.

50. Bosch AM, Bakker HD, van Gennip AH, et al. Clinical features of galactokinase deficiency: a review of the literature. *J Inherit Metab Dis* 2002;25:629–634.

51. Gitzelmann R. Hereditary galactokinase deficiency, a newly recognized cause of juvenile cataracts. *Pediatr Res* 1967;1:14–23.

52. Sardharwalla IB, Wraith JE, Bridge C, et al. A patient with severe type epimerase deficiency galactosemia. *J Inherit Metab Dis* 1988;11:249–251.

53. Goldstein JL, Hobbs HH, Brown MS. Familiar hypercholesterolemia. In: Scriver CR, Beaudet AL, Sly WS, et al., eds. *The metabolic and molecular basis of inherited disease*, 8th Ed. New York: McGraw-Hill, 2001:2863–2913.

54. Berge KE, Tian H, Graf GA, et al. Accumulation of dietary cholesterol in sitosterolemia caused by mutations in adjacent ABC transporters. *Science* 2000;290:1771–1775.

55. Lee MH, Lu K, Hazard S, et al. Identification of a gene, *ABCG5*, important in the regulation of dietary cholesterol absorption. *Nat Genet* 2001;27:79–83.

56. Kane JP, Havel RJ. Disorders of the biogenesis and secretion of lipoproteins containing the B lipoproteins. In: Scriver CR, Beaudet AL, Sly WS, et al., eds. *The metabolic and molecular basis of inherited disease*, 8th Ed. McGraw-Hill: New York, 2001:2717–2752.

57. Garcia CK, Wilund K, Arca M, et al. Autosomal recessive hypercholesterolemia caused by mutations in a putative LDL receptor adaptor protein. *Science* 2001;292:1394–1398.

58. Fredrickson DS, Levy RL. Familiar hyperlipoproteinemia. In: Stanbury JB, Wyngaarden JB, Fredrickson DS, eds. *The metabolic basis of inherited disease*, 3rd Ed. New York: McGraw-Hill, 1972:545.

59. Macaraeg PVJ Jr, Lasagna L, Snyder B. Arcus not so senilis. *Ann Intern Med* 1968;68:345–354.

60. Oram JF. Molecular basis of cholesterol homeostasis: lessons from Tangier disease and ABCA1. *Trends Mol Med* 2002;8:168–173.

61. Francis GA, Knopp RH, Oram JF. Defective removal of cellular cholesterol and phospholipids by apolipoprotein A-I in Tangier Disease. *J Clin Invest* 1995;96:78–87.

62. Brooks-Wilson A, Marcil M, Clee SM, et al. Mutations in *ABC1* in Tangier disease and familial high-density lipoprotein deficiency. *Nat Genet* 1999;22:336–345.

63. Assman G, von Eckardstein A, Brewer HB Jr. Familial high-density lipoprotein deficiency: Tangier disease. In: Scriver CR, Beaudet AL, Sly WS, et al., eds. *The metabolic and molecular basis of inherited disease*, 7th Ed. New York: McGraw-Hill, 1995:2053–2072.

64. Chu FC, Kuwabara T, Cogan DG. Ocular manifestations of familiar high-density lipoprotein deficiency (Tangier disease). *Arch Ophthalmol* 1979;97:1926–1928.

65. Pressley TA, Scott WJ, Ide CH, et al. Ocular complications of Tangier disease. *Am J Med* 1987;83:991–994.

66. Wetterau JR, Aggerbeck LP, Bouma ME, et al. Absence of microsomal triglyceride transfer protein in individuals with abetalipoproteinemia. *Science* 1992;258:999–1001.

67. Sharp D, Blinderman L, Combs KA, et al. Cloning and gene defects in microsomal triglyceride transfer protein associated with abetalipoproteinemia. *Nature* 1993;365:65–69.

68. Muller DPR, Lloyd JK. Effect of large oral doses of vitamin E on the neurologic sequelae of patients with abetalipoproteinemia. *Ann N Y Acad Sci* 1982;393:133–144.

69. Runge P, Muller DPR, McAllister J, et al. Oral vitamin E supplements can prevent the retinopathy of abetalipoproteinemia. *Br J Ophthalmol* 1986;70:166–173.

70. Dieckert JP, White M, Christmann L, et al. Angioid streaks associated with abetalipoproteinemia. *Ann Ophthalmol* 1989;21: 173–175.

71. Yee RD, Cogan DG, Zee DS. Ophthalmoplegia and dissociated nystagmus in abetalipoproteinemia. *Arch Ophthalmol* 1976;99:571–575.

72. Cohen DA, Bosley TA, Savino PJ, et al. Primary aberrant regeneration of the oculomotor nerve. *Arch Neurol* 1985;42:821–823.

73. Santamarina-Fojo S, Hoeg JM, Assman G, et al. Lecithin cholesterol acyltransferase deficiency and fish eye disease. In: Scriver CR, Beaudet AL, Sly WS, et al., eds. *The metabolic and molecular basis of inherited disease*, 8th Ed. New York: McGraw-Hill, 2001:2817–2833.

74. Bethel W, McCulloch C, Ghash M. Lecithin cholesterol acyltransferase deficiency: light and electron microscopic findings from two corneas. *Can J Ophthalmol* 1975;10:494–501.

75. Carlson CA, Philipson B. Fish-eye disease: a new familial condition with massive corneal opacities and dyslipoproteinemia. *Lancet* 1979;2:921–922.

76. Gravel RA, Kaback MM, Proia RL, et al. The G_{M2} gangliosidoses. In: Scriver CR, Beaudet AL, Sly WS, et al., eds. *The metabolic and molecular basis of inherited disease*, 8th Ed. New York: McGraw-Hill, 2001:3827–3876.

77. Cogan DG, Kuwabara T. The sphingolipidoses and the eye. *Arch Ophthalmol* 1968;79:437–452.

78. Musarella MA, Raab EL, Rudolph SH. Oculomotor abnormalities in chronic G_{M2} gangliosidoses. *J Pediatr Ophthalmol Strabismus* 1982;19:80–89.

79. Optican LM, Rucker JC, Keller EL, Leigh RJ. Mechanism of interrupted saccades in patients with late-onset Tay-Sachs disease. *Prog Brain Res* 2008;171:567–570.

80. Suzuki Y, Oshima A, Nanba E. α-galactosidase deficiency (β-galactosidosis): G_{M1} gangliosidosis and Morquio B disease. In: Scriver CR, Beaudet AL, Sly WS, et al., eds. *The metabolic and molecular basis of inherited disease*, 8th Ed. New York: McGraw-Hill, 2001:3775–3809.

81. Desnick RJ, Ioannou YA, Eng CM. α-galactosidase A deficiency: Fabry disease. In: Scriver CR, Beaudet AL, Sly WS, et al., eds. *The metabolic and molecular basis of inherited disease*, 8th Ed. New York: McGraw-Hill, 2001:3733–3774.

82. Johnson DL, Del Monte MA, Cotlier F. Fabry's disease: diagnosis by α-galactosidase A activity in tears. *Clin Chim Acta* 1975;63:81–90.

83. Rolfs A, Fazekas F, Grittner U, Dichgans M, et al.; Stroke in Young Fabry Patients (sifap) Investigators. Acute cerebrovascular disease in the young: the stroke in young fabry patients study. *Stroke* Feb 2013;44(2):340–349.

84. Weingeist TA, Blodi FC. Fabry's disease: ocular findings in a female carrier. *Arch Ophthalmol* 1971;85:169–176.

85. Sher NA, Reiff W, Letson RD, et al. Central retinal artery occlusion complicating Fabry's disease. *Arch Ophthalmol* 1978;96:815–817.

86. Allen LE, Cosgrave EM, Kersey JP Fabry disease in children: correlation between ocular manifestations, genotype and systemic clinical severity. *Br J Ophthalmol.* Dec 2010; 94(12):1602

87. Eng CM, Guffon N, Wilcox WR, et al., for the International Collaborative Fabry Disease Study Group. Safety and efficacy of recombinant human alpha-galactosidase A—replacement therapy in Fabry's disease. *N Engl J Med* 2001;345:9–16.

88. Desnick RJ, Brady R, Barranger J, et al. Fabry disease, an under-recognized multisystemic disorder: expert recommendations for diagnosis, management, and enzyme replacement therapy. *Ann Intern Med* 2003;138:338–346.

89. Polten A, Fluharty AL, Fluharty CB, et al. Molecular basis of different forms of metachromatic leukodystrophy. *N Engl J Med* 1991;324:18–22.

90. von Figura K, Gieselman V, Jaeken J. Metachromatic leukodystrophy. In: Scriver CR, Beaudet AL, Sly WS, et al., eds. *The metabolic and molecular basis of inherited disease*, 8th Ed. New York: McGraw-Hill, 2001:3695–3724.

91. Quigley HA, Green WR. Clinical and ultrastructural ocular histopathologic studies of adult-onset metachromatic leukodystrophy. *Am J Ophthalmol* 1976;82:472–479.

92. Libert J, van Hoof F, Toussaint D. Ocular findings in metachromatic leukodystrophy: an electron microscopic and enzyme study in different clinical and genetic variants. *Arch Ophthalmol* 1979;97:1495–1504.

93. Krivit W, Shapiro E, Kennedy W, et al. Treatment of late infantile metachromatic leukodystrophy by bone marrow transplantation. *N Engl J Med* 1990;322:28–32.

94. Bateman JB, Philipart M, Isenberg S. Ocular features of multiple sulfatase deficiencies and a new variant of metachromatic leukodystrophy. *J Pediatr Ophthalmol Strabismus* 1984;21: 133–139.

95. Suzuki K, Suzuki Y, Suzuki K. Galactosylceramide lipidosis: globoid-cell leukodystrophy (Krabbe disease). In: Scriver CR, Beaudet AL, Sly WS, et al., eds. *Metabolic and molecular basis of inherited disease*, 7th Ed. New York: McGraw-Hill, 1995: 2671–2692.

96. Brownstein S, Meagher-Villenure K, Polomero RC, et al. Optic nerve in globoid leukodystrophy (Krabbe's disease)—ultrastructural changes. *Arch Ophthalmol* 1978;96:864–870.

97. Krivit W, Shapiro EG, Peters C, et al. Hematopoietic stem-cell transplantation in globoid-cell leukodystrophy. *N Engl J Med* 1998;338:1119–1126.

98. Beutler E, Grabowski GA. Gaucher disease. In: Scriver CR, Beaudet AL, Sly WS, et al., eds. *The metabolic and molecular basis of inherited disease*, 8th Ed. New York: McGraw-Hill, 2001: 3635–3668.

99. Cogan D, Chu EC, Gittinger J, et al. Fundal abnormalities in Gauchers disease. *Arch Ophthalmol* 1980;98:2202–2203.

100. Sasaki T, Tsukahara S. A new ocular finding in Gauchers disease: a report of two brothers. *Ophthalmologica* 1985;191: 206–209.

101. Harris CM, Taylor DS, Vellodi A. Ocular motor abnormalities in Gaucher disease. *Neuropediatrics* 1999;30:289–293.

102. Barton NW, Brady RO, Dambrosia JM, et al. Replacement therapy for inherited enzyme deficiency—macrophage targeted glucocerebrosidase for Gaucher's disease. *N Engl J Med* 1991;324:1464–1470.

103. Charrow J, Andersson HC, Kaplan P, et al. Enzyme replacement therapy and monitoring for children with type 1 Gaucher disease: consensus recommendations. *J Pediatr* 2004;144: 112–120.

104. Andersson H, Kaplan P, Kacena K, Yee J. Eight-year clinical outcomes of long-term enzyme replacement therapy for 884

children with Gaucher disease type 1. *Pediatrics* Dec 2008;122(6): 1182–1190

105. Schuchman EH, Desnick RJ. Niemann-Pick disease types A and B: acid sphingomyelinase deficiencies. In: Scriver CR, Beaudet AL, Sly WS, et al., eds. *The metabolic and molecular basis of inherited disease*, 8th Ed. New York: McGraw-Hill, 2001:3589–3610.

106. Walton DC, Robb RM, Crocker AC. Ocular manifestations of group-A Niemann-Pick. *Am J Ophthalmol* 1978;85:174–180.

107. Cogan DG, Chu FC, Barranger JA, et al. Macular halo syndrome: variant of Niemann-Pick disease. *Arch Ophthalmol* 1983;101:1698–1700.

108. Carstea ED, Morris JA, Coleman KG, et al. Niemann-Pick C1 disease gene: homology to mediators of cholesterol homeostasis. *Science* 1997;277:228–231.

109. Davies JP, Chen FW, Ioannou YA. Transmembrane molecular pump activity of Niemann-Pick C1 protein. *Science* 2000;290: 2295–2298.

110. Naureckiene S, Sleat DE, Lackland H, et al. Identification of *HE1* as the second gene of Niemann-Pick C disease. *Science* 2000;290: 2298–2301.

111. Patterson MC, Vanier MT, Suzuki K, et al. Niemann-Pick disease type C: a lipid trafficking disorder. In: Scriver CR, Beaudet AL, Sly WS, et al., eds. *The metabolic and molecular basis of inherited disease*, 8th Ed. New York: McGraw-Hill, 2001:3611–3633.

112. Cogan DG, Chu EC, Reingold DB, et al. Ocular motor signs in some metabolic diseases. *Arch Ophthalmol* 1981;99: 1802–1808.

113. Walterfang M, Abel LA, Desmond P, Fahey MC, Bowman EA, Velakoulis D. Cerebellar volume correlates with saccadic gain and ataxia in adult Niemann-Pick type C. *Mol Genet Metab*. Jan 2013;108(1):85–89.

114. Moser HW, Linke T, Fensom AH, et al. Acid ceramidase deficiency: Farber lipogranulomatosis. In: Scriver CR, Beaudet AL, Sly WS, et al., eds. *The metabolic and molecular basis of inherited disease*, 8th Ed. New York: McGraw-Hill, 2001: 3573–3585.

115. Vormoor J, Ehlert K, Groll AH, et al. Successful hematopoietic stem cell transplantation in Farber disease. *J Pediatr* 2004;144:132–134.

116. Zarbin MA, Green WR, Moser HW, et al. Farber's disease: light and electron microscopic study of the eye. *Arch Ophthalmol* 1985;103:73–80.

117. Neufeld EE, Muenzer J. The mucopolysaccharidoses. In: Scriver CR, Beaudet AL, Sly WS, et al., eds. *The metabolic and molecular basis of inherited disease*, 8th Ed. New York: McGraw-Hill, 2001:3421–3452.

118. Canton LB, Disseler JA, Wilson EM II. Glaucoma in the Maroteaux-Lamy syndrome. *Am J Ophthalmol* 1989;108: 426–430.

119. Caruso RC, Kaiser-Kupfer ML, Muenzer J. Electroretinographic findings in the mucopolysaccharidoses. *Ophthalmology* 1986;93: 1612–1616.

120. Collins MLZ, Traboulsi EL, Maumenee IH. Optic nerve swelling and optic atrophy in the systemic mucopolysaccharidoses. *Ophthalmology* 1990;97:1445–1449.

121. Kenyon KR, Topping TM, Green WR, et al. Ocular pathology of the Maroteaux-Lamy syndrome (systemic mucopolysaccharidosis type VI): histologic and ultrastructural report of two cases. *Am J Ophthalmol* 1972;73:718–741.

122. Wraith JE, Clarke LA, Beck M, et al. Enzyme replacement therapy for mucopolysaccharidosis I: a randomized, double-blinded, placebo-controlled, multinational study of recombinant human alpha-L-iduronidase (laronidase). *J Pediatr* 2004;144:581–588.

123. Krivit W, Peters C, Shapiro EG. Bone marrow transplantation as effective treatment of central nervous system disease in globoid cell leukodystrophy, metachromatic leukodystrophy, adrenoleukodystrophy, mannosidosis, fucosidosis, aspartyl-glucosaminuria, Hurler, Maroteaux-Lamy, and Sly syndromes, and Gaucher disease type III. *Curr Opin Neurol* 1999;12: 167–176.

124. Staba SL, Escolar ML, Poe M, et al. Cord-blood transplants from unrelated donors in patients with Hurler's syndrome. *N Engl J Med* 2004;350:1960–1969.

125. Gullingsrud EO, Krivit W, Summers CG. Ocular abnormalities in the mucopolysaccharidoses after bone marrow transplantation. Longer follow-up. *Ophthalmology* 1998;105: 1099–1105.

126. Pitz S, Ogun O, Bajbouj M, Arash L, Schulze-Frenking G, Beck M. Ocular changes in patients with mucopolysaccharidosis I receiving enzyme replacement therapy: a 4-year experience. *Arch Ophthalmol* Oct 2007;125(10):1353–1356.

127. Tzetzi D, Hamilton R, Robinson PH, Dutton GN. Negative ERGs in mucopolysaccharidoses (MPS) Hurler-Scheie (I-H/S) and Hurler (I-H)-syndromes. *Doc Ophthalmol* May 2007;114(3): 153–158.

128. Thomas GH. Disorders of glycoprotein degradation: α-mannosidosis, β-mannosidosis, fucosidosis, and sialidosis. In: Scriver CR, Beaudet AL, Sly WS, et al., eds. *The metabolic and molecular basis of inherited disease*, 8th Ed. New York: McGraw-Hill, 2001:3507–3534.

129. Goldberg MF, Cotlier E, Fischenschler LG. Macular cherry-red spot, corneal clouding and beta-galactosidase deficiency. *Arch Intern Med* 1971;128:387–398.

130. Sogg RL, Steinman L, Rathien B, et al. Cherry-red spot-myoclonus syndrome. *Ophthalmology* 1979;86:1861–1874.

131. Pshezhetsky AV, Richard C, Michaud L, et al. Cloning, expression and chromosomal mapping of human lysosomal sialidase and characterization of mutations in sialidosis. *Nat Genet* 1997;15:316–320.

132. Lukong KE, Landry K, Elsliger MA, et al. Mutations in sialidosis impair sialidase binding to the lysosomal multienzyme complex. *J Biol Chem* 2001;276:17286–17290.

133. d'Azzo A, Andria G, Strisciuglio P, et al. Galactosialidosis. In: Scriver CR, Beaudet AL, Sly WS, et al., eds. *The metabolic and molecular basis of inherited disease*, 8th Ed. New York: McGraw-Hill, 2001:3611–3633.

134. Rudenko G, Bonten E, Hol WG, et al. The atomic model of the human protective protein/cathepsin A suggests a structural basis for galactosialidosis. *Proc Natl Acad Sci U S A* 1998;95:621–625.

135. Usui T, Sawaguchi S, Abe H, et al. Late-infantile type galactosialidosis. Histopathology of the retina and optic nerve. *Arch Ophthalmol* 1991;109:542–546.

136. Usui T, Abe H, Takagi M, et al. Electroretinogram and visual evoked potential in two siblings with adult form galactosialidosis. *Metab Pediatr Syst Ophthalmol* 1993;16:19–22.

137. Arbisser AI, Murphree AL, Garcia CA. Ocular findings in mannosidosis. *Am J Ophthalmol* 1976;82:465–471.

138. Letson RD, Desnick RI. Punctate lenticular opacities in type II mannosidosis. *Am J Ophthalmol* 1978;85:218–223.

139. Kornfeld S, Sly WS. I-cell disease and pseudo-Hurler polydystrophy: disorders of lysosomal enzyme phosphorylation and localization. In: Scriver CR, Beaudet AL, Sly WS, et al., eds. *The metabolic and molecular basis of inherited disease*, 8th Ed. New York: McGraw-Hill, 2001:3469–3482.

140. Libert J, van Hoof F, Farriaux JP, et al. Ocular findings in Icell disease (mucolipidosis type II). *Am J Ophthalmol* 1977;83: 617–628.

141. Raas-Rothschild A, Cormier-Daire V, Bao M, et al. Molecular basis of variant pseudo-Hurler polydystrophy (mucolipidosis IIIC). *J Clin Invest* 2000;105:673–681.

142. Bargal R, Avidan N, Ben-Asher E, et al. Identification of the gene causing mucolipidosis type IV. *Nat Genet* 2000;26: 118–123.

143. Sun M, Goldin E, Stahl S, et al. Mucolipidosis type IV is caused by mutations in a gene encoding a novel transient receptor potential channel. *Hum Mol Genet* 2000;9:2471–2478.

144. Amir N, Zlotogora J, Bach G. Mucolipidosis type IV: clinical spectrum and natural history. *Pediatrics* 1987;79:953–959.

145. Chitayat D, Meunier CM, Hodgkinson KA, et al. Mucolipidosis type IV: clinical manifestations and natural history. *Am J Med Genet* 1991;41:313–318.

146. Wakabayashi K, Gustafson AM, Sidransky E, Goldin E Mucolipidosis type IV: an update. *Mol Genet Metab* Nov 2011; 104(3):206–213.

147. Goldin E, Caruso RC, Benko W, Kaneski CR, Stahl S, Schiffmann R. Isolated ocular disease is associated with decreased mucolipin-1 channel conductance. *Invest Ophthalmol Vis Sci* Jul 2008;49(7):3134–3142.

148. Riedel KG, Zwaan J, Kenyon KR, et al. Ocular abnormalities in mucolipidosis IV. *Am J Ophthalmol* 1985;99:125–136.

149. Smith JA, Chan CC, Goldin E, et al. Noninvasive diagnosis and ophthalmic features of mucolipidosis type IV. *Ophthalmology* 2002;109:588–594.

150. Pradhan SM, Atchaneeyasakul LO, Appukuttan B, et al. Electronegative electroretinogram in mucolipidosis IV. *Arch Ophthalmol* 2002;120:45–50.

151. Jaeken J, Stibler H, Hagberg B. The carbohydrate-deficient glycoprotein syndrome. A new inherited multisystemic disease with severe nervous system involvement. *Acta Paediatr Scand Suppl* 1991;375:1–71.

152. Jaeken J, Artigas J, Barone R, et al. Phosphomannomutase deficiency is the main cause of carbohydrate-deficient glycoprotein syndrome with type I isoelectrofocusing pattern of serum sialotransferrins. *J Inherit Metab Dis* 1997;20:447–449.

153. Petersen MB, Brostrom K, Stibler H, et al. Early manifestations of the carbohydrate-deficient glycoprotein syndrome. *J Pediatr* 1993;122:66–70.

154. Stark KL, Gibson JB, Hertle RW, et al. Ocular motor signs in an infant with carbohydrate-deficient glycoprotein syndrome type Ia. *Am J Ophthalmol* 2000;130:533–535.

155. Andreasson S, Blennow G, Ehinger B, et al. Full-field electroretinograms in patients with the carbohydrate-deficient glycoprotein syndrome. *Am J Ophthalmol* 1991;112:83–86.

156. Thompson DA, Lyons RJ, Liasis A, Russell-Eggitt I, Jägle H, Grünewald S. Retinal on-pathway deficit in congenital disorder of glycosylation due to phosphomannomutase deficiency. *Arch Ophthalmol* June 2012;130(6):712–719.

157. Funke S, Gardeitchik T, Kouwenberg D, et al. Perinatal and early infantile symptoms in congenital disorders of glycosylation. *Am J Med Genet A* 2013; Epub 2013 Feb 7.

158. Gould SJ, Raymond GV, Valle D. The peroxisome biogenesis disorders. In: Scriver CR, Beaudet AL, Sly WS, et al., eds. *The metabolic and molecular basis of inherited disease*, 8th Ed. New York: McGraw-Hill, 2001:3181–3217.

159. Moser AB, Rasmussen M, Naidu S, et al. Phenotype of patients with peroxisomal disorders divided into sixteen complementation groups. *J Pediatr* 1995;127:13–22.

160. Reuber BE, Germain-Lee E, Collins CS, et al. Mutations in *PEX1* are the most common cause of peroxisome biogenesis disorders. *Nat Genet* 1997;17:445–448.

161. Cohen SMZ, Green WR, De la Cruz ZC, et al. Ocular histopathologic studies of neonatal and childhood adrenoleukodystrophy. *Am J Ophthalmol* 1983;95:82–96.

162. Hittner HM, Kretzer FL, Mehta RS. Zellweger syndrome: lenticular opacities indicating carrier status and lens abnormalities characteristic of homozygotes. *Arch Ophthalmol* 1981;99:1977–1982.

163. Garner A, Fielder AR, Primavesi R, et al. Tapetoretinal degeneration in the cerebro-hepato-renal (Zellweger's) syndrome. *Br J Ophthalmol* 1982;66:422–431.

164. Noguer MT, Martinez M. Visual follow-up in peroxisomal-disorder patients treated with docosahexaenoic Acid ethyl ester. *Invest Ophthalmol Vis Sci* Apr 2010;51(4):2277–2285.

165. Weleber RG, Tongue AC, Kennaway NG, et al. Ophthalmic manifestations of infantile phytanic acid storage disease. *Arch Ophthalmol* 1984;102:1317–1321.

166. Refsum S. Heredopathia atactica polyneuritiformis. Phytanic acid storage disease (Refsum's disease) with particular referral to ophthalmological disturbances. *Metab Ophthalmol* 1977;1:73–79.

167. Hansen E, Bachen NL, Flagge T. Refsum's disease: eye manifestations in a patient treated with low phytol, low phytanic acid diet. *Acta Ophthalmol (Copenh)* 1979;57:899–913.

168. Dickson N, Mortimer JG, Faed JM, et al. A child with Refsum's disease: successful treatment with diet and plasma exchange. *Dev Med Child Neurol* 1989;31:92–97.

169. Moser HW, Moser AE, Singh I, et al. Adrenoleukodystrophy: survey of 303 cases: biochemistry, diagnosis and therapy. *Ann Neurol* 1984;16:628–641.

170. Moser HW, Smith KD, Watkins PA, et al. X-linked adrenoleukodystrophy. In: Scriver CR, Beaudet AL, Sly WS, et al., eds. *The metabolic and molecular basis of inherited disease*, 8th Ed. New York: McGraw-Hill, 2001:3257–3301.

171. Moses J, Douar AM, Sarde CO, et al. Putative X-linked adrenoleukodystrophy gene shares unexpected homology with ABC transporters. *Nature* 1993;361:726–730.

172. Mahmood A, Raymond GV, Dubey P, Peters C, Moser HW. Survival analysis of hematopoietic cell transplantation for childhood cerebral X-linked adrenoleukodystrophy: a comparison study. *Lancet Neurol* Aug 2007;6(8):687–692.

173. Traboulsi EI, Maumenee IH. Ophthalmologic manifestations of X-linked childhood adrenoleukodystrophy. *Ophthalmology* 1987;94:47–52.

174. Glasgow BJ, Brown HH, Hannah JB, et al. Ocular pathologic findings in neonatal adrenoleukodystrophy. *Ophthalmology* 1987;94:1054–1060.

175. Kori AA, Robin NH, Jacobs JB, et al. Pendular nystagmus in patients with peroxisomal assembly disorder. *Arch Neurol* 1998;55:554–558.

176. Gess A, Christiansen SP, Pond D, Peters C. Predictive factors for vision loss after hematopoietic cell transplant for

X-linked adrenoleukodystrophy. *J AAPOS* June 2008;12(3): 273–276.

177. Herndon JH Jr, Steinberg D, Uhlendorf BW. Refsum's disease: defective oxidation of phytanic acid in tissue cultures derived from homozygotes and heterozygotes. *N Engl J Med* 1969;281:1034–1038.

178. Jansen GA, Hogenhout EM, Ferdinandusse S, et al. Human phytanoyl-CoA hydroxylase: resolution of the gene structure and the molecular basis of Refsum's disease. *Hum Mol Genet* 2000;9:1195–1200.

179. van den Brink DM, Brites P, Haasjes J, et al. Identification of *PEX7* as the second gene involved in Refsum disease. *Am J Hum Genet* 2003;72:471–477.

180. Wanders RJ, Jakobs C, Skjeldal OH. Refsum disease. In: Scriver CR, Beaudet AL, Sly WS, et al., eds. *The metabolic and molecular basis of inherited disease*, 8th Ed. New York: McGraw-Hill, 2001:3303–3321.

181. Bull P, Thomas GR, Rommens JM, et al. The Wilson's disease gene is a putative copper transporting P-type ATPase similar to the Menkes gene. *Nat Genet* 1993;5:327–337.

182. Petrukhin K, Fischer SG, Piratsu M, et al. Mapping, cloning and genetic characterization of the region containing the Wilson disease gene. *Nat Genet* 1993;5:338–343.

183. Walker JM, Huster D, Ralle M, et al. The N-terminal metal-binding site 2 of the Wilson's disease protein plays a key role in the transfer of copper from Atox1. *J Biol Chem* 2004;279:15376–15384.

184. Culotta VC, Gitlin JD. Disorders of copper transport. In: Scriver CR, Beaudet AL, Sly WS, et al., eds. *The metabolic and molecular basis of inherited disease*, 8th Ed. New York: McGraw-Hill, 2001:3105–3126.

185. Goldberg MF, Van Noorden GK. Ophthalmologic findings in Wilson's hepatolenticular degeneration. *Arch Ophthalmol* 1966;75:162–170.

186. Kirkham TH, Kamin DF. Slow saccadic eye movements in Wilson's disease. *J Neurol Neurosurg Psychiatry* 1974;37: 191–194.

187. Ingster-Moati I, Bui Quoc E, Pless M, et al. Ocular motility and Wilson's disease: a study on 34 patients. *J Neurol Neurosurg Psychiatry* Nov 2007;78(11):1199–1201.

188. Klingele TG, Newman SA, Burde RM. Accommodation defect in Wilson's disease. *Am J Ophthalmol* 1980;90: 20–24.

189. Albrecht P, Müller AK, Ringelstein M, et al. Retinal neurodegeneration in Wilson's disease revealed by spectral domain optical coherence tomography. *PLoS One* 2012;7(11):1–8.

190. McCrary JA III. Magnetic resonance imaging diagnosis of hepatolenticular degeneration. *Arch Ophthalmol* 1987; 105:277.

191. Brewer GJ, Hedera P, Kluin KJ, et al. Treatment of Wilson disease with ammonium tetrathiomolybdate. III. Initial therapy in a total of 55 neurologically affected patients and follow-up with zinc therapy. *Arch Neurol* 2003;60:379–385.

Pediatric Neuroophthalmology

Nagham Al-Zubidi • *Arielle Spitze* • *Sushma Yalamanchili* • *Andrew G. Lee*

NEUROOPHTHALMIC DISORDERS IN the pediatric population, although not as common as in their adult counterparts, are equally crucial to patients' ultimate visual and neurologic health. Very subtle initial symptoms may indicate major intracranial pathology. Prompt diagnosis and management is the best method to prevent permanent visual and neurologic sequelae.

The diseases encountered in pediatric neuroophthalmology are similar to those in adult situations in that the same broad categories like neoplastic, infectious, inflammatory, vascular, metabolic, and congenital must be considered. However, in pediatric neuroophthalmology, the frequency of the various diseases is weighted toward congenital, postinfectious, and neoplastic entities.

The clinician evaluating these patients must define the onset and progression of the present problem, and secure detailed prenatal, birth, growth and development, and family histories. The amount of history obtained directly from the child obviously depends on his or her age and mental status. Primary and secondary historical details must always be elicited from mothers, fathers, grandparents, and siblings who may have witnessed the patient's behavior.

In this chapter, pediatric neuroophthalmic problems are approached as the patients and their parents report them to clinicians by their symptoms. Each symptom complex is analyzed anatomically so that a coherent comprehensive differential diagnostic approach may be formulated.

VISUAL LOSS

Children may not complain of loss of vision (especially if mild or unilateral), and usually adapt to the deficit rather than admitting to any interference with their activities. A decrease of visual acuity in one or both eyes is often detected on routine screening examinations performed by pediatricians, school nurses, and general ophthalmologists.

After the more common problems of refractive error and strabismic or anisometropic amblyopia have been excluded, and if no anterior segment pathology can be found, concern must arise that a neuroophthalmic disorder is present. The optic nerve is the initial neuroanatomic structure of the afferent visual system and should occupy the first position in the differential diagnostic analysis.

The physical findings of unilateral optic nerve disease are identical for children and adults including decreased central visual acuity often associated with an optic nerve type visual field defect, an acquired dyschromatopsia, and a relative afferent pupillary defect (RAPD) or Marcus Gunn pupil depending on the severity of the optic neuropathy.

Bilateral optic neuropathies in some ways present a more difficult diagnostic challenge as the RAPD may be minimal or absent. Also, with bilateral optic neuropathies, dyschromatopsias may be symmetric, mimicking congenital color blindness. Finally, with bilateral, symmetric disease, the only pupillary finding is a sluggish reaction to direct light stimulation and a better near reaction, which is more difficult to appreciate than a RAPD.

Once the diagnosis of a unilateral or bilateral optic neuropathy has been established, the exact etiology must be determined. Optic nerve abnormalities can be isolated, associated with other ocular pathologies disorders of the central nervous system (CNS), part of a systemic disease, or syndromes. Toxic exposure during pregnancy (e.g., medications, illicit drugs, alcohol) and systemic maternal disorders (e.g., diabetes, seizure disorder) should be sought in the history. In addition, congenital defects of the optic nerve should be considered high in the differential diagnosis.

CONGENITAL OPTIC NERVE ABNORMALITIES: OPTIC NERVE HYPOPLASIA

Optic nerve hypoplasia may present to the pediatric ophthalmologist during the evaluation of unilateral or bilateral visual loss or during the assessment of strabismus or nystagmus. Sometimes the patient is referred for further evaluation because of the unusual appearance of the optic disk. This disk anomaly may be the harbinger of associated significant CNS and endocrinologic abnormalities.

Hypoplastic optic nerves may be unilateral or bilateral, may affect central visual acuity minimally or profoundly, and may produce any nerve fiber type visual field changes ranging from nasal defects to more typical nerve fiber layer defects, diffuse depression, or generalized constriction (1). When the optic nerve is strikingly hypoplastic (Fig. 22.1),

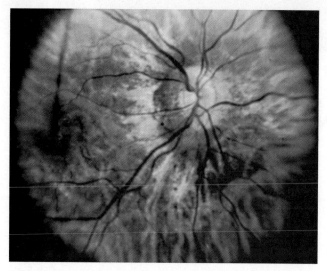

FIGURE 22.1. Marked optic disk hypoplasia. The optic disk is approximately one-half the normal size and is surrounded by a peripapillary yellowish border.

Table 22.1

FUNDOSCOPIC CRITERIA FOR DIAGNOSIS OF OPTIC NERVE HYPOPLASIA

Small optic disk

Peripapillary halo surrounds disk ("double-ring" sign)

Combined size of small disk and halo roughly approximates size of a normal disk

Normal or slightly tortuous, nondilated vessels

Decreased foveal reflex

Decreased thickness of retinal nerve fiber layer

Adapted from Rangwala LM, Liu GT. Pediatric idiopathic intracranial hypertension. Surv Ophthalmol 2007;52(6):597–617.

the fundoscopic diagnosis is relatively easy. However, detailed evaluation of the optic nerve with higher magnification may be necessary to evaluate subtle findings of optic nerve hypoplasia (Fig. 22.2).

Six fundoscopic features (Table 22.1) should be sought in optic nerve hypoplasia. First, by definition, the disk must be small. Second, the disk is typically surrounded by a peripapillary yellowish border that encircles the entire disk to form a halo. This halo constitutes the "double-ring" sign that has been invariably associated with this diagnosis. On the basis of the histopathologic study of Mosier and colleagues (2), the outer portion of the double-ring is the junction between sclera and lamina cribrosa where the choroid is discontinuous. The inner ring is demarcated by termination of the retinal pigment epithelium, with the whitish appearance of the inner ring attributed to glial and connective tissue around the retinal vessels.

The third criterion for the fundoscopic diagnosis is that the dimensions of the hypoplastic nerve and peripapillary halo roughly approximate the size of a normal optic disk. The remaining three criteria involve the retina and include (a) normal or slightly tortuous, nondilated retinal vessels; (b) decreased foveal reflex; and (c) decreased thickness of the retinal nerve fiber layer. Pathologic studies have revealed decreased numbers of retinal ganglion cells, as well as thinning of the nerve fiber layer, thereby confirming the ophthalmoscopic observations of the retina (3).

It is important to remember that the appearance of the optic nerve is not always predictive of the ultimate visual acuity and can range from 20/20 to no light perception (4). In unilateral or asymmetric disease, there can be a superimposed component of amblyopia which may be amenable to conventional amblyopia treatment (5,6).

Etiology

No single, unifying pathophysiologic concept has evolved to explain optic nerve hypoplasia, up to 45% of optic nerve hypoplasia are sporadic but many environmental factors have been reported associated with optic nerve hypoplasia including maternal insulin-dependent diabetes mellitus, epilepsy, and younger maternal age, and the use of a variety of therapeutic and "recreational" drugs including lysergic acid diethylamide and ethanol (fetal alcohol syndrome) (7). In the therapeutic category, anticonvulsants, corticosteroids, diuretics, isoretinoin, meperidine (4,8–10), protamine, zinc, and insulin have all been reported to be associated with this optic nerve abnormality (11). Histologically, the number of optic nerve axons is reduced with normal supporting glial tissue. One proposed pathogenesis is supranormal regression of optic nerve axons in utero rather than a primary failure of differentiation (4,12,13). Recent genetic studies have

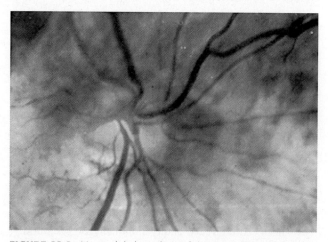

FIGURE 22.2. More subtle hypoplasia of the optic disk than shown in Figure 22.1. The lower border of the disk is truncated. The patient presented with a superior visual field defect that was initially believed to represent a chiasmal lesion.

implicated the homeobox gene *HESX1/hesx1* in septooptic dysplasia. The data suggest that this gene plays an important role in forebrain and pituitary development (14–17).

Ocular and Central Nervous System Associations

Optic nerve hypoplasia may exist as a totally isolated congenital defect, but it has also been reported with almost every other congenital ocular abnormality ranging from ocular motor palsies to microphthalmos to blepharophimosis. Moreover, a variety of neurologic abnormalities and syndromes have been associated with hypoplastic optic nerves. Some of these disorders, such as hydranencephaly and anencephaly, preclude continued growth and development.

The septo-optic dysplasia or de Morsier (18,19) syndrome has been described as optic nerve hypoplasia, brain midline defects including agenesis of the anterior commissure and septum pellucidum, as well as malformation of the chiasm (Figs. 22.3 and 22.4), and pituitary hormone abnormalities (20). de Morsier coined the term "septo-optic dysplasia" for these defects, but it was Hoyt and coworkers (21) who stressed the syndrome of septo-optic dysplasia with growth retardation secondary to hypopituitarism. Magnetic resonance imaging (MRI) of the brain and orbits should be considered in patients with optic nerve hypoplasia (22). Detection of this syndrome is critical because the endocrine abnormalities can be life threatening. In addition, growth retardation is reversible if growth hormone therapy is initiated before epiphyses close. Likewise, encephaloceles

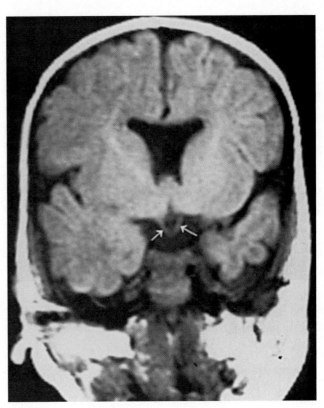

FIGURE 22.4. Coronal magnetic resonance imaging (MRI) scan of the patient in Figure 22.3. *Arrows* denote hypoplastic optic nerves.

are more common in these patients, and this brain tissue in the sphenoid sinus might be mistaken for an abnormality and even inadvertently biopsied.

OPTIC NERVE DYSPLASIA

Dysplasia of the optic nerve refers to a collection of clinical entities ranging from the morning glory syndrome and optic disk coloboma and other cavitary disk anomalies to megalopapillae and tilted optic disks. Of these, the morning glory syndrome and disk coloboma are discussed here because they may produce central visual loss in the pediatric-age group. The other disorders usually are associated with visual field defects and are discussed in the section concerning visual field abnormalities, but it is well known that tilted optic disks can produce a pseudobitemporal hemianopsia.

The morning glory syndrome (Fig. 22.5) is a rare disk anomaly first described by Kindler (23). It is comprised of a funnel-shaped excavation of the optic disk, distorted disk architecture, and a larger size than normal. The disk is surrounded by elevated, prominent, chorioretinal pigment in the shape of an annulus. There is typically a white tuft of glial tissue over the central portion of the disk. The blood vessels are a nomalous and arise from the periphery of the disk and often branch at acute angles. The term reflects the morphological similarity to the flower of the morning glory plant. The pathogenesis of the condition is unknown but there are

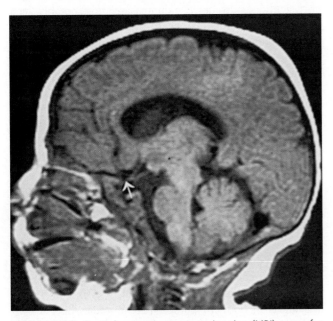

FIGURE 22.3. Sagittal magnetic resonance imaging (MRI) scan of a patient with de Morsier syndrome (septooptic dysplasia). The pertinent neuroradiologic features are hypoplastic optic nerves (*arrow*), as well as agenesis of the anterior commissure and septum pellucidum (courtesy of Dr. Robert Grossman).

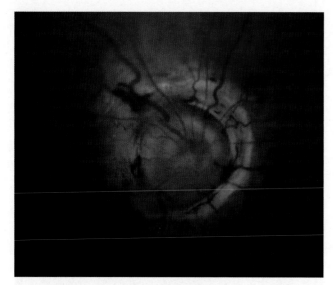

FIGURE 22.5. Morning glory syndrome of the optic disk. The disk is funnel shaped, distorted, and larger than normal size. The chorioretinal pigment surrounding the disk is shaped like an annulus.

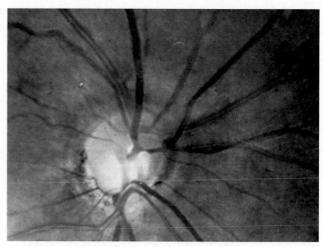

FIGURE 22.6. Optic disk coloboma, which was not associated with a corresponding colobomatous defect in the retina and choroid.

different hypotheses including failure of closure of the fetal fissure or primary mesenchymal abnormality or dilation due to dysgenesis of the terminal optic stalk. Patients can present with transient visual loss episodes or chronic visual loss. An anomalous communication between the subretinal and subarachnoid space permits fluid to produce serous retinal detachments. Patients (24,25) often are neurologically and ophthalmologically normal but basal encephaloceles have been associated with the morning glory syndrome.

Patients with this syndrome may lose vision because of both serous and rhegmatogenous retinal detachments (25). The prognosis for visual rehabilitation with traditional vitreoretinal surgical procedures is poor. However, Irvine and coworkers (26) and Chang and associates (27) reported some success in repairing these detachments when optic nerve sheath decompression surgery was performed simultaneously with vitreoretinal surgery.

Coloboma is the other major variety of dysplastic optic disk anomaly that may present in childhood with visual loss (Fig. 22.6). A coloboma is a developmental malformation with bowl-shaped excavation of the optic disk, which is deeper inferiorly resulting from partial or anomalous closure of the two sides of the proximal end of the embryonic fissure. An optic nerve coloboma may exist independently or be associated with colobomatous defects in the retina and choroid, depending on which portion of the embryonic fissure fails to close. If the proximal portion of the fissure fails to close in the correct manner, the retina and choroid are involved primarily. When the more distal segment of the fissure remains open, the nerve and its meningeal sheath are affected with a colobomatous defect. Optic nerve coloboma may occur sporadically or be inherited in an autosomal dominant pattern. It has been shown to be associated with *PAX2* gene mutations as part of the renal-coloboma syndrome (25,28–31).

Patients with optic disk coloboma frequently have reduced visual acuity but the only feature that relates to visual outcome is the degree of foveal involvement by the coloboma. The visual field defects in coloboma however are variable. Significant refractive errors and anisometropia are also common in optic nerve coloboma and should be addressed (32,33). Patients with optic nerve coloboma are also at risk for retinal detachment, which has been reported to occur as early as 5 months of age (34). Peripapillary choroidal neovascularization has been described too (35).

As in optic nerve hypoplasia, optic nerve coloboma may occur in isolation or associated with other neurologic or systemic syndromes. Coloboma are most notably seen in CHARGE (*c*oloboma, *h*eart disease, *a*tresia choanae, *r*etarded growth and development, *g*enitourinary abnormalities, and *e*ar abnormalities) association and renal-coloboma syndrome (36).

Early intervention is essential for children with poor visual acuity due to any of these conditions, and these conditions are managed by treating refractive errors, occlusion therapy, and optimizing the conditions at home and at school in an attempt to ensure that impaired vision does not impede development or education (25).

HEREDITARY OPTIC ATROPHY: DOMINANT OPTIC ATROPHY

Dominant optic atrophy (DOA) is the most common bilateral hereditary condition of the optic nerve encountered in the pediatric population. The prevalence of DOA is 1 in 35,000 individuals in northern Europe. Recent studies have shown that mutations in the nuclear-encoded dynamin-like GTPase nuclear gene *OPA1*, which is involved in mitochondrial fusion, are responsible for the majority of DOA cases. The *OPA1* gene causes DOA linked to chromosome 3q27–q29 (37–40). Patients often present in childhood after failing school screening examinations. Acute visual loss has not been described in this disease. Some patients may not come to medical attention until adulthood. A patient with a DOA mutation has a 50% probability of transmitting the pathogenic allele to each of the siblings. DOA demonstrates incomplete penetrance and children with the mutant allele have a 66% to 88% chance of manifesting the disease (41,42).

Because the visual deficits may be mild (20/40 to 20/200 range), visual acuity typically decreases over the first two decades of life. Thinning of the neuroretinal rim is a universal finding (43,44) and because children frequently do not report visual changes, the exact incidence and onset of DOA remains uncertain. Classically, DOA is detected during primary school vision screening (45) and 58% to 84% of patients report visual impairment by age of 11 years (46,47).

The degree of vision loss varies among the same family members and could be asymmetric in affected individuals. Although most patients with DOA had isolated optic neuropathy, up to 20% are associated with neurological manifestations such as sensorineural hearing, myopathy, peripheral neuropathy, ataxia, ptosis, and/or ophthalmoplegia (48,49).

In 1959, Kjer (50) published his classic monograph describing 19 Danish families with DOA. He attempted to use the presence of nystagmus as a distinguishing feature between what he believed were two forms of DOA. However, Waardenburg and coworkers (51) considered that the nystagmus was too nonspecific a finding to be used reliably to separate these two supposed entities. Review of the literature favors the position of Waardenburg. Kline and Glaser (52) described 24 individuals in 4 pedigrees without nystagmus or other extraocular motility abnormalities.

This study may represent the best description of the clinical profile of DOA. In this series, best corrected visual acuity ranged from 20/25 to 20/400. In 6 of the 12 patients, the two eyes had identical acuity, and there was a one line difference between the two eyes in two patients. The remaining four patients had greater than a two-line difference between eyes, one individual having 20/30 in the right and 20/200 in the left.

Visual field deficits for DOA are noteworthy for four characteristics: (a) elongated blind spots, (b) cecocentral scotoma, (c) mild temporal depression to central isopters (I-2-E and I-3-E) are rarely encountered, and (d) normal peripheral isopters (I-4-E or larger). Progressive loss of acuity and visual field have been described rarely in DOA. Such deterioration is so unusual that thorough diagnostic investigation is advocated in this circumstance, so that "progressive DOA" becomes a diagnosis of exclusion.

The color vision deficits in DOA are fascinating and often provide a helpful diagnostic point in distinguishing DOA from other optic neuropathies. Ishihara and Hardy-Rand-Rittler provide excellent screening methods for detecting dyschromatopsias for DOA, but only the Farnsworth-Munsell 100 hue examination precisely defines the defects. In Kline and Glaser's (52) series, a tritan (yellow-blue) error

was found in 15 of 22 eyes. In 5 of these 15 eyes, a deutan or protan axis was also identified with the tritan abnormality. The remaining seven eyes displayed a generalized dyschromatopsia without an identifiable axis. This tritan dyschromatopsia for DOA is significant because it violates Koellner's rule (i.e., disease of receptor and bipolar layer of the retina results in decreased blue-yellow sensitivity and disease of the retinal ganglion cells and visual pathways anterior to the lateral geniculate body produces red-green dyschromatopsia). To date, no explanation for the unusual tritan axis in DOA has been provided.

The appearance of the optic nerve in DOA has been controversial. There is agreement that pallor of the temporal segment of the disk occurs routinely and that diffuse pallor does not occur, but no consensus has been reached regarding other features of the optic nerve appearance. Kline and Glaser (52) believed strongly that most eyes (16 of 22 in their series) demonstrate focal temporal excavation (Fig. 22.7). This excavation can be so pronounced that the temporal portion of the disk may be on a different plane compared with the nasal aspect. The degree of temporal excavation is highly variable, and this variability may explain why different clinicians have had the strong opinions that no "pathognomonic" disk appearance exists.

Kline and Glaser (52) modified the criteria for the diagnosis of DOA as first proposed by Smith. These criteria are listed in Table 22.2. No reports on the treatment of DOA have been published to date, DOA might benefit from idebenone, but further studies are needed (47).

LEBER HEREDITARY OPTIC NEUROPATHY

Leber hereditary optic neuropathy (LHON) rarely has its onset in adulthood, the disease being found predominantly in pediatric- and adolescent-age groups. Although Leber initially described the disease as appearing between the ages of 18 and 23 years, numerous reports now exist documenting its occurrence before age 10 and essentially at any age.

LHON is a maternally inherited disorder and has a 9:1 male-to-female ratio. Approximately 50% of males and 10% of females with the genetic defect develop the optic neuropathy. The majority of cases are associated with point mutations in the mitochondrial genome responsible for complex 1 (NADH:ubiquinone oxidoreductase). These genes are referred to as the ND genes, and the point mutations are as follows: G11778A in ND4, G3460A in ND1, and T14484C in ND6. Testing is important because different mutations have different rates of spontaneous improvement in LHON. Not all LHON patients however have one of these common mutations. Currently, *ND6* is considered a hot spot because at least seven different point mutations in this gene have been found in pedigrees with LHON (53,54).

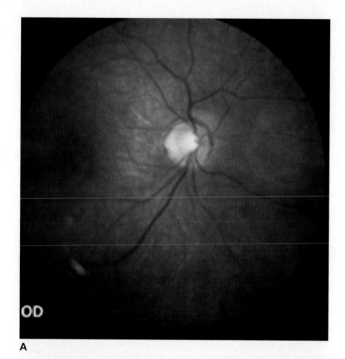

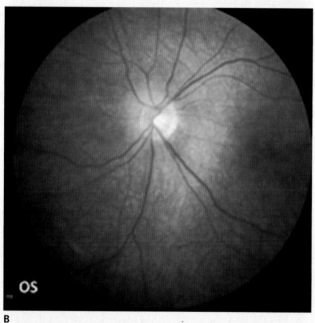

FIGURE 22.7. A and **B:** Dominant optic atrophy (DOA) demonstrating pallor of the temporal aspect of both disks with focal excavation of the temporal portion of the nerves (courtesy of Dr. Joel S. Glaser).

Table 22.2
DIAGNOSTIC CRITERIA FOR DOMINANT OPTIC ATROPHY (DOA)
Autosomal-dominant inheritance pattern (may benecessary to examine asymptomatic family members)
Insidious onset, often around 10 years of age
Bilateral, symmetric visual loss, although asymmetric loss can occur
Mild-to-moderate reduction in visual acuity
Central and cecocentral scotomata with normal peripheral isopters OU
Tritan dyschromatopsia with possibly superimposed protan and deutan defects; rarely, generalized dyschromatopsia may be present
Temporal disk pallor with possible triangular temporal excavation of disk

Adapted from Kline LB, Glaser JS. Dominant optic atrophy: the clinical profile. Arch Ophthalmol 1979;97:1680–1686; and from Smith DP. The assessment of acquired dyschromatopsia and clinical investigation of the acquired tritan defect in dominantly inherited juvenile atrophy. Am J Optom 1972;49:574–588.

Smith and colleagues (55) postulated that a typical fundoscopic picture exists for acute LHON. They described pronounced telangiectatic microangiopathy in the circumpapillary region associated with hyperemia of the disk and swelling of the nerve fiber layer surrounding the disk (Fig. 22.8). Fluorescein angiography reveals that the peripapillary disk vasculature is dilated but does not leak dye. The disks eventually become pale, with subsequent loss of the retinal nerve fiber layers.

Most patients with LHON have only optic nerve disease, but there are well-documented cases of more diffuse neurologic involvement (56). However, no specific pattern of involvement elsewhere in the CNS has yet emerged. Two patients with electrocardiographic abnormalities have also been described (57), but again this seems more the exception than the rule.

Presentation

The presenting symptoms of LHON are virtually indistinguishable from those of optic neuritis (ON). Patients report a blur or shadow in their central vision. The onset may be unilateral or bilateral. When one eye is first involved, the second eye invariably becomes affected within several days to weeks; exceptional cases are described with intervals of 3, 8, 12, and 14 years before the second eye became involved.

Treatment

A small percentage of patients with LHON demonstrate spontaneous visual improvement. To date, it is impossible to predict who will regain visual function and to what degree. At the present time, no therapeutic regimen has been documented to be effective.

Pfeffer et al. reviewed eight which showed no clear evidence supporting the use of any intervention in

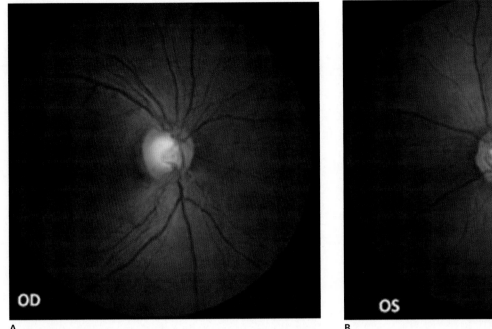
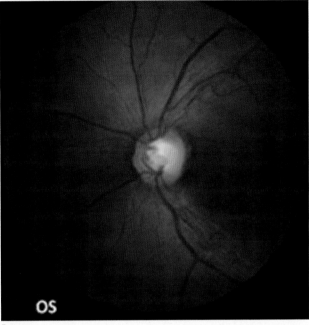

A   **B**

FIGURE 22.8. **A** and **B:** Optic atrophy involving papillomacular bundle (temporal pallor) in left and right eyes in Leber hereditary optic neuropathy.

mitochondrial disorders. Further research is needed to establish the role of a wide range of therapeutic approaches (47,58). General therapies for mitochondrial diseases have been proposed, including vitamins and cofactors (coenzyme Q10 [CoQ10], folic acid, vitamin B12, thiamine, riboflavin, L-carnitine, L-arginine, and creatine); electron acceptors (vitamin C, menadiol); free radical scavengers (CoQ10, idebenone, α-lipoic acid, minocycline, cyclosporine A, glutathione, and vitamin E); and inhibitors of toxic metabolites (dichloroacetate) (59,60).

OPTIC NEURITIS

Optic neuritis (ON) refers to an idiopathic or demyelinating condition of the optic nerve. In contrast with the adult form of this disease, ON in children has three differentiating characteristics: (a) bilateral simultaneous involvement is much more common in children than in adults, (b) between 70% and 80% of children demonstrated optic disk edema compared with approximately 30% of adults with this disorder (Fig. 22.9), and (c) association with multiple sclerosis

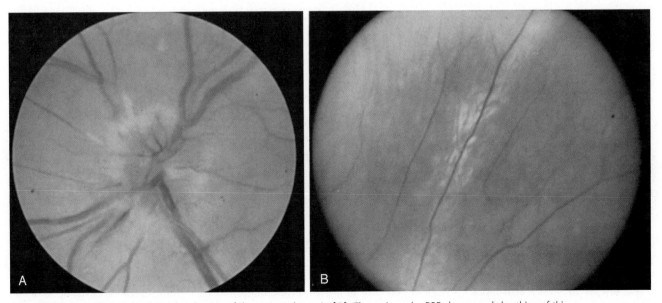

A   **B**

FIGURE 22.9. **B:** The temporal peripheral retina of the patient shown in **(A)**. The perivascular RPE change and sheathing of this retinal vessel developed 3 months after the acute papillitis.

(MS) is much lower in children than in adults. It is unclear whether this difference related that environmental or genetic risk factors in children compared with adults. There are no published studies comparing incidence rates or prevalence ratios from population-based multiethnic cohorts in either children or adults with MS or other forms of acquired demyelinating syndromes (ADS) (61).

The incidence of acquired demyelination of the CNS (ADS) in children is unknown. The annual incidence of pediatric ADS was between 0.3/100,000 and 1.66/100,000. ON was one of the most common subtypes of ADS accounting for 23% to 36% with an estimated prevalence of 3.2/100,000 (62–64).

ON in children is most often associated with postinfectious etiology with symptoms of febrile or flu-like illness preceding the ON by days to weeks. In addition, infectious, systemic inflammatory, and postimmunization causes are all possible (65,66,67).

In the pediatric population, an accurate history of visual loss is often difficult to determine and the vision loss frequently bilateral (33% to 86%) and profound (<20/200 in 90% to 95% of children) (62,68).

Visual improvement starts within 3 weeks of the visual loss, and continues up to 6 months. Younger children (<6 years of age) have a better visual prognosis than older children. Optic disk appearance was abnormal in 83.3% of the eyes in the acute phase. At presentation, RAPD was detected in 67%, visual field defects in 58.5%, and color vision defects in 50% of eyes (69).

Visual evoked potentials (VEP) are of value in confirming clinical suspicion of ON, VEP signal is initially absent in eyes with acute ON, latency remains abnormal in 45% to 65% of children up to 6 to 12 months (62,70).

If ON is suspected clinically, then neuroimaging should be performed to rule out demyelination, inflammatory disease, or less likely an intracranial mass or evidence of hydrocephalus. Underlying infectious causes, as well as increased intracranial pressure (ICP), are ruled out by performing a lumbar puncture. Pediatric ON conversion to MS ranges from 0% to 33%. Bilateral sequential or recurrent ON was associated with a higher rate of MS conversion (62,71,72). A positive MRI scan for demyelinating white matter lesions at ON onset is a strong predictor for development of MS (68,73).

Treatment of ON in the pediatric population remains controversial. To date, there has been no prospective randomized trial to determine the role of systemic corticosteroids in the treatment of pediatric ON. On the basis of the adult Optic Neuritis Treatment Trial (74,75), which showed faster visual recovery with high-dose intravenous steroids followed by oral steroids, ON is often treated with steroids (76).

DEVIC DISEASE

Devic disease (neuromyelitis optica [NMO]) is a variety of CNS demyelinating disease confined as severe acute transverse myelitis (TM), ON, or both. Recurrent NMO is 3 to 9 times more prevalent in women than in men, while in the monophasic form the female/male gender ratio is 1:1. NMO can be a fulminant monophasic or a polyphasic disease with multiple relapses and clinical remissions and with varying degrees of recovery (77,78). NMO-IgG, firstly identified by indirect immunofluorescence in patients with opticospinal variant of CNS demyelinating disorders, is an autoantibody of an IgG isotype specific for Aquaporin4 (AQP4). AQP4 is the most abundant water-channel protein in the CNS (79).

In adults, the sensitivity of NMO-IgG is 73% and specificity of 91%, and in children sensitivity ranges from 67% to 80%.

The high specificity of NMO-IgG for NMO, is coincident with clinical relapse. Children and adults may be affected with this disorder, which produces bilateral visual loss and TM. The visual loss is always bilateral, but it may begin in one eye and involve the second eye several days later (80). Paraplegia from TM quickly follows. In addition to white matter lesions, the gray matter of the spinal cord may be involved. Compared with those who have MS, patients with Devic disease demonstrate a much more elevated cerebrospinal fluid (CSF) protein concentration, as well as increased numbers of inflammatory cells in the spinal fluid. The treatment outcome of NMO is variable, unpredictable, and in many cases unsuccessful. No specific protocols are there regarding the optimum treatment regimen. IV corticosteroids are commonly used for an acute attack of ON or TM. For resistant cases, plasmapheresis, immunosuppressive therapy with (azathioprine, mitoxantrone) IV immunoglobulin, mycophenolate mofetil, and rituximab are recommended to reduce the risk of relapses (81–86).

NMO prognosis is poor. Significant physical and visual disabilities occur in more than half of adult patients within 5 years of disease onset (79).

SCHILDER DISEASE

Bilateral ON without visual improvement may be the first manifestation of Schilder disease, a rare and relentlessly progressive widespread demyelinating disease (myelinoclastic diffuse sclerosis) (87). Schilder disease may present as an intracranial mass, mimicking tumor or abscess on MRI (88–90). The disease usually develops before 10 years of age and is rapidly fatal within 1 to 2 years. However, there have been several reported cases which have responded to corticosteroid treatment (88,91,92). The disease is not inherited and has an equal male-to-female incidence. The neuropathologic features are indistinguishable from those of MS.

PAPILLITIS AND MACULAR STAR

During the past several years, there has been growing recognition and interest in a syndrome of edema of the optic nerve head (papillitis) associated with macular exudate ("macular star," "hemimacular star," or "neuroretinitis") (Fig. 22.10).

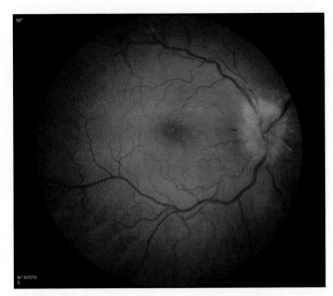

FIGURE 22.10. Papillitis associated with hemimacular star.

This entity actually dates back to 1916 and Leber's original report (93). Although Leber incorrectly hypothesized that the disorder was a primary retinal disease, he provided an exceedingly accurate clinical profile and description.

Using fluorescein angiography, Gass (94) demonstrated that the optic disk changes developed prior to or simultaneously with the macular exudate. Children and teenagers usually present with unilateral loss of vision, although cases of bilateral involvement have been described. Approximately 50% of patients present with retrobulbar pain worsened by eye movement, similar to ON associated with MS. However, patients with papillitis and neuroretinitis do not have an increased risk of MS or future episodes of clinically significant demyelination (95).

Most cases of papillitis with a macular star are "idiopathic" and are theorized to be "postviral." In contrast, several specific causes have been found, and the clinician should investigate the patient for these diagnoses. Even though some of these specific diagnoses are systemic diseases, the papillitis and neuroretinitis may be a unilateral rather than bilateral process. The differential diagnosis includes (a) cat-scratch fever (96), (b) Epstein-Barr virus (97), (c) mumps (98), (d) hepatitis B (99), (e) Lyme disease (100), (f) syphilis (101), (g) toxoplasmosis (102), and (h) sarcoidosis (103).

PAPILLEDEMA

The diagnosis and management of papilledema in pediatric neuroophthalmology should be made on an emergent basis. We recommend that the term "papilledema" be used for optic disk edema caused by increased ICP (Fig. 22.11) and that the more generic term of optic disk edema be used for other causes of disk.

In children, the most common cause of papilledema is an intracranial mass lesion producing obstructive hydrocephalus

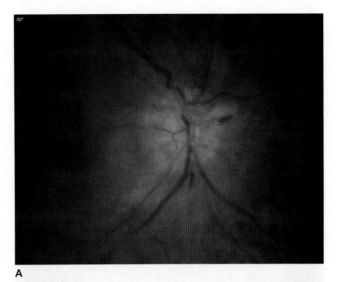

A

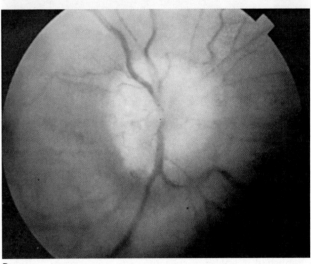

B

FIGURE 22.11. A: Acute papilledema with distention of the retinal venous system and marked optic disk edema. Note the absence of a central cup. **B:** Chronic papilledema represents one of the most difficult fundoscopic diagnoses. As the papilledema becomes more chronic, the disk begins to resemble the appearance of a congenitally anomalous disk. The disk is elevated without a central cup, and the peripapillary hemorrhages and exudates have disappeared.

(Fig. 22.12). Because such lesions may result in sudden transtentorial herniation and death, it is vital to initiate prompt and proper management for these children. Moreover, chronic bilateral papilledema of any cause may progress to optic atrophy and bilateral blindness. Papilledema is therefore a neuroophthalmic finding that has both life- and vision-threatening implications.

Symptoms

Headache caused by increased ICP and transient obscuration of vision (TVO) is the most common presenting symptom of papilledema. The headaches are of a dull, aching quality

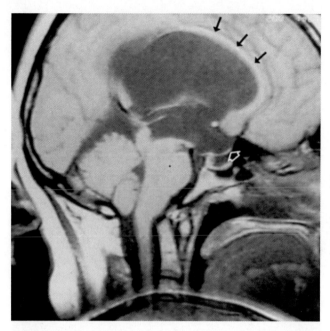

FIGURE 22.12. Sagittal magnetic resonance imaging (MRI) scan of obstructive hydrocephalus. The lateral ventricles are massively distended, resulting in thinning of the corpus callosum (*black arrows*). The third ventricle is distended, producing distortion of the optic chiasm (*white arrowhead*).

involving the entire head, although sometimes more discomfort is felt at the posterior aspect of the skull and upper cervical area. The headaches are usually worse on awakening in the morning and subside in the evening. Nausea and vomiting may accompany increased intracranial-pressure headaches, but usually only after the headache pattern has been established. Coughing, sneezing, and any type of Valsalva maneuver exacerbate the headaches.

TVOs are the most common visual symptoms produced by papilledema. These events occur without warning, and vary from blurring of the environment to total blindness. TVOs usually involve both eyes simultaneously, but unilateral events occur in some patients. Increasing frequency and severity of TVOs have been a forewarning of impending permanent visual deficits, according to Meadows (104). Rush (105) and Miller (106) do not believe that increasing TVOs necessarily foreshadow permanent visual loss. The mechanism of TVO is unknown, although the observation by Cogan (107) of precipitation of these events by change in posture suggests some role for alteration of blood flow or optic nerve CSF fluid dynamics in their etiology.

Double vision because of unilateral or bilateral sixth nerve palsies is another disturbance related to increased ICP and papilledema. The sixth nerve palsy is a non-localizing finding of increased ICP. Relief of the increased ICP produces resolution of the sixth nerve palsy.

No specific histopathologic type of mass lesion or intracranial abnormality invariably produces papilledema. The specific and varied pediatric neurooncologic and neurosurgical problems that may have papilledema as one of their presenting manifestations are discussed later.

On occasions, it has been theorized that infants may not develop papilledema because of their distensible skulls and open fontanelles. However, there are numerous examples of papilledema in infants, and thus the histologic development of the skull does not preclude the development of papilledema.

Papilledema Diagnosis by Ultrasonography

In children with head trauma and metabolic disorders, the examination of the optic nerve may be difficult. Helmke and Hansen (108) demonstrated that ultrasonography can detect dilation of the optic nerve sheath meninges caused by acute elevations of ICP. Therefore, in pediatric patients with suspected increased ICP in whom the optic nerve cannot be visualized, ultrasonography may help to establish the diagnosis of papilledema.

Treatment

Pediatric ophthalmologists confronted with a patient who has papilledema have a dual challenge. First, they must ensure that immediate high-resolution neuroradiologic studies (computed tomography [CT] and MRI scans) are performed. If an intracranial mass is discovered, appropriate inpatient neurologic and neurosurgical care must be initiated. Increased ICP is first reduced medically with acetazolamide and corticosteroids, provided that the elevated ICP has not produced significant vomiting.

Whether or not a ventriculoperitoneal shunting procedure should be performed to reduce the ICP before direct operative attack on the mass lesion remains a neurosurgical decision. Successful reduction of the ICP does not ensure that the papilledema will not permanently damage the patient's vision. Thus, the second part of the dual challenge to the pediatric ophthalmologist involves trying to protect against visual loss (109). As mentioned earlier, reduction in ICP does not prevent permanent loss of vision. Some patients even lose vision suddenly after neurosurgical decompression of the primary intracranial process (postdecompression blindness) (110). The mechanism of this phenomenon is unknown.

Some intracranial mass lesions are not totally resectable, but these children may survive for extended periods with advanced chemotherapeutic and radiation therapy regimens. However, the quality of their lives may be significantly impaired because of visual loss due to chronic papilledema. Because of the possibility of seeding distant sites with the primary tumor, CSF shunting procedures are not usually recommended. Surgical decompression of the meningeal sheath of the intracranial optic nerve may offer an effective treatment for vision in children with a good survival prognosis, despite a nonresectable central nervous mass lesion producing chronic papilledema (109).

PSEUDOTUMOR CEREBRI

Pseudotumor cerebri (PTC) is a clinical syndrome of unknown etiology; it is a term used when a patient has signs and symptoms of increased ICP, which include headache, double vision, tinnitus, transient visual obscuration, and vertigo. A set of diagnostic criteria was formulated (modified Dandy criteria) which include symptoms and signs of ICP, elevated ICP with normal CSF composition; a nonlocalizing neurologic sign except for abducent nerve palsy and negative neuroimaging except for empty sella (Fig. 22.13), with no evidence of ventriculomegaly, cerebral mass, or venous sinus abnormality; and absence of secondary causes of ICP such as the use of certain medications. The clinical characteristics of pediatric PTC are different compared to the typical syndrome in adult. Rangwala et al. and Friedman reported modification of modified Dandy criteria of Idiopathic Intracranial Hypertension (IIH) in pediatrics (Table 22.3) (111).

PTC in children is rare. Hereditary basis has been suggested but the genetic mechanism is not clear. PTC in prepubescent children differs from the adult form in several important ways. The male:female ratio is equal in these children. Obesity is not associated with PTC in young children, spontaneous remission is more common, and finally, response to oral corticosteroids is possibly better. PTC in pubescent and postpubescent children seems to follow adult disease in that there is a female predominance and it appears

Table 22.3
PSEUDOTUMOR CEREBRI

1. Symptoms or signs attributable to increased intracranial pressure (ICP)

2. Documented increased ICP (age appropriate)
   Neonates: 76 mmH$_2$O
   Age less than 8 with papilledema: 180 mmH$_2$O
   Age 8 or above or less than 8 without papilledema: 250 mmH$_2$O

3. Normal CSF composition except in neonates (32 WBC/mm^3 and protein as high as 150 mg/dL).

4. Normal MRI of brain with and without contrast, and MR venography. (Narrowing of the junction of the transverse and sigmoid sinuses is acceptable.)

5. No other signs not attributable to increased ICP (e.g., abducens nerve palsy, papilledema)

6. No other identified cause of intracranial hypertension

to have a relationship with obesity (112,113). ICP can occur at any age in childhood but 60% over age of 10 years (114). This might be related to increase in obesity in adolescence (111,115). There is no sex predilection. The incidence of ICP in the overall population is 1 out of 100,000.

PTC can be in two separate categories: idiopathic versus secondary. Although secondary causes of PTC are less identified in adults (53.2% to 77.7%) of pediatrics, cases have been associated with identifiable diseases, which include dural sinus thrombosis, malnutrition, anemia, lupus, Addison disease, exogenous hormone use/withdrawal, medication/vitamin ingestion, and Lyme disease.

Just like adults, children with chronic papilledema are at risk for permanent vision loss. Because of the risk of vision loss, these children must be treated and followed carefully.

The ophthalmoscopic diagnosis of chronic papilledema may be one of the most difficult in the whole field of ophthalmology (see Fig. 22.11B). Because of the lack of hemorrhages and exudates, the casual observer may overlook this physical finding. An awareness of the possibility of chronic papilledema is especially critical since testing to confirm severe constriction of the visual fields is difficult in younger children. Here again, much reliance has to be placed on the family's observations of the patient's visually oriented behavior.

When progressive loss of visual function can be documented in a patient with chronic papilledema, medical and/or surgical intervention is indicated. Obviously, if an underlying cause is present, it must be treated. It is important to initiate medical intervention until the underlying etiology is resolved. If corticosteroids and diuretics are ineffective,

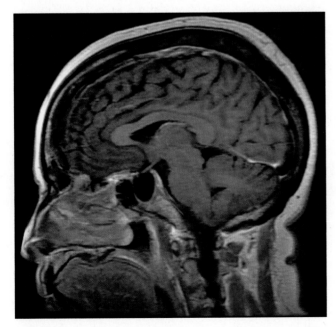

FIGURE 22.13. Sagittal magnetic resonance imaging (MRI) scan of the brain demonstrating the empty sella (*arrowhead*).

surgery with a shunt or optic nerve sheath decompression may be necessary. Both procedures are effective in treating papilledema (116–118).

OPTIC NERVE GLIOMA

Optic pathway gliomas (OPG) are childhood tumors and usually occur before the age of 20 years. Seventy-five percent of these lesions are presented before the patient is 10 years of age (119). More than 90% of optic nerve glioma are diagnosed by the age of 20 years.

OPG can present with loss of vision, strabismus, and optic nerve pallor or swelling. Sometimes there is a compressive central retinal vein obstruction and rarely even ocular ischemic syndrome with corneal edema, iritis, iris neovascularization, and glaucoma. Many patients with OPG have neurofibromatosis type 1 (NF1). The incidence of optic nerve glioma and NF1 may range from 10% to 80%.

CT and MRI scans establish the diagnosis of OPG (Figs. 22.14 and 22.15). Unfortunately, OPG has an extremely variable natural history with some patients experiencing a very benign course in contrast to others who have rapidly growing neoplasms (119–121).

The treatment of OPG is confounded by this variable natural history. For optic nerve glioma, a complete surgical excision can be a cure but sacrifices the vision and is not recommended for seeing eyes. Chemotherapy is often the first line for radiographically and clinically progressive OPG, especially in growing brains where radiation therapy might cause endocrinologic, intellectual, or developmental problems. The precise role of observation, chemotherapy, radiation therapy, or surgery remains controversial for all OPG.

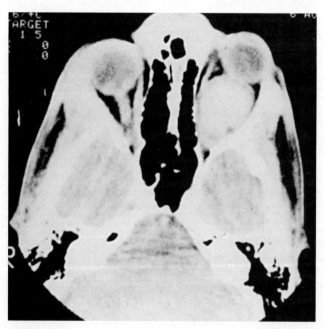

FIGURE 22.14. Axial computed tomography (CT) scan demonstrating a left retrobulbar mass that proved to be a glioma.

CHIASMAL SYNDROMES

Pathologic processes in and around the optic chiasm may present with decreased visual acuity or more typically bitemporal visual field loss. Patients with chiasmal syndromes classically develop a temporal hemianopic defect in one (junctional) or both visual fields. However, it is often difficult to demonstrate these defects in young children even by confrontation techniques. On rare occasions, parents may report that the child "bumps into objects" or consistently on one side or ignores toys in the temporal hemifield.

Disorders of the optic chiasm in children are often compressive tumors. Inflammatory, ischemic, traumatic, or demyelinating diseases of the chiasm are uncommon in children and must be a diagnosis of exclusion. The most common tumors that produce chiasmal syndromes are considered next.

Craniopharyngioma

In the general population, craniopharyngioma make up 3% of all intracranial tumors. In contrast, these tumors are the most common tumors not originating from glial cells in children and adolescents. In the pediatric population, they constitute between 8% and 13% of all intracranial tumors (122,123).

Developing from squamous cells in the vicinity of the infundibular stem and adenohypophysis, these tumors are believed to be remnants of the Rathke pouch, a structure usually destined for atrophy in prenatal life. Because of their histologic source, craniopharyngioma are often found in the suprasellar cistern, although they may invade any surrounding structures. When the tumors infiltrate and extend into the third ventricle, the flow of CSF is blocked, resulting in papilledema and obstructive hydrocephalus.

Although ophthalmologists rarely see children with craniopharyngioma without visual problems, some patients initially present with failure to maintain growth and development, diabetes insipidus, precocious puberty, or obesity. These associated findings may be crucial diagnostic clues to the pediatric ophthalmologist evaluating the patient with subtle visual findings and may guide the diagnostic investigation toward craniopharyngioma.

Optimal management of craniopharyngioma remains controversial. Surgical resection is still the mainstay therapy, but the issue of total resection versus subtotal resection followed by radiotherapy has not been answered. A recent study showed that local recurrence rates were halved with subtotal resection plus postoperative radiotherapy at 10 years, but there was no significant difference in overall survival (124). Despite the benign histologic appearance of these neoplasms, they frequently demonstrate locally invasive malignant behavior. Local recurrences are common but with current surgical, stereotactic, and local chemotherapy techniques, survival is good (125–129).

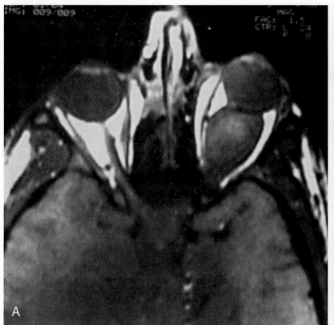

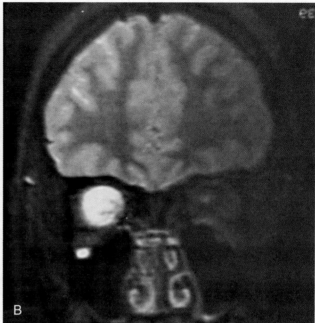

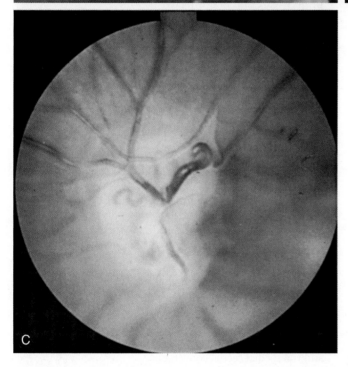

FIGURE 22.15. A: T1-weighted magnetic resonance imaging (MRI) scan of the optic glioma illustrated in Figure 22.14. The mass involves the entire intraorbital optic nerve. **B:** T2-weighted MRI scan demonstrating the high-intensity glioma tissue enveloping the entire optic nerve. Note the faint shadow of the optic nerve in the opposite orbit. **C:** Chronic optic disk edema with a retinochoroidal venous collateral (i.e., "optociliary shunt vessel") associated with an optic glioma.

Optic Chiasmal Glioma

As noted above, OPG constitute the other main neoplasm of the optic chiasm in the pediatric-age group. Histologically, these lesions are similar to optic nerve glioma and are associated with NF1. However, compared with their counterparts within the optic nerve, the chiasmal lesions are more likely to display an exophytic component. As discussed earlier, glioma of the visual pathways in children make up 3% to 5% of all childhood brain tumors, with a median age of onset at less than 5 years. Boys and girls are equally affected. About 10% to 20% of these patients have neurofibromatosis.

Perhaps because of the young age at onset and initial subtle symptoms, a long diagnostic delay is common. Patients frequently present with strabismus, and the diagnosis of chiasmal glioma often is not established until several surgical procedures for strabismus have failed to correct the ocular misalignment. Several clinicians reported monocular nystagmus similar to spasmus nutans as the presenting sign of patients with chiasmal glioma (130–132). Because of this association, detailed neuroimaging studies of the chiasm should be considered in any patient with unilateral ocular oscillatory movement. It may be impossible to distinguish clinically between "benign" spasmus nutans and the eye movement disorder associated with these tumors. Eye movement recording techniques are usually impractical in very young children.

The older the patient, the more likely are the presenting signs of chiasmal glioma to be related to decreased visual function rather than to strabismus or monocular nystagmus. The visual loss is usually of slow onset, but abrupt unilateral and bilateral loss of vision due to hemorrhage into the glioma has been described by Maitland and associates (133). Optic disk hypoplasia has been reported in 10% to 20% of patients with chiasmal glioma.

CT and MRI scans are the mainstay in the diagnosis of chiasmal glioma. Whether or not the lesion is solely intrinsic within the chiasm is the crucial question that must be answered by neuroradiologists (Fig. 22.16). For purely intrinsic lesions, surgical biopsy is not required. In comparison, intrinsic lesions with an extrinsic component usually should be biopsied because: (a) it may be difficult to determine whether the lesion is indeed a glioma by neuroimaging studies, and (b) removal of a large exophytic component or surgery for an extrinsic cyst may improve vision.

The treatment of chiasmal glioma has been controversial because the natural history of these lesions is not as well understood as once thought. Hoyt and Baghdassarian (134) described 18 patients with chiasmal glioma and found progressive visual loss in only 8 of 36 eyes. A subsequent report on the same patients confirmed the relatively benign visual course of these lesions (135). It appears that glioma associated with neurofibromatosis have a more indolent course and often do not require treatment (136,137).

A long-term mortality analysis of patients with chiasmal glioma disclosed that 54% died during a median follow-up period of 20 years (138). The five patients in this series who died of the tumor had done so by 1969, the date of the original study. Only one patient died between 1969 and 1986 from the effects of the chiasmal glioma. Radiation therapy was used for 11 of the 16 patients who died. Only 3 of the surviving 12 patients received radiation therapy.

However, some patients with chiasmal glioma clearly have a grim visual and systemic prognosis. The children who seem to have the worst prognosis are those who have

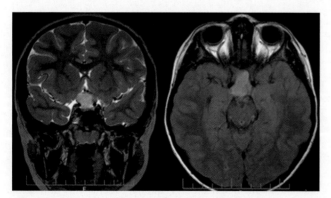

FIGURE 22.16. T1-weighted MRI of the brain (coronal and axial view) illustrate chiasmal glioma lesion is solely intrinsic within the chiasm.

hypothalamic and/or thalamic involvement (139). Children with chiasmal glioma must be followed carefully, both clinically and with serial neuroimaging. Treatment options include observation, resection of exophytic component, radiation, and chemotherapy.

NYSTAGMUS

Any intermittent or continuous new-onset nystagmus requires neuroimaging studies. In this section, the most important types of nystagmus that provide localizing neurooophthalmic diagnostic information are considered.

Seesaw Nystagmus

Seesaw nystagmus is characterized by a conjugate, pendular, alternating torsional movement, and superimposed vertical movements of each eye. The extorting eye rises and the contralateral, intorting eye falls. The nystagmus is seen best in primary gaze and in downgaze.

Seesaw nystagmus localizes to the diencephalon owing to lesions within the pathway from the zona incerta to the interstitial nucleus of Cajal (140). Large parasellar tumors producing bitemporal hemianopsias and compression in the area of the third ventricle are the most common causes of seesaw nystagmus. This variety of nystagmus may also be seen after major craniocerebral trauma and with lesions in the upper midbrain.

Convergence-Retraction Nystagmus

Convergence–retraction nystagmus is an exquisitely localizing type of eye movement abnormality that indicates a pathologic condition in the midbrain. There may be an associated complete or partial paralysis of upgaze, light near dissociation of the pupils, eyelid retraction, or skew deviation. Convergence–retraction nystagmus is often best elicited by attempted upgaze (e.g., an OKN drum rolling downward) and is believed to be produced by cofiring of extraocular muscles innervated by the third nerve in the dorsal midbrain, resulting in eyelid and extraocular muscle retraction and the medial rectus convergence.

When convergence–retraction nystagmus coexists with large pupils that are poorly or unreactive to direct light stimulation but have a better near reaction (i.e., light-near dissociation) and upper eyelid retraction (Collier sign), this constellation of clinical findings is known as Parinaud syndrome (141).

In the pediatric-age group, the most common cause of convergence–retraction nystagmus is a pineal gland tumor. The other most important cause is failure of a ventriculoperitoneal shunt (142). In shunt failure, convergence–retraction nystagmus and the other manifestations of Parinaud syndrome may develop before pronounced ventricular enlargement is evident on neuroimaging studies.

Upbeat Nystagmus

The upbeat on upgaze variety (type I) is a large-amplitude nystagmus present in the primary position and increasing with upgaze. Type I is associated with midline cerebellar findings and is localized to the anterior vermis of the cerebellum (143). In contrast, type II consists of small-amplitude upbeat nystagmus that decreases in upgaze and increases in downgaze. Type II upbeat nystagmus is associated with intrinsic medullary disease (144).

Downbeat Nystagmus

Localizing the disease process to the cervicomedullary junction, downbeat nystagmus is defined as nystagmus in primary position with the fast phase beating downward (145). MRI scan of the posterior fossa, brainstem, and cervical spinal cord is the diagnostic procedure of choice for patients with downbeat nystagmus.

Downbeat nystagmus is most frequently associated with Arnold-Chiari malformations, platybasia with basilar impression, and lower brainstem demyelination or ischemia (146,147). When downbeat nystagmus occurs with generalized cerebellar findings, the diagnosis of spinocerebellar degeneration must be considered.

Periodic Alternating Nystagmus

Periodic alternating nystagmus (PAN) is a horizontal jerk nystagmus that periodically changes directions. Usually, the eyes beat in one direction for approximately 90 seconds and then go into a null phase before beginning to move in the opposite direction. This process is continuous while patients are awake and often persists during sleep.

PAN may coexist with downbeat nystagmus, and the differential diagnosis and anatomic localization for these types of nystagmus are virtually identical. PAN has been described with primary cerebellar tumors, demyelinating disease, Arnold-Chiari malformation, ischemia (148,149), and albinism (150,151).

OPSOCLONUS

Opsoclonus defines back-to-back saccades going in various directions and composed of varying amplitudes. The saccades frequently have a multivectorial curved or oblique paths. Opsoclonus is believed to be caused by a disorder of inhibitory control of "pause neurons" within the pons. The pause neurons are thought to inhibit "burst neurons" within the pause. Therefore, opsoclonus seems to represent chaotic saccades caused by unchecked burst cells (152). Ocular flutter has the same pathogenesis as multivectorial opsoclonus but is characterized by horizontal plane back-to-back saccades. Although opsoclonus may very rarely be observed in otherwise healthy infants, it must be considered a sign of posterior fossa dysfunction until proved otherwise.

Coxsackie B, cytomegalovirus, and *Haemophilus influenzae* meningitis in children have all been associated with opsoclonus. However, the most important cause in apparently healthy children is occult neuroblastoma, and this should be the first diagnostic concern (153).

NEUROOPHTHALMIC DISORDERS OF OCULAR MOTILITY

Bilateral Ophthalmoplegia

When the patient is unable to move both eyes completely, the ophthalmologist should consider an anatomically based differential diagnostic scheme (154) (Table 22.4). The astute clinician must examine eye movements and search for associated findings such as eyelid abnormalities, proptosis, and pupillary asymmetries in order to arrive at the correct diagnosis. Often the associated physical findings rather than the eye movements themselves represent the critical clinical observations. The differential diagnosis for an acute bilateral and symmetric ophthalmoplegia includes brainstem lesion, myasthenia gravis (MG), botulism, Miller-Fisher variant of Guillain Barre syndrome, Whipple disease, and Wernicke syndrome. For the chronic, bilateral, and symmetric ophthalmoplegia, chronic progressive external ophthalmoplegia (CPEO), chronic MG, severe global thyroid ophthalmopathy, and bilateral brainstem or cavernous sinus lesions should be considered.

MYASTHENIA SYNDROMES

Myasthenia in children resembles MG in adults but there are some unique syndromes in childhood that should be considered including transient and congenital MG.

Transient Neonatal Myasthenia

This syndrome is defined as a myasthenic condition developing temporarily from transmission of maternal MG antibodies to newborn infants of mothers with MG (155). The condition affects approximately 12% of infants of mothers with MG.

Almost 80% of patients manifest weakness during the first day of life, and symptoms often develop a few hours after birth. Limited eye movements, ptosis, and orbicularis oculi weakness occur in 15% of patients. The most common initial symptoms are weakness, poor feeding, and hypotonia.

The syndrome usually persists for about 15 to 20 days, but occasionally lasts only 1 week or lingers for almost 2 months. If the diagnosis is not made and proper treatment is not instituted, death may occur from respiratory failure.

Improvement of symptoms after intramuscular or subcutaneous injection of 0.1 mg of edrophonium chloride can help to establish the diagnosis. Orally administered pyridostigmine bromide, provided that swallowing is not

Table 22.4

BILATERAL OPHTHALMOPLEGIA: DIFFERENTIAL DIAGNOSIS

Anatomic Site	Etiology	Pupil	Pain	Diagnostic Aids	Comments
Neuromuscular junction	Myasthenia Botulism	N	−	Edrophonium test, ice test, rest test, anti-acetylcholine receptor antibodies	Orbicularis weakness, transient signs
Muscles	Graves ophthalmopathy	N	Foreign body sensation	Forced ductions, CT scan of orbit, thyroid function tests	Eyelid retraction, proptosis, congestion
	Chronic progressive external ophthalmoplegia	N	−	Diplopia, rare	Family history
	Mucormycosis	±	+	Culture, CT scan of sinuses, MRI scan	Life threatening, diabetics
Cranial nerve	Diabetic-vascular	Usually NS	±	Glucose tolerance test	Pain limited, 10 d
	Multiple sclerosis	±	−	CSF electrophoresis	Cranial neuropathies, rare
	Polyradiculitis (Fischer-variant-Guillain Barre)	±	−	CSF protein	Postinfectious, subacute ataxia
	Neurosyphilis	±	−	CSF and serum VDRL	History of syphilis
	Diphtheria	±	−	Culture	
Cavernous sinus	Pituitary apoplexy	+	++	Skull series, CT or MRI scans of sella	Field defects variable, mimics optic neuritis
	Metastasis	±	+	CSF protein, cells	Severe persistent pain
Interpeduncular cistern	Basilar artery				
	a. Aneurysm	+	±	CT/CTA, catheter arteriogram	May mimic posterior fossa tumor
	b. Occlusion	+	−	Clinical signs	Coma
Skull base	Tumor, primary	±	±	CT or MRI scans, CSF	Slow evolution
	Chronic inflammation	−	−	CT or MRI scans, CSF	Slow evolution
	Meningeal carcinomatosis	±	−	MRI scan, CSF	Consecutive palsies
Brainstem	Wernicke encephalopathy	−	−	Alcoholism, bariatric surgery, eating disorders, dietary deficiency	Thiamine administration

(continued)

| Table 22.4 | | | | | |
| **(continued)** | | | | | |
Anatomic Site	**Etiology**	**Pupil**	**Pain**	**Diagnostic Aids**	**Comments**
	Dorsal midbrain syndromes	+	−	MRI scan	Eyelid retraction, convergence retraction nystagmus
	Whipple disease	±	−	CSF protein, cells	Uveitis, peripheral neuropathy, gastrointestinal symptoms

CSF, cerebrospinal fluid; CT, computed tomography; MRI, magnetic resonance imaging; N, normal; VDRL, venereal disease research laboratory. Modified for pediatric population from Sergott RC, Glaser JS, Berger LJ. Simultaneous, bilateral diabetic ophthalmoplegia: report of two cases and discussion of differential diagnosis. Ophthalmology 1984;91:18–22.

too severely impaired, may be necessary until spontaneous remission occurs.

Congenital Myasthenia

In contrast to transitory neonatal myasthenia, congenital myasthenia affects infants whose mothers do not have MG (156). Symptoms are often predominantly ophthalmic, with bilateral ophthalmoplegia, ptosis, and orbicularis oculi weakness usually developing shortly after birth. The systemic musculature is often spared clinically evident weakness. However, electromyography often detects evidence of impaired systemic neuromuscular transmission.

Although mothers may not be affected with MG, siblings in the same family often demonstrate similar findings, and congenital myasthenia is believed to have at least a partial genetic basis. Forty-two percent of patients present with the disease before 2 years of age, and more than 60% before the age of 20 years (157).

Congenital MG results from functional or structural abnormalities at the myoneural junction (158). Unlike juvenile MG, the congenital form is not immune mediated and therefore, plasmapheresis immunosuppression and systemic immunosuppression are not beneficial. Some types of congenital MG respond to anticholinesterase inhibitors, while other types fail to respond.

In addition to diagnosing congenital myasthenia, the pediatric ophthalmologist must monitor these patients for amblyopia due to paralytic strabismus. Standard occlusion therapy should be instituted when amblyopia is suspected.

Juvenile Myasthenia

Juvenile MG refers to the syndromes of ocular or generalized MG that are virtually identical in presentation, pathogenesis, course, and treatment to the adult form of MG (159). Patients present after 1 year of age, and more than 75% of cases develop after age of 10 years. Ptosis, diplopia, and

facial diplegia are common presentations, and ophthalmologists should consider MG and refer patients to neurology for evaluation of the potentially life-threatening bulbar symptoms of dysarthria, dysphagia, fatigue, shortness of breath, or nocturnal regurgitation of salivary secretions and generalized MG (Fig. 22.17A, B). Some children, usually between 2 and 10 years of age, develop an acute "malignant" variety of MG with acute bulbar symptoms progressing to acute respiratory failure within 24 hours (160).

The weakness and fatigue produced by autoimmune MG result from impaired neuromuscular transmission because of alteration of acetylcholine receptors (AChR) at the neuromuscular junction. Abnormalities of the thymus gland occur in up to 75% of MG patients, and there are other common autoimmunity-mediated associations such as Graves disease, Hashimoto thyroiditis, rheumatoid arthritis, pernicious anemia, and systemic lupus erythematosus.

Three different mechanisms for antibody-mediated damage and the eventual reduction of AChR have been postulated: (a) blockage of the receptors' active sites, (b) destruction of the AChRs in a complement-dependent reaction, and (c) enhancement of the degradation rate of AChRs by crosslinking of the receptors with antibodies (161,162). Testing for the antibodies, consideration for a referral to neurology for evaluation of generalized MG, and chest imaging (e.g., CT chest) to exclude thymoma are recommended for children with ocular MG. Consultation with a neurologist is recommended for the further evaluation and treatment of generalized MG in children.

INFANTILE BOTULISM

Because infantile botulism may present predominantly with ptosis before the development of paralysis and respiratory failure, it is possible to misdiagnose the ptosis and/or ophthalmoplegia as MG. The critical differentiating diagnostic feature is pupil involvement which does not occur

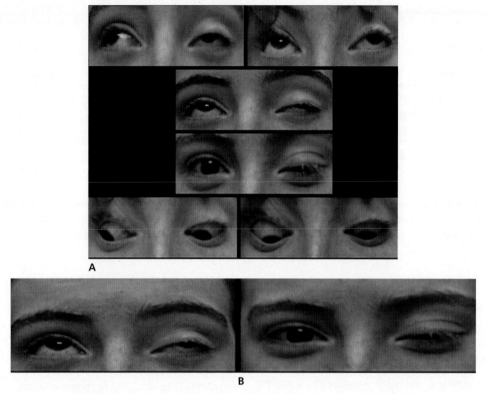

FIGURE 22.17. A-B: Juvenile myasthenia with left ptosis and ophthalmoplegia.

in MG. Fortunately, ophthalmoplegia is relatively rare with botulism and since the disease has such a fulminant onset, patients rarely present initially to a pediatric ophthalmologist. However, because of the combination of ptosis and pupillary dilation, an eye doctor may be the first physician to consider the diagnosis, even in the intensive care unit setting.

In adults, botulism develops from ingested food contaminated with toxin of *Clostridium botulinum*. A different pathogenesis exists for infants, for whom a history of honey ingestion or soil eating is obtained from the family. The honey and soil contain *C. botulinum* organisms that colonize the immature gut and produce toxin which is absorbed into the circulation (163). Diffuse autonomic dysfunction and hypotonia develop and progress to coma within 6 to 8 hours of the onset of symptoms. If proper respiratory support and intensive care are provided, the infants often improve spontaneously.

THIRD NERVE PALSY

Paralysis of the third cranial nerve in children demands a different diagnostic approach from that for the same clinical condition in adults (164,165).

Congenital third nerve palsies are usually indicative of a developmental anomaly or birth trauma, although rare cases of third nerve neuroma have been reported (166). On the other hand, acquired third nerve palsies are often an ominous sign of underlying disease. Miller (164) found that the etiology of third nerve palsy includes congenital (43%), trauma (20%), infection/inflammation (13%), tumor (10%), aneurysm (7%), and ophthalmic migraine (7%). Although aneurysm is a much less common cause of a third nerve palsy in children, the incidence is not zero and therefore consideration for some type of noninvasive angiography should be considered especially in the pupil involving third nerve palsy (e.g., CTA or MRA). Some patients with a sufficiently high pretest likelihood of aneurysm may still require a catheter angiogram to exclude aneurysm.

In congenital oculomotor nerve palsy, the pupil may or may not be involved, and both studies found a high incidence of aberrant regeneration developing in these patients. Three of the patients with congenital third nerve palsies in Miller's study developed cyclic oculomotor palsy. This condition is usually diagnosed in the first year of life. It is characterized by complete oculomotor palsy with cyclic spasm of the affected muscles. During the spastic phase, the eye adducts, the eyelid elevates, and the pupil constricts. The spastic phase usually lasts less than 1 minute and is followed by the paretic phase. The alternating spasms and paralysis usually continue during sleep (167). In addition to being associated with congenital third nerve palsy, patients may have a history of an orbital or basilar skull fracture or meningitis.

About 7 of Harley's 32 patients developed third nerve palsies in association with migraine headaches (ophthalmoplegic migraine), but we would consider this to be a diagnosis of exclusion. In very young patients, no history of migraine is available from the child but should be sought from parents or siblings.

The ophthalmoplegia is clinically indistinguishable from any other third nerve palsy and may develop at any time during the course of the headache, including the period after the pain has resolved. A history of cyclic vomiting, motion sickness, and vertigo suggests the diagnosis of ophthalmoplegic migraine. The ophthalmoplegia usually resolves within several weeks, although permanent ptosis, mydriasis, and oculomotor defects are described. When the pupil is involved and no definitive migraine history can be elicited, neuroimaging including possibly cerebral angiography may be necessary to exclude an aneurysm.

FOURTH NERVE PALSY

As for oculomotor paresis, Harley's series provides some of the best data regarding trochlear nerve palsies in children (165). Twelve of the 18 patients had congenital fourth nerve palsies, 7 being unilateral and 5 bilateral fourth nerve paralysis. Five patients demonstrated a trochlear nerve palsy after head trauma, and one manifested this problem after encephalitis. Patients with a congenital or clearly traumatic fourth nerve palsy do not typically require neuroimaging, but unexplained, bilateral, nonisolated, or progressive fourth nerve palsies probably require neuroimaging (e.g., MRI). The risk of a serious underlying condition for a neurologically isolated fourth nerve palsy is not the same as patients with the sixth cranial nerve palsy which can occur as a nonlocalizing finding of increased ICP or the less commonly seen pediatric third nerve palsy which also might be the harbinger of underlying serious disease.

SIXTH NERVE PALSY

The most common isolated cranial nerve palsy affecting ocular motility in childhood is a sixth nerve paresis. Harley (165) and Robertson and associates (168) found 33% and 10% incidence, respectively, of neoplastic disease presenting with an isolated sixth nerve palsy. In general, unexplained, progressive, nonisolated, or unresolved sixth nerve palsy in children should be imaged as many are due to brainstem glioma other supratentorial and cerebellar lesions. Evaluation for pediatric sixth nerve palsy should be directed at the accompanying signs and symptoms and might need to include serologic evaluation for infectious etiologies, and radiographic or other studies including lumbar puncture for neoplastic, inflammatory, or demyelinating postinfectious etiologies may be necessary.

When a sixth nerve palsy is associated with ipsilateral ear and facial pain, a diagnosis of Gradenigo syndrome may be made. This condition is usually caused by middle ear infection, but in the postantibiotic era tumors may mimic this presentation and therefore imaging is recommended.

MISCELLANEOUS NEUROOPHTHALMIC SYNDROMES IN CHILDREN

Kearns-Sayre Syndrome

Kearns-Sayre syndrome is a form of CPEO with many associated abnormalities, including heart block and pigmentary degeneration of the retina (169). In addition to the symmetric ophthalmoplegia, ptosis, and orbicularis oculi weakness, patients have short stature, a myopathy of skeletal muscle (ragged-red fibers on pathology), and elevated CSF protein. Other associated abnormalities may include hearing loss, peripheral neuropathy, cerebellar ataxia, pendular nystagmus, corticospinal tract dysfunction, corneal opacity, and problems with corticosteroid glucose and calcium metabolism.

Defects in pyruvate metabolism within the muscular and neural tissues of these patients have been suggested as a possible underlying etiology to explain the widespread problems. In contrast to adults with CPEO who are relatively healthy, children with Kearns-Sayre syndrome may be ill owing to the diffuse myopathy, neuropathy, encephalopathy, and endocrine disturbances. Moraes and coworkers (170) reported mitochondrial DNA deletions in both the adult CPEO syndrome and pediatric Kearns-Sayre disorder.

Ocular Motor Apraxia

Ocular motor apraxia is defined as the ability to initiate saccades in response to certain visual reflexes (such as vestibular or optokinetic stimulation), but inability to initiate saccades on command (i.e., "apraxia"). Cogan (171) first described congenital ocular motor apraxia. Initially the patient may appear to show visual attention but after several months, the child develops typical compensatory horizontal thrusting head movements for the eyes to change their object of fixation. The congenital syndrome is confined to horizontal eye movements, but the acquired condition involves both horizontal and vertical saccades. As the patient with congenital ocular motor apraxia becomes older, the eye movements may improve and the head movements become less noticeable (172). This spontaneous improvement led Cogan to postulate that this entity may represent a developmental delay rather than a total absence of the pathways for horizontal voluntary saccades. Acquired ocular motor apraxia has been associated with virtually any disorder known to affect the initiation of voluntary saccades including Huntington chorea, Gaucher disease, olivopontocerebellar degeneration, atypical Niemann-Pick disease, Mobius syndrome, ataxia-telangiectasia, posterior fossa tumors, and bilateral frontoparietal lesions (173).

Spasmus Nutans

The triad of nystagmus, head nodding, and an anomalous head position constitutes the syndrome of spasmus nutans (174). This poorly understood entity typically begins before

1 year of age and usually resolves spontaneously within 1 to 2 years. However, using eye movement recordings, Gottlob and colleagues (175) found that the nystagmus persisted in some patients of age up to 12 years. The nystagmus is frequently asymmetric, and unilateral forms have been described. The typical eye movement abnormality is a high-frequency, small-amplitude horizontal nystagmus. Unfortunately, the nystagmus of spasmus nutans is clinically indistinguishable from that associated with glioma of the afferent visual system. Therefore, many ophthalmologists obtain neuroimages for all patients before establishing the diagnosis of idiopathic spasmus nutans. Young and associates (176) report a relatively high incidence of strabismus and amblyopia in the eye with the greater nystagmus and therefore these children should be followed carefully and treated appropriately.

Mobius Syndrome

The concurrence of congenital facial diplegia with a horizontal eye movement problem should raise the possibility of Mobius syndrome. The horizontal eye movement difficulties range from an isolated sixth nerve paralysis to a complete horizontal gaze palsy. In addition, there may be tongue atrophy, head and neck deformities, and chest and extremity abnormalities. A developmental defect in and around the abducens nuclei has been suggested as a cause (177,178).

Cerebral Ataxia and Optic Atrophy

Although cerebellar ataxia has been associated with numerous neurologic syndromes, Nicolaides and coworkers (179) described ataxia with optic atrophy, as well as several other manifestations. All three patients demonstrated early normal development until cerebellar ataxia occurred following a febrile illness in infancy. In addition, the patients had generalized hypotonia, areflexia, flexor plantar responses, pes cavus, and progressive optic atrophy, as well as sensorineural hearing loss. The syndrome of cerebellar ataxia, areflexia, pes cavus, optic atrophy, and sensorineural deafness has been designated as CAPOS syndrome. It has been postulated that CAPOS syndrome has either an autosomal dominant or maternal mitochondrial inheritance pattern (179).

NONORGANIC VISUAL LOSS IN CHILDREN

Nonorganic visual loss (NOVL) is defined as visual dysfunction that is not attributable to an organic pathology; it is a relatively common problem for the comprehensive ophthalmologist. The incidence of NOVL has been reported to be 1.75% in school-aged children and can comprise 1% to 5% cases of a general ophthalmologist's practice (180,181). The exact etiology of NOVL in children is controversial and often remains unknown even with detailed histories or formal psychiatric consultation; most patients do not have any defined triggering event and often, related generalized stress. Vision loss is the most common complaint in NOVL and most children report bilateral symptoms. Visual field loss is the second most common complaint in NOVL and is seen in up to 48% of cases. The diagnosis of NOVL requires exclusion of other organic causes. The clinical examination is sufficient to establish the diagnosis of NOVL and electrophysiology may be helpful in some cases (70,182). Reassurance is necessary for most children with NOVL, but some may need formal psychiatric evaluation (183). Nonorganic overlay should be considered in children with NOVL; however, the combination of organic and NOVL is relatively common (70).

REFERENCES

1. Frisen L, Holmegaurd L. Spectrum of optic nerve hypoplasia. *Br J Ophthalmol* 1978;62:7–15.
2. Mosier MA, Lieberman MF, Green WR, et al. Hypoplasia of the optic nerve. *Arch Ophthalmol* 1978;96:1437–1442.
3. Whinery RD, Blodi FC. Hypoplasia of the optic nerve: a clinical and histopathologic correlation. *Trans Am Acad Ophthalmol Otolaryngol* 1963;67:733–738.
4. Al-Mohtaseb Z, Foroozan R. Congenital optic disc anomalies. *Int Ophthalmol Clin* 2012;52(3):1–16.
5. Kushner BJ. Functional amblyopia associated with organic ocular disease. *Am J Ophthalmol* 1981;91:39–45.
6. Kushner BJ. Functional amblyopia associated with abnormalities of the optic nerve. *Arch Ophthalmol* 1984;102:683–685.
7. Hoyt CS. Optic disc anomalies and maternal ingestion of LSD. *J Pediatr Ophthalmol* 1978;15:286–289.
8. Kim RY, Hoyt WF, Lessell S, et al. Superior segmental optic hypoplasia. A sign of maternal diabetes. *Arch Ophthalmol* 1989;107:1312–1315.
9. Margalith D, Jan JE, McCormick AQ, et al. Clinical spectrum of congenital optic nerve hypoplasia: review of 51 patients. *Dev Med Child Neurol* 1984;26:311–322.
10. Stromland K. Ocular abnormalities in the fetal alcohol syndrome. *Acta Ophthalmol Suppl* 1985;171:1–50.
11. Hoyt CS, Billison FA. Maternal anticonvulsants and optic nerve hypoplasia. *Br J Ophthalmol* 1978;62:3–6.
12. Mosier MA, Lieberman MF, Green WR, et al. Hypoplasia of the optic nerve. *Arch Ophthalmol* 1978;96:1437–1442.
13. Lambert SR, Hoyt CS, Narahara MH. Optic nerve hypoplasia. *Surv Ophthalmol* 1987;32:1–9.
14. Tajima T, Hattorri T, Nakajima T, et al. Sporadic heterozygous frameshift mutation of HESX1 causing pituitary and optic nerve hypoplasia and combined pituitary hormone deficiency in a Japanese patient. *J Clin Endocrinol Metab* 2003;88:45–50.
15. Thomas PQ, Dattani MT, Brickman JM, et al. Heterozygous HESX1 mutations associated with isolated congenital pituitary hypoplasia and septo-optic dysplasia. *Hum Mol Genet* 2001;10:39–45.

16. Dattani ML, Martinez-Barbera J, Thomas PQ, et al. Molecular genetics of septo-optic dysplasia. *Horm Res* 2000;53:26–33.

17. Dattani MT, Martinez-Barbera JP, Thomas PQ, et al. Mutations in the homeobox gene HESX1/Hesx1 associated with septo-optic dysplasia in human and mouse. *Nat Genet* 1998;19: 125–133.

18. de Morsier G. [Studies on malformation of cranio-encephalic sutures. III. Agenesis of the septum lucidum with malformation of the optic tract.] *SchweizArch Neurol Psychiatr* 1956;77:267–292.

19. de Morsier G. Median cranioencephalic dysraphias and olfacto-genital dysplasia. *World Neurol* 1962;3:485–500.

20. Signorini SG, Decio A, Fedeli C, et al. Septo-optic dysplasia in childhood: the neurological, cognitive and neuro-ophthalmological perspective. *Dev Med Child Neurol* 2012; 54(11):1018–1124.

21. Hoyt WG, Kaplan SL, Grumbach MM, et al. Septooptic dysplasia and pituitary dwarfism. *Lancet* 1970;1:893–894.

22. Brodsky MC, Glasier CM, Pollock SC, et al. Optic nerve hypoplasia. Identification by magnetic resonance imaging. *Arch Ophthalmol* 1990;108:1562–1567.

23. Kindler P. Morning glory syndrome: unusual congenital optic disc anomaly. *Am J Ophthalmol* 1970;69:376–384.

24. Pollock S. The morning glory disc anomaly: contractile movement, classification, and embryogenesis. *Doc Ophthalmol* 1987;65: 439–460.

25. Dutton GN. Congenital disorders of the optic nerve: excavations and hypoplasia. *Eye (Lond)* 2004;18:1038–1048.

26. Irvine AR, Crawford JB, Sullivan JH. The pathogenesis of retinal detachment with morning glory disc and optic pit. *Retina* 1986;6:146–150.

27. Chang S, Haik BG, Ellsworth RM, et al. Treatment of total retinal detachment in morning glory syndrome. *Am J Ophthalmol* 1984;97:596–600.

28. Oppezzo C, Barberis V, Edefonti A, et al. Congenital anomalies of the kidney and urinary tract. *GItal Nefrol* 2003;20:120–126.

29. Chung GW, Edwards AO, Schimmenti LA, et al. Renal-coloboma syndrome: report of a novel PAX2 gene mutation. *Am J Ophthalmol* 2001;132:910–914.

30. Salomon R, Tellier AL, Attie-Bitach T et al. PAX2 mutations in oligomeganephronia. *Kidney Int* 2001;59:457–462.

31. Eccles MR, Schimmenti LA. Renal-coloboma syndrome: a multi-system developmental disorder caused by PAX2 mutations. *Clin Genet* 1999;56:1–9.

32. Olsen TW. Visual acuity in children with colobomatous defects. *Curr Opin Ophthalmol* 1997;8:63–67.

33. Olsen TW, Summers CG, Knobloch WH. Predicting visual acuity in children with colobomas involving the optic nerve. *J Pediatr Ophthalmol Strabismus* 1996;33:47–51.

34. Daufenbach DR, Ruttum MS, Pulido JS, et al. Chorioretinal colobomas in a pediatric population. *Ophthalmology* 1998;105: 1455–1458.

35. Dailey JR, Cantore WA, Gardner TW. Peripapillary choroidal neovascular membrane associated with an optic nerve coloboma. *Arch Ophthalmol* 1993;111:441–442.

36. Kosaki K. Role of rare cases in deciphering the mechanisms of congenital anomalies: CHARGE syndrome research. *Congenit Anom (Kyoto)* 2011;51(1):12–15.

37. Thiselton DL, Alexander C, Taanman JW, et al. A comprehensive survey of mutations in the OPA1 gene in patients with autosomal dominant optic atrophy. *Invest Ophthalmol Vis Sci* 2002;43:1715–1724.

38. Pesch UE, Leo-Kottler B, Mayer S, et al. *OPA1* mutations in patients with autosomal dominant optic atrophy and evidence for semi-dominant inheritance. *Hum Mol Genet* 2001;10: 1359–1368.

39. Johnston RL, Seller MJ, Behnam JT, et al. Dominant optic atrophy. Refining the clinical diagnostic criteria in light of genetic linkage studies. *Ophthalmology* 1999;106:123–128.

40. Maresca A, la Morgia C, Caporali L, Valentino ML, Carelli V. The optic nerve: a "mito-window" on mitochondrial neurodegeneration. *Mol Cell Neurosci* 2013;55:62–76.

41. Cohn AC, Toomes C, Potter C, et al. Autosomal dominant optic atrophy: penetrance and expressivity in patients with OPA1 mutations. *Am J Ophthalmol* 2007;143(4):656–662.

42. Toomes C, Marchbank NJ, Mackey DA, et al. Spectrum, frequency and penetrance of OPA1 mutations in dominant optic atrophy. *Hum Mol Genet* 2001;10(13):1369–1378.

43. Vaphiades MS, Brodsky MC. Pediatric optic atrophy. *Int Ophthalmol Clin* 2012;52(3):17–28

44. Lenaers G, Hamel CP, Delettre C, et al. Dominant optic atrophy. *Orphanet J Rare Dis* 2012;7(1):46

45. Hoyt CS. Autosomal dominant optic atrophy. A spectrum of disability. *Ophthalmology* 1980;87(3):245–251.

46. Cohn AC, Toomes C, Hewitt AW, et al. The natural history of OPA1-related autosomal dominant optic atrophy. *Br J Ophthalmol* 2008;92(10):1333–1336.

47. Newman NJ. Treatment of hereditary optic neuropathies. *Nat Rev Neurol* 2012;8(10):545–556.

48. Yu-Wai-Man P, Griffiths PG, Gorman GS, et al. Multi-system neurological disease is common in patients with OPA1 mutations. *Brain* 2010;133(Pt 3):771–786.

49. Ranieri M, Del Bo R, Bordoni A, et al. Optic atrophy plus phenotype due to mutations in the OPA1 gene: two more Italian families. *J Neurol Sci* 2012;315(1–2):146–149.

50. Kjer P. Infantile optic atrophy with dominant mode of inheritance: a clinical and genetic study of 19 Danish families. *Acta Ophthalmol (Copenh)* 1959;164(suppl 54):1–147.

51. Waardenburg PJ, Franceshetti A, Klein D, eds. *Genetics and ophthalmology*, Vol. 2. Assen, Netherlands: Van Gorcum, 1953:1623.

52. Kline LB, Glaser JS. Dominant optic atrophy: the clinical profile. *Arch Ophthalmol* 1979;97:1680–1686.

53. Luberichs J, Leo-Kottler B, Besch D, et al. A mutational hot spot in the mitochondrial ND6 gene in patients with Leber's hereditary optic neuropathy. *Graefes Arch Clin Exp Ophthalmol* 2002;240:96–100.

54. Fauser S, Luberichs J, Besch D, et al. Sequence analysis of the complete mitochondrial genome in patients with Leber's hereditary optic neuropathy lacking the three most common pathogenic DNA mutations. *Biochem Biophys Res Commun* 2002;295:342–347.

55. Smith JL, Hoyt WF, Susac JO. Ocular fundus in acute Leber's optic neuropathy. *Arch Ophthalmol* 1973;90:349–354.

56. McLeod JG, Low PA, Morgan JA. Charcot-Marie-Tooth disease with Leber's optic atrophy. *Neurology* 1978;28:179–184.

57. Rose FC, Bowden AN, Bowden PMA. The heart in Leber's optic atrophy. *Br J Ophthalmol* 1970;54:388–393.

58. Pfeffer G, Majamaa K, Turnbull DM, et al. Treatment for mitochondrial disorders. *Cochrane Database Syst Rev* 2012;4: CD004426.

59. Klopstock T, Yu-Wai-Man P, Dimitriadis K, et al. A random-ized placebo-controlled trial of idebenone in Leber's hereditary optic neuropathy. *Brain* 2011;134(Pt 9):2677–2686.

60. DiMauro S, Mancuso M. Mitochondrial diseases: therapeutic approaches. *Biosci Rep* 2007;27(1–3):125–137.

61. Langer-Gould A, Zhang JL, Chung J, et al. Incidence of ac-quired CNS demyelinating Syndromes in a multiethnic cohort of children. *Neurology* 2011;77:1143–1148.

62. El-Dairi MA, Ghasia F, Bhatti MT. Pediatric optic neuritis. *Int Ophthalmol Clin* 2012;52(3):29–49

63. Banwell B, Kennedy J, Sadovnick D, et al. Incidence of acquired demyelination of the CNS in Canadian children. *Neurology* 2009;72:232–239.

64. Pohl D, Hennemuth I, von Kries R, et al. Paediatric multiple sclerosis and acute disseminated encephalomyelitis in Germany: results of a nationwide survey. *Eur J Pediatr* 2007;166:405–412.

65. Kennedy C, Carroll FD. Optic neuritis in children. *Arch Ophthalmol* 1960;63:747–755.

66. Meadows SP. Retrobulbar and optic neuritis in childhood and adolescence. *Trans Ophthalmol Soc UK* 1969;89:603–638.

67. Rollinson RD. Bilateral optic neuritis in childhood. *Med J Aust* 1977;2:50–51.

68. Absoud M, Cummins C, Desai N, et al. Childhood optic neu-ritis clinical features and outcome. *Arch Dis Child* 2011;96:860–862.

69. Tekavcic-Pompe M, Stirn-Kranjc B, Brecelj J. Optic neuritis in children—clinical and electrophysiological follow-up. *Doc Ophthalmol* 2003;107(3):261–270.

70. Suppiej A, Gaspa G, Cappellari A, et al. The role of visual evoked potentials in the differential diagnosis of functional visual loss and optic neuritis in children. *J Child Neurol* 2011;26:58–64.

71. Wilejto M, Shroff M, Buncic JR, et al. The clinical features, MRI findings, and outcome of optic neuritis in children. *Neurology* 2006;67:258–262.

72. Lucchinetti CF, Kiers L, O'Duffy A, et al. Risk factors for de-veloping multiple sclerosis after childhood optic neuritis. *Neurology* 1997;49:1413–1418.

73. Mikaeloff Y, Suissa S, Vallee L, et al. First episode of acute CNS inflammatory demyelination in childhood: prognostic factors for multiple sclerosis and disability. *J Pediatr* 2004;144:246–252.

74. Beck RW, Cleary PA. Optic neuritis treatment trial. One-year follow-up results. *Arch Ophthalmol* 1993;111:773–775.

75. The Optic Neuritis Study Group. Visual function 5 years after optic neuritis. Experience of the Optic Neuritis Treatment Trial. *Arch Ophthalmol* 1997;115:1545–1552.

76. Waldman AT, Gorman MP, Rensel MR, et al. Management of pediatric central nervous system demyelinating disorders: con-sensus of United States neurologists. *J Child Neurol* 2011;26:675–682.

77. Collongues N, Marignier R, Zéphir H, et al. Neuromyelitis op-tica in France: a multicenter study of 125 patients. *Neurology* 2010;74(9):736–742.

78. Pittock SJ. Neuromyelitis optica: a new perspective. *Semin Neurol* 2008;28:95–104.

79. Matà S, Lolli F. Neuromyelitis optica: an update. *J Neurol Sci* 2011;303:13–21.

80. Scott GI. Neuromyelitis optica. *Am J Ophthalmol* 1952;35:755–764.

81. Bonnan M, Valentino R, Olindo S, et al. Plasma exchange in severe spinal attacks associated with neuromyelitis optica spec-trum disorder. *Mult Scler* 2009;15(4):487–492.

82. Llufriu S, Castillo J, Blanco Y, et al. Plasma exchange for acute attacks of CNS demyelination: Predictors of improvement at 6 months. *Neurology* 2009;73(12):949–953.

83. Mandler RN, Ahmed W, Dencoff JE. Devic's neuromyelitis op-tica: a prospective study of seven patients treated with predni-sone and azathioprine. *Neurology* 1998;51(4):1219–1220.

84. Jacob A, Weinshenker BG, Violich I, et al. Treatment of neu-romyelitis optica with rituximab: retrospective analysis of 25 patients. *Arch Neurol* 2008;65(11):1443–1448.

85. Okada K, Tsuji S, Tanaka K. Intermittent intravenous immu-noglobulin successfully prevents relapses of neuromyelitis optica. *Intern Med* 2007;46(19):1671–1672.

86. Weinstock-Guttman B, Ramanathan M, Lincoff N, et al. Study of mitoxantrone for the treatment of recurrent neuromyelitis optica (Devic disease). *Arch Neurol* 2006;63(7):957–963.

87. Poser CM, Van Bogaert L. Natural history and evolution of the concept of Schilder's diffuse sclerosis. *Acta Psychiatr New Scand* 1956;31:285–331.

88. Kurul S, Cakmakci H, Dirik E, et al. Schilder's disease: case study with serial neuroimaging. *J Child Neurol* 2003;18:58–61.

89. Fitzgerald MJ, Coleman LT. Recurrent myelinoclastic diffuse sclerosis: a case report of a child with Schilder's variant of multiple sclerosis. *Pediatr Radiol* 2000;30:861–865.

90. Garell PC, Menezes AH, Baumbach G, et al. Presentation, management and follow-up of Schilder's disease. *Pediatr Neurosurg* 1998;29:86–91.

91. Afifi AK, Follett KA, Greenlee J, et al. Optic neuritis: a novel presentation of Schilder's disease. *J Child Neurol* 2001;16:693–696.

92. Pretorius ML, Loock DB, Ravenscroft A, et al. Demyelinating disease of Schilder type in three young South African children: dramatic response to corticosteroids. *J Child Neurol* 1998;13:197–201.

93. Leber T. Die pseudonephritischen netzhauterkrankungen die tetinitis dtellata: die purtschershe netzhautaffektron nach schwerer dchadelverletzung. In: Graef AC, Saemisch T, eds. *Graefe-saemisch handbuch der gesamten augenheilkundle*, 2nd Ed. Leipzig, Germany: Ergelmann, 1916:1319–1339.

94. Gass JD. Diseases of the optic nerve that may simulate macu-lar disease. *Trans Am Acad Ophthalmol Otolaryngol* 1977;83:763–770.

95. Parmley VC, Scheffman JS, Maitland CG, et al. Does neu-roretinitis rule out multiple sclerosis? *Arch Neurol* 1987;44:1045–1048.

96. Dreyer RF, Hapen G, Gass JD, et al. Leber's idiopathic stellate neuroretinitis. *Arch Ophthalmol* 1984;102:1140–1145.

97. Frey T. Optic neuritis in children: infectious mononucleosis as an etiology. *Doc Ophthalmol* 1973;34:183–188.

98. Maitland CG, Miller NR. Neuroretinitis. *Arch Ophthalmol* 1984;102:1146–1150.

99. Farthing CF, Howard RS, Thin RN. Papillitis and hepatitis B. *Br Med J (Clin Res Ed)* 1986;292:1712.

100. Lesser RL, Kormehl EW, Pachrer AR, et al. Neuroophthalmologic manifestations of Lyme disease. *Ophthalmology* 1990;97:699–706.

101. Fewell AG. Unilateral neuroretinitis of syphilitic origin with a striate figure in the macula. *Arch Ophthalmol* 1932;8:615.

102. Roach ES, Zimmerman CF, Troost BT, et al. Optic neuritis due to acquired toxoplasmosis. *Pediatr Neurol* 1985;1:114–116.

103. Miller NR. *Walsh and Hoyt's clinical neuro-ophthalmology*, 4th Ed. Baltimore, MD: Williams & Wilkins, 1995:4487–4489.

104. Meadows SP. The swollen disc. *Trans Ophthalmol Soc UK* 1959;79:121–143.

105. Rush JA. Pseudotumor cerebri. *Mayo Clin Proc* 1980;55: 541–546.

106. Miller NR, ed. *Walsh and Hoyt's clinical neuro-ophthalmology*, 4th Ed. Baltimore, MD: Williams & Wilkins, 1982:193.

107. Cogan DG. Blackouts not obviously due to carotid occlusion. *Arch Ophthalmol* 1965;73:461–462.

108. Helmke K, Hansen HC. Fundamentals of transorbital sonographic evaluation of optic nerve sheath expansion under intracranial hypertension. II. Patient study. *Pediatr Radiol* 1996;26:706–710.

109. Sergott RC. Diagnoses and management of vision-threatening papilledema. *Semin Neurol* 1986;6:176–184.

110. Beck RW, Greenberg HS. Post-decompression optic neuropathy. *J Neurosurg* 1988;63:196–199.

111. Rangwala LM, Liu GT. Pediatric idiopathic intracranial hypertension. *Surv Ophthalmol* 2007;52(6):597–617.

112. Balcer LJ, Liu GT, Forman S, et al. Idiopathic intracranial hypertension: relation of age and obesity in children. *Neurology* 1999;52:870–872.

113. Cinciripini GS, Donahue S, Borchert MS. Idiopathic intracranial hypertension in prepubertal pediatric patients: characteristics, treatment, and outcome. *Am J Ophthalmol* 1999;127:178–182.

114. Babikian P, Corbett J, Bell W. Idiopathic intracranial hypertension in children: the Iowa experience. *J Child Neurol* 1994; 9(2):144–149.

115. Marton E, Feletti A, Mazzucco GM, Longatti P. Pseudotumor cerebri in pediatric age: role of obesity in the management of neurological impairments. *Nutr Neurosci* 2008;11(1): 25–31.

116. Lee AG, Patrinely JR, Edmond JC. Optic nerve sheath decompression in pediatric pseudotumor cerebri. *Ophthalmic Surg Lasers* 1998;29:514–517.

117. Burgett RA, Purvin VA, Kawasaki A. Lumboperitoneal shunting for pseudotumor cerebri. *Neurology* 1997;49:734–739.

118. Eggenberger ER, Miller NR, Vitale S. Lumboperitoneal shunt for the treatment of pseudotumor cerebri. *Neurology* 1996;46:1524–1530.

119. Chutorian AM, Schwartz JF, Evans RA, et al. Optic gliomas in children. *Neurology* 1964;14:83–95.

120. Miller NR, Iliff WJ, Green WR. Evaluation and management of gliomas of the anterior visual pathways. *Brain* 1974;97: 743–754.

121. Kanamori N, Shibuya M, Yoshida J, et al. Long-term follow-up of patients with optic glioma. *Childs Nerv Syst* 1985;1:272–278.

122. Banna M, Hoore RD, Stanley P, et al. Craniopharyngioma in children. *J Pediatr* 1973;83:781–785.

123. Koos WT, Miller MH. *Intracranial tumors of infants and children*. Stuttgart, Germany: Georg Thieme Verlag, 1971.

124. Stripp DC, Maity A, Janss AJ, et al. Surgery with or without radiation therapy in the management of craniopharyngiomas in children and young adults. *Technol Int J Radiat Oncol Biol Phys* 2004;58:714–720.

125. Selch MT, DeSalles AA, Wade M, et al. Initial clinical results of stereotactic radiotherapy for the treatment of craniopharyngiomas. *Med Cancer Res Treat* 2002;1:51–59.

126. Kalapurakal JA, Goldman S, Hsieh YC, et al. Clinical outcome in children with craniopharyngioma treated with primary surgery and radiotherapy deferred until relapse. *Pediatr Oncol* 2003;40:214–218.

127. Varlotto JM, Flickinger JC, Kondziolka D, et al. External beam irradiation of craniopharyngiomas: long-term analysis of tumor control and morbidity. *Int J Radiat Oncol Biol Phys* 2002;54:492–499.

128. Isaac MA, Hahn SS, Kim JA, et al. Management of craniopharyngioma. *Cancer J* 2001;7:516–520.

129. Fisher PG, Jenab J, Goldthwaite PT, et al. Outcomes and failure patterns in childhood craniopharyngiomas. *Childs Nerv Syst* 1998;14:558–563.

130. Donin JF. Acquired monocular nystagmus in children. *Can J Ophthalmol* 1967;2:212–215.

131. Kelly TW. Optic glioma presenting as spasmus nutans. *Pediatrics* 1970;45:295–296.

132. Schulman JA, Shults TA, Jones JR. Monocular vertical nystagmus as an initial sign of chiasmal glioma. *Am J Ophthalmol* 1987;87:87–90.

133. Maitland CG, Ahiko S, Hoyt WE, et al. Chiasmal apoplexy: report of four cases. *J Neurosurg* 1982;56:118–122.

134. Hoyt WF, Baghdassarian SA. Optic glioma of childhood: natural history and rationale for conservative management. *Br J Ophthalmol* 1969;53:793–798.

135. Glaser JS, Hoyt WF, Corbett J. Visual morbidity with chiasmal glioma. *Arch Ophthalmol* 1971;85:3–12.

136. Tow SL, Chandela S, Miller NR, et al. Long-term outcome in children with gliomas of the anterior visual pathway. *Pediatr Neurol* 2003;28:262–270.

137. Allen JC. Initial management of children with hypothalamic and thalamic tumors and the modifying role of neurofibromatosis-1. *Pediatr Neurosurg* 2000;32:154–162.

138. Imes RK, Hoyt WF. Childhood chiasmal gliomas: update on the fate of patients in the 1969 San Francisco study. *Br J Ophthalmol* 1986;70:179–182.

139. Khafaga Y, Hassounah M, Kandil A, et al. Optic gliomas: a retrospective analysis of 50 cases. *Int J Radiat Oncol Biol Phys* 2003;56:807–812.

140. Daroff RB. See-saw nystagmus. *Neurology* 1965;15:874–877.

141. Gay AJ, Brodkey J, Miller JE. Convergence-retraction nystagmus: an electromyographic study. *Arch Ophthalmol* 1963;70. 453–458.

142. Cobbs WH, Schatz NJ, Savino PJ. Midbrain eye signs in hydrocephalus. *Trans Am Neurol Assoc* 1978;103:130.

143. Daroff RB, Troost BT. Upbeat nystagmus. *JAMA* 1973;225:312.

144. Schatz NJ, Schlezinger NS, Berry RG. Vertical upbeat nystagmus on downward gaze: a clinical pathologic correlation. *Neurology* 1975;25:380.

145. Cogan DG. Downbeat nystagmus. *Arch Ophthalmol* 1968;80: 757–768.

146. Cogan DG, Barrows JL. Platybasia and the Arnold-Chiari malformation. *Arch Ophthalmol* 1954;52:13–29.

147. Zee DS, Friendlech AR, Robinson DA. The mechanism of downbeat nystagmus. *Arch Neurol* 1974;30:227–237.

148. Baloh RW, Honrubia V, Konrad HR. Periodic alternating nystagmus. *Brain* 1976;99:11–26.

149. Towle PA, Romanul F. Periodic alternating nystagmus: first pathologically studied case. *Neurology* 1970;20:408.

150. Gradstein L, Reinecke RD, Wizov SS, et al. Congenital periodic alternating nystagmus. Diagnosis and management. *Ophthalmology* 1997;104:918–928.

151. Abadi RV, Pascal E. Periodic alternating nystagmus in humans with albinism. *Invest Ophthalmol Vis Sci* 1994;35: 4080–4086.

152. Cogan DG. Ocular dysmetria: flutter-like oscillations of the eyes and opsoclonus. *Arch Ophthalmol* 1954;51:318–335.

153. Ellenberger C Jr, Keltner JL, Stroud MH. Ocular-dyskinesia in cerebellar disease: evidence for the similarity of opsoclonus, ocular dysmetria, and flutter-like oscillations. *Brain* 1972;95:685–692.

154. Sergott RC, Glaser JS, Berger LJ. Simultaneous bilateral diabetic ophthalmoplegia: report of two cases and discussions of differential diagnosis. *Ophthalmology* 1984;91:18–22.

155. Namba T, Brown SB, Grob D. Neonatal myasthenia gravis: report of two cases and review of the literature. *Pediatrics* 1970;45:488–504.

156. Levin PM. Congenital myasthenia in siblings. *Arch Neurol* 1949;62:745–748.

157. Namba T, Brunner NG, Brown SB, et al. Familial myasthenia gravis: report of 27 patients in 12 families and review of 164 patients in 73 families. *Arch Neurol* 1971;25:49–60.

158. Engel AG, Walls TJ, Nagel A, et al. Newly recognized congenital myasthenic syndromes. I: congenital paucity of synaptic vesicles and reduced quantal release. II: high-conductance fast-channel syndrome. III: abnormal acetylcholine receptor (AChR) interaction with acetylcholine. IV: AChR deficiency and short channelopen time. *Prog Brain Res* 1990;84:124–137.

159. Millichap JG, Dodge PR. Diagnosis and treatment of myasthenia gravis in infancy, childhood, and adolescence. *Neurology* 1960;11:1007–1014.

160. Finnis MF, Jayawant S. Juvenile myasthenia gravis: a paediatric perspective. *Autoimmune Dis* 2011;2011:404101.

161. Drochman DB. Present and future treatment of myasthenia gravis. *N Engl J Med* 1987;316:743–745.

162. Fambrough DM, Drochman DB, Satyamurti S. Neuromuscular junction in myasthenia gravis: decreased acetylcholine receptors. *Science* 1973;182:293–295.

163. Arnon SS, Midura TF, Clay SA, et al. Infant botulism: epidemiological, clinical and laboratory aspects. *JAMA* 1977;237:1946–1951.

164. Miller NR. Solitary oculomotor nerve palsy in childhood. *Am J Ophthalmol* 1977;83:106–111.

165. Harley RD. Paralytic strabismus in children: etiology, incidence, and management of the third, fourth, and sixth nerve palsies. *Ophthalmology* 1980;87:24–43.

166. Norman AA, Farris BK, Siatkowski RM. Neuroma as a cause of oculomotor palsy in infancy and early childhood. *J AAPOS* 2001;5:9–12.

167. Loewenfeld H, Thompson HS. Oculomotor pareses with cyclic spasms: a critical review of the literature and new case. *Surv Ophthalmol* 1975;20:81–124.

168. Robertson DM, Hanes JD, Rucker CW. Acquired sixth nerve pareses in children. *Arch Ophthalmol* 1970;83:574–579.

169. Kearns TP, Sayre GP. Retinitis pigmentosa, external ophthalmoplegia, and complete heart block. *Arch Ophthalmol* 1958;60:280–289.

170. Moraes CT, DiMauro S, Zeviani M, et al. Mitochondrial DNA deletions in progressive external ophthalmoplegia and Kearns Sayre syndrome. *N Engl J Med* 1989;320:1293–1299.

171. Cogan DG. A type of congenital ocular motor apraxia presenting jerky head movements. *Trans Am Acad Ophthalmol* 1952;56:853–862.

172. Cogan DG, Chu FC, Reingold D, et al. A long-term follow-up of congenital ocular motor apraxia. *Neuroophthalmology* 1980;1:145–147.

173. Leigh RJ, Zee DS. *The neurology of eye movement.* Philadelphia, PA: FA Davis Co., 1983.

174. Norton EWD, Cogan DG. Spasmus nutans: a clinical study of 20 cases followed two years or more since onset. *Arch Ophthalmol* 1954;152:442–446.

175. Gottlob I, Wizov SS, Reinecke RD. Spasmus nutans. A long-term follow-up. *Invest Ophthalmol Vis Sci* 1995;36:2768–2771.

176. Young TL, Weis JR, Summers CG, et al. The association of strabismus, amblyopia, and refractive errors in spasmus nutans. *Ophthalmology* 1997;104:112–117.

177. Slimani F, Hamzy R, Allali B, et al. [Möbius syndrome]. *Rev Stomatol Chir Maxillofac* 2010;111(5–6):299–301.

178. Carta A, Mora P, Neri A, Favilla S, Sadun AA. Ophthalmologic and systemic features in möbius syndrome an Italian case series. *Ophthalmology* 2011;118(8):1518–1523.

179. Nicolaides P, Appleton RE, Fryer A. Cerebellar ataxia, areflexia, pes cavus, optic atrophy and sensorineural hearing loss (CAPOS): a new syndrome. *J Med Genet* 1996;33:419–421.

180. Mantyjarvi MI. The amblyopic schoolgirl syndrome. *J Pediatr Ophthalmol Strabismus* 1981;18:30–33.

181. Toldo I, Pinello L, Suppiej A, et al. Nonorganic (psychogenic) visual loss in children: a retrospective series. *J Neuroophthalmol* 2010;30:26–30.

182. Massicotte EC, Semela L, Hedges TR. Multifocal visual evoked potential in nonorganic visual field loss. *Arch Ophthalmol* 2005;123:364–367.

183. Moore Q, Al-Zubidi N, Yalamanchili S, Lee AG. Nonorganic visual loss in children. *Int Ophthalmol Clin* 2012;52(3):107–123.

23

Nystagmus

Mitchell B. Strominger

NYSTAGMUS IS A rhythmic oscillation of one or both eyes. It can be transiently evoked voluntarily or be constantly present as a nonspecific sign of abnormality. Developmental, hereditary, or acquired anomalies of the eye and central nervous system can all be associated with nystagmus.

HISTORY

When patients with nystagmus are evaluated, the history is extremely important to determine the etiology. The history should detail when the nystagmus was first noted, if it has changed over time, is constant throughout the day, changes depending on visual attentiveness, or is associated with a face turn or head movement. The prenatal history is explored for intrauterine infections, especially toxoplasmosis or rubella. A maternal history of anticonvulsant or psychogenic drug use, or gestational diabetes may suggest optic nerve hypoplasia (ONH). The birth history is directed towards prematurity, hypoxic ischemic encephalopathy, intraventricular hemorrhage, hydrocephalus, or developmental delay.

The family history gives information as to a possible hereditary factor. A family history of night blindness or color deficiency suggests congenital stationary night blindness (CSNB) or achromatopsia. For the latter condition, the family history may be especially important, because not every child with achromatopsia shows photophobia in the first few months of life (1). The family's ethnic background may suggest a metabolic condition, such as Tay-Sachs disease, or a lipofuscinosis.

EXAMINATION

Examination of the symmetry of the face, the position of the ears, dental anomalies, skin tags, and pigmentation is helpful in identifying a developmental syndrome or albinism. The visual acuity is tested binocularly first and then monocularly, at distance and near fixation, and with and without any idiosyncratic head position. In infants, the ability to fixate on and follow moving objects and the use of visual clues is noted. The ability to optically elicit ocular movements using an optokinetic nystagmus tape or drum should also be noted. In the absence of the latter, there is a high likelihood that vision is grossly defective.

The characteristic of the nystagmus waveform should be noted, although this can change during the first year of life (2). It is described by its plane, amplitude, frequency, and symmetry. The plane of oscillation may be principally horizontal, vertical, oblique, or rotary (torsional). The amplitude may be fine (less than 5 degrees), medium (5 to 15 degrees), or large (greater than 15 degrees). If the oscillations are of similar speed in either direction, it is classified as a pendular nystagmus. A nystagmus is considered jerk if there is a biphasic rhythm with a fast phase in one direction, followed by a slow phase in the opposite direction. The frequency should be noted as high, low, or in cycles per second (Hz). A slit lamp or ophthalmoscope can be used to magnify ocular movements. Electronystagmography allows a more exact and permanent objective recording.

The nystagmus is observed for an extended period to determine whether it regularly changes direction with time, suggesting periodic alternating nystagmus (PAN); if both eyes move conjugately; if the pattern changes with eye position; and if the frequency or amplitude varies. Nystagmus that remains horizontal on vertical gaze suggests infantile nystagmus syndrome (INS), fusion maldevelopment nystagmus syndrome (FMDS), PAN, or peripheral vestibular nystagmus.

Examination of the eye should detect any severe bilateral ocular abnormality such as anterior segment dysgenesis, congenital cataracts, or congenital glaucoma. The irides are examined for transillumination defects that would suggest albinism. The posterior pole is evaluated for abnormalities, such as cicatricial retinopathy of prematurity (ROP), retinoblastoma, or coloboma. A blunted foveal reflex suggests albinism. Finally, the optic nerve is examined for pallor, hypoplasia, or increased cupping.

A clinical dilemma arises when an ocular malformation either does not exist or is very subtle. Retinal conditions such as leber congenital amaurosis (LCA), achromatopsia, CSNB, and ocular albinism may be difficult to detect on clinical examination alone. In such cases, an electroretinogram (ERG) should be performed.

NYSTAGMUS ASSOCIATED WITH NEUROLOGIC DISORDERS

Convergence-Retraction Nystagmus

Variable bursts of sustained convergence and retraction of the eyes on attempted upgaze suggest a midbrain disorder. Co-contraction of all the extraocular muscles causes retraction with convergence because of the greater strength of the medial rectus muscles. In infants, one would suspect congenital aqueductal stenosis, in children a pinealoma or obstructive hydrocephalus, and in older adults a vascular accident in the tectal or pretectal area. Parinaud syndrome is convergence-retraction nystagmus in association with vertical eye movement palsies, pupillary abnormalities, lid retraction, and accommodative spasm (3).

Seesaw Nystagmus

Seesaw nystagmus is a unique vertical-torsional oscillation of both eyes in which one eye rises and intorts and its fellow eye falls and extorts. The disjunctive vertical movement alternates to provide the seesaw effect. This disorder may be congenital, but most patients have suprasellar tumors expanding within the third ventricle and compressing the brainstem. Acquired oscillopsia and bitemporal hemianopsia are associated findings (4). Other causes include a lesion in the lateral medulla or pons, syringobulbia, or severe vision loss (5).

Periodic Alternating Nystagmus

PAN is a horizontal jerk nystagmus in which the direction of the fast phase changes spontaneously and cyclically with an intervening neutral period. A typical cycle lasts 1 to 6 minutes. A sequence of jerk waveforms in one direction converts to a neutral period of pendular waveforms, followed by jerk waveforms in the opposite direction. Alternating head turns may accompany the jerk nystagmus periods. PAN appears to result from a spatial and temporal shift in the null zone (6). PAN usually remains horizontal in vertical gaze and is hypothesized to arise from an instability of the optokinetic-vestibular system. It may coexist with downbeat nystagmus, both of which suggest an abnormality in the caudal medulla (7). PAN was found on eye movement recordings of patients with idiopathic infantile nystagmus who had mutations on the FRMD7 gene on Chromosome Xq26 (NYS 1 locus) (8). Up to one-third of patients with albinism also demonstrate PAN (6). Acquired PAM occurs most commonly with disease involving the midline cerebellum. Inhibitory pathways that use gamma-aminobutyric acid (GABA) in the nodulus and uvula control the time course of rotationally induced nystagmus and therefore Baclofen, a GABA agonist, can be effective in its treatment (9).

Downbeat Nystagmus

Downbeat nystagmus is recognized by a deficit in downward pursuit whereby the eyes drift upward, and a corrective saccade returns the eyes to the primary position. It is maximal in downgaze, lateral gaze and when the head is erect or hyperextended. A rare congenital hereditary form has been identified that is usually self limited, and associated with good vision and a normal neurologic examination. A compensatory chin-down head posture is sometimes noted (10). More commonly, downbeat nystagmus is acquired and signifies an abnormality of the cerebellum (flocculus or paraflocculus). The commonest causes are cerebellar degenerations and structural lesions at the craniocervical junction such as Chiari malformation (Fig. 23.1). Alcohol, lithium, anticonvulsants, and thiamine, magnesium, and B12 deficiency may also give rise to this condition (11).

Upbeat Nystagmus

A vertical vestibular or smooth pursuit deficit similar in type but opposite in direction to downbeat nystagmus is thought to cause upbeat nystagmus, which may increase or convert to downbeat nystagmus with convergence. It may occur congenitally as a variant of congenital nystagmus (CN) with anterior visual pathway disease (12). Acquired forms occur with lesions of the brainstem (mainly the pontomesencephalic junction, rostral medulla, or caudal pons), cerebellar vermis, or after meningitis (13).

Peripheral Vestibular Nystagmus

Lesions of the labyrinth or eighth nerve cause a horizontal and rotary jerk nystagmus on lateral gaze opposite the side of the lesion. Vertigo may be marked, and tinnitus and deafness occur in concert. Visual fixation decreases

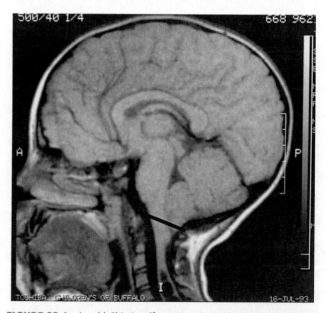

FIGURE 23.1. Arnold-Chiari malformation. Sagittal magnetic resonance imaging scan of type I Arnold-Chiari malformation with mild cerebellar tonsillar herniation below line. Note associated syrinx in cervical cord.

the intensity of the nystagmus and vertigo, which lasts minutes, days, or weeks. Central pathways eventually compensate even if the underlying cause remains. Common causes are Meniere disease, infectious or vascular disorders, and trauma (14).

NYSTAGMUS ASSOCIATED WITH VISUAL LOSS

Visual loss, or the lack of visual development, within the first 2 years of life is usually associated with nystagmus. Acquired monocular visual loss, due to an anterior visual pathway tumor or other ocular disorder, may be associated with a fine, rapid, monocular nystagmus (15). Nystagmus is usually not present in patients with cortical visual impairment because of the retention of visual input to the brain via the extrageniculostriate visual system.

Any congenital or perinatal condition that results in occlusion of the visual axis, distortion of the retinal image, or malformation of the sensory retina or optic nerve can result in nystagmus. Although electronystagmography may show complex or varied waveforms, the type of nystagmus is often related to the severity of the visual impairment. A moderate disruption in vision may result in pendular nystagmus, whereas a more severe form of the same disorder may produce a searching nystagmus. Although this may be helpful prognostically, some ocular malformations usually are readily recognized. The more common ocular malformations in which nystagmus may be a prominent sign include bilateral coloboma, congenital cataracts, congenital glaucoma, bilateral cicatricial ROP, aniridia, persistent fetal vasculature,

bilateral retinal dysplasia, and congenital toxoplasmosis with macular involvement. Other abnormalities that may be more difficult to recognize and will be further discussed include Leber congenital amaurosis, optic nerve hypoplasia, albinism, achromatopsia, congenital stationary night blindness, and X-linked juvenile retinoschisis.

Leber Congenital Amaurosis

This autosomal-recessive disorder is characterized by diminished vision starting at or shortly after birth and can be divided into eleven subtypes depending on gene locus and defect. LCA2 results from RPE65 (retinal pigment epithelium-specific 65 KDa) deficiency that disrupts the retinoid cycle. Recent studies of subretinal gene therapy using recombinant adeno-associated virus to carry the RPE65 gene have shown promising results (16).

Acuity is less than 20/200 in up to 95% of affected individuals, and a searching nystagmus is present in 75%. The pupils are poorly reactive, and many children exhibit the oculodigital sign (habitual eye rubbing). The fundus is usually normal in infancy. Pigmentary disturbances of the peripheral retina develop during childhood in most patients, along with optic disk pallor and arteriolar attenuation. A markedly reduced or absent response to the ERG is noted in virtually all patients (Fig. 23.2). A variety of ocular conditions, including keratoconus, keratoglobus, macular coloboma, disk edema, cataract, and strabismus, have been associated with LCA. As many as 15% of patients may have mental retardation. Other systemic associations include medullary cystic kidney disease, cardiomyopathy, and skeletal abnormalities.

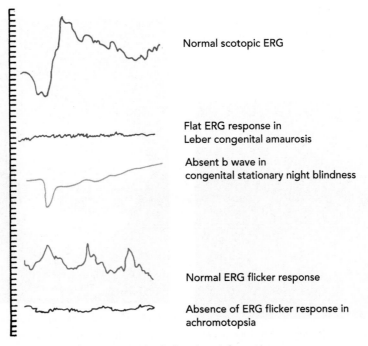

Normal scotopic ERG

Flat ERG response in
Leber congenital amaurosis

Absent b wave in
congenital stationary night blindness

Normal ERG flicker response

Absence of ERG flicker response in
achromotopsia

FIGURE 23.2. Electroretinographic findings in an infant with nystagmus.

Optic Nerve Hypoplasia

Optic nerve hypoplasia (ONH) is a congenital, nonprogressive condition characterized by a paucity of axons within the optic nerve and a diminished ganglion cell layer of the retina. Ophthalmoscopically, ONH is recognized by a small, pale nerve head. Classically, it is surrounded by a ring of white sclera and a second pigmented or nonpigmented ring outlining the scleral rim, giving rise to the term double-ring sign (Fig. 23.3). The retinal vessels usually appear relatively normal, but the retina may be deep red in color because of the thinness of the nerve fiber layer.

Severe bilateral ONH results in a searching nystagmus, whereas mild, unilateral ONH may not have visual symptoms. In one study, 78% of those with bilateral involvement, poor vision, and nystagmus had additional ocular abnormalities, compared with 21% of patients with unilateral ONH (17). Delayed development is the most frequent nonocular disorder, followed by hypopituitarism, cerebral palsy, and epilepsy. Other associations include midline facial defects and abnormalities of the cerebral cortex, brainstem, and cerebellum including absence of the septum pellucidum and agenesis of the corpus callosum (18). Associated ocular malformations include microphthalmos, coloboma, aniridia, and strabismus.

ONH is believed to result from a defect in the differentiation of retinal ganglion cell axons. It has been associated with embryonic insults at or after 6 weeks of gestation with maternal ingestion of quinidine and with anticonvulsants. It is more common in children of severely diabetic and of adolescent mothers.

Neuroimaging with MRI is recommended in all children with ONH. Cerebral hemispheric abnormalities, along with posterior pituitary ectopia, are predictive of hypopituitarism and neurodevelopmental delays (19). Endocrine consultation should also be obtained to monitor growth.

Albinism

Albinism is a genetically determined disturbance in melanogenesis with hypopigmentation of the skin, hair, and eyes. All forms of true albinism are characterized by reduced visual acuity, hypoplasia of the macula, nystagmus, and excessive decussation of most temporal retinal ganglion cell axons through the chiasm to the contralateral geniculate and cortex. (Figs. 23.4 and 24.5). Multiple inheritance patterns (autosomal recessive and X-linked) have been noted. It is apparent that there are multiple abnormal alleles of the genes responsible for melanogenesis. The result is that several different genotypes may have a similar phenotypic expression for albinism.

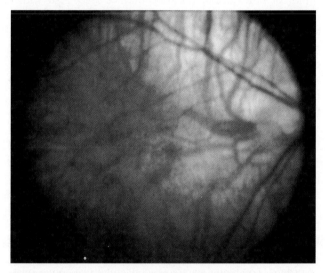

FIGURE 23.4. Fundus of a patient with albinism. Note the hypopigmented appearance of the background and the absence of a clearly defined fovea (foveal hypoplasia).

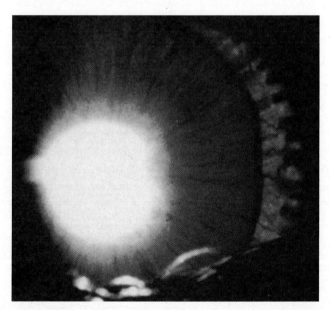

FIGURE 23.5. Iris transillumination in a patient with albinism as demonstrated by slit-lamp retroillumination. Note the lens edge as seen through the hypopigmented iris.

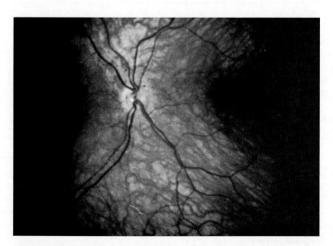

FIGURE 23.3. Optic nerve hypoplasia. Note the small optic nerve head and the surrounding ring outlining the scleral rim (double-ring sign).

Tyrosinase is the enzyme responsible for the initial steps of melanin synthesis. The autosomal-recessive form of oculocutaneous albinism (OCA) has a defect in the gene, which produces an inactive form of the enzyme. This gene is located on chromosome 11q14–21 (20). The hair bulb incubation test demonstrates the presence or absence of tyrosinase activity and provides biochemical evidence for heterogeneity, but alone it cannot separate the various forms of albinism known to exist. Clinical, biochemical, and ultrastructural criteria are now used to distinguish each form of albinism. Tyrosinase-negative OCA is considered type 1 and has four subtypes. Tyrosinase-positive OCA is type 2, which is caused by separate mutations at the P locus on chromosome 15q11.2–q12 (21). Type 3 OCA is described in African and African-American individuals. It is characterized by light brown skin and hair, moderate tanning ability, and blue-gray irides with transillumination defects. Tyrosinase is found in normal quantity but exhibits reduced tyrosine hydroxylase activity. A precise diagnosis is essential for counseling the family about the implications of the disease and the heritable pattern.

Clinical management relates to protecting the skin and maximizing vision. Affected individuals may have delayed visual maturation, only gradually becoming visually attentive after 2 to 3 months of age. They also often have high refractive errors and may benefit significantly from correction. Near acuity is relatively better than far secondary to convergence dampening the nystagmus.

It is important to recognize two special subtypes of albinism because they may have life-threatening complications. The Chédiak-Higashi syndrome (chromosome 1q43) is a lethal condition in which albinism is associated with a defect in cellular immunity (T cells) as well as leukocytes. Neutrophils show reduced migration and deficient chemotaxis and bactericidal capacity. Children have an increased susceptibility to gram-positive infections. Patients surviving infections often die of malignant lymphoreticular infiltration of the tissues (22). Hermansky-Pudlak syndrome (chromosome 10q23.1–q23.3) is an association of OCA with hemorrhagic diathesis and a ceroid-like accumulation in the reticuloendothelial cells; it is unusually prevalent in Puerto Ricans. The bleeding tendency is low, but there have been reported deaths from hemorrhage. There is a qualitative defect in platelets, and aspirin and cyclooxygenase inhibitors should be avoided because they may convert a mild bleeding disorder into a severe one. Additional associations include the development of restrictive lung disease in the third and fourth decades, ulcerative colitis, kidney disease, and cardiomyopathy.

Achromatopsia (Rod Monochromatism)

Achromatopsia is a rare congenital, autosomal-recessive disorder with a prevalence of only 3 in 100,000. The locus for this disorder has been mapped to chromosome 2q11 (23) and chromosome 8q (24). It is characterized by a complete loss of color vision, diminished visual acuity of 20/100 to 20/400, photophobia, and typically an oblique pendular nystagmus of small amplitude and high frequency. Because of severe photophobia, children with this disorder may prefer to play outside at dusk and may have better vision in dim illumination (hemeralopia). The photophobia and nystagmus may diminish and even disappear after the age of 15, but the visual acuity does not improve.

Histopathology has demonstrated that the cone photoreceptors in the retina are either missing or severely maldeveloped. The most reliable diagnostic test for infants is the ERG. In achromatopsia, the ERG flicker response is absent (Fig. 23.2) and the photopic single-flash response is reduced. The scotopic response is normal.

A form of incomplete rod monochromatism also exists. Because blue cones are involved minimally or not at all, this has also been called blue-cone monochromatism. The inheritance appears to be X-linked. Visual acuity is in the 20/60 range, nystagmus is minimal, and photophobia is absent. Unlike achromatopsia, this condition appears to progress slowly to macular scarring and cone dysfunction. It is distinguished from achromatopsia by color-plate discrepancies in which blue-cone monochromats can distinguish between blue-green and purple-blue, but achromats cannot. In addition, differences in the eye movement response to optokinetic stimuli moving from the nasal to temporal field (achromats respond poorly) can be used to distinguish these two conditions. Since blue cones probably represent only a small portion of all retinal cones, the ERG is just as abnormal in this disorder as in complete achromatopsia. However, patients with blue-cone monochromatism show a peak illumination sensitivity near 440 nm, whereas patients with rod monochromatism demonstrate a peak sensitivity near 504 nm (25).

Congenital Stationary Night Blindness

CSNB is a heritable disorder in which the predominant complaint of affected individuals is night blindness. It is characterized by a normal fundus appearance, normal daylight visual fields, absence of rod dark adaptation, and lack of progression. Multiple inheritance patterns have been identified in CSNB: autosomal dominant, autosomal recessive, and X-linked. Decreased vision, myopia, and nystagmus is seen only in some autosomal-recessive variants and never in patients with autosomal-dominant CSNB.

In X-linked CSNB, visual acuity ranges between 20/30 and 20/100. Myopia of between 3.50 and 11.0 diopters is usually present. Patients with acuities worse than 20/60 have an obvious pendular nystagmus, but electronystagmography can occasionally detect nystagmus when the acuity is better. Color vision is normal or, at worst, only mildly abnormal, differentiating this disorder from achromatopsia. The prime diagnostic tool in infants is the ERG, in which there is a reduction or absence of any positive response (b-wave) to scotopic testing (see Fig. 23.2). Clinically and genetically, two subtypes have been defined with the distinction being a mildly abnormal cone function with undetectable rod activity in type 1, and residual rod activity with a more significantly abnormal cone ERG in type 2 (26). The elucidation of the molecular basis has identified the matrix protein nyctalopin in type 1, and a subunit of a retina-specific calcium channel in type 2 (27). Both are predicted to function at various levels of retinal signal transduction. In addition, some young patients with X-linked CSNB demonstrate an initial "paradoxic" pupillary constriction in darkness (28).

Oguchi disease is a related autosomal-recessive congenital stationary disorder with diminished night vision. Unlike CSNB, there is a peculiar homogeneous yellow to grayish white discoloration of the fundus, and only occasionally mildly abnormal vision in the range of 20/25 to 20/50. The abnormal coloration usually disappears after 2 to 3 hours of dark adaptation and begins to reappear after about 10 minutes of light exposure. The appearance and reappearance of abnormal coloration with light suggests a disorder of retinal pigment kinetics. Normal rhodopsin kinetics, however, have been found in one patient. The ERG in Oguchi disease is similar to that in CSNB in demonstrating an absent b wave. In Oguchi disease, however, the ERG picture may become less abnormal after prolonged dark adaptation.

X-Linked Juvenile Retinoschisis

This recessive disorder is characterized by a cleavage of the retina at the level of the nerve fiber layer. Its prevalence ranges from 1 in 5,000 to 1 in 25,000 and is considered the most common cause of juvenile macular degeneration in males. Therefore, examination of male relatives is important to help confirm the diagnosis and provide genetic counseling. Typically, the vision is between 20/50 and 20/100 and gradually diminishes to about 20/200 with increasing age. Vitreous veils with or without retinal vessels occur in less than 50%. Vitreous hemorrhage from rupture of these vessels may be the presenting symptom. Although bilateral elevated bullous schisis cavities involving the fovea may occur in infancy, the most frequent finding is a stellate maculopathy representing foveal schisis. Clinically, this maculopathy can look very similar to cystoid macular edema (CME) but is differentiated by the lack of leakage on fluorescein angiography. A high rate of spontaneous reattachment with retinal pigment demarcation lines is reported (29). On ERG the b-wave, both scotopic and photopic, is usually reduced. The gene has been localized to the Xp22 region (30). The abnormality appears to be a dysfunctional adhesive protein secreted by the photoreceptor and bipolar cells, and transported by Müller cells into the inner retina (31). At present, no effective treatment is available.

FUSION MALDEVELOPMENT NYSTAGMUS SYNDROME

Previously characterized as latent and manifest latent nystagmus, http://www.nei.nih.gov/news/statements/cemas. pdf, fusion maldevelopment nystagmus syndrome (FMDS) describes an infantile onset, dual-jerk, nystagmus that is associated with strabismus. Associated findings include esotropia and dissociated vertical deviation. It typically is decreased with binocular fusion thus becoming clinically evident upon monocular occlusion. The fast phase is toward the viewing (nonoccluded) eye while the slow phase has decreasing velocity away from the fixating eye (32). Alternate occlusion of the eyes results in reversal of the nystagmus direction. The amplitude of the nystagmus increases with gaze directed to the side of the fixating eye (Alexander's law). Nystagmus intensity (amplitude times frequency) is greater when viewing with the amblyopic eye. Binocular vision is always better than monocular vision. It is currently hypothesized that FMDS is due to an imbalance in the input to a defective nucleus of the optic tract. Occasionally, it may be acquired spontaneously or following minor head trauma in adulthood causing oscillopsia.

INFANTILE NYSTAGMUS SYNDROME

Infantile nystagmus syndrome (INS), previously called congenital nystagmus http://www.nei.nih.gov/news/statements/cemas.pdf, is characterized by a conjugate, mainly horizontal, nystagmus even on up- and downgaze that can progress from pendular to jerk. Although difficult to identify clinically, a torsional component may be present. The nystagmus may be present at birth but typically develops during infancy. The waveform can be age dependent. Most commonly, it is of large-amplitude "triangular" in the first few months of life, then pendular, and eventually jerk at about 1 year of age (33). There is often a position of least nystagmus that is called the null zone, which may be straight ahead or in any position of gaze. Away from the null zone, the fast phase is in the direction of gaze (Alexander's law). If the null zone is in eccentric position, a compensatory face turn or abnormal head position may present. Convergence can dampen the nystagmus (nystagmus blockage syndrome, NBS). Visual prognosis is dependent upon whether a primary sensory system abnormality is present (e.g. albinism, achromatopsia). In the familial non-sensory deficit form the vision is relatively good, from 20/20 to 20/70. This is probably secondary to a foveation period during which the waveform is "flattened" when the eye is closest to the target. A common associated finding is inversion of the optokinetic reflex. With optokinetic drum testing, the quick phase is directed in the same direction as the drum rotates rather than in the opposite direction.

SPASMUS NUTANS

The classic triad of signs in spasmus nutans includes (a) monocular or dissociated, pendular, small-amplitude, rapid (high-frequency) nystagmus; (b) head nodding; and (c) an anomalous head position. However, there are numerous reports of children who have spasmus nutans without head nodding or head tilt. Spasmus nutans is usually acquired between 4 and 8 months of age and clinically ceases spontaneously by 3 years of age. It can, however, be variable in its onset and duration. Nystagmus may persist subclinically into the first decade of life; eye movement recordings in older children have demonstrated persistent asymmetric, fine, pendular nystagmus. Approximately one third of patients may develop normal acuity and stereopsis (34). The head nodding is a compensatory vestibuloocular reflex to suppress the nystagmus. A similar clinical presentation has been noted in children with chiasmatic glioma, subacute necrotizing encephalopathy, achromatopsia, CSNB, and rod dystrophy, and need to be excluded via neuroimaging and electroretinography.

NYSTAGMUS TREATMENT

Regardless of the type of nystagmus, the goal of treatment is to improve vision, eliminate anomalous (compensatory) head positions, and abolish any oscillopsia. Dampening the nystagmus amplitude, increasing the foveation period, and broadening the null zone can improve acuity in some CN patients. Using optical, medical, and surgical modalities, some of these goals have been achieved, and ongoing research continues to improve upon the armamentarium.

Optical treatment begins by obtaining the best refraction and spectacle prescription. Contact lenses have been reported to increase foveation time by increasing convergence and accommodative effort or by a sensory feedback mechanism on the eyelids leading to reduced nystagmus. Prisms can be used to shift the null zone if there is a small turn or can be used to "fine tune" surgical results. Base-out prisms can also induce accommodative convergence and sometimes need to be combined with myopic correction. In those cases in which a convergent mechanism is spontaneously maintained, base-out prisms can help realign the visual axis or improve head posture.

Several medications have made an impact on specific nystagmus types (9,11). A decrease in the oscillopsia of acquired pendular with improved acuity has been reported with Gabapentin and Memantine. Upbeat nystagmus responds to Memantine, 4-aminopyridine, and Baclofen. Downbeat nystagmus can improve with clonazepam, 4-aminopyridine and 3,4 aminopyridine. Baclofen and Memantine have been used successfully to abolish periodic alternating nystagmus and oscillopsia, although the congenital form is less responsive. Seesaw nystagmus has improved with alcohol, clonazepam, and Memantine. With all of these agents, their benefit must be weighed against the potential CNS side effects, especially drowsiness.

Botulinum toxin can be used to achieve a "pharmacoparesis" with improved vision in CN (35) and to decrease oscillopsia in acquired nystagmus (36). Approaches include retrobulbar injection or direct injection into the horizontal muscles of one or both eyes. Injections need to be repeated every few months, and potential complications include ptosis, diplopia, continued oscillopsia, and patient acceptance. Success has been mixed, with some patients requiring multiple consecutive injections (36) and others not obtaining satisfactory results (37).

Anderson (38) and Kestenbaum (39) originally described the surgical management of congenital motor nystagmus to shift the null zone to the primary position and eliminate a compensatory head posture. Dell'Osso and Flynn (40) demonstrated visual improvement using this technique by broadening the null region and reducing the nystagmus intensity (amplitude times frequency) on motility recordings. With the early surgical amounts, however, there still existed a residual head posture, and "augmented" surgery (larger bilateral recession/resection on the horizontal muscles) was advocated (41). A gaze deficit can be created with aggressive surgery, but it is accepted by most patients. When strabismus is present with an abnormal head posture, surgery on the fixating eye is performed to eliminate the head position, and the fellow eye is surgically compensated for the strabismic angle.

Large retroequatorial recessions of all four horizontal rectus muscles have been proposed for patients with a central null zone to improve vision and decrease the nystagmus amplitude (42). Some patients report an improvement in their visual function, although objective change using eye movement recordings have been minimal. Dell'Osso (43) suggested and then demonstrated in patients (44) that simply detaching the extraocular muscle, dissecting the perimuscular fascia, and then reattaching to the original site on the globe (Tenotomy and reattachment procedure) can improve foveation times and subjective visual acuity in patients with CN. This is thought to be due to an alteration in proprioceptive input from palisade organs that lie in proximity to the attachment points of the extraocular muscles.

Most cases of acquired nystagmus with oscillopsia are not amenable to neurosurgery with one notable exception. Downbeat nystagmus due to Arnold-Chiari malformation responds to suboccipital decompression and can also prevent further neurologic deficits.

SUMMARY

Nystagmus is a nonspecific sign that may occur physiologically or pathologically. The approach to diagnosing and managing infants presenting with nystagmus includes family, perinatal, and nystagmus history; ophthalmologic examination; and when appropriate, electrophysiologic and neuroradiologic examinations. If there is an obvious ocular abnormality severe enough to impair visual function, management and counseling specific for the disorder are appropriate.

In the absence of obvious ocular malformation, the workup is governed by the nature of the predominant ocular oscillation. If the nystagmus is asymmetric, rapid, and pendular, CT or MRI scan is usually indicated to rule out an intracranial process. If no CNS disorder is present, the presumptive diagnosis for asymmetric, high-frequency nystagmus is spasmus nutans. Searching nystagmus implies a severe retinal or optic nerve disorder, and the first step is to obtain an ERG to rule out LCA, along with careful inspection of the optic nerves. If the disks appear pale or other CNS signs are present, neurologic examination and neuroradiologic imaging are performed. If the nystagmus is symmetric and pendular, a careful search is made for foveal hypoplasia and iris transillumination, which would suggest albinism. In the absence of these, electrophysiologic studies and careful ophthalmoscopy may detect an isolated cone or macular abnormality. Infantile nystagmus syndrome is essentially a diagnosis of exclusion with a relatively good visual prognosis.

ACKNOWLEDGMENTS

This chapter is modified from a previous chapter on nystagmus by Robert A. Catalano MD from edition 4 of Harley's Pediatric Ophthalmology.

REFERENCES

1. Hoyt CS. The apparently blind infant. *Trans New Orleans Acad Ophthalmol* 1986;34:478–488.
2. Jan JE, Farrell K, Wong PK, et al. Eye and head movements of visually impaired children. *Dev Med Child Neurol* 1986;28:285–293.
3. Smith JL, Zieper I, Gay AJ, et al. Nystagmus retractorius. *Arch Ophthalmol* 1959;62:864–867.
4. Daroff RB. See-saw nystagmus. *Neurology* 1965;15:874–877.
5. Halmagyi GM, Hoyt WF. See-saw nystagmus due to unilateral mesodiencephalic lesion. *J Clin Neuroophthalmol* 1991;11:79–84.
6. Abadi RV, Pascal E. Periodic alternating nystagmus in humans with albinism. *Invest Ophthalmol Vis Sci* 1994;35:4080–4086.
7. Baloh RW, Honrubia V, Konrad HR. Periodic alternating nystagmus. *Brain* 1976;99:11–26.
8. Thomas MG, Crosier M, Lindsay S, et al. The clinical and molecular genetic features of idiopathic infantile periodic alternating nystagmus. *Brain* 2011;134:892–902.
9. Thurtell MJ, Leigh RJ. Therapy for nystagmus. *J Neuroophthalmology* 2010;30:361–371.
10. Brodsky MC. Congenital downbeat nystagmus. *J Pediatr Ophthalmol Strabismus* 1996;33:191–193.
11. Straube A, Leigh RJ, Bronstein A, et al. EFNS task force—therapy of nystagmus and ascillopsia. *Euro J Neurology* 2004;11:83–89.
12. Good WV, Brodsky MC, Hoyt CS, et al. Upbeating nystagmus in infants: a sign of anterior visual pathway disease. *Binoc Vis Q* 1990;5:13–18.
13. Fisher A, Gresty M, Chambers B, et al. Primary position upbeating nystagmus: a variety of central positional nystagmus. *Brain* 1983;106:949–964.
14. Reker U. Peripheral-vestibular spontaneous nystagmus: analysis of reproducibility and methodologies. *Arch Otorhinolaryngol* 1980;226:225–237.
15. Donin JF. Acquired monocular nystagmus in children. *Can J Ophthalmol* 1967;2:212–215.
16. Jacobson SG, Ciedicyan AV, et al. Gene therpy for Leber congenital amaurosis caused by RPE65 mutations. *Arch Ophthalmol* 2012;130(1):9–24.
17. Skarf B, Hoyt CS. Optic nerve hypoplasia in children. Association with anomalies of the endocrine and CNS. *Arch Ophthalmol* 1984;102:62–67.
18. Frisen L, Holmegaard L. Spectrum of optic nerve hypoplasia. *Br J Ophthalmol* 1978;62:7–15.
19. Brodsky MC, Glasier CM. Optic nerve hypoplasia: clinical significance of associated central nervous system abnormalities on magnetic resonance imaging. *Arch Ophthalmol* 1993;111:66–74.
20. Barton DE, Kwon BS, Francke U. Human tyrosinase gene, mapped to chromosome 11 (q14–21), defines second region of homology with mouse chromosome 7. *Genomics* 1988;3:17–24.
21. Ramsay M, Colman M, Stevens G, et al. The tyrosinase-positive oculocutaneous albinism locus maps to chromosome 15q11.2–q12. *Am J Hum Genet* 1992;51:879–884.
22. Blume RS, Wolff SW. The Che'diak-Higashi syndrome: studies in four patients and a review of the literature. *Medicine* 1972;51:247–280.
23. Abour NC, Zlotogora J, Knowlton RG, et al. Homozygosity mapping of achromatopsia to chromosome 2 using DNA pooling. *Hum Mol Genet* 1997;6:689–694.
24. Milunsky A, Huang X-L, Milunsky J, et al. A locus for autosomal recessive achromatopsia on human chromosome 8q. *Clin Genet* 1999;56:82–85.
25. Yee RD, Farley MK, Bateman JB, et al. Eye movement abnormalities in rod monochromatism and blue cone monochromatism. *Graefes Arch Clin Exp Ophthalmol* 1985;223:55–59.
26. Miyake Y, Yagasaki K, Horiguchi M, et al. Congenital stationary night blindness with negative electroretinogram. A new classification. *Arch Ophthalmol* 1986;104:1013–1020.
27. Pusch CM, Zeitz C, Brandau O, et al. The complete form of Xlinked congenital stationary night blindness is caused by mutations in a gene encoding a leucine-rich repeat protein. *Nat Genet* 2000;26:324–327.
28. Barricks MF, Flynn JT, Kushner BJ. Paradoxical pupillary responses in congenital stationary night blindness. *Arch Ophthalmol* 1977;95:1800–1804.
29. George NDL, Yates JRW, Bradshaw K, et al. Infantile presentation of X-linked retinoschisis. *Br J Ophthalmol* 1995;79:653–657.
30. Sieving PA, Bingham EL, Roth MS, et al. Linkage relationship of X-linked juvenile retinoschisis with Xp22.1–p22.3 probes. *Am J Hum Genet* 1990;47:616–621.
31. Mooy CM, van den Born LI, Paridaens DA, et al. Hereditary X linked juvenile retinoschisis: a review of the role of Muller cells. *Arch Ophthalmol* 2002;120:979–984.
32. Dell'Osso LF, Schmidt D, Darroff RB. Latent, manifest latent, and congenital nystagmus. *Arch Ophthalmol* 1979;97:1877–1885.

33. Reinecke RD, Guo S, Goldstein HP. Waveform evolution in infantile nystagmus: an electro-oculo-graphic study of 35 cases. *Binoc Vis* 1988;31:191–202.

34. Gottlob I, Wizov SS, Reinecke RD. Spasmus nutans: a long-term follow-up. *Invest Ophthalmol Vis Sci* 1995;36: 2768–2771.

35. Carruthers J. The treatment of congenital nystagmus with botox. *J Pediatr Ophthalmol Strabismus* 1995;32:306–308.

36. Repka MX, Savino PJ, Reinecke RD. Treatment of acquired nystagmus with botulinum neurotoxin A. *Arch Ophthalmol* 1994;112:1320–1324.

37. Tomsak RL, Remler BF, Averbuch-Heller L, et al. Unsatisfactory treatment of acquired nystagmus with retrobulbar injection of botulinum toxin. *Am J Ophthalmol* 1995;119: 489–496.

38. Anderson JR. Causes and treatment of congenital eccentric nystagmus. Br J Ophthalmol 1953;37:267–281.

39. Kestenbaum A. [New operation for nystagmus.] *Bull Soc Ophtalmol Fr* 1953;6:599–602.

40. Dell'Osso LF, Flynn JT. Congenital nystagmus surgery: a quantitative evaluation of the effects. *Arch Ophthalmol* 1979;97:462–469.

41. Nelson LB, Ervin-Mulvey LD, Calhoun JH, et al. Surgical management for abnormal head position in nystagmus: the augmented modified Kestenbaum procedure. *Br J Ophthalmol* 1984;68:796–800.

42. Helveston EM, Ellis FD, Plager DA. Large recession of the horizontal recti for treatment of nystagmus. *Ophthalmology* 1991;98:1302–1305.

43. Dell'Osso LF. Extraocular muscle tenotomy, dissection, and suture: an hypothetical therapy for congenital nystagmus. *J Pediatr Ophthalmol Strabismus* 1998;35:232–233.

44. Hertle RW, Dell'Osso LF, FitzGibbon EJ, et al. Horizontal rectus tenotomy in patients with congenital nystagmus: results in 10 adults. *Ophthalmology* 2003;110:2097–2105.

24

Ocular Trauma and Its Prevention

Robert A. Catalano

A SIGNIFICANT PROPORTION of ocular injuries occur in children. According to the Agency for Healthcare Research and Quality, approximately 28% of Emergency Department visits related to eye injuries in 2008 were for patients younger than 18 years of age. Further, the 2010 Annual Eye Injury Snapshot Project estimated that approximately 12% of all eye injuries occur in children 12 years of age or younger (1,2). The more recent U.S. data is consistent with previously published European data that the highest proportion of severe eye injuries in children occurs in the home (40% to 45%), followed by injuries sustained while playing sports or due to a motor vehicle accident (approximately 15%). In children younger than age 6 years, domestic accidents (scissors, pencils, or other sharp objects) were the principal cause; in older children, toy, stone, and ball injuries predominated (3). This study and others (4–6) revealed a substantial male preponderance and noted that most severe injuries in children are accidental and caused by another child.

In contrast with other causes of childhood visual loss, such as from congenital and/or hereditary diseases in which current treatments may be less effective, victims of ocular trauma can often benefit greatly by prompt treatment. Even greater benefit can be had if ocular trauma is prevented, which is readily attainable in the pediatric population.

HISTORY

Although most ophthalmologic office examinations for children require only a brief history, when ocular trauma is apparent or suspected, a complete and detailed history is essential, especially when a responsible adult did not observe the injury. In many cases, the initial history is the most accurate and unbiased. Extra care and attention to detail is required to detect prevarication or other attempts at deception; for example, the child may have sustained the trauma engaged in a proscribed behavior, a "supervising" adult may have been involved in the injury, or the visual loss, if any, may have predated the injury. In addition, careful documentation of all historical and objective findings, with detailed drawings or photographs, if indicated, can be crucial for purposes of determining civil liability and/or suspected child abuse.

When the patient's chief complaint is trauma, the usual sequence of questions for history taking must be greatly expanded. Precise determination of the time and place of the onset of symptoms or signs must be made. A foreign body sensation that began when the child was near a construction site prompts a search for a different type of object than if the symptoms began in a wooded area. When the inciting event is not obvious, and the symptoms and signs did not begin at a distinct time, inquiry must be made of activities in the preceding hours, days, or even weeks.

The child's precise activity at the time of injury and the site where it occurred must be determined. Whether or not the child was wearing glasses, using high-speed motorized equipment, and whether or not anyone was hammering are examples of the level of detail that must be documented. If a wild animal inflicted the injury, the animal should undergo pathologic examination of its brain to look for signs of rabies infestation. When such examination is impossible, consultation with local health officials should be sought to determine the need for rabies prophylaxis.

The general medical history must also be determined. Known medical problems, hospitalizations, prior ocular and nonocular surgeries, current medications of all types, medicinal allergies, and family history must all be explored. In addition, patients with open wounds must have their tetanus prophylaxis history reviewed and reimmunization administered, if necessary.

EXAMINATION

Despite the critical need for as complete an examination as possible to make an accurate diagnosis, initial efforts must be directed to the more important goal of preventing further injury. In the case of a ruptured globe, a more complete examination is always obtained with the child anesthetized in the operating room, which significantly reduces the risk of further injury. Complicating an already difficult situation is pain and discomfort, reducing what may be an already low level of cooperation. Extra efforts at cajoling or bribery, additional pairs of strong hands, a papoose board, local nerve block, sedation, or even anesthesia may be required alone or in combination for proper diagnosis and treatment.

Protection from Further Injury

When definitive treatment for the injury will occur later, the injured eye and adnexa should be protected from further inadvertent trauma. Lid retraction, forced opening of the eyelids and removal of a protruding foreign body is absolutely contraindicated, and topical drops of any kind should not be applied. With lid lacerations, foreign bodies, and suspected ruptured globes, a standard eye shield should be taped to the orbital rim to protect the globe and eyelids, and the head of the bed should be elevated to 30 degrees. When ophthalmic supplies are unavailable, a disposable Styrofoam coffee cup can be cut about 2.5 cm (1 inch) from its base and used for the same purpose.

From a systemic standpoint, a child with a possibly ruptured globe may be agitated, nauseated (from a vasovagal reflex), or both. Mild sedation, along with an antiemetic, may be indicated to prevent further damage. The child should be kept NPO for possible surgery, and ambient light should be reduced. If there is concern that the child may pull off a protective eye shield, elbow or other restraints may be necessary.

When a ruptured globe is repaired under general anesthesia, a nondepolarizing agent should be used (7). Depolarizing agents (e.g., succinylcholine) transiently raise intraocular pressure with possible further extrusion of intraocular contents.

Special Studies

Additional modalities of examination may be required in some instances. When motorized equipment or high-speed impacts (e.g., hammering) were involved at the time of the injury, a foreign body, either in the globe or orbit, must be suspected. An intraocular foreign body should also be considered whenever a ruptured globe is suspected. Plain radiographic films and/or noncontrast computed tomography (CT) with 1 to 2 mm axial and coronal cuts through the orbits (8,9) should be taken for accurate and precise localization. Magnetic resonance imaging (MRI) should never be used if there is any possibility of a metallic foreign body.

CT scanning is not sufficiently sensitive or specific when an occult open-globe injury is suspected. When an occult injury is suspected a formal surgical examination should be performed in the operating room (10).

If a clear view of the fundus is not obtained, ultrasonography should be considered to assess retinal integrity. However, the diagnostic possibility of a ruptured globe is a contraindication to the use of ultrasound. In this instance, any pressure on the globe may further disrupt the anatomy and cause retinal and/or uveal prolapse, and the nonsterile probe raises the risk of infection. For closed-globe injuries, ultrasound biomicroscopy is particularly superior to other

methods in the evaluation of the zonular status, angle recession, cyclodialysis, and the detection of small superficial and intraocular foreign bodies (11).

Prognosis

Open-globe injuries result in the worst visual outcomes in children with ocular trauma (12). Particularly unfavorable outcomes are also related to an initial presentation of hyphema, vitreous hemorrhage, retinal detachment, and/or a corneal wound across the pupil (13). The presence of a relative afferent pupillary defect and poor initial visual acuity are the most predictive indicators of complete loss of vision and the presence of lid laceration and posterior wound location also predict poor visual outcome (14). Children with an ocular injury sustained during major trauma (multiple injuries with an Injury Severity Score > 15) are more likely to have a basilar skull fracture and/or orbital wall fracture (15). The subsequent development of endophthalmitis also portends a poor visual prognosis. A standardized protocol of 48 hours of intravenous vancomycin and ceftazidime upon admission resulted in a posttraumatic endophthalmitis rate of less than 1% in a recent study (16).

BIRTH AND PRENATAL TRAUMA

Significant ocular injuries occur in approximately 0.2% of deliveries, particularly forceps-assisted deliveries (17). The most widely recognized finding associated with birth trauma is a vertically oriented rupture of Descemet's membrane, which is often accompanied by a hazy cornea (17). Horizontal Descemet's ruptures (Haab's striae) result more commonly from the high intraocular pressure of congenital glaucoma. Although direct contact of forceps with the cornea is usually implicated, periocular compression is also a possible mechanism of injury (18).

With time, epithelial edema fades, leaving a vertical line at the level of Descemet's membrane. This line is visually insignificant. However, true ruptures of Descemet's membrane can lead to very large degrees of astigmatism that can result in anisometropic amblyopia (19). The initial corneal haziness can also act as a form of occlusion, which can induce axial myopia and exacerbate the anisometropia (20). The use of a rigid contact lens to neutralize the astigmatism and aggressive occlusion therapy can possibly improve the visual prognosis (21).

Perinatal periocular ecchymoses (22), lid (23) or canalicular (24) lacerations, ptosis (25), corneal edema (22), hyphema (22), and multiple retinal hemorrhages (22) have also been reported. Small retinal hemorrhages usually resolve in 1 to 5 days and subconjunctival hemorrhages within 2 weeks (17). Injuries to the lid that cause ptosis are potentially very serious because the ptosis may cause an axial myopia (20), which can lead to an anisometropic amblyopia.

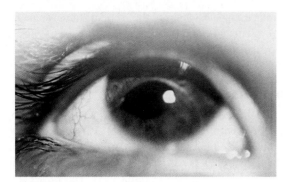

FIGURE 24.1. Penetrating injury from amniocentesis.

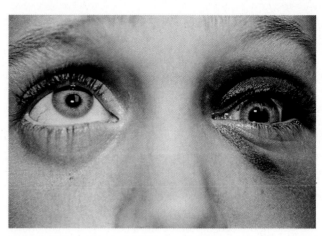

FIGURE 24.2. Eyelid and periorbital ecchymosis and limitation of upward gaze resulting from a blowout fracture.

In addition to corneal injury, forceps delivery may rarely result in choroidal ruptures, even in the absence of external signs of injury (26). Finally, ocular adnexal birth injury by a fetal monitoring scalp electrode has been reported occasionally (27).

Ocular injury can also occur prenatally, during amniocentesis. Despite ultrasound control, injury to the fetus occurs in 3% of cases (28), usually resulting in cutaneous scars. Ocular perforation may also occur, with varying degrees of visual disability (Fig. 24.1) (29,30).

INJURIES TO THE LIDS AND ADNEXA

Ecchymosis of the Eyelid

Most orbital contusions, due to blunt injuries, cause soft tissue damage with little or no disability. Blunt trauma, however, can be associated with a blowout or other orbital fractures, hyphema, angle recession, iridodialysis, retinal edema, and retinal breaks. Deep orbital bleeding can cause compression of the optic nerve or ophthalmic artery. Examination of the peripheral retina, using scleral depression, may have to wait until orbital edema subsides. The examination should not be delayed, however, in patients with symptoms suggestive of a retinal tear.

The distribution of hemorrhage can occasionally foretell a serious orbital injury. Blood under the superior conjunctiva suggests an orbital roof fracture, especially when accompanied by significant eyelid edema and ecchymosis (31). Basilar skull fractures are sometimes associated with a ring-like distribution of periorbital blood. Hemorrhage in the lower lid and inferior orbit may signal an orbital floor fracture (Fig. 24.2).

Blunt trauma can also result in ptosis secondary to a hematoma of the eyelid or levator palpebrae muscle. A permanent ptosis can result if the aponeurosis is stretched or torn. Fingers or hooks caught under the upper eyelid often result in this type of injury.

Treatment of lid ecchymosis consists of cold compresses for the initial 24-hour period, followed by warm compresses as needed.

Lid Laceration

In addition to obvious causes of lacerations from injury with sharp objects and animal bites, lid lacerations can be caused by strong blows with blunt objects, such as an elbow in a competitive basketball game. The initial evaluation of a lid laceration of any etiology is directed at the integrity of the globe; vision-threatening ocular injuries take precedence over those involving only the lids, where delayed repair may still give an excellent cosmetic and functional result. With lacerations involving the medial portion of the lid, the status of the canaliculi should be determined to the greatest extent possible without risking further injury.

There is no clear consensus concerning prophylactic treatment with antibiotics for lid lacerations. Although standard surgical practice may suggest use of antibiotics in other injuries, they may not be necessary with lid lacerations due to the rich blood supply of the lids.

Most children who sustain ophthalmic trauma are not sufficiently cooperative to allow for local or regional anesthetic techniques. Regardless of the level of cooperation, general anesthesia is mandatory whenever related injuries require its use, as in an ocular laceration.

Primary, edge-to-edge closure remains the mainstay of treatment for lid lacerations. Nonrepair of a torn canaliculus may be considered when only one canaliculus is involved (32), but when both canaliculi are involved, intubation of the canaliculi with Silastic tubing looped and brought out through the lower opening of the nasolacrimal duct increases the chance of functional success. Subsurface absorbable sutures are then used around the cut edges of the canaliculi before the cutaneous edges are repaired. Even with a complete history, a thorough search for a retained foreign body should be made at the time of repair of any laceration. The reader is referred elsewhere for detailed, specific recommendations on treatment, which are beyond the scope of this chapter.

ORBITAL TRAUMA

Blowout Fracture of the Orbital Floor

Orbital apex, lateral wall, and Le Fort type III fractures have a greater association with severe ocular injuries than blowout fractures of the orbital floor, but they occur less commonly (33). The term *direct orbital floor fracture* describes an orbital floor fracture associated with an orbital rim fracture. Much greater force is needed to fracture the orbital rim than to fracture the orbital floor. The term *indirect orbital floor fracture* describes an isolated orbital floor fracture and is known more commonly as a *blowout fracture*. Two theories have been developed to explain the pathogenic mechanism of a blowout fracture. The first maintains that these fractures result when the intraorbital pressure is suddenly elevated by a nonpenetrating blunt force. The orbital tissues are compressed, and the weakest part of the orbit, the 0.5- mm-thick orbital floor just below the inferior rectus muscle, becomes the avenue of decompression (Fig. 24.3). A more recent theory suggests that a blunt force applied to the inferior orbital rim compresses the bone and causes a buckling of the orbital floor. Orbital floor fractures are common when objects larger than the orbital opening, such as a ball, a fist, or the dashboard of an automobile, impact the orbit, particularly the inferior lateral orbit. *Macaca* monkey experiments have suggested that forces greater than 2 joules (J) are needed to produce an orbital floor fracture, and that orbital wall fractures fail to protect the globe from rupture (34).

The most apparent clinical sign of an orbital floor fracture is a limitation of upward gaze (Figs. 24.2 and 24.4). A concomitant limitation of downward gaze, however, is a more certain indication of inferior rectus or oblique muscle entrapment. Entrapment is more likely to occur when an articulated bone fragment acts like a trap door, restricting the movement of the inferior rectus or oblique muscle. This occurs most frequently with small, indirect orbital floor fractures, and most com-

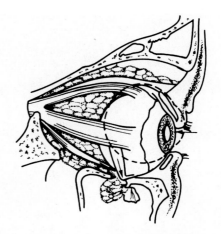

FIGURE 24.3. Schematic to demonstrate a blowout fracture of the orbital floor. The *dotted line* indicates the normal position of the globe. The small opening into the maxillary sinus entraps the inferior rectus and oblique muscles. (From Catalano RA, ed. *Ocular emergencies.* Philadelphia, PA: WB Saunders Co, 1992, with permission.)

monly the inferior rectus muscle, posterior to its adventitial connection to the inferior oblique muscle, is involved. Additional signs are lid ecchymosis, epistaxis, orbital emphysema, and hypesthesia of the ipsilateral cheek and upper lip, which results from disruption of the infraorbital nerve as it traverses the orbital floor. Enophthalmos results from expansion of the orbital volume and is an overt sign of an orbital floor fracture. It occurs more commonly with direct orbital floor fractures but it may not become apparent until orbital edema resolves. Exophthalmos from orbital edema, hematoma, or inflammation is more likely to be present acutely.

The best imaging techniques to visualize an orbital floor fracture are plain film radiography and CT scanning. The optimal plain film projection is the Waters' view because it demonstrates the orbital floor and maxillary sinus best (Fig. 24.5). An orbital floor fracture is suggested by the prolapse of orbital contents into the maxillary sinus, an air–fluid level in the

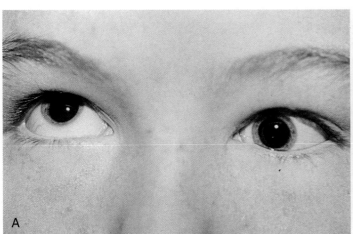
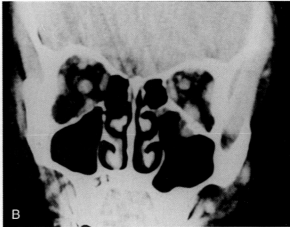

FIGURE 24.4. Blowout fracture of the left eye in a 12-year-old girl who was kicked in the eye by a classmate. **A:** Limitation of upgaze. **B:** Coronal CT scan showing tissue entrapment.

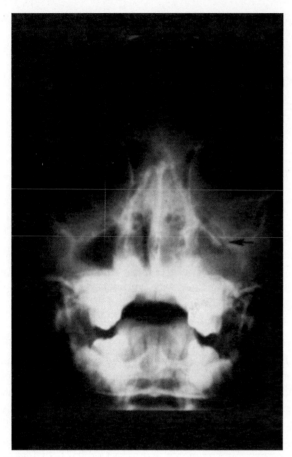

FIGURE 24.5. Waters' view demonstrating blowout fracture of the orbital floor. (From Catalano RA, ed. *Ocular emergencies.* Philadelphia, PA: WB Saunders Co, 1992, with permission.)

sinus, or orbital emphysema. Although the Waters' view is suggested for screening, direct, coronal 1.5- to 2-mm CT scanning should be obtained, if surgical repair is contemplated, because this provides more soft tissue and bone fragment detail.

The indications for and timing of surgical repair of a blowout fracture continue to evolve (35,36). The radiographic presence of fracture alone is not an indication for surgery nor is the sole finding of infraorbital hypesthesia. Generally accepted indications for repair include a motility disturbance due to extraocular muscle entrapment (within 30 degrees of the primary position) or enophthalmos. In pediatric patients, symptoms of entrapment of the inferior rectus muscle include pain, nausea, and vomiting. Surgical repair rapidly relieves these symptoms (37). Surgical intervention for a limitation of motility is based on true mechanical restriction, suggested by persistent positive forced traction testing and confirmed radiographically. It should be remembered, however, that techniques other than floor fracture repair (prisms, strabismus surgery) might be effective in relieving diplopia. Enophthalmos of greater than 2 mm generally requires repair, because it is usually cosmetically unacceptable. Because the necessary exposure of an orbital floor fracture places pressure on the globe, the presence of a penetrating ocular injury is an absolute contraindication to orbital floor repair.

The timing of surgical repair is also controversial. A blowout fracture never needs emergent treatment. Most ophthalmologists agree that surgery can be safely delayed for 10 to 14 days without risking the development of scarring or fibrosis. The passage of several days is usually needed to allow orbital swelling to subside enough to perform an adequate clinical examination. An indication for early surgical repair is the presence of enophthalmos greater than 2 mm or hypoglobus in the acute stage of an orbital floor fracture. Orbital edema and hematoma usually mask the early appearance of enophthalmos; its acute presence indicates a substantial extrusion of orbital contents into the maxillary sinus. Surgery within 2 weeks is recommended in cases of symptomatic diplopia with positive forced ductions and evidence of orbital soft tissue entrapment on CT Scan (38).

Additional therapeutic measures in the acute setting are antibiotic prophylaxis to prevent an orbital cellulitis, nasal decongestants, and ice packs.

INJURIES TO THE GLOBE

Injuries to the Conjunctiva and Sclera

A *subconjunctival hemorrhage* commonly accompanies blunt trauma (Fig. 24.6). In the absence of other injury, an affected patient is treated with reassurance alone. The hemorrhage may appear to become larger over the first several days. This occurs as gravity and the weight of the eyelid smooth out blood clots that can dissect under normal conjunctiva. Rarely, if ever, does a subconjunctival hemorrhage rebleed. The blood gradually resorbs over 2 to 3 weeks.

Conjunctival edema (*chemosis*) can accompany a minor injury. However, its presence raises the suspicion of scleral rupture or a retained foreign body. Air under the conjunctiva (*emphysema*) suggests fracture through the ethmoid

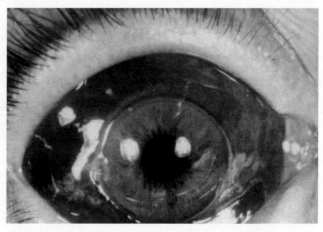

FIGURE 24.6. Traumatic subconjunctival hemorrhage. (From Catalano RA, ed. *Ocular emergencies.* Philadelphia, PA: WB Saunders Co, 1992, with permission.)

or maxillary sinus. Emphysema appears cystic and causes crepitus on palpation.

A *laceration of the conjunctiva* is especially common when a sharp object, such as a fingernail or glass, strikes the eye. In addition to conjunctival hemorrhage, prolapse of whitish-appearing Tenon's tissue or orbital fat may be evident. A complete examination to rule out a retained foreign body or an occult scleral laceration or is necessary. Ophthalmoscopy through maximally dilated pupils and ultrasound can be used to rule out the former. If sliding the conjunctiva does not allow adequate visualization to rule out a scleral laceration, the physician should not hesitate to conduct an examination under anesthesia or obtain imaging studies. Small conjunctival lacerations do not need suturing, but lacerations greater than 6 mm should be closed with absorbable suture (e.g., 7-0 plain gut), taking care not to incorporate Tenon's tissue in the wound. One should also respect the normal anatomical relationship of the caruncle and semilunar fold in the repair. The unrepaired conjunctival defect heals within 2 to 3 weeks.

Occult scleral rupture can occur with blunt trauma, especially at the limbus and just posterior to the rectus muscle insertions, where the sclera is weakest (39). In addition to a bullous conjunctival hemorrhage and chemosis, signs of rupture include an asymmetrical reduction in intraocular pressure, shallowing or deepening of the anterior chamber, irregularity or peaking of the pupil, hyphema, decreased visual acuity, and subconjunctival pigmentation. The last is due to prolapsed uveal tissue at the site of rupture. In suspected cases, as much as a 360-degree conjunctival peritomy should be performed (incising the conjunctiva at the limbus and retracting it posteriorly to expose the underlying sclera), with particular attention directed to the area under the rectus muscle insertions.

Corneal Foreign Bodies and Abrasions

Corneal and conjunctival foreign bodies are very common causes of acute ocular pain and foreign body sensation. Patients typically present with excruciating pain and a reflexive inhibition to opening their eye. They may or may not recall an object falling or flying into their eye, and their pain may or may not be immediate or may wax and wane. Although inert objects may cause little or no secondary changes, organic material can produce a severe reaction (Fig. 24.7).

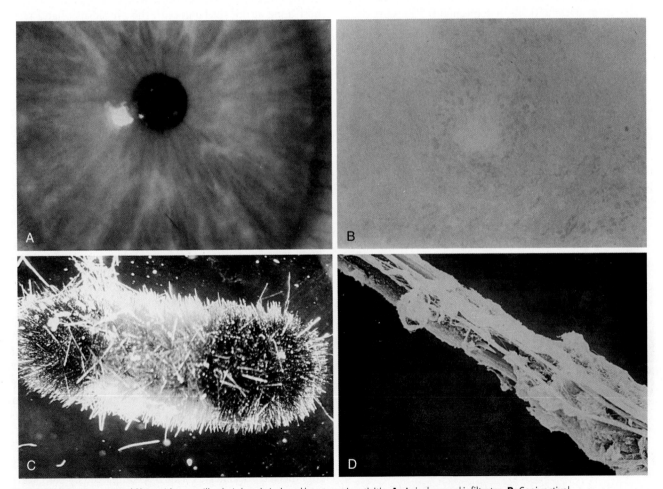

FIGURE 24.7. Four-year-old boy with caterpillar-hair (seta)–induced keratoconjunctivitis. **A:** Apical corneal infiltrates. **B:** Conjunctival foreign body granuloma (hematoxylin-eosin stain). **C:** Caterpillar with setae. **D:** Seta (scanning electron micrograph >1,000). (Courtesy of George G. Hohberger, MD, Mayo Clinic, with permission.)

The cornea and bulbar conjunctiva are examined directly with or without magnification. The palpebral conjunctiva of the lower eyelid and the inferior cul-de-sac can be examined by pulling down the lower eyelid and having the patient look up. Examination of the palpebral conjunctiva of he upper eyelid and the upper cul-de-sac is more difficult. "Double eversion" of the upper eyelid may be required. A single eversion of the upper eyelid can be achieved by gently grasping the eyelid at the lash line and pulling it down while placing minimal counterpressure at the upper border of the eyelid with a cotton-tipped applicator. The patient should be instructed to look down during the procedure. Elevation of the lid margin, counterpressure at the upper border, and gentle lid rotation usually everts the lid (Fig. 24.8). "Double eversion" of the upper eyelid is accomplished by substituting a Desmarres retractor for the cotton-tipped applicator and pulling the eyelid forward as it is rolled around the retractor (Fig. 24.9). A careful search for a foreign body is then made of both the palpebral conjunctiva and the cul-de-sac. Upper lid eversion produces discomfort, which can be minimized by instructing the patient to look down continually.

If a foreign body is found, it can usually be easily removed. Adequate anesthesia is obtained with topical anesthetics (proparacaine 0.5% or tetracaine 0.5%). One drop is usually adequate, but additional applications at intervals of 3 to 5 minutes may be necessary. Young children may require generous amounts of vocal reassurance, or, if it is unsuccessful, sedation or a brief general anesthesia.

Before the removal of a foreign body in the conjunctiva, the underlying sclera should be examined to rule out a penetrating injury. If the conjunctiva, as well as the retained foreign body, is not easily movable over the underlying sclera, or, if the foreign body appears fixed to deeper structures of the globe, an accompanying scleral injury should be suspected. Further manipulations and treatment should be carried out in the operating room, under the operating microscope.

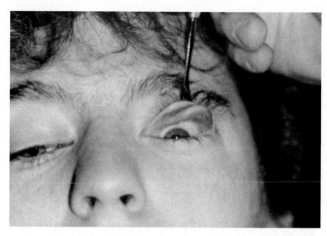

FIGURE 24.9. "Double" eversion of upper eyelid with Desmarre's retractor. (From Catalano RA, ed. *Ocular emergencies*. Philadelphia, PA: WB Saunders Co, 1992, with permission.)

If the foreign body appears to be adherent to only the cornea or conjunctiva, it can be removed with a foreign body spud, fine forceps (jewelers or tying forceps), or the edge of a medium-bore needle (22-gauge). This is best done at the slit lamp with the physician's hand resting on the patient's cheekbone. This position lessens the chance of striking the globe with a sharp object; any movement of the patient is automatically followed by the physician's hand (Fig. 24.10). Many foreign bodies can also be removed by applying a bland ophthalmic ointment (Lacri-Lube, Duratears) to the end of a cotton-tipped applicator and swabbing the foreign body, a safer approach to use when a slit lamp is not available. Although this technique removes loose or recently occurring foreign bodies, it is less effective with foreign bodies that have been present for a longer duration and have become more adherent. Once a conjunctival foreign body is removed, further treatment is usually not indicated. Once a corneal foreign body is removed, the treatment should follow the guidelines outlined later for corneal abrasions. Iron-containing corneal foreign bodies often leave a deposit of rust that may spread into the deeper layers of the cornea. The residual rust often resolves with time but can cause persistent foreign-body-like complaints. The rust ring can be scraped with a dull object, like a foreign body spud, or removed with a mechanical corneal bur (a battery-operated low-speed drill).

A corneal abrasion is one of the most common ocular complaints seen in an emergency setting. The epithelium covering the cornea is distinct in morphology and function from the conjunctival epithelium, with which it is continuous. When the corneal epithelium is scratched, abraded, or denuded, it exposes the underlying basement layer and superficial corneal nerves. This is accompanied by pain, tearing, and photophobia. Extensive abrasions can also cause a significant drop in visual acuity because the underlying layers do not offer the same smooth, reflective surface as

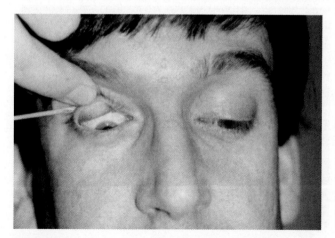

FIGURE 24.8. Eversion of upper eyelid with cotton applicator. (From Catalano RA, ed. *Ocular emergencies*. Philadelphia, PA: WB Saunders Co, 1992, with permission.)

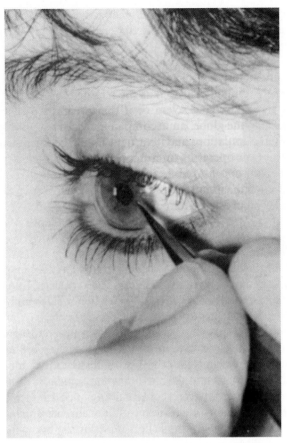

FIGURE 24.10. Method to remove foreign body at the slit lamp. The foreign body is approached obliquely from the side, lessening the chance of striking the globe with a sharp object. (From Catalano RA, ed. *Ocular emergencies.* Philadelphia, PA: WB Saunders Co, 1992, with permission.)

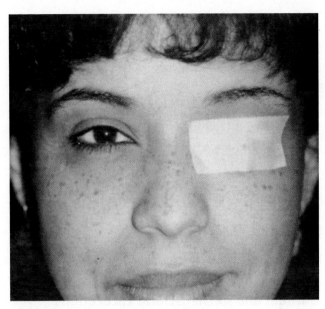

FIGURE 24.11. Immobilization of eyelids with 1-inch tape across eyelid margins. (From Catalano, RA, ed. *Ocular emergencies.* Philadelphia, PA: WB Saunders Co, 1992, with permission.)

the normal corneal epithelium. The diagnosis can usually be made by penlight alone, when the usual smooth, glistening tear film overlying the epithelium is disrupted. If possible, slit-lamp confirmation to determine the depth of the abrasion is indicated. Minute amounts of fluorescein dye, with or without the use of a cobalt-60 filtered light source, can also be used for confirmation and exact delineation.

The treatment of corneal abrasions is directed at promoting healing and relieving pain. Small abrasions can be treated with frequent applications of topical antibacterials (drops or ointment) with or without immobilization of the lid with a patch. In children, an antibiotic ointment is generally preferred because it does not have to be administered as frequently and stings less than drops. Steroid preparations are contraindicated as they slow epithelial healing and increase susceptibility to secondary infection.

Larger abrasions usually require lid immobilization for comfort, but controlled studies have not demonstrated any difference in the rate of healing or in reported discomfort with or without eye patching (40,41). Applying a small ribbon of 2.5-cm (1-inch) tape horizontally across the lash margin may be a simpler yet effective method of stabilizing

the lid (Fig. 24.11) without patching. In young children, pressure patches should be avoided as they are typically quickly pulled off by the child. In addition, patients with contact-lens-related abrasions should never be patched because they are much more susceptible to infectious keratitis from pathogens initially residing on the contact lens or in lens solutions. It is theorized that the increased temperature under the patch and patient's decreased ability to monitor their visual acuity also contribute to the increased risk of infection in these patients (42).

Most corneal abrasions completely heal within 24 to 72 hours. Patients with larger abrasions should be followed until epithelial healing has occurred, and antibiotics should be continued until the eye is symptom free for 24 hours. If a patch is used, it should not be left in place longer than 24 hours. Topical anesthetics result in almost immediate relief of pain but are toxic to the epithelium. There is no indication for their prolonged use. Ophthalmic nonsteroidal anti-inflammatory drugs and cycloplegia are better choices to reduce the pain associated with simple corneal abrasion, and they do not delay healing (43).

Thermal and Chemical Burns of the Cornea

Almost all foreign substances that enter the eye cause a burning sensation, but heat and chemicals can produce a sustained burn injury to the eye. Alkalis saponify phospholipid membranes leading to epithelial cell death and deep penetration into the eye. Acids damage the eye by causing a coagulation necrosis that can result in corneal scarring and ulceration (44). The ultimate vision with a burn to the eye is highly dependent on the initial treatment rendered. Immediate irrigation with copious amounts of moderately warm water at low pressure for at least 30 minutes is the mainstay of the initial (in the field) treatment of chemical burns. In the hospital, amphoteric buffer solutions, Ringer's lactate or normal saline is typically used as the irrigant, and a Morgan lens may be used to keep the flow directed onto the eye (45). The "normal" pH of the eye ranges from 6.5 to 8.0. During irrigation, the pH should be reassessed every 15 minutes using pH paper and if only one eye is affected, the pH of the uninvolved eye should be measured for comparison. Depending on the chemical, irrigation may need to be continued for hours and the pH should be assessed 5 and 30 minutes after irrigation to ensure that the chemical has been flushed completely. Topical analgesia with proparacaine or tetracaine is often used adjunctively, and the eyelids should be everted and fornices should be swept to dislodge any retained chemical.

Corneal and Corneoscleral Lacerations

Lacerations of the globe can be caused by injuries with sharp objects or by high-energy blunt objects smaller than the orbital opening. Many injuries of the latter type occur in sports and recreation (e.g., with a fast-moving ball in a racket sport) and are entirely preventable.

The goals of therapy are the restoration of normal anatomy and the prevention and treatment of complicating factors, such as infection and glaucoma. In young children, however, a significant complicating condition can be amblyopia, and the ultimate visual outcome is heavily dependent on its management (46,47).

Standard ophthalmic surgical practices prevail in the management of pediatric corneal and corneoscleral lacerations. A complete systemic evaluation to look for other injuries should be undertaken, especially if other injuries would preclude prompt treatment of the ocular injury or require concomitant treatment while the patient is anesthetized. Treatment with broad-spectrum antibiotics as a prophylactic measure should be initiated immediately.

Fibrin glue and cyanoacrylate tissue adhesive are both effective in closing corneal perforations up to 3 mm in diameter (48). Because tissue adhesive only adheres to dry surfaces devoid of epithelium, polymerizes on contact, and creates a rough surface, it should be applied sparingly under microscopic visualization. In addition, the aqueous chamber should be reformed with viscoelastic substance if necessary to prevent iris incarceration into the wound. A loose fitting, low water content disposable soft contact lens is placed on top of the glue for patient comfort (49). If surgery is required, small-filament nonabsorbable suture (e.g., 10-0 nylon) is used to obtain watertight edge-to-edge closure. Uncontaminated extruded uveal tissue should be repositioned in most cases. Retinal detachments and tears are generally repaired secondarily. Specific recommendations of surgical technique are beyond the scope of this chapter.

Obvious lenticular injury strongly suggests primary lensectomy, although restoring ocular integrity is of primary importance. Subsequent cataract extraction with intraocular lens implantation, even when combined with a penetrating keratoplasty, may still allow for excellent results (47).

Repair of a corneal or corneoscleral laceration should be undertaken as soon as possible. However, in a general hospital, careful consideration must be given to whether or not repair is scheduled as an emergency in the middle of the night or as an urgent case the next day. When the usual complement of a skilled ophthalmic operating room staff is not available for an emergency repair, delaying the repair until skilled staff is available may provide the best results. A delayed repair (up to 36 hours) has not been shown to be a poor prognostic factor (50).

Injuries to the Iris

A blunt ocular contusion can injure the iris sphincter muscle, resulting in pupillary constriction (*traumatic miosis*) during the first several hours, followed by dilation (*traumatic mydriasis*). Patients present with pain, photophobia, perilimbal conjunctival injection, and anisocoria. An accommodative spasm or paralysis may be associated, resulting in blurred vision and difficulty with near tasks. Signs include inflammatory or pigment cells in the anterior chamber (*traumatic iritis*) and iris sphincter tears, both of which are recognizable on slit-lamp examination. Additionally, the pupil does not constrict to light stimulation as briskly as the unaffected eye or dilate as rapidly when the illumination is reduced. Pharmacologic testing with pilocarpine 1% usually demonstrates reduced sensitivity, which is useful in distinguishing traumatic mydriasis from parasympathetic denervation (e.g., Adie's pupil), in which the iris is suprasensitive.

In addition to direct contusion injury to the iris, mydriasis can be caused by traumatic injury to the ciliary ganglion (a rare complication of orbital floor fractures). Miosis can be a component of traumatic Horner's syndrome, due to injury of the carotid plexus, cervical ganglion, cervical spine, or brainstem. Accompanying features of this syndrome are ipsilateral ptosis (lid droop), anhidrosis (decreased sweating), and relative enophthalmos (recession of the eye within the orbit).

A direct blow to the eye may also cause a cellular reaction in the anterior chamber (traumatic iritis), which may be difficult to distinguish from a microhyphema. A hyphema is characterized by red blood cells in the anterior chamber, as opposed to the white blood cells of iritis. Allowing the patient to sit quietly for several minutes allows the cells, which can be dispersed with patient movement, to layer, possibly making correct identification easier. The diagnosis is always hyphema when both red and white blood cells are present in the anterior chamber, which is actually typical. Other disorders in the differential diagnosis of traumatic iritis include long-standing, untreated corneal abrasions and traumatic retinal detachments, both of which can result in a secondary anterior chamber reaction. Pigment in the anterior vitreous (tobacco dust) is seen also in retinal detachments.

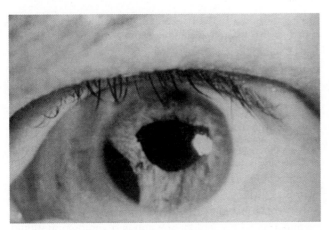

FIGURE 24.12. Iridodialysis. (From Catalano RA, ed. *Ocular emergencies.* Philadelphia: WB Saunders Co, 1992, with permission.)

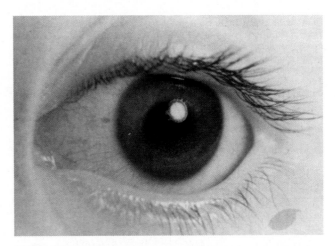

FIGURE 24.13. Hyphema. (From Catalano RA, ed. *Ocular emergencies.* Philadelphia, PA: WB Saunders Co, 1992, with permission.)

The treatment of traumatic mydriasis or miosis is supportive. Mild degrees of traumatic iritis may be treated with cycloplegia alone (e.g., cyclopentolate 1% or 2%, 4 times a day) for relief of spasm and pain. More severe iritis should also be treated with a topical corticosteroid (e.g., prednisolone acetate 0.125% or 1%, 3 or 4 times a day). Corticosteroids reduce the formation of anterior and posterior synechiae (abnormal adhesions of the iris to the cornea and lens, respectively). Both medications are tapered over several days.

Disinsertion of the iris at its root (*iridodialysis*) is characterized by polycoria (the appearance of multiple pupils) and a D-shaped pupillary aperture (Fig. 24.12). Its occurrence is usually accompanied by hyphema. Rare iris injuries include iris atrophy and iridoschisis (a split within the iris stroma). Patients with an iris injury often experience glare and photophobia and may have diplopia. A tinted contact lens or a dyed lens with an artificial pupil (available through *CIBA Vision Special Eyes Program*) can reduce these symptoms and conceal the cosmetic deformity. Sphincterotomy with the neodymium:yttrium-aluminum-garnet (Nd:YAG) laser (in aphakic and pseudophakic eyes) or argon laser (phakic eyes) may clear the central visual axis and improve visual acuity in patients with an eccentric pupil. Surgical repair of sphincter lacerations and tears can be accomplished by using the suture technique described by McCannel (51) or by using a scleral tunnel incision and double-armed 10-0 polypropylene suture (52).

Any iris abnormality should be clearly documented because other physicians may mistake pupillary asymmetry or irregularity as a sign of third cranial nerve dysfunction, related to uncal herniation.

Traumatic Hyphema

Blunt ocular injury causing a tear in the face of the anterior ciliary body is the most common cause of hyphema (bleeding into the anterior chamber) (Fig. 24.13). If a history of trauma is not elicited in a child with hyphema, one should suspect leukemia, hemophilia, juvenile xanthogranuloma, retinoblastoma, a fictitious history by the child, or child abuse. Hyphemas that occur following intraocular surgery resorb usually within days without sequelae, but the physician should be cognizant of a potential consequent rise in intraocular pressure.

Most patients with hyphema present with pain, photophobia and decreased visual acuity. The latter may improve remarkably if the blood is allowed to settle below the visual axis. Young children may be somnolent (53). The history should elicit the mechanism of injury and any complicating factors, such as a bleeding disorder, anticoagulant therapy, kidney or liver disease, or sickle cell disease or trait. A careful examination is mandatory, because one-third of hyphema patients have other ocular injuries (54). The intraocular pressure (IOP) may initially be low due to ciliary body shutdown, but it rises to elevated levels (>21 mmHg) in approximately one-third of patients within several days and should be closely monitored (53). Patients with sickle cell disease or trait are at high risk of elevated IOP within the first 24 hours (55,56). Hyphemas are graded at presentation based on the amount of blood present in the anterior chamber (Table 24.1). Gonioscopy in the early stages may reveal the site of bleeding and can confirm the presence of angle recession.

The management of traumatic hyphema is variable and controversial (54,57). There is no consensus as to whether patients should be at strict bed rest or allowed limited ambulation and whether they can watch television or read. There is also no agreement as to the efficacy of hospitalization, occlusion of one or both eyes, patching of the traumatized eye, cycloplegics, topical or systemic corticosteroids, and antifibrinolytic agents (58). Community standards often dictate hospitalization policies. Randomized trials comparing treatment modalities have not been performed, although there are reports in the literature that the outpatient management of traumatic hyphemas, even in the pediatric population,

Table 24.1

GRADING OF HYPHEMA

Grade	Percentage of Anterior Chamber Grade Filled with Blood
Microscopic	Circulation of red blood cells only, no layering
I	<33%
II	33–50%
III	50–95%
IV	100% (total or "eight ball" hyphema)

results in rebleed rates within the range reported for hospitalized children (59,60).

Hospitalization should be considered based on the patient's age (toddlers are unlikely to be easily constrained at home), probability of noncompliance (immature patients or those without assistance at home), and the likelihood of developing complications (patients with sickle cell disease or trait or those with elevated intraocular pressure at presentation). Patients with a rebleed are more likely to develop complications and should be hospitalized. Risk factors for this may be the presence of high intraocular pressure and low vision at the time of first examination (61). In one study, African-American children appeared to be at greater risk for developing a secondary hemorrhage, unrelated to the presence of sickle cell hemoglobinopathy (62). In another study, the presence of posterior segment injuries was more directly related to a poor visual outcome than the occurrence of secondary hemorrhage (63).

Antifibrinolytic agents (aminocaproic acid, tranexamic acid) may be used in populations with high rebleed rates (lower socioeconomic status, urban, younger age, delayed time from injury to admission) (64,65), although in one study their use did not result in a significantly lower incidence of rebleeds than the use of topical steroids alone (66). The side effects of nausea, vomiting, postural hypotension, tinnitus, lethargy, raised intraocular pressure (67), and hematuria should also be considered when making this decision. Contraindications include pregnancy and a cardiac, hepatic, renal, or intravascular clotting disorder. Relative contraindications include sickle cell disease or trait and total hyphema, because these agents reduce the rate of resorption of blood.

Suggested treatment of traumatic hyphema is presented in Table 24.2, and indications for surgical evacuation of the clot, which is required in approximately 5% of patients (55,57), are reviewed in Table 24.3.

Rebleeds usually occur from the second to the fifth day following injury. They are frequently of greater magnitude than the original hemorrhage and more likely to be associated with elevated intraocular pressure. An increase in size of the hyphema, particularly the presence of bright red blood over darker, clotted blood, confirms this occurrence. Secondary hemorrhage significantly reduces the visual prognosis (68). If rebleeding does not occur, cycloplegic agents and steroids are tapered beginning on the sixth day after injury, with the rapidity of tapering based on the presence of anterior chamber inflammation. Antiglaucoma medication may have to be continued indefinitely. The patient should continue to refrain from strenuous exercise and wear an eye shield at night for an additional 2 weeks. Normal activities can resume 1 month after injury. A dilated fundus examination with scleral depression and gonioscopy should be performed 1 month after injury. Recession of the anterior chamber angle occurs in up to 85% of patients with hyphema (68); these patients should be examined annually as they are at an increased risk for glaucoma, which can occur years after the injury.

Injuries to the Lens

Cataract or lens subluxation secondary to ocular contusion injuries is often associated with severe posterior segment sequelae and poor visual outcomes (69). Trauma is the most common cause of *dislocation of the lens* (Fig. 24.14). Other causes include congenital dislocation, systemic syndrome (e.g., Marfan's, homocystinuria), inflammation, and buphthalmos.

Traumatic dislocation results when contusion-induced equatorial expansion of the eye disrupts the zonule. A complete rupture results in a free-floating ("luxated") lens; partial severance results in a "subluxated" lens. Symptoms of dislocation are fluctuating vision, glare, monocular diplopia, and decreased vision, the last resulting from functional aphakia or induced astigmatism.

A partial dislocation is occasionally difficult to diagnose. The pupil should be dilated and the lens examined using retroillumination at the slit lamp. The zonules can often be seen with a gonioscopy lens. Visualization of vitreous between broken zonules or seeing the edge of the lens within the pupil confirms the diagnosis. Additional signs are shallowing (or deepening) of the anterior chamber, iridodonesis (movement of the iris with ocular movement), and phacodonesis (fine movement of the lens on ocular movement). Patients with a dislocated lens are always evaluated for other signs of ocular injury.

Complications of dislocated lenses include refractive disorders, pupillary block glaucoma, and lenticular-corneal touch. Incomplete rupture of the zonule causes the lens to be drawn to the side of the intact zonular fibers. If the lens is dislocated out of the visual axis, functional aphakia results. If the edge of the lens lies on the visual axis, astigmatism and monocular diplopia can result. Pupillary block occurs when the dislocated lens occludes the pupillary aperture. An anteriorly dislocated lens can also touch the posterior cornea, damaging the endothelial cells. Rarely, nonpupillary block glaucoma

Table 24.2

TREATMENT OF HYPHEMA

Suggested Orders	Comment
Hospitalization	Young children and elderly; all patients with rebleeds.
Bed rest	Reliable adults and older children with microhyphema may be treated with bed rest at home, if community standards allow. They should be examined daily for 5 additional days, refrain from any activity, and return immediately, if any pain or decrease in vision occurs. With the head of the bed elevated 30°; bathroom privileges with assistance.
Sedation as needed	Lorazepam (Ativan): *Adults and older children:* 2–3 mg/dL q8–12h PO. Chloral hydrate: *children:* 50 mg/kg tid. *Younger children:* consult with pediatrician.
Laxative of choice	Adults only.
Shield involved eye	Patch only if there is an associated corneal abrasion.
Eye rest	May watch television at a distance, no prolonged reading or near visual tasks.
Cycloplegia	Atropine 1% or Cyclopentolate 1% topically tid to qid.
Topical steroids	Prednisolone acetate 1% q2–6h, if a fibrinous anterior chamber reaction develops.
No aspirin products	Use acetaminophen with or without codeine for analgesia.
Antiemetic, as needed	Prochlorperazine (Compazine): *Adults:* 10 mg IM q8h, or 25-mg suppository q 12 h; *children:* 0.13 mg/kg body weight IM, or 2.5-mg suppository bid to tid. Promethazine hydrochloride (Phenergan): *Adults:* 25-mg IM, or suppository q4–6h; *children:* 1.1 mg/kg (maximum dose, 25 mg). The safety of these medications in children < 9 kg or < 2 y in age has not been established.
Antiglaucoma medications	For elevations of intraocular pressure >40 mmHg at presentation, or >30 mmHg for 2 wk or more subsequently (20 mmHg in those with sickle cell trait or disease): *First-line:* Topical β-blocker (e.g., levobunolol or timolol 0.25% tid). *Second-line:* Acetazolamide 5 mg/kg PO 3–4 times daily. (In sickle cell use, methazolamide [Neptazane] 50 mg bid to tid.) *Third-line:* Mannitol 1–2 g/kg IV over 45 min once every 24 h
Antifibrinolytic agents	Aminocaproic acid (Amicar): Use based on community standards and patient presentation (see text); dose is 50 mg/kg PO q4h (maximum 30 g/dL). *If no rebleeding occurs:* halve dose on day 3 and discontinue on day 4. Be cognizant that intraocular pressure may rise suddenly on cessation of use. *If rebleeding occurs:* continue Amicar for 5 additional days, check clotting studies, bleeding time, platelet count.
Laboratory studies	Complete blood count; clotting studies, platelet count, and liver function tests, if history of bleeding disorder. Baseline creatinine and blood urea nitrogen (BUN) if aminocaproic acid is to be used. Sickle cell prep, hemoglobin electrophoresis in black patients.
Surgical evacuation of clot	See Table 24.3 for indications.

h, hours; PO, by mouth; qid, four times a day; tid, three times a day.

can result from misdirection of aqueous humor or anterior displacement of the lens-iris diaphragm. This is suggested by shallowing of the central anterior chamber, absence of lens movement, and myopic shift in refraction. Nonpupillary block is treated with cycloplegic-mydriatic agents to relax the ciliary body and allow for posterior movement of the lens-iris diaphragm. As with any disorder simulating malignant glaucoma, iridectomy and miotics may worsen this condition.

Table 24.3

INDICATIONS FOR SURGICAL EVACUATION OF CLOT IN HYPHEMA

Indication	Comment
Elevated intraocular pressure (IOP);	IOP >50 mmHg for 5 d IOP >35 mmHg for 7 d
unresponsive to medical therapy	IOP >25 mmHg for 1 d in patients with sickle cell disease or trait or preexisting glaucoma
Corneal bloodstaining	At the first sign of bloodstaining, regardless of TOP or grade of hyphema If IOP >25 mmHg and total hyphema to prevent bloodstaining
Prolonged clot duration	Persistent total hyphema >5 d Persistent small hyphema >10 d

IOP, intraocular pressure.

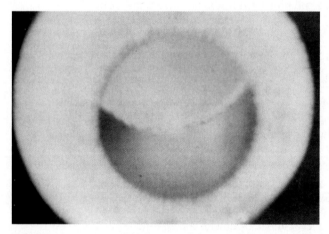

FIGURE 24.14. Traumatic dislocation of the ocular lens. (From Catalano RA, ed. *Ocular emergencies.* Philadelphia, PA: WB Saunders Co, 1992, with permission.)

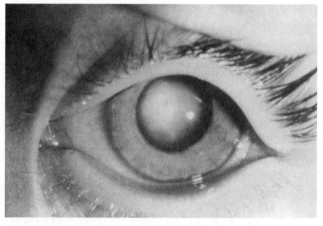

FIGURE 24.15. Contusion cataract. (From Catalano RA, ed. *Ocular emergencies.* Philadelphia, PA: WB Saunders Co, 1992, with permission.)

A noncataractous, dislocated lens may be stable and asymptomatic for years. The patient, however, should be forewarned of the symptoms of pupillary block glaucoma and advised to wear eye protection for sports and hazardous labor. Contact lenses can be used to correct an induced aphakic or astigmatic refractive error. These are preferable to spectacles because they produce less image size disparity with the normal eye (aniseikonia). Pupillary constriction or dilation occasionally improves visual acuity. Patients treated with miotics should be informed of the possibility of pupillary block glaucoma. Patients treated with mydriatics should be warned of possible dislocation of the lens into the anterior chamber and corneal decompensation. In some cases, the Nd:YAG laser can be used to lyse the remaining zonules, achieving a clear aphakic visual axis. Indications for surgical removal of a dislocated lens include pupillary block, corneal touch, inflammation, and decreased vision.

A *contusion cataract* results when the lens capsule is ruptured by a direct or contrecoup injury. In addition to lenticular opacification (Fig. 24.15), affected patients present with decreased vision, elevated intraocular pressure, and/ or intraocular inflammation. The rapidity of cataract formation depends on whether the lens capsule was ruptured. In the absence of rupture, a cataract may not develop for months; with rupture, the lens can become hydrated and cataractous within hours. Not every cataract is progressive; a small rent may self-seal with the development of a fibrous plaque at the site of the injury. When the visual acuity is not appreciably reduced and glaucoma or inflammation is not present, the preferred management is observation. Miotics may be helpful in reducing glare and diplopia may be induced by focal opacities.

As with subluxated lenses, the evaluation should include an assessment of associated injuries, as well as the location and extent of lens injury. The status of the posterior capsule and presence of any zonular rupture (dislocation of the lens) are the two most important factors in surgical planning. The lens capsule can usually be assessed at the slit lamp, but, occasionally, a fibrinous reaction in the anterior chamber, or opacification of the lens, prevents an adequate assessment. A water-bath ultrasound may be helpful in these instances. If the posterior capsule is ruptured, a pars plana approach may be prudent to minimize the risk of nuclear dislocation into the vitreous.

Any injury to the lens may also produce amblyopia from occlusion or anisometropia in very young children (under age 9). Removal of an only partially cataractous lens or a subluxated lens, whose edge is in the pupil, may become necessary if its persistence is thought to be a more potent amblyogenic factor than surgical aphakia or pseudophakia

Even in patients in their late teens, progressive axial myopia associated with traumatic glaucoma can occur (70). Lens-induced glaucoma can result from two mechanisms other than pupillary block. High-molecular-weight lens proteins liberated by trauma (lens particle glaucoma) can block the trabecular meshwork. Additionally, denatured lens material from a cataractous lens can leak through an intact lens capsule and be engulfed by macrophages that clog the anterior chamber angle (*phacolytic glaucoma*). Lens-induced glaucoma is suspected when a break in the lens capsule and fluffy white particles in the anterior chamber and chamber angle are seen on slit-lamp examination. Phacolytic glaucoma is suspected by the presence of iridescent particles, cells, and protein flare. Similar particles may be present on the surface of the lens capsule and in the anterior chamber angle, which is typically open on gonioscopic examination. Phacolytic glaucoma is confirmed by the presence of macrophages filled with lens material on microscopic examination of aqueous humor obtained by paracentesis. Both problems are treated with corticosteroids (e.g., prednisolone acetate 1% every 6 hours in lens-induced glaucoma and as frequently as every hour in phacolytic glaucoma) and antiglaucoma medications (e.g., timolol or levobunolol 0.5% every 12 hours; acetazolamide 500 mg initially, followed by 250 mg every 6 hours; or mannitol 1 to 2 g/kg intravenously over 45 minutes); and topical cycloplegia (e.g., cyclopentolate 1% every 8 hours). Cataract extraction is performed after the intraocular pressure has been brought under control (usually within 24 to 36 hours).

Injuries to the Posterior Pole of the Eye

Severe blows to the eye can result in a myriad of posterior pole injuries ranging from intraretinal hemorrhages; retinal edema, tears, detachment, and dialysis; choroidal and chorioretinal ruptures; and avulsion of the optic nerve head. The latter results usually in total loss of vision; the severity of other posterior pole injuries is correlated with involvement of the fovea.

Severe trauma can result in a concussive injury to axonal transport. This disruption in the nerve fiber layer is termed *commotio retinae* when it occurs in the retinal periphery and traumatic macular edema (Berlin's edema), if it involves the macular region. In either case, the affected retina takes on a gray, translucent appearance. With macular edema the foveal reflex is lost. Intraretinal hemorrhages may be concomitant if the retinal capillary circulation is disrupted. These may break through into the vitreous over several days, obscuring the view of the underlying retina. Mild *commotio retinae* and traumatic macular edema may resolve over a few days, but, when associated with intraretinal hemorrhages, these disorders may result in retinal atrophy, pigment scarring, and atrophic holes. In the absence of other injuries the treatment is supportive. The patient should be instructed to wear dark sunglasses to prevent exacerbating light damage to the retina. Small atrophic holes do not usually cause a retinal detachment. Even large macular holes may spontaneously resolve (71). Larger holes, however, often portend retinal tissue loss and, consequently, a less favorable prognosis (72).

Choroidal and chorioretinal ruptures are less common than traumatic macular edema and *commotio retinae*. They occur when greater force impacts the eye, causing significant distortion of the globe and stretching of the choroid. Larger ruptures result in subretinal hemorrhage, which obscures visualization of the underlying choroid. With time the hematoma resorbs, and the rupture becomes visible as a white concentric streak, which actually represents exposure of the underlying sclera. Visual disability is related to the presence or absence of foveal involvement, and a late complication is the development of choroidal neovascularization. In one study, the proximity of the rupture to the center of the fovea and the length of the rupture were associated with the subsequent development of neovascularization (73).

Retinal tears and retinal dialysis are usually consequent to severe impact directly over the retina of a small object with considerable force such as that from a pellet gun. They typically involve the ora or equator and may require cryotherapy or surgery to prevent recurrent detachment.

Traumatic optic neuropathy (TON) describes an insult to the optic nerve secondary to trauma. TON can be either "direct" or "indirect". Direct TON occurs when a fracture in the midfacial area severs the optic nerve. Indirect TON occurs when a blunt traumatic force is transmitted to the orbital apex (74). The presenting signs of the two types are often indistinguishable. In either instance, damage most commonly occurs posterior to the entrance of the central retinal vessels and the optic disk appears normal (75). Patients typically present with acute loss of vision and an afferent pupillary defect. Damage to the optic nerve anterior to this point will cause the optic nerve to appear swollen and is accompanied by retinal hemorrhage(s). Optic atrophy is a late sign of TON, typically becoming evident 6 weeks after injury (76). Neither megadose corticosteroids or optic canal decompression has been shown to be of any benefit in these patients (75,77).

Optic nerve head avulsion represents the most severe of blunt ocular injuries. It results when a blunt, small object strikes the globe from the infratemporal margin and severely compresses it against the orbital roof (78). It most commonly occurs with motor vehicle or bicycle accidents, sporting injuries, falls, or in children of approximately 135 cm in height from being struck in the eye by an opening door handle (79). The affected eye presents with a brisk afferent pupillary defect and no light perception to trace light perception in the temporal field. Widespread retinal infarction occurs, which is manifest by preretinal hemorrhages obscuring the optic disc, florid blot retinal hemorrhages, marked swelling of the retina, and a cherry red spot at the macula. Vitreous hemorrhage develops within a few hours. No treatment is useful, and recovery does not occur.

CHILD ABUSE

Despite many years of heightened awareness, both socially and politically, physical abuse and neglect of children remain an all too frequent and tragic occurrence. The National Child Abuse and Neglect Data System reported 693,174 unique cases of confirmed child abuse in 2009 (80). Physical abuse constituted 17.8% of cases, and the vast majority of perpetrators (80.9%) included a parent. Of the 1,676 fatal episodes, almost 80.8% occurred in children under age 4 years and 46.2% in children under age 1 year.

All states require health professionals to report child abuse, even if it is only suspected, and the statutes generally protect the reporting professional acting in good faith. A thorough ophthalmologic examination can often provide early evidence of child abuse. Furthermore, this condition is high on the list of systemic conditions whose successful management requires input from ophthalmologists for improved outcome. However, almost no other area of multidisciplinary management demands more caution in interpretation of findings, because *many* of the ophthalmic manifestations seen in child abuse can have other causes. A governmental agency's declaration of "confirmed" child abuse supported by an examining ophthalmologist's interpretation of typical signs can save a child's life if it is correct (81), or tragically tear a family apart, if in error (82).

Child abuse cuts across all racial and socioeconomic strata. There is no typical profile of an abusive parent or guardian, although over 80% of the perpetrators are between the ages of 20 and 49 years (80).

Forethought into the ophthalmologic examination in a suspected case of child abuse is required. When a history of trauma is omitted or denied, it is incumbent on the ophthalmologist to look for nontraumatic causes, or associated non-ocular findings that could also signal a non-traumatic condition. For example, when retinal hemorrhages are present, causes such as infection, anemia, and platelet disorders, should be investigated. A contrasting situation occurs with a "spontaneous" hyphema; in this instance the lack of cutaneous lesions consistent with juvenile xanthogranuloma should raise the index of suspicion of abuse. A more difficult situation arises when a parent or guardian gives a history of trauma, but the findings are inconsistent with the events of the admitted injury, such as a traumatic cataract allegedly sustained by being struck by another toddler.

Nonaccidental injury of children usually takes one of two forms: either the abuse results in obvious injuries (e.g., burns, bone fractures, cutaneous lacerations) or the child was violently shaken, resulting in thoracic compression as well as cranial injury from rapidly reversing head movements. Ophthalmic manifestations (e.g., hemorrhages) can occur in either case.

External and Anterior Segment Manifestations of Child Abuse

Injuries affecting the adnexae and anterior segment are noted less frequently in child abuse than vitreoretinal and optic nerve findings. However, the presence of these anterior segment abnormalities strongly suggests severe injury and poor visual prognosis (83).

Direct blows to the head and face can cause hyphema, corneal abrasion, lens subluxation and/or cataract, subconjunctival hemorrhage, lid laceration, and ecchymosis. Nonaccidental chemical injuries may cause cutaneous burns, conjunctivitis, and/or keratitis (84–86).

While periorbital injuries, such as burns, abrasions, and lacerations, can be consistent with or even suggest intentional injury, anterior segment trauma (corneal abrasion, hyphema, ectopia lentis, and some cataracts) is usually more nonspecific, prompting a careful search for other evidence of injury. Exceptions to the nonspecificity of these injuries include traumatic types of cataracts (Vossius' ring and anterior or posterior subcapsular rosettes) (87) and ectopia lentis. Lens dislocations from nonaccidental trauma have been reported in all directions except upward, which is the usual direction of displacement in Marfan's syndrome, one of the leading causes of nontraumatic ectopia lentis (88).

Posterior Segment Manifestations

Retinal and/or vitreous hemorrhages are the most commonly recognized posterior manifestations of child abuse (Fig. 24.16) (89,90). They occur in 6% to 24% of all abused

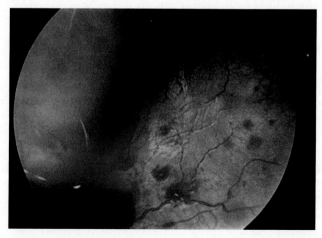

FIGURE 24.16. Retinal, preretinal, and vitreous hemorrhages in an infant with confirmed physical abuse.

children and are even more common (50% to 80%) in the shaken baby syndrome (83,91). They usually take the form of superficial (flame-shaped) hemorrhages in the posterior pole but can affect deeper layers and more peripheral locations as well. The intensity of hemorrhage correlates with the severity of neurologic injury (92) but does not appear to be related to sustained elevated intracranial pressure, elevated intrathoracic pressure, direct tracking of blood from the intracranial space, or direct impact trauma (93). Retinal hemorrhages in children under age 3 years should suggest nonaccidental trauma, because their occurrence due to true accidental trauma is uncommon (94). Further, the presence of any retinal or optic nerve sheath hemorrhage in an infant, in the absence of an appropriate explanation for these findings, should raise suspicion of child abuse (95). Cardiopulmonary resuscitation, employed in the most severe cases of child abuse or neglect, is recognized as only an infrequent cause of the retinal hemorrhages seen in some of these children (96,97). Significant vitreous hemorrhage is a poor prognostic sign for vision in abused children (98), but the major cause of vision loss in child abuse is brain injury (99).

Almost all other forms of retinal or optic nerve trauma can be seen also in child abuse. Retinal detachment, dialysis, vitreoretinal traction (100), perimacular folds (100,101), and optic nerve avulsion have all been reported in abused children. Traumatic hemorrhagic macular retinoschisis, similar in appearance to a preretinal hemorrhage but occurring in deeper layers, is common in shaken babies and is more suggestive of this etiology than the other nonspecific entities just mentioned (102,103). Optic nerve sheath hemorrhages are also possible (104) and, in fact, are indicative of trauma when found on postmortem examination (105).

SPORTS AND OTHER RECREATIONAL INJURIES

The National Electronic Injury Surveillance System estimated that there were 30,630 sports and recreational eye injuries in 2002, with more than 14,000 of them occurring in individuals younger than age 15 (106). Further, the American Academy of Pediatrics notes that most eye injuries in children aged 11 to 14 are sports related (107). The distribution of injuries among various sports is age-dependent (Table 24.4) (108). Basketball and baseball lead the list because of their widespread distribution and popularity and respective inherent risks.

Sports-related ocular injuries occur by contact with another player, contact with a ball (or puck, shuttlecock, etc.), or interaction with the playing surface. High-risk sports include those that use small, fast projectiles (e.g., air rifles and paintball), involve close contact with other players (e.g., basketball), hard projectiles (e.g., baseball/softball, cricket, racquetball, squash) or use "sticks" (e.g., hockey, lacrosse, fencing). The highest risk sports are those where eye protection is not permitted and the goal of the sport is intentional injury (e.g., boxing, full-contact martial arts) (109).

Ocular injuries from basketball occur mostly from contact with other players (110), because the ball is much too large to make direct contact with the globe. Injuries, such as corneal abrasion, lid laceration, and traumatic iritis, generally predominate (111).

In baseball, however, injuries occur mostly from the ball or related equipment (112). The ball is small enough to injure the globe and moves much more rapidly, putting the young and/or novice player at risk for significant injury,

Table 24.4						
ESTIMATED SPORTS AND RECREATIONAL EYE INJURIES BY AGE GROUP IN 2010						
		Age (years) Percent				
Activity	**Estimated Number of Injuries**	**0–4**	**5–14**	**15–24**	**25–64**	**>65**
Basketball	5,237	0.3	24.1	53.8	21.8	0.0
Baseball	2,195	1.7	59.2	9.8	29.3	0.0
Soccer	2,015	3.2	34.2	35.8	26.8	0.0
Football	1,929	0.0	45.1	47.5	7.4	0.0
Bicycling	1,661	1.3	38.4	10.4	44.8	5.1
Toys (not specified)	2,185	45.1	20.3	5.3	28.6	0.8
Fireworks	1,617	6.3	33.9	25.5	34.3	0.0
BB's or pellets	2,125	0.8	50.1	40.1	9.0	0.0

From U.S. Consumer Products Safety Commission: Product Summary Reports, All Products Body Part = 77 (Eyeball) All Diagnoses & Products. Injury Estimates for Calendar Year 2010; National Electronic Injury Surveillance System; National Injury Information Clearinghouse.

especially if the eye is unprotected. More than three-fourth of baseball-related injuries arise from batted rather than pitched baseballs, yet eye protection is often used only while at bat (113). Hyphema, orbital contusion and/ or fractures, and corneal abrasions predominate. The peak age for baseball injuries corresponds to when baseball is introduced to children in both an organized (Little League) and an ad hoc fashion. Older children are often able to hit a baseball hard, sending it to cohorts who may lack the reflexes and/or skill to safely handle it. The potential for injury from "soft" baseballs (which are 15% to 20% of major league ball hardness) is still significant, and use of these balls still requires protective eyewear (114).

Most soccer-related ocular injuries result from being struck by a kicked ball (115). Injury to the exposed superotemporal quadrant of the retina is most common, most likely because the nose protects the nasal retina. Laboratory experiments have demonstrated that soccer balls significantly deform on impact (even when underinflated), and a small "knuckle" of the ball can enter the orbit and strike the globe (116). Expansion of the eye perpendicular to the impact is believed to be pathogenic for most injuries (117). Soccer balls are also unique in that a secondary suction effect on the orbital is believed to be produced as the ball bounces off the orbit, resulting in additional distortion of the globe (116). This has been proposed as an explanation as to why soccer-related ocular injuries are disproportionately severe (118).

Because of their potential in severity, fireworks lead the list of significant injuries sustained during nonathletic recreation. The U.S. Consumer Product Safety Commission estimated that more than 8,600 firework-related injuries were treated in hospital emergency departments in 2010, with the eye being involved in approximately 1,600 (19%) of these cases (119) (see also Table 24.4). Children under the age of 15 years constitute approximately 40% of the all firework-related injuries (119). Most firework injuries occur on or around Independence Day, and 54% of the injuries took place despite adult supervision (120). Half of all fireworks-related ocular injuries and a disproportionate number of severe injuries including blindness are caused by bottle rockets (121).

Even nonstrenuous recreational activity can result in ocular injuries when insufficient care is exercised. Fishhook ocular injuries are potentially serious, because they can produce penetrating and/or perforating wounds (122,123). Finally, the incidence of injuries from certain activities changes with the activity's popularity. Ocular injuries from pellet guns are decreasing, but paintball-gun ocular injuries

are increasing. The latter are often visually devastating and the vast majority (> 95%) occur when the participants are not wearing eye protection (124,125).

Although not a sport, laser pointers are at times maliciously pointed at other individuals. Fortunately, transient ocular exposure to laser pointer beams rarely causes long-term damage. The commonest physical sign is punctate epitheliopathy, and commonest symptom is ocular discomfort (126).

PREVENTION

Ocular injuries in children are largely preventable by the use of adequate protective eyewear (6,127). The practice of many child and youth sports teams to not require eye protection contributes to the incidence of injuries. In addition, scripted television programs rarely depict the use of adequate protective eyewear during eye-risk activities, which may further influence behavior (128). According to the United States Eye Injury Registry 78% of the injuries (for all ages and all activities) occurred when no ocular protection of any kind (protective goggles or standard or prescription spectacles) was in place (129). Specifically with respect to sports and recreation it has been estimated that the universal use of protective eyewear can reduce ocular injuries during these activities by 90% (130).

In a Joint Policy Statement, the American Academy of Pediatrics and the American Academy of Ophthalmology strongly recommended protective eyewear for all sports with any risk of eyewear (131). The only sports considered "eye safe" were track and field and gymnastics. The Policy Statement further notes that protective eyewear should be mandatory for participants who are functionally one eyed or who have had prior ocular surgery and/or trauma.

"Street wear" spectacles with standard plastic lenses as well as safety eyewear that conforms only to the requirements of ANSI Z87 and is designed for industrial or educational use do not provide satisfactory protection from sports-related ocular injuries. Sports eyewear that that conforms to the requirements of the American Society for Testing and Materials (ASTM) Standard F803 is satisfactory for most sports. Eyewear that is attached to a helmet as used in certain sports, such as youth baseball, must meet other standards specific to the sport (130). All safety eyewear should be made of polycarbonate, which is lightweight, thin and the most impact-resistant material available.

REFERENCES

1. Owens PL (AHRQ), Mutter R (AHRQ). *Emergency department visits related to eye injuries, 2008*. HCUP Statistical Brief #112. May 2011. Rockville, MD: Agency for Healthcare Research and Quality, http://www.hcup-us.ahrq.gov/reports/statbriefs/sb112.pdf. Accessed September 2011.

2. When It Comes to Eye Injuries, the Men's Eyes Have It. American Academy of Ophthalmology and the American Society of Ocular Trauma. http://www.aao.org/newsroom/release/20101006.cfm. Accessed September 2011.

3. Tomazzoli L, Renzi G, Mansoldo C. Eye injuries in childhood: a retrospective investigation of 88 cases from 1988 to 2000. *Eur J Ophthalmol* 2003;13:710.

4. Kaimbo WK, Spileers W, Missotten L. Ocular emergencies in Kinshasa. *Bull Soc Belge Ophthalmol* 2002;284:49.

5. Cascairo MA, Mazow ML, Prager TC. Pediatric ocular trauma: a retrospective study. *J Pediatr Ophthalmol Strabismus* 1994;31:312.

6. Nelson LB, Wilson TW, Jeffers JB. Eye injuries in childhood: demography, etiology, and prevention. *Pediatrics* 1989;84:438.

7. Libonati MM. General anesthesia. In: Tasman W, Jaeger EA, eds. *Duane's clinical ophthalmology*. Philadelphia, PA: Lippincott-Raven Publishers, 1995;6(1):6.

8. Jankovic S, Zuljan I, Sapunar D, et al. Clinical and radiological management of wartime eye and orbit injuries. *Mil Med* 1998;163:423.

9. Davis PC, Newman NJ. Advances in neuroimaging of the visual pathways. *Am J Ophthalmol* 1996;121:690.

10. Arey ML, Mootha VV, Whittemore AR, et al. Computed tomography in the diagnosis of occult open-globe injuries. *Ophthalmology* 2007;114:1448.

11. Ozdal MP, Mansour M, Deschenes J. Ultrasound biomicroscopic evaluation of the traumatized eyes. *Eye* 2003;17:467.

12. Serrano JC, Chalela P, Arias JD. Epidemiology of childhood ocular trauma in a northeastern Columbian region. *Arch Ophthalmol* 2003;121:1439.

13. Lee CH, Lee L, Kao LY, et al. Prognostic indicators of open globe injuries in children. *Am J Emerg Med* 2009;27:530.

14. Schmidt GW, Broman AT, Hindman HB, Grant MP. Vision survival after open globe injury predicted by classification and regression tree analysis. *Ophthalmology* 2008;115:202.

15. Garcia TA, McGetrick BS, Janik JS. Spectrum of ocular injuries in children with major trauma. *J Trauma Inj Inf Crit Care* 2005;59:169.

16. Andreoli CM, Andreoli MT, Ahuero AE, et al. Low rate of endophthalmitis in a large series of open globe injuries. *Am J Ophthalmol* 2009;147:601.

17. Holden R, Morsman DG, Davidek, GM, et al. External ocular trauma in instrumental and normal deliveries. *Br J Obstet Gynaecol* 1992;99:132.

18. Hofmann RF, Paul TO, Pentelei-Molnar J. The management of corneal birth trauma. *J Pediatr Ophthalmol Strabismus* 1981;18:45.

19. Angell LK, Robb RM, Berson FG. Visual prognosis in patients with ruptures in Descemet's membrane due to forceps injuries. *Arch Ophthalmol* 1981;99:2137.

20. Hoyt CS, Stone RD, Fromer C. Monocular axial myopia associated with neonatal eyelid closure in human infants. *Am J Ophthalmol* 1981;91:197.

21. Stein RM, Cohen EJ, Calhoun JH, et al. Corneal birth trauma managed with a contact lens. *Am J Ophthalmol* 1987;103:596.

22. Jain IS, Singh YP, Grupta SL, et al. Ocular hazards during birth. *J Pediatr Ophthalmol Strabismus* 1980;17:14.

23. Sachs D, Levin PS, Dooley K. Marginal eyelid laceration at birth. *Am J Ophthalmol* 1986;102:539.

24. Harris GJ. Canalicular laceration at birth. *Am J Ophthalmol* 1988;105:322.

25. Crawford JS. Ptosis as a result of trauma. *Can J Ophthalmol* 1974;9:244.

26. Estafanous MF, Seeley M, Traboulsi EI. Choroidal rupture associated with forceps delivery. *Am J Ophthalmol* 2000;129:819.

27. Lauer AK, Rimmer SO. Eyelid laceration in a neonate by fetal monitoring spiral electrode. *Am J Ophthalmol* 1998;125:715.

28. Isenberg SJ. Ocular trauma. In: Isenberg SJ, ed. *The eye in infancy*, 2nd Ed. St. Louis, MO: Mosby, 1994:488.

29. Admoni MM, BenEzra D. Ocular trauma following amniocentesis as the cause of leucocoria. *J Pediatr Ophthalmol Strabismus* 1988;25:196.

30. Isenberg SJ, Heckenlively JR. Traumatized eye with retinal damage from amniocentesis. *J Pediatr Ophthalmol Strabismus* 1985;22:65.

31. Messinger A, Radkowski A, Greenwald MJ, et al. Orbital roof fractures in the pediatric population. *Plast Reconstr Surg* 1989;84:213.

32. Smit TJ, Mourits MP. Monocanalicular lesions: to reconstruct or not. *Ophthalmology* 1999;106:1310.

33. Read RW, Sires BS. Association between orbital fracture location and ocular injury: a retrospective study. *J Craniomaxillofac Trauma* 1998;4:10.

34. Bansagi ZC, Meyer DR. Internal orbital fractures in the pediatric age group: characterization and management. *Ophthalmology* 2000;107:829.

35. Dutton J. Management of blow-out fractures of the orbital floor. *Surv Ophthalmol* 1991;35:279.

36. Liss J, Stefko ST, Chung WL. Orbital surgery: state of the art. *Oral Maxillofac Surg Clin North Am* 2010;22:59

37. Egbert JE, Kersten RC, Kulwin DR. Pediatric orbital floor fracture: direct extraocular muscle involvement. *Ophthalmology* 2000;107:1875.

38. Burnstine M. Clinical recommendations for repair of isolated orbital floor fractures: an evidence-based analysis. *Ophthalmology* 2002;109:1207.

39. Yanoff M, Fine BS. *Ocular pathology*, 2nd Ed. Philadelphia, PA: Harper & Row, 1982:185.

40. Michael JG, Hug D, Dowd MD. Management of corneal abrasion in children: a randomized clinical trial. *Ann Emerg Med* 2002;40:67.

41. Turner A. Rabiu M. Patching for corneal abrasion. *Cochrane Database Sys Rev* 2006;(2):CD004764.

42. Schein OD. Contact lens abrasions and the nonophthalmologist. *Am J Emerg Med* 1993;11:606.

43. Weaver CS, Terrell KM. Evidence-based emergency medicine. Update: do ophthalmic nonsteroidal anti-inflammatory drugs reduce the pain associated with simple corneal abrasion without delaying healing? *Ann Emerg Med* 2003;41:134.

44. Spector J, Fernandez WG. Chemical, thermal, and biological ocular exposures. *Emerg Med Clin North Am* 2008;26:125.

45. Ratnapalan S, Das L. Causes of eye burns in children. *Pediatr Emerg Care* 2011;2:151.

46. Dana MR, Schaumberg DA, Moyes AL, et al. Outcome of penetrating keratoplasty after ocular trauma in children. *Arch Ophthalmol* 1995;113:1503.

47. Vajpayee RB, Angra SK, Honavar SG. Combined keratoplasty, cataract extraction, and intraocular lens implantation after corneolenticular laceration in children. *Am J Ophthalmol* 1994;117:507.

48. Sharma A, Kaur R, Kumar S, et al. Fibrin glue versus N-butyl-2-cyanoacrylate in corneal perforations. *Ophthalmology* 2003;110:291.

49. Macsai MS. The management of corneal trauma. Advances in the past twenty-five years. *Cornea* 2000;19:617.

50. Barr CC. Prognostic factors in corneoscleral lacerations. *Arch Ophthalmol* 1983;101:919.

51. McCannel MA. A retrievable suture idea for anterior uveal problems. *Ophthalmic Surg* 1976;7:98.

52. Brown SM. A technique for repair of iridodialysis in children. *J AAPOS* 1998;2:380.

53. Coats DK, Paysse EA, Kong J. Unrecognized microscopic hyphema masquerading as a closed head injury. *Pediatrics* 1998;102:652.

54. Crouch ER. Traumatic hyphema. *J Pediatr Ophthalmol Strabismus* 1986;23:95.

55. Brandt MT, Haug RH. Traumatic hyphema: a comprehensive review. *J Oral Maxillofac Surg* 2001;59:1462.

56. Cohen, SB, Fletcher ME, Goldberg MF, Jednock HJ. Diagnosis and management of ocular complications of sickle hemoglobinopathies: Part V. *Ophthalmic Surg* 1986;17:369.

57. Walton W, von Hagen S, Grigorian R, Zarbin M. Management of traumatic hyphema. *Surv Ophthalmol* 2002;47:297.

58. Kraft SP, Christianson MD, Crawford S, et al. Traumatic hyphema in children. *Ophthalmology* 1987;94:1232.

59. Coats DK, Viestenz A, Paysse EA, et al. Outpatient management of traumatic hyphemas in children. *Binocul Vis Strabismus Q* 2000;15:169.

60. Shiuey Y, Lucarelli MJ. Traumatic hyphema: outcomes of outpatient management. *Ophthalmology* 1998;105:851.

61. Rahmani B, Jahadi HR. Comparison of tranexamic acid and prednisolone in the treatment of traumatic hyphema. A randomized clinical trial. *Ophthalmology* 1999;106:375.

62. Lai JC, Fekrat S, Barron Y, et al. Traumatic hyphema in children: risk factors for complications. *Arch Ophthalmol* 2001;119:64.

63. Cho J, Jun BK, Lee YJ, et al. Factors associated with the poor visual outcome after traumatic hyphema. *Korean J Ophthalmol* 1998;12:122.

64. Rahmani B, Jahadi HR, Rajaeefard A. An analysis of risk for secondary hemorrhage in traumatic hyphema. *Ophthalmology* 1999;106:380.

65. Goldberg MF. Antifibrinolytic agents in the management of traumatic hyphema. *Arch Ophthalmol* 1983;101:1029.

66. Albiani DA, Hodge WG, Pan YI, et al. Tranexamic acid in the treatment of pediatric traumatic hyphema. *Can J Ophthalmol* 2008;43:428.

67. Dieste MC, Hersh PS, Kylstra JA, et al. Intraocular pressure increase associated with epsilon-aminocaproic acid therapy for traumatic hyphema. *Arch Ophthalmol* 1988;106:383.

68. Agapitos PJ, Noel L-P, Clarke WN. Traumatic hyphema in children. *Ophthalmology* 1987;94:1238.

69. Greven CM, Collins AS, Slusher MM, et al. Visual results, prognostic indicators, and posterior segment findings following surgery for cataract/lens subluxation-dislocation secondary to ocular contusion injuries. *Retina* 2002;22:575.

70. Graul TA, Kim CS, Alward WL, et al. Progressive axial myopia in a juvenile patient with traumatic glaucoma. *Am J Ophthalmol* 2002;133:700.

71. Yamada H, Sakai A, Yamada E, et al. Spontaneous closure of traumatic macular hole. *Am J Ophthalmol* 2002;134:340.

72. Yeshurun I, Guerrero-Naranjo JL, Quiroz-Mercado H. Spontaneous closure of a large traumatic macular hole in a young patient. *Am J Ophthalmol* 2002;134:602.

73. Secretan M, Sickenberg M, Zografos L, et al. Morphometric characteristics of traumatic choroidal ruptures associated with neovascularization. *Retina* 1998;18:62.

74. Anderson RL, Panje WR, Gross CE. Optic nerve blindess following blunt forehead trauma. *Ophthalmology* 1982;89:445–455.

75. McClenaghan FC, Ezra DG, Holmes SB. Mechanisms and management of vision loss following orbital and facial trauma. *Curr Opin Ophthalmol* 2011;22:426.

76. Warner N, Eggenberger E. Traumatic optic neuropathy: a review of current literature. *Curr Opin Ophthalmol* 2010;21:459.

77. Leven LA, Beck RW, Joseph MP, et al. The treatment of traumatic optic neuropathy: the international optic nerve trauma study. *Ophthalmology* 1999;106:1268–1277.

78. Hillman JS, Myska V, Nissim S. Complete avulsion of the optic nerve: a clinical, angiographic and electrodiagnostic study. *Br J Ophthalmol* 1975;59:503.

79. Chaudry A, Shamsi FA, A-Sharif A, et al. Optic nerve avulsion from door-handle trauma in children. *Br J Ophthalmol* 2006;90:844.

80. United States Children's Bureau. Child Maltreatment 2009. U.S. Department of Health & Human Services Administration for Children and Families Administration on Children, Youth and Families Children's Bureau. Washington, 2010. http://www.acf.hhs.gov/programs/cb/stats_research/index.htm#can. Accessed September 2011.

81. Marcus DM, Albert DM. Recognizing child abuse. *Arch Ophthalmol* 1992;110:766.

82. Weissgold DJ, Budenz DL, Hood I, et al. Ruptured vascular malformation masquerading as battered/shaken baby syndrome: a nearly tragic mistake. *Surv Ophthalmol* 1995; 39:509.

83. Annable WL. Ocular manifestations of child abuse. In: Reece RM, ed. *Child abuse: medical diagnosis and management.* Philadelphia, PA: Lea & Febiger, 1994:138–149.

84. Meadow R. Munchausen syndrome by proxy. *Arch Dis Child* 1982;57:92.

85. Rosenberg DA. Web of deceit: a literature review of Munchausen syndrome by proxy. *Child Abuse Negl* 1987;11:547.

86. Taylor D. Recurrent non-accidentally inflicted chemical eye injuries to siblings. *J Pediatr Ophthalmol Strabismus* 1976;13:238.

87. Cordes FC. *Cataract types.* Rochester, MN: American Academy of Ophthalmology and Otolaryngology, 1961:91–95.

88. Levin AV. Ocular manifestation of child abuse. *Ophthalmol Clin North Am* 1990;3:249.

89. Harley RD. Ocular manifestations of child abuse. *J Pediatr Ophthalmol Strabismus* 1980;17:5.

90. Kaur B, Taylor D. Fundus hemorrhages in infancy. *Surv Ophthalmol* 1992;37:1.

91. Caffee J. The whiplash shaken infant syndrome: manual shaking by the extremities with whiplash-induced intracranial and intraocular bleedings, linked with residual permanent brain damage. *Pediatrics* 1974;54:396.

92. Wilkinson WS, Han DP, Rappley MD, et al. Retinal hemorrhage predicts neurologic injury in the shaken baby. *Arch Ophthalmol* 1989;107:1472.

93. Morad Y, Kim YM, Armstrong DC, et al. Correlation between retinal abnormalities and intracranial abnormalities in the shaken baby syndrome. *Am J Ophthalmol* 2002;134:354.

94. Buys YM, Levin AV, Enzenauer RW, et al. Retinal findings after head trauma in infants and young children. *Ophthalmology* 1992;90:1718.

95. Marshall DH, Brownstein S, Dorey MW, et al. The spectrum of postmortem ocular findings in victims of shaken baby syndrome. *Can J Ophthalmol* 2001;36:377.

96. Goetting MG, Sowa B. Retinal hemorrhage after cardiopulmonary resuscitation in children: an etiologic reevaluation. *Pediatrics* 1990;85:585.

97. Kanter RK. Retinal hemorrhage after cardiopulmonary resuscitation or child abuse. *J Pediatr* 1986;108:430.

98. Matthews GP, Das A. Dense vitreous hemorrhages predict poor visual and neurological prognosis in infants with shaken baby syndrome. *J Pediatr Ophthalmol Strabismus* 1996;33:260.

99. Kivlin JD, Simons KB, Lazoritz S, et al. Shaken baby syndrome. *Ophthalmology* 2000;107:1246.

100. Massicotte SJ, Folberg R, Torczynski E, et al. Vitreoretinal traction and perimacular folds in the eyes of deliberately traumatized children. *Ophthalmology* 1991;98:1124.

101. Gaynon MW, Koh D, Marmor MF, et al. Retinal folds in the shaken baby syndrome. *Am J Ophthalmol* 1988;106:423.

102. Greenwald MJ. The shaken baby syndrome. *Semin Ophthalmol* 1990;5:202.

103. Sturm V, Landau, Menke MN. Optical coherence tomography findings in Shaken Baby syndrome. *Am J Ophthalmol* 2008;146:363.

104. Lambert SR, Johnson TE, Hoyt CS. Optic nerve sheath and retinal hemorrhages associated with the shaken baby syndrome. *Arch Ophthalmol* 1986;104:1509.

105. Budenz DL, Farber MG, Mirchandani HG, et al. Ocular and optic nerve hemorrhages in abused infants with intracranial injuries. *Ophthalmology* 1994;101:559.

106. U.S. Consumer Products Safety Commission: Product Summary Reports—Eye Injuries Only—Calendar Year 2002. US Consumer Product Safety Commission, Directorate for Epidemiology; National Electronic Injury Surveillance System; National Injury Information Clearinghouse.

107. American Academy of Pediatrics, Committee on Sports Medicine and Fitness, American Academy of Ophthalmology, Eye Health and Public Information Task Force. Protective eyewear for young athletes. *Ophthalmology* 2004; 111:600.

108. U.S. Consumer Products Safety Commission: Product Summary Reports, All Products Body Part = 77 (Eyeball) All Diagnoses & Products. Injury Estimates for Calendar Year 2010; National Electronic Injury Surveillance System; National Injury Information Clearinghouse.

109. American Academy of Pediatrics, American Academy of Ophthalmology. Joint Policy Statement. Protective eyewear for young adults. 2003.

110. Zagelbaum BM, Starkey C, Hersh PS, et al. The National Basketball Association eye injury study. *Arch Ophthalmol* 1995;113:749.

111. Zagelbaum BM. Sports-related eye trauma: managing common injuries. *Physician Sports Med* 1993;21:25.

112. Zagelbaum BM, Hersh PS, Donnenfeld ED, et al. Ocular trauma in major-league baseball players. *N Engl J Med* 1994;330:1021.

113. Berman P. Why do we need to decrease sports-related eye injuries? PowerPoint presentation at the Sports Eye Injury Meeting, June 1–2, 2006, Bethesda, MD.

114. Vinger PF, Duma SM, Crandall J. Baseball hardness as a risk factor for eye injuries. *Arch Ophthalmol* 1999;117:354.

115. Capao FJA, Fernandes VL, Barros H, et al. Soccer-related ocular injuries. *Arch Ophthalmol* 2003;121:687.

116. Capao Felipe JA. Soccer (football) ocular injuries: an important eye health problem. *Br J Ophthalmol* 2004;88:159.

117. Schepens CL. Contusion trauma. In: Schepens CL, ed. *Retinal detachment and allied diseases*, Vol 1. Philadelphia, PA: WB Saunders, 1983:71–84.

118. Capao-Felipe JA. Fern andex VL, Barros H, et al. Soccer-related ocular injuries. *Arch Ophthalmol* 2003;121:687.

119. Tu Y, Granados DV. 2010 Fireworks Annual Report: fireworks-related deaths, emergency department-treated injuries, and enforcement activities during 2006. June 2007. Consumer Products Safety commission. http://www.cpsc.gov/library/2010fwreport.pdf. Accessed September 2011

120. Smith GA, Knapp JF, Barnett TM, et al. The rocket's red glare, the bombs bursting in air: fireworks-related injuries to children. *Pediatrics* 1996;98:1.

121. Khan M, Reichstein D, Recchia FM. Ocular consequences of bottle rocket injuries in children and adolescents. *Arch Ophthalmol* 2011;129:639.

122. Aiello LP, Iwamoto M. Perforating ocular fishhook injury. *Arch Ophthalmol* 1992;119:1316.

123. Aiello LP, Iwamoto M, Guyer D, et al. Surgical management and visual prognosis of penetrating ocular fishhook injuries. *Ophthalmology* 1992;99:862.

124. Hargrave S, Weakley D, Wilson C. Complications of ocular paintball injuries in children. *J Pediatr Ophthalmol Strabismus* 2000;37:338.

125. Alliman KJ, Smiddy WE, Banta J, et al. Ocular trauma and outcome secondary to paintball projectiles. *Am J Ophthalmol* 2009;147:239.

126. Sethi CS, Grey RH, Hart CD. Laser pointers revisited: a survey of 14 patients attending casualty at the Bristol Eye Hospital. *Br J Ophthalmol* 1999;83:1164.

127. Strahlman E, Elman M, Daub E, et al. Causes of pediatric eye trauma. *Arch Ophthalmol* 1990;108:603.

128. Glazier R, Slade M, Mayer H. The depiction of protective eyewear use in popular television programs. *J Trauma* 2011;70:965.

129. United States Eye Injury Registry, Selected Data 1988–2007. *Eye trauma: epidemiology and prevention.* http://www.useironline.org. Accessed September 2011

130. Jeffers JB. An on-going tragedy: pediatric sports-related eye injuries. *Semin Ophthalmol* 1990;5:216.

131. American Academy of Pediatrics Committee on Sports Medicine and Fitness, American Academy of Ophthalmology Committee on Eye Safety and Sports Ophthalmology. Protective eyewear for young athletes. *Pediatrics* 1996;98:311.

Index

A

AACE. *See* Acute acquired comitant esotropia
Abatacept, uveitis and, 286
ABC transporters, FH and, 431
Abetalipoproteinemia, retinal degeneration and, 432–433, 433f
Ablative therapy, ROP and, 313
AC:A ratios
  intermittent exotropia and, 151
  measurement of, nonrefractive accommodative esotropia and, 148
  surgery and, 149
Accommodation, 113
Accommodative esotropia, 147–150, 148f
  congenital esotropia and, 146, 148f
  cyclic esotropia and, 149–150
  nonrefractive accommodative esotropia and, 148–149
  partial accommodative esotropia and, 149
  refractive accommodative esotropia and, 147–148
Acetazolamide (Diamox)
  dislocation of ocular lens and, 498
  pediatric glaucoma and, 271, 272t
Acetylcholine receptors (AChR), myasthenia gravis and, 471
ACHM, 20–21
AChR. *See* Acetylcholine receptors
Achromatopsia (rod monochromatism), 20–21, 309, 483
Acoustic neuromas, 412
Acquired fixation nystagmus, neurologic disorders and, 480–481
Acquired immunodeficiency syndrome (AIDS), Kaposi sarcoma and, 379
Acquired left superior oblique palsy, 157, 157f
Acquired nevi, 350, 350f
Acquired prepapillary venous loop, 318, 320f
Acquired sixth nerve palsies, treatment of, 160
Acquired third nerve palsy, 155–157, 157t
  treatment of, 155–157, 156f
Acuity test, ptosis and, 345
Acute acquired comitant esotropia (AACE), 150
  pathogenesis of, 150
  treatment of, 150
Acute conjunctivitis, 177–179, 177f
Acute follicular conjunctivitis, 177–179
  PCF and, 178, 179
Acute hydrops, keratoconus and, 226
Acute papillary conjunctivitis, 177–178
Acute phase ROP, screening guidelines for, 78–79
Acute tubulointerstitial nephritis, anterior uveitis and, 289

Acyclovir
  HSV and, 352
  HZV and, 216, 352
  neonatal HSV and, 293
  ophthalmic ointment, HSV and, 213, 214
Adalimumab, uveitis and, 286
Adenovirus, 215
  acute follicular conjunctivitis and, 178–179
  infection, loteprednol and, 215
Adrenergic agonists, pediatric glaucoma and, 273
Adrenoleukodystrophy, 446, 446f
  cerebral form of, 446
  peroxisomal biogenesis disorders and, 446
Aggrecan, sclera and, 61
Ahmed glaucoma implants, pediatric glaucoma and, 269f, 276, 278f
AIDS. *See* Acquired immunodeficiency syndrome
Alagille syndrome, pleiotropic disorders and, 10–11
Aland island eye disease, 22
Albinism, 423–426. *See also* Ocular albinism
  classification of, 424, 425t
  genetic heterogeneity and, 10
  iris transillumination in, 482f
Alexander's law, nystagmus and, 484
Alkaline injuries, calcific corneal degeneration and, 227
Alkaptonuria, 426
  HGA and, 426
Alleles, 3
Allen figure acuity testing, 124
  pediatric eye examination and, 95, 95f
Allergic conjunctivitis, 181–182
Alomide. *See* Lodoxamide
Alpha-chymotrypsin, ligneous conjunctivitis and, 184
Alport's syndrome, 241
Alternate cover test, eye examination and, 97
Alternate fixation, congenital esotropia and, 145
Ambient light exposure, ROP and, 83
Amblyopia, 106, 119–129
  classification of, 120–121
    clinical, 120–121
    mechanistic, 121
  conclusions for, 128–129
  congenital esotropia and, 145, 147
  corneal edema and, 232
  dislocation of ocular lens and, 501
  eye globe and, 64
  pathophysiology of, 121–122
  patient examination with, 123–125
    fixation preference testing, 123
    vertical prism test, 123–125

visual acuity/behavior and, 123
  prognosis of, 128
  ROP and, 88
  special issues in, 128
    concurrent ocular pathology and, 128
    older children and, 128
  therapy cessation for, 127–128
  treatment of, 125–127
    maintenance therapy in, 127, 129
    occlusion therapy and, 126
    optical correction and, 125
    penalization and, 126–127
    systemic, 127
  vision screening and, 122–123
  visual development and, 119–120
    factors in, 119–120
Amblyopia Treatment Studies
  HOTV and, 108
  PEDIG and, 126
Amblyopic eyes, 108
Amino acid metabolism, disorders of, 443–431
  albinism, 423–426
  alkaptonuria, 426
  cystinosis, 426, 427t, 428, 428f
  galactosemia, 430–431, 430t
  hyperornithinemia, 428–429, 429f, 429t
  primary hyperoxaluria, 429
Aminoglycoside antibiotics, toxic ophthalmic reactions and, 183
Amniocentesis
  prenatal ocular trauma and, 490, 490f
  single gene disorders and, 43
Amniotic fluid, prenatal diagnosis and, 43
Aneuploidy, 26
Aneurysmal bone cysts, 418
Angiogenesis, ROP and, 83
Angiokeratomata, Fabry disease and, 436, 436f
Angle in Rieger's anomaly, 196f
Animal models, myopia in, 67
Aniridia, 12, 17, 268–269
Anisometropia
  correction and, 114
  ROP and, 88
Anisometropic amblyopia, 120
Ankyloblepharon, eyelid disorders and, 340–341, 341f
Anomalous retinal correspondence, 133, 139f
Anophthalmia, 12–14
  eyelid disorders and, 358–359
Anterior chamber cleavage syndrome, 193, 194f, 200f, 269
Anterior corneal dystrophies, 221
Anterior megalophthalmos, 191–192, 191f, 192t
  differential diagnosis of, 192, 192t
Anterior polar cataracts, 246
Anterior segment dysgenesis, 17–18

509